THE ROUTLEDGE HISTORY
OF MONARCHY

The Routledge History of Monarchy draws together current research across the field of royal studies, providing a rich understanding of the history of monarchy from a variety of geographical, cultural and temporal contexts.

Divided into four parts, this book presents a wide range of case studies relating to different aspects of monarchy throughout a variety of times and places, and uses these case studies to highlight different perspectives of monarchy and enhance understanding of rulership and sovereignty in terms of both concept and practice. Including case studies chosen by specialists in a diverse array of subjects, such as history, art, literature, and gender studies, it offers an extensive global and interdisciplinary approach to the history of monarchy, providing a thorough insight into the workings of monarchies within Europe and beyond, and comparing different cultural concepts of monarchy within a variety of frameworks, including social and religious contexts.

Opening up the discussion of important questions surrounding fundamental issues of monarchy and rulership, *The Routledge History of Monarchy* is the ideal book for students and academics of royal studies, monarchy, or political history.

Elena Woodacre is a Senior Lecturer at the University of Winchester, UK, and a specialist in queenship and royal studies. Elena is the founder of the Royal Studies Network and the 'Kings & Queens' conferences and editor of the *Royal Studies Journal*, the *Gender and Power in the Premodern World* and the *Queens of England* series.

Lucinda H.S. Dean is a Lecturer at the Centre for History at the University of the Highlands and Islands, Scotland, and a specialist in late medieval and early modern ritual and ceremony of the Scottish monarchy. She has published widely in this area and co-edited a volume on *Medieval and Early Modern Representations of Authority in Scotland and the British Isles* (2016).

Chris Jones is an Associate Professor at the University of Canterbury, New Zealand. His work focuses upon medieval France and political thought. Among his publications is the monograph *Eclipse of Empire? Perceptions of the Western Empire and Its Rulers in Late Medieval France* (2007). He is Director of the Canterbury Roll Project and President of the Australian & New Zealand Association for Medieval & Early Modern Studies Inc. (ANZAMEMS).

Russell E. Martin is Professor of History at Westminster College, USA. He is widely published and the author of *A Bride for the Tsar: Bride-Shows and Marriage Politics in Early Modern Russia*. He is Editor-in-Chief of *Canadian-American Slavic Studies*, President of the Early Slavic Studies Association and a member of the Chancellery of the Head of the Russian Imperial House of Romanoff (Moscow).

Zita Eva Rohr is a Political Historian of the late Medieval and Early Modern periods and has published widely in the field of gendered political and diplomatic history, including her monograph *Yolande of Aragon (1381–1442): Family and Power* (2016). She is an Honorary Fellow at Macquarie University, Australia, in the Department of Modern History, Politics, and International Relations.

THE ROUTLEDGE HISTORIES

The Routledge Histories is a series of landmark books surveying some of the most important topics and themes in history today. Edited and written by an international team of world-renowned experts, they are the works against which all future books on their subjects will be judged.

THE ROUTLEDGE HISTORY OF MONARCHY

*Edited by Elena Woodacre,
Lucinda H.S. Dean, Chris Jones,
Russell E. Martin and Zita Eva Rohr*

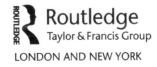

Routledge
Taylor & Francis Group

LONDON AND NEW YORK

First published 2019 by Routledge

2 Park Square, Milton Park, Abingdon, Oxon, OX14 4RN
605 Third Avenue, New York, NY 10017

Routledge is an imprint of the Taylor & Francis Group, an informa business

First issued in paperback 2020

British Library Cataloguing-in-Publication Data
A catalogue record for this book is available from the British Library

Library of Congress Cataloging-in-Publication Data
Names: Woodacre, Elena, editor. | Dean, Lucinda H. S., editor. | Jones, Chris, 1977- editor. | Martin, Russell, 1963- editor. | Rohr, Zita Eva, editor.
Title: The Routledge history of monarchy / edited by Elena Woodacre, Lucinda H.S. Dean, Chris Jones, Russell E. Martin and Zita Eva Rohr.
Description: Abingdon, Oxon ; New York, NY : Routledge, 2019. | Series: The Routledge histories | Includes bibliographical references and index.
Identifiers: LCCN 2019005332| ISBN 9781138703322 (hardback : alk. paper) | ISBN 9781315203195 (ebook)
Subjects: LCSH: Monarchy—History. | Kings and rulers—History.
Classification: LCC JC375 .R67 2019 | DDC 321/.609—dc23
LC record available at https://lccn.loc.gov/2019005332

ISBN: 978-1-138-70332-2 (hbk)
ISBN: 978-0-367-72757-4 (pbk)

Typeset in Baskerville
by Swales & Willis, Exeter, Devon, UK

Visit the companion website: www.routledge.com/cw/woodacre

TO OUR FRIENDS, FAMILIES, AND
LOVED ONES.

CONTENTS

CONTENTS

CONTENTS

xi

CONTENTS

CONTENTS

ILLUSTRATIONS

Figures

Table

ACKNOWLEDGEMENTS

This collection has only been possible through the collaborative efforts of a large group of scholars who have generously given their time and shared their research with us. We particularly want to thank the members of the wider editorial team whose names may not be on the cover but have been a very important part of the process and deserve credit for the many hours they have put into creating this collection. This includes our website editors, Cathleen Sarti and Kristen Geaman, who have put in countless hours developing our companion website, working with Routledge on the concept and design and with our contributors to build up the content. As the companion website has been an essential part of this project from the start but was new technical territory for all of us, we appreciate their hard work to bring this from an idea to reality. We also want to thank our editorial sub-teams who have given many hours of time over to the project to review and edit the papers, working closely with each of the subeditors. A huge thanks to these fantastic colleagues: Charlotte Backerra, Hélder Carvalhal, Danna Messer, Aidan Norrie, Matthias Range and Charles Reed as well as Cathleen and Kristen who also worked as subeditors. We are very grateful as well to the dozens of peer reviewers who generously gave their time to read and review chapters for us to make the collection as strong as possible. Thanks also to Alice Hancock whose copyediting skills were much appreciated as we finalized the manuscript to submit to the publisher. Finally, we want to thank the team at Routledge who have been enthusiastically supportive and very patient with unanticipated delays and flurries of queries over the course of the project, particularly Laura Pilsworth, our fantastic editor, and Morwenna Scott who has worked closely with us and been a huge help throughout.

CONTRIBUTORS

Charlotte Backerra is an Assistant Professor of Early Modern European History at the University of Göttingen, having previously taught Early Modern and Modern History at the universities of Mainz, Stuttgart and Darmstadt. Her projects cover the role of dynasties in politics, economics, and culture as well as premodern international relations and intelligence. Her doctoral thesis *Wien und London: Internationale Beziehungen im frühen 18. Jahrhundert* was published with Vandenhoeck & Ruprecht in 2018. She co-edited a volume on *Transnational Histories of the 'Royal Nation'* with Palgrave in 2017.

Henric Bagerius received his PhD in History from the University of Gothenburg, Sweden, in 2009. He is an Associate Professor of History at Örebro University, Sweden. He has published extensively on gender and sexuality in Iceland and Sweden. He has recently published a monograph on the dress reform movement in late nineteenth-century Sweden.

Kim Bergqvist is a PhD candidate in the Department of History at Stockholm University, Sweden. He currently teaches at DIS Stockholm. His research is centred on political, cultural and comparative history, medieval history writing, and the history of gender and emotions, with a particular focus on the high and late Middle Ages in Scandinavia and the Iberian Peninsula. His work has appeared in *The Medieval Chronicle*.

Sarah Betts is a doctoral candidate at the University of York, UK, where she is working on a thesis examining the cultural representations and afterlife of Civil War royalists and royalisms in England from the 1640s to the present day. She has broader interests in the history of monarchy, cultural memory and public history. She has published on Stuart matriarchy and queenship, civil war memorials and memorial practice in England, and representations of seventeenth-century history and monarchy in popular culture and television drama.

Susan Broomhall is Professor of Early Modern History at the University of Western Australia. She researches women and gender, power, emotions, material culture and knowledge practices from late medieval to nineteenth-century Europe, although the focus of much of her work is early modern France and the Low Countries. Her edited collection, *Women and Power at the French Court, 1483–1563*, was published by Amsterdam University Press in 2018.

Pascal Buresi is Research Professor at the Centre National de la Recherche Scientifique, Lyon, France and Professor at the École des Hautes Études en Sciences Sociales, Paris. He is the author of several books including *Governing the Empire: Provincial Administration in the Almohad Caliphate (1224–1269)* (Brill, 2012) and *La Frontière entre chrétienté et Islam dans la péninsule Ibérique* (Publibook, 2004). Currently, he is the Scientific Coordinator of MSCA-H2020-ITN 813547 Mediating Islam in the Digital Age (2019–2023).

Hélder Carvalhal is a PhD candidate in Early Modern History at the InterUniversity Doctoral Programme (PIUDHist). He is an integrated member of CIDEHUS, University of Évora, Portugal. His research interests and publications are divided between royal and court studies, gender and men's studies, war and labour history.

Lucinda H.S. Dean is Lecturer at the Centre for History at the University of the Highlands and Islands, Scotland (since November 2016) and is a specialist in late medieval and early modern ritual and ceremony of the Scottish monarchy with a keen interest in material culture. She has published a number of articles and book chapters on connected themes and co-edited a volume on *Medieval and Early Modern Representations of Authority in Scotland and the British Isles* (Routledge, 2016).

Chad Denton received his PhD in History and a graduate minor in women's and gender studies from the University of Missouri, USA. His specializations are in the seventeenth and eighteenth centuries, France and northern Italy, the history of gender and sexuality, and the history of emotions. Recently he published his dissertation, *The Enlightened and Depraved: Decadence, Radicalism, and the Early Modern French Nobility*, through Rowman & Littlefield.

Stephen Donnachie received his PhD in Medieval History from Swansea University, UK. He has taught Medieval and Early Modern history at Swansea University and is the Book Reviews Editor for the *Royal Studies Journal*. His research interests include the crusades, the history of the Latin East and the medieval Mediterranean world.

Anna M. Duch received her PhD in History at the University of York, UK. She is an Assistant Professor of History at Columbia State Community College, USA. She is currently the faculty lead for world history courses. Her research interests include medieval royal bodies and concepts of sanctity.

Theresa Earenfight is Professor of History at Seattle University, USA, and focuses her teaching and research on queens and queenship in medieval and early modern Europe. She is the author of *The King's Other Body: Maria of Castile and the Crown of Aragon* (University of Pennsylvania Press, 2010) and *Queenship in Medieval Europe* (Palgrave, 2013), and is currently at work on a study of Queen Catherine of Aragon.

Christine Ekholst received her PhD in History from Stockholm University, Sweden, in 2009. She has taught at several Canadian universities and is now an Assistant Professor of Medieval History at Uppsala University, Sweden. Her research focuses on sexuality, gender, legal history and the history of crime. She is currently researching gender and crime in late medieval Swedish towns.

Laura Fábián is a PhD candidate at Eötvös Loránd University, Faculty of Humanities, Institute of History Medieval and Early Modern World History Doctoral Program,

Hungary. She is the author of several articles on medieval kings and the biblical king Solomon, which have appeared in *Világtörténet* and *Micae Mediaevales VI: Fiatal történészek dolgozatai a középkori Magyarországról és Európáról*, among other publications.

Kristen L. Geaman received her PhD in Medieval History from the University of Southern California, USA. She currently teaches medieval and pre-modern world History at the University of Toledo, USA. She is interested in women's and gender history, and her work has appeared in *English Historical Review* and *Social History of Medicine*.

Mikolaj Getka-Kenig received his PhD in Modern History from the University of Warsaw, Poland. He currently works as a post-doctoral researcher at the Jagiellonian University in Cracow, Poland. His area of research is the socio-cultural history of art and architecture in Poland and Europe ca. 1800. He recently published a book on early nineteenth-century Polish public memorials and their engagement with the political discourse of merit.

Trond Norén Isaksen is an independent scholar and author of more than 250 articles and 5 books, including a study of Norwegian coronations from the twelfth to the twentieth century, *Norges krone: Kroninger, signinger og maktkamper fra sagatid til nåtid* (Forlaget Historie & Kultur, 2015). His most recent book is *Korsfareren: Sigurd Jorsalfare og hans verden* (Forlaget Historie & Kultur, 2018), a biography of King Sigurd the Jerusalemite of Norway, the first king to go on a crusade to Jerusalem.

Frank Jacob received his PhD in Japanese Studies from the University of Erlangen, Germany. He is currently Professor of Global History at Nord University, Norway. His main research focuses on modern East Asian History, especially Japan and Korea, and the history of transnational anarchism.

Chris Jones is an Associate Professor at the University of Canterbury, New Zealand. His work focuses upon France and political thought. Among his publications is the monograph, *Eclipse of Empire? Perceptions of the Western Empire and Its Rulers in Late Medieval France* (Brepols, 2007). He is Director of the Canterbury Roll Project and is the serving President of the Australian & New Zealand Association for Medieval & Early Modern Studies Inc. (ANZAMEMS).

Lloyd Llewellyn-Jones is Chair of Ancient History at University of Cardiff, UK. He is a noted specialist on rulership and court society in the Ancient Near East and has published extensively in this area including *King and Court in Ancient Persia 559–331 BCE* (Edinburgh University Press, 2013; Persian translation, 2015), *The Hellenistic Court* (Classical Press of Wales, 2017) and articles on royal women of Persia, Egypt and the Near East. Future publications include monographs on Kleopatra III and Kleopatra Thea (Routledge), and a study of Achaemenid Iran (Routledge). He also works on reception studies, having published *Designs on the Past: How Hollywood Created the Ancient World* (Edinburgh University Press, 2018), and his new project looks at ancient imagery in court portraiture and theatricals c.1550–1800.

David M. Malitz received his PhD in Japanese Studies from Ludwig-Maximilians University in Munich, Germany. He is currently teaching on the Bachelor of Arts Program in Language and Culture at the Faculty of Arts of Chulalongkorn University in Bangkok, Thailand. He is interested in and has published about modern Japanese and Thai history.

Russell E. Martin is Professor of History at Westminster College, USA. He is the author of *A Bride for the Tsar: Bride-Shows and Marriage Politics in Early Modern Russia*, which won the 2014 W. Bruce Lincoln Book Prize, and has co-written or edited seven other books on early modern and modern Russian history as well as producing over seventy peer-reviewed articles and book chapters. He is Editor-in-Chief of *Canadian-American Slavic Studies*, President of the Early Slavic Studies Association, and a member of the Chancellery of the Head of the Russian Imperial House of Romanoff (Moscow).

David Mednicoff received a JD in Law and a PhD in Political Science from Harvard University. He is Associate Professor of Middle Eastern Studies and Public Policy and Chair of the Department of Judaic and Near Eastern Studies at the University of Massachusetts-Amherst, USA. He researches and teaches on the intersection of law, politics and policy in the contemporary Middle East. Recent publications discuss post-2011 comparative Arab constitutional politics, the thick meanings of the rule of law in Arab Gulf states, the legal politics of migration regulation in Qatar and the UAE, and the legal and political ideology of Arab monarchies.

Catriona Murray is Lecturer in History of Art at the University of Edinburgh, UK. A historian of early modern British visual and material culture, her research focuses on the intersections of art and propaganda during the seventeenth and early eighteenth centuries.

Aidan Norrie is a historian of monarchy and a Chancellor's International Scholar in the Centre for the Study of the Renaissance at The University of Warwick, UK. He researches royal authority in cultures across the globe, with a particular focus on female kingship. Aidan is the editor, with Lisa Hopkins, of *Women on the Edge in Early Modern Europe* (Amsterdam University Press); with Marina Gerzic, of *From Medievalism to Early-Modernism: Adapting the English Past* (Routledge, 2018); and with Mark Houlahan, of *On the Edge of Early Modern English Drama* (Medieval Institute Publications, 2020).

Estelle Paranque is Lecturer in Early Modern History at the New College of the Humanities and Research Fellow within the Centre for the Study of the Renaissance at The University of Warwick, UK. She received her PhD in Early Modern History from University College London in 2016. She has co-edited and contributed to a number of volumes and recently published her monograph, *Elizabeth I Through Valois Eyes: Power, Representation, and Diplomacy in the Reign of the Queen, 1558–1588* (Palgrave Macmillan, 2018).

Joanne Paul is Lecturer in Early Modern History at the University of Sussex, UK, and has published widely on humanism and politics in sixteenth-century England. Her book, *Thomas More*, was published by Polity in 2016 and she has upcoming book projects with Palgrave, Cambridge University Press and Penguin. She has also published in *Renaissance Quarterly, Hobbes Studies, Renaissance Studies* and in other journals, volumes and magazines.

Matthias Range studied Art History and Musicology at the Philipps-Universität Marburg/Lahn, Germany, before gaining a DPhil in Music at the University of Oxford, UK, followed by a postdoctoral position in Early Modern History at Oxford Brookes University, UK. He currently works as a researcher at the University of Oxford. He has published widely in his main research areas: seventeenth- to twentieth-century sacred music and culture, and the history of the monarchy.

Eugénia Rodrigues is a Researcher at the Centro de História da Universidade de Lisboa, Portugal, and teaches History of Africa and History of empires at the Faculdade de Letras at the same university. She specializes in East African history during the early modern period with a focus on gender, slavery, landed property and knowledge circulation. She is the author of *Portugueses e Africanos nos Rios de Sena. Os Prazos da Coroa em Moçambique nos Séculos XVII e XVIII* (Imprensa Nacional-Casa da Moeda, 2013).

Manuel Alejandro Rodríguez de la Peña is Senior Lecturer in Medieval History at the Universidad CEU San Pablo, Spain. His research focuses on the cultural history of rulership in medieval Europe. He is the author of *Los reyes sabios. Cultura y poder en la Antigüedad Tardía y la Alta Edad Media* (Scribd, 2008) and editor of several volumes including *Carlomagno y la civilización carolingia. Estudios conmemorativos en el 1200 aniversario (814–2014)*.

Zita Eva Rohr is a specialist political historian of the late medieval and early modern periods and has published widely in the field of gendered political and diplomatic history of this rich, diverse and turbulent period of European political and diplomatic transformation. She is an Honorary Fellow at Macquarie University, Australia, in the Department of Modern History, Politics and International Relations, a chevalier in the *Ordre des Palmes Académiques* and a Fellow of the Royal Historical Society. She has published a monograph, *Yolande of Aragon (1381–1442): Family and Power* (Palgrave, 2016), based upon her PhD thesis, and has edited several collections on various aspects of queenship and the gendered history of monarchy.

Manuela Santos Silva is an Associate Professor of Medieval History at the Faculdade de Letras, Universidade de Lisboa, Portugal, with a large experience in research, teaching, and Master's and PhD supervision. She is a specialist on Portuguese history and queenship. With two other colleagues she coordinated a series of biographies of the Portuguese queens of Portugal and wrote the biography of Philippa of Lancaster, queen of Portugal. More recently, she coordinated with two other colleagues on a series on the marriages of the Portuguese royal households.

Cathleen Sarti is a Postdoctoral Researcher on Political Culture in Northern Europe, c.1400–1700. Her doctoral thesis focused on depositions of monarchs in England, Scotland, Sweden and Denmark-Norway. Her new research project asks about the role and influence of non-elite political counsellors. She is interested in political culture, history of political thought, new political history, cultural history, and methods and theories of the historical sciences. Her publications include several edited volumes on cultural history and monarchical studies, as well as book chapters on early modern depositions, or history of political thought.

Matthias Schnettger is Professor of Early Modern History at the Johannes Gutenberg University, Germany. His research interests embrace the Holy Roman Empire and small principalities and republics in Germany and Italy as well as diplomacy and processes of exchange in early modern Europe.

Valerie Schutte earned her PhD in History at the University of Akron, USA. She has published widely on books related to the Tudor monarchs, including her monograph *Mary I and the Art of Book Dedications* (Palgrave Macmillan, 2015).

Jonathan Spangler is Senior Lecturer in History at Manchester Metropolitan University, UK, specializing in courts and elites in France in the early modern period, and in particular on dynastic identity. He is the Senior Editor of *The Court Historian*, the journal for the Society for Court Studies, and has published widely on the court of Louis XIV, the Guise family and the Duchy of Lorraine. His current research projects focus on the role of the second son in the French monarchy and perceptions of same-sex relationships in early modern court societies.

Christoph De Spiegeleer received his PhD in Modern History from the Vije Universiteit Brussel, Belgium. He is currently active as Research Fellow of Liberas in Ghent, Belgium. His research interests relate to the history of the Belgian monarchy and modern funerary culture, with a particular focus on the connections between these subjects and political culture and national identity on a European level. His work on the Belgian monarchy, liberalism, socialism and funerary culture has appeared in several international journals.

Beverly J. Stoeltje received her PhD degree in Anthropology/Folklore at the University of Texas, USA, in 1979 and taught there for six years. She was a member of the faculty at Indiana University, USA, from 1986 until her retirement in 2013. She has published on Asante queen mothers, the Asante courts, the integration of chieftaincy with modernity, ritual and festival, rodeo, women of the west, beauty contests and gender in numerous journals, books and other publications.

Emily Joan Ward studied for her PhD in Medieval History at the University of Cambridge, UK. She held a Scouloudi Doctoral Fellowship at the Institute of Historical Research in London in 2016/17 and is currently a Moses and Mary Finley Research Fellow at Darwin College, University of Cambridge. She is interested in child kingship, boyhood and male adolescence, and comparative European history more generally. She has published articles in *Historical Research* (2016) and *Anglo-Norman Studies* (2018).

Paul Webster received his PhD from the University of Cambridge, UK, in 2007. He now works at Cardiff University, UK, where he coordinates the Exploring the Past adult learners progression pathway to degrees in the School of History, Archaeology and Religion. His research focuses on kingship and piety in the twelfth and thirteenth centuries, and his principal publications include monographs on *King John and Religion* (Boydell Press, 2015) and a collection, co-edited with Dr Marie-Pierre Gelin (UCL) on *The Cult of St Thomas Becket in the Plantagenet World* (Boydell Press, 2016).

Derek Whaley received his PhD in History from the University of Canterbury, UK, in 2018. His research focuses on medieval and early modern European dynasties and how they are presented within royal chronicles. He also maintains an interest in the local railroading history of Santa Cruz County, California, USA.

Benjamin Wild received his PhD in Medieval History from King's College London, UK. He has worked for a number of cultural institutions, including the Victoria & Albert Museum and the Royal Academy. He has published widely on the subject of material culture, particularly on the history of dress, and is interested, broadly, in how inanimate objects become imbued with meaning. His latest book, *Carnival to Catwalk: Global Reflections on Fancy Dress Costume*, is forthcoming from Bloomsbury Academic.

Elena Woodacre is a Senior Lecturer in Early Modern European History at the University of Winchester, UK. She is a specialist in queenship and royal studies and has published extensively in this area. Elena is the organizer of the 'Kings & Queens' conference series, founder of the Royal Studies Network, the editor-in-chief of the *Royal Studies Journal* as well as the editor of the *Gender and Power in the Premodern World* series with ARC Humanities Press and the *Queens of England* series with Routledge.

Philippa Woodcock received her PhD in History from the University of London, UK. She is a Lecturer in Early Modern European History at the University of the Highlands and Islands, UK. She is interested in military, political and landscape history, and her work has appeared in *French History, Church History and Religious Culture* and the *Royal Studies Journal*, as well as publishing *The Dictionary of Fashion* (Carlton, 2015).

UNDERSTANDING THE MECHANISMS OF MONARCHY

Elena Woodacre

Monarchy is one of our oldest and most enduring political entities. It has existed in many forms and permutations over all areas of the globe and under many names and guises, including Polynesian *ari'i rahi* and *ariki*, the *Yang di-Pertuan* of Malaysia, *Sapu* of the Inca, the *Oba* in West Africa and the Muslim *Padishahs*, and temporally from the ancient era to today's constitutional monarchs. While there are those who would seek to put an end to monarchy, as 'an outmoded and outdated institution' or would even label it, as Jeremy Paxman famously did as 'mumbo-jumbo', there is little doubt of its significance in terms of academic study, as a central element of civilizations around the globe from its earliest societies until the present day.[1] Monarchy has been scrutinized by specialists from multiple disciplines, particularly historians, anthropologists, sociologists, archaeologists, art historians, literary specialists and through the lens of gender studies.

Too often this work has been isolated by discipline or presented as oppositional to the work of specialists from other academic areas. David Cannadine noted that sociologists were interested in 'the power of ceremonial and the ceremonial of power', while anthropologists were more concerned with societal hierarchy, and historians often struggled to deal with time and change or became bogged down in context.[2] Declan Quigley also divided the work of historians and anthropologists, arguing that 'The emphasis on the comings and goings and doings of particular kings and queens contrasts sharply with the rather abstract, timeless idea of kingship set out in anthropological writing.'[3] Yet we must bring these perspectives on monarchy together. In order to understand this timeless institution we must examine both the theory and concept alongside illustrations from historical case studies of the practice and realities of rulership. We must also examine monarchy across time and place to bring together studies of ancient monarchies with modern ones, and move beyond the Eurocentric comfort zone of many western historians to compare our understanding of monarchy in a European, Christian context to the experience of it in other continental, societal and religious frameworks.

1

This global, interdisciplinary ethos underpins the present collection. What it aims to do is bring together a wide-ranging set of case studies on various aspects of monarchy in various times and places in order to enhance our knowledge of rulership and sovereignty in terms of both concept and practice. These case studies, largely drawn from historical, artistic, literary and gender specialists, complement earlier collections with a more sociological or anthropological focus like the aforementioned works edited by Cannadine or Quigley, as well as more theoretical works such as Jeroen Duindam's excellent work on dynasty and Francis Oakley's study of kingship.[4] While we do not aim to offer a comprehensive history or overview of monarchy in a textbook style manner, taken together, these studies offer an extensive historical foundation to give the reader a understanding of how monarchy operated in various societies and the ideas which underpin the institution itself. Despite the limitations of space, we have endeavoured to bring together the most expansive and diverse set of case studies possible to represent monarchy in different temporal, geographical and cultural settings.

Bringing together a wide variety of case studies sheds light on whether there are universals in rulership across time and place, and enables us to ask questions about fundamental issues: How great is cultural influence on the theory and practice of rulership? How did rulership develop in different times and places? How does monarchy operate? What does it need to function successfully? What undermines monarchy? We seek to add to the conversation in the field, asking and answering these questions about monarchy and opening a forum for further discussion that other volumes can add to with further case studies from periods and places that we were unable to include here. Ultimately, we hope that the global trend in royal studies exemplified in this collection will continue to develop, breaking down temporal, geographic and disciplinary barriers.

This introductory piece aims to complement the case studies of this collection, which are focused on particular figures, monarchies or thematic concepts by providing a more open ended theoretical consideration of monarchy as a whole. A detailed discussion of the contents of the collection and the key ideas underpinning each part of the volume will follow in introductions written by my fellow editors. I want to begin by positing a theory or a way of conceptualizing monarchy, which is illustrated in the Venn diagram in Figure 0.1.

The three areas in Figure 0.1 comprise the key elements which create the framework within which monarchy rests. All nine elements are key components. Power, law and religion are the fundamental aspects of rule which define the monarch's role. The monarchy is located within their dynasty, court and realm. Ceremonial, representation and display are the means through which the ruler demonstrates or affirms their role with regard to aspects of power, law and religion to the dynasty, court and realm. The nexus at the centre wherein the crown sits represents that intense locus wherein all the elements meet. The lines of all three circles intersect, creating the prerogatives – and boundaries – of the monarch's position.

The elephant in the room in Figure 0.1 – something that is both nowhere to be seen and yet suffuses everything – is gender. An attempt is being made here to consider monarchy in a theoretical sense, beyond gender as it were, by using neutral terms like ruler, sovereign and rulership. Yet we must acknowledge

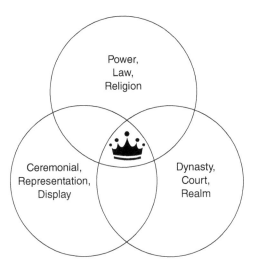

Figure 0.1 Venn diagram of the key elements of monarchy

the assumption that rulers are necessarily male and that monarchy is a innately patriarchal institution where only men can access and exercise power. However, even when the ruler is male, we must not assume that they were the sole locus of power, as discussions of the concept of corporate monarchy will demonstrate in due course. Theresa Earenfight has been an inspiration in this regard, pushing for reconsiderations of gender and power, and urging caution in the vocabulary that we use to describe the activities of male and female rulers and royal figures to avoid minimizing or devaluing the impact of women.[5] A conscious decision was made early on to avoid grouping this collection in terms of 'kingship' and 'queenship', and indeed to avoid a chronological framework so that we could break down the barriers of gender, period and place which have so often constrained our ability to fully understand the mechanisms of monarchy in their broadest possible sense.

Thus, the four parts of our volume link instead to the theoretical framework set out in this chapter. 'Models and concepts of rulership' covers aspects of power, law and religion to consider how we create, define and idealize the monarch's role. 'Ritual and representation' takes in the ideas of ceremonial, representation, display and how the monarch creates and broadcasts their image to the dynasty, court, realm and beyond. 'Dynasty and succession' clearly speaks to dynasty, court and realm with particular consideration of how a ruler is drawn from their dynasty to rule. Finally, 'Exercising authority and exerting influence' brings all of these elements together, highlighting the activity of particular agents within the wider framework of monarchy. This chapter will continue by examining the key areas (power, law and religion; ceremonial, representation and display; dynasty, court and realm) in turn before turning to the wider context and considering monarchical continuity, change and comparison in the final section.

Power, law and religion

The exercise of power is intimately and consistently associated with any discussion of monarchy. In the most fundamental form, a ruler can be defined as one who has recognized authority over a group of people and their territory.[6] A ruler is, in theory, the most important and visible person in the realm – there is an assumption that they are also the most politically powerful individual in the realm. Yet, is that always the case? This section will explore the power of the monarch, from figurehead to absolute ruler, and the basis from which that power derives.

Again, while the assumption is that the office of ruler automatically confers great power upon the holder, we can also easily think of monarchs who are effectively powerless, like today's constitutional monarchs. However, the notion of a figurehead ruler who reigns instead of rules is hardly a modern phenomenon. The *Huai Nan Tzu*, a Chinese text from c.140 BCE, emphasizes the importance of *wu-wei* or nonaction to the point of placid stillness on the part of the emperor:

> The art of the ruler is to deal with things through nonaction and to disseminate wordless instructions (*chiao*).
> Limpid and still he does not move; even when moved he is not agitated (*yao*):
> taking advantage of the course of things he delegates
> responsibility to subordinates and, holding them to account, he does not wear himself out (*lao*).[7]

At the other extreme is the nearly unlimited power wielded by monarchs such as the Tsars of Russia; Catherine II of Russia (r.1762–96) stated that 'The Sovereign is absolute; for there is no other authority but that which centers in his single Person'.[8] While Catherine defended the necessity of the absolute power of the Tsar and the utility of monarchy as a means to govern her vast realm, political theorists from the ancient world to the modern era have debated the extent of power that a ruler can exercise and the limitations of the royal prerogative.

Before considering the boundaries and extent of the monarch's power, it is important to examine where the power of the ruler comes from. While there are several means which arguably provide the basis of the monarch's power, all of them can be traced back to either law, such as being the rightful heir under the laws of succession, or religion, such as one who has been divinely selected to rule, or both. These legal and religious elements are vital tenets that confer legitimacy on the ruler and provide the cornerstone of their power and authority.[9] This section will explore both legal and religious elements of monarchical power in detail, starting with the latter.

One element linked to the power of the monarch is charisma, which has been particularly discussed with regard to the rule of the Roman emperors, from Augustus onwards.[10] Yet charisma has a distinct link to the divine. Max Weber, in his intensive discussion of charisma and authority, defined charisma as:

> [a] certain quality of an individual personality by virtue of which he is set apart from ordinary men and treated as endowed with supernatural, superhuman or at least specifically exceptional powers or qualities. These are such

as are not accessible to the ordinary person but are regarded as of divine origin or as exemplary, and on the basis of them the individual concerned is treated as a leader.[11]

The notion that a ruler is 'set apart' is one that also resonates with Declan Quigley who argues that 'The fundamental idea underlying kingship is the separation of one human being from others'.[12] This idea of separateness or difference can be seen in one form through the concept of a 'stranger king' who is perceived as a foreigner or outsider, which can be found in African, Polynesian, Indonesian and pre-Columbian societies.[13]

Part of this 'separateness' derives from the sacral nature of monarchy – a sense that the sovereign has a connection with the divine. Here too there is a spectrum between rulers: from those who were considered to be divine or living gods on one extreme, like the Egyptian pharaohs, to a religious association that does not (necessarily) mark the sovereign out as divinely appointed or sacred, such as Elizabeth II of Great Britain and Northern Ireland's role as the titular Head of the Church of England. The line between divinity and humanity for rulers could well be blurred. In South Asia, for example, while the divine aspect of monarchy was boosted in some areas by an association with the god Rama and the cult of Devaraja, Morrison has noted that 'truly deified rulers are rare'.[14] However, Kershaw has noted that in Cambodia, there was an idea that the ruler was a 'being who was himself, or could eventually become, divine'.[15] Another way of blurring these lines was by claiming divine dynastic ancestry, as can be seen in the genealogies of Aztec and Polynesian kings or even the Julio-Claudians' claim to be descended from the goddess Venus.[16] Yet another method of linking monarchy to the divine was through their claim to be divinely appointed or a representative of the divine on Earth. James VI & I of Scotland and England (r.1567/1603–25) used this notion of divine selection or appointment to claim an almost god-like status, using a biblical rationale: 'Kings are called gods by the prophetical King David because they sit upon God his throne in the earth and have the count of their administration to give unto him.'[17] Finally, rulers could be seen as blessed by the gods with supernatural abilities or magic, particularly in Africa, with examples such as the Lovedu queens who represented the Earth and had a mystical ability with regard to controlling rain.[18] In a similar vein, ancient Japanese rulers were credited with the ability to 'solicit supernatural power' to ensure a successful rice harvest.[19]

Indeed, part of a ruler's responsibilities may be to use their status somewhere in between divine and human to mediate between both worlds, currying favour with the gods and thus ensuring the prosperity of their people.[20] Oakley has argued a ruler's role was a 'primarily religious one, involving the preservation of the cosmic order and the "harmonious integration" of human beings with the natural world'.[21] Yet this responsibility to maintain the cosmic order and balance between gods and humanity carried great responsibility and even personal risk to the ruler. Calamities such as adverse weather conditions, natural disasters or crop failures could be attributed to poor rulership or the ruler's failure to please the divine and could lead to the dethronement of the ruler or the collapse of the monarchy itself.[22] The Chinese emperor Wen (r.180–157 BCE) reflected upon this perceived burden of rulership asking himself during a time of crisis, 'is there some fault in Our way of government or is there some defect in Our conduct? Or is it that We have not obeyed the Way of Heaven?'[23] Mediating between the human and divine could even require the ritual sacrifice of the ruler themselves to expel evil or to regain the approbation of the gods – this notion of 'scapegoating' or ritual regicide has been much studied and debated by anthropologists from Sir James George Frazer to the present day.[24]

Given this deep and persistent connection between the divine and rulers, there follows that there is also an enduring link between monarchy and religion. A monarch can be both a religious head as well as a secular one, such as the aforementioned current British monarch who is head of both church and state. Yet Quigley argues that there is a clear line between rulers and religion: 'Kings cannot be priests (or ministers) and priests cannot be kings. Kings are made by priests, who represent both the people and some divine or transcendent force.'[25] There has also been conflict, particularly in Christian Europe, over whether the power of the Church or the ruler was supreme. Alain Boureau reflects on this duality between church and monarchy in the Middle Ages:

> According to an ancient pattern of ecclesial doctrine, there exist in this world only two kinds of universal power, *regnum* and *sacerdotium*, both directly or indirectly ordained for the purpose of salvation. Secular power, *regnum*, followed the same pattern of lieutenancy, based on the royalty of Christ. Kings could only aspire to the prosperity that justified their power by submitting to ecclesial control.[26]

Another challenge to the relationship between monarchy and religion is modernity and secularity. At the time of writing, it remains to be seen if the eventual accession of Prince Charles will provoke a reappraisal of the monarch's role as head of both church and state in Britain or if the new Thai king Maha Vajiralongkorn will be able to attain or maintain the semi-divine status that his father King Bhumibol possessed.[27] Deploige and Denekere have explored the desacralization of modern monarchy, arguing that the French Revolution was a key watershed in this process, at least in a European sense, marking 'the transition of monarchy as a divine investiture to a monarchy legitimized by the nation'.[28]

The other key cornerstone of monarchical power is law. Burns has gone so far as to argue that 'Law is inseparable from kingship' and the fundamental aspect of the ruler's role is to uphold law and justice.[29] Indeed, oaths to uphold the laws and mete out justice to their subjects are frequently found at the heart of ceremonies to install new monarchs. For example, the accession ceremony of medieval Navarrese rulers, common to Iberian practice, was a *juramento* or oathswearing, for the ruler to swear to uphold the *Fueros*, or the law and custom of the realm and the rights of their subjects.[30] Medieval European political theorists argued that law was the foundation of rulership, that monarchy was 'derived from natural law and from the law of nations'.[31] They ruminated on the monarch's relationship with the law and their subjects as well as the ruler's role as the defender of law and justice. Adherence to the law, these theorists argued, separated monarchs from tyrants. John of Salisbury contrasted the two by noting that unlike tyrants, a ruler was 'obedient to law' and 'rules by the laws'.[32] John Wyclif explicitly linked law and religion, noting that 'The king must, therefore, establish just laws and as a consequence the rule of the law of the Lord, so that as a result of this he as well as his subjects are servants of God in His justice.'[33] Thus in Wyclif's rationale, the king served God by defending and administering the laws of the realm.

This fixation on the idea of the 'just king' and the ruler as the upholder of justice was hardly unique to a European or Christian concept of monarchy. Islamic 'mirrors for princes' also focused on the role of the ruler as the upholder of justice and linked this function closely to religion. These texts demonstrate that 'the embodiment of justice is the ruler' and that administering justice was 'instrumental to successful rule'.[34] The practical application of upholding the law and giving justice are also discussed in admonitions for the Sultan to regularly attend court hearings and decide cases according to Islamic law.[35]

While the extent to which the ruler was subject to, rather than just obliged to uphold, the law has been greatly debated and has varied significantly in different temporal and societal contexts, it is important to recognize that the royal prerogative was always limited to some extent by law and custom. In addition, rulers were always subject to a restrictive set of rules and expectations regarding how they should behave and rule. The aforementioned 'mirrors for princes' genre is an ideal example of how these ideals and expectations were transmitted to monarchs, as a veritable guidebook – or even rulebook – of rulership. They were normally written by authors who were grounded in both law and religion, and these tracts discussed the boundaries of the royal prerogative and expressed the qualities which rulers were expected to possess. These lists of qualities expected of rulers were hardly brief and perhaps reflected the idea that a ruler was meant to be superhuman or quasi-divine, as the expectations were higher than mere mortals could conceivably meet. Jeroen Duindam has noted: 'The duties of rulership as outlined in moral tracts were not only almost impossible to fulfil for most persons, they were also contradictory.'[36] Neither were these 'mirrors for princes' the only works which advised princes. Additional guidance or proscriptions for royal behaviour were given by those who wrote works on the education of rulers, slotted into dedications of various literary works and were sometimes even written by their predecessors.[37]

The often incredibly restrictive confines of court protocol also hedged monarchs with rules for their behaviour and a tight framework for their activities. The combination of meeting the expectations of kingly behaviour and adhering to court protocol made ruling itself even more challenging. Yet rulers who failed to meet the lofty expectations of their subjects or adhere to the strictures of appropriate behaviour for a monarch risked removal from power by being dethroned – leading to potential incarceration, exile or regicide as Cathleen Sarti's chapter in this collection will discuss. Rulers could also be killed when they were felt to no longer possess the qualities essential for rulership. Luc de Heusch provides the example of the Shilluk kings; a central tenet of their rule was to be the 'guarantor of fertility', thus once their own fertility was believed to be lost or compromised, they were ritually strangled.[38]

This highlights the perpetual danger that rulers faced – their power was supported by and subject to both law and religion. Their connection to the divine made them more than the average human but placed great pressure on them to mediate between worlds and ensure (cosmic) order. Rulers were charged with upholding the laws of God and the realm as well as being subject to extremely high expectations and prescriptions for their behaviour. Failing to keep the balance between the human world and the divine or failing to meet the perceived requirements of the role could lead to a fall from power. Ultimately, the power of monarchs is both supported and tightly bound by law and religion.

Ceremonial, representation, display

Without doubt, ceremonial is a central aspect of monarchy and is often deeply tied to the role of the ruler in maintaining harmony both within the realm and between the divine and human worlds. In some societies, the monarch's ceremonial actions were perceived as pivotal to their subjects' survival as in the previous discussion of the early Japanese rulers' role in ensuring the rice harvest or the elaborate rituals that Mayan rulers undertook to intercede with the gods for the rain needed to grow crops.[39] At the far extreme, ceremonial could be seen as the central impetus of not only monarchy but of the realm itself, as in the example of the 'theatre state' of Bali, where Geertz famously noted that 'Power served pomp, not pomp power.'[40]

Ceremonial and ritual underpin and affirm the monarch's role. As Quigley has noted 'The purpose of all ritual is either to transform a person from one status to another or maintain him in that status.'[41] Clearly coronations, or the ceremonies that mark the accession of a new monarch, are a key moment, when the heir transitions into that 'separate' status – positioned outside the normal society to which their peers and subjects belong. This separation from the ruler's previous, entirely human, body could involve an element of ritual regicide, if only in a symbolic sense or via a sacrificial stand-in for the king as in the case of the Maya, so that the ruler could be 'reborn' in a new monarchical, semi-divine form.[42]

While not containing an element of regicide, many European coronation ceremonies marked the ruler as divinely blessed and sanctioned as the religious officiant anointed the new ruler with holy oil. These ceremonies became increasingly elaborate over the course of the Middle Ages, as documented in lengthy *ordo* which set out the exact framework for the ritual. These manuals, such as the fourteenth-century English *Liber Regalis* or the *Ordines Coronationis Franciae* which built on earlier Carolingian and Ottonian practice, set both a pattern for later monarchs in their own realms to follow as well as a model that rulers in other realms could copy. Indeed, Sergio Bertelli has noted the spread of ceremonial practice through intermarriage and imitation, or even by the advent of new dynasties who may seek to make their own mark on the realm by making adaptations to previous rituals, as in the case of the Champenois and Evreux dynasties of Navarre who brought French ideas of royal ceremonial to the Iberian kingdom.[43] The influence of a powerful neighbour can also affect ceremonial, as Holtom demonstrated in his discussion of Chinese influence on Japanese enthronement ceremonies.[44]

The ceremonial element of the ruler's role was part of the expectations and ideals of rulership. It was not only a means of ensuring cosmic or merely courtly order but also the harmonious functioning of the realm according to a prescribed set of ritual behaviour and protocol to which all levels of society were meant to ascribe. Correct observance of ritual was not only a way for rulers to ensure celestial and terrestrial harmony but also served as a model to their subjects, according to the eighteenth-century Chinese writer Wang Youpu who argued that the ruler 'must first set an example for them [i.e. his subjects] of ceremonial behaviour and deference'.[45]

The amount of time that a monarch was required to spend performing rituals could impact their ability to function politically, turning them into more of a reigning monarch whose primary task was to oversee ceremonial, instead of being an active ruler. For example, the Japanese emperors were responsible for observing the *nenju gyoji*, the annual calendar of ceremonies. They were required by the Ritsuryō Code of 757 to perform thirteen different types of rituals.[46] One means of avoiding the strictures of ceremonial was the practice of the Tahitian *ari'i rahi* who abdicated in favour of their heir as soon as they were born – in this way the baby could become the focus of ritual and ceremonial while the parent was freed up to rule as their regent.[47]

Court ceremony could also be a means of underpinning the authority of the monarch by making them the focus of all daily ritual. Louis XIV of France (r.1643–1715) used this to great effect in the court system that he created at Versailles – from the *levée* to the *coucher du roi* all ceremonial focused on the king; if he was not physically present, the rituals were still observed with objects which stood in for the king.[48] Royal power can also be underlined by occasional, rather than daily ceremonial, as Maurice Bloch demonstrates in his discussion of the elaborate ritual of the royal bath in Madagascar.[49] Ceremonial and ritual were also a means of image creation, both justifying their power and demonstrating how rulers exemplified the virtues that monarchs were expected to possess. For example, the Nepalese ruler Prithvi Narayan Shah (r.1743–75) used religious ritual and the ceremonial of royal land donations to secure divine support for his rule and military campaigns, and also to fashion an image of himself to his subjects as a pious model ruler.[50]

Ceremonial is still a fundamental aspect of monarchy today. Indeed Jaap van Osta has argued that:

> [i]t seems clear that the role of monarchy as an institution in our present postmodern era is basically ceremonial . . . the reappearance of the 'ceremonial monarchy', i.e. a monarchy based essentially upon royal performance, is the outcome of the desacralization of the monarchy and the democratization of politics.[51]

Deploige and Deneckere affirm this idea, pointing to modern rituals such as the monarch's annual speech to their subjects, noting this is 'essentially symbolic, in the sense that the pact between the monarch and the nation was renewed and ratified every year'.[52] Modern media has made royal ceremonial more accessible – it is estimated that nearly two billion people in more than 180 countries across the globe engaged with the wedding of Prince William and Catherine Middleton in 2011 via television and media reports.[53] Likewise, in October 2017, the funeral of the Thai king Bhumibol Adulyadej was broadcast live to 177 countries in full colour (as Thai television and internet sites had previously gone into black and white in mourning for the king). It could be argued then that, following van Osta, the ceremonial aspect of monarchy has been amplified by modern media, reaffirming the centrality of ritual to the practice of rulership.

Representation and display are two important means of communicating majesty, visually underlining the power and authority of the monarch. This can not only be done through ceremonial but also via the outward appearance of the monarch, both in person and as commemorated in portraits, statues, seals, coins and tombs. The monarch's dress, as demonstrated by Benjamin Wild's contribution to this collection and Philip Mansel's *Dressed to Rule*, is a key means of royal image creation.[54] It could be used to enhance the monarch's special 'separate' status as in sumptuary laws or the use of the purple dye derived from murex which was the especial preserve of Roman and later Byzantine emperors. However, if not chosen carefully, dress and display could also undermine a ruler, just as the criticism of Marie Antoinette's extravagant dress and elaborate coiffure added fuel to the republican fire which ultimately consumed the *Ancien Regime* monarchy in France.[55]

More important than dress perhaps was regalia, the symbols of the monarch's power and authority. The ceremonial of coronation not only normally involves some element of ritual purification and blessing but the investiture of the monarch with the regalia or the symbols of their office. While regalia take many forms in different places, times and societal contexts, the sovereign's possession and use of these often sacred items visually displays their right to rule. These symbols of rulership, including crowns, orbs, sceptres or staffs of office, can often be found in images of monarchs. This imagery can be subtly inserted in the wearing of a coronation ring or the discreet placement of a crown on a table next to the ruler, or presented in a very direct way. This was demonstrated by the portrait of Charles II commemorating the Restoration of the English monarchy in 1660 by portraying him on his throne, under the cloth of state, wearing all of his (newly minted) regalia.[56] It is no accident that many coins, a visible and tangible reminder of the monarch's authority accessible to every subject on a constant basis, bore the image of the ruler enthroned or at least crowned, often with a list of their titles around the edge.[57] Even today's British coinage and stamps bear the image of Elizabeth II wearing a tiara or diadem, as pictured in Matthias Range's chapter, demonstrating the enduring power of the crown as a representation of monarchical authority.[58] Coinage offers monarchs the ability to represent themselves individually as the face of the realm as well as representatives of their dynasty through heraldic shields which are often present on the reverse of their coins and on their seals.

Display and representation were also not confined to the monarch's lifetime as their tomb could display not only the power that they wielded while living but commemorate how they lived up to the ideals of rulership. One example is the impressive double tomb of Louis XII of France (r.1498–1515) and Anne de Bretagne in the royal necropolis of Saint Denis which emphasizes the couple's piety both in being pictured as cadavers in the 'transi' underneath and as they kneel at *prie-dieu* atop the tomb. Louis' military victories are also pictured on the base highlighting his success as a general, while 'the reliefs around the tomb express the concept of worldly glory'.[59] While a monarch's plans for their tomb could be derailed by their successors or destroyed by successive generations, memorials provide the opportunity at least for a ruler to make a lasting statement of the position and authority that they possessed in life. Indeed, it is in these physical representations of individual monarchs, from the smallest coin to Cheops' pyramid, which offer enduring examples of the utility of representation and display to communicate the power of the monarch to the subjects of their realm and beyond.

Dynasty, court and realm

In recent years, there has been an increasing focus on dynasty in the field of royal studies. Studies have focused on the definition and composition of dynasty and the relationship between the monarch and their dynastic members. Jeroen Duindam's excellent study *Dynasties* posits a model of concentric circles which places the monarch at the centre, with the layers of dynasty, court and realm radiating outwards.[60] Geevers and Marini have wrestled with how to define dynasty. They argue that it is more than just a family or kin group, putting forward the interesting concept of dynasty as an iceberg where 'a minority of living family members are visible, while a host of deceased and unborn ones remain hidden'.[61] This concept is quite useful in considering the eternal aspect of dynasty – that it is about more than its current members or the ruler on the throne, who can be seen in this way as merely caretakers of the dynasty's fortunes and titles.

Dynasty forms a key bulwark of support for monarchy, and yet intradynastic rivalry can also cause the destruction of the family, allowing another dynasty to usurp their position.[62] This rivalry stems from the notion that many, or all, of the members of the dynasty are also potential claimants to the throne, which can increase tension within the kin group. It also ties in with the notion of how a dynasty self-defines, who is considered to be part of the group and who is considered to be eligible for the throne. Whether or not women were eligible successors for the throne, they have always played a central part in the creation of dynasty. In her analysis of the Aztec dynasties, Susan Gillespie demonstrates that women played a key role in legitimating kings and the royal line throughout its history, going right back to the foundation of the Tenochtitlan dynasty as its first king, Acamapichtli (r.1375–95), gained his status through being the son and husband of Toltec princesses.[63] Royal women could function as dynastic progenitors both through creating heirs of their own body or by designating heirs, as Seokyung Han's study of the women of the Choson dynasty of Korea (1392–1910) has shown.[64]

The designation of heirs or potential successors from the pool of dynastic members then is not only vital in determining the next monarch, it is crucial to maintaining dynastic harmony. They can be selected out of a pool of potential claimants, by ability, age or favour; however, the system of designation of the heir by the current ruler, as practised in many current Arab monarchies, can lead to discord within the dynasty due to disagreement over who is believed to be the most appropriate or able successor.[65] Creating clear laws or custom for succession is a means of ensuring dynastic harmony by limiting the pool of eligible successors and regulating the order of accession. There are several principles which have been applied to the succession in order to achieve this regulation, which normally include some method of reckoning based on proximity of blood to the current ruler or a common dynastic ancestor. These can include models based on birth order such as (male) primogeniture or ultimogeniture; porphyrogeniture, where only children born to the monarch during their reign are eligible successors; and succession along collateral lines rather than parent to child and favouring either agnatic or matrilineal lines of descent.[66] It is also important to recognize that there are means of selecting a monarch beyond a pool of dynastic members, as election is another means of choosing a monarch. However, as Matthias Schnettger's study of the Habsburgs in this volume demonstrates, it was still possible for a dynasty to ensure its continued hold on power in an elective monarchy by controlling the mechanism of election to favour members of its own kin group.[67]

However, while competition can be an element that can divide a ruling family, dynastic members can also work and rule cooperatively in order to ensure the harmony of the kin group and the realm. The idea of corporate monarchy, that the ruler is only the most visible part of a group which works together to rule, draws on the notion that dynastic members, including mothers, daughters, wives, brothers, uncles and cousins, have a vested interest in the dynasty's hold on power and will work together to achieve that end and the smooth rule of the realm. Earenfight has urged us to consider rulers, consorts and dynasty together, conceptualizing monarchy as a 'flexible sack' which could accommodate a group of people working together to exercise power.[68] Some dynasties, including those in Africa, Hawaii and pre-Colombian America, practised endogamy or royal incest, encouraging rulers to marry their siblings to keep power firmly within the kin group. However, as the history of the Ptolemaic dynasty of Egypt clearly demonstrates, this strategy was not necessarily effective in terms of preserving dynastic harmony or their hold on the throne as sisters and brothers dethroned and killed one another with startling frequency.[69] Another means of corporate rule within the dynasty is by splitting the duties of office. Claessen notes the example of the *tui tonga* or kings of Tonga who gradually split the royal duties and prerogative among various branches of the royal family, including the king's younger brother who started the line of the *tui haa takalaua* and took on key aspects of rule while the king retained many sacred duties. The *tui haa takalaua* later named his own son as his hereditary deputy or *tui kanokopulu*, dividing the duties of rule yet further, and finally the position of *tui tonga fefine* was created for the eldest sister of the *tui tonga*, which gave a greater role in the realm for herself and her children.[70]

Moving out 'a layer' from dynasty to court, we can start to focus on the wider setting of monarchy. Court studies have been a very active area of scholarship, from Norbert Elias' classic and much debated work *The Court Society* to the present day.[71] While it is impossible to effectively summarize these works here, it is useful for our purposes to note the models they present of the interaction or relationship between the monarch and the personnel of the court, from the highest nobility to the lowliest servant. Tracing networks both within and between courts has been a recent fruitful approach to both royal and court studies.[72] Social network analysis has also been used as a useful tool to study connections between the ruler and the members of their dynasty and court, and between courtiers. One excellent example of the potential of this type of analysis can be seen in a doctoral thesis on the household of the late medieval queens of Castile. In it, Diana Pelaz Flores was able to demonstrate the wealth of interconnections between the queens and their household members, highlighting families in service to the queens and intermarriage between them.[73] It is vital to realize the impact of wider societal structures on the formation and working of the court, for example the monogamous nature of western Christian societies radically alters the position of court women to those of polygamous societies as reflected in Islamic, Asian and African courts. Given this variety, in order to truly understand the functioning of courts, and by extension monarchy, in a wider perspective, comparison across time and place is necessary. One recent collection which takes this approach, in a similar fashion to the current volume, is Duindam, Artan and Kunt's *Royal Courts in Dynastic States and Empires: A Global Perspective.*[74]

Moving further outwards still, the physical structure of the palace provides the setting for both the monarch and their court as well as serving as a key locus of ceremonial. The creation, renovation or decoration of a palace and its surrounding landscape could also be a means of self-fashioning or projecting a particular image of monarchy. Seventeenth-century Europe offers two compelling examples of this in the 'Sun King' Louis XIV's Versailles and the Count-Duke Olivares' creation of the Palace of Buen Retiro to complement the idea of Felipe IV of Spain's role as the *Rey Planeta*.[75] The location of the palace was incredibly significant in terms of the relationship between the monarch, court and realm. More particularly, whether the palace was cited within or outside the capital was important to understanding how monarchy was framed. The capital was the theoretical centre of the realm, but as Kershaw notes, it could have an even deeper meaning in South East Asia where the 'capital stood for the whole country, being not just the nation's political and cultural centre but indeed the magic centre of the empire'.[76] Thus by situating themselves and their court in this 'magic centre', the monarch could theoretically amplify their own power. The particular placement of the palace within the capital city could be significant as well. Jacobsen notes that the palaces of Mexica rulers were strategically placed in the central precinct of Tenochtitlan in 'a zone with sacred structures and religious activity', underlining their connection to the divine, which supported their power and authority.[77]

Yet other rulers deliberately chose to cite their palaces in an extra-urban setting. Mitchell and Melville use the example of the Saljuq (Seljuk) rulers of central Asia (eleventh to fourteenth centuries) who situated themselves in camps either just outside their cities or well beyond them during the summer months to demonstrate how 'space is used not to create intimacy in the power relationship, but to emphasize distance'.[78] Indeed, the Saljuq rulers also provide an example of itinerant rulership, monarchs who kept themselves and their court on the move. This, as the *iter* of medieval German kings and the progresses of Elizabeth I of England demonstrate, can be an effective tool for a monarch to engage with the realm, by showing themselves to their subjects and engaging in ritual and ceremonial in urban and religious sites across their lands.[79] Maintaining this connection to the realm at large can be seen as a vital element of monarchy, for whether seen or unseen, as Quigley notes, 'The king is that individual who is uniquely connected to everyone in that society. That is the king's function . . . The essence of kingship, however, is that everyone is united by his or her common relation to the king.'[80]

Continuity, change and comparison

In the present age, monarchy is caught in a strange dichotomy. It is perceived by some as a relic of a backward age and has long been under threat from republicanism, and yet it continues to persist, forming a focus for popular culture, nationalism and tourism. Many monarchies have disappeared entirely due to overthrow from internal political pressures or external forces such as war or colonial expansion. The majority of today's sovereigns are constitutional monarchs who reign instead of rule – the abrupt or gradual loss of their power and prerogatives has been a central development of monarchy into the modern era. But those monarchies which remain have endured or emerged, it could be argued, because modern monarchy is about much more than the ruler themselves. Monarchy is a system, a societal mechanism, where a ruler can be more than a figure or figurehead – they can become the face of the nation, or even of an age as the British queens Elizabeth I and Victoria have demonstrated.

Jaap van Osta has discussed the means by which monarchy became an increasing focus for nationalistic sentiment and unity at the turn of the twentieth century: 'Vested with all the splendor of monarchical ritual, the monarch would be presented as the vivid symbol of continuity and consensus to which the whole nation might defer.'[81] The personal aspect of monarchy is another consideration – the greater openness and visibility of monarchy can lead to the impression that we 'know' monarchs and have a connection with them and an awareness of their personal lives that would have been unthinkable a few generations ago. This raises Kantorowicz's discussion of the body politic and body natural; how much of monarchy's endurance today is down to the personal element of monarchy vs reverence for the office itself?[82] Quigley also cautions that the increasingly personal element of monarchy can erode the 'separateness' which forms a crucial aspect of the monarch's role, that today's royals still need to 'set themselves apart in order to be identified as regal'.[83] Deploige and Deneckere also note this difficult tension between modern monarchy's need to 'move among the people' and still 'stay on [their] pedestal'.[84]

To survive then, monarchy must strike a delicate balance between continuity and change, preserving the traditions which underpin the framework of their role while adapting to stay in step with modern society and meet the expectations of their subjects as to what appropriate behaviour for today's ruler should be. One demonstration of how monarchy has adapted to follow societal change can be seen in regard to changes to the succession practices of many European monarchies with regard to gender. Between 1980 and 2013 seven European monarchies changed the law with regard to the succession to allow for equal or absolute primogeniture, that the eldest child inherits the throne regardless of their sex.[85] This move reflected greater societal change in Europe and beyond, which has resulted in increased equality for women in terms of legal and political rights, working conditions and pay. While the monarch's role cannot be equated simply to being a 'job', it is still significant that European monarchies and governments felt that the laws of succession needed to reflect societal attitudes to gender equality. However, this trend has not been universal in modern monarchies; in spite of having ruling empresses in its history, the Japanese monarchy banned the possibility of female heirs in the late nineteenth century, ironically via European influence.[86] Although there has been considerable controversy about changing this law to include female claimants to the throne, particularly prior to the birth of Prince Hisahito in 2006 when there was a near total lack of male heirs, there has to date been no official change to favour the claim of Princess Aiko, the daughter of Crown Prince Naruhito, over her male cousin. Thus, just as in society at large, women have not achieved equality in all areas and places – in this way monarchy still reflects the modern world which surrounds and supports it.

***

While contributions in our volume such as those from David Mednicoff and Beverly Stoeltje engage with monarchy right up to the present day, our authors also offer case studies of historical monarchy which extend back in time to ancient Egypt. Again, our case studies aim to increase our understanding of monarchy in a global context through our exploration of these key themes of models and concepts of rulership, ritual and representation, dynasty and succession, and exercising authority and exerting influence. The chapters that follow, taken together, also illustrate the theory posited here on the interaction between power, law and religion, ceremonial, representation and display, and dynasty, court and realm as being the core elements which make up the theory and practice of monarchy.

Notes

1 Nasim Zakaria, *The British Political System* (Lahore: Indus Publishing House, 1966), 31. Jeremy Paxman, *On Royalty* (London: Penguin, 2007), 13.
2 David Cannadine, "Introduction: Divine Rites of Kings," in *Rituals of Royalty: Power and Ceremonial in Traditional Societies*, eds., David Cannadine and Simon Price (Cambridge: Cambridge University Press, 1987), 2–5.
3 Declan Quigley, "Introduction: The Character of Kingship," in *The Character of Kingship*, ed. Declan Quigley (Oxford: Berg, 2005), 11.
4 David Cannadine and Simon Price, eds, *Rituals of Royalty: Power and Ceremonial in Traditional Societies* (Cambridge: Cambridge University Press, 1987); Declan Quigley ed., *The Character of Kingship* (Oxford: Berg, 2005); Jeroen Duindam, *Dynasties: A Global History of Power, 1300–1800* (Cambridge: Cambridge University Press, 2015); Francis Oakley, *Kingship: The Politics of Enchantment* (Oxford: Blackwell, 2006).
5 Theresa Earenfight, "A Lifetime of Power: Beyond Binaries of Power and Gender" (conference paper given at Verbis et Exemplis, London, April 26, 2018). See also her seminal article "Without the Persona of the Prince: Kings, Queens and the Idea of Monarchy in Late Medieval Europe," *Gender and History* 19, no. 1 (2007): 1–21.
6 The definition of a ruler or rulership has been much debated. Francis Oakley offers a discussion and a few working definitions in *Kingship*, 1–2.
7 Liu An, "Huai Nan Tzu," in *The Art of Rulership: A Study of Ancient Chinese Political Thought*, trans. Roger T. Ames (Albany: State University of New York Press, 1994).
8 Catherine II of Russia, *The Grand Instruction to the Commissioners Appointed to Frame a New Code of Laws for the Russian Empire: Composed by Her Imperial Majesty Catherine II* (London: T. Jefferys, 1768).
9 See Lynette Mitchell and Charles Melville, "'Every Inch a King': Kings and Kingship in the Ancient and Medieval Worlds," in *Every Inch a King: Comparative Studies on Kings and Kingship in the Ancient and Medieval Worlds*, eds. Lynette Mitchell and Charles Melville (Leiden: Brill, 2013), 11.
10 One study which looks at the transfer of Augustus' personal charisma to the office of emperor is Rebecca Edwards' doctoral thesis: "Divus Augustus Pater: Tiberius and the Charisma of Augustus," University of Indiana, PhD Thesis, 2003. See also Mitchell and Melville, "Every Inch a King," 7–8.
11 Max Weber, *On Charisma and Institution Building*, ed. S.N. Eisenstadt (Chicago: University of Chicago Press, 1968), 48.
12 Quigley, "Introduction," 4.
13 Marshall Sahlins has published extensively on this idea. For an example of his work see Marshall Sahlins, "The Stranger-King or Elementary Forms of the Politics of Life," *Indonesia and the Malay World* 36, no. 10 (2008): 177–199 (note that this is a special issue of the journal dedicated to the idea of stranger kings). On this phenomenon in the Aztecs see Susan D. Gillespie, *The Aztec Kings: The Construction of Rulership in Mexica History* (Tucson: The University of Arizona Press, 1989), 219–221.
14 Kathleen D. Morrison, "When Gods Ruled: Comments on Divine Kingship," in *Religion and Power: Divine Kingship in the Ancient World and Beyond*, ed. Nicole Brisch (Chicago: The Oriental Institute of the University of Chicago, 2008), 268.
15 Roger Kershaw, *Monarchy in South-East Asia: The Faces of Tradition in Translation* (London: Routledge, 2001), 175–182.

16 Henri J.M. Claessen, "Chiefs and Kings in Polynesia," in *The Character of Kingship*, ed. Declan Quigley (Oxford: Berg, 2005), 235–237; Gillespie, *Aztec Kings*, 216.

17 James VI & I of England and Scotland, *The True Law of Free Monarchies: Or the Reciprock and Mutual Duty Betwixt a Free King and His Natural Subject*, eds. Daniel Fischlin and Mark Fortier (Toronto: Centre for Renaissance and Reformation Studies, 1996), 54–55.

18 Luc de Heusch, "Forms of Sacralized Power in Africa," in *The Character of Kingship*, ed. Declan Quigley (Oxford: Berg, 2005), 26, 32.

19 Emiko Ohnuki-Tierney, "Japanese Monarchy in Historical and Comparative Perspective," in *The Character of Kingship*, ed. Declan Quigley (Oxford: Berg, 2005), 209.

20 See Gillespie's discussion of this with relation to the Aztec rulers in Gillespie, *Aztec Kings*, 215.

21 Oakley, *Kingship*, 7.

22 See Morrison, "When Gods Ruled," 269.

23 Emperor Wen of China, "An Edict of Emperor Wen (163 B.C.E)," in *The Establishment of the Han Empire and Imperial China*, eds. Grant Hardy and Anne Behnke Kinney (London: Greenwood Press, 2005), 147.

24 Quigley's collection *The Character of Kingship* is an excellent example of the ongoing debate and study in this area. See particularly the following chapters: Lucien Scubla, "Sacred King, Sacrificial Victim, Surrogate Victim or Frazer, Hocart, Girard," 39–62; Luc de Heusch, "A Reply to Lucien Scubla," 63–66; and Simon Simonse, "Tragedy, Ritual and Power in Nilotic Regicide: The Regicidal Daramas of the Eastern Nilotes of Sudan in Comparative Perspective," 67–100.

25 Quigley, "Introduction," 19.

26 Alain Boureau, "How Christian Was the Sacralization of Monarchy in Western Europe (Twelfth-Fifteenth Centuries)?" in *Mystifying the Monarch: Studies on Discourse, Power and History*, eds. Jeroen Deploige and Gita Deneckere (Amsterdam: Amsterdam University Press, 2006), 31.

27 See Peter A. Jackson, "Markets, Media, and Magic: Thailand's Monarch as a 'Virtual Deity'," *Inter-Asia Cultural Studies* 10 no. 3 (2009), 361–380, and Harriet Sherwood, "Prince Charles Accession Could Trigger Debate on Disestablishment," *The Guardian*, 10 December 2017, www.theguardian.com/world/2017/dec/10/prince-charles-ascension-time-for-debate-on-disestablishment-says-report.

28 Jeroen Deploige and Gita Deneckere, "The Monarchy: A Crossroads of Trajectories," in *Mystifying the Monarch: Studies on Discourse, Power and History*, eds. Jeroen Deploige and Gita Deneckere (Amsterdam: Amsterdam University Press, 2006), 17.

29 J.H. Burns, *Lordship, Kingship, and Empire: The Idea of Monarchy, 1400–1525* (Oxford: Clarendon Press, 1992), 154–155.

30 For an extended discussion of the coronation practice of the high medieval Navarrese rulers see Jose Maria Lacarra, *El Juramento de los Reyes de Navarra (1234–1329)* (Madrid: Real Academia de la Historia, 1972).

31 John of Paris, "On Royal and Papal Power," in *Medieval Political Theory-A Reader: The Quest for the Body Politic, 1100–1400*, eds. Cary J. Nederman and Kate Langdon Forhan (London: Routledge, 1993), 161, 163.

32 John of Salisbury, "Policratus: Of the Frivolities of Courtiers and the Footprints of Philosophers," book 4, chapter 1, in *Medieval Political Theory-A Reader: The Quest for the Body Politic, 1100–1400*, eds. Cary J. Nederman and Kate Langdon Forhan (London: Routledge, 1993), 30, 53.

33 John Wyclif, "On the Duty of the King," in *Medieval Political Theory: A Reader – The Quest for the Body Politic, 1100–1400*, eds. Cary J. Nederman and Kate Langdon Forhan (London: Routledge, 1993), 222.

34 Hinrich Biesterfeldt, "Ibn Farighun's *Jawami' al-'ulum*: Between Classification of Sciences and Mirror for Princes," in *Global Medieval: Mirrors for Princes Reconsidered*, eds. Regula Forster and Neguin Yavari (Cambridge, MA: Harvard University Press, 2015), 21; and Stefan Leder, "Sultanic Rule in the Mirror of Medieval Political Literature," in *Global Medieval: Mirrors for Princes Reconsidered*, eds. Regula Forster and Neguin Yavari (Cambridge, MA: Harvard University Press, 2015), 105.

35 Leder, "Sultanic Rule," 102.

36 Duindam, *Dynasties*, 54.

37 See Desiderius Erasmus, *The Education of a Christian Prince*, trans. Neil M. Cheshire and Michael J. Heath (Cambridge: Cambridge University Press, 1997) and Juan Luis Vives, *The Education of a Christian Woman: A Sixteenth-Century Manual*, trans. Charles Fantazzi (Chicago: University of Chicago Press, 2000). For book dedications see Valerie Schutte, *Mary I and the Art of Book Dedications: Royal Women, Power and Persuasion* (New York: Palgrave Macmillan, 2015). See also the examples of Charles V and James VI & I in writing manuals for their heirs; James VI & I of Scotland and England, *Basilikon Doron: Or His Maiesties Instructions to His Dearest Sonne, Henry the Prince* (Edinburgh: Felix Kyngston, 1603); Rachael Ball and Geoffrey Parker, eds., *Cómo ser rey. Instrucciones del emperador Carlos V a su hijo Felipe, Mayo de 1543* (Madrid: Centro de Estudios Europa Hispánica, 2014).

38 Luc de Heusch, "Sacralized Power," 28.

39 See Lisa J. Lucero, *Water and Ritual: The Rise and Fall of Classic Maya Rulers* (Austin: University of Texas Press, 2006).

40 Clifford Geertz, *Negara: The Theatre State in Nineteenth Century Bali* (Princeton: Princeton University Press, 1980), 13.

41 Quigley, "Introduction," 4.

42 Gillespie, *Aztec Kings*, 223. See also Quigley, "Introduction," 3 on the symbolic 'killing' of new monarchs on their accession.

43 Sergio Bertelli, *The King's Body: Sacred Rituals of Power in Medieval and Early Modern Europe*, trans. R. Burr Litchfield (University Park: University of Pennsylvania Press, 2001), 3–4. See also Íñigo Mugueta Moreno and Pascual Tamburri Bariain, "Coronación juramentada. Navarra 1329," *Príncipe de Viana* 68, no. 240 (2007): 169–190.

44 D.C. Holtom, *The Japanese Enthronement Ceremonies: With an Account of the Imperial Regalia*, vol. 2 (London: Routledge, 1996), 71–74.

45 Wang Youpu, "Exhortations on Ceremony and Deference," in *Chinese Civilization: A Sourcebook*, ed. Patricia Buckley Ebrey (New York: The Free Press, 1993), 298–300, accessed via http://afe.easia.columbia.edu/ps/china/wang_youpu_exhortations.pdf.

46 Elizabeth Lillehoj, *Art and Palace Politics in Early Modern Japan, 1580s to 1680s* (Leiden: Brill, 2011), 106.

47 Claessen, "Chiefs and Kings," 240.

48 Edward Muir, *Ritual in Early Modern Europe* (Cambridge: Cambridge University Press, 1997), 256. It is worth noting that there has been significant debate about the purpose and impact of Louis XIV's court ceremonial. For some discussion of this and a wider discussion of the development of court ceremonial in France see Olaf Mörke, "The Symbolism of Rulership," in *Princes and Princely Culture 1450–1650*, vol. 1, eds. Martin Gosman, Alasdair Macdonald and Arjo Vanderjagt (Leiden: Brill, 2003), 44–45.

49 Maurice Bloch, "The Ritual of the Royal Bath in Madagascar: The Dissolution of Death, Birth and Fertility into Authority," in *Rituals of Royalty: Power and Ceremonial in Traditional Societies*, eds. David Cannadine and Simon Price (Cambridge: Cambridge University Press, 1987), 271–297.

50 Richard Burghart, "Gifts to the Gods: Power, Property and Ceremonial in Nepal," in *Rituals of Royalty: Power and Ceremonial in Traditional Societies*, eds. David Cannadine and Simon Price (Cambridge: Cambridge University Press, 1987), 237–270.

51 Jaap van Osta, "The Emperor's New Clothes. The Reappearance of the Performing Monarchy in Europe, c.1870–1914," in *Mystifying the Monarch: Studies on Discourse, Power and History*, eds. Jeroen Deploige and Gita Deneckere (Amsterdam: Amsterdam University Press, 2006), 181.

52 Deploige and Deneckere, "The Monarchy," 19.

53 Martin Beckford and Graeme Paton, "Royal Wedding Facts and Figures," *The Guardian*, 29 April 2011, www.telegraph.co.uk/news/uknews/royal-wedding/8483199/Royal-wedding-facts-and-figures.html.

54 Philip Mansel, *Dressed to Rule: Royal and Court Costume from Louis XIV to Elizabeth II* (New Haven: Yale University Press, 2005).

55 See Caroline Weber, *Queen of Fashion: What Marie Antoinette Wore to the Revolution* (New York: Henry Holt and Company, 2007) and Kimberly Chrisman-Campbell, *Fashion Victims: Dress at the Court of Louis XVI and Marie Antoinette* (New Haven: Yale University Press, 2015).

56 John Michael Wright, *Portrait of Charles II* (c.1671–76), oil on canvas, Royal Collection Trust RCIN 404951.

57 Examples of enthroned monarchs on coins include silver tetradrachm coins of Vologases IV of Parthia (r.147–91), British Museum Object reference number: COC258647 and gold triple sovereign of Edward VI of England (r.1547–53), British Museum Object reference number: CMB222667.

58 See Figure 6.1, page 141 in this volume.

59 Kathleen Cohen, *Metamorphosis of a Death Symbol: The Transi Tomb in the Late Middle Ages* (Berkeley: University of California Press, 1973), 137.

60 See his diagram, Duindam, *Dynasties*, 5.

61 Lisbeth Geevers and Mirella Marini, "Introduction: Aristocracy, Dynasty and Identity in Early Modern Europe, 1520–1700," in *Dynastic Identity in Early Modern Europe: Rulers, Aristocrats and the Formation of Identities*, eds. Liesbeth Geevers and Mirella Marini (Farnham: Ashgate, 2015), 12.

62 For a recent case study on the dynamics of the late medieval Navarrese dynasty see Elena Woodacre, "Ruling and Relationships: The Fundamental Basis of the Exercise of Power? The Impact of Marital and Family Relationships on the Reigns of the Queens Regnant of Navarre (1274–1517)," *Anuario de Estudios Medievales* 46 no. 1 (2016), 167–201.

63 Gillespie, *Aztec Kings*, 25. See especially chapter 1, "The Woman of Discord."

64 Seokyung Han, "Dowager Queens and Royal Succession in Premodern Korea," in *A Companion to Global Queenship: An Examination of Female Rule and Political Agency in the Premodern World*, ed. Elena Woodacre (Bradford: Arc Humanities Press, 2018), 195–208.

65 For a comprehensive study see Joseph A. Kéchichian, *Power and Succession in Arab Monarchies: A Reference Guide* (Boulder: Lynne Rienner Publishers, 2008), particularly p. 4.

66 While there is insufficient space to discuss this in full here, an effective overview is given in Duindam, *Dynasties*, 127–154.

67 See Matthias Schnettger, 'Dynastic Succession in an Elective Monarchy: The Habsburgs and the Holy Roman Empire', 112–129 in this volume.

68 Earenfight, "Without the Persona," 10.

69 For an overview of this dynasty see Gunther Hölbl, *A History of the Ptolemaic Empire*, trans. Tina Saavedra (London: Routledge, 2001).

70 Claessen, "Chiefs and Kings," 241–242.

71 Norbert Elias, *The Court Society* (Oxford: Blackwell, 1983). For a useful overview of European historiography see Hannah Smith, "Court Studies and the Courts of Early Modern Europe," *The Historical Journal* 49, no. 4 (2006), 1229–1238.

72 For example see Lucy Pick, "Social Networks and the Power of Elite Women in León-Castilla c.925" (conference paper given at Verbis et Exemplis, London, April 27, 2018).

73 Diana Pelaz Flores, "'Reynante(s) en vno': Poder y representación de la reina en la Corona de Castilla durante el siglo XV," PhD Thesis, Universidad de Valladolid (2015).

74 Jeroen Duindam, Tülay Artan and Metin Kunt, eds., *Royal Courts in Dynastic States and Empires: A Global Perspective* (Leiden: Brill, 2011).

75 See Andres Úbeda de los Cobos, *El palacio del Rey Planeta: Felipe IV y el Buen Retiro* (Madrid: Museo Nacional del Prado, 2005) and Jonathan Brown and J.H. Elliott, *A Palace for a King: The Buen Retiro and the Court of Philip IV* (New Haven: Yale University Press, 1986).

76 Kershaw, *South-East Asia*, 175.

77 Casper Jacobsen, "The Centre of Power: Tasks and Strategies of the Mexica Court," in *Palaces and Courtly Culture in Ancient Mesoamerica*, eds. Julie Nehammer Knub, Christophe Helmer and Jesper Nielsen (Oxford: Archaeopress, 2014), 51–64.

78 Mitchell and Melville, "Every Inch a King," 15.

79 Mitchell and Melville, "Every Inch a King," 14, and see Mary Hill Cole, *The Portable Queen: Elizabeth I and the Politics of Ceremony* (Amhurst: University of Massachusetts Press, 1999).

80 Quigley, "Introduction," 5.

81 Van Osta, "Emperor's New Clothes," 182.

82 Ernst Kantorowicz, *The King's Two Bodies: A Study in Mediaeval Political Theology* (Princeton: Princeton University Press, 1957). Note that Princeton University Press released a new edition of this classic work in 2016 with an introduction by Conrad Leyser.

83 Quigley, "Introduction," 20.
84 Deploige and Deneckere, "The Monarchy: A Crossroads of Trajectories," 17.
85 Christine Alice Corcos, "From Agnatic Succession to Absolute Primogeniture: The Shift to Equal Rights of Succession to Thrones and Titles in the Modern European Constitutional Monarchy," *Michigan Law Review* 5 (2012), 1587–1670.
86 See a full list of Japan's reigning empresses in Jerrold Packard, *Sons of Heaven: A Portrait of the Japanese Monarchy* (London: Queen Anne Press, 1988), 351–356.

Key works

Cannadine, David and Simon Price, eds., *Rituals of Royalty: Power and Ceremonial in Traditional Societies* (Cambridge: Cambridge University Press, 1987).

Deploige, Jeroen and Gita Deneckere, eds., *Mystifying the Monarch: Studies on Discourse, Power and History* (Amsterdam: Amsterdam University Press, 2006).

Duindam, Jeroen, *Dynasties: A Global History of Power, 1300–1800* (Cambridge: Cambridge University Press, 2016).

Earenfight, Theresa, "Without the Persona of the Prince: Kings, Queens and the Idea of Monarchy in Late Medieval Europe," *Gender and History* 19, no. 1 (2007): 1–21.

Oakley, Francis, *Kingship: The Politics of Enchantment* (Oxford: Blackwell, 2006).

Quigley, Declan, ed., *The Character of Kingship* (Oxford: Berg, 2005).

PART I

MODELS AND CONCEPTS OF RULERSHIP

INTRODUCTION

Chris Jones

In a collection that consciously seeks to establish that the 'history of monarchy' is more – much more – than an episode in some whiggish history of civilization's progress along the road to western-style democracy, this first part of the volume might appear to be an anomaly.[1] As Elena Woodacre's general introduction has demonstrated, this is a volume dedicated to monarchy on a global scale. Yet in this first part of the book Europe appears to stare down from its throne – serenely or smugly, depending on your point of view – surveying the court of chapters assembled before it. Capetians and Plantagenets mingle there with Castilian kings and German emperors. Of the court's future visitors, most will, doubtless, look away from the throne itself preferring to focus their attention on those in attendance. Others – inevitably the minority in an age of chapter downloads – will consider the assembly as a whole. Some, less inclined to either politeness or deference, and finding there to be a 'wrinkled lip, and sneer of cold command' emanating from the throne, will express outrage.[2] Taken as a whole, does Part I of this volume not embody not-so-subtle traces of a division, to borrow Niall Ferguson's characterization, between the west and 'the rest'?[3] Such an approach to exploring models of rulership would seem particularly at odds with a growing interest in applying the 'global turn' to the discipline of history.[4] The latter approach, which informs this volume as a whole and is exemplified in relation to monarchy in the work of historians such as Jeroen Duindam, seeks, at the very least, to place Europe in its wider context, and to remind us more generally that there is a history beyond the continent's shores.[5]

The Ottomans, with some justification, might claim to have re-invented the model of monarchy in the Muslim world. The sixteenth-century sultan Suleiman the Magnificent (r.1520–66), who, as part of a broader claim to universal sovereignty, declared himself to be 'Caesar of all the lands of Rome', represents the pinnacle of Ottoman success.[6] Yet neither he nor any other members of the dynasty of Orhan, appear as part of this discussion. Where is the Mughal emperor Akbar (r.1556–1605) who attempted to create new arguments for the legitimacy of rulership by blending Islam, Hinduism and countless other religions into what was arguably his own unique 'faith of God' (Dīn-i Ilāhī)?[7] The worlds of the Ottomans and the Mughuls offer only two stunning examples of alternative models of monarchical rulership that are not discussed here. One could easily find others. The unique challenges offered by models of monarchy in China are not explored.[8] And where are the Mongols? The emperors of Ethiopia?

The first point to make, then, is that for all Europe's tendency to dominate, this part is actually conceived as *two* case studies: western Europe is one; the Muslim world is the other. Two of the eight chapters address the world beyond western Europe, even if the continent's shadow is hard to escape entirely. Pascal Buresi's discussion of the Almohads involves, at least in part, Iberia, while David Mednicoff considers modern Arab kingship as a reaction to western colonialism. Secondly, however, it is worth underlining that Part I is intended to be read in the context of the volume as a whole; it was not conceived with the intention of making a case for exceptionalism, western European or otherwise. It is worth noting that Kim Berqvist and Trond Isaksen's chapters, which follow in later parts of the book, are among those that encourage us to consider western Europe itself within a broader European context.[9] This is not, in short, a part of the volume in search of Ferguson's 'killer apps'.[10] And it might be noted that the fate of Shelley's Ozymandias awaits every civilization; western Europe, whose throne has, in any case, appeared more painted plasterboard than granite of late, is unlikely to prove an exception in the long run. Why, then, is Europe allowed such prominence here? In essence, a narrow focus is an attempt to both avoid tokenism and to enable the drawing of meaningful comparisons.

The chronological focus, although covering the last 1000 years, is, in a certain sense, as narrow as the geographical. Those in search of discussion of the *bretwalda*, a – possibly mythical – conception of royal overlordship associated with the early medieval Anglo-Saxon world, will find it as disappointingly absent as an exploration of the process by which Isma'il I (r.1501–24) lay the foundations for Safavid Persia.[11] Instead, the eight chapters that comprise this part provide an opportunity to delve deeply into three key themes that are critical to shaping monarchical rule, and that illustrate its vibrancy and adaptability as a model of rulership. All three overlap and are interwoven throughout, although some themes feature more prominently in some chapters than others. Europe's transition from the later Middle Ages into the early modern era, marked by seismic shifts in the structures of society, politics and the economy, offers, in this context, a perfect Petri dish for examining these themes. The same is true of the Almohad caliphate and the modern Arab monarchies, both of which emerged amid a staccato burst of bewildering social, political and economic changes.

The first theme concerns the image of the 'ideal' ruler. Or, to put it another way, it concerns the question of the template on which rulership was modelled. This was as complex an issue in the medieval and early modern west as it was – and is – in the Muslim world. The ideal ruler was never a fixed concept; his or her features ebbed and flowed as they underwent a constant process of readjustment to suit contemporary society. What constituted the model ruler evolved over time and responded to a range of changing factors. The image of the ruler shared this characteristic with the institutional framework within which rulership operated. The second theme explored here, then – aspects of which are also considered in Part II 'Ritual and representation' – is the way in which the institution of monarchy underwent a process of constant evolution to accommodate the demands of these ever-changing social, political and economic factors.

Monarchy, as a normative model, is commonly envisioned in the twenty-first century as incorporating hereditary succession, usually via primogeniture, to the rule of one people in one, clearly defined, contiguous territory; other forms are, by definition, departures from the norm. The precise mechanisms by which succession could operate are explored in more detail in Part III 'Dynasty and succession'. It is worth highlighting, however, that what has come to be regarded as the normative model was particularly suited to those in the nineteenth and twentieth centuries whose interest lay in establishing the 'naturalness' of modern nation-states. It not only drew a distinct contrast with the empires those states often replaced but imbued what was essentially a new type of political organization with the useful trappings of historical roots: nation-states 'restored' peoples to their 'natural' kingdoms while simultaneously rebooting their political formats from an autocratic and hereditary model to a representative, if not necessarily democratic, one.[12] As Trond Isaksen, Christoph de Speigeleer and Mikolaj Getka-Kenig's chapters in Part II 'Ritual and representation' illustrate, this process left nineteenth-century monarchies facing a number of challenges when it came to ceremonies such as coronations and funerals or architectural representation.[13] As late medieval and early modern Europe demonstrate *par excellence*, the reality that had inspired the original ceremonies and architecture was far from the normative model beloved of modernity's nationalists. In fact, monarchy enjoyed a bewildering variety of structures. More often than not, kings and queens inherited composite monarchies while dynasts succeeded in a hereditary manner to theoretically elective positions.

As the institutions of monarchy and the image of the ideal ruler continuously developed to meet the needs of changing circumstances, monarchs and those they ruled were presented with a paradox. How could supposedly timeless, unchanging institutions evolve? Part I's third theme concerns the perennial challenge of how the legitimacy of the monarchical model was established. The success with which the legitimacy of monarchical power was sustained in the face of continual societal change is one of the most remarkable features of both the case studies examined here. There exists in each a fundamental tension between the dominant intellectual framework, informed by, respectively, interpretations of Christianity and Islam, and the very concept of temporal rulership. It is a tension that borders on incompatibility. Consequently, at the heart of this part is an examination of the astonishing ability of monarchy to function as an effective method of government in an intellectual environment that considered it either irrelevant or, worse still, was openly hostile to the very concept of kingship.

The intellectual framework in which medieval and early modern Europeans considered models of secular rule, monarchical or otherwise, was not a promising one. It was, in essence, a key legacy of the Early Church Fathers, a loose grouping of Christian intellectuals who succeeded to the leadership of the Christian community after the death of Christ's first followers. In its earliest days, there had been a sense of 'immediacy' to Christianity: Christ's return, and the subsequent end of the world, were imminent. Consequently, the Fathers did not devote a lot of time to worldly politics. Early Christians came to two basic views of government: government was simply a punishment from God, or, at best, it might have some small, remedial value in that it enabled the spread of the Christian message by maintaining peace. The conversion of the fourth-century Roman emperor Constantine (r.312–37), and the subsequent adoption of Christianity as the religion of the Roman Empire, did little to improve the standing of worldly government among theologians. The North African bishop Augustine of Hippo (d.430) set the tone that dominated the Middle Ages and that echoed into later centuries when he divided the world between the city of God and the earthly city. The interests of the Christian lay with the former; temporal government was a part of the latter and the good Christian simply had to put up with it. At best, in Augustine's assessment, government existed not only to punish and coerce but to establish justice and peace.[14] Echoing Cicero, he believed that it was justice, above all other characteristics, that was the key to legitimizing rulership in this world: 'Justice removed, then, what are kingdoms but great bands of robbers? What are bands of robbers themselves but little kingdoms?'[15] Earthly justice would, however, always remain a pale imitation of the justice on offer in the city of God.

Augustine's influential assessment meant that an intrinsic tension governed the relationship between society, and the western Church in particular, and the rulers who emerged in the polities that replaced the Roman Empire across the west. Yet a point of agreement was that if worldly government was a necessity, the best form for that government was monarchy. Towards the end of the thirteenth century, this idea was given one of its more influential forms – and certainly its clearest expression – by the University of Paris master Giles of Rome (d.1316). Giles's *On the Rule of Princes* (*De regimine principum*; before 1282) was the second most widely disseminated 'mirror for princes' of the later Middle Ages.[16] The broader context for such mirrors, which were as common in the Islamic world as the Christian west, is explored in the general introduction to this volume.[17] *On the Rule of Princes* itself argues strongly that the ideal model for political units is the kingdom. For Giles, the ideal king should be unshackled from any limitations. Kingship should be 'regal', in which the ruler makes the law, as opposed to 'political', in which those governed make the law.[18] Government by a regal ruler, who is distinguished from the despot by his focus on the common good, is the most perfect form of government because the position of such a ruler is a more perfect reflection of the natural ordering and hierarchy of the universe.[19]

On the Rule of Princes was presented to its original audience, the son of the French king, as a vulgarization of Aristotle. While its robust argument in favour of the ruler's unrestricted power made this far from true, Giles was part of a wave of thinkers influenced by a thirteenth-century revival of interest in Aristotelian thought. Indeed, his contemporary at the University of Paris, Thomas Aquinas (d.1274), employed Aristotle's *Politics*, in particular, in order to offer a re-evaluation of the Augustinian view of earthly government. While conserving Augustine's model of the two cities, Aquinas's observation that some form of government would have existed in mankind's natural state became the starting point for a more positive re-evaluation of worldly politics.[20] In terms of the development of western political thought, Aquinas's views are often treated as a critical turning point. Whether or not they were seen as such by his contemporaries, they, like Giles's Aristotelian-inspired 'mirror', are indicative of a period in which western Europeans began to devote considerably more thought to the theory of government and to justifying the forms of it under which they lived. The roots of this change lie in the revival of interest in classical learning commonly known today as the 'Twelfth Century Renaissance'.[21]

The intellectual revival of the twelfth and thirteenth centuries took place in the context of broader social and economic changes that involved, in particular, growing urbanization, developing trade networks and renewed interaction between western Europe and the wider world.[22] Part I begins with two chapters by Manuel Alejandro Rodríguez de la Peña and Laura Fábián that consider some of the ways in which Europeans responded to an environment that was undergoing rapid change on both an intellectual and a material level. Both concentrate on the way in which western Europeans constructed their model of the 'ideal' ruler in this period. Yet in doing so they eschew the traditional 'political' theorists such as Giles and Thomas or their twelfth-century predecessors, men such as John of Salisbury (d.1180), author of the influential *Policraticus*.[23] In adopting this approach, they highlight the fact that while classical ideas would add important new facets to European reflections, they were only one of the sources to shape the model of the ideal ruler in the later Middle Ages.

As Cecilia Gasposchkin has aptly demonstrated in a recent examination of the Capetian court in the second quarter of the thirteenth century, the Bible itself remained a significant 'mirror for princes'. During the early years of the reign of the French king Louis IX (r.1226–70), pictorial Bibles were used to promote 'an ideal of Augustinian kingship, specific to the challenges of the early part of the thirteenth century, and informed by ecclesiastical priorities'.[24] In a wide-ranging chapter, Rodríguez de la Peña opens Part I by exploring one of the most influential models for western kingship with biblical roots: the 'wise king'. He considers the way in which the model flourished under the Carolingians and their Ottonian successors in East Francia before declining in an age in which royal authority faced significant challenges. Strikingly, the model was, however, revived in the atmosphere fostered by the Twelfth Century Renaissance. The idea that the ruler should be both interested in, and the patron of, learning became a hallmark of late medieval and early modern kingship. It proved particularly important to new dynasties, such as the Hauteville rulers of southern Italy, as they sought to establish themselves.

It is one particular aspect of the reviving interest in the sapiential model that Laura Fábián explores in her own contribution. Fábián's examination of the biblical king Solomon as a royal *exempla* takes us from the early medieval world of Carolingian Francia to the thirteenth- and fourteenth-century courts of France, England and Castile. Stepping beyond western Europe to embrace Byzantium, Fábián highlights, in particular, the ambivalence of the Solomonic model in medieval thought. Solomon was the Bible's most striking example of a wise king, but he was also a king who turned away from God at the end of his reign and who indulged in magic. How could such a ruler function as an ideal of kingship in a Christian society? While it was undoubtedly the most important source, the Bible was not, however, the *only* alternative to an Aristotelian model when Europeans sought to construct the 'ideal' ruler in this period.

A particularly notable legacy of the twelfth century was a new interest in law and its relationship with the ruler. It was jointly symbolized by the revived study of Roman law in the form of the emperor Justinian's sixth-century code, the *Corpus iuris civilis*, and the linked production of what became the foundation stone of the western Church's legal system, Gratian's *Decretum*.[25] As Elena Woodacre highlights in her introduction, law is a critical factor in the construction of monarchy.[26]

It proved a potent tool in the later Middle Ages. In the twelfth century, rulers such as the English king Henry II (r.1154–89) and the Hohenstaufen emperor Frederick Barbarossa (r.1152–90; emperor from 1155) sought to use law to craft an image of kingship and to project their practical authority.[27] In Sicily, the *Constitutions of Melfi* (1231) provided Frederick's grandson, Emperor Frederick II (r.1197–1250 as king of Sicily; king of the Romans from 1212; emperor from 1220), with a means not only of governing his realm but of asserting the independence of his authority from the papacy.[28] A few decades later, Louis IX issued the so-called *grande ordonnance* of 1254, a legislative programme intended to reform both general morality and royal administration in France. It signalled a new tone to Louis's kingship and lay the groundwork for a future crusade.[29] In every case where kings sought to employ law to extend and define their authority, law, in turn, shaped and redefined royal power and the nature of a ruler's relationship with his or her subjects. Of all the attempts to use law to define – and redefine – kingship in the later Middle Ages, one of the most ambitious and conscious is that explored by Manuela Santos Silva in the third contribution to this part.

In the second half of the thirteenth century, Alfonso X (r.1252–84), ruler of the Iberian kingdoms of Castile and León, oversaw the production of not one but three law codes aimed at uniting the laws and customs of both his kingdoms and providing a legal template for newly conquered territories. Two of these, the *Mirror of Laws* (*Espéculo de las leyes*) and the *Seven Parts* (*Siete Partidas*), provide a window into Alfonso's new model of normative kingship. They define the characteristics of the king and show, in particular, the way in which royal power was conceptualized as something that involved the whole of the king's family and those that comprised the royal court. Some of the generic concerns that informed his treatment of one aspect of that court, the role of the queen, are explored and placed in their wider context in Chapter 33 'For better or for worse: royal marital sexuality as political critique in late medieval Europe', Henric Bagerius and Christine Ekholst's contribution to the final part of this volume, 'Exercising authority and exerting influence'.[30] Among the many facets of Iberian kingship revealed by Alfonso's codes, two of the most notable are the emerging preference for hereditary succession and the king's efforts to balance the needs of what remained, technically, two independent kingdoms. Both highlight Alfonso's efforts to ensure the model kept pace with rapid change. The problem of ensuring their models matched reality was not one that escaped contemporary theorists, often for quite pragmatic reasons.

John of Paris (d.1306), a Dominican theologian at the University of Paris and part of the generation that followed Aquinas and built on his ideas, was one of those who reflected upon the relationship between the ideal and the real.[31] John considered the problem of whether there should, by right, be one universal ruler in temporal matters or whether the actual situation, a multiplicity of independent polities, was justified. At the time he compiled his tract *On Royal and Papal Power* (*c*.1302), the issue had become a particularly pressing one: the contemporary conflict between the French king Philip IV (r.1285–1314) and Pope Boniface VIII (r.1294–1303) saw the pope support the theoretical claims of the German-Roman emperor to authority over France.[32] John was the first to draw on Aristotle to offer a comprehensive rebuttal. He argued:

It does not follow that all the faithful should be united in one political community. Rather there are different ways of life and constitutions adapted to the different climates, languages and conditions of peoples, and what is virtuous in one people is not virtuous in another.[33]

This undoubtedly offered Philip IV a far better justification for his claims to independence in temporal matters than existing arguments based on either historical accident or legal technicalities.[34] John's Aristotelian-derived argument also had a particularly strong resonance for twentieth-century historians of political thought, who tended to see it as an important milestone on the road to the development of the nation-state.[35] Yet an argument for the 'naturalness' of territorially limited independent kingdoms was, as Charlotte Backerra illustrates in her contribution to this volume, sorely challenged by reality in both John's own time and in subsequent centuries. The principle that underpinned John's case against universal temporal authority – the need for independent rulers who could adapt to the specific conditions facing those they ruled – appeared well tailored to the needs of France's kings in the early fourteenth century. Perhaps the most striking feature of his argument, however, is how poorly it fitted the needs of virtually every other ruler in western Europe. Indeed, from English Gascony to Aragonese Sicily, far from reinforcing royal authority, an argument that emphasized the importance of a connection between rulership and 'local' conditions positively undermined it. How, in such circumstances, could English kings justify rule by 'remote control' over the southern French duchy or their Aragonese contemporaries defend their claims to what was, from an Aragonese perspective, the far-flung island of Sicily?

Alfonso X's kingship blurred the boundaries between a personal union of the crowns of Castile and León with an emerging composite monarchy in which the two kingdoms remained distinct but were inextricably linked. As Backerra makes clear in Chapter 4, the tendency of one king to rule in multiple kingdoms was the norm, rather the exception, in the late medieval/early modern European world. Personal unions, if maintained beyond the earliest generations, frequently led to the establishment of composite monarchies. Such was the case in the British Isles following the personal union of Scotland and England under James VI & I. A remarkable feature of this development, however, is the extent to which the resulting polities continued to be moulded by regional concerns. Few successful attempts were made to introduce universal laws and customs; diversity flourished. Frederick II's empire was, for example, made up of a bewildering mix of composite kingdoms to which were added personal unions, such as the kingdoms of Jerusalem and Sicily. Each was governed according to its own particular customs, and Frederick seems to have done little to change this. The *Constitutions of Melfi*, for example, were laws created to address circumstances specific to Sicily, not with universal applicability in mind.[36] In this respect, it is the Hohenstaufen empire that represents monarchy's 'norm' in the late medieval and early modern world, rather than the Capetian kingdom. It is also worth remarking that the France of Louis IX or Philip IV could, given the diversity of its customs, legal arrangements and languages, actually be considered a composite monarchy in all but name. As Backerra establishes, the composite model of monarchy had a lasting legacy on European society, one that continues to echo down to the present day.

If John of Paris's Aristotelian model of rulership stimulated modern historians of political ideas rather more than it aroused the interest of medieval and early modern kings, his comments concerning how rulers were created, while less remarked upon today, undoubtedly enjoyed a strong contemporary resonance. John offered a solution to the problem of how the ruler was established that sought to square a particularly challenging theoretical circle with contemporary reality. A few decades earlier, Giles of Rome had recognized that, as an ideal, election was the preferable means of selecting a king: it ensured the best candidate would obtain the job.[37] However, hereditary succession was fast becoming the preferred custom in western Europe. Where it did not already exist, rulers, such as Frederick II's father, Emperor Henry VI (r.1190–7), sought to introduce it if they could.[38]

John's solution to the theoretical dilemma was that royal power comes from 'God and the people who choose a king either as an individual or as a member of a dynasty, as was in fact done formerly'.[39] The relationship between dynasty and royal power is a key focus of the third part of this volume, 'Dynasty and succession'. For now, it is worth noting that John's argument reflected contemporary understanding of the nature of kingship in his native France. Here, the ruling Capetian dynasty needed to justify the removal and replacement of two former dynasties of French kings while simultaneously accounting for the uninterrupted succession of members of the Capetian family since 987. The problem became more pressing as a more sophisticated society became more interested in the problem of legitimacy.[40] John's solution is similar to Alfonso X's understanding of the origins of kingship, as Santos Silva makes clear in her analysis of the king's new law codes. Ultimately, as Giles of Rome had established, it was possible to recognize the significance of election while, paradoxically, displaying an unreserved preference for hereditary kingship. The basis for this was, as Giles explains, that all practical experience indicated that hereditary kingship offers greater stability, both because the people will more easily accept the sons of previous rulers and because the knowledge that his progeny will succeed him will ensure the quality of a king's rule.[41] As Matthias Schnettger illustrates in Chapter 5, the problem of balancing the perceived advantages of hereditary succession against the theoretical virtues of the elective principle continued to shape European dynasties throughout the early modern era.

Between 1438 and 1806, with one brief exception, the Holy Roman Empire consistently put a variation of John of Paris's theory into practice. While the principle that the Empire was an elective monarchy was never forgotten, the Habsburg dynasty became, in effect, its hereditary rulers. Schnettger traces the evolution of this process, considering the ways in which negotiation and balance became the hallmarks of dynastic success. In this particular case, the Empire's constitutional arrangements, which enshrined the emperor's position as supreme judge, feudal overlord and the source of important privileges, enabled the Habsburgs to ensure the continued survival of the imperial office and their own position as its incumbents despite the developing influence of the Empire's estates and the sheer diversity of their particular composite monarchy. The relationship between elective and hereditary succession and the challenges it posed are ones that we will return to in Part III 'Dynasty and succession'. It is worth, however, drawing particular attention to the fact that in the Habsburg case the title of 'Holy Roman Emperor' undoubtedly worked to the advantage of the dynasty, playing, as it did, a role as a powerful legitimizing instrument for their authority.

The western imperial office had been constantly reimagined following its re-emergence with Charlemagne's coronation in 800. One of the reasons for its continued survival was its flexibility. For the Ottonians, it had helped to strengthen their authority over the dukes of East Francia; for the Hohenstaufen, it cemented their claim to authority over the rebellious cities of northern Italy; for the Habsburgs, it created a focus for unity within the otherwise disparate principalities that comprised the German lands of the Empire.[42] Like Aristotelian thought, law codes, or biblical *exempla*, titles were one more weapon in the armoury of legitimization that western rulers could draw upon in the late medieval and early modern era. Amid the plethora of options available, the idea that monarchical power was authorized by the divine remained particularly significant. The link between the divine and monarchy, a topic explored by Elena Woodacre in her introduction to this volume, lent itself to arguments in favour of monarchy as the most natural form of government:[43] monarchy was, after all, as Giles of Rome had noted, a reflection of the way the universe was ordered.

By John of Paris's day some disagreement existed among the theorists of the west concerning the extent to which royal power was mediated by the Church. Giles of Rome offered the most extreme argument in favour of ecclesiastical mediation when he argued that all temporal power is, ultimately, vested in the pope, who delegates its use to kings and emperors.[44] Yet all agreed that political power, whatever its form, ultimately originated with God. While John of Paris disagreed profoundly with Giles's interpretation of the relationship between kings and the Church, God remained, for example, the first of the two components through which he suggested any king was established.[45] The idea of God as the ultimate source of legitimization is the focus of Chapter 6 by Matthias Range.

Range considers the complex history of *Dei gratia* ('by the Grace of God') as a legitimizing formula. In the early modern period, this formula frequently became associated with the concept of the 'divine right' of kings and was used as a tool to authorize near unlimited authority. Range situates the title in its wider historical context, examining its evolution. He suggests that it originated in quite different circumstances to those with which it became associated: originally, it encapsulated both a warning and an obligation on the part of the ruler. What became a quintessential component in the legitimization of monarchical authority across western Europe began its life as a means of emphasizing the monarch's humility before God, the source of his or her authority. The Christian kings and queens of western Europe were not, of course, the only rulers for whom the divine was perceived to be the ultimate source of their authority. In the second of this part's case studies, Pascal Buresi turns, in Chapter 7, to consider another instance where the divine played a key role in the shaping and legitimization of models of rulership: the Muslim world.

Like western Europe, the Muslim world struggled with the question of how the reality of monarchy could be reconciled with religious precepts, albeit the source of the struggle had different foundations. In Islamic polities the issue was not the basic irrelevance of the worldly, the problem posed by Augustine and the Church Fathers. For the Christian west, this had created a tension that was never resolved fully even when the rediscovery of Aristotle enabled more positive assessments of this worldly government. Ultimately, it was a perceived incompatibility that both eased the separation of the secular from the ecclesiastical in the west while simultaneously hastening a tendency for monarchy to appear irrelevant. As Christianity's tide receded from public life in post-Enlightenment Europe, monarchies, which had rooted their legitimacy in their relationship with the divine, often became stranded leviathans; they were left gasping on an otherwise secular shoreline. In the Muslim world, however, the issue was, and remains, different. It is not a question of a tension between worldly government and an unworldly religion; it is, instead, the problem of whether a religion with a worldly component is compatible with the institution of kingship.

When they came to power in 750, the 'Abbāsid dynasty built their reputation on the grounds that the Umayyad, whose position they had violently usurped, had enjoyed kingship (*mulk*), rather than legitimate rulership as caliphs.[46] A true caliph was a deputy of the Prophet Muhammed and a leader of the community (*Umma*). In the following century, the Persian scholar Al-Ṭabarī (839–923) got to the heart of the issue in a supposed dialogue that appeared in his *History of the Prophets and Kings* (*Ta'rīkh al-Rusul wa'l-Mulūk*):

> 'Umar said to Salmān: 'Am I a king or a Caliph?' and Salmān answered: 'If you have levied from the lands of the Muslims one dirham, or more, or less, and applied it unlawfully, you are a king, not a Caliph.' And 'Umar wept.[47]

Whatever the historical truth of Umayyad rule,[48] from 750 it became deeply ingrained in the Islamic world that, whatever else he was, the caliph was most assuredly *not* a king. Yet, 'royal' dynasties appeared to proliferate in the Muslim world, many of which, not least among whom were the 'Abbāsids themselves, appeared to embrace hereditary succession. What, then, distinguished a legitimate ruler from a mere king in an Islamic context? And could the two be reconciled?

Between the twelfth and the thirteenth centuries, the Almohad caliphate became the first polity to unite the Maghreb region of North Africa under a single indigenous political authority. In the first of two chapters that make up this second case study, Pascal Buresi explores the way in which the Almohads provide not only an instructive example of an attempt to resolve the tensions around legitimate rulership but a useful point of reflection on the nature of Islamic government in its earliest centuries. As Buresi illustrates, this topic remains a source of considerable debate. Was Islam, from its emergence, a theocratic regime, in which political power and religious authority merged in a single individual? Or was there a division between the role of the caliph, as a political figure, and the exercise of religious authority? The repercussions of this unresolved problem echo down to the present day.

In the final contribution to this part, David Mednicoff examines the way in which a model of kingship has come to dominate much of the modern Arab world. Indeed, the Arab world is one of few areas where examples of absolute royal authority remain common place. Given Islam's historical relationship with kingship, this may, at first glance, appear puzzling. And yet, as Mednicoff shows, the institution of monarchy has played a key role in enabling the Arab world to address post-colonial issues. In particular, monarchy is the mechanism by which these states have sought to integrate Islam smoothly into their governmental structures while simultaneously avoiding the adoption of the institutions of the former colonial powers. Monarchy became the means by which a unique Arab political identity could be created in regions where independent Arab government had not existed since the emergence of the early modern Turco-Mongol empires.

***

The case studies that comprise this section do not pretend to offer – either chronologically or geographically – an overview of all of the many and varied models of monarchical rulership available. There is, to take just one example, no attempt here to explore the Kingitanga, or King Movement, in Aotearoa New Zealand. The crowning of the first Māori king in 1858, eighteen years after Māori tribes ceded authority to the British Crown in the Treaty of Waitangi, was, like modern Arab kingship, a response to colonization. It was – and is – shaped by unique concerns over land and sovereignty.[49] Neither do the three themes considered – the changing face of the ideal ruler; the evolution of institutional frameworks; and the problem of legitimacy – represent all the possible approaches to, and issues raised by, the case studies themselves. In the wake of the deposition of the English king Richard II (r.1377–99; d.1400), the question of when rulers might be legitimately removed was, for example, one that vexed the anonymous compiler of the Canterbury Roll, the fifteenth-century genealogy whose image adorns the cover of this volume.[50] The issue of whether the ruler who was a tyrant, or simply useless, could be resisted or even killed was one that received considerable attention in Europe, both during the later Middle Ages and beyond.[51] The relationship between deposition and succession is explored in Chapter 30 by Cathleen Sarti in the context of Europe's northern monarchies.[52] While Part I can thus make no claims to be exhaustive, the case studies examined here do have something important to tell us: monarchy has proved remarkably successful as a system of government in societies where religion plays a key role in public life. For the European Middle Ages, the point echoes in Anna Duch's study of the relationship between royal representation and sainthood (Chapter 17 in Part II).[53] David M. Malitz's discussion of the monarchies of Meiji Japan (1868–1912) and post-war Thailand (1946–73) in Chapter 10 in Part II, on the other hand, provides an example of the continuing link between monarchy and the divine in the nineteenth and twentieth centuries.[54]

That the contemporary west, in particular, tends to view monarchy as intrinsically archaic is, perhaps, a reflection of the fact that the issues that this model of rulership is well suited to addressing have come to be regarded as less and less relevant in western society. In a world where political authority is legitimated by plebiscite and God is not accorded the right to vote, it is not difficult to understand why monarchy is so often reduced to soap opera. As Elena Woodacre notes in her general introduction, 'modernity and secularity' are a challenge to monarchy.[55] In the contemporary world, monarchy's role in government becomes little more than colourful ceremony; its processes for ensuring continuity and stability become mere headlines. One example is the 2018 wedding of Prince Harry and Meghan Markle, a case discussed in Lucinda Dean's introduction to Part II 'Ritual and representation'.[56] With function removed, monarchy struggles to be more than an occasionally entertaining distraction in the west.

Examining models of rulership formulated in societies where monarchy was deeply relevant – indeed necessary – can offer new insights into not only *how* monarchical institutions operated but *why* they proved so effective and long-lasting. Indeed, monarchy is so flexible and adaptive that it has been able to accommodate religious doctrines that have either little place for the worldly or that tend to subsume government within their doctrinal framework. Western Europe, where an Augustinian interpretation of Christianity reduced worldly government to little more than an irrelevance, provides one of the most extreme examples of the former; the Muslim world, where Islam has, at times, been interpreted to remove the autonomy of secular politics, offers a good example of the latter. Both case studies illustrate not only the vibrancy of monarchy as a concept but its elasticity as a model of rulership.

Notes

1 For the whig interpretation of history, an approach first critiqued by Herbert Butterfield, see Michael Bentley, *Modern Historiography: An Introduction* (London: Routledge, 1999), 62–70. Butterfield castigated the tendency of nineteenth-century British historians to pick out constitutional milestones and assemble them into a coherent narrative that justified the present.
2 The quotation is a line from Percy Bysshe Shelley's poem "Ozymandias," first published in *The Examiner* (1818).
3 Niall Ferguson, *Civilization: The West and the Rest* (London: Penguin, 2011).
4 For some recent thought-provoking reflections on the 'global turn', see G. Balachandran, "History after the Global Turn: Perspectives from Rim and Region," *History Australia* 14, no. 1 (2017): 6–12. For a survey of recent key literature see Jeremy Adelman, "Review Essay: Global History or the History of Globalization?" *Journal of World History* 27, no. 4 (2016): 701–708. The importance of this approach for scholars of the Middle Ages is underlined by the fact the theme selected for the 2019 meeting of the Medieval Academy of America is 'The Global Turn in Medieval Studies'.
5 Jeroen Duindam, *Dynasties: A Global History of Power, 1300–1800* (Cambridge: Cambridge University Press, 2015). For a further notable example of this approach applied to the study of monarchy see Elena Woodacre, ed., *A Companion to Global Queenship* (Bradford: ARC-Humanities Press, 2018).
6 On Suleiman's claims see Stephen F. Dale, *The Muslim Empires of the Ottomans, Safavids, and Mughals* (Cambridge: Cambridge University Press, 2010), 181–182. Suleiman's title is cited from Andrew Wheatcroft, *The Enemy at the Gate: Habsburgs, Ottomans and the Battle for Europe* (New York: Basic Books, 2009), 85. Ottoman-Habsburg diplomacy was increasingly marked by Ottoman claims to the titles associated with the Holy Roman Empire; see Colin Imber, *The Ottoman Empire, 1300–1650: The Structure of Power*, second edition (Basingstoke: Palgrave Macmillan, 2009), 113–114.
7 For Akbar's reign see Dale, *Muslim Empires*, 96–105, and for the Dīn-i Ilāhī in particular, 101–103.
8 Notable examples where Chinese case studies are addressed alongside European and Islamic ones include Richard van Leeuwen, *Narratives of Kingship in Eurasian Empires, 1300–1800* (Leiden: Brill, 2017); and, with particular reference to the court, the essays in Jeroen Duindam, Tülay Artan and Metin Kunt, eds., *Royal Courts in Dynastic States and Empires: A Global Perspective* (Leiden: Brill, 2011).
9 Respectively in this volume, see: Kim Bergqvist, "Kings and nobles on the fringes of Christendom", 622-635; Trond Norén Isaksen, "A useless ceremony of some use", 249–264.
10 'The Six Killer Apps of Western Power', which appears as a sub-title to certain editions of Ferguson's 2011 *Civilization*, are defined as 'six identifiably novel complexes of institutions and associated ideas and behaviours . . . that allowed a minority of mankind originating on the western edge of Eurasia to dominate the world for the better part of 500 years', Ferguson, 12.
11 For an introduction to the term *bretwalda*, an office that may have been more aspirational than real and possibly little more than a chronicler's 'flight of fancy', see Simon Keynes, "*Bretwalda* or *Brytenwalda*," in *The Wiley Blackwell Encyclopedia of Anglo-Saxon England*, eds. Michael Lapidge, John Blair, Simon Keynes and Donald Scragg, second edition (Chichester:

Wiley-Blackwell, 2014), 76–77 at 77. As Stephen Dale puts it, Isma'il adopted a 'legitimizing propaganda [that] reflected the extraordinarily variegated and unstructured religious environment of his audience' Dale, 65–70, quotation at 68.

12 This is not to suggest that the concept of the 'nation' and 'national' identity are exclusively linked to modernity. See the essays in Len Scales and Oliver Zimmer, eds., *Power and the Nation in European History* (Cambridge: Cambridge University Press, 2005). It can even be argued that 'nationalism' has a pre-modern history, Caspar Hirschi, *The Origins of Nationalism: An Alternative History from Ancient Rome to Early Modern Germany* (Cambridge: Cambridge University Press, 2012).

13 Respectively, in this volume, see: Isaksen, "A useless ceremony of some use", 249–264 in this volume; Christoph de Spiegeleer, "The nationalization and mediatization of European monarchies", 229–248; Mikolaj Getka-Kenig, "In pursuit of social allies", 374–389.

14 For an excellent summary of the issue in the thought of Augustine and the Fathers see Joseph Canning, *A History of Medieval Political Thought 300–1450* (London and New York: Routledge, 1996), 39–43.

15 Augustine, *The City of God Against the Pagans*, ed. and trans. Robert W. Dyson (Cambridge: Cambridge University Press, 1998), 4.4, 147.

16 For a summary of the argument and its influence see Chris Jones, "Giles of Rome, Political Thought," in *Encyclopedia of Medieval Philosophy: Philosophy between 500 and 1500*, ed. Henrik Lagerlund, 'Living' online edition (Dordrecht: Springer, 2018). https://link.springer.com/referenceworkentry/10.1007/978-94-024-1151-5_191-2 (last accessed 11 November 2018). The most successful 'mirror' was the pseudo-Aristotelian *Secret of Secrets* (*Secretum secretorum*).

17 Elena Woodacre, "Understanding the mechanisms of monarchy" in this volume.

18 For the distinction see Giles of Rome, *De regimine principum libri tres* (Rome: Bartholomæum Zannettum, 1607; repr. Aalen, 1967), 2.1.14. For detailed analysis see Roberto Lambertini, "Political Thought," in *A Companion to Giles of Rome*, eds. Charles F. Briggs and Peter S. Eardley (Leiden: Brill, 2016), 258–265.

19 For the importance of the common good in Giles's thought see Thomas Renna, "Aristotle and the French Monarchy, 1260–1303," *Viator* 9 (1978): 312–314.

20 Aquinas's conclusion that 'it was not contrary to the dignity of the state of innocence that one man should be ruled by another' is grounded in the existence of diversity in the state of nature: *Summa theologiae* Ia 96 art. 3–4 in *Aquinas Political Writings*, ed. and trans. Robert W. Dyson (Cambridge: Cambridge University Press, 2002), 1–4, quotation at 3. For an overview see Canning, *History*, 129; Antony Black, *Political Thought in Europe 1250–1450* (Cambridge: Cambridge University Press, 1992), 22–24.

21 The phrase was first coined by Charles Homer Haskins, *The Renaissance of the Twelfth Century* (Cambridge, MA: Harvard University Press, 1927). Whether or not the revival constituted a 'Renaissance' has been the subject of much subsequent debate. See, notably, the essays in *Renaissance and Renewal in the Twelfth Century*, eds. Robert L. Benson and Giles Constable (Cambridge, MA: Harvard University Press, 1982). For an overview see Anna Sapir Abulafia, "Intellectual and Cultural Creativity," in *The Central Middle Ages*, ed. Daniel Power (Oxford: Oxford University Press, 2006), 149–177; for a note of caution on the use of the term 'Renaissance', ibid., 175.

22 As a starting point for the vast literature on the growth of trade and urbanization in this period see Derek Keene, "Towns and the Growth of Trade," in *The New Cambridge Medieval History IV, c.1024–c.1198*, Part I, eds. David Luscombe and Jonathan Riley-Smith (Cambridge: Cambridge University Press, 2004), 47–85.

23 For an introduction to John see Cary J. Nederman, "John of Salisbury," in *Encyclopedia of Medieval Philosophy*. https://link.springer.com/referenceworkentry/10.1007/978-94-024-1151-5_276-2 (last accessed 11 November 2018).

24 M. Cecilia Gaposchkin, "Kingship and Crusade in the First Four Moralized Bibles," in *The Capetian Century, 1214 to 1314*, eds. William C. Jordan and Jenna R. Phillips (Turnhout: Brepols, 2017), 71–112, quotation at 77. The Bibles were 'littered with images of kings and lessons for kings', ibid., 72.

25 For an introduction see Stephan Kuttner, "The Revival of Jurisprudence," in *Renaissance & Renewal in the Twelfth Century*, 299–323. Joseph Canning has highlighted the importance

of the *Corpus iuris civilis* in particular in shaping political thought: "Ideas of the State in Thirteenth and Fourteenth-Century Commentators on the Roman Law," *Transactions of the Royal Historical Society* series 5, 33 (1983): 1–2.

26 Woodacre, "Understanding the mechanisms of monarchy", 6–7.

27 For a detailed account of Henry's reform of English law see W.L. Warren, *Henry II*, paperback edition (Los Angeles: University of California Press, 1977), 317–361; Paul Brand, "Henry II and the Creation of the English Common Law," in *Henry II: New Interpretations*, eds. Christopher Harper-Bill and Nicholas Vincent (Woodbridge: Boydell, 2007), 215–241; and for the motivations behind individual legal reforms, which Brand concludes 'fit into an overall picture of an activist king, interested in justice and the law, and determined to find a more active role for the monarchy in their provision', 234–241, quotation at 241. For Frederick's use of law see Robert L. Benson, "Political *Renovatio*: Two Models from Roman Antiquity," in *Renaissance & Renewal in the Twelfth Century*, eds. Robert L. Benson and Giles Constable (Cambridge, MA: Harvard University Press, 1982), 360–369; Kenneth Pennington, *The Prince and the Law, 1200–1600: Sovereignty and Rights in the Western Legal Tradition* (Los Angeles: University of California, 1993), 8–37.

28 *The Liber Augustalis or Constitutions of Melfi, promulgated by the Emperor Frederick II for the Kingdom of Sicily in 1231*, trans. James M. Powell (Syracuse: Syracuse University Press, 1971); David Abulafia, *Frederick II: A Medieval Emperor*, new edition (London: Pimlico, 1992), 202–214. For the role of the *Constitutions* in establishing the independence of royal from papal authority, ibid., 207. See also Wolfgang Stürner, *Friedrich II., 2: Der Kaiser 1220–1250* (Darmstadt: Wissenschaftliche Buchgesellschaft, 2000), 189–210.

29 For reform of royal administration see Jean Richard, *Saint Louis: Crusader King of France*, ed. and abridged Simon Lloyd, trans. Jean Birrell (Cambridge: Cambridge University Press, 1992), 156–158; for morality, 160–163. See also Jacques Le Goff, *Saint Louis* (Paris: Gallimard, 1996), 216–220.

30 Henric Bagerius and Christine Ekholst, "For better or for worse: royal marital sexuality", 636–654 in this volume.

31 For an overview of John's thought see Roberto Lambertini, "John of Paris," in *Encyclopedia of Medieval Philosophy: Philosophy Between 500 and 1500*, ed. Henrik Lagerlund, 2 vols (Heidelberg: Springer, 2011), vol. 1, 631–633. For in-depth discussion see the essays in *John of Paris: Beyond Royal and Papal Power*, ed. Chris Jones, Disputatio 23 (Turnhout: Brepols, 2015). For the context in which John's ideas developed see Chris Jones, "John of Paris: Through a Glass, Darkly?" in ibid., 1–31.

32 For the dispute see Thomas S.R. Boase, *Boniface VIII* (Oxford: Constable, 1933), 297–351; Joseph R. Strayer, *The Reign of Philip the Fair* (Princeton: Princeton University Press, 1980), 260–279. For the most recent detailed study see Guillaume de Thieulloy, *Le pape et le roi: Anagni (7 septembre 1303)* (Paris: Gallimard, 2010). For perceptions of papal claims in France see Chris Jones, *Eclipse of Empire? Perceptions of the Western Empire and Its Rulers in Late-Medieval France*, Cursor mundi 1 (Turnhout: Brepols, 2007), 231.

33 John of Paris, *John of Paris: On Royal and Papal Power*, trans. J.A. Watt (Toronto: Pontifical Institute of Mediaeval Studies, 1971), chapter 3, 86.

34 For an overview of the legal and historical arguments see Jones, *Eclipse*, 232–238.

35 For modern assessments of John's importance see Chris Jones, "Historical Understanding and the Nature of Temporal Power in the Thought of John of Paris," in *John of Paris: Beyond Royal and Papal Power*, 77 n. 1.

36 Abulafia, *Frederick II*, 202–203. Stürner, *Friedrich II*, 201–210, considers the extent to which the *Constitutions* were actually applied.

37 Giles of Rome, *De regimine principum*, 3.2.5.

38 For Henry's – ultimately failed – efforts see Abulafia, *Frederick II*, 83. For the question of election and heredity in the thought of late medieval theorists more generally see Black, 146–148.

39 John of Paris, *On Royal and Papal Power*, chapter 10, 124. The origins of emperors, were, according to John, somewhat different from those of kings. See Jones, "Historical Understanding," 80.

40 Chris Jones, "Understanding Political Conceptions in the Later Middle Ages: The French Imperial Candidatures and the Idea of the Nation-State," *Viator* 42, no. 2 (2011): 107–109.

41 Giles of Rome, *De regimine principum*, 3.2.5.
42 For a significant and wide-ranging recent survey of the history of the Holy Roman Empire see Peter. H. Wilson, *The Holy Roman Empire: A Thousand Years of Europe's History* (London: Penguin, 2017).
43 Woodacre, "Understanding the Mechanisms of Monarchy", 4–6.
44 The argument appears in Giles's *On Ecclesiastical Power: Giles of Rome's On Ecclesiastical Power. A Medieval Theory of World Government*, ed. and trans. Robert W. Dyson (New York: Columbia University Press, 2004), 1.7–9, 38–60. For an overview see Jones, "Giles of Rome." For detailed analysis see Robert W. Dyson, *Normative Theories of Society and Government in Five Medieval Thinkers: St Augustine, John of Salisbury, Giles of Rome, St. Thomas Aquinas, and Marsilius of Padua* (Lewiston: Edwin Mellen Press, 2003), 141–185; Lambertini, "Political Thought," 267–271.
45 John of Paris, *On Royal and Papal Power*, chapter 10, 124.
46 For the revolution that brought the 'Abbāsids to power: Hugh Kennedy, *When Baghdad Ruled the Muslim World: The Rise and Fall of Islam's Greatest Dynasty* (Cambridge, MA: Da Capo Press, 2005), 1–11.
47 Cited from Bernard Lewis, *The Arabs in History*, sixth edition (Oxford: Oxford University Press, 1993), 65.
48 The nature of government in the caliphate's first century is much debated. For traditional overviews of its development see Albert Hourani, *A History of the Arab Peoples*, new edition (London: Faber & Faber, 2005), 22–32; Bernard Lewis, *The Middle East: 2000 Years of History from the Rise of Christianity to the Present Day*, paperback edition (London: Phoenix, 2000), 54–74. For challenges to the traditional account see Patricia Crone and Martin Hinds, *God's Caliph: Religious Authority in the First Centuries of Islam* (Cambridge: Cambridge University Press, 1986); Fred Donner, *The Expansion of the Early Islamic State* (Aldershot: Ashgate Variorum, 2007).
49 For the most recent contribution to the historiography of the Kingitanga see Michael Belgrave, *Dancing with the King: The Rise and Fall of the King Country, 1864–1885* (Auckland: Auckland University Press, 2017), but see Martin Fisher, "Review: *Dancing with the King: The Rise and Fall of the King Country, 1864–1885*, (review no. 2267)," *Reviews in History*, www. history.ac.uk/reviews/review/2267 (accessed 26 October 2018).
50 Maree Shirota, "Royal Depositions and the 'Canterbury Roll'," *Parergon* 32, no. 2 (2015): 39–61.
51 On the response of the medieval theorists to this problem see Black, *Political Thought*, 148–152. For the useless king specifically in medieval thought see Edward Peters, *The Shadow King: 'Rex Inutilis' in Medieval Law and Literature, 751–1327* (New Haven: Yale University Press, 1970).
52 Cathleen Sarti, "Deposition of monarchs in northern kingdoms, 1300–1700", 581–594 in this volume.
53 Anna M. Duch, "Chasing St Louis", 330–351.
54 David M. Malitz, "The nation as a ritual community", 213–228 in this volume.
55 Woodacre, "Understanding the Mechanisms of Monarchy", 6.
56 Lucinda H.S. Dean, "Introduction" (to Part II), 183–184 in this volume.

Key works

Black, Antony, *Political Thought in Europe 1250–1450* (Cambridge: Cambridge University Press, 1992).
Canning, Joseph, *A History of Medieval Political Thought 300–1450* (London and New York: Routledge, 1996).
Dale, Stephen F., *The Muslim Empires of the Ottomans, Safavids, and Mughals* (Cambridge: Cambridge University Press, 2010).
Hourani, Albert, *A History of the Arab Peoples*, new edition (London: Faber & Faber, 2005).
Jones, Chris, ed., *John of Paris: Beyond Royal and Papal Power*, Disputatio 23 (Turnhout: Brepols, 2015).

1

THE 'WISE KING' *TOPOS* IN CONTEXT

Royal literacy and political theology in medieval western Europe (*c.*1000–1200)

Manuel Alejandro Rodríguez de la Peña

Introduction

It was the German historian Wilhelm Berges who first identified the sapiential royal *topos* and coined the concept of the 'ideal of the learned kings' (*Ideal des Gelehrtenkönigs*) to refer to it in his seminal study of medieval 'mirrors of princes' literature first published in 1938.[1] Applying the same approach to late medieval political thought, Antony Black coined the expression 'the sapiential idea'. Black pointed out that:

> The case for giving the wise an important place in government was virtually unanswerable given the belief in rationality endemic in European culture, or at least the literate culture which produced political theory. This belief stemmed from Platonism, Stoicism and their Christianised variations which came to dominate the mental perspectives of late Rome, Byzantium and the Early and High Middle Ages in the West. It was the way to keep the myth of the monarch as the seat of wisdom.[2]

Indeed, royal learning was considered by many medieval intellectuals to be just another dimension of good rulership. This is best understood if we take into consideration the judgement of William of Malmesbury, who stated that the learning of the English king, Henry I Beauclerc, was of great help to him 'for the science of government' (*ad regnandum scientiae*).[3]

The Italian Renaissance may have been the apogee of the cult of the learned prince, but it was not a unique phenomenon and had deep medieval roots. The remarks of Sergio Bertelli concerning the Renaissance court, that 'shielded from the outside world . . . [it] projects an image of itself as mysterious and inaccessible; its power is enhanced by [the] double aim of seeming both very learned and very glorious',[4] can be equally transposed onto many medieval courts. And the royal patron, even when not personally implicated in scholarship, remained a decisive figure. Until relatively recently, however, the medieval royal court was barely spared a thought in the history of western culture or science. Today, by contrast, the juxtaposition of 'science' and the 'royal court' in the Middle Ages no longer strikes the academic reader, at least, as something odd.

While royal patronage of culture was a universal phenomenon in the Latin west after 1100, there are plenty of examples of artistic, literary and scholarly patronage throughout medieval history. Indeed, if we pay attention to the context of the successive medieval renaissances, we realize that there was always a decisive royal impulse. The impact of royal patronage of learning was felt far beyond the rulers' entourages and had a lasting impact on social and cultural structures. That is certainly the case for the Carolingian (c.790–870), Alfredian (c.870–900) and Ottonian (c.960–1000) renaissances in the early Middle Ages. But we may also recall later examples such as Norman and Hohenstaufen Sicily (c.1130–1270), the Plantagenet empire (c.1150–1200), Alfonsine Castile (c.1250–1300), Angevin Naples (c.1260–1350), Valois France (c.1350–1400), or Ricardian England (c.1380–90), among many others, some of which are dealt with in Laura Fábián's chapter in this volume.

The purpose of this chapter is to explore a number of closely interrelated elements of Latin medieval civilization in order to establish a genealogy of what can be termed 'sapiential rulership'. These elements include Christian kingship, political theology, literacy, courtly culture and royal patronage of learning. In part, all were shaped by the role of the royal court as a cultural institution, particularly with regard to its patronage of learning and the arts.[5] Literacy and high culture in the mentalities and exercise of power by the governing élites equally played a significant role in their development.[6] However, the present chapter will focus on two additional critical factors: first, the manner in which court intellectuals shaped political mentalities as advocates of royal wisdom, or, we might say, as propaganda agents,[7] and, second, the contents and aims of their political theology, particularly their discourse on sapiential kingship.[8]

The chapter will argue that, following the splendour of the Carolingian and Ottonian ages, royal wisdom came to occupy a secondary position in the political theology of the succeeding centuries. One consequence of both the Feudal Revolution and the Gregorian Reform movement was that the new discourse on kingship did not have much place for royal learning. However, the twelfth-century Renaissance completely changed this trend and brought the sapiential *topos* back to the frontline of political thought. The medieval royal court not only attracted scholars but also became a place of science, and the king could not seem to be less intelligent that his household. As Martin Aurell puts it:

> It was on this that a great part of his authority rested if he wanted to make himself obeyed promptly. If he possessed no culture, his prestige would fade among the clerks of his court. The king was to excel in wisdom if he were to govern effectively.[9]

The sapiential image of kingship

A fundamental problem in analysing any act of royal patronage of learning is tracing its motivation. According to Rosamond McKitterick, medieval patronage of culture 'is emphatically not random aesthetic pleasure or arcane intellectual curiosity, but an organised and determined assembly and deployment of resources to carry out what appears to be specific aims and objectives'.[10] Further, she points out that for the Carolingians 'the patronage of book production and intellectual culture was primarily for the promotion of their royal power as Christian kings and for the consolidation of the Christian faith by disseminating the key texts on which that faith was based'.[11] Indeed, the extant evidence permits us to say that in the medieval period the chief motivation for artistic or intellectual royal patronage was rooted in Christian theology. Time and again the documents and chronicles that record medieval rulers' actions of patronage show them as moved by something we may label a 'sapiential political theology'. This political theology was wisdom-centred, this being another dimension of Christ-centred kingship.

Sapiential rulership had been, since the origins of civilization, just one of the many shapes in which sacral authority (priestly or royal) was embodied. It is true that in classical antiquity political wisdom was not always religiously based, but the early Middle Ages opted for the Platonic *sophia* and the Solomonic *hokhmá* as the sources of Christian *sapientia*. Until the western reception of Aristotelian *phronesis* in the thirteenth century, sapiential kingship remained mainly a theological issue. It is in this ideological context that we can fully understand Georges Duby's statement about kingship:

> The king in the year 1000 had this in common with the bishops: he was sacred. Since the middle of the eighth century, the Frankish king's body, like the bishop's, had been impregnated with holy oil. And therefore, his spirit was impregnated with *sapientia*. He was a sage, mysteriously informed of the intentions of the Providence, as one of the *oratores*.[12]

An early medieval ideal with lasting popularity – above all for royal wisdom and sanctity – was the cult of King David and King Solomon's biblical models for kingship.[13] This started with Carolingian mirrors for princes and continued through the centuries until the fourteenth century, when Robert the Wise of Naples was proclaimed 'the new Solomon'. In this regard, Gabor Klaniczay has stressed that:

> [a]t first it was the figure of King David, which was the most prominent among these ideals. Subsequently, Solomon was added to him as a second model with increasing frequency, joining the appreciation of peacefulness and wisdom to the triumphant and victorious image represented by David.[14]

It has also been pointed out, referring to Carolingian rulership, that 'the king began to represent a type of ruler modelled on David. He was the *novus Moyses*, the *novus David*. He was the priestly king, the *rex et sacerdos*.'[15] Thus, Pepin the Short, Charlemagne, and Louis the Pious were each praised for being a 'new David'.[16] Similarly, Walter Ullmann has stressed that it is only when 'due emphasis is given to the views which Charlemagne held in regard to the value of the Bible for purposes of government'[17] that one can understand this dimension of Carolingian kingship. Accordingly, in one of his many letters to Charlemagne, Alcuin of York recommended to his royal disciple the building of a 'new Athens', a model city in which the Liberal Arts would support Christian learning according to the principles of the 'true philosophy'.[18] In his *De rhetorica*, Alcuin upholds the ideal of a civil society whose philosopher-king orders his government according to Christian moral philosophy.[19] In a similar vein, in his *De dialectica* Alcuin also cast Charlemagne in the role of Solomon, the ideal philosopher-king and chief advocate of the 'true philosophy'.[20]

Besides this key biblical legitimation, Charlemagne's impressive patronage of learning on a grandiose scale also 'served to enhance his dignity by linking him with Roman imperial practices, and Carolingian propagandists stressed this feature of his reforms'.[21] In fact, Charlemagne's own awareness of the importance of learning at court was nurtured by neo-Roman models of active learning centres in Byzantium and in some Germanic kingdoms such as the Ostrogothic under Theoderic the Great.[22]

Sapiential rulership in the Ottonian and Salian empire

As happened in the Carolingian period, ecclesiastical ideals determined the Ottonian and Salian concept of royal authority. The image of the king as the representative of Christ (*vicarius Christi*) 'was of central importance in Salian royal theology'.[23] Ottonian and Salian sacral kingship was also expressed in the Davidic and Solomonic images of rulership that we find in the writings of the court intellectuals. For instance, Hrotsvitha of Gandersheim, who professed in an abbey patronized by the Ottonians, praised Otto the Great as a new David and his son, Otto II, as 'our Solomon' (*Salomon noster*).[24]

In the following century Abbot Bern of Reichenau and other authors compared Henry III to King David. Such Davidic images were not new, of course, yet, as Stefan Weinfurter has pointed out, 'their increased frequency in reference to Henry III is striking'.[25] Indeed, David's kingship associated the Salian ruler with the royal house of Christ, and just as David in his person had preceded Christ, the German emperor now appeared as an *imitatio* of Christ. Such allusions became even more explicit when Henry III ended the papal schism during his stay at Rome in 1046.[26]

It is no coincidence that the Ottonian-founded system of cathedral-school education was the most important element in the process of 'Romanizing' Germany in the tenth and eleventh centuries. The founding of this system is traceable to an Ottonian remarkable for his learning, his pedagogy and his statesmanship: Bruno, archbishop of Cologne (953–65).[27] In this regard, Stephen Jaeger has pointed out that Bruno:

> [h]ad a pedagogic bent that made itself felt in the documentary style of Otto's administration and, if we are to believe his biographer, in the intellectual life of the court itself. Under his influence the court was transformed into a kind of school of philosophy and the liberal arts.[28]

There is, however, no evidence for the exercise of royal patronage under the Ottonian emperors comparable to what we have for its exercise under the Carolingians.[29] It is not until the very end of the tenth century that a group of manuscripts can be associated with an Ottonian ruler with any certainty. This group, dated to the very last years of Otto III's reign (r. 983–1002), is a famous quartet of codices, all produced by scribes and artists trained at Reichenau, and are thought to have been made for the ruler's personal use.[30] Compared to Carolingian book production, this is far from impressive. Rosamond McKitterick has highlighted the shortcomings of Ottonian cultural patronage, pointing out that:

[t]here is no systematic patronage of particular centres, no group of scholars associated with the court, no royal role in the dissemination of particular texts, no cultivation of contemporary scholarship, no court atelier, no sign even of occasional sponsorship of individual scholars or craftsmen.[31]

Be that as it may, the Ottonian patronage of culture, although clearly inferior to that of the Carolingians, was highly significant if we compare it with the rest of royal-sponsored cultural activity in the tenth century. Yet, it can be said that in Otto III we find a truly Solomonic ruler. He was tutored in Greek by a Byzantine cleric and grammarian, Johannes Philagathos (*c.*945–1001).[32] Later, in 997, the most learned man of the Latin west, Gerbert of Aurillac, entered the imperial circle as Otto III's tutor and expanded the young emperor's familiarity with a range of foundational works connected with ancient Roman philosophy and history.[33]

A further potential source of information concerning Otto III's sapiential profile is to be found in the large number of books that Florentine Mutherich has suggested were once part of his personal library.[34] The forty-four books she discusses reflect Otto's education and intellectual tastes and are a 'wonderfully diverse and scholarly collection'.[35]

In Gerbert of Aurillac's introduction to his *Libellus de rationali et ratione uti*, written during the winter of 997–8, Gerbert surpassed himself as both a royal encomiast and a theorist of sapiential rulership. This is the last portion of extant writing which he addressed to Otto III. It fittingly holds a place at the height of a crescendo of sapiential discourse. Gerbert begins in the following manner:

> While we were tarrying in Germany during the warmer season of the year, occupied with imperial duties, as we always are and always shall be, I do not know what of secret import your divine mind, meditating silently with itself, may release in words when the spirit moves; and what things written by Aristotle and the greatest men in extremely difficult sentences, your god-like intellect might bring forth into the light of ordinary understanding so that, between the intervals of wars which were under way against the Slavs, it should be remarkable that anyone of mortal birth could have such mental resources from which knowledge should flow forth as keen and as clear as indeed from the purest fountain.[36]

This sapiential discourse on kingship similarly pervaded the Ottonian rulers' letters. Otto III addressed a famous letter to Gerbert in the latter part of 997, full of sapiential rhetoric:

> To Gerbert, the most erudite of teachers, laureate in the three branches of philosophy, Otto writes as to himself . . . We desire you to remove our Saxon crudeness and call forth our Greek subtlety with all the more earnestness because if there is a spark of the Greek genius to be found in us, it is you who will rekindle it. Accordingly, we ask in humble prayers that by putting the flaming torch of your learning to our little flame, you may, with God's help, revive the lively genius of the Greeks and teach us your book of Arithmetic so that, fully instructed in its lessons, we may understand something of the subtlety of the ancients.[37]

The spectres of both the Constantinian imperial ideal and Charlemagne's own reputation as the Germanic political successor to a Roman legacy informed the appearance of Otto III's ritual discovery of Charlemagne's tomb at Pentecost in 1000, which he performed in direct imitation of Augustus' own 'discovery' of Alexander the Great's grave. This is an indication of the lengths to which Otto was willing to go in order to display his internalization of antique history and his concomitant embodiment of imperial ideals.[38] And, as stated previously, Charlemagne's was one of the most influential sapiential images of royal power offered to the tenth century. For instance, in his *Res Gestae Saxonicae*, Widukind of Corvey acclaimed Charlemagne as a *rex fortissimus* who was also a seeker of wisdom (*non minori sapientia vigilabat*) and 'the most prudent of the mortal men of the age'.[39]

With the above in mind, the last Ottonian emperor, Henry II (r.1002–24), was, however, one of the few medieval German rulers who took a personal interest in biblical exegesis: 'Originally headed for a career in the Church, he had studied in the cathedral school at Hildesheim, not far from Magdeburg, where he would have acquired at least a passing knowledge of rhetoric, grammar, theology and canon law.'[40] Henry II was also said 'to have been an admirer of St Ambrose and was familiar with Gregory the Great's *Moralia*'.[41] So accomplished was his mastery of Latin 'that he could dictate his own *diplomata* and play practical jokes on members of the clergy whose linguistic skills were of a distinctly lesser order'.[42] As an example of these concerns it was said that Henry took pleasure in making Bishop Meinwerk of Paderborn look ridiculous for his deficient knowledge of Latin at a public celebration of Mass.[43]

But sapiential political theology went much further than liturgical literacy. According to Ernst Kantorowicz, no medieval political theology could work without some fiction or some 'metaphor of perfection', and there is every reason to conclude that the political metaphor of Lady Wisdom (*Imago Sapientiae*) as both a sign of God's grace and a dispenser of sapiential royal virtues was a particularly powerful one in the Middle Ages.[44]

In connection with this *imago* of Lady Wisdom, attention has been called to a miniature of an earlier date showing an Ottonian emperor as a mediator in legal matters. The miniature is found in the magnificent Gospel book that Henry II donated to the Abbey of Monte Cassino in 1022 or 1023.[45] Where a representation of St John would normally be expected, the miniature shows instead a full-page image of the emperor with a number of theological personifications. In the centre, within a large circle the emperor is enthroned in full *regalia*. In the upper corners we recognize *iustitia* and *pietas*; to the right and left, placed in smaller circles, are *sapientia* and *prudentia*, attendants and throne-companions of kingship since earliest times.

Henry II's will is directed by inspiration from above. In the circle above the emperor's head we recognize the Holy Spirit descending from heaven in the shape of a dove, a symbol of divine Wisdom.[46] As Ernst Kantorowicz has pointed out:

> In this scene of judgment Henry II clearly functions as mediator between divine Reason and human law. But, as behoves an Ottonian prince, the emperor's mediatorship is expressed liturgically, that is, by the *epiklesis* of the Spirit . . . The picture's language is theological, and not jurisprudential: the emperor is mediator and executor of the divine will through the power of the Holy Spirit, and not through the secular spirit of legal science.[47]

Therefore, to bring it to a simple formula, the Ottonian sapiential discourse had more to do with royal wisdom (*sapientia*) than with royal science (*eruditio*) or even personal literacy.

In contrast with the last Ottonians, the first ruler of the Salian Age, Conrad II, was completely illiterate. He did not even know the letters of the alphabet, and the Italian *Chronicon Novalicense* describes him as an illiterate ruler (*rex idiota*).[48] Yet the latest biographer of Conrad, Herwig Wolfram, has underlined the 'overpowering symbolism' of the imperial crown commissioned by the first Salian ruler (probably using a previous Ottonian model). This crown displays four plates interspersed between the jewels: two of them depict King David and King Solomon, and a third represents a figure of an enthroned Christ supported by an inscription: 'By me kings reign' (*Per me reges regnant*) taken from Proverbs 8:15.[49] This is, of course, the famous biblical saying of Lady Wisdom which established her as the true source of royal legitimacy. The fact that such a remarkable insignia of Salian imperial sovereignty was linked to this sapiential principle of legitimacy – be it of ultimately Ottonian origin or not – is remarkable to say the least.

How far this image conformed to reality is another matter. However, there is every indication that Conrad II's son and successor, Henry III (r.1039–56), was indeed a cultivated prince. He was portrayed by many sources not only as a Davidic ruler but also as a Solomonic lover of wisdom. He was praised by the court chaplain Wipo as a bookish and learned king, a *rex peritus*,[50] in spite of his youth (he came to the throne at the age of twenty-two and died when he was thirty-nine). Other contemporary sources tell us that 'Henry III often joined the clergy at court in reading the Scriptures or in pursuing learned discussions.'[51] Furthermore, according to the *Augsburger Annals*, Henry III's enthusiasm for learning and active promotion of the arts and sciences led to a flourishing intellectual life in Germany.[52]

With regard to the Salians, it has been pointed out that:

> Each of these monarchs was noted for an educational level far above that of most contemporary rulers; each was noted for an interest in church art, architecture, and building programmes; each was noted for a concern with scrupulous legality in their actions; each was recorded by their contemporaries as personally pious.[53]

Stefan Weinfurter has stressed in this regard that 'The spiritual and scholarly interests that bonded the king to his chaplains and other men in his following had a far-reaching impact and were instrumental in transforming the court into *the* intellectual centre of the realm.'[54] In other words, royal piety was the way by which learning entered the Salian court. This is a trend that we find in other early medieval courts, but in this case, it is particularly true.

Sapiential rulership in early Capetian France

The maintenance of the Carolingian tradition of sacral kingship was one of the main aims of the early Capetians, devoid as they were of real political power. In order to obtain the royal *auctoritas* of their prestigious predecessors, the Capetian kings found a new source of image-making in the monastic reform movement inspired by Cluny. The abbey of Fleury, a house under Cluniac protection since the 930s, became particularly linked to the new royal dynasty. And it was precisely at Fleury that a new vision of kingship was systematically expressed around the *topos* of royal sanctity.[55] Capetian kingship was reimagined portraying rulers as peaceful and wise holy men more akin to praying monks than to warring laymen.[56]

Helgaud of Fleury's openly hagiographical rendering of Robert the Pious's life (r.996–1031) is in fact 'an account of his private life and, as presented, this is almost exclusively his religious life'.[57] It was entirely conservative, in that it followed Carolingian traditions to fuse a Frankish ruler with the Old Testament David. Yet, as Jean Dunbabin has pointed out, Helgaud also innovated by making King Robert truly 'a saint of the Church'[58] and in so doing changed the very image of kingship in France.

Yet, significantly, Helgaud also described Robert II's magnificent education and related that he had studied with Gerbert of Aurillac at the cathedral school of Reims.[59] In fact, Robert the Pious is the only Capetian king to whom we can definitely attribute full Latin literacy before the reign of Louis VII (r.1137–80).[60] He was also musically inclined and was said to have enjoyed choral music. Having studied with the greatest mind in tenth-century Europe, the Capetian ruler was 'knowledgeable enough to debate the meaning of rhetorical terminology with Adalbero of Laon'.[61] An important Cluniac chronicler, Raoul Glaber, proclaimed Robert II to be *eruditum* in the liberal arts and a prudent ruler,[62] while Richer of Reims, who knew the king as a fellow student, says that he was 'well versed in divine and canon law, and applied himself to the liberal arts'.[63] Another monk-chronicler, Hariulf of Saint-Riquier, described Robert as 'a king who never failed to derive solace from books, and even carried them about with him on his travels'.[64] Also related to the sapiential *topos* is the significant fact that certain documents of this period are dated 'in the reign of the philosopher king' (*regnante rege philosopho*),[65] thus showing, points out James Thompson, 'that his contemporaries esteemed Robert not only as a pious but also as a learned king'.[66]

The old Carolingian conception of kingship was undoubtedly at work here. One of the main defenders of its legacy, Adalbero, bishop of Laon, put it to King Robert in the following manner: 'The capacity (*facultas*) of the *orator* is given to the king.'[67] Thus Adalbero acknowledged that kings had the (ecclesiastic) *facultas oratoris*, the right to pray, the right to preach. Yet given their 'youthful' ignorance, it was also important that they receive episcopal instruction and advice in the law (*legibus edocti*: v. 361).[68] These words were incorporated into a political poem addressed by Adalbero to Robert around the year 1027, the *Carmen ad Rodbertum regem*, one of the main sources of the 'feudal' schema of the three orders, but also of deep interest for scholarship on medieval political theology.

If we take into account the *Carmen ad Rodbertum*, we must conclude that the position of the king in Capetian France was far more ambiguous in sapiential terms than that of the Ottonian and Salian emperors. German and Italian bishops were members of a *Reichskirche* under royal tutelage. In eleventh-century France, however, bishops like Adalbero of Laon aspired to put Capetian kings under their own intellectual tutelage. As Georges Duby put it:

The king therefore knew how to read from a Latin book, and could chant his prayers. But he did not know enough to take full advantage of the illumination coming to him from heaven. He had need of assistants to help him decipher the message. This necessary assistance was provided by the other *oratores*, who unlike the king himself were not distracted from meditation upon things sacred by military concerns.[69]

There is one further passage of the *Carmen ad Rodbertum* which is highly significant. Here Adalbero states that the king's *vera sapientia* (true wisdom) is a gift from the king of kings, consisting in knowledge of the immutable mysteries of heaven (*scire potes quae sunt caelestia semper*), that is, the secret architecture of the Heavenly Jerusalem.[70] This may refer to a kind of spiritual wisdom without any connection to secular learning.

Sapiential references in the eleventh century in Europe could easily be multiplied, but these should suffice to show the general trend. To name just one other case, in late Anglo-Saxon England we may find the same ideological developments as in the post-Carolingian world. Simon Keynes has argued 'that Alfred was brought up on the biblical stories of David and Solomon' and, therefore, it 'requires little further imagination to see what effect their example might have had on his own exercise of kingship'.[71] This points to the various ways in which Alfred's exercise of kingship recalls the biblical accounts of the kingship of Solomon, most obviously that remarkable king's personal pursuit of wisdom.[72] However, as happened in early Capetian France, in tenth-century England Benedictine reformers reshaped the royal 'Dream of Solomon'. The latter stressed the subordinate role of the secular ruler in matters of divine wisdom. Wulfstan of York, archbishop and Benedictine monk (d.1023) said:

> The king must listen eagerly to the doctrine of the Bible, he must obey God's commandments, and furthermore he must ask for wisdom to be taught to him by his counsellors with whom he has to discuss wisdom – if he wants to be obedient to God.[73]

With these various distinctions in mind, it can be argued that while a strong Carolingian tradition of Christian sapiential rulership was influential after 1000, it was reinterpreted according to different political contexts. While in Salian Germany there was a strong continuity of the Carolingian *topos* of the wise ruler, in early Capetian France and tenth-century England there was, however, a hierocratic reinterpretation which minimized the scope of royal wisdom. Despite this hierocratic reception, it must be said that, taken as a whole, a general picture emerges from the year 1000 that sustains the idea that the sapiential *topos* of the Carolingian renaissance was echoed again and again in the following centuries.

The twelfth-century Renaissance and Plantagenet kingship

It is surely not a coincidence that the famous maxim *rex illiteratus est quasi asinus coronatus* first appeared in Europe in Anglo-Norman England, where administrative kingship was born.[74] It originated in the writings of the historian William of

Malmesbury (*c*.1080–*c*.1142).[75] In all probability, this is just a rhetorical *topos*: 'In the light of William I's illiteracy and shortness of temper, one cannot seriously believe Malmesbury's account of young, bookish Henry remarking in his father's hearing that an illiterate king is a crowned ass.'[76] Be that as it may, what is clear is that, influenced by the rivalry with the Capetians, this sapiential maxim was used as a barely disguised criticism of the unlearned kings of France by English and Angevin clerks, who took pride in the wisdom of their sovereigns. For instance, Breton d'Amboise, a chronicler of the Plantagenets working early in Henry II's reign, puts the same words in the mouth of the Angevine count Fulk the Good (940–60), whom he praises for his 'wisdom, eloquence and literacy'.[77]

While the *rex litteratus* theme fits the mould created by Henry I Beauclerc, a bureaucrat-king, it only reached its apogee during the reign of Henry II Plantagenet. Not coincidentally, John of Marmoutier described Henry II's father, Geoffrey Plantagenet (1129–51) in his *Historia Gaufredi* (*c*.1180) as 'dedicated to the practice of arms and equally to liberal studies'.[78] In much the same way Gerald of Wales asserted that Henry II devoted himself 'as much to the business of arms as to the toga; to war as much as to books'.[79]

This combination of learning and knighthood, embodied respectively in the Middle Ages by the ecclesiastical and knightly classes (*clergie et chevalerie*), reflected the ancient Roman theme of *fortitudo* and *sapientia* in feudal disguise.[80] As Martin Aurell puts it, for the clerks who built up the royal image of the Plantagenets:

> [t]he prince seemed as learned and wise as he was ready and courageous in battle. The prince achieved in his person a perfect synthesis of clerk and knight. He had become a *miles litteratus*: the prestigious model already emulated by so many of the lay courtiers.[81]

Henry II's culture and taste for literature was soon identified by the clerks of his court, who found him to be the very embodiment of a Christian learned king, a 'second Solomon' (*Salomon alter*) to quote a phrase of Gerald of Wales.[82] To incarnate Solomonic kingship was something that even someone as proud of his ancestry as a Plantagenet would appreciate.

Sometimes, the discourse on Solomonic kingship could originate in unexpected sources. Such is the case of the *Treatise on the Astrolabe* (1149) of the famous mathematician Adelard of Bath (*c*.1091–*c*.1160). This treatise on astronomy begins with a long prologue praising the intellectual qualities of the future Henry II, encouraging him to explore the astronomical lore of the Arabic East, and significantly enough, also quoting the Platonic proverb on philosopher-kings:

> Henry, I know that you, the king's grandson, were educated in all aspect of philosophy. It is said that the commonwealth is happy when ruled by philosophers and its people pursue the subject . . . This is why you must learn not only what Latin texts have to tell but also what the Arabs have to teach us about the movement of the earth and the orbits of the stars.[83]

Through all these literary and scholarly works the Plantagenet rulers were aptly linked to an ancient sapiential tradition which portrayed them as a lineage of learned counts and kings, who embodied, from the tenth century, the figure of the *miles litteratus*. It is not, therefore, surprising that it was in the *Gesta Comitum Andegavorum* that the saying *rex illiteratus est quasi asinus coronatus*[84] is first recorded in France. As a matter of fact, the taunt that a French king was 'an illiterate king' and was to be equated with a 'crowned ass' was 'a cliché much favoured in twelfth-century Angevin circles, for it sprang from a sense of family superiority – the counts of Anjou were, by any standards, learned men'.[85]

The Cistercian writer, Helinand of Froidmont (1160/70–*c.*1229) also quotes the saying in a mirror for princes, the *De bono regimine principis* (*c.*1200), not hesitating to quote a phrase that pokes fun at the French kings, despite the fact he had been employed as a poet at the court of Philip II Augustus.[86] Gerald of Wales insinuated the same maxim into the first preface of his *De principis instructione*, another mirror for princes.[87] Finally, in his *Polycraticus* (1159), John of Salisbury used the phrase as a way of promoting the superiority of an education that was intellectual and biblical rather than simply military. He uses it by way of a moralizing story in an imaginary letter in which a German emperor advises the king of the Franks to get his children well educated.[88]

Through John's much-read work this sapiential maxim spread throughout Europe. For John of Salisbury, as for the rest of these authors, the aphorism *rex illiteratus est quasi asinus coronatus* served, as Martin Aurell points out, 'to confirm that every king needs to acquire the experience and knowledge built up as century succeeded century, so as not to repeat the errors made in Antiquity'.[89] We find a variation of the aphorism in a letter Peter of Blois sent to the king on behalf of Rotrou of Rouen and the other bishops of his realm encouraging Henry II to give his son, the Young Henry (then aged six), an education as thorough as the one he had received. Here we find a phrase that (although less often quoted that the *crowned ass* maxim) was no less effective: 'an illiterate king is a ship without oars and a bird without feathers'.[90] Later, Peter of Blois gave examples of wise rulers of the past that included Julius Caesar, a master of literature, civil law and philosophy, and Alexander the Great, who had been educated by Aristotle, alongside the learned rulers of the Old Testament (Solomon, David, Hezekiah and Josiah) and the Christian Roman Empire (Constantine, Theodosius, Justinian and Leo). All were as good scholars as they were soldiers.[91] Here we find again the *topos* of *clergie* and *chevalerie*, *fortitude* and *sapientia* applied to rulers.

Nevertheless, it may be asked, as Philippe Buc does, if the fashion for this maxim was stimulated solely by the ambitions of the clergy to insinuate themselves into a place in the sun near the king, as payment for the learning which they had acquired in the schools.[92] Martin Aurell has answered this question negatively:

> Ambition was not the chief motive of those intellectuals who, once at court, got nostalgic for the spiritual life under the pressure of the harsh acquisitiveness of their new jobs. It would seem that the popularity of the maxim was a symptom of a rather wide double phenomenon, of the rise of the State (which led to the technical advances in the royal bureaucracy) and of the intellectual renaissance.[93]

V.H. Galbraith's words on this subject are particularly relevant:

The metaphor of an illiterate king being a crowned ass, which William of Malmesbury had attributed to young Henry, was repeated by writers of the next generation – John of Salisbury, Gerald of Wales, Breton d'Amboise – until it became a cliché and a growing embarrassment to unlettered monarchs.[94]

***

The *topos* of royal wisdom came to dominate the political theology of late Rome, Byzantium, and the early and high Middle Ages in the west. However, after the short-lived splendour of the Carolingian and Ottonian ages, the prince's wisdom was relegated to a secondary position in the royal ideology of the eleventh century. This was, to a certain extent, logical: a consequence of the Feudal Revolution and the Gregorian Reform movement was that the new discourse on kingship did not have much place for royal learning. The twelfth-century Renaissance completely changed this trend and brought the sapiential *topos* to the frontline of political thought once again. In Norman Sicily and Plantagenet England, the medieval royal court not only attracted scholars but also became a place of science, and the royal patron, when not personally implicated in scholarship, played a key role in the advancement of learning.

Twelfth-century rulers are notable for the way in which many literary and scientific works linked them to an ancient sapiential tradition, portraying them as the legitimate heirs of Roman, Carolingian and Byzantine wise rulers of the past. In this respect, these works suggest that the year 1000 did not prove to be any form of mental 'barrier': authors always found their sources in the earlier centuries. Indeed, to obtain the political legitimacy attached to the Solomonic ideal was crucial for newcomers like the Houses of Plantagenet and Hauteville. The influence of Carolingian models cannot be overestimated here. Yet, we also find new developments such as, for example, the bureaucrat-king or the literate knight *topoi*. By 1200, the ideological foundations were already in place for the thirteenth-century apogee of brilliant learned rulers such as Frederick II of Sicily and Alfonso X of Castile. By then, the Platonic philosopher-king was no longer a political myth; it had become a political reality.

Notes

1 Wilhelm Berges, *Die Fürstenspiegel des hohen und späten Mittelalters*, Schriften der Monumenta Germaniae Historica, 2 (Hannover, 1938). The same sapiential *topos* is analysed by Hans Hubert Anton in *Fürstenspiegel und Herrscherethos in der Karolingerzeit* (Bonn: Bonner Historische Forschungen, 1968).

2 Anthony Black, *Political Thought in Europe, 1250–1450* (Cambridge: Cambridge University Press, 1992), 160.

3 William of Malmesbury, "*Gesta Regum Britanniae*," in *Deeds of the English Kings of England*, eds. M. Winterbottom and R.M. Thomson (Oxford: Oxford University Press, 2002), vol. 2, 467; C. Warren Hollister, *Henry I* (New Haven: Yale University Press, 2001), 34, n. 27.

4 Sergio Bertelli, "The Courtly Universe," in *The Courts of the Italian Renaissance*, eds. S. Bertelli, F. Cardini and E. Garbero (London: Sidgwick & Jackson, 1986), 17.

5 Yitzhak Hen, *Roman Barbarians. The Royal Court and Culture in the Early Medieval West* (New York: Palgrave Macmillan, 2007); David R. Pratt, *The Political Thought of King Alfred the Great* (Cambridge: Cambridge University Press, 2007), 151–165; Rosamond McKitterick, "Royal Patronage of Culture in the Frankish Kingdoms under the Carolingians: Motives

and Consequences," in *Committenti e produzione artistico-letteraria nell'alto medioevo occidentale*, ed. E. Artifoni (Spoleto: Centro Italiano di Studi sull' Alto Medioevo, 1992), 93–129.

6 Charles F. Briggs, "Knowledge and Royal Power in the Later Middle Ages: From Philosopher-Imam, to Clerkly King, to Renaissance Prince," in *Power in the Middle Ages*, ed. S.J. Ridyard (Sewanee, TN: The University of the South, 2010), 81–97; Alexander Murray, *Reason and Society in the Middle Ages* (Oxford: Clarendon Press, 1979); Herbert Grundmann, "Litteratus-Illitteratus," *Archiv für Kulturgeschichte* 40 (1958): 1–65; idem, "*Sacerdotium-Regnum-Studium*: Zur Wertung der Wissenschaft im 13. Jahrhundert," *Archiv für Kulturgeschichte* 34 (1951): 5–21.

7 Gabor Klaniczay, "The Ambivalent Model of Solomon for Royal Sainthood and Royal Wisdom," in *The Biblical Models of Power and Law: Papers of the international conference*, ed. I. Biliarsky (Frankfurt am Main: Peter Lang, 2008), 75–92. Important studies on Christian mentalities regarding wisdom can also be found in Carlo Ginzburg, "High and Low: The Theme of Forbidden Knowledge in the Sixteenth and Seventeenth Centuries," *Past and Present* 73 (1976): 28–41; Wolfgang Edelstein, *Eruditio und Sapientia: Weltbild und Erziehung in der Karolingerzeit. Untersuchungen zu Alcuins Briefen* (Freiburg: Verlag Rombach & Co, 1965). Two outstanding studies on the symbolic implications of the iconography of Lady Wisdom are: Fairy Von Lilienfeld, "Frau Weisheit: In byzantinischen und karolingischen Quellen des 9. Jahrhunderts – allegorische Personifikation, Hypostase oder Typos?" in *Typus, Symbol, Allegorie*, ed. M. Schmidt, Eichstätter Beitrage, 4 (Ratisbon: Friedrich Pustet, 1982), 146–186; Marie Therese d'Alverny, *Études sur le symbolisme de la Sagesse et sur l'iconographie* (Aldershot: Ashgate, 1993).

8 Manuel Alejandro Rodríguez de la Peña, *Los reyes sabios. Cultura y poder en la Antigüedad Tardía y la Alta Edad Media* (Madrid: Actas, 2008); Jean-Patrice Boutet, "Le modèle du roi sage aux XIIIᵉ et XIVᵉ siècles: Solomon, Alphonse X et Charles V," *Revue Historique* 310, no. 3 (2008): 545–566; Samantha Kelly, *The New Solomon. Robert of Naples (1309–1343) and Fourteenth-Century Kingship* (Leiden: Brill, 2003); Jeannine Quillet, *Charles V: Le Roi lettré – Essai sur la pensée politique d'un règne* (Paris: Perrin, 1984).

9 Martin Aurell, *The Plantagenet Empire 1154–1224*, trans. D. Crouch (London: Pearson-Longman, 2007), 95.

10 McKitterick, "Royal Patronage of Culture," 112; Hen, *Roman Barbarians*, 22.

11 Rosamond McKitterick, "Ottonian Intellectual Culture in the Tenth Century and the Role of Theophanu," *Early Medieval Europe* 2, no. 1 (1993), 57.

12 Georges Duby, *The Three Orders. Feudal Society Imagined*, trans. A. Goldhammer (Chicago: University of Chicago Press, 1980), 17.

13 Hugo Steger, *David rex et Propheta. König David als Vorbildlicher Verkörperung des Herrschers und Dichters im Mittelalter, nach Bilddarstellungen des achten bis zwölften Jahrhunderts* (Nuremberg: Hans Karl, 1961); Adrian Mettauer, *David sanctissimus rex: Ein frühmittelalterliches Herrscher-ideal im Strittpunkt klerikaler und laikaler Interessen* (Tübingen: ICLS, 2002), 25–38.

14 Klaniczay, "The Ambivalent Model," 75–76; Ernst H. Kantorowicz, *The King's Two Bodies: A Study in Medieval Political Theology* (Princeton: Princeton University Press, 1957), 81.

15 Ernst H. Kantorowicz, *Laudes Regiae: A Study in Liturgical Acclamations and Mediaeval Ruler Worship* (Berkeley: University of California Press, 1958), 57.

16 Klaniczay, "The Ambivalent Model," 76.

17 Walter Ullmann, *The Carolingian Renaissance and the Idea of Kingship* (London: Methuen & Co, 1969), 19.

18 Alcuin of York, "*Epistolae*," in *Epistolae Karolini Aevi*, ed. E. Dümmler, MGH Epistolae 4 (Berlin: Weidmann, 1895), Epistle 170, lines 20–26, 279; Mary Alberi, "The Better Paths of Wisdom: Alcuin's True Philosophy and the Worldly Court," *Speculum* 76, no. 4 (2001): 907.

19 Alberi, "The Better Paths of Wisdom," 908–9; Claudio Leonardi, "Alcuino e la retorica," in *Dialektik und Rhetorik im früheren und hohen Mittelalter: Rezeption, Uberlieferung und gesellschaftli-che Wirkung antiker Gelehrsamkeit vornehmlich im 9. und 12. Jahrhundert*, ed. J. Fried, Schriften des Historischen Kollegs, 27 (Munich: R. Oldenbourg Verlag, 1997), 171–174.

20 Alberi, "The Better Paths of Wisdom," 909.

21 Hen, *Roman Barbarians*, 2–3.

22 Hen, *Roman Barbarians*, 2–3.

23 Ian S. Robinson, *Henry IV of Germany (1056–1106)* (Cambridge: Cambridge University Press, 1999), 13–14.

24 Hrosvitha of Gandersheim, "*Gesta Ottonis*, Prologus," in *Opera omnia*, ed. W. Berschin (Munich: Teubner, 2001), 275. Klaniczay, "The Ambivalent Model," 77.

25 Stefan Weinfurter, *The Salian Century: Main Currents in an Age of Transition*, trans. Barbara M. Bowlus (Philadelphia: University of Pennsylvania Press, 1999), 89; Paul Gerhard Schmidt, "Heinrich III: Das Bild des Herrschers in der Literatur seiner Zeit," *Deutsches Archiv* 39 (1983): 582–590.

26 Weinfurter, *The Salian Century*, 89.

27 C. Stephen Jaeger, *The Origins of Courtliness: Civilizing Trends and the Formation of Courtly Ideals (939–1210)* (Philadelphia: University of Pennsylvania Press, 1985), 8.

28 Jaeger, *The Origins of Courtliness*, 4; Josef Fleckenstein, "Königshof und Bischofschule unter Otto den Grossen," *Archiv für Kulturgeschichte* 38 (1956): 38–62.

29 McKitterick, "Ottonian Intellectual Culture," 55.

30 Munich, Bayerische Staatsbibliothek, Clm 4453 (Gospels); Bamberg Staatsbibliothek Bibl. 22 (Song of Songs, Proverbs of Solomon, glossed Book of Daniel), Bamberg Staatsbibliothek Bibl. 76 (glossed Book of Isaiah); Bamberg Staatsbibliothek Bibl. Lit. 5. McKitterick, "Ottonian Intellectual Culture," 59.

31 McKitterick, "Ottonian Intellectual Culture," 62–63.

32 Gerd Althoff, *Otto III*, trans. P.G. Jestice (University Park, PA: Pennsylvania University Press, 2003), 50, 55–56, 73–75.

33 Percy Ernst Schramm, *Kaiser, Rom und Renovatio* (Darmstadt: Wissenschaftliche Buchgesellschaft, 1957), 97–99.

34 Florentine Mütherich, "The Library of Otto III," in *The Role of the Book in Medieval Culture*, ed. P. Ganz (Turnhout: Brepols, 1986), 11–26.

35 McKitterick, "Ottonian Intellectual Culture," 61.

36 Gerbert of Aurillac, *Libellus de rationali et ratione uti*, ed. Jacques-Paul Migne. *Patrologia Latina*, vol. 139 (Paris, 1853), prologue; O.G. Darlington, "Gerbert, *obscuro loco natus*," *Speculum* 11, no. 4 (1936): 518.

37 Darlington, "Gerbert, *obscuro loco*," 517–518.

38 Eliza Garrison, "Otto III at Aachen," *Peregrinations* 3, no. 1 (2010): 114; Althoff, *Otto III*, 148–152.

39 Widukind of Korvey, *Res Gestae Saxonicae*, eds. P. Hirsch and H.E. Lohmann, MGH Scriptores 60 (Hannover, 1935), 425, I: 15.

40 David A. Warner, "Saints, Pagans, War and Rulership in Ottonian Germany," in *Plenitude of Power. The Doctrines and Exercises of Authority in the Middle Ages*, ed. R.C. Figueira (Aldershot: Ashgate, 2006), 29; Stefan Weinfurter, *Heinrich II (1002–1024)* – Herrscher am Ende der Zeiten (Regensburg: Friedrich Pustet, 1999), 25–26; Hartmut Hoffmann, *Mönchskönig und 'rex idiota': Studien zur Kirchenpolitik Heinrichs II. und Konrads II.*, MGH Studien und Texte 8 (Hannover: Hahn Verlag, 1993), 117–120.

41 Warner, "Saints, Pagans, War," 29.

42 Warner, "Saints, Pagans, War," 29; Hartmut Hoffmann, "Eigendiktat in den Urkunden Ottos III. und Heinrichs II.," *Deutsches Archiv* 44 (1988): 390–423, at 402–410.

43 Horst Fuhrmann, *Germany in the High Middle Ages (c. 1050–1250)*, trans. T. Reuter (Cambridge: Cambridge University Press, 1986), 39.

44 Manuel Alejandro Rodríguez de la Peña, "*Imago Sapientiae*: los orígenes del Ideal sapiencial medieval," *Medievalismo* 7 (1997): 11–39.

45 Kantorowicz, *The King's Two Bodies*, 113.

46 Kantorowicz, *The King's Two Bodies*, 114.

47 Kantorowicz, *The King's Two Bodies*, 114–115.

48 "Per omnia litterarum inscius atque idiota," *Chronicon Novaliciense*, ed. G.H. Pertz. In *Chronica et Gesta Aevi Salici*, MGH Scriptores 7 (Hannover, 1846), 128. James W. Thompson, *The Literacy of the Laity in the Middle Ages* (New York: Burt Franklin, 1960), 88.

49 Herwig Wolfram, *Conrad II, 990–1039: Emperor of Three Kingdoms*, trans. D.A. Kaiser (University Park, PA: Pennsylvania University Press, 2006), 150–151.

50 "Haec operam dederat, quod rex in lege studebat; / Illa sibi libros persuasserat esse legendos, / Ut varios ritus diiudicet arte peritus," Wipo, *Tetralogus, Carmen Legis*, ed. G.H. Pertz, MGH Scriptores 11 (Hannover, 1854), 250, verses 158–162. Fuhrmann, *Germany in the High Middle Ages*, 39; Thompson, *The Literacy of the Laity*, 88.

51 Weinfurter, *The Salian Century*, 97.

52 Weinfurter, *The Salian Century*, 97.

53 James H. Forse, "Bruno of Cologne and the Networking of the Episcopate in Tenth-Century Germany," *German History* 9, no. 3 (1991): 269.

54 Weinfurter, *The Salian Century*, 98.

55 Frederic S. Paxton, "*Abbas* and *Rex*: Power and Authority in the Literature of Fleury, 987–1044," in *The Experience of Power in Medieval Europe, 950–1350*, eds. R.F. Berkhofer III et al. (Aldershot: Ashgate, 2005), 198–200.

56 Paxton, "Abbas and Rex," 199–203, 211–212.

57 Joel T. Rosenthal, "Edward the Confessor and Robert the Pious: 11th Century Kingship and Biography," *Mediaeval Studies* 33 (1971): 12.

58 Jean Dunbabin, *France in the Making: 843–1180* (Oxford: Oxford University Press, 1985), 135.

59 Helgaud of Fleury, "*Epitome Vitae Regis Rotberti Pii*," in *Vie de Robert le Pieux*, eds. R.H. Bautier and G. Labory (Paris: CNRS, 1965), 60.

60 Thompson, *The Literacy of the Laity*, 127; Laurent Theis, *Robert le Pieux. Le roi de l'an mil* (Paris: Perrin, 1999), 28–29.

61 J. C. Lake, "Truth, Plausibility, and the Virtues of Narrative at the Millennium," *Journal of Medieval History* 35, no. 3 (2009), 238.

62 Raoul Glaber, *Historiarum Libri Quinque*, II, 1, in *Rodulfus Glaber Opera*, ed. J. France (Oxford: Clarendon Press, 1989); Thompson, *The Literacy of the Laity*, 127.

63 "et divinis ac canonicis institutes clarissimus haberetur; liberalibus studiis incumberet," Richer of Reims, in *Historiarum Libri Quatuor*, IV, 13, ed. G. Waitz, MGH Scriptores 51 (Hannover, 1877), 634. Thompson, *The Literacy of the Laity*, 127.

64 "ut librorum nunquam indiguerit juravi solamine," Hariulf of Saint-Riquier, *Chronicon Centulense*, IV, 2, in *Chronique de l'abbaye de Saint-Riquier*, ed. F. Lot (Paris: Picard, 1894), 181. Thompson, *The Literacy of the Laity*, 127.

65 Charles Pfister, *Études sur le règne de Robert le Pieux (996–1031)* (Paris: F. Vieweg, 1885), 16, 34 n. 3, 35–36; Thompson, *The Literacy of the Laity*, 127.

66 Thompson, *The Literacy of the Laity*, 127.

67 Adalbero of Laon, "*Carmen ad Rodbertum Regem*," in *Poème au roi Robert*, Les classiques de l'histoire de France au moyen âge 32, ed. Claude Carozzi (Paris Les Belles Lettres, 1979), 14–15, verse 366; Duby, *The Three Orders*, 17.

68 Duby, *The Three Orders*, 17.

69 Duby, *The Three Orders*, 18, 46.

70 Adalbero of Laon, *Carmen ad Rodbertum*, 14–15, verses 189–193; Duby, *The Three Orders*, 45.

71 Simon Keynes, "A Tale of Two Kings: Alfred the Great and Aethelred the Unready," *Transactions of the Royal Historical Society*, fifth Series, 36 (1986): 210. Regarding the role of wisdom in Alfred's political ideas, see Pratt, *Political Thought*, 151–165.

72 Keynes, "A Tale of Two Kings," 210. Asser makes the comparison explicit in his "*De rebus Gestis Alfredi*," in *Life of King Alfred*, ed. William H. Stevenson (Oxford: Oxford University Press, 1959), c. 76; see also c. 99.

73 Wilhelm G. Busse, "The Self-Understanding of the Reformers as Teachers in Late Tenth-Century England," in *Schriftlichkeit im fruhen Mittelalter*, ed. U. Schaefer (Tubingen: Gunther Narr Verlag, 1993), 68.

74 C. Warren Hollister and John Baldwin, "The Rise of Administrative Kingship: Henry I and Philip Augustus," *American Historical Review* 83, no. 4 (1978): 867–905.

75 William of Malmesbury, *Gesta Regum Anglorum*, v, 390; Aurell, *The Plantagenet Empire*, 94.

76 Hollister, *Henry I*, 33.

77 Aurell, *The Plantagenet Empire*, 94.

78 John of Marmoutier, "*Historia Gaufredi Ducis*," in *Chroniques des Comtes d'Anjou et des seigneurs d'Amboise*, eds. L. Halphen and R. Poupardin (Paris: Picard, 1913), 176; Jim Bradbury, "Geoffrey V of Anjou. Count and Knight," in *The Ideals and Practice of Medieval Knighthood*,

eds. C. Harper-Bill and R. Harvey (Woodbridge: Boydell Press, 1990), vol. 3, 23; Aurell, *The Plantagenet Empire*, 94.

79 "Tan armata quam togata, tam martia scilicet quam litterata," Gerald of Wales, *De principis instructione*, ed. Robert Bartlett. In *Instruction for a Ruler* (Oxford: Oxford University Press, 2018), 7. Aurell, *The Plantagenet Empire*, 94.

80 Aurell, *The Plantagenet Empire*, 94.

81 Aurell, *The Plantagenet Empire*, 94.

82 Gerald of Wales, "*Topographia Hibernica*," in *The History and Topography of Ireland*, ed. John J. O'Meara (Harmondsworth: Penguin, 1982), book 3, 48.

83 Charles H. Haskins, "Adelard of Bath and Henry Plantagenet," *English Historical Review* 111 (1913): 515–16; Aurell, *The Plantagenet Empire*, 98.

84 "rex illiteratus est quasi asinus coronatus," *Gesta Comitum Andegavorum*, eds. L. Halphen and R. Poupardin, *Chroniques des Comtes d'Anjou et des seigneurs d'Amboise* (Paris: Picard, 1913), 140. Aurell, *The Plantagenet Empire*, 94.

85 Dunbabin, *France in the Making*, 249.

86 Helinand of Froidmont, *Flores*, in PL, vol. 212, col. 736; Aurell, *The Plantagenet Empire*, 95.

87 Aurell, *The Plantagenet Empire*, 95.

88 John of Salisbury, *Policraticus*, trans. Cary Nederman (Cambridge: Cambridge University Press, 1990), book 4, 6; Aurell, *The Plantagenet Empire*, 94.

89 Aurell, *The Plantagenet Empire*, 95.

90 Peter of Blois, *Epistulae*, no. 67, in PL, vol. 207, col. 211; Reto R. Bezzola, *La cour d'Angleterre comme centre littéraire sous les rois Angevins (1154–1199)* (Paris: Honoré Champion, 1963), 45–46; Aurell, *The Plantagenet Empire*, 95.

91 Peter of Blois, *Epistulae*, no. 67, col. 211.

92 Philippe Buc, *La ambiguité du livre : Prince, pouvoir et peuple dans les commentaires de la Bible au Moyen Age* (Paris: Beauchesne, 1994), 184–185; Aurell, *The Plantagenet Empire*, 95.

93 Aurell, *The Plantagenet Empire*, 95.

94 V.H. Galbraith, "The Literacy of the Medieval English Kings," *Proceedings of the British Academy*, 21 (1935): 91.

Key works

Aurell, Martin, *The Plantagenet Empire 1154–1224* (London: Pearson-Longman, 2007).

Hen, Yitzhak, *Roman Barbarians: The Royal Court and Culture in the Early Medieval West* (New York: Publisher, 2007).

Jaeger, Stephen C., *The Origins of Courtliness: Civilizing Trends and the Formation of Courtly Ideals (939–1210)* (Philadelphia: University of Pennsylvania Press, 1985).

Kantorowicz, Ernst H., *The King's Two Bodies: A Study in Medieval Political Theology* (Princeton: Princeton University Press, 1957).

Klaniczay, Gabor, "The Ambivalent Model of Solomon for royal sainthood and royal wisdom," in *The Biblical Models of Power and Law: Papers of the International Conference*, ed. I. Biliarsky (Frankfurt am Main: Peter Lang, 2008), 75–92.

Murray, Alexander, *Reason and Society in the Middle Ages* (Oxford: Clarendon Press, 1979).

2

THE BIBLICAL KING SOLOMON IN REPRESENTATIONS OF WESTERN EUROPEAN MEDIEVAL ROYALTY*

Laura Fábián

King Solomon, the famously wise ruler of the Old Testament and successor to King David, was a popular model for kings from the early centuries of Europe's Middle Ages. He was the presumed author of four biblical books, the *Book of Proverbs*, *Ecclesiastes*, the *Song of Songs* and the *Book of Wisdom*, which served as ethical and political guides for kings as well as lay people. An ambivalence surrounded his character that derived partly from the fact that he was influenced by his wives and lovers, and became idolatrous and turned away from God at the end of his life. Moreover, an ancient tradition held that Solomon acquired his knowledge thanks to magical practices.[1] David, alongside Solomon, was one of the most favoured biblical exemplars for rulers, especially in the early Middle Ages.[2] Yet, Solomon became increasingly viewed in the thirteenth and fourteenth centuries as the example to emulate. Varied associations, some negative, meant it was impossible, however, for medieval authors to create a fixed image of him.

The highlighted aspects of the Solomonic ideal varied through the ages as Solomon was intermittently associated with peace,[3] justice (1 Kings 3:16–28), wealth (1 Kings 10:14, 23), wisdom[4] and, not without potentially negative connotations, involvement in magical practices.[5] From the Bible, we know of several famous episodes concerning the king, such as 'Solomon's Judgement', an incident in which he resolved a dispute between two women who both claimed to be the mother of the same child. Moreover, his rich kingdom and his famed knowledge were said to have drawn the attention of the Queen of Sheba, who travelled to meet with the king. Legendary objects as well as virtues were connected with him, ranging from the temple he built (1 Kings 6) and his palace (1 Kings 7), to his throne (1 Kings 10:18–20), key[6] and ring.[7] Solomon's Temple in Jerusalem became an archetype, one which many medieval rulers sought to imitate.

This chapter will examine the way in which King Solomon was employed as a royal *exempla* in the medieval west between the ninth and fourteenth centuries. A Solomonic typology was certainly not attached to every medieval ruler's image. The instances selected in this study are, however, particularly notable examples. First, the chapter will touch on the early instances of so-called 'new Solomons', particularly among Carolingian and Byzantine rulers. The analysis will then focus on a thirteenth-century group of kings: Saint Louis IX of France, Henry III of England and Alfonso X the Wise of Castile. Finally, it will consider a quintessentially Solomonic king, the fourteenth-century French ruler Charles V the Wise in contrast with one of his near contemporaries, the English king, Richard II. The following questions will be discussed: Which aspects of Solomon were selected and promoted for emulation? When and how did a monarch engage consciously in imitating Solomon as a strategy to increase his reputation through the use of biblical typology?

The tradition of Solomon incorporates scriptural and theological sources, vernacular literature, folklore, Islamic culture, magical treatises, the visual arts and political writings. Besides clerical writings, vernacular literature sought to fill the gap and interpret the mystery around the way in which the figure of Solomon develops in the Bible. In this respect, good examples of vernacular texts include the entertaining dialogue *Solomon and Marcolf*, which appeared in various languages, the closely related English text *Solomon and Saturn II*, or popular legends like that of King Solomon and Alexander the Great, and an episode in the legend of Edward the Confessor in which two pilgrims met with Solomon during their travels.[8] This chapter will, however, restrict itself to exploring political, liturgical, poetical and iconographical sources connected with royalty.

In most cases, citations of the Solomonic books in the sources have no intended message about kingship and political thought. It was, of course, common for medieval authors to quote the Bible in support of their arguments,[9] the words of Solomon from Proverbs being only one example. Methodologically, it is important, therefore, to separate specific allusions to the ruler as a new Solomon – which always depend on the historical context and the genre of the source – from the general citations. Those examples that feature Solomon as a supporting actor, that is, for example, as son of David or father of Rehoboam, can be discounted. Similarly, many cases in which citations associated with Solomon appear to have no particular significance need not be considered. However, caution is required: in some cases – for example in a mirror for princes that contains indirect references to biblical figures[10] – such citations might help to convey the author's general opinion about Solomon if the king was referred to on multiple occasions or other Old Testament kings were conspicuous by their absence. This study focuses primarily on those instances when a direct comparison can be drawn between Solomon and a specific ruler with the exception of instances in which an author placed particular emphasis on Solomon. This comparison is not evident in every example, but as Elka Bakalova put it: 'It is much more common to find a complex system of implicit guidelines which aims at activating certain associations.'[11] We need to keep in mind that the use of the biblical typology could be mixed, and the rulers' contemporaries sometimes applied numerous models at the same time, including David, Joshua,[12] Melchizedek, the Magi[13] or the negative example of a king like Saul.[14]

Early medieval kingship: the example of the Carolingian rulers and the Byzantine tradition

The use of the Bible for political purposes was already current in the Merovingian period and is evident in the works of Gregory of Tours and Sulpicius Severus. The Carolingian rulers together with their advisors followed this earlier practice.[15]

Not only did the leading clerics of the Carolingian court compare their kings to Old Testament figures, but popes also relied on this method of parallelism.[16]

By way of a brief illustration, we can refer to some examples from Carolingian circles. First, it is worth mentioning Charlemagne because it was commonplace that in his court he was called – among other things – 'David'. This demonstrates the tendency to use biblical figures in courtly rhetoric.[17] Charlemagne, as a conqueror, was definitely not a peaceful Solomon-like king, but the Solomon analogy emerged in a letter. Alcuin wrote to Charlemagne that the chapel in Aachen 'is being constructed by the art of the most wise Solomon',[18] invoking the builder-aspect of Solomon and drawing a clear parallel between them. According to this interpretation, Charlemagne's building in Aachen was created as a second Jerusalem.[19] On the other hand, Einhard, writing in his *Vita Caroli Magni*, did not refer to Solomon as a named biblical personage at all. This was the result of his general preference for the classical antique tradition over the biblical quotations relied on by other medieval authors. In the Bible, when the Temple was finished but prior to its consecration, God promised that if Solomon kept God's commandments and the faith, his heir would rule. However, if Solomon was idolatrous, his heirs would be wiped from the Earth (1 Kings 9:6). As Mary Garrison noted, Einhard mentioned that Charlemagne took care of his church and the correct observance of the rites at Aachen.[20] While not a concrete comparison between the two rulers, this could be taken as a subtle analogy between the temple building of Solomon and Charlemagne's similar activity.[21] Despite the letter of Alcuin and Einhard's possible allusion, Charlemagne, however, was mostly a Davidic ruler in the eyes of his contemporaries.[22]

Charlemagne, as David, embodied another typology: his son, Louis the Pious, was openly praised as a new Solomon, drawing on the biblical 'father-son' identification. Following his conquering father, Louis was proclaimed a pious king, and his kingship was characterized as a more irenic period in which the Solomonic model played a heightened role in court circles.[23] The poet Ermoldus Nigellus's *In honorem Hludowici* (*c*.826–9) described Louis as a fine example to his son, Pipin II of Aquitaine. Ermoldus's biography and the reason for his exile by Louis are unclear; certainly he created his poem during his banishment in the hope of rehabilitation.[24] The poem was an imaginary dialogue between Louis and Pope Stephen IV during their meeting in 816. Despite the fact that Ermoldus's biblical language was not prominent in this work, the Solomonic comparison is important. In the conversation, the Pope not only compared Louis to Solomon, but he also stressed that the Frankish king was more powerful in his heart; he lived more chastely and while Solomon ruled only Israel, Louis was able to rule all the kingdoms in Europe.[25] In two other examples, the authors draw an analogy between Solomon and Louis's peaceful reigns. After Louis's death, the monk Notker the Stammerer in his work about Charlemagne (*Gesta Karoli Magni*) stated that Louis was as peaceful as Solomon while Charlemagne was as warlike as King David.[26] Amalarius of Metz (*c*.820), in the preface to his *Liber officialis*, emphasized the peaceful aspect of Solomon's character and evidently connected it to Louis.[27]

The parallel between a Carolingian ruler and Solomon was employed in the case of Louis's successor, Charles the Bald, as well. The cultural milieu of his court – including the activity of Hincmar of Reims and Sedulius Scottus – was susceptible to the rhetoric of peace, and Charles was a particularly well-educated king among the Carolingian rulers.[28] Sedulius composed an *adventus* verse in 869, dedicated to Charles, and formulated an illustrious parallel for his arrival at Metz: 'Holding the paternal sceptre, a peacemaker, like Solomon'. In the historical context, Charles the Bald, after expanding his power to Lorraine in 869, was able to reunite two of the three kingdoms.[29] In the eyes of Sedulius, Charles – in this typology – became the Solomon who ruled over Israel and Juda; only such a peaceful monarch could prevail in two Carolingian kingdoms.[30] In addition, the sumptuous *S. Paolo Bible* was produced under the patronage of Charles the Bald and contains a portrait of both the king and Solomon. William Diebold pointed out that a parallel could be drawn between the two compositions because the two rulers' appearances are similar. However, Charles's depiction might also be likened to that of other royal figures in the Bible, such as Pharaoh or Saul.[31]

Naturally, this idealized image of kingship was familiar in the Byzantine court. The Greek antecedents go back to Eusebius who invoked several Old Testament models. For example, he pictured Constantine as a new Moses in the fourth century. In the Byzantine tradition, Solomon appeared mostly as an example of a royal builder. In Constantinople the Throne of Solomon[32] and the *templum Salomonis*[33] were also a celebrated aspect of the biblical king. This tendency was exemplified by the sixth-century emperor Justinian's famous exclamation – uttered in relation to Hagia Sophia – 'Solomon, I have outdone thee.'[34] Beyond the symbolic significance of Hagia Sophia, the church was also a location for Solomonic relics. According to ninth- and tenth-century sources, these included the chalice and golden table from the Temple of Jerusalem.[35] The most famous object, however, was Solomon's legendary throne. The *Book of Ceremonies* alludes to a mechanical throne (*automata*) in the hall of the Magnaura in Constantinople, but it is unclear whether the Byzantines considered it Solomon's original throne or just a reproduction.[36] While, as Shaun Tougher observes, competition between the Byzantine and Carolingian courts was certainly real, in the specific case of Old Testament models the origins and direction in which influence flowed cannot be determined with certainty.[37]

As with the Frankish royal family, the Byzantines adopted the tradition in the ninth and tenth centuries that while the father was a new David, his son was known as a new Solomon. The most prominent example of this custom was Basil I and his son Leo VI the Wise. Basil, the founder of the Macedonian dynasty, was referred to as David, and this fact could also have influenced his son's link to Solomon. It was well known that Basil I was descended from the lower ranks of society, and he was attentive to the education of his son. Emperor Leo VI was unusual among Byzantine rulers to the extent he built an ideology focused on the virtue of wisdom.[38] Several writers connected Leo's reign to Solomon in that he was concerned for the law, interested in church building and possessed great knowledge. He was a classic example of an early new Solomon, both during his lifetime and after his death, when his reign came to be remembered as a 'golden age'.[39] In 907, the diplomat Leo Choirosphaktes wrote that Leo could be counted in the company of Solomon and other wise men. A few years later, in 912, the patriarch Nicholas wrote to the pope to say that Leo had received his wisdom as a gift from God, like Solomon.[40]

The Franks and the Byzantine emperors were not the only ones to use this typological pairing. The Holy Roman Emperor Otto I was called a new David and his son was viewed as another Solomon. This conception of the Saxon dynasty was reflected in the works of Hrotsvitha von Gandersheim, a secular canoness who used the Old Testament typology for political purposes.[41] As Manuel Alejandro Rodríguez de la Peña discusses in his chapter in this volume, the crown of the Holy Roman emperors was made in the tenth century and includes four plates decorated with biblical figures. Between Christ, King David, King Hezekiah and the prophet Isaiah, Solomon appears as part of the composition. This image functioned as an important model for the emperors, both at their coronation and during their rule.[42]

Saint Louis, Henry III of England and Alfonso X

From the twelfth – but especially from the thirteenth – century, the use of Old Testament figures and stories as models for kings began to flourish. Emphasis shifted away from popular ancient historical characters, such as legendary Greek heroes,[43] to Old Testament figures, particularly kings.[44] Three thirteenth-century kings offer particularly good examples of the different ways in which Solomon came to be used to strengthen royal authority in court circles.

The piety of the French king – and later saint – Louis IX informed the way in which the Capetian ruler was presented as one particular type of Solomonic model. As Jacques Le Goff noted, the Old Testament models employed in creating an image of Louis's rulership are complex, especially in regard to the king's holiness.[45] Louis was like King David and Solomon or Josiah, but was also sometimes presented as a new Abraham, Moses or Joshua.[46] Old Testament language was a common instrument employed by authors of mirrors of princes at Louis's court. Vincent of Beauvais and Guibert of Tournai frequently used biblical characters to express their viewpoint about good or bad kings. Vincent cited Solomon thirteen times, mostly in the *De morali principis institutione* because of his wisdom.[47] Guibert of Tournai highlighted Solomon's justice mainly in *Eruditio regum et principum*, but Solomon's wives and lovers were also mentioned as deterrent examples.[48]

One way to understand the role of the biblical stories for the Capetians, particularly for Louis and his mother Blanche of Castile, is to single out a few examples from the visual arts. Meredith Cohen analysed the windows of the cathedral of Reims, where, with the exception of Adam, Solomon was the only Old Testament figure to appear in the medieval windows (*c.*1245–55). Meredith Parsons concluded that the 'Solomon in Bed' window referred to Louis IX.[49] The iconography of the stained-glass windows of the Sainte-Chapelle, completed in 1248, summarized the political and cultural aspirations of Louis. It was a royal programme with an emphasis on the Old Testament.[50] The chapel is a pictorial composition of biblical books from Genesis to the Book of Kings presented in a narrative form. In the mid-nineteenth century, the panels were restored and a number replaced. Alyce A. Jordan has reconstructed their hypothetical arrangement while following, principally, Louis Grodecki's older numbering system.[51] The last window departs from the biblical cycle and is generally considered to depict the story of Louis himself, who carried the relics of the Passion to Paris.[52] Solomon appears at the top of the Book of Kings lancet as an idolatrous king, praying to an idol. This lancet is placed, as Jordan has noted, in *oppositio* to the lancet featuring Louis: Solomon's failure and the subsequent collapse of his dynasty (God's punishment for his sin) is contrasted with Louis's dynastic continuity. This arrangement suggests that the deliberate intention was to draw a comparison that implied that Louis was a better king than Solomon. Louis in this context carried the relics of the True Cross, while, in contrast, Solomon was shown adoring an idol.[53] This schema was echoed in the earlier example from Ermoldus, who wrote that Louis the Pious had surpassed Solomon.

About twenty-seven years after the death of Louis, Old Testament typology came to feature prominently in commemorative sermons relating to the king's canonization process. The Dominican preacher Jacob of Lausanne created five sermons for the canonization feast of Louis, of which two are significant, the *Videte regem Salomonem* and the *Rex sapiens*.[54] The *Videte regem* begins by drawing a clear parallel between Solomon and St Louis. Following the form of a scholastic sermon, the point of departure is a biblical verse, in this case the Song of Songs 3:11, which notes the richness and wisdom of Solomon who surpassed all kings. According to the two extant versions of the sermon, God gave wisdom to Solomon for secular government and did the same for Louis IX. The conception of wisdom as a holy gift appeared in the B version where Jacob emphasized that Louis bore two types of wisdom, *sapientia* and *prudentia*. This version established that for the 'divine things' (*divinorum*) wisdom was necessary while the secular offices required prudence.[55] The *Rex sapiens* (Wisdom 6:23) also referred to the wisdom of Solomon,[56] but here Solomon appears as a guilty figure who abandoned the true faith unlike Louis who always ruled with justice and divine wisdom, the same connotation implied in the stained glass of the Sainte-Chapelle.

Throughout the Middle Ages it was a conventional expectation that rulers follow the tenets of Christianity, particularly those relating to ruling in peace and showing mercy. Following John of Salisbury's influential *Policraticus*, authors of mirrors of princes started, from the mid-thirteenth century, to prioritize the virtue of *sapientia*. This virtue was described as a gift from God, as in the sermon of Jacob of Lausanne. While *sapientia* was mostly a theoretical and contemplative virtue, to be prudent was a practical skill of increasing political importance.[57] Aristotelian language influenced conceptions about royal knowledge: besides theology, rulers had to complete their learning with other scientific disciplines and acquire scholarly learning (*prudentia*). This virtue's importance increased and the emphasis shifted to *prudentia*: it was not only the product of divine knowledge but also an obtainable skill, and for fourteenth-century rulers it became a crucial aspect to be better educated.[58] Louis IX and his period marked the transition towards this outlook.

King Solomon could also be used in concrete political situations, as was the case in the sermon Pope Boniface VIII delivered as part of Louis's canonization process on 11 August 1297 in Orvieto. He began the sermon with an Old Testament reference: 'And King Solomon exceeded all the kings of the earth in riches and wisdom' (1 Kings 10:23) (*Magnificatus est ergo rex Salomon, super omnes reges terrae, divitiis et sapiential*). The pope transformed the citation so that St Louis surpassed the greatness of Solomon. Both of them were called *rex pacificus*. The political reason for this allusion was the earlier conflict between the French king, Philip IV the Fair, and Boniface. It is clear that the pope was using this analogy as a condemnation of Philip who lacked those virtues in contrast to his grandfather. Although the canonization itself was a sign of the rapprochement between the pope and the French king, as M. Cecilia Gaposchkin has pointed out, Boniface's criticism was observable in this process.[59]

Louis's contemporary, Henry III of England, showed a greater personal predilection for the figure of Solomon. Henry was not only drawn towards the biblical king, but he supported the cult of an earlier 'new Solomon': the saintly king Edward the Confessor who was a crucial model of the wise ruler available to Henry.[60] The ideological and dynastic rivalry between France and England continued for centuries, and until the canonization of St Louis, the Capetian dynasty lacked any saint-king. Nonetheless, the English royal house had a national saint from the twelfth century, Edward, who was compared to Solomon in hagiographical literature. Henry was one of the most generous English royal patrons, a tendency which is reflected in the lost images of Winchester and in the Painted Chamber of Westminster. The Painted Chamber's structure and the arrangement of frescoes was established by Paul Binski.[61] Henry's interest in biblical kingship appeared in the Old Testament stories and the painting of the two militant guardians of Solomon in Bed (Song of Songs 3:7–8) in a complex composition (c.1263–72).[62] The most striking feature in the Westminster and Winchester paintings is that King Solomon does not appear, yet the composition alludes to him. Behind Henry's bed was depicted the coronation of Edward the Confessor surrounded by the guardians. Henry himself completed the depicted scene and was shown to be the next new Solomon. The king also ordered a new throne, the iconography of which invoked the Throne of Solomon: the leopards of Henry's throne invoking the lions of Solomon.[63]

The magical part of the Solomonic image also came to the fore in royal image-making in the thirteenth and fourteenth centuries, and appeared spectacularly in the reign of the Castilian king Alfonso X the Wise. Alfonso strongly emphasized his cultural patronage via commissions of magical treatises and translations such as the *Picatrix* (1256–8) and the *Liber Raziel* (c.1259). The pseudo-Solomonic books – like the *Liber Raziel* – contain allusions to Solomon, and legends attributed their authorship to him.[64] However, the *Cantigas de Santa Maria* collection of poems, traditionally attributed to Alfonso himself, implied that it contained several citations of Solomon. The king's iconographical programme referred to Solomon as well.[65] The *Siete Partidas* statutory code cites Solomon several times.[66] In one sense this is not surprising because Solomon was a general symbol of justice and law, yet allusions to Solomon in law books were certainly not universal, which makes this case notable. Alfonso X ordered the translation of nineteen magical books, and in the *Liber Raziel*'s prologue Solomon is portrayed as an expert in science and nature. This was an evident allusion to Alfonso as the wise, Solomonic king.[67] However, the increasing role of Solomonic wisdom can be found especially among 'wise kings' of the fourteenth century.

The widespread image of learned kings: the wise kings of the fourteenth century

It is essential to mention the most Solomonic ruler of the fourteenth century, Robert the Wise of Naples. Samantha Kelly's detailed analysis proves how important Solomon was to Robert: the Angevin ruler deliberately used this model in speech and referred to himself as Solomon's successor.[68] This self-conscious and extensive use of King Solomon in Robert's self-representation is a distinctive case. It is not necessary to go very far, however, to find other rulers from this period who compared themselves – or were compared – to Solomon. Among them was the Emperor Charles IV of Luxemburg. Pope Clement VI and in 1378 the archbishop of Prague in the funeral of the emperor drew the comparison with the latter in his sermons.[69]

To show how the Solomonic ideal crystallized, we will examine the third ruler of the Valois dynasty, Charles V the Wise. Jean-Patrice Boudet drew a parallel between Alfonso X and Charles V on the basis of the translation of astrological treatises at court, something which characterized the rule of both kings.[70] Many of the astrological works translated at Charles's court, were attributed to Solomon.[71] Other manuscripts where Solomon was an active figure were also commissioned. Charles inherited political conflicts at the beginning of his rule that included the revolt of Étienne Marcel and the Jacquerie, in addition to the Hundred Years War. In dealing successfully with this difficult situation, Charles increased his reputation.[72] He made an effort to increase Valois' prestige with his royal library and via the activity of the scholars, philosophers, translators and artists at his court. After his death, his reign came to be regarded as a 'golden age'.

Solomon appears in the prologues dedicated to the French king or in connection with his portrait in manuscripts. Hence, the Solomonic image was presented to Charles's inner circle and of course directly to the king himself. Charles ordered a translation of the work *De proprietatibus rerum* by Bartholomaeus Anglicus from Jean Corbechon in 1372. In his preface – which preceded the text of Bartholomeus – Corbechon cited the words of Solomon,[73] and, after enumerating other ancient sages (Aristotle, Charlemagne, Alexander the Great, etc.), he returned to a particular emphasis on Solomon and wisdom, and highlighted that Charles V was a well-educated king. On this basis he labelled him a new Solomon.[74] In another work commissioned by Charles, a translation of Guillaume Durand's *Rationale divinorum officiorum*, the translator who was the Carmelite theologian Jean Golein, wrote a prologue about the ideal of the *rex sapiens* where his central figure was Solomon.[75] Mentions of Solomon by name in this latter exceeded any other paragon of intelligence seven fold.[76] Citing Solomon could be meaningful, especially if the author neglected other model figures: Charlemagne appears in only one paragraph and Alexander the Great only three times. The only biblical figure cited in addition to Solomon is Josephus. Thus, the central wise king in this introduction is evidently Solomon. In justifying his work, Jean drew a direct comparison between Charles V and Solomon.[77] At the end of the translation he added his own tract (*Traité du sacre*), which was a commentary on the coronation rite and an explanation of French ideology. Here Jean drew further attention to Solomon, the latter appearing as a model, again, seven times more than other figures.[78]

Charles V is also notable for the portrait images that appear in the codices he commissioned. The king was depicted several times in dedication portraits as a learned ruler debating with scholars or reading a book.[79] In the example in Figure 2.1, taken from a translation of the *Policraticus*,[80] King Solomon appears in the miniatures alongside Charles himself.[81]

In the *Policraticus*'s (1372) dedication portrait Charles is reading a book, a reference to the message of the manuscript: a king had to be literate. In folio 12r, Charles is depicted sitting in front of the Latin Church fathers and philosophers, a group of wise men among whom is to be found Solomon. Charles is sitting on his throne; he is crowned and wears distinctive blue clothing to indicate he is a king. Solomon is also depicted wearing a crown and similar blue clothing, while the other figures do not wear crowns or distinctive blue garments. Below, a crowd of people stare upward at the two rulers and at Christ at the top of the image. The miniature is accompanied by the inscription: 'Blessed is the land whose king is a wise man.'[82] Both Charles and

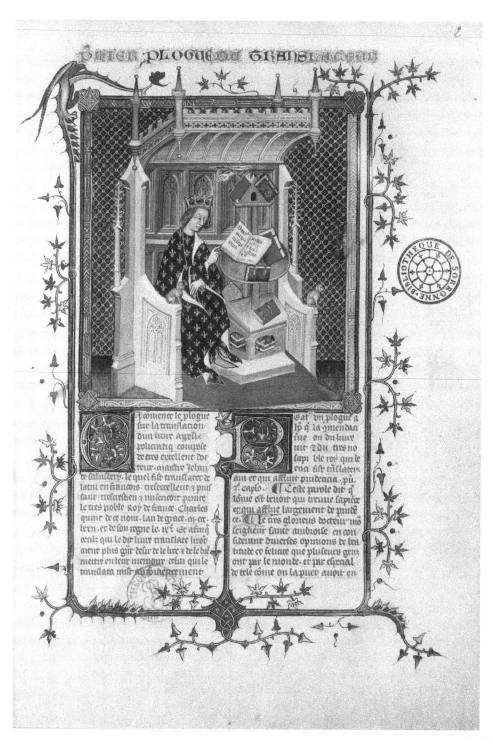

Figure 2.1 Charles V of France, called the Wise. King of France (r. 1364–80), member of the Valois dynasty. Representation of Charles V in his library. Mary Evans/Iberfoto

Solomon appear as wise rulers and as the only kings. They are positioned on the same level, and Charles, sitting on his throne with lions (the throne of Dagobert), gazes at the masters collecting their knowledge (symbolized by books) in a basket. He appears an educated king and a successor to the learned Solomon.[83] If we compare this miniature with the preface, written by the translator, Denis Foulechat, it is apparent that Solomon is the central figure.[84] Here Foulechat highlighted the importance of a king's knowledge, which show the ideological background of the royal court. He enumerates several wise models (such as Plato and Saint Ambrose), but Solomon and his words are cited six times, more than any other exemplars. As Iva Rosario has pointed out, Emperor Charles IV, Charles V's uncle, is depicted resembling the priest-king Melchizedek in two manuscripts, the Vyšehrad Antiphonal and the Missal of John of Středa.[85] The miniature of Solomon and Charles V suggests, by contrast, that the French king did not aspire to create a similar 'crypto-portrait' of himself *as* Solomon; he was content to draw a clear comparison.

The development of Charles V's image as a 'new Solomon' after his death is similar to the growth of St Louis's post-mortem reputation: both rulers became the subject of explicit comparisons with the biblical ruler. The memory of Charles was tinged by a certain nostalgia, which transformed his reputation at the court a few decades after his death. This reassessment was owed in part to the madness of his successor, Charles VI, and, in particular, to what was, from a French perspective, a disastrous phase in the Hundred Years War. Philippe de Mézières, one of Charles' most important former advisers, praised his wisdom and labelled the king 'the wise Solomon' (*le saige Salomon*) in his *Songe du vieil pèlerin* in 1389.[86] Around 1380, the court poet Eustache Deschamps also mentioned this idea, citing Charles alongside the illustrious exemplars of the past. Charles could be compared to Solomon with regard to his learning. The idea also appeared in another ballade, written for Charles's funeral.[87] In this nostalgic era, contemporaries started to draw explicit comparisons between Charles and the wise Solomon; Charles thus became similar to the Old Testament king in his talents and activities.

The long-term impact of Charles V's Solomonic legacy can, as Nigel Saul highlighted, be seen at the court of Richard II of England. Saul noted that Richard was familiar with the wisdom-related image making of Charles. Richard's epitaph, with the inscription 'prudence', and the *De quadripartita regis specie* (Oxford, Bodley MS 581) manuscript both demonstrate an awareness of the importance of Solomonic image making in the king's self-representation.[88] The family connections are also significant: Richard's second wife was Isabelle of Valois, grandchild of Charles V. Despite the ambivalent character of Richard's rule, contemporaries used biblical typology to refer to the king. Evidently, Richard was not a typically wise Solomonic-king like Charles V. He was certainly not as interested in the patronage of books and education. However, in some cases we can find Richard as Solomon in contemporary writings.

It is important to recognize that in Richard's case, the magi typology was more common, a famous example being the Wilton diptych's iconography.[89] Only his commission of the *De quadripartita regis specie* represents Richard as possessing Solomonic wisdom;[90] other sources tended to exclude any mention of wisdom on Richard's part. We can however note a specific and repeated use of the Solomon-image. This was applied to Richard's sumptuous court, which led to a comparison with the wealth of Solomon. For instance, Roger Dymmok, a Dominican friar, writing in his *De duodecim errores et hereses Lollardum* (1395), a work dedicated to Richard, referred to him as a *rex sapiens.*[91] He told the story of Solomon and the Queen of Sheba (1 Kings 10:4–7). In terms of the political usage of the Old Testament, this was not a conventional story to employ, especially in this period.[92] The Queen of Sheba travelled to Jerusalem to meet Solomon and ascertain the truth regarding rumours of his knowledge. She brought numerous presents to fascinate Solomon. When the Queen saw the luxury of Solomon, she was convinced. Surprisingly, the final part of Dymmok's description highlighted Solomonic wealth in the context of courtly art, food and clothes.[93] Thus Dymmok, by comparing the wealth of Richard to that of Solomon, 'protected' his king by drawing a positive biblical parallel. Here, we see the curious use of a biblical citation to interpret and defend a contemporary political situation, even though the reality of Richard's extravagance was distasteful in the eyes of many contemporaries.[94] Richard's immense household was famous for its luxury – one example being its extravagant clothing, something that was regarded as wasting the kingdom's money.[95] On other occasions biblical comparisons focusing on Richard II seem more ambivalent. The chronicler Adam of Usk called Richard 'Rehoboam', Solomon's son, who lost his kingdom after the death of his father.[96] Rehoboam (1 Kings 12) was a symbol of a king who did not want to follow good counsel and was the archetype of the child-king.[97] This comparison is all the more significant if we remember the fact that Richard was deposed in 1399. The parallel between Solomon and Richard could be described as inconsistent: lacking Solomon's wisdom, Richard at least matched his luxury.

***

The role of King Solomon as a royal exemplar changed through the centuries. Nevertheless, he remained, among other things, the quintessence of the wise king archetype. This chapter has aimed to present the diverse and analogic features of this model. Solomon appeared in several aspects of royal representation: in connection with coronations, courtly art and literature, political writings and canonization.

Why did Solomon become such a popular model in the thirteenth and fourteenth centuries? It is quite impossible to determine the origins, but the increasing role was connected with the recovery of Old Testament imagery that took place from the twelfth century and the increasing importance of the *rex sapiens* ideal, specifically, which took place from the thirteenth century. Medieval rulers started to imitate Solomon – alongside King David especially in the early period – when they found that, with the help of their courtiers, his figure could increase their prestige. Which aspect of Solomon was accentuated depended on the personal characteristics of the king and the current political situation. Sometimes the ruler's desire to come across as a wise and Solomonic king was only achieved posthumously: knowledge, status as a sacral king and wise decisions became more important than any failure in the king's lifetime.

The Solomonic ideal for rulers did not disappear after 1400. For example, in the early modern period Solomon appeared in the east in Suleiman the Magnificent's rule in the sixteenth century. Suleiman was associated with Solomon by many Islamic scholars, both because he was named after him – first among the Ottomans to be so – and because of his wisdom.[98] The Tudors and the Stuarts also knew of the use of Solomon to increase their power in a symbolic way. Henry VIII employed references to him as did James VI & I.[99] Solomon was a popular model for rulers for centuries. It is not as easy to determine the end of his symbolic role as it is in a case such as the magi typology.[100]

Notes

* The author is preparing a study of King Solomon as a royal model in the late Middle Ages for her PhD dissertation project.

1 Concerning the ambivalent character of King Solomon in medieval culture: Gábor Klaniczay, "The Ambivalent Model of Solomon for Royal Sainthood and Royal Wisdom," in *The Biblical Models of Power and Law. Les modèles bibliques du pouvoir et du droit*, eds. Ivan Biliarsky and G. Radu Păun (Frankfurt am Main: Peter Lang Verlag, 2008), 75–92; Mishtooni Bose, "From Exegesis to Appropriation: The Medieval Solomon," *Medium Aevum* 65 (1996): 187–210.

2 Hugo Steger, *David rex et Propheta. König David als vorbildliche Verkörperung des Herrschers und Dichters im Mittelalter, nach Bilddarstellungen des achten bis zwölften Jahrhunderts* (Nuremberg: Hans Karl, 1961); Colum Hourihane, *King David in the Index of Christian Art* (Princeton: Princeton University, 2002).

3 Paul J.E. Kershaw, *Peaceful Kings. Peace, Power, and the Early Medieval Political Imagination* (Oxford: Oxford University Press, 2011), 56.

4 In addition to the four biblical books already mentioned see, for example: 1 Kings 4:29–34; 1 Kings 10:1–13.

5 Pablo A. Torijano, *Solomon the Esoteric King. From King to Magus, Development of a Tradition* (Leiden: Brill, 2002).

6 Julien Véronèse and Jean-Patrice Boudet, "Le secret dans la magie rituelle médiévale," *Micrologus, Natura, Scienze e Società Medievali*, 14 (2006): 101–150.

7 Allegra Iafrate, "Opus Salomonis: Sorting Out Solomon's Scattered Treasure," *Medieval Encounters* 22 (2016): 328 n. 3.

8 Jean-Patrice Boudet, "La chronique attribuée à Jean Juvénal des Ursins, la folie de Charles VI et la légende noire du roi Salomon," in *Une histoire pour un royaume, XIIe–XVe siècle*, eds. Anne-Hélène Allirot et al. (Paris: Perrin, 2010), 299–309.

9 Pierre Riché, "La Bible et la vie politique dans le haut Moyen Age," in *Le Moyen Age et la Bible*, eds. Pierre Riché and Guy Lobrichon (Paris: Beauchesnes, 1984), 385–400.

10 Wilhelm Berges, *Die Fürstenspiegel des hohen und späten Mittelalters*. Schriften des Reichsinstituts für ältere deutsche Geschichtskunde (Leipzig: Monumenta Germaniae Historica,1938).

11 Elka Bakalova, "King David as a Model for the Christian Ruler: Some Visual Sources," in *The Biblical Models of Power and Law. Les modèles bibliques du pouvoir et du droit*, eds. Ivan Biliarsky and G. Radu Păun (Frankfurt am Main: Peter Lang Verlag, 2008), 96.

12 M. Cecilia Gaposchkin, "Louis IX, Crusade and the Promise of Joshua in the Holy Land," *Journal of Medieval History* 34 (2008): 245–274.

13 Doina-Elena Craciun, *Les Rois mages, images du pouvoir des rois en Occident (XIIe–XVIe siècles)* (unpublished PhD dissertation, EHESS: Paris, 2016).

14 Benjamin Zweig, "Picturing the Fallen King: Royal Patronage and the Image of Saul's Suicide," in *Patronage. Power and Agency in Medieval Art*, ed. Colum Hourihane (Princeton: The Index of Christian Art, Department of Art and Archeology, Princeton University, in association with Penn State University Press, 2013), 151–174.

15 Riché, "La Bible et la vie politique," 385–388.

16 Mary Garrison, "The Franks as the New Israel? Education for an identity from Pippin to Charlemagne," in *The Uses of the Past in the Early Middle Ages*, eds. Yitzhak Hen and Innes Matthew (Cambridge: Cambridge University Press, 2000), 123–124.

17 Garrison, "The Franks as the New Israel?" 153.

18 Alcuin, Ep. 145, *Monumenta Germaniae Historica Epistolae*, IV, ed. Ernst Dümmler (Berlin: Weidmann, 1895), 231–35 at 235.

19 Garrison, "The Franks as the New Israel?" 154–156. Allegra Iafrate subscribes to an earlier interpretation of the throne of Charlemagne, suggesting that the six steps alluded to the biblical Throne of Solomon: Allegra Iafrate, *The Wandering Throne of Solomon: Objects and Tales of Kingship in the Medieval Mediterranean* (Leiden: Brill, 2016), 225.

20 Einhard, *Vita Karoli Magni*, eds. O. Holder-Egger, G.H. Pertz and G. Waitz, MGH SRG 25 (Hannover, 1911), 30–31.

21 Garrison, "The Franks as the New Israel?" 156.
22 For a summary of Charlemagne as a new David see, Thomas F.X. Noble, *Images, iconoclasm, and the Carolingians* (Philadelphia: University of Pennsylvania Press, 2009), 234–35; Steger, *David rex*, 126–127.
23 Kershaw, *Peaceful Kings*, 174–189.
24 Peter Godman, *Poets and Emperors: Frankish Politics and Carolingian Poetry* (Oxford: Clarendon Press, 1987), 111.
25 This is an allusion to 1 Kings 10:1–13, the meeting of the Queen of Sheba and Solomon. The pope was recalling the words of the queen: *Charlemagne and Louis the Pious: The Lives by Einhard, Notker, Ermoldus, Thegan, and the Astronomer*, trans. Thomas F.X. Noble (University Park, PA: Pennsylvania State University Press, 2009), 148–149.
26 *Taten Kaiser Karls des Grossen [von] Notker der Stammler*, ed. Hans F. Haefele, MGH SRG 12 (Berlin, 1959), 89; *Charlemagne and Louis the Pious*, trans. Noble, 115.
27 Symphosius Amalarius, *De ecclesiasticis officiis libri quatuor*, Patrologia Latina, vol. 105, col. 988; Kershaw, *Peaceful Kings*, 181–182.
28 Janet L. Nelson, *Charles the Bald* (London: Longman, 1992), 15, 83. For a more detailed analysis see Kershaw, *Peaceful Kings*, 212–219; Samantha Kelly, *The New Solomon: Robert of Naples (1309–1343) and Fourteenth-Century Kingship* (Leiden: Brill, 2003), 260.
29 Nelson, *Charles the Bald*, 219–220.
30 Anton emphasized that this resemblance was unique because Charles the Bald was compared to David as well as Solomon: Hans Hubert Anton, *Fürstenspiegel und Herrscherethos in der Karolingerzeit*, Bonner historische Forschungen, 32 (Bonn: Wissenschaftliche Buchgesellschaft, 1968), 430–432.
31 William J. Diebold, "The Ruler Portrait of Charles the Bald in the S. Paolo Bible," *The Art Bulletin* 76 (1994): 12–14.
32 Allefrate, *The Wandering Throne*, 55–105.
33 Robert Ousterhout, "New Temples and New Solomons: The Rhetoric of Byzantine Architecture," in *The Old Testament in Byzantinum*, eds. Paul Magdalino et al. (Washington, DC: Dumbarton Oaks Research Library and Collection, 2010), 223–253.
34 Shaun Tougher, "The Wisdom of Leo VI," in *New Constantines: The Rhythm of Imperial Renewal in Byzantium, 4th–13th Centuries*, ed. Paul Magdalino (Aldershot: Ashgate Variorum, 1994), 173.
35 Tougher, "The Wisdom of Leo VI," 174; Allegra, *The Wandering Throne*, 35–38, 41–43.
36 Shaun Tougher, *The Reign of Leo VI (886–912)* (Leiden: Brill, 1997), 124–125.
37 Tougher, *The Reign of Leo VI*, 126 n. 109.
38 Tougher, *The Reign of Leo VI*, 110.
39 Claudia Rapp, "Old Testament Models for Emperors in Early Byzantinum," in *The Old Testament in Byzantinum*, eds. Paul Magdalino and Robert S. Nelson (Washington, DC: Dumbarton Oaks, 2010), 175–197; Tougher, *The Reign of Leo VI*, 122–131.
40 Tougher, "The Wisdom of Leo VI," 177.
41 Manuel Alejandro Rodríguez de la Peña, "Sapiential rulership in the Eleventh Century: The Political Theology of Royal Wisdom," in *Political Theology in Medieval and Early Modern Europe: Discourses, Rites, and Representations*, eds. Jaume Aurell, Monserrat Herrero and Angela Concetta Miceli Stout (Turnhout: Brepols, 2017), 92.
42 Herwig Wolfram, *Conrad II, 990–1039: Emperor of Three Kingdoms*, trans. Denise A. Kaiser (Pennsylvania: Pennsylvania University Press, 2006), 148–153.
43 On the shifting emphasis from warrior king to wise king see Laura Fábián, "L'image du roi sage en Occident au XIVe siècle et un exemple concernant la Hongrie à l'époque angevine: le *Secretum secretorum* de Louis le Grand de Hongrie," in *"M'en anei en Ongria". Relations franco-hongroises au Moyen Âge II*, eds. Attila Györkös and Gergely Kiss (Debrecen: MTA, 2017), 83–103.
44 Concerning the background to this, see Jacques Le Goff, *Saint Louis* (Paris: Gallimard, 1996), 452; Harvey Stahl, *Picturing Kingship. History and Painting in the Psalter of Saint Louis* (University Park, PA: The Pennsylvania State University Press, 2008), 154–167.
45 Le Goff, *Saint Louis*, 448–463, 813.
46 Laura Fábián, "IX. Lajos bibliai királymodellje: Salamon király," *Világtörténet* 4 (2014): 579–604.

47 *Vincentius Belvacensis: De morali principis institutione*, ed. Robert J. Schneider (Turnhout: Brepols, 1995), 9, 59–64.

48 *Le Traité "Eruditio regum et principum" de Guibert de Tournai*, ed. Alphonse de Poorter (Louvain: Institut de philosophie de l'université, 1914), 17–18.

49 Meredith Parsons Lillich, "King Solomon in Bed, Archbishop Hincmar, the 'Ordo' of 1250, and the Stained-Glass Program of the Nave of Reims Cathedral," *Speculum* 80 (2005), 764–801.

50 Meredith Cohen, *The Sainte-Chapelle and the Construction of Sacral Monarchy* (New York: Cambridge University Press, 2015).

51 Alyce A. Jordan, *Visualizing Kingship in the Windows of the Sainte-Chapelle* (Turnhout: Brepols, 2002), 80–83.

52 Jordan, *Visualizing Kingship*, 124–126.

53 Jordan, *Visualizing Kingship*, 25–26; Daniel H. Weiss, "Architectural Symbolism and the Decoration of the Ste.-Chapelle," *The Art Bulletin*, 77 (1995): 317; Daniel H. Weiss, *Art and Crusade in the Age of Saint Louis* (Cambridge: Cambridge University Press, 1998), 54–74; Daniel H. Weiss, "The Three Solomon Portraits in the Arsenal Old Testament and the Construction of Meaning in Crusader Painting," *Arte Medievale* 2 (1992): 15–38.

54 For the texts see M. Cecilia Gaposchkin, *Blessed Louis, the Most Glorious of Kings* (Notre Dame, IN: University of Notre Dame Press, 2012), 228–245, 248–299.

55 Gaposchkin, *Blessed Louis*, 288; Fábián, "IX. Lajos bibliai királymodellje," 585–586.

56 Gaposchkin, *Blessed Louis*, 239.

57 Jacques Krynen, *L'empire du roi. Idées et croyances politiques en France, XIIIe–XVe siècle* (Paris: Gallimard, 1993), 179–187, 208–224, especially 217–224; Kelly, *The New Solomon*, 259–269; Chris Jones, "Giles of Rome, Political Thought," in *Encyclopedia of Medieval Philosophy: Philosophy Between 500 and 1500*, ed. Henrik Lagerlund, 2 vols (Heidelberg: Springer, 2011), vol. 1, 417–423.

58 Krynen, *L'empire du roi*, 217–224; Kelly, *The New Solomon*, 261–263. Naturally, this did not exclude the earlier use of the notion *prudentia*.

59 M. Cecilia Gaposchkin, *The Making of Saint Louis* (Ithaca, NY: Cornell University Press, 2008), 57.

60 The comparison dates back to the eleventh century, and was noted for the first time in the *vita* of Edward written in 1065–67: *The Life of King Edward Who Rests at Westminster*, ed. Frank Barlow (Oxford: Clarendon Press, 1992), 6–7, 18–19.

61 Paul Binski, *The Painted Chamber at Westminster* (London: The Society of Antiquaries of London, 1986).

62 Binski, *The Painted Chamber*, 42–43; Parsons, *The Gothic*, 254–255.

63 Francis Wormald, "The Throne of Solomon and St. Edward's Chair," in *Essays in Honour of Erwin Panofsky. De Artibus opuscula*, 40 (New York: New York University Press, 1961), 537–539; Parsons, *The Gothic*, 257.

64 Jean-Patrice Boudet, *Entre science et nigromance: astrologie, divination et magie dans l'Occident médiéval (XIIe–XVe siècle)* (Paris: Publications de la Sorbonne, 2006), 187–197.

65 Jean-Patrice Boudet, "Le modèle du roi sage aux XIIIe et XIVe siècles," *Revue Historique* 647 (2008), 547.

66 Manuel Alejandro Rodríguez de la Peña, "*Rex strenuus valde litteratus*: Strength and Wisdom as Royal Virtues in Medieval Spain (1085–1284)," in *Princely Virtues in the Middle Ages 1200–1500*, eds. Cary Nederman and István Bejczy (Turnhout: Brepols, 2007), 48–49.

67 Alfonso X el Sabio, *Astromagia (Ms. Reg. lat. 1283a)*, ed. Alfonso D'Agostino (Naples: Liguori, 1992), 40–42.

68 Kelly, *The New Solomon*, 222.

69 Eva Schlotheuber, "Drugi Salomon i 'mądry król': 'Teologia władzy' i praktyka władania cesarza Karola IV (zm. 1378)," *Prace Historyczne* 141 (2014): 629.

70 Boudet, "Le modèle du roi sage," 545–66; Boudet, *Entre science*, 303–304.

71 *Recherche sur la librairie de Charles V*, ed. Léopold Delisle, 2 vols (Paris: H. Champion, 1907), vol. 1, 38. For example, Charles possessed several astrological manuscripts, including the *Liber Razielis*, the *Ars Notoria* and the *De quattuor annulis* (*les Anneaux Salmon*), which were connected to Solomon by the astrological tradition. Boudet, "Le modèle du roi sage," 556–557, 560–561.

72 Françoise Autrand, *Charles V, le sage* (Paris: Fayard, 1994).

73 *Le Livre des propriétés des choses : Une encyclopédie au XIV* siècle, ed. and trans. Bernard Ribémont (Paris: Stock, 1999), 53–56.

74 Ribémont, *Le Livre des propriétés*, 53, 55; Donal Byrne, "*Rex imago Dei*: Charles V of France and the Livre des propriétés des choses," *Journal of Medieval History* 7 (1981): 102.

75 Boudet, "Le modèle du roi sage," 558. For Jean Golein's prologue: Paris, Bibliothèque nationale de France, MS français 437, fols 1r–3v. For the digitized manuscript: http://gallica.bnf.fr/ark:/12148/btv1b8447301s (last accessed 10 October 2016).

76 For example, "[e]t aussi Salemon non mie tant seulement estudioit en divers livres mais en ordena pluseurs par son estude." BnF, MS fr. 437, fol. 2r.

77 "[c]ommande mon dit souverain seigneur a moy son tres petit clerc frere Jehan Golein de lordre de Nostre Dame du carme . . . que je li mette et translate de latin en francois le livre que on appele le racional des divins offices. car il considerant que Salemon vouloit enquerir de toutes choses par les queles il se gouvernoit temporelment, de quoy la royne de Sabba s'esbahi forment pour lordenance des minstrans mais plus se peust esmerveillier se elle veist la noblesce de France et lordre des ministrans a Dieu ordenez par les roys de France." BnF, MS fr. 437, fol. 2v.

78 Richard A. Jackson, "The Traité du sacre of Jean Golein," *Proceedings of the American Philosophical Society* 113 (1969): 308–324.

79 Claire Richter Sherman, "Representations of Charles V of France (1338–1380) as a Wise Ruler," *Medievalia et Humanistica*, new series 2 (1971): 83–96; Claire Richter Sherman, *The Portraits of Charles V of France (1338–1380)* (New York: University Press, 1969), 18–32.

80 BnF fr. MS 24287. See François Avril, *La Librairie de Charles V, exposition à la Bibliothèque Nationale* (Paris: Bibliothèque nationale, 1968), 119–120. For the digitized manuscript: http://gallica.bnf.fr/ark:/12148/btv1b8449687z (last accessed 10 October 2016).

81 Laura Fábián, "Egy 14. századi új Salamon: V. (Bölcs) Károly (1364–1380) francia király," in *Micae Mediaevales VI. Fiatal történészek dolgozatai a középkori Magyarországról és Európáról*, eds. Laura Fábián, Dorottya Uhrin et al. (Budapest: ELTE BTK Történelemtudományok Doktori Iskola, 2017), 67–86.

82 Ibid.

83 Sherman, *The Portraits*, 76.

84 Denis Foulechat cited Solomon six times, Aristotle and Saint Ambrose three times, and others only once. Denis Foulechat, *Le Policratique de Jean de Salisbury (1372), livres I–III*, ed. Charles Brucker (Geneva: Droz, 1994), 81–87.

85 Iva Rosario, *Art and Propaganda, Charles IV of Bohemia (1346–1378)* (Woodbridge: Boydell Press, 2000), 98–100.

86 Philippe de Mézières, *Le songe du vieil pèlerin I–II*, ed. G.W. Coopland (Cambridge: Cambridge University Press, 1969), vol. 2, 296.

87 "A Salomon puet estre comparez pour son savoir." Eustache Deschamps, *Oeuvres complètes*, eds. Queux de Saint-Hilaire and G. Raynaud (Paris: Société des Anciens Textes Français, 1878–1904), vol. 3, 239, balade 432, verses 9–12.

88 Nigel Saul, *Richard II* (New Haven: Yale University Press, 1999), 357.

89 Doina, *Les Rois mages*, 302–305.

90 *Four English Political Tracts of the Later Middle Ages*, ed. Jean-Philippe Genet (London: Offices of the Royal Historical Society, University College London, 1977), 31–39.

91 *Roger Dymmok, Liber contra XII errores et hereses Lollardorum*, ed. H.S. Cronin (London: Wyclif Society, 1921).

92 Patricia J. Eberle, "The Politics of Courtly Style at the Court of Richard II," in *The Spirit of the Court: Selected Proceedings of the Fourth Congress of the International Courtly Literature Society*, eds. G.S. Burgess and R.A. Taylor (Cambridge: D.S. Brewer, 1985), 175.

93 *Roger Dymmok*, 295.

94 Saul, *Richard II*, 356; Christopher Fletcher, *Richard II, Manhood, Youth, and Politics, 1377–99* (Oxford: Oxford University Press, 2008), 56.

95 Saul, *Richard II*, 336.

96 *The Chronicle of Adam Usk, 1377–1421*, ed. and trans. Chris Given-Wilson (Oxford: Clarendon Press, 1997), 76. A comparison between Richard and Rehoboam was justified

by the king's inexpert advisers. Philippe Buc, *Pouvoir royal et commentaires de la Bible (1150–1350). Annales. Économies, Sociétés, Civilisations* 44 (1984): 707.

97 Buc, "Pouvoir royal," 692–693.

98 Ágnes Drosztmér, "The Good Fowler as a World Conqueror: Images of Suleyman the Magnificent in Early Modern Hungarian Literary Practice," in *Practices of Coexistence: Constructions of the Other in Early Modern Perceptions*, eds. Marianna D. Birnbaum and Marcell Sebők (Budapest-New York: Central European University Press, 2017), 6–8.

99 William Carroll Tate, *Solomonic Iconography in early Stuart England* (Lewiston; Lampeter: Edwin Mellen Press, 2001), 4.

100 Doina, *Les Rois mages*, 46.

Key works

Boudet, Jean-Patrice, "Le modèle du roi sage aux XIIIe et XIVe siècles," *Revue Historique* 647 (2008): 545–566.

Fábián, Laura, "Egy 14. századi új Salamon: V. (Bölcs) Károly (1364–1380) francia király [A 14th-century new Solomon: Charles V the Wise]," in *Micae Mediaevales VI. Fiatal történészek dolgozatai a középkori Magyarországról és Európáról*, eds. Laura Fábián, Dorottya Uhrin, Csaba Farkas and András Ribi (Budapest: ELTE BTK Történelemtudományok Doktori Iskola, 2017), 67–86.

Gaposchkin, M. Cecilia, *The Making of Saint Louis* (Ithaca: Cornell University Press, 2008).

Kelly, Samantha, *The New Solomon. Robert of Naples (1309–1343) and fourteenth-century Kingship* (Leiden: Brill, 2003).

Krynen, Jacques, *L'empire du roi: Idées et croyances politiques en France, XIIIe–XVe siècle* (Paris: Gallimard, 1993).

Sherman, Claire Richter, "Representations of Charles V of France (1338–1380) as a Wise Ruler," *Medievalia et Humanistica* (1971): 83–96.

Tougher, Shaun, "The Wisdom of Leo VI," in *New Constantines: The Rhythm of Imperial Renewal in Byzantium, 4th–13th Centuries*, ed. Paul Magdalino (Aldershot: Ashgate Variorum, 1994), 171–179.

3

REGAL POWER AND THE ROYAL FAMILY IN A THIRTEENTH-CENTURY IBERIAN LEGISLATIVE PROGRAMME

Manuela Santos Silva

Introduction

Two of the legal codes produced during the reign of the thirteenth-century Iberian king, Alfonso X (r.1252–84), ruler of Castile and León, contain whole sections dedicated to the king, his family and the court, as well as to the households of both the king and the queen. The *Especulo* and the *Siete Partidas* were compiled at a time when both political thought and the ambitions of thirteenth-century rulers were transforming. Each code was produced in notably different political circumstances. Consequently, a careful comparative analysis can reveal the significant changes that took place in a period when concepts of monarchy were still very much under construction on the Iberian Peninsula.

The chronology of the various legal compilations written by jurists during Alfonso X's reign demonstrates that the king's primary objective was to merge old Leónese laws with Castilian customary practice, thereby creating an ideal framework for their adoption in his newly conquered lands.[1] This was clearly the aim of the legal compilation known today as the *Especulo* ('The Mirror of Laws'), a pragmatic and systematic code of the realms' laws; it was equally the intention of the contemporaneous *Fuero Real* ('Customs of the Kingdom'), which sought to synthesize all customary local legislation.[2] Within a short space of time, however, Alfonso recalibrated his initial aim. A new legal code was devised, one that was divided into seven different parts that corresponded to religious, political, administrative, judicial and social determinations. This new code followed a more 'mirrors of princes'-like model and became known from the fourteenth century as the *Siete Partidas* ('The Seven Parts').[3] Unlike the earlier compilations, the new code incorporated clauses and legal arguments drawn from Justinian's sixth-century *Corpus iuris civilis* into the Iberian legal tradition, and validated these additions by recourse to biblical and philosophical writings, especially those of Aristotle. The *Siete Partidas* also corresponded to a secondary development: it was justified by Alfonso's – ultimately failed – candidacy for the position of Holy Roman Emperor following the death of Frederick II in 1250.[4]

The evolution of monarchical ideas is apparent when the *Especulo* and the *Siete Partidas* are compared with specific attention paid to each of their underlying concerns regarding key topics, such as the court. An analysis of both codes offers, in particular, an ideal framework within which to explore the importance of the different members of the royal family within a medieval monarchy.

The Iberian legal tradition

From the sixth to the eleventh centuries, institutions and laws on the Iberian Peninsula evolved autonomously vis-à-vis other regions of western Europe that had once been part of the Roman Empire. In response to Islamic dominance further south, the territories of kingdoms established in northern Iberia after the eighth century were formed in pragmatic ways according to diverse historical situations. These generated differences in the legal and institutional apparatus that evolved in each.

The kingdom of Asturias-León was founded upon the ideal of the reconstruction of the old Visigothic kingdom that had been defeated by the Muslim invasion in the eighth century.[5] During the reign of Alfonso II (r.791–842), the legislative code that had been elaborated previously by Hispanic Visigoths in the seventh century – the *Liber Judiciorum* – was adopted.[6] In this code, the new Christian kingdom found a consistent body of laws for guidance.[7] However, from the ninth until at least the eleventh century, the expansionary project of the Asturian-Leónese kingdom towards western and south-western territories (Galicia and northern Portugal) and south-eastern lands (Castile) would favour the emergence of regulations that stemmed both from local jurisprudence and from the customs of its indigenous peoples as well as those of immigrants from other parts of Iberia.[8]

Even if local regions tended to influence the development of territorial laws, the Visigothic code continued to be applied in the kingdom of León, possibly in some of the conquered territories governed by vassals of its king, and even among the *hispani* of some Catalan counties.[9] This legal framework, known as Receswinth's law code of 654, was later revised into several short versions, and, in 1241, during the reign of Fernando III, king of Castile (r.1217–52), León (r.1230–52) and Galicia (r.1231–52), it was translated into the vernacular *romance* language.[10]

Regardless of the historical connections between León and Castile, the latter could almost be considered 'a lawless land'. It was a striking example of customary diversity due to the people from different territories and cultures who had occupied the region, and the abuse of power by the local noble retinues who demanded either the maintenance of ancient laws or the establishment of new discretionary rules.[11] Eastern Iberia, by contrast, had different legal traditions. There, the influence of the Franks, mixed with ancestral customs, was felt strongly. Navarre, Aragon and the Catalan counties shaped their institutions and cultural mentality on Frankish models rather than upon western Iberian traditions.[12]

During the twelfth century, the re-emergence of Roman law in the form of the Christian law code completely revised in the sixth century by the Byzantine emperor Justinian I and later reintroduced to western Europe by legal scholars at Bologna, reiterated the ideal of a well-structured state governed by a firm power.[13] In north-western Iberia, this ideal was buttressed in the thirteenth century during the reigns of Fernando III and Alfonso X, kings of both Castile and León, which had been reunited and were joint kingdoms.[14] It seemed that a new occasion had arisen for stating a Leónese-Castilian dominance in relation to the other

Iberian kingdoms, as had earlier been the case under Alfonso VI (r.1065–1109) and Alfonso VII (r.1126–57) of León and Castile, both of whom had claimed for themselves the title of emperors of *Hispania* following the Leónese tradition, initiated by Alfonso III.[15]

The task of compiling Iberian local and regal legislation, translating it into the vernacular and the elaboration of new legal codes started in Fernando III's reign but was infused with much greater dynamism in the reign of Alfonso X. It reveals a process that was clearly influenced by political developments both within and beyond the realms of Castile and León, and one that profited from the recent renewal of the study of Roman law that had provided western Christianity with a more universally applicable *ius commune*.[16] In the same way as the Bolognese scholars had combined canon and civil law, the Castilian court fused the Visigothic *Fuero Juzgo*, the canon and the Roman laws and the local customs (*fueros*).[17]

In 1981, Jerry Craddock, whose chronology of Alfonso X's legislative work is closely followed in this chapter, established that the first compilation of Alfonso's laws was the *Especulo*, completed in 1255.[18] Julio Valdeón acknowledged that this work can be matched to Germanic texts of the same period known as 'Mirror of Laws' and recognized that its aim should be understood as that of providing the Castilian-Leónese realm with a summary of its law.[19] The five different books (*libros*) of the *Especulo* included many enacted laws of Iberian provenance. The intention here was that they be used to judge 'all people of our kingdoms and our seigneurie',[20] an approach that added strength to the notion that the king was the source of all laws, even though he needed to summon his parliament (*cortes*) to enact them.[21] Almost contemporaneous with the drafting of the *Especulo*, *fueros* were compiled to establish a single *fuero real* that could replace a wide array of local customs, usages and determinations.[22]

Yet even before the *Especulo* was completed, a much lengthier enterprise was begun by Alfonso. Its purpose was to prepare a new code, one strongly influenced by canon and Roman civil law. It took a dozen years to complete. Finessing and improving the code, however, continued until the end of the thirteenth century.[23] The origin of its name, the *Siete Partidas*, lies in its division into seven parts. Each *partida* had a specific main subject and was divided into titles (*títulos*) containing more than 2500 laws (*leyes*).

Alfonso's legal reforms were received with protest by the nobility of the kingdoms of Castile and León, and many years were to pass before the legal precepts contained in his codes were enforced fully by his great-grandson, Alfonso XI (r.1313–50).[24] This issue notwithstanding, Alfonso X's key legislative works proved influential on the Iberian Peninsula: they were adopted in Portugal, from the reign of his grandson King Dinis (r. 1279–1325), and at a very early stage of their development the Alfonsine legal codes were translated into Portuguese.[25]

Regal authority

Both codes strengthened the role of the king over his territory and subjects, framing the monarch as the maker of laws and positioning the law as the main pillar of the royal system that was now starting to be implemented.[26] It might be expected that the *Especulo* and the *Partidas*, the latter begun while the five books of the *Especulo* were still being written, would be conceptually similar. However, as several historians have already stressed, the *Especulo* aimed to unite Iberian legal heritage for practical reasons, that is for use in courts and in the royal court, while the *Siete Partidas* became in effect the ethical and political legacy of Alfonso X. This legacy was solidly supported by the *auctoritas* of the canon and the Roman civil law and by other classical rationale, which were reflected in the introductions to each new title or section.[27]

The first book of the *Especulo* begins by stating that no one can be exempt from sanction merely because they do not know the law; ignorance of the law was not an acceptable excuse.[28] Yet only the subsequent two titles match the opening statement of the *Siete Partidas* (I–II, I–III), that is that both king and kingdom are subject to divine justice because everything belongs to God according to the commandments and teachings of the Church.[29] Book two of the *Especulo* begins by reiterating how advisable it is to have faith in the laws and sacraments of the Church and to obey them because Jesus Christ is at the beginning and end of all things, administering them always with justice and according to the law. Reigning above all kings, as their overlord, Christ himself brought kings into the world to govern His terrestrial kingdoms and administer justice on His behalf.[30]

In keeping with these notions that terrestrial rulers depend on and were subject to God, both works – book two of the *Especulo* and the second part of the *Siete Partidas* – are dedicated to temporal justice. *Especulo* II–I begins by defining the substance and nature of a king.[31] According to this title, the king represents 'the soul of the people' and his mission is 'to rectify mistakes made in his territory', to protect his subjects and to keep the peace by administering natural justice. Making use of the classical metaphor of the human body – popularized in the twelfth century by John of Salisbury – the legislator explains that it is by the soul (i.e. the king) that the body (i.e. the realm or his subjects) survives and is vouchsafed, even if the people's approval of the king's rule is essential.[32]

One of the most interesting aspects to consider concerning regal authority is the way in which the *Especulo* and the *Partidas* treat the mechanism of succession with regard to both kings and emperors. In order for the king to possess all the essential attributes of rulership, the *Especulo* explains that he must be elected from among the best in his community.[33] To ensure his fitness to be the 'governor of the people', the lord of his kingdom and even its 'ruler' (*regla*),[34] a king must have exceptional qualities of leadership, combined with outstanding and demonstrable military competence. Moreover, since a king was ranked highest in his land as overlord, with the responsibility and duty to act righteously in the defence of all his subjects, he must be honoured by them.[35] Thus, the construction of his realm should be understood as a yearning to amalgamate the diversity of people who live in his territories, linked to his obligation to ensure the well-being and protection of his people.[36]

The regulations in use prior to the adoption of the Alfonsine legislation – the so-called *Fuero Juzgo* code, based on Visigothic laws – directed that kings should be elected, just as contemporary Holy Roman Emperors were. The same law that codified the election of a new king prevented the children of the deceased monarch from acceding to the royal patrimony.[37] Nevertheless, in the *Especulo*, after election had been identified as the legitimate route by which a ruler should reach the throne, a new law was introduced declaring that the first-born child – normally a boy but a girl in a case where no sons had been born – should inherit the kingdom.[38]

This implies that, by the mid-thirteenth century, it was believed that election was only to be used to select the founder of the dynasty and that once the king had become the overlord of his territory and the point of reference for his people, his family was linked to that same realm and the crown would become hereditary.[39] The idea recurs in the second *Partida*.[40]

The idea of an existing divinely appointed dynasty had always been present in monarchical ideology. To be favoured with leadership qualities presupposed coming from ancestors with the same attribute.[41] This identification of rulership with the inheritance of the realm represents a revised conception of royal power in western kingdoms, one that corresponds to an overall tendency towards the emergence of hereditary monarchies.[42] Yet, a tension existed: as Jeroen Duindam has stressed, for late medieval monarchies, as a general principle, the ideal of kingship 'stipulated personal qualifications as much as it glorified pedigree'.[43]

The content of the second *Partida* appears, at first glance, to be organized similarly to the second book of the *Especulo*. Yet the important geopolitical juncture at which the *Partidas* corpus was drafted – a time at which Alfonso X was toying with the possibility of becoming Holy Roman Emperor – is evident in the fact that kingship is not the *Partida*'s only concern: the role of the emperor and other forms of temporal justice are also explored.[44]

In the *Partidas*, the image of an emperor is that of an elected dignitary, one whom all subjects in his empire must obey and who recognizes no higher temporal authority but has nonetheless to yield to the pope in spiritual matters. There was no similarity between this understanding of the imperial office, which was rooted in contemporary German models of rulership, and the Iberian tradition of an Hispanic empire as Alfonso X's ancestors from the eleventh and twelfth centuries had conceived it. The latter was an empire headed by León (now united with Castile) but that also comprised all the other Christian *regna* (kingdoms, counties, etc.) within the Peninsula.[45] By the thirteenth century, the *imperator totius Hispaniae* could not aspire to be more than a king whose political power was of any greater authority than that of his Iberian counterparts, thus it was a title with no practical consequences.[46] And whatever the ambitions of Alfonso X towards the Iberian Peninsula's *imperium*, he acknowledged his power was that of a king.

In both codes, references to the pope as an intermediary between God and royal power are completely absent.[47] In the second *Partida*, a parallel is drawn between the divine sphere and the earthly sphere, with kings taking the place of God with the aim of securing justice and law in their kingdoms, just as an emperor would in his empire.[48] This means that both kings and emperors were conceived of as vicars of God on earth, enforcing justice and providing each person with what was rightfully theirs.[49] This image undoubtedly strengthened the power of rulers, while the guiding principles proposed in the remaining laws further defined regal power.

A more striking detail of the second *Partida* when comparing the power of emperors and kings is that the power exercised by the latter is arguably more extensive than that exercised by the former. As the emperor was elected while the king was lord of his kingdom by right of inheritance, the emperor's authority ended with his death, while that of the king did not. Indeed, the *Partidas* value the power of kings precisely *because* they could leave their kingdoms to their offspring, having governed them according to their will and with a view to the continuation of their dynasties. In addition, based on feudal tradition, kings could make use of the territories of their kingdoms to reward individuals for their loyalty. Such vassals could be co-opted to husband and safeguard the inhabitants of their territories in keeping with the inclinations and policies adopted by their royal predecessors.

It is almost paradoxical that an imperial candidate presents the power of a king as more flexible and potentially greater than that of an emperor. In fact, the line of argument seems to imply that in the case of the latter, in addition to being subject to the pope as an intermediary between God and himself in spiritual matters, an emperor had to submit to electoral scrutiny and therefore theoretically had little room to manoeuvre in adapting his governance to ever-changing circumstances. By contrast, when someone met the requirements to succeed to the throne as a blood relative of a defunct king, the possibility of an elected king was not even envisaged. The second *Partida* (I, ix) argues that the most natural way to rise to kingship is for the throne of the deceased king to pass to his first-born son or to one of his closest blood relatives.[50] The door remained open, however, to female succession, allowing a man of any social rank who had married an heiress to the throne – as had sometimes occurred in Asturias and León, and remained possible in Iberian countries – to obtain the title of king as the queen's husband. The other possible avenues to kingship were only valid in truly exceptional situations. If no such male or female relative could be found, then another likely male contender could be called upon, even if he did not meet the criteria of being part of the royal bloodline. Finally, Alfonso X envisaged the possibility of ascension to the throne by the approval of a pope or an emperor 'in those lands where they have the right to do so'.[51]

Any of these forms of attaining kingship were considered to be lawful. As a function of his high status, elevation to the kingship came with the obligation that the king love and honour all his subjects, regardless of their position in society, and that he promote harmony and justice among all inhabitants of his lands.[52] However, the reality was that, from the earliest times of monarchy, the highest-ranking nobles should be rewarded with gifts of land for services rendered or to ensure their loyalty.[53] Though they were neither emperors nor kings, they likewise enjoyed the benefits of lordship and were therefore entitled to hold a share of the kingdom. In return, they ought to honour their king as they were his favoured vassals and auxiliaries within the royal court.[54]

The court

The *Especulo* and the second *Partida* agree on their explanation of the word 'court'. According to the *Especulo*, this word is applicable to the place where all the people in charge of guarding, honouring and helping their lord gather.[55] The *Partidas* give a more concrete, perhaps more didactic, definition, while keeping the basic elements of the earlier work. The 'court' is the physical space where the king is present and resides, as well as the institution of his vassals and officials who serve and advise him on a daily basis.[56] His subjects, from all parts of his kingdom, visit this space and institution to pay tribute to, seek justice from, or to take care of other business with the king. The word 'court' is said to derive from two Latin words: *cohors*, a meeting place for those who must honour and defend the king, and, *curia*, a place for solving problems where all are apportioned a legal right according to status. Reference should also be made to an explanation given in the *Especulo*: the court was a space wherein one could find the sword that 'cut' injustice.[57] This sword, the sword of the king, must be used to maintain order and justice in his territories, and that is the reason why the vicar of God assumes the power of making laws on Earth as indeed happened during Alfonso X's reign.[58]

All subjects are welcome at court decrees the second *Partida*.[59] Consequently, the court had to be so arranged as to be capable of housing everybody, as a place where any-one could have their issues addressed. Furthermore, the court should be a place where every visitor felt assured of their own personal safety. For that purpose, a five-league radius around the place where the court was based was declared secure ground.[60]

During the Middle Ages, courts were peripatetic. Consequently, the *Especulo* states that the king belongs to no predetermined place within his territory.[61] The court was the place where the king was in residence, and everyone within a one-league radius of this place was said to be at court.[62] According to fifteenth-century Castilian and Portuguese chronicles, it was frequently the case that a city could not house all mem-bers of the court, so individuals or groups of courtiers were required to secure their lodgings in villages, monasteries and in other venues, in areas surrounding where the king had established his court.

As he progressed throughout his realm, the king was accompanied by a vast reti-nue, the officials who served him and often by the queen, his children (of age and under-age) and, in these cases, by the 'households' of each member of the royal family. Small wonder that, according to certain estimates, approximately 500 to 1000 people joined the king in his perambulations across the territory of the kingdom.[63]

The queen and the king's mistresses

The *Especulo* (II–III) offers clear evidence that among the members of the court the king's wife enjoyed an exceptional status. The compilation states that, having referred to the position and honour of the king, in all fairness, it should make mention of the position and honour of the queen, his wife, who was the closest person to him.[64] This principle, that those closest to the king could share in his regal aura and power, is evident in many monarchies at particular moments and in specific contexts; it is closely linked to the transition from elective to hereditary systems of succession. This was because only the king, regardless of his origins, possessed the superior qualities of leadership capable of attracting God's favour, and thereby was ideally positioned to perpetuate superior qualities and skills in his offspring.[65] The importance of the king's wife derived from being his partner in generating heirs (and spares). However, unlike her progeny, the queen was not mentioned in the Visigothic *Fuero Juzgo* except in laws sixteen and seventeen that determine that a deceased king's children and wife must be respected and protected.[66] It is in the hereditary system of succession that we can better appre-hend the burgeoning relevance of the king's wife, his partner in the transmission of his kingly honour to their offspring. The primordial role played by the queen and her place within the royal family stemmed from, and indeed underpinned, the dynastic ideal of monarchy.[67]

The second *Partida* is more detailed than the *Especulo* regarding the characteriza-tion of the queen's role. It addresses the relationship between the king and his wife in title six.[68] The first requirement it posits is the need for the couple's harmony; specifically, having chosen a good queen-wife, the king had an obligation to honour, value and protect her. For her part, the queen must be his partner in both hardship and pleasure. Harmony should reign between them because the heir to the throne emerged from the offspring born to them both. The lawmaker indicates that: 'Should the king love, honour and guard his wife in this manner, then he shall be loved, honoured and guarded by her and give a good example to all the inhabitants of his land.'[69] To help the king choose a suitable wife, the *Partidas* advise him to follow a four-part model, which suggests that a prospective queen must: first, belong to a fine lineage, so as to increase her husband's honour and convey it to their offspring; second, be beautiful, so as to better seduce her husband and generate attractive offspring whose beauty would impact on other people; third, be of good conduct, not only to please her husband but also to know how to honour him and behave honourably; and finally, be rich, so as to add wealth to her husband, their children and the land. Moreover, adds the lawmaker, a king whose wife fulfils all four criteria should thank God for her having done so. If, on the other hand, a king could not find a woman who met the criteria, then at least he should make sure he considers her lineage and good habits as these are her most durable qualities and her most valuable assets.[70]

The *Especulo*'s major concern, however, is for the purity of the queen's soul and body. Its most pressing preoccupation is possible adultery on the part of the queen, a transgression that could have severe repercussions for royal succession. Adultery committed by a queen was therefore considered more grave than that of any other woman.[71] In a polity governed by Christian codes, in which the power vested in kings was born from divine will, going against God's precepts naturally added gravity to the sin of adultery. In both the *Especulo* and the second *Partida*, the founding argument against adultery is to be found in Creation itself: God created one woman for one man, and vice-versa, transforming them into a single entity.[72] The second *Partida* adds that the king must love the queen, his wife, and she must love him in return, because they become one through their marriage and cannot be separated save by death or by specific valid reasons that might lead to an annulment of their union.[73]

The *Especulo*, while holding the queen chiefly responsible for the maintenance of her virtue, does not hold back from stating that, in addition to the 'protection of the queen's soul', the 'protection of the queen's body' is imperative; the queen should not be killed, nor wounded, nor arrested, nor her intimacy violated, unless that for a justifiable reason this was ordered by her own husband, the king.[74] Nevertheless, from what is stated, nothing implies that the importance and role of the queen goes much further than being the king's companion and his partner in the generation of their future progeny.[75] However, the fact that the queen is the closest person to the king and his partner in life may open the door for situations in which the queen has a considerable share in the governance of the realm.[76]

Interestingly, the first law of *Especulo* II–III, which defines the 'Protection of the Queen', also determines 'the way in which any other woman the king may have without blessing [that is to say, out of wedlock] should be guarded'.[77] This clause, removed from the text of the second *Partida*, demonstrates that, among those practices and laws considered in the drafting of the *Especulo* there was included, and deemed relevant, the idea that the aura protecting the king's person could be extended to those enjoying his intimacy even if such intimacy was not sanctioned by the ecclesiastical authorities.

Having concubines was a common practice for kings in the first centuries of the Middle Ages, and it speaks to a tradition governed by rules established during the Roman era.[78] It was considered a temporary phase in a man's life, usually corresponding to his youth, especially in the upper layers of society. Even if children were born from such liaisons, the man could later marry, with the previous relationship having been annulled, so that the new relationship was not deemed adulterous.[79] It was a practical solution for unions of a sentimental and sexual nature, linking people of different social ranks who would never be allowed to marry otherwise.[80] It was not before the twelfth century that the Christian religion elaborated a specific liturgy and incorporated marriage as a sacrament.[81] The evidence of Iberian kings' private lives shows that the Church's decisions in this area were not immediately taken into account, a point reinforced by the *Especulo*'s legislation for the king's relationships out of wedlock. According to the *Especulo*, for the sake of the king's honour, no one should have sexual intercourse with the king's mistress, nor kidnap her, nor force her into marriage unless the king first approved it. In fact, such crimes constituted treason and were punishable by death, the loss of assets or exile, depending upon who perpetrated them and the social status of the woman in question.[82]

The king's children

Another area touched on in the *Especulo* – yet absent in the *Siete Partidas* – governs the security of the king's children and touches directly upon those of his children born as a result of adultery (II–IV, iii). It emphasizes the gravity of adulterous relationships, particularly within the king's and queen's households.[83] This forms part of a series of regulations aimed specifically at preventing the king's sons, daughters and sisters from involving themselves in relationships of a sexual nature from which children might be born out of wedlock.[84] According to this law's rationale, the king should demonstrate irreproachable behaviour in such matters, thereby making it clear that he does not condone extramarital liaisons on the part of his relatives.

Regarding the protection of the king's and the queen's closest relatives, the laws naturally express concerns about the good reputation and good behaviour of princes (*infants*) and princesses (*infantas*), emphasizing the importance of choosing good tutors and governors for royal offspring to prevent them from exposure to avoidable dangers.[85] Extreme care needed to be devoted to the first-born son, who had the right to highest honours, identical to those enjoyed by his father, the king.[86] Although they did not benefit from the same status as their legitimate half-brothers and sisters, royal children born out of wedlock and who were killed in battle were to be given the same funerary honours as those extended to the kingdom's highest nobility.[87]

Regardless of the consideration of illegitimate children of the king given in the *Especulo*, the second *Partida* states unambiguously that 'lawfully born children (sons and daughters) are those born of rightful marriage' (II–VII). In this part of his code, Alfonso X establishes a full-fledged educational programme for legitimate offspring, both boys and girls. Clearly, the intention here was to prepare the future royal children as kings and queens through education. Earlier, the *Partida* described 'what the king should be in his deeds', establishing a moral programme and suggesting the qualities that should be displayed by a good monarch (II–V). These rules were very similar to the typology defined in other 'mirrors of princes'.[88] Emphasis is placed upon the need for a king to know how to read and to be curious to learn, which enables him to become autonomous, that is to be liberated from the need to be advised or even instructed on an ongoing basis. The king likewise needed to know how to pray to God in the most efficacious manner, as piety was a central element of kingship.[89] A further skill that the king had to perfect in order to better administer justice was to know and to understand his subjects.[90] He also needed to naturally 'be skilful in the art of arms'. At the heart of this requirement is the traditional image of a warrior-chief who skilfully masters the arts of war, simultaneously providing a model for the men whom he commands.[91] Title five of the second *Partida* also stresses that in equestrian practice the king should 'have enjoyment and pleasure, so that he can better take hardship when he has to endure it', in hunting as well as war.[92] The king should draw maximum benefit from this sport, as it 'is very helpful to appease thoughts and anger'.[93] The king is also advised to listen to songs and musical instruments and to play chess and other games, in addition to reading and listening to tales and stories and other books that talk about 'those things that bring joy and pleasure to men'.[94]

In order for this model of a well-balanced and cultivated monarch to materialize, a king at once cultured, skilful at arms and physically active, young princes needed to undertake a fully developed programme of education with their father not only as their key point of reference, but also their principal teacher and mentor.[95] The *Partidas* summarize an educational programme wherein special reference is made to the following requirements: a king's loving and protective relationship with his children, the correct ways in which to raise them, the ways in which to teach them in terms of age-appropriate pedagogical content and the rewards he will reap by applying these principles as well as how he should teach them to do good and punish their errors.

The second *Partida* structures its pedagogy both with regard to Iberian traditions and the conceptualization of monarchy as a hereditary institution (II–VII, i). It explains that, in medieval Iberia, the children of kings are called *infantes*, a word of Latin origin referring to the first age of life. The motivation for loving the children born of the married couple is defined in the following terms: 'because they come from them, they are like parts of their body', but also because they will continue the work of their parents.[96] The second *Partida* suggests that child-rearing should take into account the nature of children; it should find ways to engage them and enable them to absorb rules and teachings. The sound education of princes is beneficial not only to them, as they learn to better comply with their obligations towards other people, but also enables them to become models of correct behaviour for those who will serve them.[97]

Children's parents, in this case the king and the queen, should have the primary responsibility for their offspring's education. First, they should select healthy wet and dry nurses, honourable and of good descent, so as to contribute to the good health and rearing of the princes.[98] Later, they should appoint dedicated and loyal tutors who care about their children's eating habits, their speech and their training in correct behaviour.[99] Tutors should likewise be responsible for advising young princes not to drink too much, nor to eat in a way that could be harmful to their physical health and moral well-being and who can teach them to be wise in their discourse and in their daily habits.[100] As a result of this education programme, the *infantes* should also learn to love and fear God, and to respect their father, their mother and their elder brothers 'who are their natural lords on account of lineage'.[101] They should also love their relatives and vassals and treat them with equanimity at all times, both in praise and in punishment.

According to the second *Partida*, learning to read and write was part of any prince's education. He should also be taught to be merry, as excessive sadness could make him unhealthy. It was desirable that princes rode, hunted and played cavalry games. If reared in good habits, they would more easily come to know and understand subjects of all ranks.[102] The king's role should not be limited to the rearing of his children; he should also ensure their inheritances, seek good marriages for them and do them all the good he can while he lives, 'so as to enable them to live honourably'.[103] The king should enact a knightly educational programme with increased responsibility for his children, as the royal family acted as an example to all society.

Alfonso X did not forget to devote two items specifically to the king's daughters. He was particularly concerned: 'because males can go everywhere, and learn from everybody, but they [daughters] should learn only from their father, or their mother, or the people given by their father and mother to accompany them'.[104] Nurses and ladies-in-waiting should be selected with extreme care, with an emphasis upon their loyalty and good habits. Mothers should be particularly concerned with the rearing of their daughters, making sure they learned to read so that they could write letters and study their psalters. More than their brothers, *infantas* needed to exhibit irreproachable behaviour, particularly regarding the manner in which they dressed.[105]

The goal of this entire educational programme was to prepare the *infanta* for her future as a woman married to someone of similar rank. Political and military alliances with other kingdoms and peace treaties often depended on daughters' marriages. Alfonso understood that it was easier to achieve conjugal harmony if the groom was handsome and pleasing to the eye in order to nurture more love in his wife (as indeed the bride should be to her husband). This, in turn, would enable the couple's union to bear more children. Both husband and wife needed to be endowed with good moral habits so that they could avoid temptation and ensure a more lasting love, and of course, both should be in good physical shape so that they could generate healthy children. As soon as a princess came of age, the search for a good husband should be the top priority of her parents.[106]

Royal relatives and the household

While a king was to be very involved with providing his children with a good education such that they might continue his work, he could also call upon his relatives to assist him in the task of governing. To this end, the second *Partida* argues that 'if animals, which are dumb creatures and without understanding, love others of their kind, uniting with them and assisting them when it is necessary, especially should men, who have understanding and reason, by which they should be governed, do so' (II–VIII, i).[107] Writing in the prologue to his *Book of Lineages* in fourteenth-century Portugal, the Count of Barcelos, Don Pedro – also the author of a *General Chronicle of Hispania* – expresses the same notion of solidarity among relatives. If one has a relative in fifth or sixth degree, or even more remotely, if he is of higher rank, one ought to serve him. If he is one's equal, one ought to help him. If he is of lower rank, one ought to do him good because 'there is no friendship as pure as that which unites those who come from the same blood'.[108] Since no one can better serve a king or a queen than family members, they ought to be loved, honoured and given privilege like no other.[109] They should always have a privileged place in a king's household, in a queen's household, and in the households of princes and princesses, as long as they always remember to be loyal and to provide their benefactors with the service to which they are entitled.[110]

Title nine of the second *Partida* completes the social framework of those who, in the service of the king in his chambers, help him to administer his household and assets, and more broadly his kingdom.[111] In the popular contemporary metaphor that equated the kingdom with the body, the king's officers played a prominent role: those who helped a king to rule were the brain; those taking care of his body were the internal organs; and those in charge of his land were the external organs that guided and protected him by referring to such things as a man hears, sees, tastes, smells and touches.[112] Their importance for the success of royal governance is clear.

The second *Partida* defines the word 'office' as the service provided by a subject to a king or to a city (II–IX, prologue). It describes the ideal profile of individuals who should serve the king in his household, ending with a ranked list of the officials in royal service.[113] Giving priority to 'spiritual' offices, title nine describes the functions and qualities of the chaplain, the chancellor and the king's counsellors. In considering the structure of the kingdom's government, a definition is provided of high-ranking nobles, notaries and clerks: the members of the king's armed forces, whose role is to secure the king's defence, and then of his physicians, whose duty it is to keep the king in good health. Reference is then made to the men in charge of household supplies and their management. Last, title nine mentions those who represent the king in his territories and describes the offices most closely related to the king's government, addressing, in order of priority, questions of a military, administrative and judicial nature.

The same subject matter is dealt with in a similar way in the *Espéculo* (II–XII, XIII). The king's household officials are divided more simply into clergymen and laymen, with priority being given to clergymen, 'by virtue of the honour of the holy church and faith'. Among such clergymen, reference is made to high-ranking chaplains, chancellors, notaries and physicians with a clarification that the latter could be laymen, lesser clergy of a king's household and clerks. Laymen are hierarchically listed as military, administrative officials and judicial officials.[114] Law nine of title thirteen refers to the special care that should be paid to people who have been raised by the king, even if they occupy lower-ranking positions,[115] demonstrating that, in addition to family ties by blood, the court and its households should likewise be understood to be a family: a family of service.

The lawmakers of both compilations were keen to establish penalties for those who attempted harm against the physical integrity of members of a king's household by killing or wounding them. In the case of a queen's household, the lawmakers' primary anxiety was that attempts might be made to sully the reputation or honour of the ladies who were its members.[116] Indeed, the second *Partida* clearly explains that the maidens and ladies of the household must find the queen's chamber to be a refuge from evil women and men's influence.[117] Therefore, the queen's household must occupy the most private area of the palace or other 'hidden' quarters of the building where the court is resident.[118]

As explained in the *Especulo* (II–XV) – and in essence repeated in the *Partidas* – a queen's household was composed of women who were relatives of the king, his daughters, sisters, etc. (either single, married or widowed); ladies of high rank, such as daughters or wives of high-ranking nobles; and other ladies of knightly descent, as well as widows and nuns. Included in a queen's household were her children's wet and dry nurses, her chamber stewardesses and other servants who could either be Christian or Moors. In keeping with the same rationale behind the functioning of a peripatetic court, a queen's household and its rules not only concerned the building within which a queen might be resident but applied equally to the entire town (or any other place) where a queen might stay.[119] The rules governing the officials of a queen's household were identical to those of a king's.[120] As with her husband, the queen was served by numerous male officials – within the household and in her dominion – but neither legal text mentions these latter specifically.

Conclusion

As this chapter demonstrates, Alfonso X's legislation sought to understand and define the role of the royal family and of the royal court – as well as ideal rulership – for an Iberian context. While the *Especulo* and *Partidas* law codes are not necessarily easy sources to employ in such an examination, they reveal that Alfonso intended to set out a model of rulership strongly centred on the king himself, one that viewed the royal family and the court as extensions of the monarch. As such, both became part of the process of rulership and agents of royal power.

Among the reforms he undertook, Alfonso paid particular attention to the necessity of updating the regulations that specifically concerned royal power. Visigothic law had anticipated that kings should be elected; by the time Alfonso drafted his codes, a hereditary system had become established in nearly every kingdom in western Europe. Consequently, and even though the *Especulo* still referenced alternatives that had been used in the past, title sixteen of book two clearly established the principle that the realm should be inherited by the first-born child of the king.[121] Succession to the throne by alternate means was deemed possible, but it was envisioned that after any period of disruption, rulership by way of dynastic succession would always resume. Moreover, the fact that a new king could complete his father's unfinished work was considered to be a driver of stability. Alfonso X, who completed his father's reforms, personified this idea.

The idea that the king should rule with the assistance of his court had its origins in an older, hierarchical system of nomadic warrior societies in which all military and administrative offices were held by secular elites who were advised in turn by clerical elites. The building of a *curia* around the king, which helped him in every required task, saw his entourage comprise a majority of high-ranking nobles, but it was also made up of people from other social strata who could supply all the services due to the monarch. It was only natural that it soon became necessary to create a similar system to assist the queen, one that was dominated by women but where several tasks were also performed by men.[122] Yet the entire Alfonsine legislative structure assigned an overwhelmingly passive role to women. It would seem that a queen's household existed as a function of the king and his closest collaborators, preferably apart from or hidden away from any gaze that might potentially seek to hurt the king by injuring his queen, his daughters or the ladies and maids who served them.[123] The political structure Alfonso aimed to build in his territories was based around the king with his officials as an extension of himself. Both the queen and the royal progeny appear to represent a similar idea: they were an extension of the king's persona.

Despite this, longstanding matrimonial traditions in the western kingdoms of the Iberian Peninsula gave women significant economic autonomy that allowed them to manage their households from their wedding day until the end of their lives.[124] Additionally, queens were, critically, able to be involved in the governance of the kingdom through short- or long-term regencies, cooperation in the management of the crown's property or through informal diplomatic acts.[125] None of this, however, is reflected in the Alfonsine codes.[126] Yet, the same law code that determined an 'end' to the Hispanic tradition of partible inheritance by which the kingdom was shared among all children upon the death of their father did not, however, discard the possible inheritance of the king's throne by a first-born daughter in the absence of a male heir.[127] An acceptance of female inheritance reflects both past precedent in not only Castile but also in the other Iberian kingdoms, and indeed would happen again in the future.[128] Alfonsine legislation was adopted and adapted to the customs of neighbouring realms; the codes, in turn, acted as an essential foundation for future legal compilations, such as those of fifteenth-century Portugal.[129]

All the Iberian kingdoms shared some basic institutions and traditions and, even if there was a spirit of reform and 'modernization' in the legislative work of Alfonso X, his court could still be described as 'feudal', in that these codes sought to secure the collaboration of the entirety of 'society' in the royal court. The court's collective flavour was preserved in the Alfonsine codes, although henceforth it centred upon the king himself. In reality, both the *Especulo* and the *Siete Partidas*, particularly the chapters describing the king's and queen's households, testify to a monarchy under construction.

Notes

1 Julio Valdéon, José Mª Salrach and Javier Zabalo, *Feudalismo y Consolidación de los Pueblos Hispánicos (siglos XI-XV)*, in *História de España*, ed. Manuel Tuñon de Lara, vol. 4 (Barcelona: Editorial Labor S.A., 1982), 65.

2 Marina Kleine, "Para la guardia de la poridad, del cuerpo y de la tierra del rey: los oficiales reales y la organización de la corte de Alfonso X," in *Historia. Instituciones: Documentos*, 35 (Seville: Universidad de Sevilla, 2008), 234–235; Julio Valdéon, *Alfonso X el Sabio* (Valladolid: Junta de Castilla y León, 1986), 31.

3 Kleine, "Para la guardia de la poridad," 235.

4 José Luís Martin, *La península en la Edad Media* (Barcelona: Editorial Teide, 1980), 422; Marco Ortiz Palanques, "El concepto de rey, reino y territorio en las siete partidas," *Revista Filosofia* 23 (2012): 439; Cayetano J. Socarras, *Alfonso X of Castile: A Study on Imperialistic Frustration* (Barcelona: Ediciones Hispam, 1976), 131; José Angel García de Cortázar, *La época medieval*, third edition (Madrid: Ediciones Alfaguara, 1983), 307.

5 Miguel Angel Ladero Quesada, *La formación medieval de España. Territorios. Regiones. Reinos*, second edition (Madrid: Alianza Editorial, S. A., 2008), 51.

6 "The Visigothic Code (*Forum judicum*)," trans. S.P. Scott, http://libro.uca.edu/vcode/visigoths.htm (last accessed 20 August 2018); Valdéon, *Alfonso X*, 28; Valdéon, Salrach and Zabalo, *Feudalismo y Consolidación*, 64–65.

7 *Fuero Juzgo ó Recopilacion de las Leyes de los Wisigodos Españoles*, second edition (Madrid, 1792).

8 Valdéon, Salrach and Zabalo, *Feudalismo y Consolidación*, 64; García de Cortázar, *La época medieval*, 290–294.

9 Ladero Quesada, *La formación medieval*, 51.

10 Ladero Quesada, *La formación medieval*, 51; Vicente Ángel Álvarez Palenzuela, ed., *Historia de España de la Edad Media* (Barcelona: Ariel, 2002), 498.

11 A popular proverb called Castile "un país sen leyes": Valdéon, *Alfonso*, 28. Ortiz Palanques, "El concepto de rey," 139.

12 Martin, *La península*, 154–163, 362–371.

13 Valdéon, Salrach and Zabalo, *Feudalismo y Consolidación*, 64; Álvarez Palenzuela, *Historia*, 498; García de Cortázar, *La época medieval*, 306; Valdéon, *Alfonso X*, 30–31.

14 Valdéon, Salrach and Zabalo, *Feudalismo y Consolidación*, 64; Ortiz Palanques, "El concepto de rey," 139.

15 Socarras, *Alfonso X*, 9–10, 15–17, 20; Álvarez Palenzuela, *Historia*, 498; Ladero Quesada, *La formación medieval*, 52.

16 Valdéon, Salrach and Zabalo, *Feudalismo y Consolidación*, 65–66.

17 Antonella Liuzzo Scorpo, "Religious Frontiers and Overlapping Cultural Borders: The Power of Personal and Political Exchanges in the Works of Alfonso X of Castile (1252–1284)," *Al-Masaq* 23, no. 3 (2011): 219; Marie R. Madden, *Political Theory and Law in Medieval Spain* (New York: Fordham University Press, 1930), 69.

18 Jerry Craddock, "La cronologia de las obras legislativas de Alfonso X el Sabio," *Anuario de Historia del Derecho Español* 51 (1981): 366–417.

19 Valdéon, *Alfonso X*, 31.

20 *As Siete Partidas del Rey Don Alfonso El Sabio cotejadas con varios códices antiguos* (Madrid: La Real Academia de la Historia, 1807), vol. 1 [hence *Especulo*] I–I, i, "Por ende nos el sobre dicho rey don Alfonso . . . feziemos estas leyes que son escriptas en este libro, que es espeio del derecho porque se judguen todos los de nuestros regnos e de nuestro senhorio," 1. Citations from the *Especulo*, *Fuero Juzgo* and the *Partidas* are given in Roman numerals in the format: [book/*partida*]–[title], [law] followed by the page number in Indo-Arabic numerals in the modern edition.

21 Valdéon, *Alfonso X*, 30; García de Cortázar, *La época medieval*, 308.

22 Álvarez Palenzuela, *Historia*, 499; Valdéon, *Alfonso X*, 31.

23 Craddock, "La cronologia," 395–396.

24 Martin, *La península*, 421; Craddock, "La cronologia," 397; Valdéon, Salrach and Zabalo, *Feudalismo y Consolidación*, 66. Both the *Especulo* and the *Fuero Real* also met with protests.

25 The *Partidas* were translated into Portuguese around 1341: José Domingues, "A Tradição Medieval das Sete Partidas em Portugal," 10, https://7partidas.hypotheses.org/692 (last accessed 1 June 2017); José Mattoso, *Identificação de um País. Ensaio sobre as origens de Portugal – 1096–1325*, II: *Composição* (Lisbon: Editorial Estampa, 1985), 96; Marcello Caetano, *História do Direito Português (1140–1495)*, second edition (Lisbon: Verbo, 1985), 342.

26 Alexander Marey, "El rey, el emperador, el tirano: el concepto del poder e ideal político en la cultura intelectual Alfonsina," in *Cuadernos de Historia del Derecho* (Madrid: Universidad Complutense, 2014), 231–232; Valdéon, *Alfonso X*, 30; Álvarez Palenzuela, *Historia*, 499.

27 George Martin, "De nuevo la fecha del Setenario," *e.Spania. Revue electronique d'études hispaniques médiévales* 2 (2006), http://e-spania.revues.org/ (last accessed 20 October 2018).

28 *Especulo* I–I, "De las leyes. E fabla en él que ninguno non se puede escusar de la pena por decir que non sabe las leyes," 2.

29 *As Siete Partidas del Rey Don Alfonso el Sabio cotejadas con varios códices antiguos* (Madrid: La Real Academia de la Historia, 1807), vol. 2, [hence *Partida*] II, 3. Compare with *Especulo* I–II, "De la santa Trenidat e de la fe Catolica"; ibid., I–III, "De los articolos de Fe e de los Sacramentos de santa iglesia," 7–10.

30 *Especulo* II, 12.

31 *Especulo* II–I, "De la guarda de la persona del rey," 12; ibid., II–I, i, "Que cosa es rey," 12–13.

32 Ortiz Palanques, "El concepto de rey," 140, 150; Marina Kleine, "Os elementos do corpo político e a justiça nas *Siete Partidas* de Afonso X (1221–1284)," *Politeia* 5 (2007): 116.

33 *Especulo* II–I, iii, "Por que convino que fuese rey," 13–14.
34 *Especulo* II–I, ii, "Por que a nombre rey," 13. Kleine, "O s elementos do corpo político," 107.
35 *Especulo* II–I, v, "Por que razón debe ser el rey onrado," 14.
36 Ortiz Palanques, "El concepto de rey," 139.
37 *Fuero Juzgo*, Exórdio, ii, "estabelecemos que daqui adelantre, los Res deben ser esligidos, ó en á Cidat de roma; ó en aquel logar, ó morir el outro Rey ... mas las cosas que elos ganáren, non las debe haber nengono de sos fijos, e sos herederos," 3.
38 *Especulo* II–XVI, i, "Que deven facer al fijo mayor del rey, que es heredero del regno en sus cosas," 68–69.
39 Jeroen Duindam, *Dynasties: A Global History of Power, 1300–1800* (Cambridge: Cambridge University Press, 2016), 3–4.
40 *Partida* II–I, vii, "Porqué convino que fuse rey": "Complidas et verdaderas razones mostraron los sábios antíguos por que convino que fuese rey ... Mas el home de todo esto non há nada para si à menos de ayuda de muchos ... et por ende fue mester por derecha fuera que hobiesen uno que fuese cabeza dellos, por cuyo seso se acordasen et se guiasen ... et por esta razon convino que fuesen reyes, et los tomasen los homes por señores," 12–13.
41 Henry A. Myers and Herwig Wolfram, *Medieval Kingship* (Chicago: Nelson Hall, 1982), 4.
42 Madden, *Political Theory*, 88.
43 Duindam, *Dynasties*, 127. The same idea appears in Ruth Mazo Karras, *From Boys to Men: Formations of Masculinity in Late Medieval Europe* (Philadelphia: University of Pennsylvania Press, 2003), 35.
44 *Partida* II, "Que fabla de los emperadores, et de los reyes et de los otros grandes señores en cuyo poder es la justicia temporal," 1.
45 Socarras, *Alfonso X*, 9–20, 131–137; Álvarez Palenzuela, *Historia*, 498–499; Ladero Quesada, *La formación medieval*, 51–55.
46 Ladero Quesada, *La formación medieval*, 52–53; Socarras, *Alfonso X*, 15–20, 135–136.
47 Socarras, *Alfonso X*, 134–136; Mattoso, *Identificação*, 95–96.
48 Ortiz Palanques, "El concepto de rey," 146.
49 *Partida* II–I, v, "Qué cosa es rey, et como es puesto en lugar de Dios," 11; ibid., II–I, vii, "Por qué convino que fuese rey, et qué lugar tiene," 12–13.
50 *Partida* II–I, ix, "En quantas maneras se gana el regno derechamente," 15–17.
51 *Partida* II–I, ix, 16.
52 *Partida* II–I, x, "si el usase mal de su poderio en las maneras que dixiemos en esta ley, quel puedan decir las gentes tirano," 17–18.
53 *Partida* II–I, vii, 13; viii, 13–15.
54 *Partida* II–I, xi, "Quáles son los otros grandes et honrados señores que non son emperadores nin reyes," 18–19; xii, 20–21.
55 *Especulo* II–XIV, i, 54.
56 Strictly speaking, 'court' could mean the people who lived close to the king and who helped him govern his territory: Kleine, "Para la guardia de la poridad," 233.
57 *Partida* II–XXVII, 36–37.
58 Marey, "El rey, el emperador, el tirano," 232; Kleine, "Os elementos do corpo politico," 103–104.
59 *Partida* II–XXVIII, 37–38.
60 *Especulo* II–XIV, ii, 54–55; iii, 55–56.
61 *Especulo* II–XII, i, 42.
62 *Especulo* II–XIV, iii, 55.
63 António Resende de Oliveira, "Beatriz Afonso (1244–1300)," in *As primeiras rainhas*, eds. Maria Alegria Fernandes Marques et al. (Lisbon: Círculo de Leitores, 2012), 411; Rita Costa-Gomes, "Les déplacements de la cour portugaise. Deux axiomes et quatre hypothèses pour une comparaison des monarchies ibériques," in *e-Spania. Revue interdisciplinaire d'etudes hispaniques médiévales et modernes* 5 (2009), https://e-spania.revues.org/18853 (last accessed 20 October 2018).
64 *Especulo* II–III, 23.
65 Duindam, *Dynasties*, 14; Myers and Wolfram, *Medieval Kingship*, 4.

66 *Fuero Juzgo*, xiv, "Los hijos del rey deben ser respectados, y amparados de los Subditos, de manera, que de nadie recibon daño alguno," 19; xv, "Los hijos del Rey deben ser honrados por el Pueblo, y sus cosas guardadas," 20; xvi, "Después de muerto el Rey, no se han de hacer injurias á la mujer, hijos, ó familia del Rey," 21; xvii, "La Reyna viuda, y sus hijos, sean honrados y respectados, y no se les haga fuerza ni daño alguno en sus personas ni bienes," 22.

67 Diana Pelaz Flores, *Poder y representación de la reina en la Corona de Castilla (1418–1496)* (Ávila: Junta de Castilla y León, 2017), 14, 17.

68 *Partida* II–VI, "Qual debe el rey seer a su muger et ella a el," 47.

69 *Partida* II–VI, ii, "Como el rey debe amar, et honrar et guardar á su mujer," 49.

70 *Partida* II–VI, i, "Quáles cosas debe el rey catar en su casamento," 48.

71 *Especulo* II–III, "De la guarda de la reyna," 23.

72 *Especulo* II–III, 23.

73 *Partida* II–VI, ii, 48.

74 *Especulo* II–III, ii, "Que ninguno non mate nin fiera la reyna nin descubra su poridad," 24.

75 "La piedra angular del ser reina: la unión matrimonial," Pelaz Flores, *Poder y representación de la reina*, 96.

76 Pelaz Flores, *Poder y representación de la reina*, 15, 24, 34–41; Manuela Santos Silva, "Felipa de Lancáster, la dama inglesa que fue modelo de reginalidad en Portugal (1387–1415)," *Anuario de Estudios Medievales* 46, no. 1 (2016): 203–230.

77 *Especulo* II–III, i, "Como debe ser guardada otra mugier que el rey oviese que non fuese de bendecion," 24.

78 Ruth M. Karras, *Unmarriages. Women, Men and Sexual Unions in the Middle Ages* (Philadelphia: University of Pennsylvania Press, 2012), 11, 17; Duindam, *Dynasties*, 123–124.

79 Karras, *Unmarriages*, 12–18; Georges Duby, *Le chevalier, la femme et le prêtre: Le mariage dans la France féodale* (Paris: Hachette, 1981), 48; Manuela Santos Silva, "Reminiscências matriciais nos casamentos régios medievais," in *Casamentos da Família Real Portuguesa. Diplomacia e Cerimonial*, eds. Ana Maria S. A. Rodrigues, Manuela Santos Silva and Ana Leal de Faria (Lisbon: Círculo de Leitores, 2016), vol. 1, 19–22.

80 Duby, *Le chevalier*, 33.

81 Karras, *Unmarriages*, 3, 10, 45; Duby, *Le chevalier*, 178.

82 In the fourth *Partida*, the legislator defines a statute for the concubines as in *Especulo*, XIV, i.

83 *Especulo* II–IV, iii, "Que los fijos del rey deben ser guardados que oviere de ganancia," 26–27.

84 *Especulo* II–IV, i and ii, 25–26.

85 *Especulo* II–IV, iv, v and vi, 27–28.

86 *Especulo* II–V, 29.

87 *Especulo* II–IV, vii, "De la guarda de los fijos del rey de ganancia," 28.

88 *Partida* II–V, i, 21, 33–47. Nicholas Orme, *From Childhood to Chivalry: The Education of the English Kings and Aristocracy 1066–1530* (London & New York: Methuen, 1984), 109–110.

89 *Partida* II–V, xvi, "Cómo el rey debe seer acucioso en aprender ler, et de los saberes lo que pudiere," 44.

90 *Partida* II–V, xvii, "Cómo el rey se debe trabajar de conocer los homes," 44–45.

91 *Partida* II–V, xix, 46. Mazo Karras, *From Boys to Men*, 28, 35; Orme, *From Childhood to Chivalry*, 182–185.

92 *Partida* II–V, xx, "Cómo el rey debe ser mañoso en cazar," 46.

93 *Partida* II–V, xix, 45.

94 *Partida* II–V, xx, 47.

95 *Partida* II–VII, "Qual debe ser el rey a sus fijos et ellos a el," 49–60.

96 *Partida* II–VII, i, "Cómo el rey debe amar à sus fijos, et porque razones," 50.

97 *Partida* II–VII, ii, "Cómo el rey há de facer criar à sus fijos," 50–51.

98 *Partida* II–VII, iii, "En qué manera deben ser guardados los fijos de los reyes," 51–52.

99 *Partida* II–VII, iv, "Que los fijos de los reyes deben haber ayos, et quáles deben seer," 52–53; v, "Qué cosas deben acostumbrar los ayos à los fijos de los reyes para ser limpios et apuestos en el comer," 53–54.

100 *Partida* II–VII, vi, "Cómo los fijos de los reyes deben ser mesurados en beber el vino," 54–55; vii, "Como los ayos deben mostrar à los fijos de los reyes que fablen bien et

apuestamente," 55; viii, "Que los ayos deben mostrar à los fijos de los reyes que hayan buen contenente," 56–57.

101 *Partida* II–VII, ix, "Quáles cosas debe el rey enseñar à sus fijos," 57.

102 *Partida* II–VII, x, "Qué cosas deben mostrar à los fijos de los reyes quando comienzan à seer donceles," 58–59.

103 *Partida* II–VII, xiii, "Cómo el rey debe facer bien à sus fijos, et castigar los quando erraren," 60.

104 *Partida* II–VII, xi, "Quáles amas deben haber las fijas de los reyes, et cómo deben ser guardadas," 59.

105 *Partida* II–VII, xi, 59.

106 *Partida* II–VII, xii, "Cómo el rey et la reyna se deben trabajar en casar sus fijas," 59–60.

107 *Partida* II–VIII, i, "Cómo debe el rey amar, et honrar et facer bien à aquellos con quien ha debdo por linaje," 60. For this translation: *Las Siete Partidas* II: *Medieval Government: The World of Kings and Warriors*, ed. Robert I. Burns, trans. Samuel Parsons Scott (Philadelphia: University of Pennsylvania Press, 2001), 309.

108 *Livro de Linhagens do Conde D. Pedro*, ed. José Mattoso, 2 vols (Lisbon: Academia das Ciências, 1980), vol. 2, prologue.

109 *Partida* II–VIII, i, 60.

110 *Partida* II–VIII, i, "En qué manera debe el rey escarmentar à sus parientes quando algunt yerro ficieren," 61.

111 *Partida* II–IX, "Qual debe el rey ser a sus oficiales, et a los de su casa et de su corte, el ellos a el," 61.

112 Kleine, "Para la guardia de la poridad," 232.

113 *Partida* II–IX, 61–86.

114 *Especulo* II–XII, 41–46; II–XIII, 46–54.

115 *Especulo* II–XIII, ix, "Como devem seer onrados e guardados los de criazon del rey, e que pena merece qui los mataze o los desornase [*sic*]," 53.

116 *Especulo* II–XV, "Como devem guardar a la reyna en sus mugieres e en sus omes, e en sus heredades, e en todo lo al que ha," 60–67.

117 *Partida* II–XIV, iii, 130.

118 "The part of a house to which access is restricted or forbidden," almost as if it were an Ottoman harem: Duindam, *Dynasties*, 110.

119 *Especulo* II–XV, viii, 65.

120 *Especulo* II–XV, xii, 67.

121 *Especulo* II–XVI, i, "Que deven facer al fijo mayor del rey, que es heredero del regno en sus cosas," 68–69.

122 *Partida* II–VI, ii, "Como el rey debe amar, et honrar et guardar à su mujer," 48.

123 *Partida* II–XIV, iii, 130.

124 *Fuero Juzgo* III–I, vi, "Ninguno puede mandar en arras a su mujer, mas que la decima parte de sus bienes," 89–91; Ana Maria S.A. Rodrigues and Manuela Santos Silva, "Private Properties, Seigniorial Tributes and Jurisdictional Rents: The Income of the Queens of Portugal in the Middle Ages," in *Women and Wealth in Late Medieval Europe*, ed. Theresa Earenfight (New York: Palgrave Macmillan, 2010), 209–228.

125 Theresa Earenfight, *Queenship in Medieval Europe* (London: Palgrave MacMillan, 2013), 160–168.

126 A point noted by Theresa M. Vann, "The Theory and Practice of Medieval Castilian Queenship," in *Queens, Regents and Potentates*, ed. Theresa M. Vann (Cambridge: Academia Press, 1993), 125–147.

127 *Especulo* II–XVI, i, 69.

128 Maria do Rosário Ferreira, "Urraca e Teresa: o paradigma perdido," *Guarecer on-line* (2010), 1–16, http://ifilosofia.up.pt/gfm/seminar/docs/Urraca_e_Teresa_Marsupio_Guarecer%5B1%5D.pdf (last accessed 21 August 2018).

129 José Domingues, "As partidas de Afonso X e a natureza jurídico-política do Estado Português," in *Natura e Natureza no tempo de Afonso X, o Sábio*, eds. José Carlos Ribeiro Miranda and Maria do Rosário Ferreira (Vila Nova de Famalicão: Edições Humus, Lda, 2015), 32.

Key works

Cradock, Jerry, "La cronologia de las obras legislativas de Alfonso X el Sabio," *Anuario de Historia del Derecho Español* 51 (1981): 366–417.

Kleine, Marina, "Os elementos do corpo político e a justiça nas *Siete Partidas* de Afonso X (1221–1284)," *Politeia* 5, pmd (1/3/2007): 103–117.

Kleine, Marina, "Para la guardia de la poridad, del cuerpo y de la tierra del rey: los oficiales reales y la organización de la corte de Alfonso X," *Historia. Instituciones. Documentos* 35 (2008): 229–240.

Madden, Marie R., *Political Theory and Law in Medieval Spain* (New York: Fordham University Press, 1930).

Marey, Alexander, "El rey, el emperador, el tirano: el concepto del poder e ideal político en la cultura intelectual alfonsina," *Cuadernos de Historia del Derecho Vol. 21* (Madrid: Universidad Complutense, 2014), 229–242.

Ortiz Palanques, Marco, "El concepto de rey, reino y territorio en las siete partidas," *Revista Filosofia* 23 (2012): 139–162.

Scorpo, Antonella Liuzzo, "Religious Frontiers and Overlapping Cultural Borders: The Power of Personal and Political Exchanges in the Works of Alfonso X of Castile (1252–1284)," *Al-Masaq* 23, no. 3 (2011): 217–236.

4

PERSONAL UNION, COMPOSITE MONARCHY AND 'MULTIPLE RULE'

Charlotte Backerra

The most common form of premodern monarchical rule was the composite monarchy. In early modern Europe, the union of realms – kingdoms or principalities linked by the rule of one monarch – was a common phenomenon. And it continues to be a form that flourishes today. The House of Windsor still leads a composite monarchy encompassing large parts of the world: the UK, Canada, New Zealand, Australia and other countries continue to recognize Queen Elizabeth II as their Head of State.

This chapter traces the history of personal unions and composite monarchies from the High Middle Ages to the early nineteenth century. It will begin by exploring definitions used by historians over the last decades to show the development of this field of studies, which has been especially notable since the late 1980s. Subsequently, it will analyse the origins and endings of personal unions as well as the forces that foster both integration and separation by looking at historical examples from European history. Actors, institutions, political culture, geography and historical coincidences could contribute to or resist the development of composite monarchies. Some territories were pointedly kept separate from each other, while in other contexts, monarchs, elites, and/or the people tried to merge two or more dominions into one realm either politically, legally, economically, or via a combination of all three. It was challenging to do so when actors had to cross long distances between territories or had to speak different languages, adhere to different codes of conduct, and so on. Composite rule meant that there were flexibilities allowing the continued use of different laws, forms of financial governance, or other traditions connected with each former single kingdom within a nevertheless unified monarchy. For each element discussed, only a few examples will be mentioned. A conclusion with some consideration of the present day will complete this overview.

The analyses of these developments provide an opportunity to look at questions of rulership and statehood, of national or regional identities, and of political culture in a broader sense, to trace origins of changes in territorial and national borders, and to examine possible causes for these changes. What steps were taken in the process of a developing composite monarchy? What motivations did other social and political groups have to prevent or countenance these unified but diverse realms? Last but not least, for a Europe that has reached a crossroads in the present day, the development and structuring of a composite state in history remains an interesting template worth analysing.[1]

Definitions

Both contemporaries and historians have tried to find definitions for the rulership of one monarch over different territories since political thought turned its focus on the early modern state in the second half of the twentieth century. With respect to a legal definition, 'personal union' in terms of rulership means that one individual acts as monarch for different principalities; the only connection between the latter is the ruler. The monarch may have different ranks and titles as a ruler: for example, they may be emperor, king and duke at the same time. Emperor Charles VI's shortened title on a seal of 1725 demonstrates this perfectly:

> Charles VI, by God's Grace Roman Emperor, all times Augmenter [of the Empire], King of Germany, Spain, Hungary, Bohemia, both Sicilies, of Jerusalem and the [West] Indies, Archduke of Austria, Duke of Burgundy, Brabant, Milan, Prince of Swabia, Catalonia, Margrave of the Holy Roman Empire, Count of Habsburg, Flanders, [and] Tyrol.[2]

Some of the titles of composite monarchies – including Croatia and Slavonia as part of Hungary, Silesia and Moravia as part of Bohemia, and Carniola, Carinthia and Styria as part of Austria – are missing here. In addition, several older, contested principalities, such as the duchy of Limburg, are not mentioned. Neither are the newly integrated eastern domains conquered after the successful wars against the Ottoman Empire (Serbia, Bosnia, Walachia) and Mantua as one of the new Italian territories. Spain and Catalonia are, however, mentioned, despite being claimed by the new Bourbon dynasty of the Spanish kingdoms.

At the opposite end of the continuum, a 'real union' would be a union based on common laws and institutions but where the lands ruled were not yet considered one territory in legal terms – an example, the case of Schleswig and Holstein, will be discussed later in the chapter. While both terms continue to be used, historiographical definitions of forms of monarchical rule are mostly based on discussions about state formation processes and use either 'state' or 'monarchy' with adjectives. Most are based on specific (pre-modern) examples, thus explaining the style of rulership and government according to these cases.

Helmut Koenigsberger has worked on composite forms of government since the 1970s.[3] The most general distinction he makes is between composite states separated by sea or other realms, and composite states with adjoining territories. Koenigsberger generally prefers the term 'states' because he writes about monarchies as well as republics and uses the word as a more general descriptive.[4] He emphasizes the role of the estates and/or noble/privy councils, and therefore the difference between *dominum regale* and *dominum politicum et regale*. The first was rule without the necessity of estates or representative assemblies for levying taxes or issuing laws. The French monarchy in the seventeenth and eighteenth centuries offers the best example of this.[5] *Dominum politicum et regale*, on the other hand, meant that estates or parliaments and the monarch had to collaborate for the functioning of the monarchy.

The latter was more common: different regional assemblies were responsible for each territory in a composite state; while general assemblies could exist, they were not necessary.[6] These phenomena will be discussed further in a later section of this chapter on institutions and structures.

John Elliott differentiates more generally between two types of composite monarchies based on their origins and organizational foundations.[7] The first, an 'accessory union', involved adding one territory to another, with no distinction of laws and rights drawn between the two.[8] The second option was a union *aeque principaliter*, a union of equal realms. Each kingdom – or principality – kept its rights and privileges and was governed as if it was a singular territory ruled by one monarch. According to Elliott, this form became the dominant, yet adaptable, form of composite monarchies.[9] Besides regional estates, other elements of functioning composite monarchies were: government officials appointed according to territorial traditions; patronage systems unique to each principality; and – at least initially – separate legal systems.[10] The problem lay in the equality or independence of the principalities: as most composite monarchies included a more dominant component with regard to dynastic, political, or economic power or territorial expansion, the other part(s) might feel – or be – threatened by it, causing disquiet and insecurities.[11]

Elliott's idea of a union of equal realms fits especially the Spanish monarchy from the rule of the Catholic kings (*Reyes Católicos*), Ferdinand II of Aragon and Isabel I of Castile, in the late fifteenth century and later during the Habsburg era, and the Austrian hereditary lands of the Habsburgs from the sixteenth century. This concept, termed *zusammengesetzte Monarchie* in German and *monarquía compuesta* in Spanish, has been favoured by many Spanish, Austrian and German historians.[12] In terms of British history, Conrad Russell and Jenny Wormald speak of 'multiple kingdoms', even though the underlying concept of composite monarchies based on personal unions remains the same. The kingdoms of England, Scotland and Ireland and their intertwined history led first to the creation of personal unions and then composite monarchies between, first, England – since the Middle Ages a combined realm of England and Wales[13] – and Ireland, and of England and Scotland in 1603. As will be discussed later in the chapter, the unification of the English and the Scottish parliaments as a British parliament in 1707, to which the Irish parliament was added in 1801, strengthened the union without abolishing legal, religious, economic, or cultural differences.[14]

Looking at the monarch's relationship with his or her subjects, Harald Gustafsson points out that there existed differences in most cases.[15] Most monarchs were not only kings (or queens), but held titles as king, duke, count, baron and so on at the same time, and their subjects related to them accordingly. Gustafsson contrasts the internal rule between unitary and conglomerate states. In very few monarchies, such as England in the early modern period, the monarch held these titles without any legally differing ties to his or her subjects. Such cases might be called a singular principality, or unitary state. Gustafsson classifies most monarchies, however, as conglomerate states. One example is Denmark, whose king was also the duke of Schleswig and the duke of Holstein. Here two united duchies were ruled in personal union with the Danish kingdom; at the same time, one duchy was a fiefdom of the Danish crown, while the other was a fiefdom of the Holy Roman Empire.[16]

Coming to the same conclusions, Franz Bosbach has proposed using the term *Mehrfachherrschaft* instead of composite or conglomerate monarchies.[17] Unfortunately, the varied and multi-layered meaning of the German word does not easily translate into English: 'the rule over multiple territories and/or according to multiple types of law' is one way of unpacking this complex concept. The term can be applied to monarchies as well as republics but differs from 'composite/conglomerate state' in that it does not include any implicit reference to the modern state. As such, it is now accepted by many German-speaking historians as a way of characterizing early modern styles of rulership.

For cases originating in a dynasty's politics, Robert von Friedeburg and John Morrill suggest the term 'dynastic agglomerate'.[18] This draws attention to the fact that the initiators were part of 'princely dynasties pursuing not only dynastic ambitions and princely prestige but the consequences of dynastic chance'.[19] These agglomerates were not stable structures, but could rapidly change. Monarchs, elites and other actors had to adapt to growing numbers of dominions and peoples joined together, or to the dissolution of the whole.[20] The various examples of composite monarchies based on dynastic politics will be discussed in what follows.

The case of dominions ruled by two (or more) princes, the so-called condominium, is rarely reflected on by researchers and will not be discussed in any detail here. Andorra, for example, was ruled jointly by the Count of Foix and the Bishop of Urgell from 1278. The county was later joined by marriage with the kingdom of Navarre, so that, in 1594 when Henry king of Navarre became Henry IV of France, the rights to Foix passed to the king of France. According to the constitution of 1993, the present day co-rulers – called *Copríceps* or co-princes – of the sovereign state of Andorra are the Bishop of Urgell and the President of the Republic of France.[21]

In the following, the term 'composite monarchies' will be used when speaking about the rule of one monarch over multiple territories – kingdoms and other principalities as well as all forms of dominions – according to the respective laws and customs of each. Early modern colonial empires like Spain or England/Great Britain are most appropriately discussed within the context of such composite monarchies.[22] Their specific situations, which involved long distances between the territories and widely different cultural as well as historical backgrounds, are, however, mostly analysed without an explicit reference to 'composite monarchy'. The limitations of this chapter mean the focus here will be on developments within Europe; multi-continental issues will only be mentioned in passing.

Origins and endings of personal unions in premodern Europe

The most common origin of personal unions lay in dynastic politics; they were principally the result of marriage policies. Marriages between partners of equal standing were favoured and, when both were of ruling dynasties, dominions, titles and privileges could be combined through marriage. The Spanish kingdoms of Castile and Aragon – with the latter already being a composite monarchy – were first united by the marriage of Isabel I of Castile and Ferdinand II of Aragon in 1469. With the death of their only son John in 1497, and of their eldest daughter Isabella (married to the king of Portugal) and of her son, Miguel de la Paz, in 1498 and 1500 respectively, Charles, the son of their third child, Juana, inherited all the realms.[23]

Notably, in Spanish, this composite monarchy was called 'the Spains' (*las Españas*), signifying the multiple principalities included.[24] Juana was married to Philip, who had inherited, through his mother, the duchy of Burgundy and the Low Countries and was the son of Maximilian, emperor of the Holy Roman Empire and ruler of the Habsburg dominions. Their son, Charles, thus inherited not only the Spanish kingdoms with all their dependent territories and colonies all over the world but also Burgundy and the Netherlands, as well as the Habsburg hereditary lands in Austria and Germany; he was subsequently elected emperor after his grandfather's death in 1519.[25] With these legacies, Charles V (as he styled himself as emperor) became the single most powerful monarch in Europe in the first half of the sixteenth century, ruling over the proverbial 'empire on which the sun never sets'.

When there was no direct heir to a composite monarchy, successors were chosen according to the inheritance laws of each territory. Elizabeth I decided not to marry, so her closest royal relative James VI, king of Scotland, also became king of England (and Ireland) on her death in 1603, creating a personal union of all the kingdoms of the British Isles. In a case similar to that of James VI & I, Henry III, who ruled over the kingdom of Navarre, became King Henry IV of France after the assassination of the last Valois king in 1589. In 1620, this composite monarchy of France and Navarre became a real union, a union ruled by Louis XIII of France (and II of Navarre) as its common ruler. The union was jointly administered and possessed shared institutions, but France and Navarre remained distinct territories in legal terms.[26]

Other personal unions and composite monarchies came about because of elite decisions. In most cases, a dynastic crisis and strong estates laid the groundwork, sometimes with the added element of an electoral monarchy. One example of this was the union of the three Nordic kingdoms of Norway, Denmark and Sweden finalized in Kalmar in 1397. Based on dynastic politics, Margarete, the Danish king's daughter and Norwegian king's wife, was accepted by the elites of both countries as regent after her father, husband and son had all died. After a rebellion in Sweden, that kingdom was added to the composite monarchy. With the coronation of Margarete's relative Erik in Kalmar, measures were taken to combine the three into a true union first by the politics of Margarete as regent and later by King Erik, whose unifying policies in the end caused the first dissolution of the Union of Kalmar in 1440. From 1442, a true personal union was established under King Christoffer, who again united the Scandinavian kingdoms until his death in 1448.[27]

A third type of personal union came about through conquest. When conquest resulted in the death, deposition, or abdication of the former ruler, the conqueror could establish himself as the legitimate ruler. Most conquests of European dominions were based on alleged dynastic rights, and in many cases the victor also managed to gain the elite's and the people's support. An example is the dynastic crisis in Portugal during the 1580s, which allowed Philip II to take over on behalf of the Spanish Habsburgs.[28] With overseas territories and colonies, this was different, as former kingdoms and dominions were often not acknowledged by the European conquerors. Instead, new dominions were established, like the Spanish viceroyalties in Central and South America.

A combination of all three above-mentioned causes was the background for the personal union of England, Scotland, Ireland and Orange-Nassau under William III and Mary Stuart between 1689 and 1701.[29] Both William and Mary had a dynastic claim to the British kingdoms – Mary as the daughter of the former deposed king, James II, and William as his nephew (his sister's son) as third in line after the younger princess Anne. In a situation of political conflict, William managed to secure the support of a large proportion of the political elite, who backed Mary's claim for power against the reigning king. William, also the stadtholder of the province of Holland in the Netherlands, invaded England with his army in 1688. When James II fled to France in December 1688, William and Mary were then the logical choice for the political elite to choose as the new king and queen. With, respectively, the Bill of Rights (1689) – enshrining the Declaration of Right in statutory form – and the Claim of Right Act (1689), the parliaments of England and Scotland agreed to the continuation of the personal union of the British kingdoms as well as to their personal union with William's Dutch and German territories.[30]

Probably the most basic principle of dynastic rule was to look for the expansion of the dynasty's rights, lands and subjects, and to secure their transfer to the following generations. Consequently, most monarchs did not want to end an existing personal union.[31] If an existing composite monarchy was split because of inheritance rights, most often the dynasty tried to keep up the appearances of a coherent unit. The Habsburg dynasty, even though it seemed to be the best example for the creation of personal unions through dynastic politics, also employed the partition of territories when several sons might inherit. Examples can be found in the later Middle Ages, prior to the rule of Maximilian I, but are also notable on two occasions in the sixteenth century when the dynasty's power was at its height. Charles V decided to give the Austrian lands to his brother Ferdinand in 1521/2 when the division of the Spanish and the Austrian Habsburgs seemed the only way to appease the latter, and, later, in 1564, it proved necessary to split the Austrian hereditary lands between Ferdinand's sons.[32]

Dynastic treaties to secure reciprocal inheritance between two separated lines of a dynasty were a common phenomenon. With the Treaty of Oñate in 1617, the Spanish Habsburgs secured their rights of inheritance to the kingdoms of Bohemia and Hungary if the Austrian lines became extinct. In the same period, the Spanish king Philip IV and the Austrian monarch Ferdinand II declared there to be a reciprocal right of inheritance between the Habsburg dynasties.[33] These treaties and declarations of intent could, however, not win against the strong opposition to a new universal Habsburg composite monarchy when the very problem they should have solved occurred in reality at the end of the seventeenth century when the Spanish Habsburgs faced extinction because Charles II of Spain died without issue. This situation will be discussed later on. For another dynasty, the Wittelsbach, the dynastic treaty of Pavia of 1329, which had divided the dynasty's lands between two branches of the family into the Electorate of the Palatinate, including the Upper Palatinate in Bavaria, and the Dukedom of Bavaria, became effective in 1777. After the extinction of several other religiously diverse and territorially widespread lines, the Elector Palatine finally inherited the territories of the Bavarian line, uniting the Wittelsbach dominions for the first time since the Middle Ages.[34]

The chances of dynastic and territorial splits were lowered if there was a universal, normally male, heir. The practice of primogeniture was common, for example, in Italy, France and England from the (late) medieval period. Yet European monarchies like the Habsburgs, Wittelsbachs, Guelphs, Hessians and others continued the practice of shared or divided inheritance; it was only widely discouraged or abandoned in favour of primogeniture in the late seventeenth and eighteenth centuries.

Forces favouring integration and separation

As the idea of a personal union is, by its nature, a 'top down' concept, monarchs and the members of their families were most often responsible for the joint government of the kingdoms that were brought together. Some actively tried to integrate the territories under their rule: besides a possible expansion of the dynasty's power, a composite monarchy also often reduced the danger of wars between territories, especially if the principalities had a history of violence and conflict.[35] Such was the case with James VI & I and his push to combine the English and Scottish kingdoms with all their territories. After his accession to the English throne in 1603, he wanted not only a personal union of his kingdoms but 'an uniformitie of constitutions both of body and minde ... A communitie of the Language, the principal meanes of Civil societie, An unitie of Religion, the chiefest band of heartie Union, and the surest knot of lasting.'[36] His dominions should be united as the 'kingdom of Great Britain', symbolized by the Union Jack as a common flag and maps and orders given to 'North and South Britain'.[37]

James's 'Union of Love' did not succeed, even though he tried not only to unite councils, courts and churches but also members of the nobility in marriage. He granted the latter lands in both kingdoms and also supported legal measures such as Calvin's Case, which argued for the 'Britishness' of the people born in the combined kingdom, the so-called Post-Nati.[38] Working against James's ambition was the reluctance of the political elite – probably also of the people – of England to accept Scotland (and the Scottish) as an equal component of the union. But the decision of James VI & I to reside in London and to rule the kingdoms of the British Isles from the more dominant kingdom had long-term implications. His efforts were the basis on which the militarily enforced union of Oliver Cromwell's Commonwealth later stood. They determined that even when the end of the Stuart dynasty in the Protestant line was anticipated, the Scottish parliament's decision to set in motion a process for the selection of a separate Scottish king, via the Act of Security 1704, while a theoretical possibility, proved in practical terms impossible to implement. Instead, with the union of the parliaments in 1707, a composite monarchy became a 'real union' under the name Great Britain.[39]

For some monarchs, combining their crowns and lands was not an active policy in their own lifetime, yet they tried to keep their realm together with succession laws that passed all titles, territories and rulership to their successor. The most prominent example of the eighteenth century was Emperor Charles VI and the so-called Pragmatic Sanction of 1713, which was accepted as law in all the territories he personally ruled until 1725.[40] Charles had survived both his father and brother but had had to leave Spain – the first kingdom he claimed – as he was unable to keep the throne and crown after his election and coronation as emperor of the Holy Roman Empire in 1711. While he finally accepted the loss of Spain in 1725, Charles wanted to leave every other territory and title to any future son and heir – and lacking a male heir, to a daughter – in their totality. The Pragmatic

Sanction settled the indivisibility of the Habsburg territories. Dynastically, Charles introduced primogeniture, the right of inheritance for any eldest son, and combined it with the so-called 'contingent succession' of daughters. With this, he favoured his heirs before those of his late elder brother, making his line the dominant one in any future succession.[41]

Charles was successful in combining the territories as a de facto *monarchia Austriaca* by the legal succession of his daughter Maria Theresa in 1740. In the following decades, in both Maria Theresa's reign, as well as those of her sons, a multi-layered policy led to the establishment of the Austrian-Habsburg monarchy as a composite monarchy. With the adoption of the title of 'Emperor of Austria' in 1804, Francis II (as Holy Roman Emperor) became Emperor Francis I of Austria, ruling over Austria, Bohemia, Silesia, Romania and Hungary as well as all other remaining Habsburg territories. This made him for two years – from 1804 to 1806 – the only declared emperor of two empires in history.[42] From the mid-eighteenth century, central ministries were established, officials, officers and courtiers from the different parts of the monarchy were appointed and laws were approximated.[43] At the same time, religious, cultural and linguistic differences were maintained and supported. For example, constitutional texts were translated into the languages of the Empire, schooling continued in the local vernaculars and – later – a hymn was introduced that was sung in every spoken language of the Austrian Empire. This anthem-hymn was introduced as a folk song, not a national anthem, which, together with the free translations ordered by Emperor Francis Joseph in 1854, helped popularize it.[44]

Although the advantages of a composite monarchy were obvious to monarchs and their heirs, the rules for the political elites of such a conglomerate were not as clear. To keep monarchical unions together, the elites of every component part were needed as willing participants to help in government and administration. This was achieved, in part, by institutions such as estates or parliaments; it was also accomplished through (privy) councils, (secret) conferences and similar bodies. To the members of these and other elite circles, the benefits and rewards to be gained needed to compensate for any loss of power or say within a composite monarchy.

The composite monarchies of the kingdom of Poland and the grand duchy of Lithuania had been ruled in a personal union since the marriage of Jadwiga, Queen Regnant of Poland, with Jogaila, later known as Władysław II Jagiełło, Grand Duke of Lithuania, in 1386. But when facing a decisive defeat by Russia on the Lithuanian side, and the extinction of the dynasty of the Jagiellons and therefore the end of the personal union, the diets of both entities agreed to a real union. After separate acts in this regard, both approved it in the Union of Lublin of 1569. The Commonwealth of Poland-Lithuania, while retaining the separate dominions as kingdom and duchy, became one by the will of its elites. The treaty declared: 'The Kingdom of Poland and the Grand Duchy of Lithuania are one indivisible and uniform body and also one uniform Commonwealth, which grew and consolidated into one nation from two states and nations.'[45] By establishing an elective monarchy at the same time, the members of the nobility present in the general diet (*sejm*) gained even more power over the political future of their country.[46]

Should communication fail between monarch and elites, most often in terms of divergent political or religious opinions, this could lead to rebellions, sometimes even the deposition of monarchs and the dissolution of a composite monarchy.

In the 1560s, the Dutch elite rebelled against King Philip of Spain and his political practices in the rule of the Netherlands, which included the strong influence of the king's Spanish counsellors, the stationing of Spanish soldiers in the Netherlands and the reorganization of the episcopate as well as the restriction of bishoprics to theologians chosen by the monarch. These threatened the local elites' strong position as part of government, which had been introduced during the time of Emperor Charles V.[47] The threat involved anti-reformist measures meant to re-Catholicize the Dutch provinces. Inquisitors were, for example, sent to look for heretics in the Dutch dioceses. The conflict escalated following Calvinist iconoclasm and the subsequent passing of a thousand death sentences by the so-called Council of Blood established under the new governor, the Duke of Alba.[48] William of Orange, once one of the most influential members of the Habsburg government in the Netherlands, organized the opposition against 'some grandees of Spain', which had misled the 'trustful and good prince' in their aim to enrich themselves.[49] He could not approve 'how piteously the privileges and rights of the country with the religion of God are laying there oppressed and destroyed.'[50] The first military campaign led by William of Orange and supported by his dynasty of Nassau-Orange was unsuccessful. But the conflicts over the right to rule and the violence continued until the seven northern provinces renounced their allegiance to King Philip II in 1581 and declared, 'that the king of Spain has forfeited the sovereignty and government of the afore-said Netherlands'.[51] With this abjuration, the Dutch, as the Spanish king's subjects, had rejected the composite monarchy which had linked their country with the kingdom of Spain. For his long-term efforts in the fights against the Spanish rule, William of Orange was rewarded with the governorship of the newly founded republic. Similar cases can be seen in Scandinavian history, which led to the depositions of King Sigismund in Sweden and King Christian II in Denmark, Sweden and Norway.[52]

Institutions and structures

The above-mentioned institutions constituted, and were themselves part of, the development of composite forms of monarchy. Institutions and structures of government as well as political, religious, social, financial and legal controls contributed, alongside regents and viceroys, privy councils, estates, parliaments, Churches, legal courts and ministries, to the success or failure of the joining of formerly disjoined territories after the establishment of a union.

The vast distances between joint principalities and main residences meant that for most composite monarchies rulers needed either an itinerant court or to establish formal representatives in the form of viceroys, governors, or councils. Charles V used all of these. He himself travelled constantly from one territory to another. Life on the road, in addition to severe attacks of the gout and malaria, was detrimental to his health. The gout was a result of his unhealthy eating habits since his early adulthood.[53] At the end of his reign, even before he abdicated in favour of his brother, Charles was in constant pain and needed to be carried in a litter or sedan chair.[54] For the Holy Roman Empire, the Second Imperial Government (*Reichsregiment*) of 1521 consisted of a council of twenty under the chair of the emperor's brother, Ferdinand; it reigned whenever the ruler himself was not in the Empire. It lasted until the election of Ferdinand to the

Romano-German kingship, a position that legally made him his brother's co-ruler. In Austria, Ferdinand was first governor, and from 1522, the independent duke – it was taken for granted that he would in all matters act in the best interests of the house of Austria. Following this model, Charles appointed his wife Isabel of Portugal as regent for the Spanish kingdoms, and his aunt Margaret of Austria and later his sister Mary of Hungary as regents for the Netherlands. They were heads of government with formal councils of local elites as supporting institutions, being selected 'as regent and governor . . . to act, order, and command . . . as we ourselves do and can do in person'.[55] For the viceroyalties in the Americas, a similar system was adopted; the highest position was, however, not taken by members of the family (among other things because of the long and dangerous journey). Even though all regencies were fashioned for a specific principality, they served to bond all parts under one dynasty's rule.

Councils had been used since the Middle Ages to offer aid and support to the ruler but could also act together with a regent to govern a monarchy. In some composite monarchies these even sustained the union in times of weak or absent kings. After the Union of Kalmar fell into disarray with the death of King Christoffer in 1448, the regents and the *riksråd* (councils of the realm) preserved the kingdoms from the late fifteenth to the early sixteenth century. In Sweden, the council fashioned a new seal showing the patron saint, Erik, instead of a king. All councils, however, including those of Denmark and of Norway, acted with a clear indication that they had the Union in mind. In the end, the formerly abandoned Norwegian council even negated the Danish king's hereditary rights and insisted on the election of Frederic as king of Norway in 1524, establishing a new composite monarchy of Denmark and Norway.[56]

In the British Isles, the Council of Wales and the Marches, established in 1472 by Edward IV, acted on behalf of the Princes of Wales. Headed by the Lord President and a deputy, it consisted of twenty members selected by the king. It was responsible for the implementation of policy, civil and ecclesiastical administration as well as regional military efforts. It also acted as a criminal court, court of appeal and as a court for the poor: 'His Majesties Loving Subjects within the Dominion and Principality of Wales, and the Marches thereof, as heretofore used and accustomed, may freely repair unto the said President and Council for Relief and Justice in their lawful and necessary Suits.'[57] Similar to the Council of the North, which controlled the border region with Scotland, the Council of Wales and the Marches was a sign of the not yet fully integrated periphery of the English king's domains – after the Glorious Revolution, it was dissolved in favour of the London-based Privy Council and its sub-committees.

From the seventeenth century onwards, the role of (representative) assemblies changed in the European political systems. Parliament's growing role in the institutional context of composite monarchy is, for example, demonstrated by the establishment of Great Britain by the consecutive joining of all three parliaments of the British Isles. This first occurred for a very short time from 1654 to 1660 during the Commonwealth. It was instituted on a more permanent basis by the joining of the English and Scottish parliaments in 1707, and later of the Irish to the British parliament in 1801. The problem was that it was neither possible – nor was there a willingness – to extend this parliamentary expansion to the American colonies. The representative assemblies of the colonies did not accept the supremacy of the Westminster parliament, but insisted on their own rights, and this, among other reasons, led to the War of American Independence.[58] In contrast, in France and in the Spanish and Scandinavian kingdoms, the role of the assemblies was limited by royal control in the seventeenth century.

The constitution of the *Confoederatio Bohemica* adopted by the elites of the 'Lands of the Bohemian Crown' in 1619 made the general estates of Bohemia the heart of the confederation of the Bohemian composite monarchy. The kingdom of Bohemia, the margraviate of Moravia and the duchy of Silesia as its major constituents all had separate estates, but the *Generallandtag* should discuss and decide 'now and forever all counsel concerning the whole body'.[59] The *Confoederatio* also established the *ius incolatus*, a common citizenship for nobles in all domains, and a common board of appeal. The system favoured Protestantism: Catholics were excluded from the most important offices. All treaties of peace and alliance and of dynastic concerns were valid for all lands of the Bohemian crown, and together they were responsible for the defence of all lands. Thus, the constitution adopted a federal system, with an elected monarch at the top. Even when the Bohemian lands became part of the hereditary lands of the Habsburgs, after the defeat of the estates in the Battle of White Mountain in 1620, little changed. The Habsburg rulers appointed the Bohemian officials (though they preferred Catholics for these positions), especially for the administration of the Bohemian chancery and the position of state captain, but the structures remained until the mid-eighteenth century.[60]

Very complex, and probably unique, were the institutions integrating – but at the same time separating – the duchies of Schleswig and Holstein into the composite monarchy headed by the Danish king. The rulers were relatives of the Danish king, first three, then two dukes, who held joint overlordship of the nobility of both duchies and over territories in all parts of them. While Schleswig was a Danish fief, Holstein was imperial, and thus the duke of Holstein sat in the Imperial Diet in Regensburg – accordingly, the legal traditions and respective courts were also different. Internally, there existed one diet for both duchies, but several local institutions of self-government. With regard to Denmark, the German Chancery in Copenhagen was responsible for the duchies. Financial matters might have been the only area to be really integrated in Denmark, managed, as they were, by the Danish exchequer.[61]

One recent suggestion is that analysis of the strength of the financial markets that operated between formerly unconnected principalities is an indicator of the extent to which policies of integration were successful. In the Spanish kingdoms between 1705 and 1750, regulated by the king and the representative bodies known as the *Cortes*, the interest rates for long-term annuities were at 3 per cent in Castile, while in Aragon they stayed at 5 per cent. An interesting analysis of private borrowing shows that no one borrowed from their neighbours in the other kingdoms even though there were only minor differences in the legal framework for loans.[62] The problem lay in the different court systems. Extradition between the kingdoms was only possible in cases of capital offences, not debts, and no one could be forced before a court in another of the Iberian kingdoms:

> In accordance with the law and old traditions of these kingdoms, when someone is absent, and is [summoned to] court, we send a request [*requisitoria*] to notify him his official summons. And it seems that . . . those of the kingdom of Aragon do not consent to notify the requests which are sent to this kingdom against those who reside in it.[63]

Other institutions also signal integrated structures, for example a shared military – in the case of the union of Denmark and Norway, only the navy – or general taxes raised for war and government.[64] The same can be said for central government officials sent by the king such as the French governors and intendants, which reported directly to the king and his ministers.[65] Especially in Protestant countries, bishops could be appointed by royal command, and even a combined church system was possible as in Denmark-Norway after 1536.[66]

Political culture

The concept of 'political culture' is discussed in differing terms in the various historiographical traditions. In general, it means, 'the framework of values and attitudes regulating political actions', as they are expressed in the practices and structures of political systems.[67] Religion, language, identities and mentalities, the role of nobility, citizens, or peasants in the political system, economic values, and legal and other traditions are all elements of political culture worth discussing. In historical situations most cannot be separated but are interdependent and reciprocal. In the following, the focus will be on religion and languages as parts of the framework of values and attitudes influential for political systems.

Religious, or rather confessional, differences became highly problematic with the spread of the Reformation in Europe. It has been suggested by Daniel Nexon that the Reformation period proved problematic to dynastic rule because confessionalization reduced the possibilities of 'polyvalent signalling' in religious terms. It made it nearly impossible for rulers to 'signal different identities and values to different audiences'.[68] The consequences for Spanish rule in the Netherlands have been discussed already. But other examples from the sixteenth and seventeenth century include the end to the personal union between Sweden and Poland-Lithuania, and the Habsburgs' problems with the kingdom of Bohemia, which led to the outbreak of the Thirty Years' War in 1618. With the death of the last Jagiellon as king of Poland-Lithuania, and following the brief reigns of Stephan Báthory and Henri, duke of Anjou (later Henri III of France), his nephew Sigismund was elected to become the new king in 1587. He was brought up a Catholic by his mother, a Jagiellon, and spoke Polish. The problem lay with his paternal inheritance of Sweden, where he acceded to the throne in 1592. A formal separation of both kingdoms was not realized, and a dynastic rival, his uncle Charles, organized a synod in Uppsala, which determined that the faith of Sweden would follow the Lutheran confession. Charles used the fear of a possible re-Catholicization within a composite monarchy of Poland-Lithuania and Sweden. Sigismund's Catholic faith, the Polish legal requirement to remain primarily in Poland to keep the crown, and conflicts over the role of the Swedish assemblies led to Sigismund's deposition in Sweden in 1599 because of 'foreign rule with violence and tyranny'[69] which ended the short union of Poland-Lithuania and Sweden.[70]

A more pragmatic handling of confessional differences can be seen in the eighteenth century. The Hanoverian kings of Great Britain from 1714 were Lutherans when in their German lands. They were also heads of the English – Anglican – Church as well as of the Reformed Church of Scotland in the British Isles. One historian calls this practice 'confessional cross-dressing'.[71] In general, the dynasty had to adhere to the 'Protestant' identity of the British Isles to be accepted and to rule without fear of religiously motivated uprisings – the Act of Settlement, after all, expressly excluded the claims of the Catholic Stuarts to the throne. Contention between Protestant confessions over presbyterian and episcopal Church structures certainly led to uprisings in the seventeenth century, for example when Charles I tried to install Anglican prayer books in Scotland in 1637. His father, James VI (as king of Scotland), had already tried to formalize his influence over the presbyterian, reformed Kirk of Scotland under the heading of 'no bishop, no king' because only a hierarchical Church administration with the monarch as head of the Church offered him the possibility of ecclesiastical influence. Any policy seemingly supportive of so-called 'non-jurors' – those that could or would not pledge their allegiance to the king and Church of England (or Scotland), especially the Catholics – could lead to riots in later times, as it did with the so-called Gordon Riots after the passing of the Catholic Relief Act in 1778.[72]

More problematic was the question of religion when it was tied to linguistic differences and regional or national identities as it was in the Highlands and Islands of Scotland or in Ireland. In the early modern period, many English and Scottish settlers in Ireland spoke English rather than the Irish version of Gaelic. Following the religious transformation of the sixteenth century, the English Book of Common Prayer and the Bible had to be used in all territories. An attempt to translate these into Gaelic under Elizabeth I failed because of the resistance of English bishops in Ireland. For the most part, the Irish therefore stayed true to the Church of Rome, while the English and Scottish settlers became Protestant.[73] Over the course of the sixteenth and seventeenth centuries, the question of religion and identity became linked even more closely to Irish policy in London and in Dublin. The introduction of penal laws for Catholics excluded the majority of the Irish from the political system: roughly 200 acts were passed in this regard.[74] Together with the English Navigation Acts, which were passed against Scottish and Irish trade, the differing legal arrangements of the kingdoms were thus made obvious. Even the toleration of Catholics in all the British kingdoms and formal integration of Ireland into the composite monarchy of 'Great Britain and Ireland' in 1800/1 did not help to integrate the Catholic Irish after centuries of segregation. On the contrary, as a result of feelings of political and economic oppression, separatist tendencies grew over the centuries, leading to the Irish War of Independence, the creation of the Irish Free State in 1922 and the formal separation of the Republic of Ireland in 1937.

Since the nineteenth century, language policies were used to create unity in states with diverse ethnic groups. And today, in some countries like Belgium or Spain, linguistic differences are signs and causes of serious challenges to state integrity. Most successful with a multi-lingual (political) system, however, is Switzerland. The majority of people speak German or French, but Italian and Rhaeto-Romanic are also accepted legally and in practice. In early modern Europe, the unifying dimension of a common language was theoretically discussed and sometimes used as the basis for changes to political culture, for example in a legal context. In a grammar of the language of Castile published in 1492, the author writes: 'The language was always the companion of rulership, and in this sense followed it, since together they began, grew, and flourished, and together both found later their doom.'[75] But, in reality, multiple languages were the norm within and no deterrence to composite monarchies.

101

In legal terms, Latin had been the dominant language in most European realms because of the use of Roman law in civil as well as in religious courts and the Church more generally since Late Antiquity or the Middle Ages. In several composite monarchies, this practice, at least, was abandoned in favour of the common or regional language. In southern France, starting in the late fifteenth century, all legal acts, treaties, protocols, testimonies and reports needed to be in French or the regional dialect (langue d'oc) 'to avoid misuse and inconveniences'. This was also adapted for the region north of the Loire and, in fact, for all of France in 1539, but with the ambiguous expression to use the 'French native language' – in several commentaries over the next centuries, it was debated whether this included the southern regional languages or only the French of the Île-de-France.[76] Territorial additions in the following centuries introduced German, Dutch and Basque as well as Castilian and Catalan to the mix. A certain pragmatism helped maintain a composite language policy until the French Revolution.

In the composite monarchy of the kingdom of Denmark and the duchies of Schleswig and Holstein a similar outlook with regard to languages can be found. In the duchies, High and Low German were the main languages, while Danish was the language for governing Denmark (this included Norway from around 1500, when Old Norwegian fell out of use). The royal family and their officials used German and Danish. The growing status of Denmark in continental military matters meant that all military-related policy was conducted in German, because the main population of the composite monarchy's continental component were living in the German-speaking duchies. The opposite was true for the navy: the kingdom of Denmark largely consisted of islands, and naval personnel were recruited from these areas; consequently, Danish was the navy's main language. The preference of kings like Frederic III, who introduced Danish absolutism in 1660, and his grandson Frederick IV for the German language (and culture) increased the reach of this language within the composite monarchy. Some officials never even learnt Danish. Only from the mid-eighteenth century with the beginnings of a Danish nationalism did language become politicized.[77] Until the late nineteenth-century, however, German remained one of the two governing languages even for mainland Denmark.

In the Spanish global composite monarchy, Castilian was the language at the royal court, but Catalan, Valencian, Italian and Dutch as well as Latin where also used for pragmatic reasons. Protocols of the *Consiglio Collaterale*, counselling the Viceroy of Naples and Sicily, were written in Castilian and Italian with Latin introductions and conclusions. A difference was to be found in the Viceroyalty of New Spain in Southern America, where expatriate Spanish officials used Castilian, whereas the indigene initially retained their native languages. The missionaries sent to Christianize these latter people did not want to use their influence in the region to spread Castilian because, as translators, they held a monopoly on communication between the monarchy and its American population.[78]

Further elements: geography, historical coincidences and dynastic 'pot luck'

For the establishment of some composite monarchies, geography played a supporting role.[79] The pre-eminent example is the British Isles where water served as a boundary and border as well as a protective barrier against direct invasions. Here, the concept of a British monarchy was supported by the geographical factor of an insular situation. After the Union of the Crowns in 1707 and the Union with Ireland in 1801, the propaganda of a seafaring people (though originally more the Scottish and the Irish) surrounded by its natural habitat was expanded to all the isles and furthered the sense of a community within the former kingdoms and of otherness compared to the 'continent' or 'Europe'.[80] The geography of the Iberian peninsula similarly supported the composite monarchy of Spain and Portugal.[81] And in the seventeenth century, Louis XIV based his policy to affirm the French monarchy on the idea of a geographically rounded off territory with seas to the south, west and part of the north, and mountain ranges to the southwest and southeast, calling for a 'reunion' of France with supposedly formerly French territories.[82] The River Rhine served as a (controversial) 'natural border' to the east and remained a contested borderline as late as the nineteenth century.[83] However, an example of a composite monarchy supported by water as a line of communication was the Kalmar Union: the Swedish region of Scania with its many islands and peninsulas was always closer to Denmark than to central Sweden. Similarly, going back in time to the early medieval period, the Gaelic overkingdom of Dál Riada was situated between today's Ireland and Scotland, and its existence was only possible because of the use of the Irish Sea as a waterway between the coastline territories and islands.[84]

On the other hand, the Burgundian inheritance of the Low Countries was separated from the main Habsburg residences and lands, be they in Spain, Bohemia, or Austria, by lands not ruled by the dynasty. The practice of installing family members as regents or governors helped to keep the Dutch lands within the composite monarchy, but was not enough – as was pointed out above – in times of serious differences with the elites or over political culture.[85]

One final point: for composite monarchies, the role of historical coincidences, or rather what we might term dynastic 'pot luck', cannot be underestimated. Some of the examples of monarchical unions discussed in this chapter might well have ended quite differently were it not for untimely deaths or lack of issue. The Habsburg inheritances offer one example: after some prosperous marriages in the Middle Ages, the dynasty was comparably poor by the time one of the richest heiresses of the fifteenth century, Mary of Burgundy, married Maximilian of Habsburg. The conditions in their marriage treaty were quite strict: whoever died first left the full inheritance to the children of the marriage while the surviving partner inherited nothing.[86] Consequently, after the early death of Mary, Maximilian was only regent of Burgundy for their son Philip, who died before his father, and then for his grandson Charles. The same happened in subsequent generations with the untimely deaths of the spouses of Maximilian's children and grandchildren. The deaths of Juan, the Principe of Asturias, husband of Maximilian's daughter Margaret of Austria, and Louis II, king of Bohemia, Hungary and Croatia, husband of Maximilian's granddaughter Mary and brother-in-law of his grandson Ferdinand, eventually resulted in their respective realms and political claims falling to the Habsburg dynasty.[87] The advantageous consequences for the Habsburg composite monarchy in the time of Charles V have been discussed already.

In the sixteenth century, the children of the English and Irish king Henry VIII all died without legitimate heirs: Edward in his youth; Mary, who exhibited two false pregnancies and possibly died of ovarian cancer; and Elizabeth, who refused to marry. The closest male relative was the Scottish king, James VI, great-grandson of Henry's sister Margaret. Though born a Catholic as the son of Queen Mary I of Scotland, he was brought up a Protestant in the custody of several regents after his mother's forced abdication and his own coronation at the age of one. As a legitimate, male Protestant, his succession to the third throne of the British Isles with its overseas colonies seemed straightforward. But it could only happen because regardless of six marriages, there were only three children of Henry VIII born in wedlock and no grandchildren, and because James's mother lost her throne as a result of her policy and behaviour.[88]

But there are also cases of monarchies that did not combine – or are no longer combined – regardless of the potential lines of succession. At the turn of the eighteenth century, King Charles II of Spain, the last king of the Spanish Habsburgs, died without heirs in 1700. Several candidates were considered. The most acceptable, because he was not a member of a comparably powerful dynasty, was a grandnephew of the king of the Wittelsbach dynasty and son of the prince elector of Bavaria. But he predeceased the Spanish king in infancy. In the end, it came down to a choice between the afore-mentioned Charles (VI) – a Habsburg, second son and brother of emperors and, from 1711, himself Holy Roman Emperor – and Philip of Bourbon, grandson of the French king Louis XIV. As neither the Spanish elites nor the other European powers supported either a Bourbon universal monarchy comprising Spanish and French territories or a new Habsburg universal monarchy of the global Spanish and the Austrian territories, it was only after nearly fifteen years of war that Philip was accepted as king of Spain by most European powers and the majority of the Spanish. The Spanish inheritance in Europe was partly distributed as compensation to the last Habsburg. Charles VI there-after ruled the southern Netherlands – the so-called Austrian Netherlands or today's Belgium – the kingdoms of Naples and Sardinia – exchanged in 1718 for the kingdom of Sicily – and the Stato dei Presidi. In addition, a merging of France and Spain, both ruled by the Bourbon dynasty after the War of the Spanish Succession, was prohibited by international treaties.[89]

Conclusions and reflections: from personal unions to nation states

This chapter has shown that the process of developing a composite monarchy was, in general, supported by introducing common symbols and institutions. Flags, coats of arms and sometimes also coinage, demonstrated with minimal words, on the one hand, who the common ruler *was* while, on the other – and this was especially true where dynastic coats of arms were employed – that the individual entities had been unified under one monarch. Hymns put such ideas into words, while maps commissioned by the ruler or supporting groups presented the composite monarchy as a whole.[90]

Ruling over such a combined realm in the early modern period was difficult. The monarch needed secure ways of communication. He or she might need to travel with their court to different regions and to install representatives – for example regents or governors – for day-to-day administration. But the appointment of such representatives might lead to, rather than prevent, instability: their views might not always accord with those of the ruler, or their acts might even lead to conflict between the ruler and the ruled.

Within common or collaborating bodies such as estates, parliaments, councils, ministries and other institutions of the financial, legal, or religious system, elite actors of formerly separate dominions had to work together and became better acquainted. This could support the development of a composite monarchy but might also strengthen existing differences between peoples by verifying prejudices.

The fact that they were required to accept people of a supposedly minor or subordinate principality as their equals could lead some political actors to act to prevent the establishment of a composite monarchy, as could the fear of losing powers, rights, or privileges. The power of religion to separate people should also not be underestimated in the early modern period. However, a strong motivation to countenance a diverse, but unified realm was to gain power and might in the face of common enemies. Another aim was to establish peace between the different peoples within a composite monarchy.

This overview of European composite monarchies from the late medieval to the end of the early modern era has shown, first, that it was a phenomenon shared by nearly every realm ruled by a monarchy. The only 'political' body to ban personal unions – at least in theory – was the Catholic Church after the Council of Trent. As the high officials of the Roman Church were also the secular rulers of regions that varied in size from city-states to the vast principalities of the Rhineland, accumulating spiritual principalities meant to also accumulate territory. Even though the practice was forbidden by the Catholic Church, it continued well into the eighteenth century.[91] In fact, the only kingdom in Europe that consisted of a singular territory was Sweden between 1533 and 1561–82. Second, the specific structures and institutions of composite monarchies developed over time according to regional requirements. Third, a disparity between the laws of the various territories that made up a composite monarchy was a common characteristic.

From the late eighteenth century, the theory of the nation state gained influence over political debates.[92] The unity of territory, people, government, language and political culture was seen as a 'natural' state. According to the influential nineteenth-century scholar of international law, Georg Jellinek, a sovereign state needed a *Staatsgebiet* (state territory), a *Staatsvolk* (state people) and *Staatsgewalt* (state authority) to be a subject in international law. The unity of people, territory and law was, for example, forcefully introduced by the French Revolution and Napoleon Bonaparte to late eighteenth- and early nineteenth-century France. The interdependence of statehood and nation was thereafter taken up by historians, legal experts and politicians, leading to the spread of so-called 'nationalism' all over Europe and – via the dynastic, monarchical and colonial relations – across the world.[93]

Yet the concept of the state largely remained theoretical, as the composite empires and kingdoms, and the modern states that derive from them, illustrate to this day. Different people, different regional constitutions, different civil and electoral laws, and even different languages are still the norm in many of today's members of the European community. Looking back, one can conclude that an examination of the early modern composite monarchies as examples may be beneficial to addressing present-day challenges and to searching for acceptable solutions and compromises. Recently it has been suggested that 'while outwardly stressing unity and harmony', a composite monarchy 'in fact functioned by accepting disagreement and disgruntlement as permanent elements of its internal politics'.[94]

Accommodating legal, administrative, economic and other differences, although sometimes challenging, worked in theory and practice to form more or less cohesive unions that stood the test of time – and might also work in our own time.

Notes

1 For the discourse on a possible comparison of the EU with the Holy Roman Empire as a composite monarchical structure, see Peter H. Wilson, *The Holy Roman Empire: A Thousand Years of Europe's History* (London: Penguin, 2017), 680–686.
2 See the titles of Charles VI on the 1725 imperial seal; the inscription shows the Latin abbreviations, the transcription and translation is by the author. Seal of Charles VI, 1725, photo by Jonas Haller, 2006, https://de.wikipedia.org/wiki/Datei:Siegel_Karl_VI.jpg (last accessed 6 June 2018).
3 See in general Helmut G. Koenigsberger, "Dominium regale or Dominium politicum et regale. Monarchies and Parliaments in Early Modern Europe," in *Politicians and Virtuosi: Essays in Early Modern History*, ed. Helmut G. Koenigsberger (London: Continuum International Publishing Group, 1986).
4 See Susan Reynolds, "The Idea of the Nation as a Political Community," in *Power and the Nation in European History*, eds. Len Scales and Oliver Zimmer (Cambridge: Cambridge University Press, 2005), 56.
5 Koenigsberger, "Dominum regale," 10–11.
6 Ibid., 13–14.
7 John H. Elliot, "A Europe of Composite Monarchies," *Past & Present* 137 (1992).
8 Ibid., 52.
9 Ibid., 52–54.
10 Ibid., 55–60.
11 Ibid., 60–66.
12 See Arno Strohmeyer, "'Österreichische' Geschichte der Neuzeit als multiperspektivische Raumgeschichte. Ein Versuch," in *Was heißt "österreichische" Geschichte? Probleme, Perspektiven und Räume der Neuzeit-Forschung*, eds. Martin Scheutz and Arno Strohmeyer (Innsbruck: Studien Verlag, 2008); Peter Rauscher, "El gobierno de una 'monarquía compuesta': Fernando I y el nacimiento de la Monarquía de los Austrias en el centro de Europa," in *Fernando I, 1503–1564: Socialización, vida privada y actividad pública de un Emperador del Renacimiento*, eds. Alfredo Alvar Ezquerra and Friedrich Edelmayer (Madrid: Sociedad Estatal de Conmemoraciones Culturales, 2004); and Xavier Gil Pujol, "Visíon europea de la monarquía española como monarquía compuesta, siglos XVI y XVII," in *Las monarquías del Antiguo Régimen. ¿Monarquías compuestas?* eds. Conrad Russell and José Andrés-Gallego (Madrid: Editorial Complutense, 1996).
13 By the Laws in Wales Act 1535 and 1542, Wales was incorporated into the Kingdom of England; the English legal system and administration were expanded to include Wales. See Henry VIII, "An Act for Laws and Justice to be ministered in Wales in like Form as it is in this Realm," and "An Act for certain Ordinances in the King's Majesty's Dominion and Principality of Wales," in *The statutes at large, of England and of Great Britain. Vol. 3*, eds. John Raithby and Thomas Edlyne Tomlins (London: George Eyre, Andrew Strahan, 1811), 243–255, 407–428. The acts were repealed in 1993.
14 See Jenny Wormald, "The Creation of Britain. Multiple Kingdoms or Core and Colonies?" *Transactions of the Royal Historical Society* 2 (1992); Conrad Russell, *The Causes of the English Civil War* (Oxford: Oxford University Press, 1990), 27. Similarly, the term 'monarchie plurielle' is used in French by Bartolomé Bennassar, "Pratiques de l'État moderne en France et en Espagne de 1550 à 1715," in *Les monarchies française et espagnole. Milieu du XVIe siècle-début du XVIIIe siècle (Actes du colloque de 2000)*, ed. Jean-Marie Constant (Paris: Presses de l'Université de Paris-Sorbonne, 2001).
15 Harald Gustafsson, "The Conglomerate State. A Perspective on State Formation in Early Modern Europe," *Scandinavian Journal of History* 23, no. 3–4 (1998). Gustafsson uses 'state', even though he only talks about monarchies.

16 Ibid., 197.
17 Franz Bosbach, "Mehrfachherrschaft: Eine Organisationsform frühmoderner Herrschaft," in *Membra unius capitis. Studien zu Herrschaftsauffassungen und Regierungspraxis in Kurbrandenburg (1640–1688)*, eds. Michael Kaiser and Michael Rohrschneider (Berlin: Duncker & Humblot, 2005).
18 Robert von Friedeburg and John Morrill, "Introduction. Monarchy Transformed: Princes and their Elites in Early Modern Western Europe," in *Monarchy Transformed: Princes and their Elites in Early Modern Western Europe*, eds. Robert von Friedeburg and John Morrill (Cambridge: Cambridge University Press, 2017), 4.
19 Ibid., 4.
20 Ibid., 4–5.
21 Art. 43, François Mitterrand, Jordi Farrás Forné and Joan Martí Alanís, "Constitució del Principat d'Andorra, 28 April 1993," *Buttletí Oficial del Principat d'Andorra* 5, no. 24 (1993): 451, www.bopa.ad/bopa/005024/Pagines/7586.aspx (last accessed 6 June 2018); see also Francesco Violi, "Condominiums and Shared Sovereignty," In *50 Shades of Federalism*, http://50shadesoffederalism.com/theory/condominiums-shared-sovereignty/, 2–3 (last accessed 6 June 2018).
22 For the British empire of the eighteenth century: Helmut G. Koenigsberger, "Composite States, Representative Institutions and the American Revolution," *Historical Research* 62 (1989): 143.
23 Riita Jallinoja, *Families, Status and Dynasties, 1600–2000* (London: Palgrave Macmillan, 2017), 25.
24 Bernd Marquardt, *Universalgeschichte des Staates: Von der vorstaatlichen Gesellschaft zum Staat der Industriegesellschaft* (Berlin, Zurich: LIT Verlag, 2009), 240.
25 Jallinoja, *Families*, 25–26.
26 Klaus Malettke, *Die Bourbonen. Volume 1* (Stuttgart: W. Kohlhammer, 2008), 2–27.
27 Harald Gustafsson, "A State that Failed? On the Union of Kalmar, Especially its Dissolution," *Scandinavian Journal of History* 31, no. 3–4 (2006): 206–207.
28 Peer Schmidt, "Die Reiche der spanischen Krone: Konflikte um die Reichseinheit in der frühneuzeitlichen spanischen Monarchie," in *Zusammengesetzte Staatlichkeit in der Europäischen Verfassungsgeschichte: Tagung der Vereinigung für Verfassungsgeschichte in Hofgeismar vom 19.3.–21.3.2001*, ed. Hans-Jürgen Becker (Berlin: Duncker & Humblot, 2006), 178.
29 Jonathan I. Israel, *The Dutch Republic: Its Rise, Greatness, and Fall, 1477–1806* (Oxford: Oxford University Press, 1995).
30 "The Declaration of Right" of 13 February 1689 was included in the "Bill of Rights". 16 December, 1689, in *English Historical Documents: 1660–1714*, ed. Andrew Browning (London: Eyre & Spottiswoode, 1966), 122–128. "Claim of Right. 4 April, 1689," in Browning ed., *English Historical Documents*, 635–639.
31 A notable exception was George I/George Louis, prince elector of Hanover and, from 1714, king of Great Britain. He tried to use his wills to end the personal union of Great Britain and Hanover and to establish primogeniture for Great Britain and a system of secundogeniture for Hanover. "Testament of George I," in Richard Drögereit, "Das Testament König Georgs I. und die Frage der Personalunion zwischen England und Hannover," *Niedersächsisches Jahrbuch für Landesgeschichte* 14 (1937): 180–199. His son managed to suppress his father's will, so the union continued until 1837. For George II's instructions to redact the legal copy of the will in the emperor's archives: Secretary of State, Viscount Townshend to the British ambassador to the Court of Vienna, Earl of Waldegrave, private, London (Whitehall), 06.11.1727, The National Archives, UK, State Papers Foreign 80, 62, f. 80.
32 Winfried Schulze, "Hausgesetzgebung und Verstaatlichung im Hause Österreich vom Tode Maximilians I. bis zur Pragmatischen Sanktion," in *Der dynastische Fürstenstaat: Zur Bedeutung von Sukzessionsordnungen für die Entstehung des frühmodernen Staates*, ed. Johannes Kunisch (Berlin: Duncker & Humblot, 1982), 256–261.
33 "Cession, y Renuncia, 1617, Jun. 6," in *Coleccion de los Tratados de Paz, Alianza, Tregua, Neutralidad, Comercio, etc. de España. Vol. 2*, ed. Joseph Antonio de Abreu y Bertodano (Madrid: Diego Peralta, Antonio Marin, Juan de Zuñiga, 1740), 233–254.

34 Karl-Friedrich Krieger, "Bayerisch-pfälzische Unionsbestrebungen vom Hausvertrag von Pavia (1329) bis zur Wittelsbachischen Hausunion vom Jahre 1724," *Zeitschrift für Historische Forschung* 4 (1977): 385–413.

35 Marquardt, *Universalgeschichte*, 242.

36 James VI & I, "Proclamation of 20 October 1604," in *Stuart Royal Proclamations*, vol. 1, eds. J.F. Larkin and P.L. Hughes (Oxford: Oxford University Press), 94–95, cited from Wormald, "The Creation of Britain," 177–178.

37 Ibid., 178.

38 Ibid., 180–185.

39 Ibid., 189–194.

40 Gustav Turba, *Die Grundlagen der Pragmatischen Sanktion. Volume 2: Die Hausgesetze* (Leipzig: Franz Deuticke, 1912), 94–194; Heinrich Benedikt, *Das Königreich Neapel unter Kaiser Karl VI. Eine Darstellung auf Grund bisher unbekannter Dokumente aus den österreichischen Archiven* (Vienna: Manz Verlag, 1927), 277.

41 For the edition of the Pragmatic Sanction: Gustav Turba, ed., *Die Pragmatische Sanktion. Authentische Texte samt Erläuterungen und Übersetzungen* (Vienna: Kaiserlich-Königliche Schulbücher-Verlage, 1913), 48–53.

42 For the Holy Roman Empire, see the chapter by Matthias Schnettger in this volume.

43 Wilhelm Brauneder, "Die Habsburgermonarchie als zusammengesetzter Staat," in *Zusammengesetzte Staatlichkeit in der Europäischen Verfassungsgeschichte. Tagung der Vereinigung für Verfassungsgeschichte in Hofgeismar vom 19.3.–21.3.2001*, ed. Hans-Jürgen Becker (Berlin: Duncker & Humblot, 2006), 207, 215, 227–228.

44 Andrea Lindmayr-Brandl, "Vom patriotischen Volkslied zur nationalen Kaiserhymne. Formen der Repräsentation in 'Gott, erhalte Franz, den Kaiser!'," in *Die Repräsentation der Habsburg-Lothringischen Dynastie in Musik, visuellen Medien und Architektur, 1618–1918 [Representing the Habsburg-Lorraine Dynasty in Music, Visual Media and Architecture, 1618–1918]*, ed. Werner Telesko (Vienna, Cologne and Weimar: Böhlau, 2017), 109–110. The melody of this hymn is by Joseph Haydn, the text – based on the English "God save the King" – originally by Lorenz Leopold Haschka, was changed multiple times in the nineteenth century. For the various versions see Franz Grasberger, *Die Hymnen Österreichs* (Tutzing: H. Schneider, 1968).

45 Art. 3, *The Union of Lublin, 1569*. Cited from the online edition by the Polish Historical Society, 3, www.history.pth.net.pl/files/source_editions/The_Union_of_Lublin_1569.pdf (last accessed 6 June 2018).

46 John Robertson, "Empire and Union: Two Concepts of the Early Modern European Political Order," in *A Union for Empire: Political Thought and the British Union of 1707*, ed. John Robertson (Cambridge: Cambridge University Press, 1995), 24.

47 Dirk Maczkiewitz, *Der niederländische Aufstand gegen Spanien (1568–1609): Eine kommunikationswissenschaftliche Analyse* (Münster: Waxmann, 2005), 60, 96–110.

48 Anton van der Lem, *Opstand! Der Aufstand in den Niederlanden. Egmonts und Oraniens Opposition, die Gründung der Republik und der Weg zum Westfälischen Frieden* (Berlin: Wagenbach, 1996), 50–70.

49 "The Prince of Orange's Warning to the Inhabitants and Subjects of the Netherlands, 1 September 1568," in *Texts Concerning the Revolt of the Netherlands*, eds. E.H. Kossmann and A.F. Mellink (Cambridge: Cambridge University Press, 1974), 84.

50 Ibid., 86.

51 "Edict of the States General of the United Netherlands by which they declare that the king of Spain has forfeited the sovereignty and government of the afore-said Netherlands, with a lengthy explanation of the reasons thereof, and in which they forbid the use of his name and seal in these same countries, 26 July 1581," in ibid., 216–228.

52 See the chapter by Cathleen Sarti in this volume.

53 Jaume Ordi et al., "The Severe Gout of Holy Roman Emperor Charles V," *The New England Journal of Medicine* 355 (2006): 516–520.

54 Martin Mutschlechner, "Karl V.: Resignation und Abdankung," *Die Welt der Habsburger*, www.habsburger.net/de/kapitel/karl-v-resignation-und-abdankung (last accessed 29 May 2018).

55 Horst Rabe and Peter Marzahl, "'Comme représent nostre propre personne': Regentschaften und Regentschaftsordnungen Kaiser Karls V.," in *Karl V. Politik und*

politisches System. Berichte und Studien aus der Arbeit an der politischen Korrespondenz des Kaisers, ed. Horst Rabe (Konstanz: Universitätsverlag Konstanz, 1996), 75–83. Citation taken from the full powers of Charles's aunt Margarete by Charles in 1519, ibid. 86, n. 47.

56 Gustafsson, "A State that Failed?" 209–212.

57 Charles II, *By the King: A Proclamation Concerning the President and Council of Wales, and Marches of the Same. 28 September, 1661* (London: John Bill and Christopher Barker, 1661).

58 Helmut G. Koenigsberger, "Zusammengesetzte Staaten, Repräsentativversammlungen und der amerikanische Unabhängigkeitskrieg," *Zeitschrift für Historische Forschung* 18, no. 4 (1991): 421–423.

59 "Konfoederation des Königreichs Böhemb mit den incorporirten Ländern, als Mähren, Schlesien, Ober und Nieder Lausitz. Article 26," in *Der Beginn des Dreißigjährigen Krieges. Der Kampf um Böhmen. Quellen zur Geschichte des Böhmischen Krieges 1618–1621,* ed. Miroslav Toegel (Prague: Academia, 1972), 151–165. Cited from and trans. in Joachim Bahlcke, "Die Böhmische Krone zwischen staatsrechtlicher Integrität, monarchischer Union und ständischem Föderalismus. Politische Entwicklungslinien im böhmischen Länderverband vom 15. bis zum 17. Jahrhundert," in *Föderationsmodelle und Unionsstrukturen. Über Staatsverbindungen in der frühen Neuzeit vom 15. zum 18. Jahrhundert,* ed. Thomas Fröschl (Munich: Oldenbourg, 1994), 99.

60 Karel Malý, "Die Verfassung des Staates der Böhmischen Krone," in *Zusammengesetzte Staatlichkeit in der Europäischen Verfassungsgeschichte. Tagung der Vereinigung für Verfassungsgeschichte in Hofgeismar vom 19.3.–21.3.2001,* ed. Hans-Jürgen Becker (Berlin: Duncker & Humblot, 2006), 77–82. Bahlcke, "Böhmische Krone," 97–102.

61 Harald Gustafsson, "Conglomerates or Unitary States? Integration Processes in Early Modern Denmark-Norway and Sweden," in *Föderationsmodelle und Unionsstrukturen. Über Staatsverbindungen in der frühen Neuzeit vom 15. zum 18. Jahrhundert,* ed. Thomas Fröschl (Munich: Oldenbourg, 1994), 56.

62 Cyril Milhaud, "Fragmentation of Capital Markets in Early Modern Spain? Composite Monarchies and their Jurisdiction," (Paris: HAL archives-ouvertes, 2016), 4–11, https://hal.archives-ouvertes.fr/hal-01365882 (last accessed 6 June 2018).

63 In *Novisima Recopilacion de Navarra,* vol. 2. 1735: 681. Cited from Milhaud, "Fragmentation," 14.

64 Gustafsson, "Conglomerates," 59. Toby Barnard, "Scotland and Ireland in the Later Steward Monarchy," in *Conquest and Union. Fashioning a British State, 1485–1725,* eds. Steven G. Ellis and Sarah Barber (London and New York: Longman, 1995), 270–273.

65 Franz Bosbach, "Krieg und Mehrfachherrschaft im 17. Jahrhundert," *Prague Papers on History of International Relations* 4 (2000): 79. In this case Bosbach is writing about conquered territories incorporated into France, but the measures taken can be generalized.

66 Gustafsson, "Conglomerates," 55.

67 Birgit Emich, *Territoriale Integration in der Frühen Neuzeit: Ferrara und der Kirchenstaat* (Cologne: Böhlau, 2005), 20.

68 Daniel H. Nexon, *The Struggle for Power in Early Modern Europe: Religious Conflict, Dynastic Empires, and International Change* (Princeton: Princeton University Press, 2009), 108.

69 Anders A. Stiernman, *Alla Riksdagars och Mötens Besluth: samt arfföreningar / Regements-Former, Försäkringar och Bewillningar / som / på allmenna Riksdagar och Möten / ifrån år 1521. intil år 1727. giorde / stadgade och bewiljade äro; med the för hwart och ett Stånd utfärdade all-menna Resolutioner* (Stockholm, 1728), 481.

70 For the deposition of Sigismund: Cathleen Sarti, "Monarchenabsetzungen im frühneuzeitlichen Nordeuropa" (PhD dissertation, University of Mainz, 2017), 89–101.

71 Michael Schaich, "Introduction," in *The Hanoverian Succession: Dynastic Politics and Monarchical Culture,* eds. Andreas Gestrich and Michael Schaich (Farnham: Ashgate, 2015), 9.

72 Barnard, "Scotland and Ireland," 260–265. "Catholic Relief Act, 1778," in *The Eighteenth Century Constitution: Documents and Commentary,* ed. Ernst Neville Williams (Cambridge: Cambridge University Press, 1960), 343–345. For the Gordon riots: Ian Gilmour, *Riot, Risings and Revolution: Governance and Violence in Eighteenth-Century England* (London: Hutchinson, 1992), 342–370.

73 Ute Lotz-Heumann, "Sprachliche Übersetzung – kulturelle Übersetzung – Politische Übersetzung? Sprache als Element des politischen Prozesses auf den frühneuzeitliche

britischen Inseln," in *Politik und Sprache im frühneuzeitlichen Europa*, eds. Thomas Nicklas and Matthias Schnettger (Mainz: Philipp von Zabern, 2007), 61–62. Lotz-Heumann proves that the simultaneous establishment of rule, language and religion failed in the Scottish Highlands and Islands, as well as in Ireland, because it was associated with conquest and oppression. Ibid. 70.

74 James Kelly, "Sustaining a Confessional State: The Irish Parliament and Catholicism," in *The Eighteenth-Century Composite State. Representative Institutions in Ireland and Europe, 1689–1800*, eds. D.W. Hayton, James Kelly and John Bergin (Basingstoke: Palgrave Macmillan, 2010), 45–53.

75 Elio Antonio de Nebrija, *Gramática Castellana*, eds. Miguel Angel Esparza and Ramón Sarmiento (Madrid: Fundación Antonio de Nebrija, 1992), 99, cited from and trans. in Christian Büschges, "Politische Sprachen? Sprache, Identität und Herrschaft in der Monarchie der spanischen Habsburger," in *Politik und Sprache im frühneuzeitlichen Europa*, eds. Thomas Nicklas and Matthias Schnettger (Mainz: Philipp von Zabern, 2007), 16.

76 Rainer Babel, "Sprache und Politik im Frankreich der Frühen Neuzeit: Eine Bestandsaufnahme," in *Politik und Sprache im frühneuzeitlichen Europa*, eds. Thomas Nicklas and Matthias Schnettger (Mainz: Philipp von Zabern, 2007), 35–37.

77 Sebastian Olden-Jørgensen, "Sprache der Verwaltung, Sprache der Politik: Die politischen Sprachen in den Ländern des dänischen Königs 1536–1730," in *Politik und Sprache im frühneuzeitlichen Europa*, eds. Thomas Nicklas and Matthias Schnettger (Mainz: Philipp von Zabern, 2007).

78 Büschges, "Politische Sprachen?" 28–31.

79 Maria Baramova, "Border Theories in Early Modern Europe," *European History Online (EGO)* (Mainz 2010-12-03), 5–6, www.ieg-ego.eu/baramovam-2010-en (last accessed 6 June 2018).

80 Linda Colley, *Britons: Forging the Nation, 1707–1837* (New Haven: Yale University Press, 2005), 17–18. See also David Armitage, "The British Conception of Empire in the Eighteenth Century," in *Imperium – Empire – Reich: Ein Konzept politischer Herrschaft im deutsch-britischen Vergleich [An Anglo-German Comparison of a Concept of Rule]*, eds. Franz Bosbach and Herman Hiery (Munich: K.G. Saur Verlag, 1999), 92 for the concept of a British Empire "as Protestant, commercial, maritime and free".

81 Schmidt, "Die Reiche der spanischen Krone," 178.

82 See for Vauban's, the French military strategist's view, Michèle Virol, *Vauban. De la Gloire du Roi au Service de l'Etat* (Seyssel: Champ Vallon, 2003), 94–97.

83 Andreas Rüther, "Flüsse als Grenzen und Bindeglieder: Zur Wiederentdeckung des Raumes in der Geschichtswissenschaft," *Jahrbuch für Regionalgeschichte* 25 (2007): 39–40.

84 Ewan Campbell, *Saints and Sea-Kings: The First Kingdom of the Scots* (Edinburgh: Canongate, 1999).

85 For the regencies in the time of Charles V, see Rabe and Marzahl, "Regentschaften"; for the re-establishment of the permanent governorship after the addition of the Netherlands to the Austrian composite monarchy after the War of the Spanish Succession in the eighteenth century and the rights and limits set for Archduchess Elisabeth Maria, see Sandra Hertel, *Maria Elisabeth: Österreichische Erzherzogin und Statthalterin in Brüssel (1725–1741)* (Vienna, Cologne, Weimar: Böhlau 2014), 59–72.

86 "Marriage treaty between Maximilian and Maria, undated [18th August 1477]," in *Quellen zur Geschichte Maximilians I. und seiner Zeit*, ed. Inge Wiesflecker-Friedhuber (Darmstadt: Wissenschaftliche Buchgesellschaft, 1996), 38–39.

87 Alfred Kohler, "Die dynastische Politik Maximilians I," in *Hispania – Austria: Die katholischen Könige, Maximilian I. und die Anfänge der Case de Austria in Spanien*, eds. Alfred Kohler and Friedrich Edelmayer (Vienna: Verlag für Geschichte und Politik; Munich: Oldenbourg, 1993).

88 See Levine as early as his 1973 book, Mortimer Levine, *Tudor Dynastic Problems, 1460–1571* (London: George Allen and Unwin, 1973); for Mary Stuart's abdication, see the chapter by Cathleen Sarti in this volume.

89 See the comprehensive description of this question by Matthias Schnettger, *Der Spanische Erbfolgekrieg, 1701–1713/14* (München: C.H. Beck, 2014), 16–28.

90 See for Austrian maps of the eighteenth century Brauneder, "Die Habsburgermonarchie," 207; or for a map explicitly drawn for the new king of Prussia in 1701, see Helmut Neuhaus,

"Das Werden Brandenburg-Preußens," in *Zusammengesetzte Staatlichkeit in der Europäischen Verfassungsgeschichte. Tagung der Vereinigung für Verfassungsgeschichte in Hofgeismar vom 19.3.–21.3.2001*, ed. Hans-Jürgen Becker (Berlin: Duncker & Humblot, 2006), 239.

91 Hubert Jedin, *Die Geschichte des Konzils von Trient. Volume 2* (Freiburg i. Br.: Herder, 1978), 312–313.

92 See in general Len Scales and Oliver Zimmer, eds. *Power and the Nation in European History* (Cambridge: Cambridge University Press, 2005).

93 This is discussed in the edited volume on the "Transnational Histories of the 'Royal Nation'," Milinda Banerjee, Charlotte Backerra and Cathleen Sarti, eds. *Transnational Histories of the 'Royal Nation'* (Basingstoke: Palgrave Macmillan, 2017).

94 Wilson, *The Holy Roman Empire*, 686.

Key works

Bosbach, Franz, "Mehrfachherrschaft: Eine Organisationsform frühmoderner Herrschaft," in *Membra unius capitis: Studien zu Herrschaftsauffassungen und Regierungspraxis in Kurbrandenburg (1640–1688)*, eds. Michael Kaiser and Michael Rohrschneider (Berlin: Duncker & Humblot, 2005), 19–34.

Elliot, John H., "A Europe of Composite Monarchies," *Past & Present* 137 (1992): 48–71.

Gustafsson, Harald, "Conglomerates or Unitary States? Integration Processes in Early Modern Denmark-Norway and Sweden," in *Föderationsmodelle und Unionsstrukturen: Über Staatsverbindungen in der frühen Neuzeit vom 15. zum 18. Jahrhundert*, ed. Thomas Fröschl (Munich: Oldenbourg, 1994), 45–62.

Koenigsberger, Helmut G., "Dominium regale or Dominium politicum et regale. Monarchies and Parliaments in Early Modern Europe," in *Politicians and Virtuosi: Essays in Early Modern History*, ed. Helmut G. Koenigsberger (London: Continuum International Publishing Group, 1986), 1–25.

Pujol, Xavier Gil, "Visión europea de la monarquía española como monarquía compuesta, siglos XVI y XVII," in *Las monarquías del Antiguo Régimen. ¿Monarquías compuestas?* eds. Conrad Russell and José Andrés-Gallego (Madrid: Editorial Complutense, 1996), 65–95.

Wormald, Jenny, "The Creation of Britain: Multiple Kingdoms or Core and Colonies?" *Transactions of the Royal Historical Society* 2 (1992): 175–194.

5

DYNASTIC SUCCESSION IN AN ELECTIVE MONARCHY

The Habsburgs and the Holy Roman Empire

Matthias Schnettger

It is most remarkable – though not completely unique – that, with only one short interruption, one single dynasty managed to retain the royal or rather imperial dignity in the Holy Roman Empire for more than 350 years. The house of Habsburg ruled from 1438 to the very end of the empire, in 1806. This chapter aims to explain why this dynasty, which was often harshly criticized and was by no means characterized by an uninterrupted succession of excellent rulers, succeeded in preserving the imperial crown for a longer time than any of the preceding ruling houses.

The Habsburgs' emperorship was shaped by several basic conditions and essential factors that have to be taken into account. First of all, no emperor was just an emperor: he was a member of one of the most eminent European dynasties, the ruler of an accumulation of territories which exceeded by far the possessions of any other prince. It was an empire whose centre of gravity was usually on the periphery. The different roles of the emperors interfered with each other in different ways and with different results. And, of no little importance, their powerful position and the growing royal-imperial nimbus of their dynasty were of great advantage to the Habsburgs' imperial succession. Finally, we must not underestimate the fact that, for more than 350 years and with only one exception, the Habsburgs managed to generate a (more or less) appropriate candidate for each election for the head of the empire.

When focusing specifically on the evolution of the emperorship several aspects must be taken into consideration: on the one hand, the development of the empire's constitution from the fifteenth century tended to limit the emperor's position. At the same time, the empire's estates, that is the prince-electors, the princes and the Imperial Cities which formed the Imperial Diet, gained notable influence on the way the empire was ruled. On the other hand, the emperor retained notable room for manoeuvre as supreme judge and feudal lord and as the source of a great variety of privileges. These enabled him to maintain his clients among the empire's estates. The early modern period in the empire is marked by the negotiation of the always precarious balance of emperor and empire, that is between the estates of the empire (*Kaiser und Reich*). In this context, the prince-electors deserve special attention since their votes were indispensable for the succession of the emperor. From the sixteenth century onwards, the confessional schism played a key role in the empire, which affected the position of the emperor as well.

In order to analyse the foundations as well as the evolution of the Habsburgs' emperorship, I will follow its development chronologically over the centuries, focusing on the above-mentioned factors and contexts.[1]

Foundations and transformations of the Habsburg emperorship

When Albrecht II was elected king of the Romans in 1438, there were quite a few weighty arguments in his favour. First, he could count on a double royal and imperial tradition, being both a member of the house of Habsburg, which had produced three kings in the thirteenth and fourteenth centuries, and the son-in-law of Emperor Sigismund who had designated him eventual successor to his hereditary territories as early as 1423. While he had difficulties in maintaining his Bohemian inheritance, he had been crowned king of Hungary in 1437.[2] We can, thus, identify three factors that favoured Albrecht's success: the royal tradition of the Habsburgs, kinship with and designation by his predecessor, and the disposition of patrimonial dominions sufficient to bear the weight of the royal or imperial crown. All these factors not only kept their importance for the Habsburgs' emperorship during the following centuries but became even more important.

Though the reign of Albrecht lasted less than two years, the Habsburgs, more concretely Frederick, duke of Styria, Carinthia and Krain, managed to retain the royal crown. Frederick was elected king of the Romans in 1440.[3] Frederick turned out to be the first member of the House of Austria and at the same time the very last ruler to be crowned Roman emperor by the pope in the city of Rome, in 1452. In the eyes of contemporaries, the acquisition of the imperial nimbus notably increased the dignity of Frederick himself, but also of his descendants, making them more eligible for future royal and imperial elections. When Frederick confirmed the – falsified – *Privilegium maius* in favour of the Habsburgs (1442–53) he further strengthened his dynasty's position in its hereditary lands and in the empire.[4] From then on the title 'archduke' became generally accepted and thus the equality of the house of Austria with the electors of the empire – or even its precedence.

During the course of Frederick's long reign his reputation suffered damage as a result of the fact he did not manage to keep the kingdoms of Bohemia and Hungary under his control, even losing a part of his Austrian dominions. The concentration on his hereditary lands was responsible for a neglect of the empire's affairs. This led to harsh criticism, but Frederick was never in any real danger of being deposed. He even managed to turn the problem into an advantage when in 1486 his son Maximilian I (r. 1486/93–1519) was elected king of the Romans in order to assist his father in the government of the empire.[5] It was the first election of a king of the Romans during his predecessor's lifetime since 1376. These elections *vivente Imperatore* proved to be an important means for the Habsburgs to preserve the imperial dignity in their own house. In this way the reigning emperors were able to use their influence to drive the election in the desired direction. Although the prince-electors were, of course, conscious of this de facto restriction in their freedom of choice, they rarely resisted the emperors' advances, so that seven elections *vivente Imperatore* took place between 1486 and 1764.[6]

In several respects, Maximilian I contributed significantly to the imperial status of his family.[7] As a result of his marriage to Mary of Burgundy (1477) he had increased the Habsburg dominions considerably even before his accession to the royal throne. It is most interesting that, unlike his father, Maximilian was less criticized for his negligent government of the empire, but he was distrusted by the German princes because of his determined policies. While, for example, Maximilian declared he was acting on behalf of the empire's rights in imperial Italy (*Reichsitalien*), his adversaries suspected him of acting mainly in the interests of his own house, something that formed a *leitmotiv* for most of the criticisms raised against the Habsburgs in the following centuries.

For the evolution of the emperorship it was most important that during Maximilian's reign the so-called *Reichsreform* tended to strengthen and codify the influence of the imperial estates on the government of the empire. A crucial point was marked by the Diet of Worms (1495) when, among others, the *Reichskammergericht* as a Supreme Court, which was separated from the king's court, was established, and the Diet's competence in matters of peace and war, legislation and taxation was sanctioned. Yet Maximilian managed to preserve several prerogatives for himself. With the installation of the Imperial Aulic Council (*Reichshofrat*) as the second Supreme Court of the empire and as advisory board for all imperial matters, Maximilian founded an institution which became one of the most important instruments of the emperor's influence in the following centuries.[8]

Another new element in the reign of Maximilian gained particular importance: the creation of the title 'Roman emperor elect' (*Erwählter Römischer Kaiser*). In fact, this title, taken up by Maximilian in Trent in 1508 with the consent of the Pope, was at first merely intended as a provisional solution when the king was not able to continue on his way to Rome because of his enemies. Neither Maximilian nor Julius II planned to put an end to papal coronations. But unintentionally, they established a model for an emperorship *without* papal coronation that turned out to be acceptable even for the Protestant electors and princes who detested the papal 'Antichrist'.

Unfortunately, Maximilian had not been able to realize his design of securing the succession in emperorship for his grandson Charles, who had grown up in the Low Countries. Charles took over the rule of the Low Countries in 1515 and his maternal, Spanish inheritance in 1516–17. But when Maximilian died in 1519 Charles's origin and early fortunes turned out to be a problem. Without a doubt the election of 1519 was among the most difficult ones the Habsburgs faced. For some of the prince-electors the succession of the powerful Spanish king seemed dangerous, and King Francis I of France was a strong opponent. On the other hand, even a few of Charles's own councillors judged the acquisition of the imperial dignity an undesirable undertaking. But at last, Charles, who was labelled as a prince of German origin and did not stint on expending the necessary funds, was elected, largely due to the fact that none of the German princes risked standing as a serious candidate himself. But the electors tried to control the new head of the empire by imposing on him an electoral capitulation. From now on each king of the Romans or Roman emperor had to swear to such an instrument intended to limit his room for manoeuvre.[9]

The reign of Charles V (r. 1519–56)[10] marks both the peak of early modern emperorship and an exceptional case, too. Charles turned out to be the last emperor to occupy the position of the universal secular leader of the Christian community. But it was his Spanish inheritance that formed the main basis of his power. Within the Empire he retained only the peripheral Burgundian territories, while very soon, in 1521–2, he ceded the ancient Habsburg dominions to his younger brother Ferdinand. With Ferdinand, elected king of the Romans in 1531, Charles could count on a capable deputy in Germany. This did not mean at all that Charles neglected his imperial duties, even when he stayed far away from the empire for long periods.

In 1530 Charles was crowned king of Italy and then emperor by Pope Clement VII. He was thus the very last Roman emperor to be crowned by a Pope. Charles's coronation did not take place in Rome, but in Bologna: the papal capital had been heavily damaged by Charles's own mercenaries in the sack of Rome (1527). In spite of frequent tensions with the popes, Charles did his best to secure the unity and Catholic orthodoxy of the Christian church, thereby fulfilling one of the noblest traditional duties of emperorship. In the end neither his efforts to suppress the Lutheran 'heresy' by the Edict of Worms (1521) nor the search for a theological reunion nor the attempts to conquer the Protestant estates militarily turned out to be successful. Charles's tremendous power even provoked opposition among the Catholic German princes. Even in the house of Habsburg itself opposition arose when Charles presented his so-called *Erbreichsplan*, which envisioned an everlasting Habsburg emperorship, but discriminated against Ferdinand and his descendants. In 1552 a conjuration of several princes put an end to the emperor's position of strength, which then collapsed like a house of cards. In spite of some minor successes and of a provisional agreement with the rebellious princes (Treaty of Passau, 1552), Charles resigned in 1556. Except for Franz II he was the only early modern emperor to renounce the Holy Roman crown. His abdication marks a turning point in the history of early modern emperorship: though his successors claimed to be 'Roman' – i.e. universal – emperors, they never had the slightest chance of establishing a real universal monarchy.[11]

Consolidation at a lower level: the Roman emperorship of the Austrian Habsburgs in the second half of the sixteenth century[12]

After Charles V, concepts of emperorship seem to be reduced in several respects. With the Austrian dominions, the lands of the Bohemian Crown and the western part of Hungary (from 1526), Ferdinand's I patrimony was by no means comparable to that of his nephew Philip II of Spain who took the leading part in the dynasty. Except for accidental tensions, the relations between the two branches of the house of Austria were usually shaped by cooperation and confirmed by several dynastic marriages so that the perception of one 'house of Habsburg' prevailed. A strong relationship with Spain could mean both valuable support as well as a serious problem for the Austrian Habsburgs in general, and for the emperor in particular, especially when he was suspected of subordinating the empire's needs to Spanish desires.

Since the reign of Charles V, the confessional question constituted a tremendous challenge for the emperor. As we have seen, Charles failed to restore the unity of the Christian church. In contrast, Ferdinand I (r. 1556–64) showed a more flexible attitude. But for him, too, it was most difficult to reconcile various incompatible demands.[13] First of all, there were his personal beliefs. Like every Habsburg emperor – with the one exception of the chameleon-like Maximilian II – Ferdinand was a convinced Roman Catholic. Furthermore, in accordance with the traditional concept of emperorship, he had to act as *advocatus ecclesiae*, and that meant for Ferdinand and his successors he was an advocate of the papal church.[14] On the other hand, there was the necessity of getting along with the Protestant estates of the empire. Already by 1552 it had been Ferdinand who negotiated the Treaty of Passau, which served as the basis for the Peace of Augsburg (*Augsburger Religionsfrieden*, 1555). This settlement did not solve the doctrinal conflict but furnished the Catholic and Protestant estates of the empire with a set of juridical rules that made the lasting confessional discord manageable. It was fundamental that the Protestants were granted an unlimited inclusion in the public peace and that the princes of the empire were conceded the right to choose their own confession – and that of their subjects.

For our subject, it is most important to notice that during the Augustan negotiations Ferdinand remained committed to excluding the ecclesiastical princes from this freedom of choice by insisting on the so-called ecclesiastical reservation (*reservatum ecclesiasticum; Geistlicher Vorbehalt*) in the text of the agreement. Any ecclesiastical prince who wanted to convert to Protestantism had to resign and thus open the way for the election of a Catholic successor. By this means Ferdinand and the Catholic estates of the empire wanted to perpetuate the Catholic majority in the Imperial Diet and especially in the electoral college. Indeed, with the votes of the three ecclesiastical electors of Mainz, Cologne and Trier and of the – since 1526, Habsburg – King of Bohemia, the Catholic electors would always prevail over their Protestant colleagues, the Count Palatine, the Duke of Saxony and the Margrave of Brandenburg.[15] Without any doubt, the lasting Catholic majority in the electoral college was one of the fundamental reasons why the Habsburgs managed to retain the imperial dignity.[16] With the one exception of the Bavarian Wittelsbachs, the leading electoral and princely dynasties opted for Protestantism and thus became ineligible for the Catholic electorates. A stable alliance between the Habsburg emperor and the ecclesiastical princes of the empire was established. In general, the emperor could count on the support of the ecclesiastical clients while they could expect to be defended by their imperial patron against the aspirations of their powerful Protestant neighbours.[17]

In 1558, Ferdinand gained the imperial title when he was proclaimed 'Elected Roman Emperor' (*Erwählter Römischer Kaiser*) by the electors at Frankfurt. From now on every head of the empire bore this title. The consolidation of Ferdinand's emperorship became manifest when his eldest son Maximilian was elected king of the Romans in 1562.

Maximilian II (r. 1564–76) followed the irenic path of his father. He was able to preserve the peace within the empire though there were, of course,[18] tensions, and he obtained the support of the imperial estates for the protection of the Habsburg dominions against the Ottoman threat. In 1575, he achieved the election of his eldest son Rudolph as king of the Romans, too.

As already pointed out, a crucial prerequisite of the Habsburgs' emperorship was their hereditary dominions. It has to be noted, though, that the Habsburg rule was not unchallenged, even in their patrimonial lands, especially when a large part of the nobles and towns adopted the Protestant faith and were eager to secure their churches against the interference of their ruler. The Habsburgs' position was even weaker in Bohemia where the estates of the kingdom claimed the right to elect their king freely. Although the Habsburg candidates to the throne were always accepted, there was the risk that in case of a serious conflict the estates might opt differently. In Hungary, the Habsburg kings held only the western part of the realm while the central and eastern provinces were under direct or indirect Ottoman rule from the 1540s.

Due to a division of the estate between his younger brothers and himself, Maximilian II only ruled Hungary, the Bohemian provinces, and Lower and Upper Austria, while Tyrol and the so-called inner Austrian provinces (mainly Styria, Carinthia and Krain) had been assigned to his brothers. However, Maximilian left all his territories to his eldest son, whereas Rudolph's younger brothers did not inherit their own principalities. On the one hand, this decision prevented further fragmentation of the Habsburg dominions, but on the other, it provoked a certain dissatisfaction among the cadets.

Another challenge for Rudolph II was the confessional problem that flared up violently in the 1580s, with the War of Cologne (1583–8). This conflict marked a turning point in several respects. First, the cooperation of Bavaria, Spain, the pope and the emperor forced Gebhard of Truchsess of Waldburg, who had converted to Lutheranism, to flee his electorate, which was given to the Bavarian Prince Ernst, thus preserving the Catholic majority in the electoral college. Furthermore, it became clear that the Catholic forces were determined to compel the observance of the ecclesiastical reservation even though they had tolerated Protestants being appointed to several bishoprics in northern Germany up until that point. The Catholics were not able to drive them out, but they did not acknowledge them either, which meant that they could not occupy their seats in the Diet of the empire. Finally, the confessional conflict even affected the viability of the *Reichskammergericht*, too. Emperor Rudolph II did not play a dominant part in these conflicts, but rather than acting as an impartial judge, he was usually a member of the Catholic 'party'.

If, in spite of all these tensions, the position of the emperor remained stable until the beginning of the seventeenth century,[19] this was not due to the Ottoman threat, which had an ambivalent effect. On the one hand, it exposed the emperor to pressure from the estates of the empire and those of the Habsburg dominions. On the other, the external threat produced a certain cohesion within the empire aimed at resisting the common enemy. In fact, the erosion of Rudolph's II emperorship gathered speed only when the so-called Long Turkish War (1593–1606) was terminated with the peace of Zsitvatorok.

Emperorship in a period of crisis: the age of the Thirty Years' War

For the Roman emperorship the Thirty Years' War marked a dangerous crisis, a crisis that started with the so-called fraternal strife (*Bruderzwist*) in the house of Habsburg.[20] Rudolph II had never been a dynamic prince, but as the years passed his indolence concerning government grew notably. A most serious problem was that Rudolph never married, thus neglecting even the elementary duty of securing the dynastic succession. In the late 1590s there was a growing opposition within the Habsburg dynasty itself headed by Rudolph II's brother Matthias. But it was only in 1606 that Matthias and his allies started to put their plans into action when they declared the emperor mad. It was Archduke Matthias who negotiated the peace of Zsitvatorok in the same year, and Rudolph was coerced to appoint his hostile brother governor of Hungary. Two years later Matthias, who had secured the support of the Hungarian,

Austrian and Moravian Estates, went further, invaded Bohemia and forced Rudolph to cede Hungary, Austria and Moravia to himself.

In the same period imperial authority broke down outside the Habsburg dominions, too. In 1608, the Imperial Diet (where Rudolph had not been present himself) was dismissed without success because of the violent conflict between Catholic and Protestant estates. This conflict was linked to the case of Donauwörth, a mainly Lutheran Imperial City. After several incursions by the Protestant majority against the Catholic minority, Rudolph placed Donauwörth under the Ban of the Empire in 1607. Even more delicately, Rudolph conferred the execution of the sentence on Duke Maximilian of Bavaria who profited by the opportunity to occupy Donauwörth, to adopt the Counter-Reformation and to retain the city until the inhabitants had paid the debts incurred by the execution of the ban – which turned out to be never. This damaged Rudolph's position as supreme judge of the empire. The partiality of both the emperor and his Aulic Council in favour of Catholicism had reached an unbearable degree for several Calvinist and Lutheran estates who allied themselves in the Protestant Union in 1608. Rudolph was not even capable of profiting from the formation of the Catholic League in 1609, because it was Maximilian of Bavaria who took the leading position in this alliance and endeavoured to keep out the Habsburgs.

The last act of Habsburg fraternal strife took place in 1611 when Matthias marched into Bohemia. While Matthias was elected and crowned king of Bohemia, Rudolph was put into custody in the Hradschin where he died in January 1612. These month of imprisonment underlined the utter humiliation of early modern emperorship.

Although Matthias was elected and crowned emperor without difficulty, there was no real recovery of the emperorship during his reign (r. 1612–19). First, Matthias and his favourite minister, the bishop of Vienna and cardinal (from 1615–16) Melchior Khlesl, who had acquired the reputation of a ruthless counter-reformer of the Habsburgs' dominions, did not manage to re-establish the emperor's position as arbiter above the confessional parties in the empire. The first and only Imperial Diet of Matthias's reign was dissolved, as had happened in 1608, without success (1613). An important source of Matthias's weakness was his childlessness. It was only in 1611 that he married his cousin, Archduchess Anna of Tyrol; their union remained without progeny.

In fact, only the Styrian line of the German branch of the Habsburg dynasty had generated a male descendant, Archduke Ferdinand, who was chosen and established as Matthias' heir. Unwillingly, the estates of Bohemia and of Hungary elected Ferdinand king in 1617–18, but soon the confessional and constitutional conflict in Bohemia came to a head with the well-known defenestration of the imperial regents at Prague in May 1618.[21]

After Matthias' death Ferdinand II (r.1619–37) was elected and crowned Roman emperor in Frankfurt.[22] There were schemes for a change of dynasty, but in the end Ferdinand's election was safe though at the same time he was deposed by the Bohemian estates. Ferdinand's emperorship was substantially characterized by the Thirty Years' War. Overcoming the Bohemian crisis with the help of Spain and Bavaria, he not only subjugated the Bohemian dominions and Austria to his effective control but notably extended his imperial prerogatives and power, especially when he transferred the Palatine electorate to Maximilian of Bavaria and laid down the famous edict of restitution (*Restitutionsedikt*), which ordered the return of a large number of ecclesiastical estates to the Catholics (1629). Furthermore, with the help of Albrecht von Wallenstein, he established his own imperial army. Remarkably enough he did not summon a single Diet. But with the congress of Regensburg (1630) the limits of his authority became evident: he had to dismiss Wallenstein while the electors refused to elect Ferdinand's son king of the Romans. Military disaster followed a few months later with the advance of the Swedish. However, when Gustav Adolphus of Sweden was killed (1632), Ferdinand managed to take the initiative again and concluded the favourable Treaty of Prague (1635) which was intended to allow the expulsion of foreign troops from the empire by an army under the command of the emperor. Several historians have even attributed a factual or at least intended 'imperial absolutism' to Ferdinand.[23]

A few months before he died Ferdinand II experienced his last success when, finally, his son was elected king of the Romans. The reign of Ferdinand III (r. 1637–57) was also shaped by the Thirty Years' War, but in contrast to his father, he had to face the erosion of the imperial power when the French and Swedish forces gained ground. The imperial estates, who in 1640–1 were assembled at a Diet for the first time since 1613, wanted peace at almost any price.[24]

Without any doubt, the Peace of Westphalia (1648) is a key event in the history of the empire as well as of emperorship. Nationalist historians disparaged the Westphalian Peace as the deepest humiliation of the empire and the German nation during the early modern period, and argued that with 1648 the emperors lost any space for manoeuvre. Recent research has nuanced our understanding of the Treaties of Munster and Osnabrück. First, the balance of power between the emperor and the estates within the constitution of the empire was not altered substantially compared with the period before the war. Some Protestant princes, supported by Sweden and France, intended to restrict the emperor's influence radically, but their schemes evaporated to a large extent.[25]

Furthermore, the political and confessional status quo in the Habsburg dominions was maintained so that the basis of imperial power was even consolidated. At the same time, and even since the time of Matthias, the characteristics of the baroque Habsburg emperorship began to evolve. On the one hand, the emperors appeared outside their dominions less frequently. They went to Frankfurt for their royal or imperial election and coronation and attended a few Diets. Consequently, the society of presence (*Präsenzgesellschaft*) with its more or less frequent and immediate personal contacts between the emperor, the electors and the princes that had shaped the reigns of Ferdinand I and Maximilian II, evaporated. In fact, personal enfeoffments had ceased by the sixteenth century.[26]

On the other hand, the emperors started to transform Vienna into a suitable – and determinedly Catholic – imperial capital and thus into a stage perfectly appropriate for the glorification of the Roman emperor and his august family. For example, Matthias' wife Empress Anna founded the *Kapuzinergruft*, which turned out to be the Habsburgs' family grave.[27]

Leopold I and his sons: the re-ascent of the emperorship – and its limits[28]

After 1648, Ferdinand III managed to consolidate his position by the ostentatious adoption of the terms of Westphalia. In 1653 he secured the imperial dignity for the next generation of the Habsburgs when his eldest son was elected king of the Romans before an Imperial Diet took place, which was intended to address the problems and questions that had remained unsolved in 1648. Among others, there was the question of the faculty of an election *vivente Imperatore*. During the Diet, Ferdinand enacted a new regulation for the Imperial Aulic Council on his own authority, instead of giving a share to the imperial estates. With such measures, he skilfully took advantage of the spaces for manoeuvre that the treaties of Munster and Osnabrück had left to him. The Diet was dissolved in 1654 with most of the delicate *negotia remissa* not yet settled.

But soon the situation altered dramatically: just a few months after the dissolution of the Diet the newly elected king of the Romans Ferdinand IV died suddenly (1654). At the same time, Ferdinand III lost his nimbus as emperor of peace when he entered the Northern War against Sweden, restarted to support his Spanish relatives in their enduring war. This reproduced the antagonisms of the final phase of the Thirty Years' War. Finally, in 1657, Ferdinand himself died suddenly leaving his seventeen-year-old son and heir Leopold (Ignaz) in a very difficult situation.[29]

The election-diet of 1657–8 was the most difficult one for the house of Habsburg since 1519. A strong party of the imperial estates under the guidance of the influential elector of Mainz, Johann Philipp of Schönborn, was suspicious of Leopold's aims and looked for alternatives. Several opposing pretenders were discussed, among others the young Louis XIV of France. In the end, Leopold I (r. 1658–1705) was elected and crowned in July 1658,[30] but under rather unpleasant circumstances: a severe electoral capitulation was imposed on him, which inhibited any support for Spain, and several important electors and princes, with the participation of France and Sweden, formed the first so-called Rhenish Confederation aimed at forcing Leopold to keep his promises.

The distrust between the emperor and a great part of the estates of the empire induced Leopold to delay the convocation of the Imperial Diet as long as possible, although he urgently needed the estates' support against the newly arising Ottoman threat. At last, the Diet was opened in January 1663, the estates – and the Rhenish Confederation – gave their military assistance, and the Turkish army was defeated. But instead of exploiting the victory, Leopold, who distrusted Louis XIV and his allies, immediately concluded the peace of Eisenstadt (1664).

It is most interesting that the detested Diet became a very useful instrument of influence for Leopold I. Leopold himself and some electors and princes of the empire were personally present in Regensburg for only a few short months. The Diet did not dissolve but was transformed into an assembly of envoys that first continued to discuss the *negotia remissa*, but later conferred on any matter that affected the empire. After a while, Leopold learned to use the so-called Perpetual Diet as a public forum of the empire and as an instrument for uniting the estates behind their emperor.[31]

This evolution was facilitated by the changing external situation of the empire. From the 1670s onwards, it was no longer Leopold, but Louis XIV who was perceived as a threat to peace. In the 1680s and 1690s this perception increased thanks to the so-called French Reunions and the Nine Years' War (1688–97). At the same time the Habsburg dominions were menaced by an Ottoman attack that again culminated with the siege of Vienna (1683). This double threat enabled Leopold – despite his total lack of military virtues – to occupy the position of the defender of the Holy Empire against the 'infidels' and their equally detestable French counterparts.[32] Not least thanks to the support of the empire, Leopold acquired the major part of Hungary with the Treaty of Karlowitz (1699). Two years earlier, with the Peace of Rijswijk, Louis XIV had been forced to abandon at least a part of the Reunions of the 1680s. In the 1690s, a revival of the imperial policy towards *Reichsitalien* took place as well.

The external consolidation went along with the strengthening of Leopold's position within the Habsburg dominions and in the empire. In 1687, the Hungarian Diet acknowledged the Habsburgs' hereditary claim to the Crown of St Stephen. In 1690, Leopold's eldest son Joseph I was elected and crowned king of the Romans. And, in 1692, the emperor promoted the Duke of Brunswick-Hannover, Ernst August, to the electoral rank on his own authority in order to gain his assistance in the running wars.

In the time of Leopold, the evolution of the Habsburgs' self-fashioning as the most august house of Austria and as the one and only imperial dynasty, went on. One of the most remarkable ingredients of the imperial image was the venerable age and origin of the Habsburgs' dynasty with its uninterrupted succession of Roman kings and emperors since 1438, with its first crowned head Rudolph I and with its mythological roots in Troy. Another tradition with a great importance for the Habsburgs was that of the ancient Roman emperors: Leopold was not only a descendent of Rudolph I but also of Charlemagne, Constantine the Great and Augustus. Likewise important for the conception of himself and of his dynasty was the indubitable and ostentatious commitment to the Catholic faith. While he had to respect the equal status of the Protestant estates guaranteed by the Peace of Westphalia, Leopold took very seriously his position as an *advocatus ecclesiae* and eagerly promoted Catholicism in the Habsburg dominions. During his reign several attempts for a reunion of the German Protestants with the Catholic Church took place.[33] Since the time of Ferdinand II and Ferdinand III there was an increasing Italian influence in Vienna which promoted the transalpine transfer of devout practices, works of art, eruditeness, music and opera, and led to the ascent of the imperial court. It became an alternative to Louis XIV's Versailles. With liberation from the Ottoman threat the cityscape of Vienna changed fundamentally: only then could Vienna become an adequate capital for the Roman emperor.[34]

Leopold's reputation was strengthened considerably when almost all estates of the empire followed him into the War of the Spanish Succession (1701–13/14), a conflict of a mainly dynastic nature which hardly affected the empire directly. At the height of the war Leopold died and was followed by Joseph I (r. 1705–11) whose reign in several respects marked a turning of the tide in Habsburg emperorship.[35] Joseph's accession to the throne was welcomed enthusiastically given the heaviness that had characterized Leopold's style of government, especially during his later years. Indeed, Joseph achieved several military and political successes. In 1708, he solved the question of the ninth Hanoverian electorate with the readmission of the Bohemian electorate, thereby strengthening notably his own position.[36] Only then did the Habsburgs themselves occupy a seat in the electoral curia of the Imperial Diet. In the same year, the emperor's position as supreme head was underlined when Joseph put several German and Italian princes under the Ban of the Empire because of their alliance with France.

At the same time, the limits of the re-ascent of the imperial position became visible: on the one hand, Joseph's rather dynamic politics raised suspicion that the efforts of the empire were being abused for the sole profit of the house of Austria, and indeed, in case of conflict, Joseph and his leading ministers tended to favour the Austrian interests instead of the concerns of the empire. On the other, not only Austria, but several other major princes of the empire began to 'outgrow' the empire and thus the emperor's sphere of influence. Already in 1697, the elector of Saxony had been elected king of Poland; in 1701, with imperial assent, the elector of Brandenburg adopted the dignity of a king in Prussia; and in 1714 the Hanoverians ascended the British throne.[37]

It was Joseph's brother Charles VI (r. 1711–40) who had to face the rising problems.[38] His election and coronation in 1711 went off smoothly. With the treaties of Rastatt and Baden (1714), of Passarowitz (1718) and of London (1718–21) the dominions of the Austrian Habsburgs reached their maximum extent. But the lack of a male heir constituted a serious threat and rendered the Habsburg position vulnerable. This was notwithstanding Charles's law of succession, the famous Pragmatic Sanction of 1713, and his efforts to obtain the consent of the estates of the Habsburg dominions, of the empire and of the European powers to the succession of his eldest daughter Maria Theresia. In the empire, a renewal of confessional dissent took place and was exploited by the elector-kings of Brandenburg-Prussia and of Hannover-Great Britain in accordance with their political aims. At the same time, with the reconciliation of the branches of Bavaria and the Palatinate the Wittelsbach, who temporarily held four electorates, formed a new and probably opposing power bloc in the empire.

This vulnerability was not visible prima facie. For example, during the reign of Charles VI recourse to the Imperial Aulic Council increased notably.[39] The emperor intervened in internal conflicts in several principalities and Imperial Cities. In several Imperial Abbeys the so-called 'Kaisersäle' were built and underlined the allegiance of the *Reichskirche* towards the emperor. But in the 1730s two disastrous wars, the War of the Polish Succession (1733–5/8) and the Turkish War of 1736–9, caused notable territorial losses and undermined the military reputation of the Habsburg monarchy. When Charles VI died unexpectedly in 1740, the succession to the imperial throne was unsettled. Maria Theresia as a woman could not be elected and schemes for electing her husband, Franz Stephan of Lorraine, the Grand-Duke of Tuscany, as king of the Romans had not yet been realized.

Permanence and change: the Habsburg-Lorraine emperors[40]

With the death of Charles VI, the Habsburg emperorship in a narrow sense came to an end, but after two years of interregnum (1740–2) and the disastrous experiment of the Wittelsbach emperorship of Charles VII (r. 1742–5),[41] it was obvious that the imperial crown should return to the house of Habsburg, now Habsburg-Lorraine, in the person of Maria Theresia's husband Franz Stephan of Lorraine. Because of the enduring War of the Austrian Succession (1740–8) the election and coronation of Franz I (r. 1745–64) in Frankfurt had to be consummated under the protection of Austrian military forces, but no major problems occurred despite the withdrawal of the elector of Brandenburg(-Prussia) and of the Count Palatine, both of whom acknowledged the new emperor subsequently.[42]

Prima facie, the situation seemed nearly unaltered compared to the period before 1740. The emperor resided in Vienna again, and a great part of the personnel of the imperial institutions that had worked for Charles VI were re-engaged. But there were quite a few differences. First, Franz I was not the king, but the husband of the queen of Hungary and Bohemia while his own dominions were situated at the very periphery of the empire. The authority of the Roman emperor was diminished notably, and the Bavarian intermezzo had shaken the relations between the court of Vienna and the traditional imperial clients. Furthermore, with the rise of Prussia, the internal balance of the empire changed significantly. From now on, imperial politics were substantially shaped by the Austro-Prussian relationship. It is most interesting that, probably in 1746, a discussion took place in Vienna concerning whether or not the imperial crown was still of any use to the house of Austria. The question was answered in the affirmative; nevertheless it is remarkable that the question had been asked at all.[43]

During the Seven Years' War (1756–63) Franz I was successful in mobilizing the majority of the imperial estates for a military venture against the peace-breaker Frederick II, but in 1757 this attempt turned out to be a complete failure. Moreover, the Prussian king was keen on representing the power conflict as a confessional quarrel caused by the court of Vienna. Thus, Frederick styled himself as defender of the empire's constitution against the emperor. He did not aspire to the imperial crown but reached the position of a kind of counter-emperor.[44]

This was facilitated unwillingly by Joseph II (r. 1765–80) who had been elected king of the Romans in 1764 and followed his father in 1765. At first, the young and brilliant emperor was greeted with hope, even enthusiasm. Indeed, he set about addressing several deficiencies in the imperial constitution. While he was successful with a reform of the Imperial Aulic Council, his efforts to reform the Imperial Chamber as well failed as a result of Prussia's obstruction. His expansionistic foreign policies turned out to be even more fatal for the emperor's reputation. The first partition of Poland (1772), the War of the Bavarian Succession (1778–9) and his schemes for exchanging Bavaria with the Austrian Netherlands led to profound uncertainty among the smaller estates of the empire who had formed the Habsburgs' clientele to date. After the death of his mother and co-regent Maria Theresia (1780), Joseph alarmed the prince-bishops with his radical ecclesiastical reforms. A fundamental distrust of Joseph provoked the formation of a structured anti-imperial opposition, for the first time since the 1660s. The so-called *Fürstenbund* was under the guidance of Prussia and included, among others, the electors of Saxony and Hanover and even a few ecclesiastical princes.

When Joseph died in 1790 his brother Leopold II (r. 1790–2) was elected and crowned emperor. He tried to regain lost faith but, unfortunately, he died almost immediately and was followed by his son Franz II (r. 1792–1806), who turned out to be the last Roman emperor.[45] For a final time the time-honoured ceremonies of the election and coronation took place in Frankfurt, but in the face of the French Revolution they seemed even more out of date than they had been judged by enlightened contemporaries in 1764. Obviously, the solemnities of the empire no longer fitted with the sobering realities.[46]

The end of the Roman emperorship[47]

Although the weakening cohesiveness of the empire had become apparent and the Roman imperial crown had lost a part of its importance for the Habsburgs by the 1790s, there was no sign of an imminent end to the empire. It was the French Revolution and the following Coalition Wars which led to the final crisis and to the eclipse of the Holy Roman empire and its emperorship.

Soon, it became obvious that the imperial war against revolutionary France (since 1792) could not easily be won. With the withdrawal of Prussia from the war in 1795, victory became even less probable. While the northern part of Germany left the war under the tutelage of Prussia, the southern estates of the empire were forced by Austria to continue the war. Finally, in 1797, Franz II himself was coerced into peace negotiations. With the Treaty of Campo Formio he not only abandoned the Habsburg dominions in the Netherlands and Lombardy but also renounced the parts of the empire on the left bank of the Rhine and claims to *Reichsitalien*. He did so as head of the Habsburg monarchy (and not as Roman emperor), but obviously, this decision marked a precedent for the following peace treaty of the empire. Indeed, the Peace of Lunéville, concluded after the Second Coalition War in 1801, confirmed the cessions of 1797.[48]

Most remarkably, the court of Vienna did not even try to control the negotiations for the implementation of the decisions of 1801. This allowed the greater part of the traditional imperial clientele to be eliminated with the so-called *Reichsdeputationshauptschluss*, which determined the extinction of almost all ecclesiastical principalities and most of the Imperial Cities in order to compensate the secular princes for their losses on the left bank of the Rhine. Furthermore, the college of the prince-electors was re-composed and, for the first time, the Protestants prevailed. Thus, the future of the Roman emperorship of the Habsburgs became extremely uncertain.

It is no wonder that Franz II followed the example of Napoleon Bonaparte by creating a new, Austrian emperorship (1804). For about two years, he was at the same time the Roman emperor Franz II and the emperor of Austria Franz I. His new (and hereditary!) imperial dignity differed substantially from the older one, because it was not linked with the universal Roman empire and thus did not claim any supremacy over the other Christian monarchs, but only marked Austria's position as a great power among others.

It was no surprise when the Roman emperorship of the Habsburgs came to an end two years later. With the Peace of Pressburg (1805), the Habsburg position was further weakened and the end of the empire became conceivable. After the withdrawal of sixteen leading estates of the empire in July 1806 and an ultimatum from Napoleon, Franz did not hesitate very long and resigned his Roman imperial crown (8 August). In doing so he ended not only (at least de facto) the millennial Holy Roman Empire but also a period of 350 years of the Habsburg Roman emperorship.[49]

Conclusion: the characteristics of the Habsburgs' Roman emperorship

It is quite remarkable that the Habsburg dynasty held the electoral office of the Roman emperor nearly without interruption for more than 350 years. In contrast to many other German dynasties, they had the advantage of a tradition as Roman kings reaching back to the thirteenth century. And, every member of the family elected and crowned as Roman king or emperor respectively reinforced the nimbus of the Habsburg as *the* dynasty of kings and emperors. The house of Austria, due to its territorial acquisitions from the late fifteenth century onwards, seemed the only German dynasty capable of wearing the burden of the imperial crown. The dynasty never failed to emphasize this in their self-representation. Eventually, the Habsburgs were considered to be 'born' candidates for the imperial throne without the principle of electoral monarchy even being questioned formally.

Several factors supported this development. One of the most important elements to secure dynastic succession even for the electoral office of the emperor was the election of the Roman king *vivente Imperatore*. Another beneficial factor was the low number of prince-electors, which was more easily managed than bigger electoral colleges like the Polish Sejm. Furthermore, the Habsburg emperors and the prince-electors shared an interest in limiting German princes' demands for more influence in the realm. Moreover, not only in the electoral college but also elsewhere in the empire, Habsburg rulers could establish a stable, pro-Habsburg party and clientele. They could, after all, use imperial rights and privileges to achieve this, not least with their ability to give various privileges and to act as supreme judge. Those actors who had less power and influence in the empire compared to the mighty princes and dynasties were especially supportive of the imperial rule of the Habsburgs due to their hope that the rulers would in turn defend their endangered positions. Their support enhanced the influence of the Habsburgs in institutions of the estates, especially the Imperial Diet. This way, the emperors could creatively and flexibly use the possibilities open to them under the constitution. In doing so, the art of striking a compromise was much more effective than an over-emphasis on imperial prerogatives which usually led to resistance by the imperial estates.

Since the sixteenth century, the importance of confession grew. Due to the Roman Catholic majority in the electoral college and the Habsburgs' representation as a firm Catholic dynasty, they secured their claim to the imperial office. Moreover, the emperors of the house of Habsburg contributed to the fact that large parts of the imperial church remained Catholic, including the ecclesiastical electors: imperial church and Habsburgs emperors upheld each other. Then again, despite several collaborations, a structural opposition developed among the Protestant imperial estates against the Catholic emperor. It became one of the biggest challenges for emperors to support Catholic interests and respect constitutionally guaranteed Protestant rights at the same time.

Ambivalent in a similar way was the significant power imbalance between the Habsburgs and the less powerful German dynasties. At first, territorial acquisitions were an advantage. However, the centre of the Habsburg dominions shifted more and more to the border of the Holy Roman Empire. The house of Austria even outgrew the realm: the Habsburgs had become a European dynasty. This in turn led to territorial and dynastic interests dominating the interests of the empire at the court in Vienna.

Critique of the early modern emperors was usually based on their exceeding their jurisdiction, oppressing German freedoms and/or the interests of the empire in favour of their own dynastic interests. However, (nearly) every search for an alternative candidate for the office of the emperor turned up empty. German dynasties lacked the necessary resources while foreign candidates, especially the French king, while considered from time to time, were never realized. In contrast, the Habsburgs were, until the end of the empire, accepted as 'German' dynasty.

It is no coincidence that the only election of a non-Habsburg emperor in the early modern period occurred in the eighteenth century when circumstances of the Habsburgs' emperorship changed due to both the dynastic succession crisis in the house of Austria and the rise of Brandenburg-Prussia as a second, German great power. After the failure of the experiment of a Wittelsbach 'emperorship of the estates' (1742–5), the now Habsburg-Lorraine dynasty once again gained the emperor's title. The relationship between the house of Austria and the Roman-German realm, however, was obviously looser. Nonetheless, the Holy Roman Imperial Crown was only lost to the Habsburgs when that realm itself ended in 1806.

Notes

1 For an overview see Anton Schindling and Walter Ziegler, eds., *Die Kaiser der Neuzeit: Heiliges Römisches Reich, Österreich, Deutschland* (Munich: Beck, 1990); Peter H. Wilson, *Heart of Europe: A History of the Holy Roman Empire* (Cambridge: Harvard University Press, 2016), 60–63.

2 Paul-Joachim Heinig, "Albrecht II. (1438–1439)," in *Die deutschen Herrscher des Mittelalters: historische Portraits von Heinrich I. bis Maximilian I. (919–1519)*, eds. Bernd Schneidmüller and Stefan Weinfurter (Darmstadt: WBG, 2004), 486–494; Karl-Friedrich Krieger, *Die Habsburger im Mittelalter: Von Rudolf I. bis Friedrich III.* (Stuttgart: Kohlhammer, 2004).

3 Paul-Joachim Heinig, *Kaiser Friedrich III. (1440–1493): Hof, Regierung, Politik*, 3 vols (Cologne: Böhlau, 1997).

4 Cf. Günther Hödl, "Die Bestätigung und Erweiterung der österreichischen Freiheitsbriefe durch Kaiser Friedrich III.," in *Fälschungen im Mittelalter. Internationaler Kongreß der Monumenta Germaniae Historica, München 1986* (Hannover: Hahn, 1988), vol. 3:1, 225–246.

5 Susanne Wolf, *Die Doppelregierung Kaiser Friedrichs III. und König Maximilians (1486–1493)* (Cologne: Böhlau, 2005).

6 1486: Maximilian I; 1531: Ferdinand I; 1562: Maximilian II; 1575: Rudolph II; 1636: Ferdinand III; 1653: Ferdinand IV; 1690: Joseph I; 1764: Joseph II. Helmut Neuhaus, "Die Römische Königswahl vivente imperatore in der Neuzeit: Zum Problem der Kontinuität in einer frühneuzeitlichen Wahlmonarchie," in *Neue Studien zur frühneuzeitlichen Reichsgeschichte*, ed. Helmut Neuhaus (Berlin: Duncker & Humblot, 1997), 1–53.

7 Hermann Wiesflecker, *Kaiser Maximilian I.: Das Reich, Österreich und Europa an der Wende zur Neuzeit*, 5 vols (Munich: Oldenbourg, 1971–1986); Manfred Hollegger, *Maximilian I., 1459–1519: Herrscher und Mensch einer Zeitenwende* (Stuttgart: Kohlhammer, 2005).

8 Eva Ortlieb, "Vom Königlichen/Kaiserlichen Hofrat zum Reichshofrat: Maximilian I., Karl V., Ferdinand I.," in *Das Reichskammergericht: Der Weg zu seiner Gründung und die ersten Jahrzehnte seines Wirkens (1451–1527)*, ed. Bernhard Diestelkamp (Cologne: Böhlau, 2003), 221–289; Leopold Auer, "The Role of the Imperial Aulic Council in the Constitutional Structure of the Holy Roman Empire," in *The Holy Roman Empire, 1495–1806: A European Perspective*, eds. J.W. Evans, Michael Schaich and Peter H. Wilson (Oxford: Oxford University Press, 2012), 63–76.

9 Wolfgang Burgdorf, ed., *Die Wahlkapitulationen der römisch-deutschen Könige und Kaiser 1519–1792* (Göttingen: Vandenhoeck & Ruprecht, 2015).

10 Harald Kleinschmidt, *Charles V: The World Emperor* (Stroud: Sutton Publishing, 2004); Alfred Kohler, *Karl V., 1500–1558: Eine Biographie* (Munich: Beck, 2014); Luise Schorn-Schütte, *Karl V.: Kaiser zwischen Mittelalter und Neuzeit*, third edition (Munich: Beck, 2006); Joachim Whaley, *Germany and the Holy Roman Empire*, 2 vols (Oxford: Oxford University Press, 2011), vol. 1, 155–336.

11 Wilson, *Heart*, 295–352.

12 Whaley, *Germany*, vol. 1, 339–417.

13 Alfred Kohler, *Ferdinand I., 1503–1564: Fürst, König und Kaiser* (Munich: Beck, 2003); Ernst Laubach, *Ferdinand I. als Kaiser: Politik und Herrscherauffassung des Nachfolgers Karls V.* (Munich: Aschendorff, 2001).

14 Albrecht P. Luttenberger, "Kirchenadvokatie und Religionsfriede, Kaiseridee und kaiserliche Reichspolitik im 16. und 17. Jahrhundert," in *Legitimation und Funktion des Herrschers: Vom ägyptischen Pharao zum neuzeitlichen Diktator*, eds. Rolf Gundlach and Hermann Weber (Stuttgart: Steiner, 1992), 185–232.

15 Until 1708, the Bohemian vote at the Imperial Diet was suspended.

16 Schemes for a Protestant emperorship were never realized. Heinz Duchhardt, *Protestantisches Kaisertum und Altes Reich: Die Diskussion über die Konfession des Kaisers in Politik, Publizistik und Staatsrecht* (Wiesbaden: Steiner, 1977).

17 Eike Wolgast, *Hochstift und Reformation: Studien zur Geschichte der Reichskirche zwischen 1517 und 1648* (Stuttgart: Steiner, 1995).

18 Maximilian Lanzinner, *Friedenssicherung und politische Einheit des Reiches unter Kaiser Maximilian II. (1564–1576)* (Göttingen: Vandenhoeck & Ruprecht, 1993); Albrecht P. Luttenberger, *Kurfürsten, Kaiser und Reich: Politische Führung und Friedenssicherung unter Ferdinand I. und Maximilian II.* (Mainz: Zabern, 1994).

19 Karl Vocelka, *Rudolf II. und seine Zeit* (Vienna: Böhlau, 1985); for the confessional aspect Stefan Ehrenpreis, *Kaiserliche Gerichtsbarkeit und Konfessionskonflikt. Der Reichshofrat unter Rudolf II., 1576–1612* (Göttingen: Vandenhoeck & Ruprecht, 2006).

20 Whaley, *Germany*, vol. 1, 418–74; Václav Bůžek, ed., *Ein Bruderzwist im Hause Habsburg (1608–1611)* (České Budějovice: Filozofická fakulta, 2010).

21 Peter H. Wilson, *Europe's Tragedy: A History of the Thirty Years War* (London: Allen Lane, 2009); Peter H. Wilson, "The Thirty Years War as the Empire's Constitutional Crisis," in *The Holy Roman Empire, 1495–1806: A European Perspective*, eds. J. W. Evans, Michael Schaich and Peter H. Wilson (Oxford: Oxford University Press, 2012), 95–114; Whaley, *Germany*, vol. 1, 563–644.

22 Thomas Brockmann, *Dynastie, Kaiseramt und Konfession: Politik und Ordnungsvorstellungen Ferdinands II. im Dreißigjährigen Krieg* (Paderborn: Schöningh, 2011).

23 Heiner Haan, "Kaiser Ferdinand II. und das Problem des Reichsabsolutismus. Die Prager Heeresreform von 1635," *Historische Zeitschrift* 207 (1968): 297–345.

24 Mark Hengerer, *Kaiser Ferdinand III. (1608–1657): Vom Krieg zum Frieden* (Vienna: Böhlau, 2012); Lothar Höbelt, *Ferdinand III. (1608–1657): Friedenskaiser wider Willen* (Graz: Ares, 2008).

25 Leopold Auer, "Die Ziele der kaiserlichen Politik bei den Westfälischen Friedensverhandlungen und ihre Umsetzung," in *Der Westfälische Friede. Diplomatie – politische Zäsur – kulturelles Umfeld*, ed. Heinz Duchhardt (Munich: Oldenbourg, 1998), 143–173.

26 Barbara Stollberg-Rilinger, *Des Kaisers alte Kleider. Verfassungsgeschichte und Symbolsprache des Alten Reiches* (Munich: Beck, 2008).

27 Magdalena Hawlik-van de Water, *Die Kapuzinergruft. Begräbnisstätte der Habsburger in Wien*, second edition (Freiburg: Herder, 1993).

28 Volker Press, "Die kaiserliche Stellung im Reich zwischen 1648 und 1740 – Versuch einer Neubewertung," in *Stände und Gesellschaft im Alten Reich*, ed. Georg Schmidt (Stuttgart: Steiner, 1989), 51–80; Whaley, *Germany*, vol. 2, 1–183.

29 Matthias Schnettger, *Der Reichsdeputationstag 1655–1663: Kaiser und Stände zwischen Westfälischem Frieden und Immerwährendem Reichstag* (Munich: Aschendorff, 1996).

30 Karl Otmar Freiherr von Aretin, *Das Alte Reich 1648–1806*, 4 vols (Stuttgart: Klett-Cotta, 1993–2000), vol. 1, 184–362, vol. 2, 15–137.

31 Anton Schindling, *Die Anfänge des Immerwährenden Reichstags zu Regensburg: Ständevertretung und Staatskunst nach dem Westfälischen Frieden* (Mainz: Zabern, 1991); Karl Härter, "The Permanent Imperial Diet in European Context," in *The Holy Roman Empire, 1495–1806: A European Perspective*, eds. J.W. Evans, Michael Schaich and Peter H. Wilson (Oxford: Oxford University Press, 2012), 115–135.

32 Martin Wrede, *Das Reich und seine Feinde: Politische Feindbilder in der reichspatriotischen Publizistik zwischen Westfälischem Frieden und Siebenjährigem Krieg* (Mainz: Zabern, 2005).

33 Matthias Schnettger, "Kirchenadvokatie und Reichseinigungspläne, Kaiser Leopold I. und die Reunionsbestrebungen Rojas y Spinolas," in *Union, Konversion, Toleranz*, eds. Heinz Duchhardt and Gerhard May (Mainz: Zabern, 2000), 139–169.

34 Maria Goloubeva, *The Glorification of Emperor Leopold I in Image, Spectacle, and Text* (Mainz: Zabern, 2000); Jutta Schumann, *Die andere Sonne. Kaiserbild und Medienstrategien im Zeitalter Leopolds I.* (Berlin: Akademie-Verlag, 2003); Jeroen F. J. Duindam, *Vienna and Versailles: The Courts of Europe's Dynastic Rivals, 1550–1780* (Cambridge: Cambridge University Press, 2006); Herbert Karner, ed., *Die Wiener Hofburg 1521–1705: Baugeschichte, Funktion und Etablierung als Kaiserresidenz* (Vienna: Verlag der Österreichischen Akademie der Wissenschaften, 2014); Hellmut Lorenz and Anna Mader-Kratky, eds., *Die Wiener Hofburg 1705–1835: Die kaiserliche Residenz vom Barock bis zum Klassizismus* (Vienna: Verlag der Österreichischen Akademie der Wissenschaften, 2016).

35 Charles W. Ingrao, *In Quest and Crisis: Emperor Joseph I and the Habsburg Monarchy* (West Lafayette, Indiana: Purdue University Press, 1979); Aretin, *Das Alte Reich*, vol. 2, 139–219; Matthias Schnettger, "A Turn of Tide: The War of the Spanish Succession and its Impact on German History," in *The Transition in Europe between XVII and XVIII Centuries: Perspectives and Case Studies*, eds. Antonio Álvarez-Ossorio, Cinzia Cremonini and Elena Riva (Milan: Franco Angeli, 2016), 35–52.

36 After 1708 there were seven Catholic electors – Mainz, Cologne, Trier, Bohemia, Bavaria, Saxony (Catholic since the conversion of Frederick August I in 1697), Palatine (re-created in 1648, Catholic since 1685) – and only two Protestant ones – Brandenburg and Hanover. Even when the Bavarian and Palatine electorate were united in 1777 the Catholics held a majority of 6:2.

37 Whereas the Bavarian aspirations for Spain or a kingdom in Italy and the schemes of an Armenian crown for the Elector-Palatine failed.

38 Aretin, *Das Alte Reich*, vol. 2, 221–412; Bernd Rill, *Karl VI.: Habsburg als barocke Großmacht* (Graz: Styria, 1992).

39 Eva Ortlieb und Gert Polster, "Die Prozessfrequenz am Reichshofrat (1519–1806)," *Zeitschrift für Neuere Rechtsgeschichte* 26 (2004): 189–216.

40 Whaley, *Germany*, vol. 2, 347–444.

41 Aretin, *Das Alte Reich*, vol. 2, 413–69; Peter Claus Hartmann, *Karl Albrecht – Karl VII.: Glücklicher Kurfürst – unglücklicher Kaiser* (Regensburg: Pustet, 1985).

42 Aretin, *Das Alte Reich*, vol. 3, 19–111.

43 Ibid., 32–34.

44 Ibid., 113–361; Karl Otmar Freiherr von Aretin, *Heiliges Römisches Reich 1776–1806: Reichsverfassung und Staatssouveränität*, 2 vols (Wiesbaden: Steiner, 1967), vol. 1, 11–241; Derek Beales, *Joseph II*, 2 vols (Cambridge: Cambridge University Press, 1987–2009).

45 Aretin, *Das Alte Reich*, vol. 3, 361–531; id., *Heiliges Römisches Reich*, vol. 1, 242–506.

46 Stollberg-Rilinger, *Des Kaisers alte Kleider*, 227–46.

47 Whaley, *Germany*, vol. 2, 557–644.

48 Matthias Schnettger, "'Abschied von Germania'. Italienische Perspektiven auf das Ende des Alten Reiches," in *Epochenjahr 1806? Das Ende des Alten Reichs in zeitgenössischen Perspektiven und Deutungen*, eds. Christine Roll and Matthias Schnettger (Mainz: Zabern, 2008), 41–59.

49 Bettina Braun, "Das Reich blieb nicht stumm und kalt. Der Untergang des Alten Reiches in der Sicht der Zeitgenossen," in *Epochenjahr 1806? Das Ende des Alten Reichs in zeitgenössischen Perspektiven und Deutungen*, eds. Christine Roll and Matthias Schnettger (Mainz: Zabern, 2008), 7–29; Lothar Höbelt, "Die Wiener Sicht: der Kaiserhof und Österreich," in *Epochenjahr 1806? Das Ende des Alten Reichs in zeitgenössischen Perspektiven und Deutungen*, eds. Christine Roll and Matthias Schnettger (Mainz: Zabern, 2008), 31–39.

Key works

Evans, R.J.W., Michael Schaich and Peter H. Wilson, eds., *The Holy Roman Empire, 1495–1806: A European Perspective* (Oxford: Oxford University Press, 2012).

Schindling, Anton and Walter Ziegler, eds., *Die Kaiser der Neuzeit: Heiliges Römisches Reich, Österreich, Deutschland* (Munich: Beck, 1990).

Stollberg-Rilinger, Barbara, *Des Kaisers alte Kleider: Verfassungsgeschichte und Symbolsprache des Alten Reiches* (Munich: Beck, 2008).

Volker Press, "Die kaiserliche Stellung im Reich zwischen 1648 und 1740: Versuch einer Neubewertung," in *Stände und Gesellschaft im Alten Reich*, ed. Georg Schmidt (Stuttgart: Steiner, 1989), 51–80.

Von Aretin, Karl Otmar Freiherr, *Das Alte Reich 1648–1806* (Stuttgart: Klett-Cotta, 1993–2000), 4 vols.

Whaley, Joachim, *Germany and the Holy Roman Empire*, 2 vols (Oxford: Oxford University Press, 2011).

6

DEI GRATIA AND THE 'DIVINE RIGHT OF KINGS'

Divine legitimization or human humility?

Matthias Range

The idea of rule *Dei gratia,* 'by the grace of God', was one of the core concepts of almost all European monarchies. As part of rulers' titles *Dei gratia* was important in European history for at least 1100 years, from the eighth to the nineteenth centuries. At the beginning of the second millennium, the phrase is still in use by at least some European monarchs: those of the United Kingdom, Denmark, the Netherlands, Liechtenstein, Monaco and (if not actively) of Spain, as well as in numerous Commonwealth realms.

With its fundamental historical importance, there have been discussions of and writings about *Dei gratia* and the appertaining interpretations and context for centuries. Notwithstanding its significance, however, Jack Autrey Dabbs's *Dei Gratia in Royal Titles* from 1971 has so far remained the only dedicated, if somewhat sketchy, study on the use in rulers' titles.[1] Indeed, the topic has not met with much interest recently, with the relevant core studies on it remaining valid but dating from some time ago. More recent research on *Dei gratia* has focused on the early Middle Ages, especially on the Carolingians. The neglect may result not least from a controversial understanding of the phrase. In particular, the common understanding of *Dei gratia* indicating a 'divine right' of monarchs has led to the phrase's original meaning being widely ignored and unexplored. Re-examining this will be worthwhile as an addition to discussions on rulers' sacrality and their subjects' right to resistance – topics that have received more attention in recent historiography.

Overall, notwithstanding France, most research has been concerned with Germany and Britain – the two countries in which the so-called theory of the 'divine right of kings' was most distinctly and influentially developed and where it has long been the issue of discussions. Focusing on these two countries, this short study will present an introduction to the main issues.

Dei gratia

The addition of *Dei gratia* to rulers' titles is obviously linked with Christianity and Christian kings: the 'deo' referred to is the God of the Bible. The origins of the phrase are almost certainly biblical.[2] Most probably, the phrase is taken from the

Latin translation of St Paul's First Letter to the Corinthians 15:10: 'Gratia autem Dei sum id quod sum' – 'But by the grace of God I am what I am.'[3]

The main issue with the phrase *Dei gratia* has been, and still is, its political and socio-cultural meaning and interpretation. Claus Richter explains that the phrase often allows two valid interpretations for the early Middle Ages.[4] In fact, one could easily argue that these interpretations are more generally valid. One interpretation is that the bearer wanted to express humility ('Demut'), by showing that an office is held by God's grace and not through one's own merit. The other interpretation is that the phrase – especially when used by rulers – expresses the belief that the bearer has received the office not from another human and is thus free from human judgement; the office-holder's independence is thereby increased significantly.

At first, the *Dei gratia* phrase was included not in rulers' but in clerics' titles, and Karl Schmitz, in his still very valuable study from 1913, has pointed out that the Council of Nicaea in 325 called itself 'Dei gratia congregatum'.[5] Heinrich Fichtenau, in his similarly important study, has mentioned that around the turn of the sixth to the seventh century, the addition of *Dei gratia* to the title had been common (*geläufig*) among 'the bishops in the Lombard Kingdom and its neighbours'.[6] There were similar phrases in the titles of the Roman popes from as early as the late fifth century, and they used *Dei gratia* by the late sixth century – and Merovingian bishops used it soon afterwards.[7]

It is not clear exactly when and why the *Dei gratia* phrase was incorporated into secular rulers' titles. The connection between rulers and religious authority is of course much older than Christianity, reaching back as far as Ancient Egypt, and has long been discussed.[8] Schmitz has highlighted that specific title formulas already existed in pre-Christian times.[9] However, as Richter pointed out, a phrase akin to *Dei gratia* was rarely used in antiquity – as far as he can determine the only cases involve Darius the Great, Xerxes and Artaxerxes.[10] The reason for this is assumed to be that in antiquity the interpretation of the ruler as actually being God-like and divine was the stronger and more common view. For the Christian context, Joseph Canning has observed that the earliest use in a ruler's title seems to date from the time of the Lombard king Agilulf (590–616) and that it was 'also applied' to the Visigothic king Svinthila (621–31).[11] Agilulf had it prominently encrusted in the inscription of a votive crown, which no longer exists but which is well documented: *gratia Dei vir gloriosus, rex totius Italiae.*[12] Canning observes that 'by the end of the seventh century the Anglo-Saxon kings were employing it or similar titles'.[13] At the same time, he points out that 'The idea of kingship by divine favour was, however, older than the formula itself and can be discerned as early as the reign of the Vandal king, Huniric (d. 484).'[14] In any case, the crucial moment for the history of the phrase was probably its adoption in the ruler's title in Carolingian times.

The Carolingian use of the *Dei gratia* phrase had been developing since Pippin the Younger, also known as 'Pepin the Short', who ruled as king of the Franks from 751 until 768.[15] However, Canning notes that 'it only became part of normal chancellery usage after his death from 769'.[16] Indeed, it is by now well accepted that Pippin's successor Charlemagne was the first Western monarch who added *Dei gratia* to his title.[17] Bernard S. Bachrach has pinpointed that 'no later than Sunday, 5 June 774, Charlemagne already styled himself "Carolus Dei gratia rex Francorum et Langobardorum"'.[18]

In 800, Charlemagne was famously crowned emperor by Pope Leo III. As Ildar Garipzanov has observed, however, 'the formula *gratia Dei* disappeared from his intitulature after 800'; and neither Louis the Pious nor Lothar I, anointed as emperors in 816 and 823 respectively, used *Dei gratia* in their imperial titles.[19] It was only Louis II (r.844–75) who introduced the phrase into the imperial title, being styled *Dei gratia imperator Augustus* in his diplomas.[20] At the same time, as J. Rufus Fears has noted, *Dei gratia* first appeared as part of the inscription on coins in around 864, for Charles the Bald, king of West Francia.[21] From the late ninth century onwards, the use of the *Dei gratia* formula became wide-spread among princes all over Europe.[22]

The 'divine right of kings'

Dei gratia and the so-called 'divine right of kings' are often linked – at least in historiography and modern understanding. Notwithstanding precursors in the deified rulers of antiquity, the Christian idea of a 'divine right of kings' developed from a holistic appreciation of biblical references to the ruler's authority. Most directly, in Rom. 13:1, St Paul specifies 'Let every soul be subject unto the higher powers. For there is no power but of God: the powers that be are ordained of God.' Canning has paired this passage with John 19:11, where Jesus said to Pilate 'You would have no power over me if it had not been given you from above.'[23] Canning explains that:

> None of these passages mentioned kings as such, but taken together, and understood in a *milieu* in which kingship was the current form of government, they provided a mental context for perceiving royal power as being derived from God's goodwill or favour.[24]

Moreover, 1 Sam 8.11ff., with the Prophet Samuel's definition of a king for Israel, was one of the most important passages used to explain rulership.[25] As Annette Weber-Möckl explains, this passage was important in sixteenth- and seventeenth-century political writings because it links to the issue of whether absolute government is ordered or at least tolerated by God, or whether such government contradicts both tradition and divine order.[26]

The ground-breaking work on 'divine right' was John Neville Figgis's seminal study from 1896, with an extended second edition from 1914.[27] Figgis provided a useful definition of the 'propositions' that make up the 'theory of the divine right of kings in its completest form':

> (1) Monarchy is a divinely ordained institution. (2) Hereditary right is indefeasible . . . (3) Kings are accountable to God alone . . . (4) Non-resistance and passive obedience are enjoined by God.[28]

Figgis argued that the theory had been developed into its full bloom by the late sixteenth-century French writer Jean Bodin.[29] Similarly, referring to Charles Howard McIlwain's opinion that 'the Divine right of kings is a modern and not a medieval theory', Paul W. Fox specified that 'it was in sixteenth-century France that the elements in the theory, mingled with absolutism, began to be asserted clearly and publicly'.[30] Most prominently, perhaps, 'divine right' ideas were publicly referred to by a reigning king himself: James VI & I, of Scotland and England. Andreas Pečar has shown how the king's ideas were derived from several passages in the Bible.[31] Notwithstanding the king's published writings – such as the 1589 tract *The Trew Law of Monarchies* – James I famously made some strong claims in a speech to Parliament in 1610. In that, he postulated that 'kings are not only God's lieutenants upon earth, and sit upon God's throne, but even by God himself they are called gods.'[32]

Providing examples for both England and France, Fox concludes: 'It was in the seventeenth century that the doctrines of absolutism and divine right reached their zenith.'[33] Hence, much literature that has looked at *Dei gratia* and the 'divine right' has done so in the context of so-called 'absolutism'.[34] Horst Dreitzel summarized: 'The titular formula "By the Grace of God" is retrospectively often seen as representative of the absolutism of Christian politics.'[35] As Georg Flor states with a critical undertone in his more recent, significant study on the concept, the monarchical rule 'by the Grace of God' came to be taken as the 'questionable legitimisation of a ruler's claim to unlimited power'.[36] More directly, W.H. Greenleaf explained that it was 'the theory of the divine right of kings by which was maintained the notion of non-resistance to monarchs whether they observed the law or not'.[37] The same interpretation is taken on by Wolfgang Reinhard who argues that the autonomous medieval sacrality of the monarch continued in the idea of the sovereign being beyond human jurisdiction.[38] Indeed, as Pečar has worked out, historically one of the issues discussed in relation to the theory of the divine right was how far monarchs had to follow the law or were above it.[39]

The link between divine right and absolutist claims became so strong that, when absolutism became less prominent, this entailed more and more criticism of 'divine right' ideas. The theory lost more or less any wide support. By 1813, an anonymous Irish writer could refer to 'the absurd doctrine of the divine right of Kings'.[40] Similarly, Figgis opened his comprehensive study with the words: 'That the theory is absurd, when judged from a standpoint of modern political thought, is a statement that requires neither proof nor exposition.'[41] This judgement, however, does not necessarily apply to the concept of *Dei gratia*. For a better understanding of this concept it is instructive to discuss Richter's two aforementioned possible strands of interpretation.

Human humility

Richter explains that, when the phrase from St Paul's First Letter to the Corinthians was eventually taken up by clerics in late antiquity, they did so 'as a simple expression of humility', added to their names to point out their meekness and devotion.[42] The phrase's emphasis on 'grace' was inherent in the aforementioned Vulgate translation: 'Gratia autem Dei sum id quod sum.' Not only does 'Gratia' open the sentence, but its importance is furthermore heightened by the word 'autem' ('however'). In his still important 1929 study on *Dei gratia*, Willy Staerk summarized that 'one can hardly go wrong' in seeing 'an expression of humility as the perpetual basic tone of *Dei gratia*'.[43] Following the emphasis on humility, Staerk advocated the term of *Devotionsformel*, which is widely used in German historiography. This can be roughly translated as 'devotional formula', but it has the implication of a 'formula pointing out devotion' or 'humility'. When the *Dei gratia* phrase is called *Devotionsformel*, the term itself strongly indicates its interpretation. As Schmitz has explained, through the *Devotionsformel* 'the writer wants to express the feeling of his own lowliness or dependence on a higher authority, namely God'.[44] Notably, *Dei gratia* is just one of several such formulas, another very famous one being *Servus Servorum Dei* ('Servant of the Servants of God') that has become part of the papal intitulature.[45]

Regarding the incorporation of *Dei gratia* into rulers' titles, Walter Ullmann has suggested that the clerics who directed the Carolingian chancery 'probably applied to royal intitulature the formula known from their clerical documents'.[46] More directly, Richter assumed that the formula was added to the titles of Charlemagne and his brother Carloman because they had the desire to express their 'christliche Gesinnung', their 'Christian spirit'.[47] When Percy Schramm asked whether Charlemagne himself took the initiative to add the phrase to the royal title, he concluded that his motivation originated in its connotations of humility.[48] Moreover, Schramm summarized that 'it is sure that he [Charlemagne] took the meaning expressed in the formula seriously for the rest of his life'.

Schmitz has interpreted the *Dei gratia* phrase very much in the sense of expressing humility, as emphasizing that 'every Christian should always endeavour to be aware of his own powerlessness, of not being able to do anything without God's support'.[49] As he explains, this understanding of the *Dei gratia*-phrase 'is an obvious one, since it agrees completely with Christian teaching that all of man's possessions are a gift, received through God's grace'.[50] In Rom. 11:6, St Paul had straightforwardly explained that if something is received by 'grace', then it is not received 'of works', or through merit.[51] In this sense, grace is something obtained without any effort – while at the same time being unobtainable through even the greatest effort. On the other hand, however, there was uncertainty about when or why God would grant his grace. As Fichtenau explained, the *Dei gratia*-phrase received great relevance ('große Actualität') through the teachings of Pelagius and the resulting responses by St Augustine from 412 onwards: while Pelagius argued that God grants grace to the deserving, as he had granted it to St Paul, Augustine opined that this would degrade it to a mere reward for a service; rather, Augustine explained, grace was granted to the undeserving.[52]

Walther Kienast has provided numerous examples, from the mid-ninth to the early twelfth century, where the formula's meaning as a 'sign of mere piety' is clarified by words such as 'humilis'.[53] Similarly, Dreitzel has pointed out that the later 'absolutist interpretation of *Dei gratia* did not correspond with the medieval origins of the formula and its use in the Empire up to the sixteenth century'.[54] At the same time, he emphasizes that its origins were an 'expression of humility' that was 'meant to signify that a special status had not been achieved by one's own merits but merely thanks to God'. Dreitzel shows that this interpretation always persisted in the background, as it was used in a polemical way up until the nineteenth century.

G.R. Elton has found a good way of summarizing the phrase's meanings when he observed how kings since Charlemagne were 'kings by the grace of God, by God's gift and permission'.[55] Incidentally, with its inherent stressing of human humility, *Dei gratia* corresponds very much with the famous phrase 'remember you are a man' at Roman triumphal processions.[56] Indeed, *Dei gratia* highlights an intriguing, otherwise blurred dichotomy: the monarch is, as it were, on the same side as his or her human subjects in the face of the Divine omnipotence. If the monarch were to reign by 'divine *right*', then he or she would, in a way, be on God's side – but since it is merely by 'Divine *grace*', the monarch is on the same side as all other humans.

Divine legitimization

Richter has argued that *Dei gratia* in several of St Paul's letters is not merely a sign of his humility, but rather that St Paul used this phrase also 'to fight off attacks on the legitimacy of his apostolate' – he had to justify himself as an apostle, since he had not personally known Jesus.[57] All the same, Richter concludes that the *Dei gratia* formula 'for St Paul is a theological statement, not an ecclesiastical one [*kirchenrechtliche*]', thus reducing the stress on its legitimizing character.[58] Nevertheless, as alluded to in the context of divine right, legitimization was to become one of the phrase's main aspects. It is surely possibly that Charlemagne added *Dei gratia* to his royal title out of humility, in an act of devotion. However, the phrase could also have been added for political reasons. Fichtenau went so far as to propose that the idea of 'God-given kingship' could have been Charlemagne's main reason for adopting *Dei gratia* in his title.[59] Similarly, Ullmann observed:

> By combining the two fundamental Pauline principles – 'all power comes from God' and 'What I am I am by the grace of God' – and shaping them into a governmental principle of the first order by means of adoption of the royal grace formula, Charlemagne by a single brilliant stroke made concrete in the realm of government what had hitherto been a rarefied abstract concept.[60]

Staerk concedes that 'the idea of human humility before divine omnipotence may have been part of the understanding of this phrase in the pious awareness of the Middle Ages', but he concludes that the 'decisive fact for taking on this formula [in titles] was the legitimization of the ruler, whose actions had founded the new dynasty'.[61] Therefore, he suggests that *Dei gratia* was no longer a *Devotionsformel* but a *Legitimationsformel*, a 'legitimization formula'.[62] Staerk's terminology has become widely accepted and has proven to be very useful in historiography. Flor summarizes that apart from the '*Dei gratia* as humility formula', there is also 'the *Dei gratia* as legitimization formula', concluding that 'divine affirmation can become more important than humility towards God'.[63]

Herwig Wolfram argued along the same lines but suggested a reading that subtly differentiated between the two interpretations. He interpreted *Dei gratia* not as expressing a straightforward Divine legitimization, but rather that it is the monarch's devotion expressed in *Dei gratia* that is rewarded by God through his legitimization.[64] Nonetheless, referring to the work of Lothar Bornscheuer, Wolfram also supported the notion that *Dei gratia* and its variants ought not to be called *Devotionsformel*, as this term 'captures only half the essence and nothing of the constitutional theory'.[65] As Flor has summarized, while nobody could foresee such a development when the phrase was first added to rulers' titles, *Dei gratia* was going to become 'the immortal byword of an absolutist-legitimistic form of government'.[66] In fact, Volker Sellin has shown how the reading as a 'legitimization' lost its political significance only during the revolutions of the nineteenth century.[67]

In the context of 'legitimization' one must address the reading of the *Dei gratia* phrase as meaning 'instituted by God'. Fichtenau has noted that the Byzantine imperial title had not included *Deo gratia*.[68] Rather, as Richter mentioned, the Byzantine emperor's title included the 'respectful addition' of *Deo coronatus*, 'crowned by God', to be used 'when the emperor is addressed'.[69] This was also taken on by Charlemagne once he was crowned emperor: 'Serenissimus augustus a Deo coronatus . . . imperator . . . per misericordiam Dei rex Francorum et Langobardorum.'[70] Notwithstanding the fact that in this example *gratia* (grace) is changed to *misericordia* (mercy), Kienast has deduced that the *Deo coronatus* phrase 'leaves no doubt about [Charlemagne's] being sent by God'.[71] While *Deo coronatus* is much stronger in its wording than *Dei gratia*, the latter eventually came to be interpreted as meaning more or less the same thing. The direct crowning by God has been depicted in many works of art. One of the clearest and most famous examples is the image of the enthroned Otto III from the Liuthar Gospels, from around 1000. Here, the emperor is crowned directly by God's hand coming from above. In his study on royal rule and Divine grace, Ludger Körntgen includes a detailed discussion of this image and its historical context, observing that this illustration 'depicts the essence of the idea of the sacred rulership'.[72] Herbert von Borch had gone so far as to suggest that the *Dei gratia* phrase in general 'expressed the claim . . . to be a deputy for God'.[73] It would thus have matched the phrase of 'vicarius Christi', deputy of Christ, which was another popular addition to rulers' titles in the early Middle Ages.[74]

Nonetheless, Flor emphasizes that *Dei gratia* does not negate the 'worldly foundations of power' and does not constitute 'a claim to the throne based exclusively on God's Grace'; indeed, he goes so far as to suggest that *Dei gratia* also comprises 'the involvement of the people through election or acclamation'.[75] The latter is still strongly emphasized in the Recognition ceremony at the beginning of British coronations. These 'elections' or 'acclamations', however, are nothing more than a mere confirmation of the assumed Divine choice.

'Divine right' vs Gottesgnadentum

In the context of the 'divine right of kings', it is interesting to note that in modern German the term used to describe the concept, in no matter what historical era, is *Gottesgnadentum* – literally meaning something like 'the state of being through God's grace'. Whereas the term 'divine right' in British history came 'into specific use' in the seventeenth century, in the context of the Stuart kings, the term *Gottesgnadentum* dates only from the nineteenth century.[76]

As mentioned above, the theory of the 'divine right of kings' is based on several biblical passages.[77] The term is not, however, derived from *Dei gratia*. The German term of *Gottesgnadentum*, on the other hand, seems to be much more linked to *Dei gratia* – even if only semantically. In contrast to 'divine right', *Gottesgnadentum* by the mere word itself, points out that the important factor is grace, it is a 'Gottes-*Gnaden*-tum'. The term thus intrinsically expresses humility and is not a legitimization. Fichtenau has explained that this term is 'used only in German', possibly referring to the fact that in many other languages the equivalent term refers to 'right'.[78] For instance, in English and French, a ruler's actual title would still read 'by the *grace* of God' / 'par la *grace* de Dieu'; nevertheless, the naming of the concept as 'divine *right*', or '*Droit* Divin', introduces some abstract 'right' that the bearer of the title appears to have. Stefan Ruppert opens his article on '*Gottesgnadentum*' in the *Enzyklopädie der Neuzeit* with the words that 'Generally, *Gottesgnadentum* means the legitimization of power through the will of God.'[79] This, however, is already a strong interpretation, based on historical usage and reality – not on actual 'meaning' based on semantics and ideals.

In any case, in German historiography, the term *Gottesgnadentum* has indeed been used very much to the same effect as the English 'divine right'.[80] When Staerk, in the late 1920s concluded that the phrase 'von Gottes Gnaden' ('by the grace of God') expressed the 'göttliche Recht', or 'divine right' of the king, he could already refer back to F.J. Stahl's work on law and constitutional law from 1856.[81] However, there remains at least a clear semantic difference between *Gottesgnadentum* and 'divine right'. Flor indicated a difference when he summarized that over the centuries 'the *Gottesgnadentum* turns into the divine Right of kings'.[82] Similarly, Otto Brunner has pointed out that the 'divine right of kings' that was discussed controversially in seventeenth-century England was not the same as the *Gottesgnadentum* in its original understanding of a rule through the grace of God.[83] Importantly, at the time, there was no notable discussion of whether there actually was a 'right', in contrast to a 'grace' bestowed on the monarch.

The different interpretations of the word caused Fichtenau to conclude that *Gottesgnadentum* is 'unfortunately a rather imprecise' (*recht unpräziser*) term.[84] Indeed, whereas its literal meaning reflects well the early medieval understanding of a monarch *Dei gratia*, submitting himself in humility to the higher authority, the use of *Gottesgnadentum* for later forms of monarchical government – especially for absolutist ones – is not a good fit. Recognizing the semantic clash, Brunner argued for a thorough distinction. Referring to James I's aforementioned speech to Parliament, Brunner explains that this *Jure-Divino-Königtum*, or 'divine right kingship', must not be mixed with the kingship of earlier centuries (*dem älteren Gottesgnadentum*), since it is 'an extreme development of princely sovereignty'.[85]

A legitimizing interpretation would arguably be in accordance with a phrase from Proverbs 8:15, the famous 'per me reges regnant', or 'by me the kings reign'.[86] It is questionable, however, how far any such legitimization could be interpreted into the *Dei gratia* phrase. Given its original, verbatim meaning, with the stress on 'grace', any sort of legitimization must appear like a perversion of the original sense. After all, any political Divine legitimization in a Christian context would probably have contradicted Jesus's own division between the religious and the secular, temporal world. In Matthew 22:21 he had taught 'Render unto Caesar the things that are Caesar's, and unto God the things that are God's', and in John 18:36 he had explained 'My kingdom is not of this world.'

Obligation

Apart from humility and legitimization, there is a third, possibly even more important, aspect to consider in relation to *Dei gratia*. Lutz E. von Padberg explained that the *Gottegnadentum* of the early Middle Ages had 'nothing to do with high-handedness/vainglory [*Selbstherrlichkeit*], but with duty, even the submission to God's will', and that in this sense 'sacred kingship meant also a limitation of earthly power'.[87]

Regarding the 'divine right', J.W. Allen, in his seminal study on *English Political Thought*, pointed out the 'ambiguity of the term' at the times of James I and Charles I. He concluded that 'belief in the King's divine right implied no particular belief as to the extent of a King's rights in England or elsewhere. The content of the belief was, in fact largely negative.'[88] Burgess supported this and argued that the theory of 'divine right' was 'not solely absolutist, but could also imply some sort of limitation on royal authority'; indeed, that it was 'a theory of *obligation*, concerned primarily with the need to demonstrate to both rulers and subjects their duties before God'.[89] Similarly, Brunner observed that the 'Christianization of kingship' had put a stronger emphasis on the 'ruler who received his office from God', but had also bound him 'to the common, obligatory Christian ethos'.[90]

The aspect of 'obligation' received heightened attention in the sixteenth century. The idea of salvation through God's grace was one of the core issues of Luther's Reformation – indeed triggering the whole movement. Nonetheless, there was no discussion on the wording of royal titles.[91] Hellmuth Mayer has emphasized that Luther as such 'never taught the *Gottesgnadentum* of kings'.[92] Other reformers, such as Calvin or Zwingli, did not noticeably comment on the concept either. All the same, referring to the research of James Estes and Wolfgang Sommer, Robert von Friedeburg observed that 'Luther reminded princes that good administration, good servants and other elements of good rule were gifts of God and not due to their own abilities.'[93] Thus one could argue that Luther, willingly and knowingly or not, highlighted and supported the earlier reading of *Dei gratia*. Dreitzel summarized that Protestantism generally interpreted *Dei gratia* 'in the context of similar biblical verses as a particular obligation of princes to keep God's laws and also as a special dependence on his protection and judgment'.[94]

In earlier centuries the aspect of the monarch's obligation had been heightened by another fact: subjects had, at least theoretically, a right to resistance. This has been discussed in Fritz Kern's still significant study on *Gottesgnadentum* and the right to resistance in the early Middle Ages.[95] The idea of a right to resistance was present for a long time. Fox has noted that the Sunking's own chaplain, Bishop Jacques Bossuet 'and a few others even left room for the resistance of subjects where private conscience revealed that God commanded it'.[96] However, as Lothar Schilling has pointed out more recently, Bossuet allowed merely 'passive resistance'.[97]

Coming back to James VI & I's famous claim that kings are like gods, it is often overlooked that, in the same speech, he also spoke about obligation. With this analogy, the king was merely referring to Psalm 82, and this also brought him to put a clear limitation on this idea: he emphasized that kings are still mortal humans who 'will be glad to bind themselves within the limits of their laws'.[98] A similar 'obligatory' character applied – at least theoretically – even to French absolutism. Fox states that it was 'tempered by obligation', since churchmen 'insisted that though the monarch had a divine right to govern, he had no less a divine duty to rule justly'.[99] At the same time, Fox points out that while Louis XIV reminded his heir of 'les obligations que vous avez à Dieu' – the 'obligations that you have towards God' – he 'continued to insist that the king alone could interpret the royal obligation to the Deity'.[100]

The aspect of obligation implied in the *Dei gratia* phrase became relevant, prominently, during the controversies in the revolutionary year of 1848. A huge majority in the Prussian national assembly had voted to omit the phrase 'Von Gottes Gnaden' ('by the Grace of God') from the king's title, since it was supposed to be reminiscent of absolutism and of subjects' having to follow the divinely ordained authorities. In the end, however, this vote was revised under the pressure of the conservative groups, and the phrase remained in the title until the end of the monarchy in 1918.[101] The straightforward justification was that the formula 'merely showed a tradition hallowed by centuries, without any practical significance'.[102] However, as Dreitzel has highlighted, the assembly also emphasized that the *Dei gratia* phrase:

> should always remind our princes that, even though we declare them not to be responsible to us, they are still responsible to the higher authorities, of which responsibility neither we, nor our constitution, nor any other earthly power can dissolve them.[103]

Thus, it was through this very phrase that the assembly at least attempted to put some sort of limitation on the monarch.

Brunner has pointedly observed that 'The fight against the "divine right of kings" has not prevented the King of Great Britain from continuing to bear "by the Grace of God" in his title.'[104] However, one could ask, provocatively, why this fight should have resulted in the removal of this phrase from the royal title: after all, the phrase and the concept denote rather different ideas. While the *Dei gratia* phrase beautifully sums up the complex concept of monarchs ruling 'by the grace of God', it has very little to do with the rather different concept of the 'divine right of kings'. Just like *Gottesgnadentum*, the phrase *Dei gratia* does not originally imply any sense of a 'right'. There is at best a historical link in the questionable interpretation of the phrase. In the end, whether *Dei gratia* is read as expressing 'human humility' or as referring to 'divine legitimization', in either case there remains for the bearer of the title a distinct 'obligation'. It is the obligation to show himself/herself worthy – either of the grace received without precondition or of the power at his/her disposal.

(Modern) implications

Brunner has argued that 'in this modern world since 1760, since the Enlightenment, *Gottesgnadentum* seems like a myth, which is not believed in, at least not literally, and which is at best a symbol'.[105] However, it is precisely because it has not been believed in 'literally' that the appreciation of *Gottesgnadentum*, and of the *Dei gratia* phrase, has long suffered as a result of the questionable link to a supposed 'divine right'. In fact, what critics in the English-speaking world have challenged over the centuries was this concept, but not as such the phrase *Dei gratia*.

The phrase *Dei gratia* is still present in several monarchs' titles; and even when it is not part of the title of a head of state, and even when the state is not a monarchy, the phrase and its ideas or implications remain influential and significant. For instance, Mayer has argued that Luther's understanding that those in power are responsible in conscience only to God, one aspect of *Dei gratia*, has been preserved to some extent in the constitutional laws of Germany.[106]

A meaningful way of interpreting this phrase for the 21st century is certainly a return to its roots: the observation that the phrase is *sui generis* an expression of humility with a strong aspect of obligation. With its Christian origins, one might think that the significance of the phrase depends on a Christian context. However, although the phrase *Dei gratia* is so clearly linked to Christian rulers, it could be questioned whether any established religious belief is a necessary, relevant factor. After all, God, the 'Dei' that qualifies the origins of grace, could meaningfully be read as neutral 'providence' or 'destiny', if not simply as 'chance'. In any case, the more important aspect of the phrase is that of *gratia*, of a 'grace' that has come upon someone as a complete gift, deservingly or not. If the aspect of 'grace' is appropriately stressed, then the *Dei gratia* phrase can be very meaningful. Even in modern, largely secularized, non-religious societies, this, or a similar phrase, can have an undeniable attractiveness with its pointing towards human limitation and obligation.

In 1872, an anonymous 'Republican' wrote a sarcastic attack on 'divine right' in a small, provincial publication. This incorporated a noteworthy argument. With regard to William the Conqueror's becoming king of England, the writer remarked that 'divine right . . . would have been of little use in founding his title, had his own sword not carved out the crown for him'.[107] While this paradox may apply to the idea of a 'divine right of kings', it does not exist with the *Dei gratia* phrase. In this case, if William had not been born into his position, he would not have had the opportunity to take his 'own sword' in the first place and to 'carve out the crown for him'. So, the first important step was grace, destiny, coincidence, good luck, or whatever one choses to call it.

For modern-day office holders – even, if not specifically, for elected politicians – one could argue that they are in their position not as such by their own doing, or at least not entirely as a result of their own efforts. Therefore, some sort of 'devotion' or 'humility' formula similar to *Dei gratia* might be a valuable addition to their titles. Immanuel Kant, in a somewhat sarcastic comment in relation to Frederik the Great, stressed that such expressions in rulers' titles should not make the sovereign 'haughty' (*hochmüthig*), but rather that they ought to 'humiliate' (*demüthigen*) him in his soul, if he has any understanding (*Verstand*) – 'which is to be presumed'.[108] It is surely as useful to point out the importance of humility and obligation to modern-day rulers as it was to the monarchs of bygone ages.

The 'original' understanding of *Dei gratia* has never disappeared – or at least it was revived in the mid-twentieth century. On the occasion of her coronation in 1953, Elizabeth II declared: 'Therefore I am sure that this, my Coronation, is . . . a declaration of our hopes for the future, and for the years I may, by God's Grace and Mercy, be given to reign and serve you as your Queen'.[109] The phrase '*D*[*ei*] *G*[*ratia*] *Reg*[*ina*]', or 'Queen by the grace of God', is still prominently embossed on every single British coin, around the head of the monarch (see Figure 6.1).[110]

Interestingly, the Queen specified the understanding of 'grace' through the addition of 'mercy' – thus preventing any ambiguity. The Queen's inclusion of the words 'by God's Grace', through which she hopes to be given a long reign, is a notable reference to her own lack of power vis-à-vis the vicissitudes of destiny. In this understanding, the phrase *Dei gratia*, 'by the grace of God', in the Queen's title is very much not a Divine legitimization of her reign, but rather a sign of her humility. It reminds both the Queen and her subjects of the fact that she is merely human.

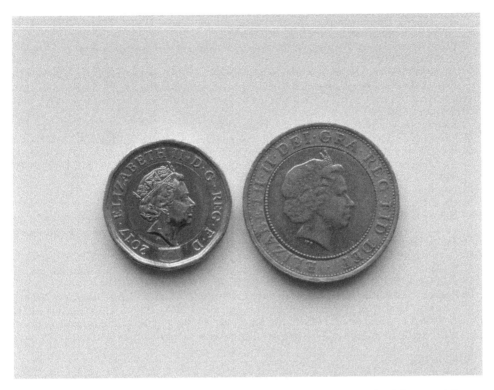

Figure 6.1 Modern British £1 and £2 coins, 2018, with the royal title (in Latin) around the monarch's head, incorporating 'D G' and 'DEI GRA'. Crown copyright.

Notes

All translations from German are by the author; relevant terms and expressions are also given in the original.

1 Jack Autrey Dabbs, *Dei Gratia in Royal Titles* (Paris: Mouton, 1971).

2 See, for instance, Joseph Canning, *A History of Medieval Political Thought: 300–1450* (London: Routledge, 1996, repr. 1998 and 2005), 18; and for a more general study Andreas Pečar and Kai Trampedach, eds., *Die Bibel als politisches Argument*, publ. as *Historische Zeitschrift. Beiheft* 43 (2007).

3 Vulgate and King James Bible translations. For definitions, literature and early occurrences of the phrase in titles see Rudolf Leeb, *Konstantin und Christus: Die Verchristlichung der imperialen Repräsentation unter Konstantim dem Großen als Spiegel seiner Kirchenpolitik und seines Selbstverständnisses als christlicher Kaiser* (Berlin: De Gruyter, 1992), esp. p. 124.

4 Claus Richter, *Der Sinn der Dei-gratia-Formel in den französischen und deutschen Dynastenurkunden bis zum Jahre 1000, untersucht mit besonderer Berücksichtigung der Geschichte dieser Formel von der paulinischen Zeit* (unpubl. Dr.-phil. diss.: Frankfurt am Main, 1974), 5f. See also the review of Richter's book by Herwig Wolfram in *Historische Zeitschrift* 222 (1976), 159–161. On the various definitions and interpretations of *Dei gratia* see also Georg Flor, *Gottesgnadentum und Herrschergnade: Über menschliche Herrschaft und göttliche Vollmacht* (Cologne: Bundesanzeiger, 1991), 72–75.

5 Karl Schmitz, *Ursprung und Geschichte der Devotionsformeln bis zu ihrer Aufnahme in die Fränkische Königsurkunde* (Stuttgart: Ferdinand Enke, 1913), 140.

6 Heinrich Fichtenau, "'Dei gratia' und Königssalbung," *Geschichte und ihre Quellen: Festschrift für Friedrich Hausmann zum 70. Geburtstag*, ed. Reinhard Härtel (Graz: Akademische Druck- u. Verlagsanstalt, 1987), 25–35, here 31.

7 Ildar H. Garipzanov, *The Symbolic Language of Authority in the Carolingian World (c. 751–877)* (Leiden: Brill, 2008), 161.

8 See still Herbert von Borch, *Das Gottesgnadentum. Historisch-soziologischer Versuch über die religiöse Herrschaftslegitimation* (Berlin: Junker und Dünnhaupt, 1934). See also Flor, 17–54.

9 Schmitz, 6–16.

10 Richter, 46. For Darius's title see also Dabbs, 17.

11 Canning, 17. For the use of *Dei gratia* in rulers' titles see also Schmitz, ch. 7, 154–180.

12 For this see Reinhard Elze, "Die Agilulfkrone des Schatzes von Monza," *Historische Forschungen für Walter Schlesinger*, ed. Helmut Beumann (Cologne: Böhlau, 1974), 348–357.

13 Canning, 17. See also Dabbs, App. IV.

14 Canning, 17f.

15 Heinrich Fichtenau, "Zur Geschichte der Invokationen und 'Devotionsformeln'," in idem, *Beiträge zur Mediävistik: Ausgewählte Aufsätze*, vol. 2: *Urkundenforschung* (Stuttgart: Anton Hiersemann, 1977), 37–61, here 55.

16 Canning, 49.

17 See lately Werner Goez, *Kirchenreform und Investiturstreit: 910–1122*, second edn, rev. by Elke Goez (Stuttgart: W. Kohlhammer, 2008), 78. See also Canning, 49.

18 Bernard S. Bachrach, *Charlemagne's Early Campaigns (768–777): A Diplomatic and Military Analysis*, "History of Warfare" vol. 82 (Leiden: Brill, 2013), 338. Bachrach refers to *Die Urkunden der Karolinger*, I, [*MGH, Dip. Karol.*] no. 80. For the use of the formula in documents of Charlemagne and his brother Carloman see also Richter, 109–110.

19 Garipzanov, 152.

20 Ibid., 151.

21 J. Rufus Fears, "Gottesgnadentum," *RAC* [*Reallexikon für Antike und Christentum*, Stuttgart 1950ff.], vol. 11: *Girlande-Gottesnamen* (Stuttgart: Anton Hiersemann, 1981), columns 1103–1159, here 1149.

22 For the addition of the formula into rulers' titles, see also Franz-Reiner Erkens, *Herrschersakralität im Mittelalter: von den Anfängen bis zum Investiturstreit* (Stuttgart: W. Kohlhammer, 2006), 133.

23 Canning, 18.

24 Ibid., 18.

25 Annette Weber-Möckl, *"Das Recht des Königs, der über euch herrschen soll": Studien zu 1 Sam 8, 11 ff. in der Literatur der frühen Neuzeit* (Berlin: Duncker & Humblot, 1984), 7, 94.

26 Ibid., 95.

27 John Neville Figgis, *The Theory of the Divine Right of Kings* (Cambridge University Press, 1896; second edn, 1914). For literature on divine right see more recently Andreas Pečar, *Macht der Schrift: Politischer Biblizismus in Schottland und England zwischen Reformation und Bürgerkrieg (1534–1642)* (Munich: Oldenbourg, 2011), esp. 241.

28 Figgis, 5f. For these 'essential ingredients', see also Paul W. Fox, "Louis XIV and the Theories of Absolutism and Divine Right," *The Canadian Journal of Economics and Political Science/Revue canadienne d'Economique et de Science politique* 26, no. 1 (1960), 128–142, here 132 and 140.

29 Figgis, 127. See also Fichtenau, "Dei gratia," 35.

30 Fox, 133. For a more detailed study on the French context see Jacques Krynen, "Rex Christianissimus: A medieval theme at the roots of French absolutism," *History and Anthropology* 4 (1989), 79–96.

31 See Andreas Pečar, "Auf der Suche nach den Ursprüngen des *Divine Right of Kings*. Herrschaftskritik und Herrschaftslegitimation in Schottland unter Jakob VI," *Die Bibel als politisches Argument*, publ. as *Historische Zeitschrift. Beiheft* 43, eds. Andreas Pečar and Kai Trampedach (2007), 295–314.

32 The whole speech is included in David Wootton (ed. and introduction), *Divine Right and Democracy: An Anthology of Political Writing in Stuart England*, originally published by Penguin Books in 1986, reprint (Indianapolis: Hacket Publishing, 2003), 107–109, here

107. For a detailed study on the king's understanding of 'divine right' see Hansjochen Hancke, "Die Lehre vom Divine Right of Kings bei Jakob I. von England und ihre Bedeutung in den englischen Verfassungskonflikten des frühen 17. Jahrhunderts," (PhD dissertation, University of Münster, 1969).

33 Fox, 134.

34 See, for instance, especially Fox and Glenn Burgess, "The Divine Right of Kings Reconsidered," *The English Historical Review* 107, no. 425 (1992), 837–861. For a critical more recent discussion of the concept of 'absolutism' see, for instance, the essays in Lothar Schilling, ed., *Absolutismus: Ein unersetzliches Forschungskonzept?* (Munich: R. Oldenbourg, 2008).

35 Horst Dreitzel, *Monarchiebegriffe in der Fürstengesellschaft: Semantik und Theorie der Einherrschaft in Deutschland von der Reformation bis zum Vormärz*, vol. 2: *Therie der Monarchie* (Cologne: Böhlau, 1991), 515.

36 Flor, 124 ("zur fragwürdigen Legitimation unumschränkter Herrschaft").

37 W.H. Greenleaf, "The Tomasian Tradition and the Theory of Absolute Monarchy," *The English Historical Review* 70 (1964), 747–760, here 747.

38 Wolfgang Reinhard, *Geschichte der Staatsgewalt: Eine vergleichende Verfassungsgeschichte Europas von den Anfängen bis zur Gegenwart* (Munich: Beck, 1999; second rev. edn 2000), 39.

39 See Pečar, *Macht der Schrift*.

40 "M—D," "Thoughts on the Divine Right of Kings," *The Belfast Monthly Magazine* 10, no. 56 (31 March 1813), 197–202, here 197.

41 Figgis, 1.

42 Richter, 139 ("als einfachen Ausdruck demütiger Gesinnung").

43 Willy Staerk, "Dei Gratia. Zur Geschichte des Gottesgnadentums," *Festschrift Walter Judeich zum 70. Geburtstag, überreicht von Jenaer Freunden* (Weimar: Hermann Böhlaus Nachf., 1929), 160–172, here 164.

44 Schmitz, 1.

45 For this see Staerk, 164

46 Walter Ullmann, *The Carolingian Renaissance and the Idea of Kingship: The Birbeck Lectures 1968–9*, first published by Methuen in 1969 (Abingdon: Routledge, 2010), 125.

47 Richter, 112. For Charlemagne's general relationship with and use of Christianity see Rosamond McKitterick, *Charlemagne: The Formation of a European Identity* (Cambridge University Press, 2008).

48 For this and the following see Percy Schramm, *Kaiser, Könige und Päpste. Gesammelte Aufsätze zur Geschichte des Mittelalters*, vol. 1: *Von der Spätantike bis zum Tode Karls des Großen (814)* (Stuttgart: Anton Hiersemann, 1968), 198.

49 Schmitz, 15.

50 Ibid., 140.

51 For this see also Fichtenau, "Dei gratia," 31, who observes that the term 'grace' also reminds us of the opposite term, 'human merit'.

52 Fichtenau, "Dei gratia," 30.

53 Walther Kienast, *Der Herzogstitel in Frankreich und Deutschland (9. bis 12. Jahrhundert) Mit Listen der ältesten deutschen Herzogsurkunden* (München: R. Oldenbourg Verlag, 1968), 355.

54 This and the following, see Dreitzel, 516.

55 G.R. Elton, *Studies in Tudor and Stuart Politics and Government*, 2 vols (Cambridge University Press: 1974), ii, 200.

56 For this phrase see Mary Beard, *The Roman Triumph* (Cambridge, MA: Harvard University Press, 2009), 85–92.

57 Richter, 48–57, quotation on 54. See also ibid., 139.

58 Ibid., 55f.

59 Fichtenau, "Dei gratia," 30 and 32.

60 Ullmann, 34.

61 Staerk, 164.

62 Ibid., 169. For this being the first use of the term 'Legitimationsformel', see Fichtenau, "Zur Geschichte," 37–61, here 56.

63 Flor, 74 ("Demutsformel" and "Legitimationsformel").

64 Wolfram, 160.

65 Ibid., 160.

66 Flor, 71f. ("unsterblichen Schlagwort einer absolutistisch-legitimistischen Regierungsform").

67 Volker Sellin, *Gewalt und Legitimität: Die Europäische Monarchie im Zeitalter der Revolutionen* (Munich: Oldenbourg Verlag, 2011), 5f. and 84–86.

68 Fichtenau, "Zur Geschichte," 54.

69 Richter, 113.

70 See Schramm, 269.

71 Kienast, 355.

72 Ludger Körntgen, *Königsherrschaft und Gottes Gnade: Zu Kontext und Funktion sakraler Vorstellungen in Historiographie und Bildzeugnissen der ottonisch-frühsalischen Zeit* (Berlin: Akademie Verlag, 2001), 178–211, here 179 ("die bildliche Verdichtung der Idee des sakralen Herrschertums"). For research and literature on this image see also Egon Boshof, *Königtum und Königsherrschaft im 10. und 11. Jahrhundert*, third rev. and extended edn (Munich: Oldenbourg, 2010), 115.

73 Borch, 104.

74 For a recent study of this see Andreas Kosuch, *Abbild und Stellvertreter Gottes: der König in herrschaftstheoretischen Schriften des späten Mittelalters* (Cologne: Böhlau Verlag, 2011), here esp. 99f.

75 Flor, 74.

76 See the entry in the *Oxford English Dictionary* (online version – www.oed.com – last accessed 22 March 2017). For the German see Fichtenau, "Dei gratia," 25, fn. 2; and Dreitzel, 522.

77 See above, fns 23–25.

78 Fichtenau, "Dei gratia," 35.

79 Stefan Ruppert, "Gottesgnadentum," *Enzyklopädie der Neuzeit Online*, ed. Friedrich Jaeger, first published online 2014, http://dx.doi.org/10.1163/2352-0248_edn_a1489000 (last accessed 19 October 2017): "Ganz allgemein bezeichnet G. die Legitimation von Herrschaft durch den Willen Gottes."

80 See, *pars pro toto*, Flor's study.

81 Staerk, 170.

82 Flor, 115: "Das Gottesgnadentum wird zum göttlichen Recht der Könige."

83 Otto Brunner, "Vom Gottesgnadentum zum monarchischen Prinzip: der Weg der europäischen Monarchie seit dem hohen Mittelalter," in ibid., *Neue Wege der Verfassungs- und Sozialgeschichte*, first publ. in 1956, second, enlarged edn (Göttingen: Vandenhoeck u. Ruprecht, 1968), 160–186, here 164. For much research on this topic see also Ronald G. Asch, *Von der "Monarchischen Republik" zum Gottesgnadentum? Monarchie und politische Theologie in England von Elisabeth I. bis zu Karl I.*, publ. as *Historische Zeitschrift. Beiheft 39* (2004), 123–148.

84 Fichtenau, "Dei gratia," 35.

85 Brunner, 172.

86 For a study of this phrase and in the context of 'sacred' kingship in the Middle Ages, see Franco Cardini and Maria Saltarelli, eds., *Per me reges regnant: la regalità sacra nell'Europa medievale* (Rimini: Il Cerchio, 2002).

87 Lutz E. von Padberg, "Das christliche Königtum aus der Sicht der angelsächsischen Missionschule," *Das frühmittelalterliche Königtum: Ideelle und religiöse Grundlagen*, ed. Franz-Reiner Erkens (Berlin: Walter de Gruyter, 2005), 190–213, here 209.

88 J.W. Allen, *English Political Thought, 1603–1660*, 2 vols planned, but only one appeared (London, 1938), i, 97.

89 Burgess, 839 (emphasis original).

90 Brunner, 165f. ("das allgemein verpflichtende christliche Ethos").

91 See Dabbs, *passim*.

92 Hellmuth Mayer, "Zur Naturrechtslehre des Luthertums," *Festschrift für Hans Welzel zum 70. Geburtstag am 25. März 1974*, eds. Günter Stratenwerth et al. (Berlin: Walter de Gruyter, 1974), 65–100, here 90. For the 'impact of the Reformation on theories of kingship in England and on the European Continent', see Burgess, 838.

93 Robert von Friedeburg, *Luther's Legacy: The Thirty Years War and the Modern notion of "State" in the Empire, 1530s to 1790s* (Cambridge University Press, 2016), 118.
94 Dreitzel, 517.
95 Fritz Kern, *Gottesgnadentum und Widerstandsrecht im früheren Mittelalter: zur Entwicklungsgeschichte der Monarchie*, first publ. in 1914, second edn (Münster: Böhlau-Verlag, 1954). See also Michael Pauen, "Gottes Gnade: Bürgers Recht – Macht und Herrschaft in der politischen Philosophie der Neuzeit," *Macht und Herrschaft: Sozialwissenschaftliche Konzeptionen und Theorien*, ed. Peter Imbusch (Wiesbaden: Springer Fachmedien, 1998), 27–44, here 40–42.
96 Fox, 136.
97 Lothar Schilling, "Bossuet, die Bibel und der 'Absolutismus'," *Die Bibel als politisches Argument*, eds. Andreas Pečar and Kai Trampedach, publ. as *Historische Zeitschrift. Beiheft* 43 (2007), 349–370, here 354.
98 See Wootton, 109 (as in fn. 32).
99 Fox, 130. See also ibid., 136.
100 Ibid., 140.
101 Flor, 143.
102 For a fuller discussion of the 1848 assembly see Sellin, 85f (here quoting from the minutes).
103 Dreitzel, 527f.
104 Brunner, 164.
105 Brunner, 174.
106 Mayer, 90.
107 *"A Republican"*, Vox dei: or *"King by the Grace of God"*, by a Republican of the Order of Reason, Religion, and Law (Middlesbrough: N. Bragg, 1872), 13.
108 Immanuel Kant, *Zum ewigen Frieden: Ein philosophischer Entwurf* (Frankfurt and Leipzig, 1796), 25.
109 Radio transmission on the evening of 2 June 1953. For a transcript see "Her Majesty's Coronation-day Broadcast," *Elizabeth Crowned Queen: The Pictorial Record of the Coronation*, first published by Odhams Press [1953], reprint (London: Bounty Books, 2006), 7–8.
110 The title also includes the letters 'F D' – for 'Fidei Defensor', or 'Defender of Faith'. This, however, has nothing to do with *Dei gratia* and need not be discussed here.

Key works

Brunner, Otto, "Vom Gottesgnadentum zum monarchischen Prinzip: der Weg der europäischen Monarchie seit dem hohen Mittelalter," in *Neue Wege der Verfassungs- und Sozialgeschichte*, first publ. in 1956, second, enlarged edn (Göttingen: Vandenhoeck u. Ruprecht, 1968), 160–186.

Canning, Joseph, *A History of Medieval Political Thought: 300–1450* (London: Routledge, 1996, repr. 1998 and 2005).

Fichtenau, Heinrich, "'Dei gratia' und Königssalbung," *Geschichte und ihre Quellen: Festschrift für Friedrich Hausmann zum 70. Geburtstag*, ed. Reinhard Härtel (Graz: Akademische Druck- u. Verlagsanstalt, 1987), 25–35.

Figgis, John Neville, *The Theory of the Divine Right of Kings* (Cambridge University Press, 1896; second edn, 1914).

Flor, Georg, *Gottesgnadentum und Herrschergnade: Über menschliche Herrschaft und göttliche Vollmacht*, "Bundesanzeiger" no. 119a (1991).

Schmitz, Karl, *Ursprung und Geschichte der Devotionsformeln bis zu ihrer Aufnahme in die Fränkische Königsurkunde* (Stuttgart: Ferdinand Enke, 1913).

Staerk, Willy, "Dei Gratia. Zur Geschichte des Gottesgnadentums," *Festschrift Walter Judeich zum 70. Geburtstag, überreicht von Jenaer Freunden* (Weimar: Hermann Böhlaus Nachf., 1929), 160–172.

7

A CASE STUDY OF PRE-MODERN ISLAMIC MONARCHY

The Almohad caliphate of the Maghreb and al-Andalus in the 12th–13th centuries[*]

Pascal Buresi

It is impossible, within the space of a few pages, to present a synthesis of the monarchies and systems of government in the Islamic world in the pre-modern era. Such a study would encompass more than a thousand years of history and include the evolution of politics, institutions, administrations and ideologies. It would downplay the infinite diversity of solutions invented by very different societies ranging from China to sub-Saharan Africa to central Asia, southeast Asia and al-Andalus, the latter the southern part of the Iberian peninsula conquered in 711 in the name of the Umayyad rulers of Damascus and an integral part of the Islamic world until the end of the fifteenth century. In addition, we must acknowledge the scarcity of sources for the earlier periods, the uncertainty of our knowledge of many situations and the vigour of historiographical debates. Indeed, any synthesis would, in fact, deny the history of these societies and apply an unduly reductionist approach to Islamic political systems.

To respond to this problem, this chapter will present a case study, that of the Almohads (*al-muwahhidûn*).[1] Between the mid-twelfth and mid-thirteenth centuries, the Almohads politically unified the Maghreb region of North Africa from Tripolitania to the Atlantic, including al-Andalus, under a single indigenous political authority for the first time in history. Unlike earlier periods of regional unification, the Almohads were not foreigners like the Romans, Byzantines, or Arabs – they were Berbers who originated in the Atlas Mountains. This case study will begin by presenting the political history of the Almohads and its context before discussing the specific nature of the Almohad political system, drawing on all the textual and material sources available including chronicles, biographical dictionaries and hagiographies, architecture, numismatics, and especially documents produced by the Almohad chancery. This will serve as a reference point to outline the rhetorical, ideological and conceptual tools that were available to the Muslims of the Maghreb at that time. These tools retrospectively illuminate the exercise of power in the early centuries of Islam, a topic on which researchers do not agree. There are a wide variety of theories and hypotheses between those who maintain that Islam was born as a theocratic regime, where political power and religious authority were concentrated in the hands of a single man, and those who believe that the Islamic royalty that appeared in the Arabian peninsula in the seventh century distinguished immediately between the political aspect of caliphal power and the religious character of prophetic authority based on the influence of pre-Islamic models. After briefly presenting the major historiographical debates surrounding the period in which Islam emerged, this chapter will end by showing how the early period can be better understood retrospectively through the lens of subsequent case studies, such as that involving the Almohads.

Towards a retrospective history

What can be deduced from the Almohad experience of Islamic monarchy during its first centuries? The historiographical debates on the beginnings of Islam are evidently due to the lack of sources for the religion's first decades. Some, such as Fred Donner, consider the Quran to be a reliable source that reflects the state of the Arabian peninsula at the end of the seventh century.[2] Others, such as Patricia Crone, Michael Cook and John Wansbrough, reject all the Islamic texts (Quran, Sunnah, the lives of the Prophet) as being late and biased.[3] This uncertainty regarding the reliability of the sources results in widely varying opinions on the nature of the political system put in place by the Prophet and his successors. Later in this chapter we will summarize some of these positions in an attempt to resolve this endless debate, a debate which focuses on the *singular* nature of a putative Islamic power. Whether such a power ever actually existed is not a given. Not all Christian countries, be they Catholic, Orthodox, or Protestant, have taken the same path over the centuries, neither have they established identical political systems. There is no reason to think that a greater unity exists among Islamic countries, which range from Indonesia to sub-Saharan Africa, from the steppes and deserts of North Africa, Turkey and Persia to the shores of East Africa and the Indian sub-continent. It would seem that the idea of non-separation between political and religious spheres in Islam is linked to the representation of the Muslim religion as an all-encompassing system and to the recurrent claims of the doctors of Islamic law, the *fuqahâ'* and the *'ulamâ'* ('the scholars'), to control the political destiny of Muslim society, rather than the actual exercise of power in Islamic countries. The case of the Almohads provides an example that illustrates that in order to explain Islamic legal systems and political thought in the Middle Ages, we need to understand the peripheries.

The following biographical summary is to be understood less as a historical account than as an expression of Almohad imperial ideology as it was gradually developed from the twelfth century on, although this does not exclude the possibility of historical truth in certain concrete elements. In any case, what interests us here is not the authentic life of Ibn Tûmart (d.1130), founder of the Almohad movement, but the narrative – the account as it was commonly accepted by pre-modern Maghrebi society and its successors. This hagiography served as a model of the exercise of power for the dynasty which later claimed Ibn Tûmart as its founder.

The Mahdi Ibn Tûmart: founder of the Almohad movement

Ibn Tûmart was born between 1076 and 1082 into the Hargha tribe of the Masmûda Berber confederation. He studied at Cordoba and then in the East, notably with the great mystic al-Ghazâlî (d.1111). Or, at least, Ibn Tûmart supposedly learned from this most celebrated savant of the age: the chronology at times contradicts this possibility. Historians, in general, accept the idea that Ibn Tûmart journeyed to the East, but dispute his meeting with al-Ghazâlî, who, at this time, lived in Khorasan.[4] Faced with the impossibility of determining the truth, we will relegate this detail to the realms of possibilities without concerning ourselves with its authenticity because, from the perspective of the narrative, biographical elements such as these, reproduced with some variation by most chroniclers, add to the framework constructed by the Almohad movement. Upon his return from the East, around 1116–17, Ibn Tûmart became a censor of morals, embracing a vehemently puritanical form of asceticism favoured by the inhabitants of the rural regions of the Maghreb.[5] From 1120, he rebuked the reigning Almoravid rulers for their corruption and anthropomorphism. The Almoravids were also Berbers but from the Sanhâja confederation who had ruled since the end of the eleventh century in the far western Maghreb (today's Morocco) and in al-Andalus.[6] The catalyst for the Almohad movement, therefore, was the reformation of morals and legal practices, as well as challenging Almoravid power, thereby establishing an austere and rigorous view of social norms on the one hand, and of legitimate authority on the other. Fearing a reaction from the authorities, Ibn Tûmart sought refuge at Igîlîz, his native town near Târûdânt. This flight is presented in the Almohad sources as 'his first hijrah', following the model of the exile of Muhammed from Mecca to Medina in 622. At Igîlîz, Ibn Tûmart proclaimed himself before his supporters – and was recognized as – imâm and the Mahdi. This was a manifestation of his aspirations, as much political as they were spiritual and religious. At the same time, he organized his troops, the conquest of Almoravid power and the ideological system of tawhîd (the 'dogma of uniqueness' or more simply, 'monotheism'). From Igîlîz, accompanied by a small escort, Ibn Tûmart gathered together the Masmûda tribes of the western High Atlas and Anti-Atlas ranges. As a result of an injury sustained while fighting around this time, he did not command his troops personally, but rather left that task to others, in particular his companion al-Bashîr. For a second time, around 1124, facing Almoravid opposition, Ibn Tûmart took refuge in southern Morocco, at Tinmâl, which would be considered a few decades later the birthplace and first capital of the Almohad movement. This is the 'second hijrah'. From this date, Ibn Tûmart had all the attributes of the Mahdi: he was a 'guide' and 'infallible', and he adopted religious forms of authority and applied them to politics. It is from this mountain location, Tinmâl, that Ibn Tûmart directed his followers to assault the Almoravids.

After several years of waiting in their fortress in the Atlas Mountains and frustrated that they could not extend their power, the Almohads proceeded to eliminate less motivated members from the tribes through a process that the sources call 'selection' (tamyîz). Once this purge – of which the victims probably numbered in the thousands – was completed, the Almohads went on the offensive and defeated the Almoravid troops at Aghmât, seizing the city and opening the road to Marrakesh. Nevertheless, they also suffered a heavy defeat in 1128 beneath the walls of Marrakesh in the so-called battle of al-Buhayra. A large part of the early followers of Ibn Tûmart were killed in the battle and Ibn Tûmart himself died a few months later.

'Abd al-Mu'min: founder of the Almohad empire

According to the sources, it was two or three years later, doubtless around 1132, that 'Abd al-Mu'min (d.1163) nominated himself as heir to the Mahdi Ibn Tûmart and seized the leadership of the Almohad movement.[7] Drawing lessons from the defeat at al-Buhayra and from the impossibility of defeating the cavalry of the Christian mercenaries hired by the Almoravids, the Almohads decided to avoid open battles in the future and instead isolated Marrakesh, staying off the plains and the foothills of the High and Middle Atlas Mountains. This strategy was called in the sources the 'Seven Years' Campaign', from 1140 to 1147. The Almohads began by ensuring the cooperation of the local populations, to whom 'Abd al-Mu'min promised the abolition of non-Quranic taxes. Then, they attacked the fortresses loyal to Marrakesh. The strategy of avoiding open battles and focusing instead on raiding allowed the Almohads to defeat or suppress many Almoravid troops by isolating them. After the conquests of Fez, Meknes, Tlemcen, Ceuta and Salé, the only city in North Africa to remain loyal to the Almoravids was Marrakesh. But, cut off from the last contingents of Almoravid troops from al-Andalus and the Atlantic plain, which supplied the city with the grain needed for its survival, Marrakesh was unable to resist the Almohad siege for long. After the conquest of Marrakesh, in 1147, the Almohads installed themselves in the old palaces of the Almoravid dignitaries located on the western side of the city. They pardoned some of the old ruling elite, but executed all the relatives of the Almoravid dynasty itself, in particular the young Almoravid emir, Ishâq. The accession to power and the conquest of Marrakesh transformed the Almohad insurrection into a state system. As the opponents of the Almoravids came together, the tactical alliances which had led to the dynasty's success collapsed. Each group sought to make a profit from the disappearance of centralized Almoravid power. As a consequence, the Almohads faced a series of revolts that challenged their own newly established power in most of the Maghreb.

The first to revolt was Ibn Hûd al-Mâssî. From Mâssa, an old *ribât* that is supposed to play an important role on the day of the Last Judgement, al-Mâssî managed to unite numerous tribes. All of the peoples of the Atlantic plain, the Middle Atlas range and a great part of the High Atlas recognized his authority. Meanwhile, certain regions in al-Andalus, such as the Gharb, regained their independence, and Ceuta, the most important port along the Straits of Gibraltar, revolted under the leadership of the charismatic qâdî 'Iyâd, who no doubt sought to re-establish the Mâliki school of law. Instead of uniting, though, the leaders of these different revolts – and innumerable local rebels, of whom only their names have survived – fought each other. In one year, thanks to discipline reinforced through two decades of struggle against the Almoravids, the Almohads managed to restore a situation that seemed hopeless. In 1148, they defeated and killed al-Mâssî and, in 1149, they forced the Almoravid rebel Yahya Ibn al-Sahrawiyya ('the son of the Saharian woman') to seek refuge in the desert that was his mother's namesake. Alternating between violence and clemency, 'Abd al-Mu'min took advantage of the division among his opponents. However, he ultimately imposed himself only through systematic repression as part of what the sources call the 'recognition [of the new power or of the mistake committed]' (*al-i'tirâf*). This was a continuation of the *tamyîz*, the internal purge led by Ibn Tûmart. A list of people to be eliminated was provided to the defeated tribes and rebels, who were responsible for conducting the executions themselves. The goal was to break tribal solidarity in favour of a higher authority and a supra-tribal ideal. It was a fundamental step towards the development of the idea of a state in the Maghreb.

Before turning his attention towards the Iberian peninsula, 'Abd al-Mu'min focused his efforts on the central Maghreb, where for several decades the Hilali Arab tribes had dominated the interior. The latter, who feared the loss of the financial and territorial advantages that had been granted to them by the princes of Bougie, opposed the Almohads fiercely. As 'Abd al-Mu'min returned to Marrakesh, they rebelled against the Almohad garrisons left in their cities, forcing the caliph to return. A decisive battle occurred at Setif in 1153, which resulted in a victory for the Almohads, who pardoned the defeated and urged them to fight on other fronts, primarily in al-Andalus and Ifriqiya. It took several more years for the Almohads to organize the conquest of the latter province. In 1159, a combined land and sea expedition was launched with the aid of the Arab tribes that were already fighting the Normans in Ifriqiya. Between 1159 and 1160, all the Norman-controlled ports were seized by the Almohads. They then advanced to Cyrenaica on the border of the Fatimid Empire, the eastern coastal region of present-day Libya. They had just created the largest natively ruled empire in the Maghreb.

Almohad centralization and the imperial administration

The Almohad empire had a very centralized politico-military structure. The caliph personally led great military expeditions, which could mobilize tens of thousands of soldiers annually. The *imâm*-caliph could not be present on all the fronts at once, though, so the use of the caliphal army in one region almost inevitably led to trouble in another. For example, while 'Abd al-Mu'min led the conquest of Ifriqiya, al-Andalus suffered devastating incursions from the Christians of the northern Iberian peninsula, as well as from the allies of Ibn Mardanîsh (d.1172), ruler of the taifa of Murcia. The Almoravids had tried to solve the problem of fighting on multiple fronts by granting a large amount of autonomy to the different provincial governors and by turning al-Andalus into a viceroyalty, but the Almohads chose a different option: temporary peace treaties. During the entire Almohad period, Ifriqiya and al-Andalus were the two most threatened borders of the empire, on one side by Arab tribes and troops sent by the Fatimids of Cairo until 1171, and on the other by the various Iberian Christian kingdoms. The extreme centralization of Almohad power and the important role played by the caliph led the Almohads to sign temporary truces with all their enemies before engaging in battle. In addition, on the Iberian peninsula the Almohads forged an alliance with Navarre, which had no borders with al-Andalus, and, from the 1170s, with León against the kingdoms of Castile and Aragon.

The administrators of this transcontinental empire adopted a number of original practices. The Almohads not only integrated into their administration a certain number of Almoravid-era functionaries, but they also retained the previous provincial divisions. Initially, the governors were chosen from the shaykhs, Ibn Tûmart's first companions, and representatives of the allied tribes, but from 1156, they were chosen from among the *sayyids*, a term that first designated the sons of the first caliph, 'Abd al-Mu'min, then their descendants, and constituted a specific rank in the Almohad hierarchy. At the same time, the autonomy of the governors decreased and they saw their authority subject to that of their ruler. In Ifriqiya, in order to fight effectively against the Banû Ghâniya, Caliph al-Nâsir (r.1199–1214) was forced to give broad authority to the governor of the province, Abû Muhammed 'Abd al-Wâhid Ibn Abî Hafs al-Hintâtî, even though he was not a member of the Mu'minid family. This essentially shielded the new governor from the game of appointments and dismissals. In fact, provincial governors acquired a certain level of independence within the empire, but only after the Almohads were defeated at the battle of Las Navas de Tolosa in 1212.

In addition to foreign threats on the eastern and northern borders, the Almohads faced numerous problems within the Sahara regions of the Maghreb and in Ifriqiya. These revolts highlight the difficulties in developing state structures in nomadic areas. In the southern territories of the Anti-Atlas, populated by tribes related to the Almoravids such as the Lamta and Gazzula, the Almohads built or reinforced numerous fortresses. However, this did not prevent approximately fifteen revolts from occurring between the mid-twelfth and mid-thirteenth centuries. These rebellions developed, in general, around a charismatic individual of Berber ancestry who sometimes claimed to be the Mahdi and sometimes a prophet, drawing on lines of tribal solidarity and the resentment created by Almohad domination. The intensity and number of the rebellions are indicative of the Almohad efficiency, in particular, in levying taxes. The most complex movement was that of the Ghumâra in the 1160s. Their leader took the honorific surname *Mazîdagh* ('he who is inhabited [by a spirit]') with the *nisba* ('surname') of al-Ghumârî, and minted his own coins.[8] The reputation of this man was so great that the Almohads, instead of putting him to death as they did with many other rebels, exiled him to Cordoba.[9] Lastly, in the 1250s, a man from Hintâta managed to declare independence in the Sûs (the mid-southern region of contemporary Morocco). By then, the Almohad empire was concentrated around Marrakesh, only a shadow of its former grandeur. The Almohad conquest, long and difficult, was considered a new conquest for Islam. The seizure of all the lands by force (*'anwat^{an}*) justified, in Almohad eyes, claiming a new legal status. Considered until then by the jurists to have been conquered in the eighth century by negotiation (*sulh^{an}*), the region had been relatively spared when it came to taxes levied by the different dynasties. From an Almohad perspective, a slate that up to that point had been marked by the Arab conquests in the first century of Islam and the status quo they had established was now wiped clean. The Almohads considered their own conquest to constitute the first and foundational *fath* ('success/victory/opening'). This, in turn, obtained through military action, allowed them to modify the legal and fiscal status of the lands, entrenched by several centuries of territorial administration, Umayyad, Fatimid, Zirid, etc. Thus, in 1159, the Almohad caliph ordered a *taksîr*, a survey for financial purposes of all the lands of the empire, from Tripolitania to Nûl Lamta in the Atlantic plain. After deducting one-third of the area, corresponding to the non-cultivable lands such as mountains, forests, rivers, lakes, roads and rocky areas, the rest of the empire was subject to a property tax (*kharâj*), for which the amount in goods and in currency was specified for each tribe. In this way, the Almohads followed through with their commitment to abolish illegal taxation while simultaneously legitimizing a high tax rate by changing the status of the lands. As Yassir Benhima put it:

This new legal situation gave the Almohads a great deal of manoeuvrability in directing the movements and migration patterns of the various tribal groups, allowing them to grant land concessions as remuneration to its soldiers and civil servants, while also granting them the ability to implement intensive state exploitation of agricultural wealth.[10]

These fiscal changes provide valuable information on the first centuries of Islamic domination, where financial issues were not regulated in this manner. Previously, control of these territories had been nominal, and rulers had been content with controlling the coastal towns and plains; they rarely ventured into the interior to impose their authority.

The brutality of the Almohad reforms (fiscal, political, ideological, legal, monetary) was made possible by the Mahdist nature of the founder of the movement. It is because Ibn Tûmart was recognized as Mahdi, that is the Messiah expected at the end of time to restore justice and equity, that the new power was able to impose a new social and political order.

Mahdism

As Maribel Fierro relates, Mahdism plays an essential role in the story of salvation in the Muslim community, because the temporal figure of the Mahdi guarantees salvation not at the end of time, but here and now.[11] The Almohad movement was not the first Mahdist movement in the Maghreb region, nor the last, but it is, however, the archetype for the extent of its political realization, the coherence of its religious dogma, and the elaboration of its ideology, developing, as it did, as an imperial polity that extended from Libya to the Atlantic and to the Iberian peninsula. Paradoxically, it is because Ibn Tûmart, the founder of the movement, was regarded by his followers as Mahdi, the predestined 'saviour' in the End Times who would show the way for humanity, and as an impeccable *imam*, a 'guide' protected from all error, that his successors, the Almohad caliphs, were able to emancipate their power from the authority of the *fuqahâ'* and the ulemas. The ulemas had been the almost unchallenged interpreters of the divine word since the Mu'tazilite crisis that took place in Baghdad in the ninth century.[12] It is difficult to know if it was during the lifetime of Ibn Tûmart or, more likely, after his death that the different titles – 'acknowledged Mahdi', 'impeccable imam' – were attributed to him. Inspired by Shiite beliefs, impeccability (*'isma*) signified that, due to divine inspiration, the *imâm* was protected from all vice, error and corruption by virtue of his genealogical relationship to the Prophet via the descendants of his daughter, Fâtima, and his son-in-law and cousin. 'Alî. Ibn Tûmart and 'Abd al-Mu'min were, therefore, given Alid genealogies that traced their ancestries back to 'Alî (r.656–61), who is considered the first *imâm* by the Shiites.[13] For all these reasons, the Almohads are sometimes portrayed as Shiites or akin to Shiites, but this is incorrect. To avoid the risk of being accused of heterodoxy and Shiism, within which Mahdism undeniably fits, the Almohads chose to celebrate the titular guardian figure of 'Uthmân b. 'Affân (r.644–56) and the legacy of the Umayyads, mortal enemies of the Alids and all Shiite sects from the seventh to the twelfth centuries. To emphasize this, they adopted on their banners the iconic white colour of the Umayyad dynasty of Damascus and later Cordoba, in contrast to the black colour of the Abbasids.[14] At the same time, the Almohads restored the city of Cordoba as capital of al-Andalus in 1161, replacing Seville, which had held that status under the late Almoravids (1070–1147). Furthermore, they invented a Quranic relic, supposedly written by 'Uthmân and stained with his blood, even though 'Uthmân was considered by all Shiites to be a usurper of the power of 'Alî and a falsifier of scriptures. This copy of the Quran (*mushaf*) attributed to 'Uthmân is mentioned systematically in the textual sources and was recognized as canonical by the dynasty alongside the book written by Ibn Tûmart.[15] During military parades, these two precious volumes were exhibited on a white she-camel and a mule. They were both kept in the sanctuary of the mosque at Tinmal where Ibn Tûmart was buried. In reference to the Quran (the Book of God) and the Sunnah (the Tradition of His Messenger), the Almohad caliphate claimed the strictest orthodoxy, and from this flowed their absolute authority over their contemporaries. Within this framework, Ibn Tûmart was only limited in his authority by the Quran and Sunnah, but because he was divinely chosen, he was a unique and perfect interpreter of these texts. The Almohad caliphs used this dogma of the impeccability of the Mahdi to justify the administrative centralization of the empire around the person of the ruler and forced the obedience of religious elites and the marginalization of the Mâliki juridical-religious school that had previously dominated the Maghreb. The Almohads' break with the ulemas and *fuqahâ'* – guarantors and transmitters of the Law – is particularly remarkable. The caliphs ordered the burning of the works of jurisprudence, which had previously been used by the ulemas to interpret the Law and define norms of governance.[16] These works practically disappeared during the period. Instead, the Almohad caliphs, 'orthodox successors' of the 'impeccable *imam*' Ibn Tûmart, imposed justice and interpreted the Law by relying on the only two foundations that were unanimously accepted: the Quran and the Sunnah. In this way, the processes of legitimizing power no longer relied upon legal consultations emanating from the *fuqahâ'*, as under the previous dynasty and under other contemporary and earlier eastern dynasties, but on specific mechanisms: the infallibility and impeccability of the founder of the dynasty; mimicry of the Prophetic model; a return to the text of the Revelation; and glorification of the Quranic text, used, in particular, as a decorative motif in inscriptions, such as the legends on coins.

The greatest scholars of the time, such as Ibn Tufayl (known in the Western Latin sources as 'Abubacer', d.1185) and Ibn Rushd ('Averroes', d.1199), were asked to elaborate on the doctrine, which was simultaneously philosophical, political and religious. Meanwhile, the entire population of the Almohad empire, including its elites, was employed to diffuse the doctrine. But it did not appear all at once; rather, it developed gradually under the rule of the first two caliphs, 'Abd al-Mu'min and Yûsuf I (r.1163–84). Modern historians speak of the 'Almohad revolution' as if the rupture with the past was profound, but the entirety of the conceptual tools used were the most 'classical' of Islamic traditions. It was the combination of different ideas which constituted a break in the tradition. The adoption of a name with religious connotations (*al-muwahhidûn*), which evokes the divine uniqueness (*tawhîd*), implicitly categorizes Muslims who do not adhere to the movement as apostates. In effect, this dogma led the Almohads to dismiss the human interpretations that the collections of law (*fatâwâ, nawâzil*) – upon which Maliki doctors relied to give their opinions – were constituted from a legal standpoint.

Almohad doctrine attempted a synthesis of all earlier Muslim theological thought. The place occupied by philosophers in the elaboration of Almohad dogma allows us to understand the contemporary glorification of philosophy, of speculative theology (*kalâm*) and of the use of reason in understanding the divine word. Support for an allegorical, rather than a literal, reading of Quranic verses and indeed the name 'Partisans of Unity' (*ahl al-tawhîd*) are both direct references to *mu'tazilism*, which developed in Iraq at the end of the eighth century and during the ninth. It led to a serious crisis between the ulemas and the Abbasid caliphs, a crisis which ended with the victory of the religious caste at the expense of the political establishment. The Almohad approach makes clear that the question of reconciliation between reason and revelation had not been definitively resolved in ninth-century Baghdad but remained a lasting topic of negotiation among scholars and between scholars and leaders. Moreover, the legitimization of violence against non-aligned Muslims and the claim to the caliphate by non-Arabs are part of the Kharijite tradition, which profoundly shaped the Maghreb from the eighth century. In addition, the importance of prayer, asceticism and proximity to God reveals the influence of Sufism and mysticism on Almohad ideology. And lastly, in the field of law, the rejection of any other basis other than the Quran and Sunnah – such as reasoning through analogies (*qiyâs*), individual appreciation (*ra'y*), the consensus of legal doctors (*ijmâ'*), all bases more or less accepted by the Maliki, Hanafi and Shafi'i law schools – brought the Almohads closer to the Hanbali school, which was otherwise very different in many respects.

The (re-)invention of the tradition of Islamic power

The Almohad empire (1130–1269) was led by an *imâm*-caliph, a title that manifested his 'universal' ambition to govern all Islamic lands (the *dâr al-Islâm*). The Almohad leader competed in titles, prerogatives, legitimacy and, more generally, ideology with the Abbasid caliphs of Baghdad (750–1258) and the Fatimid rulers of Cairo (969–1171). The religious reforms of the Almohads found their origin in a kind of 'parallel' revelation and the reproduction of Muhammad-like deeds that, in a sense, refounded the original Islamic empire and Islamic monotheism in the West. In a religion which presented itself as a culmination, Muhammad being the seal of the prophets, and in a history dominated by the weight of traditions where any innovation was perceived from the onset to be blasphemy, the only possible reform was to return as closely as possible to that which was considered to be a permanent point of reference: the first decades of the Islamic revelation and the establishment of the caliphate (612 to the end of the seventh century). Pushed to an extreme, this tendency led, with the Almohads, to a repetition of origins, which, from a cyclical and eschatological perspective, fused the contemporary history of Ibn Tûmart's followers with the beginnings of Islam.

Generally, Almohad rulers systematically applied terminology from early Islam to the history of the Muslim – now Almohad – West. This appears in the names the Almohads gave to their newly founded cities. Thus, upon the foundations of a fortress built by the last Almoravid emir, 'Abd al-Mu'min constructed a new city called both al-Mahdiyya ('the city of the Mahdi') and Ribât al-Fath ('the *ribât* of victory') – the future Rabat – which faced Salé from across the Bou Regreg River.[17] 'Abd al-Mu'min also renamed Gibraltar (Jabal Târiq, 'mountain of Tariq'), which references Târiq ibn Ziyâd, the first conqueror of the Iberian peninsula in 711, Jabal al-Fath ('mountain of victory').[18] This idea of *fath* is very much related to the first decades of the history of Islam and a literary genre known as 'books of victories' (*kutub al-futûhât*), which recounted the great successes sanctified by the tradition of the Prophet and his successors.[19] After the Mahdi, whose appearance signifies the beginning of the End Times, the era of the caliphate, which immediately follows the initial era of Muhammad's prophecies, begins again.[20] Thus, at the beginning of the thirteenth century, the first four Almohad caliphs received the qualification of 'orthodox' / 'well-guided' (*râshidûn*) on coins and in textual sources, an epithet reserved in Sunni Islam for the first four caliphs: Abû Bakr (r.632–4), 'Umar (r.634–4), 'Uthmân (r.644–56) and 'Alî (r.656–61).

A new religion, a new chosen people: the Masmûda Berbers

The capacity of Almohad thinkers to articulate all these elements into a synthesized, cohesive dogma gave the empire a completely original ideology with which its rulers could assert their independence from the mostly Andalusian ulemas and claim for the Maghreb absolute power over all the other regions of the Muslim world. Indeed, the Almohad reformation affirmed the pre-eminence of the western territories of Islam compared to all other parts of the Muslim world in the twelfth century. This idea of power was closely linked to the history of the Umayyad caliphate of Cordoba and its secession from the eastern centres of power, with the Almohad reformation succeeding in creating a synthesis from the histories of the Maghreb and al-Andalus.

The Maghreb in the Middle Ages was one of the peripheries of the Islamic world. Conquered late, the source of multiple revolts, and home of dissidents and heterodoxies until the eleventh century (notably Kharijism and Fatimid Shiism), the region did not hold the noble status of the Umayyad caliphates of Syria and al-Andalus or those of the Abbasids of Baghdad or the Fatimids of Cairo. Ibn Tûmart and, more importantly, his successors began a true revolution by claiming for the Maghreb primacy over all other Islamic regions in the world. To accomplish this, Ibn Tûmart adopted a unique perspective in his writings regarding two prophetic traditions: 'Islam began as a foreign/strange [thing] (*gharib^{an}*) and it will become foreign/strange again as it began – blessed be the foreigners (*al-ghurabâ*)!' and 'The inhabitants of the West (*ahl al-Gharb*) will always be on the side of truth until the Hour comes'. He identified the 'foreigners/strangers' (*gharib, ghurabâ*) of the first prophetic saying with the inhabitants of the West (*Gharb*) in the second, playing on the fact that these terms were formed from the same root, GH-R-B.[21]

This particular reading, which reduces the esoteric qualities of the prophecies, opens them up to numerous interpretations. However, an explicit and concrete meaning was generally adopted by the Almohads. In their understanding, the Berbers – and more particularly the Masmûda living at the extreme edge of the Maghreb – were explicitly designated by the Prophet as possessors of Truth. They would serve as a vanguard destined to enlighten and save the rest of the Muslim community on the day of the Final Judgement. After the Almohads, this reading appeared in all hagiographic dictionaries that extolled the virtues of the saints of the Maghreb or the merits of the Berbers. Ibn Tûmart and the Almohads, therefore, managed to give the leading role in the great history of Islam to the people of the

Maghreb, notably at the expense of the scholars of al-Andalus and the Arabs of the East. The place accorded to the Maghreb and the Berbers in the history of Islam has had important consequences in linguistics. Indeed, one of the rare certainties that we possess regarding the preaching of Ibn Tûmart is that he addressed his disciples in a Berber dialect. Almohad authors never sought to erase this truth even while discrediting the Almoravids for their alleged illiteracy and their lack of knowledge of the Arabic language. The two writings attributed to Ibn Tûmart, and probably completed later, the Credo ('aqida) and the Spiritual Guide (murshida) were only translated into Arabic in the reigns of his successors, several years after the death of their presumed author. The translation into Arabic was probably less a simple transfer from one language to the other than, as Madeleine Fletcher believes, an original creation that sought to canonize the origins and founder of the movement.[22]

Ibn Tûmart was, thus, also a mediator of the Arab-Muslim religion in a non-Arab environment (al-'ajam), a vital step towards the Islamization of the medieval Maghreb. Under the Almohads, the Berbers acquired, for the first time in history, a rank and a status hitherto reserved for the Arabs. The type of language written by this powerful group was called the 'western language' (al-lisân al-gharbî) rather than the 'Berber language' (al-lisân al-barbar), which was considered pejorative. This 'western language' was established as sacred since Ibn Tûmart had used it to deliver his message. The language of the 'western foreign Berbers' – the ghurabâ' of the prophetic hadîth – was promoted by the Almohads as an imperial language, with precedence over Arabic. It was based on the Berber language used in the Masmûda tribe and enriched with numerous Arabic terms borrowed primarily from religious texts. The promotion of the Berber language to the rank of sacred gave strength and cohesion to Almohad ideology, which allowed its diffusion in the little-Arabized population. In 1152, when the Almohads were about to unify the Maghreb, 'Abd al-Mu'min addressed the people of the empire from Bougie with a letter that insisted upon the role given to the 'western language' and the duty of all inhabitants of the empire to learn it.

Ultimately, Almohad ideology proposed an adaptive language for all. For the urban masses, Ibn Tûmart's message focused primarily on the censorship of morals, in other words, the Quranic duty of 'prescription of good and prohibition of evil'. This was, in fact, the first message of Ibn Tûmart who, on his return from the East, was known for breaking wine jars and musical instruments and castigating the effeminate clothing of men and the shamelessness of women wherever he went. In rural areas, the use of the Berber language as a sacred tongue equal to Arabic contributed to the success of the Almohads. For Andalusians and literate elites in general, the conceptual system was much more elaborate. It offered them the ability to free themselves from the restrictions imposed by the Maliki ulemas by encouraging speculative debate and the use of reason. Although failing to adhere to strict Almohad dogma, many scholars appreciated its openness and intellectual stimulation.

The last essential element in the Almohad system was the place of religion in the state through the cult of the founder of the movement, Ibn Tûmart, and, more generally, of the Almohad caliphs. From the conquest of Marrakesh, the caliph 'Abd al-Mu'min established the process of undertaking an official pilgrimage to the tomb of Ibn Tûmart at Tinmal.[23] This is the first example in the Muslim West of an official cult. The phenomenon of pious visits (ziyâra) to the tombs of saints already existed, but neither the Rustemids of Tahert (761–909), the Idrissids (789–985), nor the Umayyads of Cordoba (929–1031) had attempted to use these popular practices to their benefit. The visits of the Almohad caliphs to the tomb of the Mahdi at Tinmal, therefore, provided a rhythm to the life of the empire. Before leading their troops, the Almohad caliphs adopted the custom of going to the tomb of Ibn Tûmart to obtain the blessing of the founder-saint of the dynasty. They went there with their entourage, composed of their favourites, important dignitaries and their praetorian guard. Almohad sources call this a *hâjj* ('pilgrimage'), a term traditionally reserved for the fifth pillar of Islam, the pilgrimage to Mecca. Usually, one uses the word *ziyâra* ('[pious] visit') for visiting the tomb of a saint. Almohad authors were, therefore, placing Tinmal on the same level as the Holy Places of the Arabian Peninsula, with which, after the eastern journey of Ibn Tûmart, the Almohads did not seek any connection.

The influence of this pilgrimage centre outlasted the Almohad dynasty. When the Merinid vizier al-Milyânî defiled the tombs of the Almohad caliphs Abû Ya'qûb (r.1163–84) and Abû Yûsuf al-Mansûr (r.1184–99) in 1274, he did not dare attack those of Ibn Tûmart and 'Abd al-Mu'min. Furthermore, his actions were disavowed by the Merinid sultan Abû Yûsuf (r.1258–86), who doubtless feared alienating a large portion of the population.[24] This episode reveals how entrenched the cult of Ibn Tûmart had become among the rural and Berber populations, not only as an emblematic figure of the Almohad movement but also as a saint. For a long time, the influence of Tinmal extended well beyond the southern Maghreb. With the disappearance of the Almohads, the site stopped being the object of an official cult, but remained a holy site and place of pilgrimage, attracting significant crowds each year. According to Ibn al-Khatib (d.1374), several principalities emerged in the western High Atlas after 1269 and their rulers continued to venerate Tinmal.[25] Under the Saadian (1554–1660) and Alawid (1666–present) dynasties, numerous saints claimed descent from Ibn Tûmart, and certain lineages in the south continue to do so even today.

Muslim kingship: the origins and characteristics of Islamic monarchy

Although a term for king (*malik*) – and the related term 'monarchy' (*malakiya*) – existed in Arabic, historically it was, as the Almohad history shows, infrequently employed. Present in the Quran, the term is rooted in ideas of possession, property, domination and control. However, Islamic systems of government favoured other terms: caliph, emir, commander of the faithful (*amir al-mu'minin*), guide (*imâm*), and later sultan, shâh, or khân in Asia. It is revealing that the Almohads, who attempted in the twelfth century a historically unique synthesis of Muslim political concepts, never claimed the title of *malik* but adopted most of the others.

In his book *Muslim Kingship*, Aziz El Azmeh presented an overview of the question of royalty in Islam that should, in theory, have saved us from writing this section; yet, it is a book that defends controversial ideas. El Azmeh's overview addresses the first five to six centuries of Islam and concludes with the fall of the caliphate of Baghdad in 1258, not because this marks an inexorable decline, as it is considered to be by some historians, but because, according to the author, the paradigms of Islamic power were well established by this time. Subsequently, one witnesses only a development of existing structures and concepts.[26] El Azmeh's perspective is profoundly different from the traditional approach in that he considerably downplays the importance of the Prophet's generation by situating the first century of Islam in pre-Islamic political constructions of Late Antiquity as developed by Peter Brown.[27] Consequently, a rupture did not occur in 632, at the death of the Prophet Muhammed, nor in 660, at the end of the Râshidûn caliphate of Sunni Islam, but rather at the end of the eighth century. This approach breaks with that of Muslim scholars, as well as that of Orientalists of the nineteenth and twentieth centuries. Indeed, El Azmeh considers the reign of 'Abd al-Malik (r.685–705), during which a new Islamic coin was minted and Arabic was imposed as the state language, as a continuation of systems of governance established before Islam. According to El Azmeh, prophecy was not yet the foundational paradigm of the Islamic state in the early period. Models of royalty would be found in the empires that Islam had overthrown and conquered, and beyond them in the history of the Near East and the Middle East, of which Islam was the heir. This concept situates Islam within the continuity of history and views it from the perspective of the *longue durée* rather than presenting it as the result of an abrupt 'break'.[28]

Islam, like the Byzantine Empire, was eastern to the extent that the sovereign would never lose his spiritual authority, whereas in western Europe, the empire and the papacy divided the temporal and spiritual spheres between them. The difference between East and West is not related to some religious specificity, but to political and social reasons, as eastern Orthodox Christianity reveals, being closer to Islam than to western Catholicism regarding the relationship of the temporal and the spiritual spheres.

Like Jocelyne Dakhlia and Makram Abbès, El Azmeh relies on the literature of the 'mirrors of the princes' to emphasize that political references are pre-Islamic, surveying works such as Ardashir's will, the letters of Alexander to Aristotle, and the 'secret of secrets'.[29] His primary reference work is the *Kalîla wa dimna*, the first Islamic prose book, translated from Persian. Thus, political wisdom derived from Persian during the first centuries of Islam, and the art of governance transcended religious barriers. Two changes contributed to the Islamization of the art of governance. First, the pressure from the Shiites who, from the end of the ninth century, claimed for their *imâm* all spiritual and temporal privileges, from human government to the interpretation of the Quran, which would have led to a true union of church and state if the idea had prevailed. Second, the birth of a body of scholars – ulemas and *fuqahâ'* – who considered themselves collectively to be the guardians of the Revelation and the only legitimate holders of religious authority. Distancing themselves from the concrete exercise of power by the Turks, who had recently converted to Islam, the ulemas opposed the secular power of the Seljuk princes and, later, the religious character of the Zenghids and Ayyubids. During this period, the caliph retained an aura of power because he remained the symbolic leader of the ulemas, who together formed a collective incarnation of prophetic heritage.

When the Abbasid caliphate disappeared due to the Mongols in 1258, the utility of the institution was reduced to such a point that Ibn Taymiyya (d.1328) concluded that the caliphate was no longer necessary if the *sharî'a* was respected.[30] Politics were henceforth divided between the sultan, who exercised temporal power, and the ulemas, who collectively held the religious role that the caliph had claimed between

the eighth and thirteenth centuries. The ulemas, therefore, became the only counterpoint to the arbitrary power of the sultans. The Almohads, despite the important
influence they had on minds at the time, even in the East, are eventually mentioned
by El Azmeh, but only to discard their intellectual, conceptual and political autonomy: 'The Almohads and their Merinid successors instituted courtly norms directly
derived from the Baghdadian models, including drums beating outside palace gates,
albeit in a rudimentary form that reflected both provincialism and arrivism [sic].'[31]
Clearly El Azmeh considers the Maghreb too peripheral and irrelevant to affect the
Islamic heartland, where everything would have been decided. Yet one can view the
Almohad empire as an attempt to restore full caliphal power: the caliph was the only
authorized interpreter of the Revelation and tried quite successfully to dispossess the
ulemas of their religious prerogatives and incorporate them into the state bureaucracy (*dîwân*).

The peripheries are essential when explaining Islamic legal systems and political
thought in the Middle Ages. It is, however, hardly surprising that El Azmeh does
not consider them as he entirely ignores the question of ethnicity: in the East, the
sultans were Turks, foreign to the societies over which they ruled; in the West, the
rulers at the time were Berbers; and in India, they were Turco-Mongolians. All of El
Azmeh's thinking is based on an 'eastern' outlook developed by Egyptian, Syrian and
Iraqi thinkers and designed to ensure the symbolic superiority of the Arab Middle
East over all other Islamic regions.[32] Although he does not hesitate to include the
theories on history and the state formulated by the influential writer Ibn Khaldûn
(d.1406), El Azmeh notably treats his works as if they were written by simply another
eastern Islamic author.[33] And yet it was Almoravid and Almohad models that gave
this scholar from the Maghreb the basis for his theories.[34]

Contrary to those who support the idea of a 'break' symbolized by the Revelation
and the importance of the prophetic model, El Azmeh roots the first century of
Islamic monarchy in Late Antiquity. In minimizing the rupture, he underlines the
influence of the antique models of the sacred monarchies of Mesopotamia and
India. Abbès and Dakhlia subscribe to this idea of the early distinctiveness of a secular political thought in Islam, independent from religion and prophecy.[35] On the
other hand, Nabil Mouline, who also insists in his latest work on the need to focus on
the caliphal institution and long-term social phenomena instead of 'breaks', comes
closer to the conclusions of Crone, Hinds and Cook: he argues that Islamic governance was theocratic from almost the beginning.[36] At the centre of this system, the
political leader is a divine actor in the societies of the Middle East. Beginning with
the observation that the pre-Islamic Arabian Peninsula was the site of numerous
monarchical experiments in which the king was considered an agent of Heaven,
Mouline deduces that Muhammad's preaching, which challenged the social and
political balance, created a system based on links that transcended tribal and clan
differences. In the continuity of Islamic tradition and the largely reconstructed biography of the Prophet, Mouline re-adopts the idea that the Hijra constituted a major
political rupture: on this date (622), the Prophet, spiritual guide that he was, became
head of state and a warlord. Considering that neither the Quran nor the Sunnah
define a properly 'Islamic' political system, Mouline views the caliphal institution as
a break and an innovation, created *ex nihilo* and destined to perpetuate prophetic
authority. He admits, however, that it is difficult to know with precision what the

caliphate was in the early years of its development. Never called caliph (*khalīfa*) nor king (*mulk*) in the oldest sources that we have, the leader of the community carried, it seems, the title of *imām* (guide) or *amīr al-mu'minīn* ('commander of the faithful'). Following the same premise as El Azmeh – that the Muslim political system should be placed in a continuity of pre-Islamic political practices – Mouline comes to the opposite conclusions: for him, the head of the community undoubtedly had theocratic pretensions. Mouline sees in the multiple revolts that broke out at the death of Muhammed in 632 – what the Islamic tradition calls the *ridda* and considers a general apostasy of the tribes – the sign of an intractable entanglement of religion and politics.

With the establishment of the Umayyad Caliphate of Damascus (644 or 660), the symbols relating to the caliphate materialized as large-scale architectural productions such as the Dome of the Rock in Jerusalem, while the caliph reinforced the sacredness of his task. This allowed the leader of the community to reaffirm his role in the quest for salvation. With the Abbasids, who succeeded the Umayyads after a revolution in 749/750, the messianic dimension of the ruler became a fundamental basis for the exercise of power. The surnames chosen by the caliphs of Baghdad for their reigns (*laqab*-s) – for which the name al-Mahdi appears regularly – reflected the eschatological dimension of the caliphate. For Mouline, the caliphate sought to reproduce the cosmic order by placing the sovereign at the centre of the religion as the guarantor of social balance.[37] In order to strengthen the charismatic authority of the caliph, the rulers adopted *regalia*: the sceptre (*qadīb*) for justice, the seal (*khatam*) for administrative power, the cape (*burda*) of the Prophet and the colour black as symbolic of the caliphate. In addition, ceremonies helped establish the religious function of the ruler: the Friday sermon (*khutba*), in theory given by the ruler in the capital or in his name in the other towns, created a close association between religious authority and political discourse. The ceremony of allegiance (*bay'a*) demonstrated the hierarchy between the ruler and his subjects. Mouline then joins El Azmeh in considering the ninth and tenth centuries as the moment where, at the end of the mu'tazilite crisis (mid-ninth century), the caliph definitively lost his status as interpreter of the Revelation to the benefit of the ulemas. The accession to power of non-Arab military princes (Turkish or Persian) was the culmination of this division between politico-military functions exercised by foreigners and religious functions assumed collectively by the ulemas. Within this new framework, the caliph was content to serve the symbolic function of protector of the faith and guarantor of the unity of power.

Thus, according to Mouline, as well as Crone and Hinds, who rely on the successive uses of the titles 'caliph of God' (*khalīfatu Llāh*) and 'caliph of the envoy of God' (*khalīfatu rasūli Llāh*), the first caliphs would have claimed, following the example of the Prophet, all of the political, religious and moral functions, and the caliphate itself was conceived as a theocratic institution.[38] It was at the point where the body of the *ulemas* was constituted that they imposed the second title in an attempt to secularize the functions of the caliph and reserve for themselves the authority to interpret the Revelation.[39]

Given the absence of sources for the first decades of Islam, these historiographical debates will probably never end. Today, it is impossible to say exactly when the title of caliph appeared and whether it was related to God (as vicar) or the Prophet (as successor). The only thing we are certain of is that the term caliph was definitely in existence by the reign of 'Abd al-Malik at the end of the seventh century. He established this title during a period that saw the expansion of an Islamic religious language on a global scale in an attempt to bolster the authority of the Umayyads against the claims of a rival, Ibn al-Zubayr (r.681–92).[40] Political opposition, therefore, became religious deviance.

What infects some of these debates is the attempt by a certain number of scholars to define the essence of Islam by starting from a definition of an 'original' Islamic political system, one from which everything that followed was derived. What these scholars have in mind is the development of another system, one whose evolution is often held up – contestably – as normative: western European society. The evolution of western civilization is characterized – although this itself is debatable – as a progressive separation between politics and religion from the Middle Ages. These two elements, the definition of the model and its implicit comparison to the history of certain western European societies, have prevented us from paying attention to geographic diversity and the different political systems adopted in Muslim countries. In fact, as Hugh Kennedy rightly points out, the caliphate was from the beginning an evolving institution.[41] The attributes of different rulers were discussed, negotiated and challenged constantly in the pre-modern era of the Islamic 'commonwealth'. If an institution such as the papacy, which ensured a transition between Earth and Heaven and competed with temporal powers, did not exist in Islam, the ulemas, the numerous saints, and the mystics and their brotherhoods constituted individually and collectively a powerful counterpoint, sometimes participating in the exercise of power, at other times refusing it and often developing other forms of power on the margins of political systems, thereby preventing an eventual monopoly on the religion by the princes. The Almohad example reveals the capacity for different societies, periodically, to seize rhetorical tools and political or religious concepts, and adapt and reshape them in a new context. In so doing, societies both reuse tradition and lay the groundwork for its subsequent reinvention.

Notes

* Translated by Derek R. Whaley.
1 For a detailed look, see Pascal Buresi and Hicham El Aallaoui, *Governing the Empire: Appointing Provincial Officials in the Almohad Caliphate*, trans. Travis Bruce Studies in the History and Society of the Maghreb 3 (Leiden: Brill, 2012) and Pascal Buresi and Mehdi Ghouirgate, *Le Maghreb médiéval (XII*e*–XV*e* siècle)*, Cursus (Paris: Armand Colin, 2013). A simplified system for transliteration from the Arabic is used. When they exist, English forms are privileged (such as in the case of ulemas instead of *'ulamâ*).
2 Fred McGraw Donner, *Narratives of Islamic Origins: The Beginnings of Islamic Historical Writing*, Studies in Late Antiquity and Early Islam 14 (Princeton: Darwin Press, 1998).
3 Patricia Crone and Martin Hinds, *God's Caliph: Religious Authority in the First Centuries of Islam* (Cambridge: Cambridge University Press, 2003); Michael Allan Cook and Patricia Crone, *Hagarism: The Making of the Islamic World* (Cambridge: Cambridge University Press, 1980); John E. Wansbrough, *The Sectarian Milieu: Content and Composition of Islamic Salvation History* (Amherst, NY: Prometheus Books, 1978).
4 Frank Griffel, "Ibn Tûmart's Rational Proof for God's Existence and Unity of and His Connection to the Niẓâmiyya Madrasa in Baghdad," in *Los Almohades: problemas y perspectivas*,

eds. Patrice Cressier, Maribel Fierro and Luis Molina, Estudios árabes e islámicos, 11 (Madrid: CSIC-Casa de Velázquez, 2005), 2: 752–813, at 755.

5 For the career of Ibn Tûmart: Rachid Bourouiba, *Ibn Tûmart* (Alger: Soc. nationale d'ed. et de diffusion, 1982); 'Abd al-Majîd Al-Najjâr, *al-Mahdi Ibn Tûmart* (Cairo: Dâr al-Ġarb al-Islâmî, 1983).

6 María Jesús Viguera, "Los Almorávides," in *El retroceso territorial de al-Andalus: almorávides y almohades, siglos XI al XIII*, ed. María Jesús Viguera (Madrid: Espasa Calpe, 1998), 41–64.

7 For the early history of the Almohad caliphate: Évariste Lévi-Provençal, "Ibn Tumart et 'Abd al-Mu'min: le Faķih du Sûs et le Flambeau des Almohades," in *Mémorial Henri Basset: nouvelles études nord-africaines et orientales. 2* (Paris: Geuthner, 1928), 21–37; Évariste Lévi-Provençal, *Documents inédits d'histoire almohade. Fragments manuscrits du 'legajo' 1919 du fonds arabe de l'Escurial, publiés et traduits avec une introduction et des notes par E. Lévi-Provençal* (Paris: Librairie Orientaliste Paul Geuthner, 1928), 85. Al-Najjâr presents the different dates given by the sources: *al-Mahdi Ibn Tûmart*, 28–29.

8 Ibn Abi Zar', *Rawd al-qirtâs*, ed. 'A. Ibn Mansûr (Rabat: Imprimerie royale, 1999; first published in 1860), 274, cited by Mehdi Ghouirgate, *L'ordre almohade (1120–1269): une nouvelle lecture anthropologie* (Toulouse: Presses Universitaires du Mirail, 2014), 231.

9 On the treatment of the defeated in the Almohad period, see Ghouirgate, *L'ordre almohade (1120–1269)*, chapter 6: "Un souverain vengeur: l'éclat des supplices," 253–309.

10 Yassir Benhima, "Notes sur l'évolution de l'iqtâ' au Maghreb médiéval," *al-Andalus Magreb. Estudios Árabes e Islámicos* 16 (2009): 27–44.

11 Maribel Fierro, "Le mahdi Ibn Tûmart et al-Andalus: l'élaboration de la légitimité almohade," *Revue des mondes musulmans et de la Méditerranée* 91–94 (2000): 107–124. See also Michael Brett, "Le Mahdi dans le Maghreb médiéval," *Revue des mondes musulmans et de la Méditerranée* 91–94 (2000): 93–106, and more generally, Mercedes García-Arenal, ed., *Mahdisme et millénarisme en Islam, Revue des mondes musulmans et de la Méditerranée* (special issue), 91–94 (2000).

12 Mohammad Ali Amir-Moezzi and Sabine Schmidtke, "Rationalisme et théologie dans le monde musulman médiéval. Bref état des lieux," *Revue de l'histoire des religions* 4 (December 2009): 613–638.

13 Maribel Fierro, "Las genealogías de 'Abd al-Mu'min, primer califa almohade," *Al-Qantara* 24, no. 1 (June 2003): 77–107.

14 M.J. Viguera, "Las reacciones de los Andalusíes," in *Los Almohades: problemas y perspectivas*, vol. 2, eds. P. Cressier, M. Fierro and L. Molina, Collection Estudios árabes e islámicos, Monografías (Madrid: CSIC, 2006), 705–735.

15 Pascal Buresi, "Une relique almohade: l'utilisation du coran (attribué à 'Utmân b. 'Affân [644–656]) de la Grande mosquée de Cordoue," *Études d'Antiquités africaines* 1, no. 1 (2008): 273–280.

16 Janina M. Safran, "The Politics of Book Burning in Al-Andalus," *Journal of Medieval Iberian Studies* 6, no. 2 (July 2014): 148–168.

17 Alberto García Sanjuán, "La Noción de Fatḥ En Las Fuentes Árabes Andalusíes y Magrebíes (Siglos VIII al XIII)," in *Orígenes y Desarrollo de La Guerra Santa en la Península Ibérica: Palabras e Imágenes para una legitimación (siglos X–XIV)*, eds. Carlos de Ayala Martínez, Patrick Henriet and J. Santiago Palacios Ontalva Collection de La Casa de Velázquez, vol. 154 (Madrid: Casa de Velázquez, 2016), 31–50.

18 On the concept of *fath* in the Quran, see Fred M. Donner, "Arabic *Fath* as 'Conquest' and its Origin in Islamic Tradition," *Al-'Usûr al-Wustâ* 24 (2016): 1–14.

19 For specific references to the chronicle texts, see Pascal Buresi, "La réaction idéologique dans la péninsule Ibérique face à l'expansion occidentale aux époques almoravide et almohade (XIᵉ–XIIIᵉ siècles)," in *L'expansion occidentale (XIᵉ–XVᵉ siècles). Formes et conséquences*, Congrès de la société des historiens médiévistes de l'enseignement supérieur public (Madrid, 23–25 May 2002) (Paris: Publications de la Sorbonne, 2003), 229–241.

20 Mercedes García-Arenal, *Messianism and Puritanical Reform: Mahdîs of the Muslim West*, trans. by Martin Beagles, The Medieval and Early Modern Iberian World 29 (Leiden-Boston: Brill, 2006). See also Maribel Fierro, "Sobre monedas de época almohade: I. El dinar del cadí 'Iyâḍ que nunca existió. II. Cuándo se acuñaron las primeras monedas almohades y la cuestión de la licitud de acuñar moneda," *al-Qantara* 27, no. 2 (2006): 457–476, specifically 465:

'En suma, el mahdismo de Ibn Tûmart era, ante todo, una fórmula político-religiosa para crear un Estado. De hecho, este tipo de mahdismo no es sino la actualización – post-Muhammad – del modelo profético de los orígenes del islam.'

21 Maribel Fierro, "Spiritual Alienation and Political Activism: The Gurabâ' in Al-Andalus during the sixth/twelfth century," *Arabica* 47, no. 2 (April 2000): 210–240.

22 Madeleine Fletcher, "The Almohad Tawhid: Theology Which Relies On Logic," *Numen* 38, no. 1 (January 1991): 110–127.

23 Pascal Buresi, "Les cultes rendus à la tombe du mahdî Ibn Tûmart à Tinmâl (xɪɪᵉ–xɪɪɪᵉ s.)," *Comptes rendus des séances de l'Académie des Inscriptions et Belles-Lettres* 152 (2008): 391–438.

24 al-Tâsâftî Al-Marrâkushî and Ibn Khaldûn cited by Mehdi Ghouirgate, *L' ordre almohade (1120–1269): un nouvelle lecture anthropologie* (Toulouse: Presses Universitaires du Mirail, 2014), 442.

25 On the veneration of Ibn Tûmart after the disappearance of the Almohads, see Mercedes García-Arenal, *Messianism and Puritanical Reform: Mahdis of the Muslim West*, The Medieval and Early Modern Iberian World, vol. 29 (Leiden: Brill, 2006), 221.

26 Aziz Al-Azmeh, *Muslim Kingship: Power and the Sacred in Muslim, Christian and Pagan Polities* (London: Tauris, 2001), 296.

27 Peter Brown, *Le monde de l'antiquité tardive: de Marc Aurèle à Mahomet*, trans. Christine Monatte (Paris: Gallimard, 2011).

28 Ultimately, El Azmeh develops a fundamentally secular vision of Islamic history and its systems of government. He explains that, in its first century, Islam was in fact a continuation under another name of the Achaemenid empire. Everything in the structures of the first century, including ceremonies, prostration, the kissing of hands and feet, the symbolism of colours and the imposition of silence, brought the new political system closer to that of previous empires. Al-Azmeh, *Muslim Kingship*, 88–89.

29 Jocelyne Dakhlia, "Les Miroirs des princes islamiques: une modernité sourde ?" *Annales. Histoire, Sciences Sociales* 57, no. 5 (October 2002): 1191–1206; Makram Abbès, *Islam et politique à l'âge classique* (Paris: Presses Universitaires de France, 2009).

30 Nabil Mouline, *Le Califat: Histoire politique de l'islam* (Paris: Flammarion, 2016), 121–122.

31 Al-Azmeh, *Muslim Kingship*, 148.

32 We could consider the production of the eighth- to twelfth-century Eastern scholars as a reverse of Said's *Orientalism*, a kind of eastern colonial vision of the West.

33 No contextualization at all of his work, his writings and his analyses is offered by El Azmeh who uses him as an atemporal and universal expert on the Islamic world and history: Al-Azmeh, *Muslim Kingship*, passim.

34 For many decades, Ibn Khaldun's *Prolegomena* have been annexed by many researchers and authors to a universal thought on theory of power: Yves Lacoste, *Ibn Khaldoun naissance de l'histoire, passé du Tiers monde* (Paris: La Découverte, 2009); Abdesselam Cheddadi and Ibn Khaldûn, *Ibn Khaldûn: L'homme et Le Théoricien de la civilisation*, Bibliothèque des histoires (Paris: Gallimard, 2006); Gabriel Martinez-Gros, *Ibn Khaldûn et les sept vies de l'islam*, La Bibliothèque Arabe. Hommes et Sociétés (Arles: Sinbad: Actes sud, 2006); Gabriel Martinez-Gros, *Brève histoire des empires: Comment ils surgissent, comment ils s'effondrent*, La Couleur des idées (Paris: Éditions du Seuil, 2014); Gabriel Martinez-Gros, *Fascination du Djihad: Fureurs islamistes et défaite de la paix* (Paris: PUF, 2016). Yet, my future project is to deconstruct this universalization of Ibn Khaldun to reroot his work in the history of Maghreb.

35 Dakhlia, "Les Miroirs des princes islamiques"; Abbès, *Islam et politique*.

36 Mouline, *Le Califat*.

37 Mouline, *Le Califat*, 62.

38 To Watt, the title of caliph [of the envoy of God] referred to a temporal delegation of prophetic authority. William Montgomery Watt, *Islamic Political Thought* (Edinburgh: Edinburgh University Press, 1968; rev. 1998).

39 Crone and Hinds, *God's Caliph*; and Patricia Crone, *God's Rule: Government and Islam – Six Centuries of Medieval Islamic Political Thought* (New York: Columbia University Press, 2004).

40 Fred McGraw Donner, *Muhammad and the Believers: At the Origins of Islam* (Cambridge, MA: The Belknap Press of Harvard University Press, 2010).

41 Hugh Kennedy, *The Prophet and the Age of the Caliphates: The Islamic Near East from the Sixth to the Eleventh Century* (Edinburgh: Pearson, 2004); and Hugh Kennedy, *Caliphate: The History of an Idea* (London: Basic, 2016).

Key works

Al-Azmeh, ʿAzîz, *Muslim Kingship: Power and the Sacred in Muslim, Christian and Pagan Polities*. Paperback edition (London; New York: I. B. Tauris, 2001).

Buresi, Pascal, and Hicham El Aallaoui, *Governing the Empire: Provincial Administration in the Almohad Caliphate (1224–1269): Critical Edition, Translation, and Study of Manuscript 4752 of the Hasaniyya Library in Rabat Containing 77 Taqadim ('appointments')*. Studies in the History and Society of the Maghrib, vol. 3 (Leiden: Brill, 2013).

Crone, Patricia, and Martin Hinds, *God's Caliph: Religious Authority in the First Centuries of Islam* (Cambridge: Cambridge University Press, 2003).

Dakhlia, Jocelyne, *Le divan des rois: le politique et le religieux dans l'islam* (Paris: Aubier, 1998).

Dakhlia, Jocelyne, "Les Miroirs des princes islamiques: une modernité sourde?" *Annales. Histoire, Sciences Sociales* 57, no. 5 (October 2002): 1191–1206.

Kennedy, Hugh N., *The Prophet and the Age of the Caliphates: The Islamic Near East from the Sixth to the Eleventh Century* (London: Pearson Education, 2004).

Mouline, Nabil, *Le Califat: Histoire politique de l'islam* (Paris: Flammarion, 2016).

8

CONTEMPORARY KINGSHIP IN MUSLIM ARAB SOCIETIES IN COMPARATIVE CONTEXT

David Mednicoff

Ruling monarchies have been important historically and may still be important as political archetypes. Yet they have nearly disappeared as forms of actual governance in most regions of the contemporary world, with one notable exception. Kings who hold real power remain in Bahrain, Brunei, Jordan, Kuwait, Morocco, Oman, Qatar, Saudi Arabia and the United Arab Emirates. What these countries have in common is, of course, a majority Muslim population and, other than the tiny island of Brunei in the South China Sea, Arab cultural-linguistic identity.

Without advancing a quasi-teleological, orientalist, or essentialist cultural argument about Islam or Arab politics, can we make sense of how significant countries with common points of social meaning retain ruling monarchies? This chapter argues that kingship in contemporary Arab Muslim-majority countries has helped address specific post-colonial tensions around the official role of religion, a popular interest in steering a political path distinct from the formal institutional makeup of former colonial powers, and dilemmas of political continuity and change. Monarchy was hardly inevitable as a post-colonial form of rule in Arab societies. Yet it has survived for diverse reasons significantly longer than social scientists expected,[1] suggesting the possible more general viability of monarchy as a political form.

This chapter is divided into three sections. First, I discuss the basic history and post-independence adaption of contemporary Arab monarchy. Second, I look at the institutions and methods of legitimation that have allowed permutations of an 'old-fashioned' ruling dynastic monarchy to endure, while paying attention to variation among different contemporary Arab royal regimes. These legitimation methods include reference to idealized political tropes drawn from Islamic history. Finally, I conclude with reflections on what the endurance of Arab monarchies suggests for monarchies and more seemingly modern forms of government. If Arab kingship has endured largely through a combination of its help in resolving particular regional challenges around post-colonial political legitimacy and luck, the global significance of neo-traditional, status-based leadership retains some vitality.

Before proceeding, it is useful to define briefly Muslim Arab kingship. I use the term to have minimal substantive content; I refer here to a pattern of governance in which a king rules over a state in the Arab world (thus excluding Brunei from detailed further treatment), and makes reference in part to Islam as one aspect of justifying his rule (throughout the chapter, the male pronoun is used since Arab kingship has been nearly entirely male and remains so in the contemporary era). Making reference to Islam presupposes neither a qualitative external judgement about the system's religious legitimacy, nor a rigid set of criteria for what makes an Arab king connected to Islam. It merely means that the monarchy ties itself to ideas or symbols prevalent in Arab Islamic political history.

This broad generalization requires several more specific clarifications. First, while I use the term 'king' for convenience, the Arabic term for this concept, *malik*, was specifically rejected and delegitimized in mainstream Islamic political thought. This is because the term connotes ownership or possessor of a society, whereas a Muslim ruler's mandate was to execute divine law in the interest of the Muslim community. A Muslim king thus could lay no claim to ownership of his society, and Islamic political theory therefore utilizes alternative terms for *malik* to enhance this contrast.[2]

This leads to the second clarification. Contemporary Arab kings use a mix of titles that also suggests their interest in balancing traditional political identity and contemporary nationalism. As a rule, the countries with the larger populations, Saudi Arabia, Morocco and Jordan, use the term 'king' to refer to their leaders, despite its aforementioned negative image in earlier history, while the smaller countries and Oman deploy 'emir' or 'sheikh' instead. While the latter terms are derived from verbs meaning to rule, they also can be honorifics not limited to political rulers. 'Emir' has a clearer connotation of political rule, while 'sheikh' invokes local, tribal, or religious leadership status.

It is not possible to be precise about the evolution of these terms to correspond to specific political implications in the rulers of contemporary Arab monarchies. Nonetheless, the smaller countries may wish to amplify their link to traditional small-scale governance, while the larger ones may find a title for a head of state more clearly associated with large-scale political centralization and non-Islamic comparative state history useful.

Arab monarchy as a historical reference point and post-colonial reality

Like many parts of the world, Arab regions were governed mainly by kings for many centuries prior to the modern period. However, several features particular to Arab Islamic history help contextualize the resilience of monarchy in the contemporary Middle East. First, the particular intensity and pervasiveness of colonialism, though hardly unique to the Arab world, led to an experience during the colonial era and an enduring ideological resonance of a local association of hypocrisy and coercion with Western politics, including democracy as practised in Western countries.[3] Second, and connected to the first, anti-colonial nationalism on both elite (Jordan) and populist (Morocco) levels sometimes took the form of embracing dynastic monarchy. Third, the particular manner in which long-term historical monarchy in the Arab world derived from, and was justified through, classical Islamic legal and political theory facilitates its continuing resilience and nostalgic reception among contemporary Middle Easterners, sometimes even in highly degraded derivative forms, such as the contemporary Islamic State's claim of the mantle of the caliphate.

But what did the caliphate represent in classical Islamic theory, and what faint reverberations might it carry for contemporary Muslim Arab kingship? The caliphate, the initial term for Islam's sociopolitical ruler, refers to an individual meant to be an earthly deputy of God, which is a real distinction from a typical king.[4] For this reason, groups like the Islamic State likely view the caliphate as a distinct model from today's Arab kings. Nonetheless, contemporary Arab kingship is influenced by the historical values and trajectory of what a legitimate and reasonable leader should be, including the caliphate.

Of prime significance here is that in classical theory, from early figures like Ibn Muqaffâ to quite different later ones like Ibn Taymiyya, rulers should come to power by some representative choice of the community and through their fealty to shared (religious) communal values, and they should have as their primary function the execution of (divinely derived) law.[5] The idea that a ruler's legitimacy is a function of his fealty to understanding and executing (but not creating) just law provides a template for the rule of law that is rooted in Arab Islamic historical experience. Thus, Arab kingship might seem a reasonable political alternative that both is grounded in Islamic political precedents and embraces the rule of law to modern Western representative republican democracy, particularly given that the latter stood for de facto authoritarian rule packaged as the rule of law under colonialism.

Models of kingship specifically from early in Islamic history inspire commanded contemporary Arab Muslims' respect because the governing values and practices of the religion's founder and believed prophet of God's words, Muhammed, and of his immediate successors, have passed down to subsequent generations of Muslims as sacred texts that inspire emulation and respect. In other words, the practices of early Islamic communal rulers, especially Muhammed and the caliphs that followed him, have become culturally routinized as the ideal types of sociopolitical leadership.[6] Particular efforts for contemporary Arab Muslims to answer the question, 'what would Mohammed do' may be no more likely to achieve consistency than Christians' response to 'what would Jesus do'. Yet, those efforts by Muslims are grounded in a clearer template of sociopolitical government than their Christian counterparts, given Islam's immediate status on its founding of being a spiritual and self-governing sociopolitical community.[7]

Of course, the fact that a sociopolitical system led by a male leader whose claim to authority was executing divinely inspired law became a model for just Islamic governance hardly meant that Muslim Arab rulers governed in a manner free from authoritarian excess, or even consistent with legal predictability. The socio-legal underpinnings of Islamic imperial rule, after its expansion through parts of Africa, Asia and Europe, rested on legal scholars and judges serving as advisers and enforcers of the rule of law.[8] Such a system embedded the possibility that rulers would make efforts to weaken the legitimacy and authority of Islamic jurists in order to consolidate their own repressive political capacity. This occurred in many places and through many dynasties in Islamic Middle Eastern history, until the combination of imperial authoritarian techniques and even more consistently repressive colonial rule led to the end of the system of monarchical figures being supported by, or credibly serving the maintenance of, the Islamic rule of law.[9]

Yet the erosion and contentious unresolved nature of the ideal type of Muslim rulers in the service of the rule of law did not destroy the ideal type itself. Indeed, the relative abstractness and lack of concrete legacy of this ideal type in the wake of colonialism meant that the model could stand for a variety of styles of rule and connections to Islam. This, in turn, facilitated Arab Islamic kingship as a more contemporary political construct. That people in Arab Muslim-majority societies had twentieth-century experience with Western colonial repression, but vaguer, idealized, impressions of Islamic monarchy, could make the latter governance template hold continued relevance, along with other post-colonial models of nationalism, even if its specific content was unclear.

The ideal type of an Arab Islamic monarch had additional resonance because of the Middle East's and North Africa's highly regionalized political history. With the formal reality of an Arab Islamic caliphate, until the Mongol sacking of Baghdad in 1258, that linked western Africa to southwest Asia, monarchical dynasty with a sacred communal justification had centuries to install itself as a default template for governance. Even local rulers who established political autonomy from the central caliphate ruled as hereditary kings and attempted to legitimize their rule as local agents of the caliphal dynasty. This pattern largely persisted with the re-establishment of an Islamic regional monarchy in much of the Middle East and North Africa in the form of the Ottoman Empire. Until the colonial period, the default template of centralized kings deriving their authority, at least theoretically, from their service to executing Islamic law dominated politics and replicated itself in localized imitators. Given this, colonial powers often left kings in titular control during their period of imperial dominance, as in Egypt and Jordan.[10]

Arab Islamic kings re-emerged at the heads of independent nation-states more directly during the decolonialization processes of the twentieth century through two basic patterns. First was the adaption to post-colonial nation-state building of a long-standing dynasty that continued to rule in principle under colonial control. The Arab Gulf states of Bahrain, Oman and the UAE fit this pattern, as all had an emir, or monarchical ruler, whose family held political control for hundreds of years into the era of independence.[11]

Yet the true model of a long-term ruling dynasty in the Arab world is Morocco. As I have discussed elsewhere (2016), the current king hails from a dynasty dating back to 1672. French rulers kept in place the 'Alawi dynasty as nominal rulers of the bulk of Morocco that they controlled in the twentieth century, on the assumption that a traditional ruler could be controllable and legitimizing, without being a challenge to colonial rule. The French did not anticipate that Muhammed V, the titular 'Alawi Sultan, would come to symbolize Moroccan national identity for millions of Moroccans when he aligned himself with a nationalist party, was exiled by the colonial government and became a lightning rod for populist anger towards the French.[12] Morocco's nationalist struggle and restoration of a long-ruling dynasty through a mass uprising may have been a peculiarity. But continuity and renovation for an historical ruling monarchy occurred in other Arab states as well, particularly in the Gulf region.

A second pattern of Arab monarchy is the establishment of a ruling dynasty in the past several centuries, followed later by the establishment of a national unit and the consolidation of national territory. This pattern took place in Kuwait and Qatar, tiny societies prior to the growth of the oil economy, under British foreign protection in the heyday of colonialism, that had ruling families, in Kuwait's case for several centuries, before their nations emerged. Yet, a non-Gulf Arab state is again a more paradigmatic case. Jordan did not exist as a territorial unit prior to the British and French division of much of the Middle East into their respective colonial spheres of influence.

The Transjordan area, which had been linked to contemporary Syria but was separated through the Sykes-Picot Agreement 1916 into a British mandate, lacked a long-standing ruler associated with it. The British tried to address this by building a monarchy around one of the brothers of an elite family descending from the family of the Prophet Muhammed, the Hashemites. The British also placed a Hashemite on the thrones of Iraq and Syria, but only the Jordanian Hashemites survived post-colonial upheavals to build for themselves the status of a dynasty whose successive members have ruled over a relatively recently created national territorial unit. If Jordan's monarchy, or indeed, very existence, retains a recent, manufactured feel, the country's middle-aged king survived the 2011 uprisings that rocked the Arab regions around him rather well.

In short, ruling monarchical dynasties throughout the world, including the Middle East and North Africa, have by and large lost their hold on most nations' political control. However, in a set of Arab countries, such dynasties gained new life in the post-colonial period and continue to govern after decades of national independence. What common sociopolitical institutions and themes have allowed Arab kingship to buck global trends?

Arab kingship and the politics of national legitimacy

When Arab North African and Middle Eastern countries achieved political independence as nation-states, in the aftermath of World War II, ruling monarchies seemed destined for the dustbin of political history. Indeed, ruling kings in Egypt, Iraq, Libya, Syria and Tunisia had all lost power by 1970. With the exception of Oman and Saudi Arabia, Arab Gulf states were small, depended on British power in their external relations, and were not even established in some cases until 1971. This suggests that their monarchical polities could be explained by small size, comparative political under-development, a major influx of oil funds, or all three.[13] Jordan's and Morocco's monarchies could have disappeared at a variety of moments, such as the two nearly successful military coups against former Moroccan king Hassan II in the early 1970s.[14]

If the continuing survival of Arab kings is a global outlier and contingent on a variety of specific events, dynastic incumbents nevertheless benefited from the general historical context discussed earlier, as well as some specific trends in post-colonial Arab political history, including the support they may have enjoyed by Western countries seeking stable allies during the Cold War period.

In response to all of this, these monarchies made conscious efforts to keep their political systems relevant. I discuss each of these in turn presently, focusing on a model of non-Islamist post-colonial Arab political model that lost much of its appeal by the 1970s, the related renewal of Islamic political legitimacy and the persistence of contemporary Arab kings to associate themselves with tradition and history to tap into broad registers of pre-colonial legitimacy.

The failure of post-colonial Nasserism

The final destruction of the Ottoman Empire by European forces in World War I, along with the construction of a new Turkish state based on ethnic nationalism, rather than pan-Islamic identity, at its core dealt a major blow to the ideal type of ethnically inclusive Muslim religious monarchy that had dominated the history of Islam in the Middle East. The destruction of the last candidate for a regional caliphate that had emerged after the Mongol conquest of the Abbasids led different peoples of the Middle East and North Africa to formulate alternative political formulas for governance, mostly centred around territorial nation-states with a looser official affiliation with Islam than the Ottomans and earlier models embraced. Such formulas were accelerated by the European colonial domination which divided the Arab region into more rigid political units than had mostly been true under the caliphate.

At the same time, the regionalism that had been central to the caliphal structure of Middle Eastern political history did not vanish; rather, it bubbled under the surface during colonial control and re-emerged in a different form with independence. The most influential political system to prosper in the heyday of post-colonial nationalism was Gamal Abd el-Nasser's military authoritarianism in Egypt from the mid-1950s until the late 1960s. Nasser explicitly rejected both an elected secular representative democracy and an Islamist traditionalist system grounded in a quasi-caliphal monarch.[15] Nonetheless, a key element of his widespread popularity throughout the Arab world was an explicit appeal to Arab regionalism that reflected earlier Middle Eastern political history, albeit in a form denuded of explicit religious underpinnings.

Nasser's political formula of appealing to Arab regionalism without its pre-colonial, pan-ethnic, Islamic monarchical accompaniments allowed him to dominate the region's politics like no other modern Arab leader.[16] It inspired his own and neighbouring citizens in its assertive autonomy for Arabs as a global political force no longer beholden either to historical Islamic empires or Western dominance. However, Nasser's legitimation formula also included serving as the political and military ringleader in popular Arab war efforts against Israel. The 1967 Arab-Israeli war, known in Arabic as the *naksa*, 'setback' or 'upheaval', represented so monumental a defeat for Egypt and its allies that Nasser's political star faded rapidly, along with the non-religious regionalism that he popularized.[17]

Nasser died in 1970. While Arab leaders that came after him, like Muammar Qaddafi of Libya and Saddam Hussein of Iraq, mimicked aspects of his pan-Arabism and confrontationalism, and secular politics continued to be important, the 1970s in the Middle East and North Africa marked the beginning of a renewed turn towards political Islam.[18] This exploded with the Iranian revolution of 1978 and the assassination of Egyptian president Anwar Sadat in 1981 by local Islamists.

Islamist politics as the post-1970s norm in the Middle East

The fact that the most popular Arab political system soon after independence rejected excessive identification with traditional Islamic history did not mean that Egyptian Muslims, or Muslim subjects of governments similar to Nasser's, discarded their religious identity. Rather, with the resounding failure of Nasser's Arab nationalism, a political cycle began in which many Arab Muslims considered, in some cases as an urgent priority, the importance of reframing political legitimacy in a manner more consistent with the pre-colonial past.

Yet, the traditional Arab-led caliphate had been dead for centuries, the failure of the non-Arab Ottoman version of the caliphate was comparatively fresh in historical memory and national boundaries were beginning to consolidate. Therefore, it was quite unclear what a legitimate, post-colonial political system that drew on Islamic identity and tradition would look like in practice. Indeed, for this reason, outside powers, including the United States, had funded and armed Arab Islamist political movements when it suited their interests, such as the struggle to end Soviet influence in Afghanistan in the 1980s. The presumed impracticality, even possibly archaic nature, of Islamist political activism made it seem comparatively unlikely as a long-term movement that could threaten global power dynamics.[19]

It remains true that Islamist political forces have not succeeded in creating a stable, novel governing template in the Arab world. Some systems, like Sudan's government, have largely been isolated from the rest of the world, while others, like that established in Egypt in 2012 by the Muslim Brotherhood and led by Mohamed Morsi, alienated much of the local population.[20] At the same time, given the impeccable legitimacy of Islam as a product of the Arab world, and the unpopular authoritarianism that has hobbled many Arab political systems for decades, it is not surprising that much, if by no means all, of the region's struggle for a more responsive or representative government has been framed in highly diverse Islamic ideology.

For the most part, contemporary Islamist politics in Arab countries remains a major unresolved issue. Morsi's elected Islamist president was overthrown in 2013 in a very popular military coup.[21] Other Arab state leaders have intervened to crush Islamist movements, or stop them from coming to power in the rare instances in which they were on the verge of an electoral victory, as in Algeria in 1992.[22] Islamist political actors are hardly the only forces in Arab countries. Yet, they have generally succeeded in attracting members through networks easily formed through mosques and other religious spaces, and have benefited from some Arab countries' refusal to allow anti-regime political parties.[23] As Islamic political movements have been driven from lawful participation in many Arab countries, some of their adherents have joined more violent organizations such as al-Qaeda. Thus, connecting the popularity of Islamic politics with Arab political systems that appear legitimate has remained an elusive challenge.

There is one major exception to this challenge, however. This is the remaining monarchies, who never abandoned appeals to Islam as part of their efforts at political legitimation.

Monarchies as reinvented quasi-Islamic fusions of tradition and modernity

Given the above overall trajectory of Arab political legitimation in the twentieth century, the continuing relevance of Islamic kingship is clear. These monarchical systems resonated sufficiently, if vaguely, with the ideal type of a ruler grounding his authority in the realization of Islamic values at the core of the historic caliphate. This grounding could address the major challenge of connecting the popularity of Islamic identity with Arab political orders.

Yet, there was nothing inevitable or automatic about Arab monarchies revitalizing their relevance in the contemporary post-colonial world. Arab kings have made major political efforts to stay in power, including the use of carrots and sticks, alongside unceasing work to shape and control the media narratives in their countries. While all leaders do this, central to these particular efforts has been monarchs' attempts to take advantage of the indeterminacy of what Islamic kingship might mean in a world of nation-states and the embers of a transnational ruling caliphate long extinguished.

A key for contemporary Arab kings in working to maintain their relevance has been a clear positioning of themselves as linked to 'tradition' to create a balance with post-caliphal, post-colonial modernity. Tradition is a fluid and contestable term, and can even be somewhat counter-factual with reference to a particular ruler. For example, the Jordanian monarchy is hardly traditional in the sense that it, like the country itself, is less than a century old. One method today's Muslim Arab kings use to link themselves to tradition is descent from the bloodline of the Prophet Muhammed, which establishes a credible link of hereditary nobility and a mild presumption of political legitimacy. This is how Jordan's Hashemite dynasty tried to overcome its inexperience with political rule.

The strategy has been used widely by other Arab kings. Dynastic lineage charts are common in media reports associated with major national days, and these charts can go back centuries, with purported links to the Prophet that are hard to verify. Morocco's state-owned newspapers, for example, routinely featured a family tree of the ruling Alaoui dynasty on the national holiday celebrating the monarchy.[24]

Whether they use the term 'emir', 'sheikh', or 'king', Arab kings deploy a wide range of particular political tactics to back up the broad claim that they harken back to tradition, with each political system using a different mix. The tactics include associating the ruler with Islamic rituals or as the guarantor of Islamic observance, incorporating neo-traditional political forms, like the *majlis*, into contemporary governance, encouraging the ruler to be seen as above or distinct from the government, and relying on familial status or other blood-based ties to cement bureaucratic control. These tactics are particularly or uniquely available to kings and are additional to legitimation tactics employed by rulers more generally, such as coercion or fear of coercion, and internationally oriented events that can help consolidate national identity, such as hosting major events or going to war. In short, in a part of the world with fairly limited direct popular democratic political accountability by leaders, monarchy retains value as a regime form because it allows for a wider variety of government tactics to legitimize rule.

The association of kings with their country's practice of Islam is a tool available to some, but not all, Arab monarchs. It has been most often deployed in Saudi Arabia. The reason for its use in Saudi Arabia is obvious; the country is home to Mecca and Medina, the two holiest cities of Islam. The Saudi ruler therefore is referred to as the 'guardian of the two sacred sites'.

Understandably, then, Saudi Arabia represents a strong case in which the monarchy is linked to the country's practice of Islam. Indeed, the country enforces a higher level of Islamic legal criminal punishments and restrictions against Quranic moral infractions such as alcohol consumption and adultery than any other Arab state. The king genuinely presides over a particular version of the enforcement of *shari'a*. Since the core duty of a Arab Islamic monarch is the execution of *shari'a*, the Saudi royal regime can claim to replicate this central traditional function of Islamic legitimation. Of course, connecting the monarchy strongly to the enforcement of actual *shari'a* also opens it up to critiques of being inconsistent or opportunistic about its loyalty to *shari'a*, or the ethical or moral performance of key members of the royal family.

Given this, and given that *shari'a* provisions are limited in their actual legal use in post-colonial Arab monarchies besides Saudi Arabia, other royal regimes in the region do not peg their Islamic credentials so strongly to the enforcement of law. The king of Morocco has used a different strategy to identify publicly with Islam; he has presided as a largely symbolic quasi-papal figure over the country's Islamic practice. For example, *'Id el-Adha* (the 'feast of sacrifice') is a central Muslim holiday when the head of each family kills and consumes a lamb in a commemorative re-enactment of the religious story of Ibrahim's/Abraham's near-sacrifice of his son.

In Morocco, the king, robed in white, sacrifices a lamb on this day on symbolic behalf of the nation. Similarly, during the holy month of Ramadan, the king symbolically presides over varied religious symposia and rituals, connecting himself with the observance of Islam on a national basis.[25] King Mohammed VI also has an annual ceremony in which he accepts the symbolic loyalty of his country's political elite, called the *bay'a*, which is a recreation of the traditional Islamic ceremony of political leadership investiture.[26]

In this last tactic, the Moroccan king overlaps with other Arab kings who have adapted Islamic historical political ceremonies or forms to their more contemporary political systems. Chief among these is the *majlis* in smaller Arab Gulf states. Monarchies with elected parliaments like Morocco, Jordan and Kuwait use the term *majlis* as part of the official Arabic title for the body, as the term can mean 'assembly'. Yet the Arabic root actually refers to 'sitting'; a *majlis* can mean a group of people who come together to discuss and decide important issues. Though informal, the *majlis* was a key quasi-deliberative body in pre-modern Islamic societies. In this sense, countries that do not have a strong, functioning parliament, like Qatar and the UAE, deploy the *majlis* as a kind of town meeting deliberative body with important traditional historical resonance, and with the idea that it keeps rulers accountable. Legislative and political initiatives are likely to be discussed in the context of a series of *majalis*, prior to actual promulgation. This helps account for the lack of actual, formal parliamentary legislation in the smaller Gulf Arab monarchies, where this sort of consultative process continues to have the possibility of reaching significant subgroups of the overall population in a quasi-representative way. In short, whether tied to a contemporary political form, or linked to a reinvigoration of a traditional one, a term like *majlis* carries historic reverberations that link to pre-modern Arab Islamic kingship.

Contemporary Muslim Arab kings enjoy another political strategy that is not available to their non-royal non-elected Arab peers. As is true in constitutional monarchies in Europe where kings no longer actually rule, the monarch is meant to stand as a unifying political force that represents the entire nation and stands above political factions. The remaining ruling monarchies of the Arab Islamic world make use of this idea of being above the political fray to associate unpopular specific policies or bureaucrats with a government, rather than their overall rule. Given that these kings are in fact authoritarian rulers who direct most aspects of their countries' politics, the idea that these rulers are not part of actual political contestation and policy-making is a clear fiction. Yet, it can serve as an additional means to deflect unpopular sociopolitical outcomes as ephemeral and changeable.

Morocco and Jordan serve as the model here, not coincidentally because both countries have had elected governments and political parties for many decades. After constitutional reforms in 2011, the system functions through parliamentary elections in which diverse parties compete. The system is structurally similar to Western more democratic constitutional monarchies, except that, in these Arab cases, the monarchy retains much more power and controls significantly the initiation and final shaping of legislation. The winning party produces a prime minister, who then forms a cabinet, as in many Western democracies. The king appoints this prime minister. Moreover, the king can ask the prime minister or other ministers to resign in the case of a crisis.

Muhammed VI did this in the spring of 2017, when the prime minister who emerged in the 2016 elections proved unable to form a government. The politics around the formation of the cabinet that this new prime minister negotiated, on the one hand, allows for royal intervention, and, on the other, puts in place a governing coalition of diverse parties from which the king can claim distance.[27]

Jordan also has a sufficiently robust parliament for its king to deploy the strategy of placing himself above the government. However, political parties are generally less autonomous, with the major opposition party, an affiliate of the Muslim Brotherhood, refusing to take part in recent parliamentary elections. On the whole, the appearance of governmental autonomy from the king is weaker than in Morocco, although the same strategy is used. Yet, Jordanian politics also maintains a role for extended familial-geographical networks known as tribes. In a society in which non-ideological, blood-tie-grounded political units still matter, the dynastic king, whose authority connects to blood ties, may enjoy an advantage in maintaining his authority.

This applies as well to smaller Gulf Arab monarchies, with the partial exception of Kuwait, where parliaments are not well enough established for strong use of a royal strategy to appear above the fray and culpability of particular policies or politics. Indeed, the official legislative advisory bodies in Qatar and the UAE, as opposed to quasi-traditional ones like *majalis*, have not had new elections for over a decade.

Nonetheless, in addition to being at the top of a hierarchy where blood-based tribal ties continue to matter, the kings of oil-rich states make use of a related strategy that helps them maintain their rule. This is the large size of the royal family itself. By maintaining a ruling elite within an extended royal family, both continuity and a level of bureaucratic loyalty can be enhanced.[28] Members of the extended royal family may disagree or even oppose one another's influence, internally, but share a larger interest in pursuing policies and inter-tribal politics that enhance the royal family's overall influence. Particularly in Gulf Arab societies with relatively small citizen populations, the extended royal family can be important as a core of bureaucratic control and outreach to other family-based tribal organizations. At the same time, the recent restructuring of power in the Saudi royal family suggests that Arab monarchy allows for flexible political reshuffling and a linkage of modern bureaucracy and particular political office, such as control of the armed forces, with assigning and reconfiguring royal succession and other central elements of power.

To summarize, Arab countries' historical legacy of Islamic monarchy, and the comparative failure of elected, responsive political systems to flourish and move away from secularism, have combined to provide monarchies with the potential for additional resources to stabilize their rule that are less available to other non-democratic regime types. Thus, particular historical trajectories of Arab societies and an appreciation for how these trajectories present strategies of possible utility for regime endurance make sense of the survival of contemporary Muslim Arab kings. There is no reason to assume either that monarchies in these countries are inevitable, that they are grounded in an immutable or amorphous aspect of culture or that they are maintained solely by harsh repression, or, in the particular case of oil states, money alone.

In short, I have described specific historical and political reasons that ruling monarchies exist today in the form of Arab kingship in the Middle East. But what do these political systems tell us about monarchy and politics today in a broader global context in which they appear rather antiquated or anomalous?

Arab Muslim kingship in a comparatively less royal world

Monarchies have been important historically because they have addressed a variety of challenges that are central to political stability. Among these are the problem of trust in political leadership and of succession. I discuss the issue of contemporary Arab monarchy in terms of each of these political challenges in turn.

Monarchies were so common prior to the age of modern nation-states because they offered a solution to the chaotic task of choosing a community's political leader. Someone's particular personal status, generally manifested by family origin, was established, often by force, and later legitimized, to create a privilege or right to rule. Monarchies fit well within the concept of traditional legitimacy, one of the categories of Max Weber's classic sociological argument about the main sources of legitimation.[29]

Moreover, monarchs also conceivably satisfy the criteria of Weber's other two sources of legitimacy. These are charismatic leadership, which is difficult to determine precisely but include specific personal qualities that attract popular loyalty, and legal-rational legitimacy, which entails dependable procedures and rules that citizens appreciate.[30] Starting from the privileged position they occupy with respect to traditional legitimacy, monarchies have an interest in playing up the possible charisma of their incumbent to the extent this is feasible, and in appearing to follow fixed rules and procedures.[31] In this context it is helpful to recall that traditional Muslim leaders in particular derive their right to rule from their commitment to enforcing Islamic law, *shari'a.*

If the prevalence of monarchical rule has a logic in the context of the idea of traditional legitimacy, one key shorthand aspect of the transformation that the modern nation-state era represents is a shift towards rational-legal legitimacy. In this regard, the legitimation of political authority through rules and procedures need not, but does tend to favour, the regularization of determining leaders through meaningful and broad citizen input, in other words, electoral democracy. Combined with the spread of European and other industrial states' Enlightenment values of anti-aristocratic equality and civil rights, electoral mechanisms for establishing political authority replaced dynastic heredity as the basis of a right to rule in most contemporary political systems.

However, the post-colonial states of the Arab world have faced a two-fold obstacle around such electoral mechanisms for authority, one concrete and the other symbolic. The concrete obstacle is the generally poor record of Arab political systems of allowing elections in which political leadership is actually contested. To the extent that looking at such Arab countries in tandem is logical, they have generally been ruled in recent decades by non-democratic governments. Only Lebanon, to a limited extent, and Tunisia, since the 2011 uprisings, have a track record of enfranchising citizens to choose their actual leaders. Thus, a lack of general experience with elected governments provides little concrete regional confirmation of the advantages to political legitimacy of such governments.[32]

Added to this is the symbolic issue of popular cultural experience with the specific experience of Western political ideals in the wake of colonialism. The Middle East region's pre-independence experience of the reality of European professions about democracy is that they were hypocritical. Without casting doubt on many Arabs' appreciation of aspects of elected governments and other democratic ideals in general, mistrust abounds of the particular dynamics of electoral mechanisms as they have existed in Europe and the developed broader Anglo-American industrial world. The combination of a post-colonial dearth of specific history of elected leaders, and the tarnish on political practices that are implicated symbolically in past colonial domination, do not imply any inevitable conflict between elected governments and Arab countries. These factors, taken together, do leave a somewhat more open space for continuing relevance for the well-trodden political historical path of political legitimation of monarchies in the Middle East and North Africa.

In addition to legitimacy, monarchies address a common political challenge of stable leadership succession. The stability and performance of electoral systems are disrupted routinely during elections and their inherent transition periods between leaders. In the United States, for example, campaigns for chief executive typically begin at least a year prior to a general election, and the transition period to when a new chief executive assumes office takes months. The cost of such disruption can be justified as a sign that democratic popular sovereignty, and the underlying legal-rational legitimacy that puts electoral rules above individual rulers, are both vibrant. For example, that Tunisia has managed several peaceful electoral transitions since the uprisings of 2011 that overthrew its former authoritarian leader, Zine ben Ali, is a sign that the country may be realizing democratization.[33]

But the disruption of leadership succession is nonetheless disorderly. And political disruption, or at least the fear of it, has been one of the concerns that non-elected governments in the Middle East have used to justify their political stewardship. In particular, in the aftermath of the chaos and violence that emerged in post-2011 uprisings countries like Libya, Syria and Yemen, fear of political disruption in Arab politics runs strong in the region and is subject to ready exploitation.

Monarchies can offer a salve for such fear. The presumptions that leadership will remain in the royal family, that the royal family has a right to lead, and that the current monarch has the political capacity and space to plan for a smooth succession, all may ameliorate the prospects for a lengthy and overly disruptive leadership transition process. With its legacy of occupation and resource exploitation from Europe, its geostrategic importance, and its high levels of militarization fuelled by both internal governments and external pressures, the Middle East may be comparatively receptive to political tools to reduce governing instability, such as those embedded in dynastic monarchy.

The political usefulness of some of the stabilizing tools of monarchy suggests a broader point about monarchies. The presumed global, general transition away from monarchical systems may be overstated. Monarchies persist today in two clear ways. First, many elected political systems retain hereditary monarchs that provide symbolic continuity and unity. Second, many non-monarchical systems exhibit quasi-dynastic political tendencies, perhaps to simulate the stabilizing features of actual monarchies.

On the first point, forty-three (or forty-four including the quasi-state of Vatican City) contemporary nations retain monarchies, or nearly 25 per cent of the countries of the world. This considerable number highlights the more substantial symbolically legitimizing and stabilizing prospects for a titular national figurehead who represents long-term political continuity. In the UK and other Commonwealth countries, appreciation for Queen Elizabeth II continues; some analysts appreciate the soft power and standing above daily contentious politics of the monarchy.[34] Similarly, the official site for the British monarchy states that the Queen plays a key political role as a 'focus for national identity, unity and pride',[35] which is exactly the symbolic work that ruling monarchs in the contemporary Arab Middle East undertake. In short, looking beneath the surface at constitutional non-ruling monarchies reveals their ongoing political significance.

Yet we can go further with respect to the relevance of monarchies, in that many non-monarchical systems seem to exhibit quasi-dynastic tendencies in their political leadership. The current prime minister of Canada, Justin Trudeau, is the son of a former Canadian head-of-state. Presidential politics in the United States has been marked in the past thirty years by the predominance of two families, the Bushes and the Clintons. The present occupant of the White House has installed his son-in-law and daughter in central positions of power, very much in the way that ruling monarchies have done.

Outside of Arab monarchies, a similar pattern has existed, although it was disrupted by the 2011 popular uprisings. Egypt, Libya and Syria resembled monarchies in the way that their pre-2011 leaders were groomed for their roles, or in the Syrian case where political authority was passed on from a long-ruling father to a son. In important Arab and non-Arab countries alike, non-monarchies often reveal a hint of political familial rule that is one of the signal features of hereditary dynastic rule.

The broader lesson here is that distinctions among political systems, though important, may be less clear-cut than their names or basic descriptions imply. Rather than monarchy and democracy being separable through an obvious bright line, important functions and features of different political systems may well be shared. In particular, diverse political systems have to include features that boost accountability and legitimacy, along with features that enhance order and stability. This underlying logic is familiar to political philosophers and formed an important underpinning for the US Constitution framers' justification of the separation of powers system that juxtaposed a representative electoral government and entrenched forces of order, while eschewing explicit monarchy.[36]

How diverse political systems balance features of accountability and stability vary, show different trends over time and take different precise regime forms across countries and regions. That overt ruling monarchies have declined as an explicit form of government generally does not mean that the problems of legitimacy and order that they have addressed historically have gotten easier.

In the end, ruling monarchical dynasties continue to function in Arab Middle Eastern countries for a basic reason. They provide some comparatively consensual tools for political stability in a region that has mostly known it in recent decades through especially coercive local leaders that have been enabled through global complicity. Though 'old-fashioned', monarchies in the region continue to allow for slightly less repression and overall acceptance in a global moment in which authoritarian and dynastic political tendencies are on the rise.

Notes

1 For example, Samuel Huntingdon, *Political Order in Changing Societies* (New Haven: Yale University Press, 1968).
2 For example, Wael B. Hallaq, *Shari'a: Theory, Practice, Transformations* (Oxford: Oxford University Press, 2009), 198.
3 See, generally, Eugene Rogan, *The Arabs: A History* (New York: Basic Books, 2009), 1–9.
4 For example, Hugh Kennedy, *Caliphate: The History of an Idea* (New York: Basic Books, 2016), 5–7.
5 See, generally, Hallaq, *Shari'a*, chapters 2–5, and Anthony Black, *The History of Islamic Political Thought*, second edition (Edinburgh: Edinburgh University Press, 2011), chapters 2, 7 and 16, *inter alia.*
6 For example, Kennedy, "Introduction," in *Caliphate.*
7 For example, Albert Hourani, *A History of the Arab Peoples* (Warner: New York, 1991), 20–21, 69–71.
8 Hourani, *History*, 69.
9 Wael B. Hallaq, *The Origins and Evolution of Islamic Law* (Oxford: Oxford University Press, 2005), 204–206.
10 Rogan, *Arabs*, 182, 192–195.
11 See, generally, Rosemary Said Zahlan, *The Making of the Modern Gulf States* (London: Unwin Hyman, 1989), chapters 1, 2.
12 For example, Hourani, *History*, 363–365.
13 Hazem Beblawi and Giocomo Luciani, eds., *The Rentier State* (London: Croom Helm, 1987).
14 See, generally, Susan Gilson Miller, *A History of Modern Morocco* (Cambridge: Cambridge University Press, 2013), chapter 6.
15 R. Stephen Humphreys, *Between Memory and Desire: The Middle East in a Troubled Age* (Berkeley: University of California Press, 1999), 63–70.
16 Rogan, *Arabs*, 288.
17 See, generally, Fouad Ajami, *The Arab Predicament: Arab Political Thought since 1967* (Cambridge: Cambridge University Press, 1981). It can certainly be argued that Arab regionalism remains an important political *leitmotif*, despite the major blows to its political credibility that 1967 represented.
18 Adeed Dawisha, *Arab Nationalism in the Twentieth Century: From Triumph to Despair* (Princeton: Princeton University Press, 2005), 276–281.
19 See Robert Dreyfuss, *Devil's Game: How the US Helped Unleash Fundamentalist Islam* (New York: Metropolitan, Henry Holt, 2005), 1–5.
20 Steven A. Cook, *False Dawn: Protest, Democracy, and Violence in the New Middle East* (Oxford: Oxford University Press, 2017), 110–112.
21 Cook, *False Dawn*, and Robert F. Worth, *A Rage for Order* (New York: Farrar, Straus and Giroux, 2016), 135–137.
22 Hugh Roberts, *The Battlefield: Algeria 1988–2002 – Studies in Broken Polity* (London: Verso, 2003).
23 See, generally, Carrie Rosefsky Wickham, *The Muslim Brotherhood: Evolution of an Islamist Movement* (Princeton: Princeton University Press, 2013).

24 See, for example, *Le Matin du Sahara et du Maghreb*, 30 July 1993, 1.
25 See, for example, *Le Matin* (online), "S.M. le Roi, Amir Al-Mouminine, accomplit la prière de l'Aïd Al-Fitr à la Mosquée Al-Mohammadi à Casablanca et reçoit les vœux en cette heureuse occasion," 26 June 2017, https://lematin.ma/express/2017/s-m-le-roi-amir-al-mouminine-accomplit-la-priere-de-laid-al-fitr-a-la-mosquee-al-mohammadi-et-recoit-les-voeux-en-cette-heureuse-occasion/274139.html (last accessed 30 November 2017).
26 See for example, "Morocco and Its King: Popular, but Prickly," *The Economist*, 27 August 2009, www.economist.com/node/14327617 (last accessed 30 November 2017).
27 See Al-Jazira, "Morocco's King Forms New Government," 5 April 2017, www.aljazeera.com/news/2017/04/morocco-king-names-coalition-government-170405185201695.html (last accessed 1 June 2017).
28 See, generally, Michael Herb, *All in the Family* (Albany: SUNY Press, 1999).
29 Traditional legitimacy for Weber and his successors denotes authority that is linked to historically accepted patterns and customs, which includes monarchies. See Weber, *The Theory of Social and Economic Organization*, ed. Talcott Parsons (New York: Free Press, 1964). For a longer summary discussion of political legitimacy relevant to this section of this chapter, see Peter Fabienne, "Political Legitimacy," *The Stanford Encyclopedia of Philosophy*, ed. Edward N. Zalta (summer 2017 edition), https://plato.stanford.edu/archives/sum2017/entries/legitimacy/ (last accessed 31 July 2017).
30 See Max Weber, *Weber's Rationalism and Modern Society*, trans. and eds. Tony and Dagmar Waters (New York: Palgrave Macmillan, 2015), 137–138.
31 One recent account of an Arab monarchy that suggests that this remains the case in Morocco is M. Daadaoui, *Moroccan Monarchy and the Islamist Challenge: Maintaining Makhzan Power* (New York: Palgrave Macmillan, 2011), 31.
32 Note that this in no way implies that citizens of Arab countries are anti-democratic. Public opinion polling in recent years suggests that democratic political systems have support and concerns about governmental accountability are common. See, for examples, M. Moaddel, "Values and Perceptions of the Islamic and Middle Eastern Publics," ed. Mansoor Moaddel (New York: Palgrave Macmillan, 2007), and M. Tessler, *Public Opinion in the Middle East: Survey Research and the Political Orientations of Ordinary Citizens* (Bloomington: Indiana University Press, 2011).
33 See, generally, Safwan M. Masri, *Tunisia: An Arab Anomaly* (New York: Columbia University Press, 2017).
34 See, for example, Emma Barnett, "Is the Queen the Most Powerful Woman in Britain," in *The Telegraph*, 12 February 2013, www.telegraph.co.uk/women/womens-life/9862997/Is-the-Queen-the-most-powerful-woman-in-Britain.html (last accessed 31 July 2017).
35 See www.royal.uk/role-monarchy (last accessed 31 July 2017).
36 Alexander Hamilton, James Madison and John Jay, *The Federalist with Letters of "Brutus"*, ed. Terence Ball (Cambridge, Cambridge University Press, 2003).

Key works

Black, Anthony, *The History of Islamic Political Thought*, second edition (Edinburgh: Edinburgh University Press, 2011).
Daadaoui, Mohammed, *Moroccan Monarchy and the Islamist Challenge: Maintaining Makhzan Power* (New York: Palgrave Macmillan, 2011).
Hallaq, Wael B., *Shari'a: Theory, Practice, Transformations* (Oxford: Oxford University Press, 2009).
Herb, Michael, *All in the Family* (Albany: SUNY Press, 1999).
Mednicoff, David, "The Politics of Sacred Paralysis: Constitutionalism in North Africa in the aftermath of 2011," in *Constitution-Writing, Religion and Democracy*, eds. Asli Bali and Hanna Lerner (Cambridge: Cambridge University Press, 2016).
Miller, Susan Gilson, *A History of Modern Morocco* (Cambridge: Cambridge University Press, 2013).

PART II

RITUAL AND REPRESENTATION

INTRODUCTION

Lucinda H.S. Dean

'To be accepted as a king, one had to behave like a king.'[1] Grant Simpson made this statement regarding Robert I (or the Bruce) of Scotland's request that his heart go on crusade after his death: a decision made, Simpson argues, so that in death he could carry out the kingly crusade of the 'great' medieval kings on which he arguably modelled himself.[2] After coming to the throne of Scotland in rather inauspicious circumstances in 1306 during the first Scottish wars of independence, Robert I's questionable legitimacy as ruler meant that he had a great deal to prove to be 'accepted as king'. Historians have increasingly come to recognize that the Bruce propaganda machine, named by others as such despite the anachronistic modern connotations, actively shaped and modelled the royal image and successfully represented the king's authority in a range of ways. This propaganda including a range of pious activities, demonstrations of military strength, architectural patronage, written rhetoric and rituals – such as his inauguration at Scone in 1306, the consecration of St Andrews Cathedral in 1318, the marriage of his son at Berwick in 1328 and his own funeral the following year – was all undertaken to meet expectations nationally and internationally.[3] Yet, presenting a royal image that conformed with and responded to contemporary expectation was not solely a concern for Robert I and his advisers or indeed for medieval rulers. As the chapters in this part demonstrate, it is one that resonates across history and one that has arguably become ever more necessary in a modern age with an increasingly mediatized and politicized public who have unprecedented access to royalty.

The royal wedding of Prince Harry and Meghan Markle, newly created duke and duchess of Sussex, prominent in the media at the time of writing, offers a prime modern example. It emphasizes the continuing prominence of royal ritual and representation, and the necessity to retain elements deemed traditional, balanced with the concurrent need to respond to expectations and the critical voices. Approximately 110,000 people gathered in Windsor on Saturday 19 May 2018, and BBC coverage predicted that 1.9–2 billion people would watch or listen to the coverage worldwide. Over 18 million British viewers tuned in live, viewing figures in the United States topped 29 million, and approximately 3.4 million tweets about the wedding were sent during the ceremony.[4] While the internet and social media might continue to bristle with criticism of the continuation of the British monarchy and the expense of royal ceremonies (and for the royal family itself) laden upon the taxpayer, nonetheless, millions of people were transfixed by this royal display. The couple exchanged vows in a ceremony replete with symbolism designed to send very public messages about the role of this specific royal couple. For example, a bridal veil embroidered with the floral emblems of all the nations of the Commonwealth to represent the focus of their charity work: a central facet to the claims of continued relevance and engagement with the people of Britain and beyond. Equally, there were various aspects highlighted as 'traditional' in the coverage by the press, such as the use of an open carriage procession accompanied by the mounted guard, which was a recognizable form of royal display for a contemporary audience that placed the royal couple in an open-air and accessible environment to be viewed by the attending public. This particular royal wedding – with a gospel choir singing *Stand By Me*, an animated American Episcopalian minister giving a sermon about the power of love, and a guest list that rejected all politicians – seemed a particularly personal one in which the cameras seemed almost intrusive at times. Yet, arguably, the 'personal' aspects of this ceremony were as much by design as any other components. Elements such as the gospel choir and the Episcopalian minister placed alongside more traditional elements made a statement about the blending of British and American, blurring the lines and embracing the bride's nationality and ethnic roots as well as the groom's. Moreover, the intimate nature of this public ceremony brought a level of humanized normality in response to expectations understood by a younger generation of royals ever aware of the necessity to remain relevant and relatable, and fill the role of celebrity par excellence.

In many respects, the role and function of monarchy, where it survives, for the twenty-first-century social media generation has changed significantly from its pre-modern roots. Moreover, the ritualized and representative means through which monarchy communicates to its variant publics has had to adapt and develop as the institution has risen, fallen and been resurrected. What was expected of Robert the Bruce, for example, might appear a far cry from what modern audiences expect from Harry and Meghan. Yet, similarities do emerge over time and place, as the following chapters consider. One of these is the enduring need to provide a show for the 'people' – albeit that the show, audience and content are variable. Ritual and representation of monarchy was and is not an 'empty display' nor a light-hearted sideshow to political action. During the cultural turn in history of the 1960s and 1970s, scholars, including Ralph Giesey, Roy Strong, David Bergeron and Sydney Anglo, focused attention on the importance of royal ritual and representation.[5] In the wake of these early studies, the real explosion of research into the role and function of ritual and representations of monarchy has taken place since the 1990s with interdisciplinarity at the heart of many of the projects that extend and enhance these earlier explorations.[6] A seminal contribution to research on the creation, maintenance and manipulation of the royal image is Peter Burke's *Fabrication of Louis XIV* (1992), the very title of which encapsulates the ideas within about the process of image making.[7] By titling it the 'fabrication' of Louis rather than the 'image' of Louis, Burke identifies that by the age of absolutism the image, representation and rituals of the monarchy were so central that they were almost one and the same as the person of the monarch.[8] Indeed, Woodacre's introduction to this volume exemplifies this core thesis of Burke's work, emphasizing the increasing recognition of ritual and representation as a fundamental element to the functioning of monarchy across the ages.[9]

Ritual and representation are shaped and formed, invented and reinvented by context, and can offer often still underestimated insights into the societies, polities and monarchies that developed them. Moreover, a fuller engagement with context offers the historian a firmer grasp of the meaning of ritual and display.[10] Scholars such as Jacques Le Goff, Paul Binski and Philippe Buc have long since cautioned against the over-reliance of historians and others on prescriptive texts, such as coronation *ordines* for example, due to the potential pitfalls of such instructional records for understanding a particular ritualized political moment without considering relevant context.[11] Representing authority, in any medium, also requires an audience with which to have a dialogue, and research has seen a refocusing of attention from the designers of ritual and representations to the audience and public response. Kevin Sharpe argues that this owes much to the history of the book and an increased interest in readers, history from below and its focus on the consumer, and works on the rise of the public sphere, such as the translation of Jürgen Habermas' *The Structural Transformation of the Public Sphere* (1989).[12] As challenges to monarchy have proliferated, and the publics with which monarchy has had to interact have become exponentially larger, more vocal and politically self-aware, the reasons for the invention and reinvention in the developments of ritual and representations of monarchy become more obvious to historians.[13] However, monarchy has always had to be fluid in its interpretation of tradition and adapt ritual and representations. Static representations and rituals were no more likely in the medieval era than in the twentieth century.

While there have been many advancements in this field, and a veritable trove of literature now exists, there is a continued propensity for studies of rituals and representations of monarchy to focus on one person, such as Burke's study of Louis XIV, or a particular court in a specific era, such as Sharpe's work on the Tudors and Stuarts. There are comparative studies within a European context, such as John Adamson's edited collection on the princely courts of early modern Europe or MacGlynn and Woodacre's collection on image and perception of medieval and early modern monarchy, and also in the edited collections of research societies exploring facets of representation. However, these too tend to be limited – for very practical reasons – by chronology or representational type.[14] By contrast, this part offers twelve new case studies that explore the intricacies of the constant process of reinvention, renewal and realignment of monarchy through a multitude of media and ritual forms across geographies and chronologies. To avoid adherence to strict chronological progression and geographical groupings, these chapters are arranged, as much as is possible, to reveal the fluidity and continuities through time and space. There are, of course, period-specific issues that occur in contributions researching concurrent time periods, like the issues of mediatization and national identity which arise in chapters in later time periods. Yet, a conscious decision was made to highlight the ongoing necessity – across time and place – for monarchy to adapt and change in response to context and publics, and to identify continuities that span all imposed boundaries. Here, ritual and representation are interlocked and organically connected. Many chapters in this part touch on both, but the chapters are arranged with those centred on ritualized action and behaviour first, before moving to those focusing more on representation: from religious and pious ritual, via rituals of national identity, travel and diplomacy, perceptions of monarchy, use of rhetoric, the treatment of royal bodies, to the material representations of monarchy.

Conformity to a set of contemporary expectations is often a measure of the relative 'success' of a monarch as a ruler or political figure. In medieval Europe, monarchs were judged on their ritualized pious devotion, martial prowess and political ability, and monarchs had to strike a visible balance of all three. As such, the personal religious devotions of monarchs of this era were almost invariably tied to very public manifestations of private religiosity as monarchs sought to achieve their public persona. Paul Webster admits that to untangle the private and the public in this case is near impossible, particularly with little record of the personal thoughts of monarchs on this topic. He addresses, therefore, the manner in which anointed medieval monarchs publicly expressed their expected private religiosity. His chapter uses a case study of the pre-Reformation English monarchy set against the wider European context. This exploration includes almsgiving and charity offered to the poor; the commissioning, owning and gifting of the material expressions of piety, from chaplains' fine vestments to devotional objects and texts to religious foundations of grand proportions; demonstrations of orthodoxy through pilgrimage, crusades and stands against heresy; and royal ritual preparations for death. All these methods of displaying personal piety link to the salvation of the soul undertaken across medieval society in Europe in a variety of ways. As such, the upscaled public efforts of monarchs reflected contemporary expectations of the pious virtue of divinely anointed monarchs through ritualized actions, symbols and charity.

Public demonstrations of pious virtue were not only reserved for medieval kings in Europe. David M. Malitz's study of the monarchies of Meiji Japan (1868–1912) and post-war Thailand (1946–73) illustrates that – among other things – demonstrations of virtue and piety, including spending time as a Buddhist monk (for Thai monarchs) and royal progresses centred on ritual shrines, retained importance amid the rich performative palettes of monarchy in modern south-east Asia and Japan. Woodacre's introduction to this volume raises pertinent debates about the increasing challenges faced by post-revolutionary era European monarchs, whose connections with the divine were undermined through a process of desacralization. Yet, in Japan and Thailand, the virtue and divinity of the monarchy remained , and, ultimately, this became tightly bound with national authenticity.[15] Moreover, these Asian monarchs complemented traditional 'religious' ritual actions with more modern concepts, such as granting of religious freedom and the charitable support of worthy causes to reflect changing contexts, as emphasized through symbolism and guest choices at the wedding of Harry and Meghan at Windsor in May 2018. Malitz's two case studies demonstrate the unique potential of a performative monarchy in the process of nation-building and constructing national identity in regions of marked cultural diversity. Though not focusing on concurrent chronological periods, both offer comparative periods of monarchical development during a time of rapid modernization for these two respective nations. The monarchies of both nations suffered periods of obscurity due to political circumstance, which Malitz explores before analysing how the respective countries managed their monarchy's return to prominence by drawing on western European rituals and long-term national traditions rooted in the performative nature of monarchy. Malitz's research reveals monarchy as a ritual institution capable of both reconciling traditions with modernity and negotiating between the local and the international as well as how the symbolism and rituals of monarchy became a critical feature of these royal nation states.

Christoph De Spiegeleer demonstrates the importance of ritual display, royal symbolism and the performance of monarchy, which are similarly identifiable in the newly created monarchical polities seeking to consolidate national identity in the aftermath of the revolutionary era in later nineteenth-century Europe. His contribution looks at the funerals of the first monarchs of the newly founded kingdom of Belgium, Leopold I (d.1865), and the near contemporaneous unified countries of Germany and Italy: Wilhelm I (d.1888) and Vittorio Emanuel II (d.1878), respectively. The ritual performances that took place, and the manner in which they were recorded in the rapidly proliferating newspaper medium, were vital to the perceived and actual stability of the respective realms. As with the diverse cultural, religious and ethnic groups drawn together under the monarchies of Japan and Thailand, these new European nations were rife with potential conflict and contradictions. The development of these displays, drawing on past and present, offered opportunities to capitalize on re-engagement with the ceremonial splendour of pre-revolutionary times in uniting these newly formed countries around the monarch. The mediatization of these rituals and representations of monarchy witnessed in these case studies characterize the amplification of royal ceremonial through modern media as introduced by Woodacre.[16] Although far from the accessibility offered by digital media, the era of the illustrated newspaper introduced a widely accessible form of media communication offering the opportunity to enhance national solidarity and loyalty through shared experience. However, De Spiegeleer identifies that the use of display and the proliferation of media engagement also carried the potential risk of the widening of social divisions where the monarch polarized groups and opinion.

The themes of mediatization and national identity are also prominent in Trond Isaksen's chapter exploring nineteenth-century coronations in Scandinavia. As Woodacre notes, coronations were a key ceremonial moment defining monarchy in many cases, but the undertaking of the ritual was never universal or uniform across Europe even in pre-modern times.[17] By the nineteenth century, many Europeans considered the sacral nature of kingship as an outdated concept and increasingly vocal opposition criticized the ceremonial rituals of coronation, centred on the crowning and anointing which represented such concepts in a tangible form, likening them to medieval superstitions of a pre-Enlightened age. Indeed, none of the newly created countries in De Spiegeleer's case study held coronations for their monarchs.[18] The amplified challenges to the divine or religious cornerstone to monarchy are starkly apparent in such instances. Nonetheless, the coronation rituals were not universally disregarded, and a number of European kingdoms retained, restored and even introduced such ceremonies throughout the nineteenth century and beyond.[19] Isaksen's chapter explores the differing opinions on, and the reception of, the continuing coronation ceremonies in the then unified realms of Norway and Sweden from 1814 to 1905 and beyond. Drawing on a rich array of official, personal and newspaper records, this contribution argues that even in a climate of growing criticism of coronation and anointing ceremonies in Scandinavia, the significance of the ceremony endured in Norway for significantly longer and was even written into the Norwegian constitution composed at the start of the union with Sweden. The fact that the ceremony faced heavy criticism after the collapse of the union, despite its continuation in a pared back format, raises interesting questions about what the coronation offered Norway in the specific context of this union in contrast to its independent national identity.

Negotiations of national identity and the relative positions of strength between polities as demonstrated through ritual were, of course, not an issue confined to the nineteenth century. Such negotiations were front and centre in diplomatic interactions occurring long before the development of nation states as we recognize them today. Eugénia Rodrigues' chapter explores the dynamics of early modern diplomacy in the first globalization, or the first global age, c.1450–1800.[20] Such negotiations are central in this case study of the ritual interaction between Munhumutapa in Eastern Africa and Portugal, which considers three core aspects of diplomacy – ceremonial and ritual protocol, cross-cultural exchange and gift-exchange practices, and modes of legitimizing treaties – with the added complexity of intercontinental relations. Drawing examples from these interactions across the sixteenth to the eighteenth centuries, this contribution explores how different cultures negotiated ritual interactions to accommodate each other for mutual gain and to underscore the relative sovereignty of each diplomatic partner. Rodrigues' research demonstrates that ritual and representation, particularly through material and oral culture, were as central to the Karanga people of Munhumutapa and their sovereign as they were to any European royal court. For both parties, engaging with an unfamiliar ritual language meant that the potential for misinterpretation was high risk as some of the examples in this study amply demonstrate. Nonetheless, even with the presence of these challenges, rituals of diplomacy in this context offered a vital tool for the negotiation to achieve their respective goals and retain their sovereign identity. Even during Portuguese hegemony in the seventeenth century, and despite developing tastes for Portuguese-supplied luxury status symbols – such as textiles and clothing styles, silks, carpets, imported beads from India – the Karanga sovereign (the *mutapa*) did not fully forego traditional modes of display. As such, a level of adaptability and fluidity of ritual action and representations of sovereignty allowed envoys of both monarchies to navigate this diplomatic minefield.

In this example of diplomatic interaction, ambassadorial envoys represented the authority and status of the Portuguese crown. By way of contrast, Philippa Woodcock's chapter explores the manner in which monarchs themselves used royal travel beyond their realm to represent power and shape, particularly domestic, identity in the sixteenth century. There are plenty of modern examples revealing that monarchs travel for such purposes, including the international and domestic , travels of the twentieth-century Thai and Japanese monarchies discussed by Malitz. Woodcock's chapter on royal travel in sixteenth-century France demonstrates the continuing importance of monarchs' movements beyond their realms in the century before the French monarchy fixed itself within Versailles and its surrounds. This later centralization was designed to demand that nobles and others seeking royal favour came to the king in his space, but Woodcock's examples demonstrate how royal travel offered a similar occasion for controlling noble movement and eliciting favour through proximity. Using the case studies of Louis XII (r.1498–1512) and Henri III (as king of Poland-Lithuania, r.1573–75; as king of France, r.1574–89),

Woodcock's chapter offers a comparison between two quite different monarchs' use and purpose of travel beyond their kingdoms with a particular focus on its importance to the exercise of domestic authority. Three key areas of travel form the focus of the discussion: entourage and anonymity, transport, and the speed and difficulty of travel. Through examples across each of these areas, Woodcock underscores the multifaceted value of travel as a ritual activity utilized by early modern monarchs to shape perceptions of power and represent different aspects of royal authority during this period.

Perceptions of dynastic stability and royal power were a central concern of early modern monarchies across Europe and, as highlighted in Woodacre's introduction, gender 'suffuses everything' even if it has not always been recognized as so doing.[21] Scholars – such as Mark Ormrod, Christopher Fletcher, Katherine J. Lewis and Emma Levitt – have been instrumental in the growing body of research emerging around the role that contemporary understanding and expression of masculinity play in furthering perceptions of kingship.[22] The manner in which masculine models were used and reused in the later medieval and early modern eras form the core of the two chapters by Hélder Carvalhal and Estelle Paranque. Building on previous work in this area, Carvalhal looks at masculinity and monarchy through a case study of the late fifteenth- to sixteenth-century Avis dynasty in Portugal.[23] His study offers an introduction to and exploration of the hegemonic masculinity model, first proposed by Connell in a much more modern context, to explore how such concepts might be transposed onto an earlier era.[24] Carvalhal includes a valuable initial investigation into the role of subaltern non-dominant forms of masculinity – an underexplored aspect of Connell's theory in an early modern context – by focusing on the role of Moorish representations and material culture as well as the use of the concept of the 'savage' in Portugal and beyond. Carvalhal identifies evidence of cross-cultural exchange in the use of certain subaltern masculine tropes and highlights interesting avenues for further comparative research. His study also provides an analysis of the extent to which contemporary rhetoric and theory around manhood and masculinity were realized in practice by considering the developments in European didactic literature and 'mirrors for princes', with a focus on Portuguese works, and then analysing the physical manifestations of the masculine display in which the Avis dynasty took part. These included ritual performances – such as jousts, tournaments, bullfights and hunting – and action in battles, usually in the manner of crusades against the infidel in Iberia or beyond. Carvalhal demonstrates that, while rhetorical expectations of masculinity were moving away from the typical 'medieval' chivalric knight to the polite (even effeminate) courtier, the practice of monarchical masculine display in sixteenth-century Portugal still rotated around the more physical manifestations of masculine prowess. In this case, actions perhaps spoke louder than words.

In contrast, by analysing the speeches and writings of monarchs, and those directly communicating with or addressing other rulers, Paranque's chapter looks at two models of kingship, both of which are central to manhood: that of the father and the warrior. Drawing on examples from England, Spain and France across the sixteenth and seventeenth centuries, Paranque illustrates how such rhetorical tropes were used as representational tools to shape and mould the royal image across Europe in the early modern era. This work adds to Carvalhal's argument that further comparative work of the means by which cultural exchange was linked to masculine models is needed. Paranque's core case studies identify two monarchs for whom representation of typical 'kingly' or 'manly' attributes is not without challenge: Elizabeth I using the trope of the father, and Henri III using that of the warrior. For Elizabeth, as a regnant queen, there were numerous challenges to gender norms, and Paranque builds here on arguments made by Anna Whitelock and in her own work elsewhere on Elizabeth as a warrior.[25] Similarly, however, Henri III's reputation for male favourites – as noted by Carvalhal – also placed him in a potentially challenging position in terms of gender norms and expectations regarding the manly activities that composed the warrior type. Paranque's chapter demonstrates how valuable the traditional masculine tropes of 'the father' and 'the warrior' were for these monarchs' expressions of kingship, and how their manipulation by those less naturally labelled as 'father' or 'warrior' further emphasizes the necessity for monarchs to colour within expected lines, even if those lines were malleable and fluid in nature.

Representations of the king as both a father and a warrior have strong religious connotations, and Paranque notes the additional challenge for monarchs seeking to be fathers to their people, in a religious sense, during the complexities of post-Reformation divisions. Prior to the Reformation, a monarch could take part in many pious ritual activities, as explored in the opening chapter to this part by Webster. In addition to such activities, calling on saintly ancestors and the concept of *beata stirps* (holy stock or roots) was also a method used to represent the divinity and sacred nature of monarchs. Anna Duch considers late medieval European monarchical representations and the role of sainthood by offering a reassessment of English efforts to have further royal saints recognized by the papacy between the thirteenth and early sixteenth centuries. While France saw the canonization of Louis IX through the efforts of Philip IV in 1297, English royal saints were in short supply after Edward the Confessor. Reasons for the English failure to secure royal saints after Edward the Confessor usually rest with internal political crises in England and French dominance over the papacy, but Duch argues that a far wider range of issues and challenges faced the English efforts to increase their host of royal saints. Through a broad survey of European canonizations in the late medieval period, Duch's chapter demonstrates that the canonization of Louis IX was actually the anomaly by the late thirteenth century rather than England's failure to promote or produce strong saintly candidates. An examination of the attempts to canonize Henry III (d.1272), Edward II (d.1327) and Henry VI (d.1471) reveals the challenges their causes faced and uncovers notable variations in culture and tradition between England and the continent. These issues included English preference for keeping the royal body intact in death (except for removing internal organs) and the proliferation of political opposition saints who challenged royal authority (such as Thomas Beckett or Thomas of Lancaster). Moreover, the English monarchies own approach was different, with a notable lack of effort to seek canonization of female relatives and an engagement with saintly ancestors as political exemplars rather than religious ones. By offering new insights into English royal sainthood through the wider lens of European canonization, Duch indicates the variety of traditions, personalities and forces acting upon monarchical representation in the medieval era. Although Webster argues rightly against a penchant for English exceptionalism during this period, Duch's chapter identifies that one shoe certainly did not necessarily comfortably fit all in the sacral and sacred representations of monarchy.

In closing, Duch notes that despite all the medieval efforts to acquire saintly status for various medieval English monarchs in death, the only other English king to be identified as a 'blessed' saint and martyr was the Protestant monarch Charles I in the English Book of Common Prayer. Conversely, the execution of Charles I in 1649 was, as Catriona Murray suggests, an act that stripped the royal body of sacred powers and mystique. Ideas regarding the divine right of kings, espoused by James VI of Scotland and I of England (Charles's father and predecessor), and an increasing European move towards absolute kingship, demonstrate that early modern monarchs sought the elevation of the sacred and divine royal body to match or exceed the mystical qualities of their saintly medieval forebears. Yet, they lived in an era wherein the royal body was a contested icon while also increasingly accessible to the public. Through research into the use of monumental sculpture in public spaces in Stuart England, Murray addresses the neglected origins of the use of public monuments for the representation of royal authority in the early modern British Isles and the role these monuments played in the development of new forms of political communications between the public and the monarch. Murray's chapter considers the shift from the sacred recumbent tomb – reclaimed for use for political reasons by James VI & I at the start of his English reign – to upright secular monuments, placed in civic and institutional public spaces, during the reigns of Charles I and his successors to represent Stuart authority. Murray develops this analysis by exploring the public's reactions, or 'monumental interventions', to these recreations of royal bodies. Whether inspiring awe or inciting anger, the introduction of these royal bodies to public spaces in England ultimately provided a unique stage for a new kind of political dialogue between the ruler and the ruled.

The changing relationship between the ruler and the ruled that comes to the fore in Murray's work emerges elsewhere in this part, particularly with Malitz, De Spiegeleer and Isaksen's considerations of the nineteenth century and earlier in Rodrigues' chapter, continuing through to the final two chapters in this part. Mikolaj Getka-Kenig's contribution considers the political role of architectural representations of monarchical authority in post-French-Revolution continental Europe. The newly restored or created monarchies that form the basis of this study had to manage an ambiguous legacy of pre-revolutionary palaces, representative of former absolute monarchs, as tools to represent their own mediated superiority in an era marked by an increasingly self-aware political community. With examples radiating out in chronology and geographic location from Paris and the revival of the monarchical regime of Napoleon Bonaparte in 1804, to select case studies from the French satellite monarchies and then a wider survey of the post-1814–15 period, this chapter explores how new monarchs manipulated this ambiguous legacy for their new publics in post-revolutionary Europe. For example, Getka-Kenig shows how the neutrality of neoclassicism replaced the eccentricities of the Baroque and the excesses of absolutism – returning to Renaissance principles and an appreciation of the monumentality of ancient Rome and Greece. Perhaps the most notable pattern across the architectural projects analysed in this chapter, however, is the increasing democratization of access to royal palaces and architectural complexes. Monarchs demonstrated this through their return to capital cities from sites such as

Versailles,[26] by the combining of royal palaces with public and military spaces, the rearrangements of public squares around urban palaces, the use of former palaces as museums and galleries, and the creation of publicly accessible parks and gardens. As such, these royal palatial spaces were able to marry traditional aspects of majesty with key legacies of the revolution by adapting royal architectural representations to new social circumstances.

The final chapter shares a focus on the responses of monarchy to societal change through visual representations, but through a very different aspect of royal representation: dress. By taking a *long durée* approach from medieval to modern, Benjamin Wild considers how monarchical representation reflects long-term shifts and continuities to the status and role of monarchy, and demonstrates how the clothing of royal bodies can be a barometer for interpreting monarchy and its ability to respond to various publics and contexts. Wild argues that the period from 1640 to 1840 saw the most notable changes in monarchical fashions. The latter decades of this period coincide with the period discussed by Getka-Kenig in his considerations of architecture. The fact that marked changes to monarchical representation were made in both these forms of material culture during and after a time when monarchy was challenged, and even deposed and abolished, is perhaps not surprising. However, the similarities here underscore the importance of placing such changes into their historical context. Wild's analysis of the sartorial representations of monarchs in Europe and beyond, with a particular interest in Britain, demonstrate how shifts in politics, religion, society, technology, business and trade had an increasing impact on the monarchy, where it survived. By bringing the assessment up to the twenty-first century, Wild's contribution also helps in understanding how postwar monarchies (predominantly that of Britain) have responded increasingly to public expectations that they reflect their continued purpose and ongoing relevance. Overt statements about rulership, authority and majesty witnessed at various stages in the previous centuries, particularly where real or imagined power was threatened, have long since been deemed unnecessary by monarchies that have accepted their constitutional role. The clothing of modern monarchs – as with many pre-modern monarchies before them – must often strike the difficult balance between expected regality and overt excess to reflect the reasons that the monarchies retain their value to a substantial proportion of their respective citizens, as emphasized in the arguments of Deploige, Deneckere and Quigley raised in Woodacre's introduction.[27]

Wild's chapter brings this introduction, and the section itself, full circle to the opening comments about the ways in which Robert the Bruce presented himself in a manner that allowed him to be 'accepted as king'. Ultimately, this necessity has not really changed over time or geographical region, but the expectations of what must be done 'to be accepted as monarch', and the identity of those who can voice them publicly, has rarely stood still. The use of the Commonwealth floral symbols on Megan Markle's veil in 2018 certainly had origins in the use of similar symbols of Commonwealth, and before that Empire, on twentieth-century coronation robes during a time when the monarchy was renegotiating its role both nationally and internationally.[28] Yet, here the royal couple claimed no sovereignty over these peoples, instead illuminating one of their primary purposes in this time and place: reflecting their role as royal figures who will focus their energies on supporting charities within that Commonwealth to support its citizens. Across time and place, the status and authority of monarchy, both real and imagined, has never been fixed but rather constantly shifting. Thus, the rituals and representations of monarchy, too, have to be flexible – if often underpinned by notable continuities and constancies – and need to be analysed against the relevant historical context so that common symbols are not misunderstood. By considering a multitude of forms of ritual and representation, this part explores the ways in which mechanisms of monarchy were, and still are, made manifest across chronologies and geographies. From the pious ritual of the medieval monarch in a society dominated by deep-rooted religious beliefs, through to the early modern monarchs expressing contemporary understandings of masculine ideals (even where these are contradictory in changing times), to the careful fashion choices of modern monarchies walking the blurred lines between relevance and obscurity, or reverence and censure, the chapters in this part engage with and extend the ongoing explorations of how this enduring institution has used ritual and representation. In so doing, it demonstrates that, in many respects, monarchs have always been subject to contemporary opinion and expectation, even if their publics have gained manifold means to critique, challenge and undermine them over time.

Notes

1 Grant G. Simpson, "The Heart of King Robert I: Pious Crusade or Marketing Gambit?" in *Church, Chronicle and Learning in Medieval and Early Renaissance Scotland: Essays presented to Donald Watt on the Occasion of the Completion of the Publication of Bower's Scotichronicon*, ed. Barbara E. Crawford (Edinburgh: Mercat Press, 1999), 181.

2 Ibid., 172–186.

3 For various discussions on the Bruce propaganda machine, see: ibid; Fiona Watson, "The Enigmatic Lion: Scotland, Kingship and National Identity in the Wars of Independence," in *Image and Identity: the Making and Re-Making of Scotland Through the Ages*, eds. Dauvit Broun, R.J. Finlay and Michael Lynch (Edinburgh: John Donald, 1999), 18–37; Roland Tanner, "Cowing the Community? Coercion and Falsification in Robert Bruce's Parliaments," in *Parliaments and Politics in Scotland, Vol. I: 1235–1560*, eds. Keith Brown and Roland Tanner (Edinburgh: Edinburgh University Press, 2004), 50–73; Michael Penman, *Robert the Bruce: King of the Scots* (New Haven: Yale University Press, 2014); Lucinda Dean, "Projecting Dynastic Majesty: State Ceremony in the Reign of Robert the Bruce," *International Review of Scottish Studies*, 40 (September 2015): 34–60; and Michael Penman, "*Who is this King of Glory?* Robert I and the Consecration of St Andrews Cathedral, 5 July 1318," in *Medieval and Early Modern Representations of Authority in Scotland and the British Isles*, eds. Katherine Buchanan and Lucinda H.S. Dean, with Michael Penman (Abingdon: Routledge, 2016), 85–104.

4 BBC, "Royal Wedding Live Coverage," 19 May 2018; Jim Waterstone, "Royal Wedding Confirmed as Year's Biggest UK TV Event," *The Guardian*, 20 May 2018, www.theguardian.com/uk-news/2018/may/20/royal-wedding-confirmed-as-years-biggest-uk-tv-event (accessed 7 June 2018); "Over 29 Million Viewers Watch Prince Harry and Meghan Markle's Royal Wedding," *Nielsen Company*, 20 May 2018, www.nielsen.com/us/en/insights/news/2018/over-29-million-viewers-watch-prince-harry-and-meghan-markles-wedding.html (accessed 7 June 2018). Though not the first televised, Seidler argues that the wedding of Prince Charles and Princess Diana was perhaps the first arranged with a full focus on global audiences in 'a rebranding of Britain in a post-imperial age where monarchy was to affirm its importance in "selling Britain" to a global tourist market'. See Victor J. Seidler, *Remembering Diana: Cultural Memory and the Reinvention of Authority* (Houndmills: Palgrave Macmillan, 2013), 31–32.

5 Ralph Giesey, *The Royal Funeral Ceremony in Renaissance France* (Geneva: Librairie a Droz, 1960); Roy Strong, *The English Icon: Elizabethan & Jacobean Portraiture* (London: Routledge

and Kegan, 1969); Roy Strong, *Art and Power, Renaissance Festivals 1450–1650* (Woodbridge: Boydell, 1984); David M. Bergeron, *English Civic Pageantry, 1558–1642* (London: Edward Arnold, 1971); and Sydney Anglo, *Spectacle, Pageantry and Early Tudor Policy* (Oxford: Oxford University Press, 1969).

6 The bibliography of works that considers this area is now too vast and varied to do justice to in an endnote, even just for Europe alone. Notable projects that have developed include the *European Festival Research Project*, with publications such as: J.R. Mulryne, Maria Ines Aliverti and Anna Maria Testaverde, eds., *Ceremonial Entries in Early Modern Europe: The Iconography of Power* (Farnham: Ashgate, 2015); Ronnie Mulryne, Helen Watanabe-O'Kelly and Margaret Shewring eds., *Europa Triumphans: Court and Civic Festivals in Early Modern Europe* (Aldershot and Burlington VT: Ashgate, 2004). The *Palatium Project* on early modern court residences, with publications including the PALATINUM e-publications (now four volumes: www.courtresidences.eu/index.php/publications/e-Publications/); and most recent edited collection, J.R. Mulryne, Krista De Jonge, Pieter Martins and Richard L.M. Morris, eds., *Architectures of Festival in Early Modern Europe: Fashioning and Re-fashioning Urban and Courtly Space* (Abingdon: Routledge, 2017). The Royal Studies Network, its publications and its journal, *Royal Studies Journal,* have also provided an environment for such discussions to grow in a manner that attempts to break down barriers of chronology and geography.

7 For a clear example of the influence of Burke's work, see Kevin Sharpe, *Selling the Tudor Monarchy: Authority and Image in Sixteenth-Century England* (New Haven: Yale University Press, 2009), *passim,* but particularly 1–57.

8 For a discussion of the title choice, see Peter Burke, *Fabrication of Louis XIV* (New Haven: Yale University Press, 1992), 10–11.

9 Elena Woodacre, "Understanding the Mechanisms of Monarchy," 2–3, 8–10 in this volume.

10 David Cannadine, "The Context, Performance and Meaning of Ritual: The British Monarchy and the 'Invention of Tradition', c. 1820–1977," in *The Invention of Tradition,* eds. Eric Hobsbawm and Terence Ranger (Cambridge: Cambridge University Press, 1983), 104–108; Joel F. Burden, "Rituals of Royalty: Prescription, Politics and Practice in English Coronation and Royal Funeral Rituals c. 1327 to c. 1485" (unpublished thesis, University of York, December 1999), 1–28; and Andrew Brown, *Civic Ceremony and Religion in Medieval Bruges, c. 1300–1520* (Cambridge: Cambridge University Press, 2011), 27–28.

11 Jacques le Goff, "A Coronation Program for the Age of St Louis: The Ordo of 1250," in *Coronations: Medieval and Early Modern Monarchic Ritual,* ed. Janos M. Bak (Berkeley: University of California Press, 1990), 47; Paul Binski, *Westminster Abbey and the Plantagenets: Kingship and the Representation of Power, 1200–1400* (New Haven: Yale University Press, 1995), 126–140; and Burden, "Rituals of Royalty"; Philippe Buc, *The Dangers of Ritual: Between Early Medieval Texts and Social Scientific Theory* (Princeton: Princeton University Press, 2001).

12 For a detailed exploration of prominent literature on this shift, see Sharpe, *Selling the Tudor Monarchy,* particularly 20–34. See also Sharpe, *Image Wars: Promoting Kings and Commonwealth in England, 1603–1660* (New Haven: Yale University Press, 2010); Sharpe, *Rebranding Rule: The Restoration and Revolution of Monarchy, 1660–1714* (New Haven: Yale University Press, 2013), particularly 1–9.

13 Eric Hobsbawm, "Introduction: Inventing Tradition," in *The Invention of Tradition,* 1–14.

14 *The Princely Courts of Europe, 1500–1750,* ed. John Adamson (London: Seven Dials, 2000); Sean MacGlynn and Elena Woodacre, eds., *The Image and Perception of Monarchy in Medieval and Early Modern Europe* (Newcastle: Cambridge Scholar Publishers, 2014). See also endnote 6 above.

15 Woodacre, "Understanding the Mechanisms of Monarchy," 5–6 in this volume.

16 Ibid., page 9, particularly see discussions of Van Osta.

17 Ibid., 8.

18 Wilhelm I was crowned as king of Prussia, but not as king of unified Germany.

19 One of the prominent monarchies of the modern era that retained the coronation is Britain, but even here it was not without challenge during the nineteenth century, see Cannadine, "The Context, Performance and Meaning of Ritual," particularly 108–120; Roy Strong, *Coronation: A History of Kingship and the British Monarchy* (London: Harper Collins, 2005), particularly 353–419.

20 Rodrigues uses the term 'first globalization' but it is often also referred to as the first global age, and for most it begins in earnest in the fifteenth century, although this is still debated. For some examples, see Geoffrey C. Gunn, *First Globalization: the Eurasian Exchange, 1500 to 1800* (Lanham: Rowman and Littlefield, 2003); Dennis O. Flynn and Arturo Giráldez, *China and the Birth of Globalization in the Sixteenth Century* (Farnham: Ashgate, 2010); Charles Parker, *Global Interactions in the Early Modern Age* (Cambridge: Cambridge University Press, 2010); and *Goods from the East, 1600–1800: Trading Eurasia*, ed. Maxine Berg with Felicia Gottman, Hanna Hodacs and Chris Nierstrasz (Basingstoke: Palgrave Macmillan, 2015).
21 Woodacre, "Understanding Mechanisms of Monarchy," see page 2–3 this volume.
22 W.M. Ormrod, "Monarchy, Martyrdom and Masculinity: England in the Later Middle Ages," in *Holiness and Masculinity in the Middle Ages*, eds. Patricia H. Cullum and Katherine J. Lewis (Cardiff: University of Wales Press, 2004), 174–191; Christopher Fletcher, "Manhood and Politics in the Reign of Richard II," *Past and Present*, 189 (2005): 3–39; Christopher Fletcher, *Richard II: Manhood, Youth and Politics, 1377–99* (Oxford: Oxford University Press, 2008); Christopher Fletcher, "Manhood, Kingship and the Public in Late Medieval England," *Edad Media Revista de Historia*, 13 (2013): 123–142; Katherine J. Lewis, *Kingship and Masculinity in Late Medieval England* (Abingdon: Routledge, 2013); Glenn Richardson, "Boys and Their Toys: Kingship, Masculinity and Material Culture in the Sixteenth Century," in *The Image and Perception of Monarchy*, 183–206; and Emma Levitt, "The Construction of High Status Masculinity through the Tournament and Martial Activity in the Later Middle Ages" (unpublished PhD thesis, University of Huddersfield, 2016).
23 Hélder Carvalhal and Isabel dos Guimarães Sá, "Knightly Masculinity, Court Games and Material Culture in Late-medieval Portugal: The Case of Constable Afonso (c.1480–1504)," *Gender and History*, 28, no. 2 (August 2016): 387–400.
24 Raewyn Connell, *Gender and Power: Society, the Person and Sexual Politics* (Cambridge: Polity Press, 1987; reprint Oxford: Blackwell, 2003), particularly 180–190; Raewyn Connell, *Masculinities* (Cambridge: Polity Press, 1995, reprint 2005), particularly 67–86; and Raewyn Connell and James W. Messerschmidt, "Hegemonic Masculinity: Rethinking the Concept," *Gender and Society*, 19, no. 6 (2016): 829–859.
25 For example, see Anna Whitelock, "Woman, Warrior, Queen?" in *Tudor Queenship: the Reigns of Mary and Elizabeth*, eds. Alice Hunt and Anna Whitelock (New York: Palgrave Macmillan, 2010), 173–189; and Estelle Paranque, "The Representations and Ambiguities of the Warlike Kingship of Elizabeth I," in *Medieval and Early Modern Representations of Authority in Scotland and Britain*, 163–176.
26 See more of the importance of the capital city as a 'magic centre' in Woodacre, "Understanding the Mechanisms of Monarchy," see page 13 this volume.
27 Ibid., 14, notes 83–84.
28 Strong, *Coronations*, 440–442.

Key works

Bak, Janos, ed., *Coronations: Medieval and Early Modern Monarchic Ritual* (Berkeley: University of California Press, 1990).
Binski, Paul, *Westminster Abbey and the Plantagenets: Kingship and the Representation of Power, 1200–1400* (New Haven: Yale University Press, 1995).
Burke, Peter, *Fabrication of Louis XIV* (New Haven: Yale University Press, 1992).
MacGlynn, Sean and Elena Woodacre, eds., *The Image and Perception of Monarchy in Medieval and Early Modern Europe* (Newcastle: Cambridge Scholars Publishing, 2010).
Sharpe, Kevin, *Selling the Tudor Monarchy: Authority and Image in Sixteenth-Century England* (New Haven: Yale University Press, 2009).
Strong, Roy, *Art and Power, Renaissance Festivals 1450–1650* (Woodbridge: Boydell, 1984).

9

FAITH, POWER AND CHARITY

Personal religion and kingship in medieval England

Paul Webster

Edward the Confessor was buried in January 1066 in Westminster Abbey, the church he had transformed. As his earliest hagiographer described:

> [t]he funeral rites were arranged at the royal cost and with royal honour . . . They bore his holy remains from his palace home into the house of God, and offered up prayers and sighs and psalms . . . they blessed the office of the internment . . . with the singing of masses and the relief of the poor . . . They also caused the whole of the thirtieth day following to be observed with the celebration of masses and the chanting of psalms, and expended many pounds of gold for the redemption of his soul in the alleviation of different classes of the poor.[1]

The Confessor was canonized in 1161, and the abbey became a focal point of English kingship.[2] It was the site of coronation from William the Conqueror's reign onwards, provided the focus for royal religious ritual, much of it linked to the cult of the Confessor and, from the death of Henry III (1272) to that of George II (1760), it was the most frequently chosen church for royal burial.[3] Westminster's importance to kingly devotions in England is widely recognized and formed part of the religious dimension to rulership those kings sought to project. As Anna M. Duch's contribution to this volume shows, this was closely linked to royal engagement with the cult of the saints, because association with a saintly predecessor brought an aura of religiosity to the dynasty.[4]

The account quoted above reveals further aspects of the relationship between faith and the presentation of power. The prayers, psalms, masses and almsgiving for the deceased king's soul were provision expected for a royal burial. They were also religious activities in which rulers themselves engaged. This chapter explores the wider context of royal prayer and giving by kings in aid of their spiritual wellbeing and the future prospects of their souls, activity with potentially private motives often undertaken in public. Provision for the soul and engagement with religious ritual played an important part in the life of a ruler. These were central aspects of kingship between the eleventh and fifteenth centuries, even within the kingdom of England, where such activity has traditionally been underestimated in scholarly writing.

In what follows, features of royal 'personal religion' and the way monarchs ruled will often be discussed together. Without sources written by royal figures in which they set out personal beliefs, it is not possible to determine whether these were pious individuals of genuine faith. Our sources reveal 'external manifestations of the king's devotions', often framed as provision for the individual's soul and for members of their immediate kin-group.[5] This can be read in personal terms, but where kings were concerned it often took place in the context of public ceremony in which the ruler's royal office was at the forefront of the minds of all involved. Religious giving could reflect personal response, designed (and often stated) as for the wellbeing of the soul in life and salvation after death, linked to the developing doctrine of purgatory and desire to ease the soul's posthumous suffering. Meanwhile, royal participation in religious ceremonial, accompanied by largesse, was expected of a king, emphasizing royal authority and presenting 'kingship as merciful, beneficent and pious'.[6] A monarch could be judged as much on his fulfilment of such obligations as for military or governmental activity. In this context, the distinction between private faith and public devotions is often difficult, if not impossible to draw. In terms of studying kingship, reconstructing the 'external manifestations' of a king's personal religion can help in determining how far rulers conformed to expectations, in turn contributing to assessments of their effectiveness.[7]

European context

Religion as an aspect of kingship has received important consideration in studies of European rulership. Ninth- and tenth-century Frankish monarchs cultivated an image as models of Christian kingship. Charles the Bald (r.840–77, as emperor 875–7) introduced archiepiscopal anointing of the ruler and his children, promoting royal sacrality, with the anointed king as mediator between God and people. The second Capetian ruler, Robert II 'the Pious' (r.987–1031), was reputedly capable of healing the sick, a precursor for later claims (in France and England) that the so-called 'royal touch' cured the skin-disease scrofula.[8] Historians of the twelfth century have debated the significance of the abbey of Saint-Denis and the influence of Suger (abbot 1122–51). His rebuilding and promotion of his church celebrated its royal associations as the burial site of successive dynasties: Merovingians, Carolingians and Capetians. The abbey held the royal insignia and war-banner, the *Oriflamme*. Kings were encouraged to regard St Denis as their protector. Military victories by Louis VI (r.1108–37) in 1124 and by Philip II (r.1180–1223) in 1214 contributed to this narrative's success. Through the evolving concept of sacral kingship, the French rulers were seen, and portrayed themselves, as *reges christianissimi* ('most Christian kings'). This continued under Louis IX (r.1226–70) – church-builder (notably of the Sainte-Chapelle, at the heart of the Paris palace complex), crusader and, later, saint. Under Philip IV (r.1285–1314), St Louis' reign was seen as a golden age. Royal propagandists glorified the French kingdom as specially blessed by God.[9]

The creation of religious centres of dynastic memory and promotion have also been noted in the Holy Roman Empire, for instance Ottonian cultivation of the nunneries of Quedlinburg and Gandersheim, Magdeburg Abbey, established by Otto I (king of east Francia 936–73, king of Italy 951–73, emperor 962–73) in 937, and association with the Carolingian centre of power at Aachen. From coronation to burial, Ottonian ceremonial emphasized the religious dimension to rule and the link between anointing and receiving the grace of God. The Magi who attended Christ's nativity began to be portrayed as kings.[10] Such traditions continued under the Salians, who focused commemoration on their burial church, Speyer Cathedral. Henry III (r.1039–56) won a reputation for intense piety. However, his successor, Henry IV (r.1056–1105/6), was excommunicated (1076). His dramatic penance before Pope Gregory VII at Canossa (1077), and the concessions made by Henry V (r.1105/6–25) in the Concordat of Worms (1122), constituted important stages in redefining the relationship between royal and religious authority.[11] Even so, twelfth- and thirteenth-century rulers did not abandon all claims to holiness, developing 'choreographed use of liturgy for political ends', for instance in the royal (as opposed to imperial) coronation of Frederick I Barbarossa (r.1152–90). Popes might seek to exalt their position and downplay the status of the emperor when conducting imperial coronations, but had far less control away from the papal court, when royal inaugurations were held at Aachen.[12] Meanwhile, posthumous cults developed around emperors, including (briefly) Henry IV, but more enduringly at Bamberg for Henry II (d.1024, canonized 1146) and his wife Kunigunde (d.1040, canonized 1200).[13]

Seeking canonized predecessors was a hallmark of the twelfth century. The German emperors sought to outflank Capetian religious activity by claiming Charlemagne for themselves. Frederick Barbarossa secured the earlier emperor's in 1165, cultivating the royal church at Aachen as similar to Saint-Denis.[14] Frederick II (r.1215–50) also prioritized Aachen, securing coronation there and reburying Charlemagne. When his power waned, association with dynastic churches continued even during the short-lived English imperial claim of Richard, earl of Cornwall (d.1272). Like previous kings 'of the Romans', Richard hastened to Aachen for coronation in 1257. Meanwhile, Rudolf I of Habsburg (r.1273–91) ended his reign by riding to Speyer, to die and be buried alongside several of his Salian and Hohenstaufen predecessors.[15]

Royal religiosity is also considered in writings on Spanish Christian rulers. When Alfonso VI of Castile-Léon (r.1072–1109) took Toledo in 1085, he staked his claim to be seen as a defender of the faith.[16] Alfonso VIII of Castile (r.1157–1214) emphasized the Christian dimension to his rulership.[17] Historians have also focused on the religious activity of James I of Aragon (r.1213–76), on the piety of Iberian queens and their daughters, and on the royal chapel and creation of dynastic burial churches, such as Las Huelgas at Burgos (founded, in 1187, by Alfonso VIII of Castile and his wife, Eleanor of England).[18]

European dynasties shared patterns of religious military activity. From the twelfth century the emerging concept of the crusade was used to enhance their image as Christian kings. The Capetians Louis VII (r.1137–80), Philip II and Louis IX took part in crusades to the Holy Land.[19] Their late thirteenth- and early fourteenth-century successors also made commitments to continue this tradition. The emperors followed suit, for instance Conrad III in 1147–8, the abortive crusade of Frederick I in 1190 and the crusade planned by Henry VI but launched without him in 1197. Frederick II secured the title of King of Jerusalem in 1225 by marrying Isabella of Brienne. His crusade was delayed and mired in papal-imperial politics, but briefly regained Jerusalem in 1229 through the emperor's diplomacy.[20] Meanwhile, in Iberia, crusading ideology was increasingly linked with attempted reconquest of territory under Islamic control, for instance in descriptions of Christian victory at the battle of Las Navas de Tolosa (1212) and of subsequent campaigns down to the fifteenth century.[21] This could also include backing the religious military orders, which developed close links to various European courts.[22]

Action against heretics also visibly demonstrated orthodoxy and commitment to Christian rulership. Louis VIII of France (r.1223–6) joined crusades against the Albigensian heretics, before and after becoming king.[23] Moves against those framed as enemies of the Church could enhance monarchical prestige (and wealth), notably when Philip IV of France brought about the dissolution of the Knights Templar between 1307 and 1314.[24] As Given argues, in:

> [l]evelling accusations of demonology, witchcraft and heresy, a king took on enemies that were at once terrifying but defenceless . . . In the shadow realm of the fantastic and the imaginary, a king could symbolically and dramatically act out his crucial role in Christian society.[25]

Meanwhile, public demonstrations of royal orthodoxy and commitment to the Church can be seen in attitudes towards other faiths. The Jewish community fulfilled a financial role in royal service, which led rulers to tread a fine line in showing support or ambivalence towards conversion initiatives, for instance those of the thirteenth-century orders of mendicant friars.[26] Monarchs sometimes sought to protect the Jewish community from attacks provoked by crusade preaching.[27] However, as kings found themselves less able to draw money from the Jewish community, the later medieval period saw an increase in punitive inquiries, followed by expulsions.[28]

Historical writing on kingship and personal religion in England

Historiography of European rulers has had limited influence on work on the religion of England's kings, with some exceptions. Marc Bloch investigated the 'royal touch', which he argued was practised from the reigns of Louis IX (in France) and Edward I (in England), with potential earlier precursors.[29] Ernst Kantorowicz included England in exploring the difference between the mortal man crowned king and the nature of the office he entered, and in examining litany composed to praise medieval rulers.[30] Historians have compared the rulers of England and France, examining Westminster Abbey alongside Saint-Denis, comparing individuals and their courts, and kings reputed as pious and (or) who were canonized, notably Edward the Confessor, Henry III and Louis IX.[31] Modern studies of royal women draw similar comparisons, considering how dynasties influenced one another.[32]

Royal saints are considered elsewhere in this section. Here, the wider context to royal devotions will be explored. Studies of England's medieval kings often focus on 'administrative kingship' and the political, military and national dimension to royal power.[33] Biography, in particular, devotes relatively brief attention to personal religion, with England's kings consistently described as 'conventionally pious'.[34] However, 'conventional piety is not easy to define: individual taste embraced contrasts, not to say contradictions'.[35] Furthermore, such assessment makes exceptions of kings for whom there is a greater volume of religious activity, whether or not this was radically different from that of predecessors or successors. Henry III (r.1216–72) provides a prime example, although there is no published synthesis of the relationship between his piety and kingship.[36] Likewise, Henry V (r.1413–22) has been seen as 'the first king since Henry III to have shown more than conventional piety'.[37] While devotional acts by individual rulers have been considered, with the exception of work by Elizabeth Hallam there have been fewer attempts at wider comparison.[38]

Thus, the personal religion of the post-Conquest kings stands as 'a study that richly deserves to be written'.[39] Recent studies have begun to address this need. Work on King John (r.1199–1216) suggests how exploration of royal religion adds to our perception of a ruler universally condemned. Further avenues are suggested by examinations of Angevin pilgrimage, devotion to the Virgin Mary and of the religious activity of the kings of the Scots.[40] The latest biographies accord greater significance to religious acts. The piety of William the Conqueror (r.1066–87) has been characterized as 'theatrically demonstrative', while Henry Bolingbroke performed ostentatious devotions even before ascending the throne as Henry IV (1399).[41] Malcolm Vale shows how royal religion can be central to analysis of rulership, looking beyond Henry V as a warrior king to argue that 'ecclesiastical and devotional matters ranked very highly indeed', driven by desire to counter Lollardy, and by attention to detail in religious observance. This included provision for religious activity within the royal household in wartime and attempted reform of monasticism. The prevailing image of Henry is dictated by his victory at Agincourt (1415). He nonetheless cultivated the priest-like dimension to kingship. Vale explores the extent to which 'conscience' dictated royal choices, examining Henry's personal attention to services, prayers and almsgiving. As with Henry III, comparison is drawn with Louis IX of France, although the latter 'stood alone'.[42] England therefore provides a suitable case study.

Chaplains, masses, devotional texts and almsgiving

England's kings engaged in a range of religious acts. Each can be linked to projecting an image of power. Provision for devotions of the royal household, and of the king himself, occurred across the period, seen in evidence for the royal chapel and its personnel.[43] One royal chaplain, William of Poitiers, composed a panegyric biography of William the Conqueror in the 1070s.[44] In 1416–17, another (anonymous) cleric likely to have been a royal chaplain penned the *Gesta Henrici Quinti*.[45] Employment of royal chaplains is shown by payment of their wages. Their role is implicitly demonstrated by the commissioning or survival of items used daily during services, including towels, vestments, candlesticks, crucifixes and images of saints, and by supply of bread and wine for the mass. The 'Treasure Roll' of Richard II (r.1377–99) lists a striking collection of gold and silver-gilt chapel goods.[46] Perhaps the most remarkable surviving example of royal chapel equipment is the Wilton Diptych, a portable altarpiece commissioned by Richard II, probably in the final phase of his reign (1395–9). This depicts the king being presented to the Virgin Mary and Christ-child by his favoured saints: Edward the Confessor, Edmund King and Martyr, and John the Baptist.[47] This was probably used for Richard's private devotions at Westminster or when he travelled. It also made a statement of his belief that kingship and divine power were inextricably linked.

Further glimpses can be found in sources noting royal attendance at mass, for example for Richard I (r.1189–99) and John.[48] Henry III ordered mass to be held daily, even when Simon de Montfort held him captive (1264–5). He also engaged with inherent obligations of the service (almsgiving to the poor). This in turn suggests that de Montfort felt it important to ensure that what was expected of a king, including religious activity, continued even when that king was little more than a figurehead.[49]

Potentially private devotions performed in public are also seen in reports of Richard I's efforts to act as befitted a king. The Lionheart 'adorned his chaplain with costly garments', walked through the church urging the religious to greater efforts in chanting the liturgy, before respecting the silence expected during mass, no matter what business was pressed upon him.[50] The public dimension is also seen in performance of religious ritual celebrating kingship, notably the *Laudes Regiae*, which linked the hierarchies of heaven and earth, with anointed kings supported by angels and archangels.[51] Performance of the *Laudes*, probably accompanied by crown-wearing, often occurred on court occasions such as Christmas, Easter and Whitsunday, for example between *c.*1185 and *c.*1240.[52]

Kings also commissioned masses for royal souls, often performed in a public setting. The royal family was prominent in endowing chantries, which evolved from masses for named individuals on particular occasions, such as the anniversary of their death, to arrangements for services at particular altars performed by priests employed specifically for the task, to the construction of chapels with dedicated priests within churches. In the second half of the twelfth century, provision was made at Reading Abbey to commemorate Eleanor of Aquitaine (d.1204), and at Rouen Cathedral for Henry the Young King (d.1183). Courtiers also endowed chantries, including stipulations for masses for royal figures.[53] Richard II and Henry V established multiple chantries and paid for thousands of anniversary masses. Henry V specified that priests at the altar beside his tomb should be visible to the people.[54] Thus, arrangements for the individual king's soul were part of a public statement, encouraging additional prayers by the faithful while conspicuously demonstrating royal wealth and power.

Ruling families also commissioned or were given religious texts to accompany their devotions, but also high-status items reflecting their owners' position. The earliest surviving list of royal books, preserved in a letter issued by John in 1208, includes two bibles.[55] The fifteenth-century illuminated bible owned by Henry IV and his Lancastrian successors is the largest surviving example made in medieval England. Henry was also the earliest ruler known to have possessed a bible in English.[56] He may also have composed religious music, with Henry V also associated with the musical setting of services.[57] The latter owned and borrowed numerous theological works, several of which were to be given to religious communities following his death.[58]

From the Anglo-Saxon era to the Reformation, rulers owned a range of religious texts.[59] Service books were first brought to Kent by the Frankish princess Bertha, who married Aethelberht I in 581. Glimpses of royal receipt or giving of religious manuscripts can be found for seventh- and eighth-century Northumbria, East Anglia and Mercia. Gospel books, psalters and other texts can be linked to Aethelstan's court in the early tenth century, containing inscriptions requesting prayers for the king. The *Regularis Concordia*, drawn up at the request of Edgar (d.975), gave prominence to prayers for the ruler and his queen, as an established part of each monastic service.[60]

While there are no surviving religious books owned by kings between the Norman Conquest and the accession of Edward I (r.1272–1307), rulers were wealthy patrons, well placed to commission, own and give books. The written word flourished at court, both in an administrative context and in terms of literature in circulation.[61] Some of this covered religious themes, for instance the vernacular life of St Edward the Confessor, dating to the 1250s, dedicated to Eleanor of Provence (c.1223–91) and perhaps also owned by Eleanor of Castile (1241–90), or the service books acquired by Henry III for chapels around the kingdom.[62] Meanwhile, the Douce Apocalypse was commissioned by the future Edward I and Eleanor of Castile in the final years of Henry III's reign.[63] Surviving psalters were probably given to or commissioned by several of England's queens, not least Isabella of France, wife of Edward II (r.1307–27).[64] Royal children learnt the psalms as early as the reign of Alfred (r.871–99). The Alphonso Psalter (c.1284), named for the son of Edward I and Eleanor of Castile, is potentially indicative of the care taken in their teaching.[65] In the later Middle Ages, books of hours found a place in the royal collection, for example the Bedford Hours, given to Henry VI (r.1422–61 and 1470–1) by his uncle and aunt, John, duke of Bedford, and Anne of Burgundy in 1430.[66] Royal books of hours also include that of Richard III (r.1483–5).[67] We do not know how rulers used these texts, but their creation and survival implies significance, indicating expectation that kings and queens place devotions at the heart of daily activity and the exercise of their role.

Also within the royal household, the king's almoner organized distribution of charity. Largesse from the king's table and from his increasingly regular provision for the poor and sick can be traced.[68] This was linked to concern over the difficulties facing the rich man in entering the kingdom of God, and was suitable benevolence for a king to show. Henry III was a notable benefactor of the poor, usually on feast days, stipulating that this was for the souls of his relatives. He provided clothing and food, usually bread, fish or meat, and ale. Such giving took place in England even when the king was overseas. In 1242 Henry ordered 102,000 paupers to be fed for the soul of his sister Isabella (d.1241), who had been married to the emperor Frederick II. The king's agents, who could not necessarily gather so many people for a single sitting, were to 'feed them by turns from day to day till the number is completed'.[69] Henry also made substantial donations to the mendicant friars, as these orders arrived in and spread across England, providing clothing, food, wine, building materials, and items for celebration of services.[70] In 1259, the king noted that he held the Dominican friars 'in special devotion as men of the gospel and ministers of the Most High King'.[71] Although Henry III's charity continued trends from the reign of John, his father, the number of recipients increased alongside the frequency of occasions on which money and food were dispensed.[72] Regular almsgiving, recorded by the king's almoner, also featured in the devotional practices of Edward I and Edward II.[73] Sometimes, kings arranged for provision for the poor to continue after their deaths. Henry V requested involvement of paupers in ceremonies marking the anniversary of his death and for distributions to the poor in aid of his soul.[74]

Demonstration of orthodoxy

The kings of England also demonstrated power and sought the wellbeing and salvation of their souls by going on pilgrimage and giving to the churches they visited.[75]

For some, such pilgrimage included participating in and (or) supporting crusades. Richard I's deeds on the Third Crusade shaped his reputation, in the Middle Ages and beyond.[76] Henry III's eldest son, Edward, was on crusade when his father died in 1272 and, as king, took the crusaders' vow again in 1287. Here, and in other theatres of war, the crown might request prayers for the king and his campaign from bishops, religious orders and individual houses. This was an organized feature of Edward I's campaigns in Wales, Scotland and France.[77]

Several kings undertook to crusade but never set out. Twelfth-century examples include Henry II (r.1154–89) and his eldest son Henry the Young King (d.1183).[78] In the thirteenth century, John and Henry III both took the cross, while in 1313, Edward II made the vow alongside Philip IV of France in a ceremony at Nôtre-Dame Cathedral in Paris. In the early 1330s, a joint Anglo-French crusade was proposed, to be led by Philip VI (r.1328–50) of France and Edward III of England (r.1327–77).[79] Royal sons sometimes participated in crusades. Robert Curthose, eldest son of William I, was one of the leaders of the First Crusade and was said to have turned down the offer of the crown of Jerusalem.[80]

Not all rulers demonstrated commitment to their faith by mounting a crusade, but they showed support in other ways. Henry II made substantial financial contributions.[81] Henry III assembled a gold treasure from the late 1240s, intended to support a crusade but then spent subduing rebellion in Gascony in 1253–4.[82] Another means of association lay in using crusade imagery in decorating royal chambers. Depictions of the siege of Antioch during the First Crusade and of Richard I fighting Saladin during the Third Crusade were created for Henry III, perhaps at the instigation of Eleanor of Provence. Similar motivations probably inspired Edward I's pictorial additions to the Painted Chamber at Westminster.[83] Kings also commissioned or received luxury manuscripts containing histories of the crusades and of royal deeds in the Holy Land.[84]

Just as European kings demonstrated orthodoxy in their response to heresy and to other faiths, so did the rulers of England. Despite his long dispute with the church (1206–14), and his alliance with Count Raymond VI of Toulouse, later condemned as a heretic, King John ordered suppression of heresy in south-western France.[85] When required, Edward II acted against the Knights Templar.[86] Richard II and his successors faced the emergence of an English heresy: Lollardy. Richard was firmly orthodox in his response. The fight against heresy formed a regular feature of his letters in the last decade of his reign.[87] Henry IV's 1401 parliament introduced the statute known as *De Heretico Comburendo*, even if burning of heretics was not a new phenomenon in England. This emphasized royal commitment to defending orthodoxy, while buttressing efforts to maintain order and secure revenue, although Henry allowed debate about church reform. A statute against Lollards was issued in 1406. Oldcastle's rebellion prompted another under Henry V in 1414. Thus, royal actions 'effectively eliminated Lollardy as a serious threat to both Church and State'.[88]

Historians have written extensively on royal attitudes to the Jewish community which arrived in England following the Norman invasion.[89] As in Europe, there followed decades of uneasy balance between royal protection and persecution. Under Stephen (r.1135–54), Jewish presence expanded from London to areas under the king's control during the civil war, as Stephen sought to secure his political and financial position.[90] In 1218, orders were issued, in the name of the boy-king Henry III, for all Jews to wear badges. This was the first mandate of its kind in Europe, perhaps instigated by the papal legate Guala, following the Fourth Lateran Council (1215). As an adult, Henry founded the *Domus Conversorum* in London in 1232. Here, converted Jews were housed, having surrendered their money and possessions to the crown.[91] Exploitation and persecution of the Jewish community became increasingly commonplace, leading to the expulsion ordered by Edward I in 1290.[92]

Benefaction, foundation and burial

Throughout the period, churches could point to parts of their fabric and estates that were royal donations. Reciprocal expectations were increasingly formalized in arrangements for masses at specific altars. This could involve new religious practices being integrated into communities favoured by kings, as with the chantry chapels established for Henry V and Henry VII (r.1485–1509) at Westminster Abbey.[93] Subjects also promised prayers for the royal family as part of obligations agreed when the king issued licences to found chantries.[94] Commitments were honoured beyond a ruler's lifetime. For instance, at the Dissolution of the Monasteries, almsgiving was recorded at St Peter's Abbey, Gloucester linked to William the Conqueror, his eldest son Robert Curthose, Henry I, Edward II, Richard II and Anne of Bohemia.[95]

In founding religious houses, rulers made permanent statements of power in the landscape, associating themselves with the most popular religious orders: Benedictine communities in the eleventh century; Cistercians in the twelfth, thirteenth and into the fourteenth centuries.[96] Kings and queens led patronage for mendicant friars in the thirteenth and fourteenth centuries.[97] Later patterns reveal preference for colleges and communities of particularly austere orders, such as the Carthusians and Celestines.[98] Royal foundations were often substantial. John's abbey at Beaulieu (Hampshire), established in 1204, was conceived as the largest Cistercian house in England at the time. Henry V planned Carthusian Sheen on a scale not seen since Henry III's work at Westminster.[99] Gifts extended beyond lands and building-stone, as the royal family created endowments befitting their status and in search of spiritual credit. By seeking intercession from established and emerging religious orders, they continued regnal traditions and engaged with current trends. Yet royal patrons sometimes lost interest. Edward I personally laid the foundation stone at Vale Royal Abbey (Cheshire) in 1277. The community's foundation history emphasized its origins in a vow made by Edward while in peril at sea. However, the king ordered contributions to cease in 1290, instead sponsoring St Stephen's Chapel at Westminster, envisaged as a parallel for the Sainte-Chapelle of the French kings.[100] Overall, however, rulers founded religious houses to benefit their souls. Continued support for predecessors' foundations created a chain of communities performing services for the dynasty.

Finally, relationships between personal religion and display of power are seen when kings died and were buried. Rulers provided for their souls in their final testaments.[101] Henry V composed three wills. The last, written in 1421, was updated from his deathbed in 1422. In an effort to secure his claims in France, he invoked St Denis and St Rémi alongside English royal saints. Detailed provisions were made for services, including 20,000 masses across a year (around 55 per day). Almsgiving in Henry's name was to take place annually.[102]

Royal deaths gave chroniclers an opportunity to pen moralizing portraits, comparing a king's passing to characteristics of his rule.[103] Edward the Confessor's death (1066) was framed in the context of posthumous efforts to secure his canonization. Writers in the century that followed portrayed an ideal end.[104] By contrast, descriptions of Henry II's demise (1189) noted thunderstorms, sickness and suffering, with disrespectful treatment of the royal body, plundered by thieving members of the household.[105] Meanwhile, choice of burial location could be personal, and the royal funeral provided opportunities to display power and wealth, even when the successor was absent.[106] When Henry III died (1272), his heir Edward was on crusade. Nonetheless, 'the magnates . . . attended the ceremony with due reverence' and carried Henry's body, 'decked in precious garments and the royal diadem', to the grave.[107]

Funerary display also involved construction of elaborate tombs. From the thirteenth century these usually included an effigy depicting the crowned king. Several tombs were located at Westminster Abbey, which emerged as a dynastic church comparable to those of other dynasties, as England's rulers awaited the Last Judgement in proximity to the royal saint, Edward the Confessor.[108] From the later fourteenth century, evidence shows that kings gave thought to the ceremonial treatment of their bodies between death and burial, and (or) to activities before, during and beyond the funeral, in aid of their souls. Richard II constructed a joint tomb at Westminster, in which he was eventually interred alongside Anne of Bohemia. Henry V commissioned an elaborate chantry chapel to surround his tomb. His testament detailed the timing and themes of masses to be celebrated there, demonstrating his particular devotion to the Virgin Mary. Vestments for the priests and equipment for services were ordered.[109] Even in the grave, the association of royal power and the religious dimension to kingship held continued prominence.

Conclusion

This chapter has highlighted a range of religious activities of England's medieval rulers. Many could be seen as acts of personal piety by individuals seeking salvation. They were also part of what was expected of a king, linked to the religious aura surrounding his role. The two were inextricably linked, because anointing at the coronation singled out the ruler as divinely ordained. The sources do not often note this directly, but kings and chroniclers were aware of it. Richard II, when required to relinquish his kingship in 1399, allegedly commented that 'he did not wish to renounce those special dignities of a spiritual nature which had been bestowed upon him, nor indeed his anointment; he was in fact unable to renounce them, nor could he cease to retain them'.[110] It may be argued that the religious dimension to English medieval kingship deserves further attention, developing the lead shown in studies of European monarchies. There is a strong case to be made against English exceptionalism. Between the seismic shifts of the Norman invasion and the dissolution of the monasteries, the kings of England and their consorts engaged with the religious trends of their day. In addition to being 'administrative kings', these rulers stood alongside their European counterparts in engaging with religious ritual and harnessing this to demonstrate their power.

Notes

1 *The Life of King Edward Who Rests at Westminster*, trans. Frank Barlow (London: Nelson, 1962), 81.

2 Frank Barlow, *Edward the Confessor* (New Haven: Yale University Press, 1997), 229–233, 277–284, 309–324; Bernhard Scholz, "The Canonisation of Edward the Confessor," *Speculum* 36 (1961): 38–60; Paul Binski, *Westminster Abbey and the Plantagenets* (New Haven: Yale University Press, 1995).

3 The exceptions were Edward II (buried at Gloucester), Henry IV (Canterbury), Henry VI, Edward IV, Henry VIII, Charles I (Windsor) and George I (Hanover). Recent discoveries have apparently confirmed that Richard III was buried at Leicester, while Edward V disappeared in the Tower of London in 1483.

4 Anna M. Duch, Chasing St Louis: the English monarchy's pursuit of sainthood', 330–351 in this volume.

5 Nigel Saul, *Richard II* (New Haven: Yale University Press, 1997), 304.

6 Geoffrey Koziol, "Political Culture," in *France in the Central Middles Ages 900–1200*, ed. Marcus Bull (Oxford: Oxford University Press, 2001), 62.

7 Paul Webster, *King John and Religion* (Woodbridge: Boydell, 2015), 1–2; Mark Ormrod, "The Personal Religion of Edward III," *Speculum* 64 (1989): 853; Malcolm Vale, *Henry V: The Conscience of a King* (New Haven: Yale University Press, 2016), 159.

8 Bernd Schneidmüller, "Constructing Identities of Medieval France," in *France in the Central Middles Ages 900–1200*, ed. Marcus Bull (Oxford: Oxford University Press, 2001), 23, 35.

9 Elizabeth Hallam and Judith Everard, *Capetian France 987–1328*, second edition (Harlow: Longman, 2001), 239–245, 263–288, 298–304, 333–338, 357, 396–397, 401–403; Schneidmüller, "Constructing Identities," 37–41; Koziol, "Political Culture," 74–75.

10 Janet Nelson, "Rulers and Government," and Eckhard Müller-Mertens, "The Ottonians as Kings and Emperors," in *The New Cambridge Medieval History: Volume III c. 900–c. 1024*, ed. Timothy Reuter (Cambridge: Cambridge University Press, 1999), 105, 108–109, 244–246, 257–264.

11 Hanna Vollrath, "The Western Empire under the Salians," in *The New Cambridge Medieval History: Volume IV c. 1024–c. 1198, Part II*, eds. David Luscombe and Jonathan Riley-Smith (Cambridge: Cambridge University Press, 2004), 48–49, 56–60, 68, 71.

12 Johanna Dale, "Inauguration and Political Liturgy in the Hohenstaufen Empire, 1138–1215," *German History*, 34 (2016): 191–213.

13 Vollrath, "Western Empire," 68; Müller-Mertens, "Ottonians as Kings and Emperors," 265–266.

14 Benjamin Arnold, "The Western Empire, 1125–1197," in *New Cambridge Medieval History: Volume IV*, 404–405, 417, 420.

15 Michael Toch, "Welfs, Hohenstaufen and Habsburgs," in *The New Cambridge Medieval History: Volume V c. 1198–c. 1300*, ed. David Abulafia (Cambridge: Cambridge University Press, 1999), 382, 393, 397; Björn Weiler, *Henry III of England and the Staufen Empire 1216–1272* (London and Woodbridge: Royal Historical Society and Boydell, 2006), esp. 172–197.

16 Simon Barton, "Spain in the Eleventh Century," in *New Cambridge Medieval History: Volume IV*, 172.

17 Peter Linehan, "Spain in the Twelfth Century," in *New Cambridge Medieval History: Volume IV*, 499.

18 Robert Burns, "The Spiritual Life of James the Conqueror, King of Arago-Catalonia 1208–1276," in *Jaime I y su Epoca* (Zaragoza: Institución Fernando el Católico, 1979), 323–357; Miriam Shadis, "Piety, Politics, and Power: The Patronage of Leonor of England and her Daughters Berenguela of León and Blanche of Castile," in *The Cultural Patronage of Medieval Women*, ed. June McCash (Athens, GA: University of Georgia Press, 1996), 202–227; Rita Costa-Gomes, "The Royal Chapel in Iberia," *Medieval History Journal* 12 (2009): 77–111; Xavier Dectot, *Les tombeaux des familles royales de la peninsula ibérique au Moyen Age* (Turnhout: Brepols, 2009).

19 James Naus, *Constructing Kingship: The Capetian Monarchs of France and the Early Crusades* (Manchester: Manchester University Press, 2016); William Chester Jordan, *Louis IX and the Challenge of the Crusade* (Princeton: Princeton University Press, 1979).

20 Rudolf Hiestand, "Kingship and Crusade in Twelfth-Century Germany," in *England and Germany in the High Middle Ages*, eds. Alfred Haverkamp and Hanna Vollrath (London: The German Historical Institute; and Oxford: Oxford University Press, 1996), 235–265; David Abulafia, *Frederick II* (London: Pimlico, 1988), 164–201. Otto IV took crusade vows but never set out, providing on his deathbed for fulfilment by proxy: Hiestand, "Kingship and Crusade," 246.

21 Miguel Gómez, "Las Navas de Tolosa and the Culture of Crusade in the Kingdom of Castile," *Journal of Medieval Iberian Studies* 4 (2012): 53–57; John Edwards, "*Reconquista* and Crusade in Fifteenth-Century Spain," in *Crusading in the Fifteenth Century*, ed. Norman Housley (Basingstoke: Palgrave Macmillan, 2004), 163–181, 235–237.

22 For example, José Manuel Rodríguez García, "Alfonso X and the Teutonic Order: An Example of the Role of the International Military Orders in Mid Thirteenth-Century Castile," in *The Military Orders Volume 2: Welfare and Warfare*, ed. Helen Nicholson (Aldershot: Ashgate, 1998), 319–327.

23 Catherine Hanley, *Louis: The French Prince Who Invaded England* (New Haven: Yale University Press, 2016), 182–190, 212–222.

24 For example, see Julien Théry, "Une hérésie d'état, Philippe le Bel, le procès des 'perfides Templiers', et la pontificalisation de la royauté française," *Médiévales* 60 (2011): 157–185.

25 James Given, "Chasing Phantoms: Philip IV and the Fantastic," in *Heresy and the Persecuting Society in the Middle Ages*, ed. Michael Frassetto (Leiden: Brill, 2006), 272.

26 David Abulafia, "The King and the Jews," in *The Jews of Europe in the Middle Ages*, ed. Christoph Cluse (Turnhout: Brepols, 2004), 43–54; Alexander Patschovsky, "The Relationship between the Jews of Germany and the King (11th–14th Centuries): A European Comparison," in *England and Germany in the High Middle Ages*, eds. Alfred Haverkamp and Hanna Vollrath (London: The German Historical Institute; and Oxford: Oxford University Press, 1996), 193–218.

27 Hiestand, "Kingship and Crusade," 248–253.

28 William Chester Jordan's work is especially important, for example William Chester Jordan, *The French Monarchy and the Jews* (Philadelphia: University of Pennsylvania Press, 1989). See also Marie Dejoux, "Gouvernement et pénitence : Les enquêtes de réparation des usures juives de Louis IX (1247–1270)," *Annales* 69 (2014): 849–874; Elizabeth Brown, "Philip V, Charles IV, and the Jews of France: The Alleged Explusion of 1322," *Speculum* 66 (1991): 294–329.

29 Marc Bloch, *The Royal Touch*, trans. John Anderson (London: Routledge, 1973).

30 Ernst Kantorowicz, *The King's Two Bodies* (Princeton: Princeton University Press, 1957); Ernst Kantorowicz, *Laudes Regiae* (Berkeley: University of California Press, 1958).

31 For example, Geoffrey Koziol, "England, France, and the Problem of Sacrality in Twelfth-Century Ritual," in *Cultures of Power*, ed. Thomas Bisson (Philadelphia: University of Pennsylvania Press, 1995), 124–148; David Carpenter, "The Meetings of Kings Henry III and Louis IX," in *Thirteenth Century England X*, eds. Michael Prestwich, Richard Britnell and Robin Frame (Woodbridge: Boydell, 2005), 1–30.

32 For example, Colette Bowie, *The Daughters of Henry II and Eleanor of Aquitaine* (Turnhout: Brepols, 2014); Shadis, "Piety, Politics and Power."

33 Warren Hollister and John Baldwin, "The Rise of Administrative Kingship: Henry I and Philip Augustus," *American Historical Review* 83 (1978): 867–905.

34 For further discussion see Webster, *King John*, 2, fn. 6.

35 Chris Given-Wilson, *Henry IV* (New Haven: Yale University Press, 2016), 380.

36 Currently the focus of Antonia Shacklock, "Piety and Politics in the Reign of Henry III" (PhD dissertation, University of Cambridge, forthcoming). See also Sally Dixon-Smith, "The Pro-Anima Almsgiving of Henry III of England 1227–72" (PhD dissertation, University of London, 2003); Katie Phillips, "Devotion by Donation: The Almsgiving and Religious Foundations of Henry III," *Reading Medieval Studies* 43 (2017): 79–98.

37 Jeremy Catto, "Religious Change Under Henry V," in *Henry V: The Practice of Kingship*, ed. Gerald Harriss (Oxford: Oxford University Press, 1985), 106.

38 Judith Green, "The Piety and Patronage of Henry I," *Haskins Society Journal* 10 (2001): 1–16; Michael Prestwich, "The Piety of Edward I," in *England in the Thirteenth Century*, ed.

Mark Ormrod (Grantham: Harlaxton College, 1985), 120–128; Charles Farris, "The Pious Practices of Edward I, 1272–1307" (PhD dissertation, Royal Holloway College, University of London, 2013); Ormrod, "Personal Religion of Edward III," 849–877; Elizabeth Hallam, "Aspects of the Monastic Patronage of the English and French Royal Houses, c. 1130–1270" (PhD dissertation, University of London, 1976). See also the bibliography on the companion website for this volume.

39 Nicholas Vincent, "The Pilgrimages of the Angevin Kings of England 1154–1272," in *Pilgrimage: The English Experience from Becket to Bunyan*, eds. Colin Morris and Peter Roberts (Cambridge: Cambridge University Press, 2002), 12.

40 Webster, *King John*; Vincent, "Pilgrimages"; Nicholas Vincent, "King Henry III and the Blessed Virgin Mary," in *The Church and Mary*, ed. Robert Swanson, *Studies in Church History* 39 (2004): 126–146; Michael Penman, "Royal Piety in Thirteenth-Century Scotland: The Religion and Religiosity of Alexander II (1214–49) and Alexander III (1249–86)," in *Thirteenth Century England XII*, eds. Janet Burton, Phillipp Schofield and Björn Weiler (Woodbridge: Boydell, 2009), 13–30. See also the bibliography on the companion website for this volume.

41 David Bates, *William the Conqueror* (New Haven: Yale University Press, 2016), 77–78; Given-Wilson, *Henry IV*, 76, 376–381.

42 Vale, *Henry V*, xv, 8, 126–203.

43 Ian Bent, "The English Chapel Royal before 1300," *Proceedings of the Royal Musical Association* 90 (1963–64): 77–95; Webster, *King John*, 24–26; Alison McHardy, "Religion, Court Culture and Propaganda: The Chapel Royal in the Reign of Henry V," in *Henry V: New Interpretations*, ed. Gwilym Dodd (Woodbridge: Boydell, 2013), 131–156.

44 *The Gesta Guillelmi of William of Poitiers*, eds. and trans. Ralph Davies and Marjorie Chibnall (Oxford: Clarendon, 1998).

45 *Gesta Henrici Quinti*, eds. and trans. Frank Taylor and John Roskell (Oxford: Clarendon, 1975), xviii–xxiii; Vale, *Henry V*, 32–33, 126–127.

46 London, The National Archives, E 101/411/9; Jenny Stratford, *Richard II and the English Royal Treasure* (Woodbridge: Boydell, 2012).

47 London, The National Gallery, NG4451, www.nationalgallery.org.uk/paintings/english-or-french-the-wilton-diptych (accessed 18 February 2017). On the Diptych see, for example, Dillian Gordon, Lisa Monnas and Caroline Elam, eds., *The Regal Image of Richard II and the Wilton Diptych* (London: Harvey Miller, 1997).

48 *Magna Vita Sancti Hugonis*, eds. and trans. Decima Douie and Hugh Farmer, 2 vols (London: Nelson, 1961–62), vol. II, 101–102; John Brewer, James Dimock and George Warner, eds., *Giraldi Cambrensis Opera*, 8 vols (London: Longman, 1861–91), vol. III, 301–302.

49 London, The National Archives, E101/349/30, discussed in Benjamin Wild, "A Captive King: Henry III between the Battles of Lewes and Evesham, 1264–5," in *Thirteenth Century England XIII*, eds. Janet Burton et al. (Woodbridge: Boydell, 2011), 51–54.

50 *Radulphi de Coggeshall Chronicon Anglicanum*, ed. Joseph Stephenson (London: Longman, 1875), 96–97.

51 Kantorowicz, *Laudes Regiae*; Roy Strong, *Coronation* (London: Harper Collins, 2005), 40; Ian Bent, "The Early History of the English Chapel Royal, ca. 1066–1327," 2 vols (PhD dissertation, University of Cambridge, 1969), vol. I, 320–361, vol. II, 244–286.

52 *The Great Roll of the Pipe for the Thirty-Fourth Year of the Reign of King Henry the Second, A.D. 1187–1188* (London: Pipe Roll Society, 1925), 19; *The Historical Works of Gervase of Canterbury*, ed. William Stubbs, 2 vols (London: Longman, 1879–80), vol. I, 524–527; Webster, *King John*, 27–28; *Calendar of the Liberate Rolls: Henry III. Vol I. A.D. 1226–1240* (London: HMSO, 1916), for example at 311.

53 Christopher Cheney, "A Monastic Letter of Confraternity to Eleanor of Aquitaine," *English Historical Review* 51 (1936): 488–493; Judith Everard and Michael Jones, eds., *The Charters of Duchess Constance of Brittany and her Family 1171–1221* (Woodbridge: Boydell, 1999), 16 (charter Ge7), 47 (C4); David Crouch, "The Origin of Chantries: Some Further Anglo-Norman Evidence," *Journal of Medieval History* 27 (2001): 169, 171–172, 177, 179–180; Webster, *King John*, 29–30.

54 *Calendar of the Patent Rolls: Richard II. Vol. VI. A.D. 1396–1399* (London: HMSO, 1927), 452, 464–465, 477, 565, 579–580; Patrick Strong and Felicity Strong, "The Last Will and Codicils of Henry V," *English Historical Review* 378 (1981): 89–100.

55 Thomas Duffus Hardy, ed., *Rotuli Litterarum Clausarum in Turri Londinensi asservati, Vol. I, 1204–1224* (London: Record Commission, 1833), 108a; Nicholas Vincent, "The Great Lost Library of England's Medieval Kings? Royal Use and Ownership of Books, 1066–1272," in *1000 Years of Royal Books and Manuscripts*, eds. Kathleen Doyle and Scot McKendrick (London: British Library, 2013), 84–85, 98.

56 Given-Wilson, *Henry IV*, 381, 387–388. The illuminated bible is London, British Library, Royal Ms. 1 E IX, www.bl.uk/manuscripts/FullDisplay.aspx?ref=Royal_MS_1_e_ix (accessed 14 April 2017). On the bible in English see Henry Summerson, "An English Bible and Other Books Belonging to Henry IV," *Bulletin of the John Rylands Library* 79 (1997): 109–116.

57 Given-Wilson, *Henry IV*, 381, 386–387; Vale, *Henry V*, 204–213. Debate centres on the Old Hall Manuscript: London, British Library, Additional Ms. 57950,: www.bl.uk/manuscripts/FullDisplay.aspx?ref=Add_MS_57950 (accessed 4 January 2018).

58 Vale, *Henry V*, 128–129, 147–148, 224–226; Strong and Strong, "Last Will and Codicils of Henry V," 93–94.

59 Scot McKendrick et al., *Royal Manuscripts: The Genius of Illumination* (London: British Library, 2011).

60 Richard Gameson, "The Earliest English Royal Books," in *1000 Years of Royal Books and Manuscripts*, eds. Kathleen Doyle and Scot McKendrick (London: British Library, 2013), 4–6, 10, 14–19; *Regularis Concordia anglicae nationis monachorum sanctimonialiumque*, ed. and trans. Thomas Symons (London: Nelson, 1953). See also Michal Kobialka, *This Is My Body: Representational Practices in the Early Middle Ages* (Ann Arbor: University of Michigan Press, 1999), 58–59, 95.

61 Vincent, "Great Lost Library," 73–102.

62 Cambridge, Cambridge University Library, Ms. Ee. 3. 59, https://cudl.lib.cam.ac.uk/view/MS-EE-00003–00059/1 (accessed 28 April 2017); Vincent, "Great Lost Library," 89–90.

63 Oxford, Bodleian Library, Ms. Douce 180, http://bodley30.bodley.ox.ac.uk:8180/luna/servlet/view/all/what/MS.+Douce+180?sort=Shelfmark%2CDescription%2CImage_Description%2Csort_order (accessed 28 April 2017). See also Vincent, "Great Lost Library," 101–102.

64 London, British Library, Royal Ms. 2 B VII, www.bl.uk/manuscripts/FullDisplay.aspx?ref=-Royal_MS_2_b_vii (accessed 18 February 2017); Munich, Bayerische Staatsbibliothek, cod. gall. 16; Anne Stanton, *The Queen Mary Psalter* (Philadelphia: American Philosophical Society, 2001); Anne Stanton, "The Psalter of Isabelle, Queen of England 1308–1330: Isabelle as the Audience," *Word and Image* 18, no. 4 (2002): 1–27.

65 London, British Library, Additional Ms. 24686, www.bl.uk/manuscripts/FullDisplay.aspx?ref=Add_MS_24686&index=0 (accessed 28 April 2017); Gameson, "Earliest English Royal Books," 10.

66 London, British Library, Additional Ms. 18850, www.bl.uk/catalogues/illuminatedmanuscripts/record.asp?MSID=6474&CollID=27&NStart=18850 (accessed 28 April 2017); Scot McKendrick, "A European Heritage: Books of Continental Origin Collected by the English Royal Family from Edward III to Henry VIII," in McKendrick et al., *Royal Manuscripts*, 45.

67 London, Lambeth Palace, Ms. 474, http://leicestercathedral.org/about-us/richard-iii/book-hours/ (accessed 18 February 2017).

68 In records such as London, The National Archives, E101 (Exchequer Accounts Various), E361 (Exchequer: Pipe Office: Enrolled Wardrobe and Household Accounts), E373 (Exchequer: Pipe Office: Pipe Rolls), E403 (Exchequer of Receipt: Issue Rolls and Registers), E404 (Exchequer of Receipt: Warrants for Issues). See also Hilda Johnstone, "Poor-Relief in the Royal Households of Thirteenth-Century England," *Speculum* 4 (1929): 149–167; Lawrence Tanner, "Lord High Almoners and Sub-Almoners, 1100–1957," *Journal of the British Archaeological Association* 20–21 (1957–58): 72–83.

69 *Calendar of the Liberate Rolls: Henry III. Vol. III. A.D. 1240–1245* (London: HMSO, 1930), 124, 306, 324.

70 For example, *Calendar of the Liberate Rolls 1240–1245*, 85, 182, 281; *Calendar of the Liberate Rolls: Henry III. Vol. IV. A.D. 1245–1251* (London: HMSO, 1937), 182.

71 *Calendar of the Patent Rolls: Henry III. Vol. V. A.D. 1258–1266* (London: HMSO, 1910), 20.

72 Webster, *King John*, 110–130; Charles Young, "King John and England: An Illustration of the Medieval Practice of Charity," *Church History* 29 (1960): 264–274; Sally Dixon-Smith, "The Image and Reality of Alms-Giving in the Great Halls of Henry III," *Journal of the British Archaeological Association* 152 (1999): 79–96; Dixon-Smith, "Pro-Anima Almsgiving of Henry III."

73 For example, *Records of the Wardrobe and Household 1286–1289*, eds. Benjamin Byerly and Catherine Byerly (London: HMSO, 1986), 272–305. See also Prestwich, "Piety of Edward I," 120–123; Seymour Phillips, *Edward II* (New Haven: Yale University Press, 2011), 64; Arnold Taylor, "Royal Alms and Oblations in the Later Thirteenth Century," in *Tribute to an Antiquary: Essays Presented to Marc Fitch*, eds. Frederick Emmison and Roy Stephens (London: Leopard's Head, 1976), 93–126.

74 Vale, *Henry V*, 139–140, 249; Strong and Strong, "Last Will and Codicils of Henry V," 90–91.

75 For example, Stephen Marritt, "Prayers for the King and Royal Titles in Anglo-Norman Charters," *Anglo-Norman Studies* 32 (2010): 184–202; Emma Mason, "*Pro statu et incolumitate regni mei*: Royal Monastic Patronage 1066–1154," in *Religion and National Identity*, ed. Stuart Mews, *Studies in Church History* 18 (1982): 99–117; Vincent, "Pilgrimages."

76 Sources include: *Chronicle of the Third Crusade: A Translation of the Itinerarium Peregrinorum et Gesta Regis Ricardi*, trans. Helen Nicholson (Aldershot: Ashgate, 1997). See also, John Gillingham, *Richard I* (New Haven: Yale University Press, 1999), 101–253.

77 Michael Prestwich, *Edward I* (New Haven: Yale University Press, 1997), 66–85, 326–333; David Burton, "Requests for Prayers and Royal Propaganda under Edward I," in *Thirteenth Century England III*, eds. Peter Coss and Simon Lloyd (Woodbridge: Boydell, 1991), 25–35.

78 Hans Mayer, "Henry II of England and the Holy Land," *English Historical Review* 97 (1982): 721–739; Matthew Strickland, *Henry the Young King, 1155–1183* (New Haven: Yale University Press, 2016), 275–276, 297, 308.

79 Webster, *King John*, 169–170; Alan Forey, "The Crusading Vows of the English King Henry III," in *Military Orders and Crusades* (Aldershot: Variorum, 1994), 229–247; Phillips, *Edward II*, 210; Mark Ormrod, *Edward III* (New Haven: Yale University Press, 2013), 181–183. See also Christopher Tyerman, *England and the Crusades 1095–1588* (Chicago: University of Chicago Press, 1988); Timothy Guard, *Chivalry, Kingship and Crusade* (Woodbridge: Boydell, 2013), esp. 182–206.

80 William Aird, *Robert Curthose: Duke of Normandy (c.1050–1134)* (Woodbridge: Boydell, 2008), 153–190.

81 Mayer, "Henry II of England"; Alan Forey, "Henry II's Crusading Penances for Becket's Murder," *Crusades* 7 (2008): 153–164.

82 David Carpenter, "The Gold Treasure of Henry III," in *The Reign of Henry III*, (London and Rio Grande: Hambledon, 1996), 107–136.

83 Laura Whatley, "Romance, Crusading, and the Orient in King Henry III of England's Royal Chambers," *Viator* 44 (2013): 175–198; Matthew Reeve, "The Painted Chamber at Westminster: Edward I and the Crusade," *Viator* 37 (2006): 189–221.

84 For instance London, British Library, Royal Ms. 15 E I, www.bl.uk/catalogues/illuminatedmanuscripts/record.asp?MSID=7740 (accessed 11 January 2018); discussed in Erin Donovan, "A Royal Crusade History: The *Livre d'Eracles* and Edward IV's Exile in Burgundy," *Electronic British Library Journal* (2014), www.bl.uk/eblj/2014articles/article6.html (accessed 11 January 2018).

85 Thomas Duffus Hardy, ed., *Rotuli Litterarum Patentium in Turri Londinensi asservati, vol. I, pt. 1, 1199–1216* (London: Record Commission, 1835), 124a.

86 Helen Nicholson, ed., *The Proceedings Against the Templars in the British Isles* (Farnham: Ashgate, 2011); Jeffrey Hamilton, "King Edward II of England and the Templars," in *The Debate on the Trial of the Templars (1307–1314)*, eds. Jochen Burgtorf, Paul Crawford and Helen Nicholson (Farnham: Ashgate, 2010), 215–224.

87 Saul, *Richard II*, 293–303.
88 Given-Wilson, *Henry IV*, 183–186, 366–378; Vale, *Henry V*, 8, 186–190 (with the quotation at 187), 275–276.
89 Relevant works are listed on the companion website for this volume.
90 Kevin Streit, "The Expansion of the English Jewish Community in the Reign of King Stephen," *Albion* 25 (1993): 177–192.
91 John Tolan, "The First Imposition of a Badge on European Jews: The English Royal Mandate of 1218," in *The Character of Christian-Muslim Encounter*, eds. Douglas Pratt et al. (Leiden: Brill, 2015), 145–166; John Tolan, "Royal Policy and Conversion of Jews to Christianity in Thirteenth-Century Europe," in *Contesting Inter-Religious Conversion in the Medieval World*, eds. Yaniv Fox and Yosi Yisraeli (London and New York: Routledge, 2017), 101–105.
92 Prestwich, *Edward I*, 344–346.
93 On Henry VII's chantry, see Margaret Condon, "God Save the King! Piety, Propaganda, and the Perpetual Memorial," in *Westminster Abbey: The Lady Chapel of Henry VII*, eds. Tim Tatton-Brown and Richard Mortimer (Woodbridge: Boydell, 2003), 59–97.
94 For instance, *Calendar of the Patent Rolls, 1396–1399*, 452, 464–465. See also Vale, *Henry V*, 149–151.
95 *Valor Ecclesiasticus temp. Henr. VIII auctoritate regia institutus*, 8 vols, eds. John Caley and Joseph Hunter (London: Record Commission, 1810–34), vol. II, 411–418.
96 Studies include: Christopher Brooke, "Princes and Kings as Patrons of Monasteries: Normandy and England," in *Il monachismo e la riforma ecclesiastica (1049–1122), Miscellanea del centro di studi medioevali*, 6 (1971): 125–142; Marjorie Chibnall, "The Changing Expectations of a Royal Benefactor: The Religious Patronage of Henry II," in *Religious and Laity in Western Europe, 1000–1400*, eds. Emilia Jamroziak and Janet Burton (Turnhout: Brepols, 2006), 9–21; Christopher Holdsworth, "Royal Cistercians: Beaulieu, Her Daughters and Rewley," in *Thirteenth Century England IV*, eds. Peter Coss and Simon Lloyd (Woodbridge: Boydell, 1992), 139–150. See also Hallam's work in note 37.
97 A wider study has yet to appear.
98 Given-Wilson, *Henry IV*, 378–380; Vale, *Henry V*, 142–147.
99 Webster, *King John*, 66; Vale, *Henry V*, 144–145.
100 *The Ledger Book of Vale Royal Abbey*, ed. John Brownbill (Edinburgh: Record Society of Lancashire and Cheshire, 1914), 1–19; Jeffrey Denton, "From the Foundation of Vale Royal to the Statute of Carlisle: Edward I and Ecclesiastical Patronage," in *Thirteenth Century England IV*, 123–137; *The History of The King's Works, Vol I: The Middle Ages*, 3 vols, eds. Reginald Allen Brown, Howard Colvin and Arnold Taylor (London: HMSO, 1963), vol. I, 248–257, 510–527.
101 *A Collection of all the Wills, Now Known to be Extant, of the Kings and Queens of England*, ed. John Nichols (London: J. Nichols, 1780); Stephen Church, "King John's Testament and the Last Days of his Reign," *English Historical Review* 125 (2010): 505–528; Margaret Condon, "The Last Will of Henry VII," in *Westminster Abbey: The Lady Chapel of Henry VII*, eds. Tim Tatton-Brown and Richard Mortimer (Woodbridge: Boydell, 2003), 99–140.
102 Vale, *Henry V*, 240–259; Strong and Strong, "Last Will and Codicils of Henry V," 89–91.
103 Stephen Church, "Aspects of the English Succession, 1066–1199: The Death of the King," *Anglo-Norman Studies* 29 (2007): 17–34; John Gillingham, "At the Deathbeds of the Kings of England, 1066–1216," in *Herrsche- und Fürstentestamente im Westeuropäischen Mittelalter*, ed. Brigitte Kasten (Cologne, Weimar and Vienna: Bohlau, 2008), 509–530.
104 *Life of St Edward the Confessor by St Aelred of Rievaulx*, trans. Jerome Bertram (Southampton: Saint Austin Press, 1997), 93–95.
105 William Stubbs, ed., *Chronica Magistri Rogeri de Houdene*, 4 vols (London: Longman, 1868–71), vol. II, 366–367; Brewer, Dimock and Warner, *Giraldi Cambrensis*, vol. VIII, 259–262, 282–315.
106 Anna Duch, "The Royal Funerary and Burial Ceremonies of Medieval English Kings, 1216–1509" (PhD dissertation, University of York, 2016); Chris Given-Wilson, "The Exequies of Edward III and the Royal Funeral Ceremony in Late Medieval England," *English Historical Review* 123 (2009): 257–282.
107 *A Hundred Years of History from Record and Chronicle*, ed. and trans. Hilda Johnstone (London: Longman, 1912), 148–149.

211

108 See, for example, Binski, *Westminster Abbey*, esp. 90–120; David Palliser, "Royal Mausolea in the Long Fourteenth Century (1272–1422)," in *Fourteenth Century England III*, ed. Mark Ormrod (Woodbridge: Boydell, 2004), 1–16.
109 Vale, *Henry V*, 243–246, 252; Strong and Strong, "Last Will and Codicils of Henry V," 89–93.
110 *Chronicles of the Revolution 1397–1400*, ed. Chris Given-Wilson (Manchester: Manchester University Press, 1993), 188–189.

Key works

Dixon-Smith, Sally, "The Image and Reality of Alms-Giving in the Great Halls of Henry III," *Journal of the British Archaeological Association* 152 (1999): 79–96.

Green, Judith, "The Piety and Patronage of Henry I," *Haskins Society Journal* 10 (2001): 1–16.

McKendrick, Scot, John Lowden and Kathleen Doyle, eds., with Joanna Frońska and Deirdre Jackson, *Royal Manuscripts: The Genius of Illumination* (London: British Library, 2011).

Ormrod, W. Mark, "The Personal Religion of Edward III," *Speculum* 64 (1989): 849–877.

Vale, Malcolm, *Henry V: The Conscience of a King* (New Haven: Yale University Press, 2016).

Vincent, Nicholas, "The Pilgrimages of the Angevin Kings of England 1154–1272," in *Pilgrimage: The English Experience from Becket to Bunyan*, eds. Colin Morris and Peter Roberts (Cambridge: Cambridge University Press, 2002), 12–45.

10

THE NATION AS A RITUAL COMMUNITY

Royal nation-building in imperial Japan and post-war Thailand

David M. Malitz

Nationalisms can be understood as cultural systems shaped by particular histories which create collective identities through the use of symbols and myths.[1] Monarchy has long been recognized as a potent national symbol linking the present with the past and thus providing a sense of authenticity and continuity. Using Meiji Japan (1868–1912) and post-war Thailand until the fall of the Thanom dictatorship (1946–73) as case studies, it is argued here, however, that apart from being one national symbol among others, monarchy can be a uniquely powerful institution for nation-building and the creation of national identities. As a ritual institution, monarchy can negotiate social complexities and contradictions necessarily present in every imagined community.[2]

The choice of the two cases studies employed here despite the temporal, cultural and historical differences needs some explanation. The point here is not that the two countries shared fundamentally similar experiences during the time periods examined here; neither is it implied that the two 'royal nations' are both the inevitable outcomes of a presupposed cultural homogeneity centred on the monarchy.[3] Rather, and much more modestly, it is proposed that the national and royal hegemonies were the outcome of nation-building projects centred on the monarchies, which occurred against the background of profound socioeconomic and political changes. During the periods explored here, 'modern monarchies' were formed to secure the political allegiance of diverse populations within territories with fixed boundaries, fusing national identity with dynastic loyalty. Furthermore, being well versed in their own ritual traditions, and having studied the modern monarchies of Europe, nation-building elites stressed the importance of ritual for the success of their projects. The two cases can be differentiated from Europe in a twofold manner. First, in contrast to Europe, in neither country had traditionally a legitimate political authority apart from monarchy been known.[4] Second, while in the literature of nationalism studies royalty is often a symbol of 'permanence' and 'authenticity', in the Japanese and Thai cases monarchy became symbols of their nation's authenticity and modernity, proving that the first was reconcilable with the latter.[5]

The focus on two different eras can be explained by the fact that, in contrast to Meiji Japan, it was only from the late 1950s onwards that a Thai royal nation-building programme for the whole country was attempted. In addition, there are structural differences supporting this choice of time frames. Based on the nationalism studies literature, Hans-Ulrich Wehler identifies six factors which determine the success of a national project.[6] The first two are arguably the most fundamental. First, the imagined community's territory needs to be sufficiently integrated through infrastructure. Pre-modern Japan already had a well-developed network of roads which allowed for the reliable circulation of people, goods and ideas.[7] In the second half of the nineteenth century, these roads were accompanied by rail links. By the late 1880s, the main trunk lines were complete.[8] In pre-modern Thailand, in contrast, canals and rivers were the main form of transportation, which made travel to the outlying regions arduous and lengthy. A rail connection to the second-largest city of Chiang Mai was only completed in 1921.[9] Investment in highways began in earnest in the 1930s but accelerated in the 1950s through US aid.[10] Second, for a majority of a population to embrace a national identity, they have to be literate. Due to a well-established network of temple schools, literacy rates in pre-Meiji Japan were relatively high and have been estimated at 40 to 50% for men and 15% for women. Compulsory education was introduced in 1872. By the end of Emperor's Meiji reign, approximately 90% of all children received a primary education.[11] The late nineteenth century also saw the beginnings of modern education in Thailand; nonetheless, the expansion of the system progressed much more slowly than in Japan.[12] US state agencies estimated a literacy rate of 30 to 40% for Thailand in 1953.[13]

These nation-building projects were not conducted in free marketplaces of ideas, but rather against the background of state repression. To explain their success and durability by repression alone, however, rejects the audiences' agency and would thus be far from convincing. After all, these projects were undertaken to support the building of modern and centralized states rather than to legitimize existing strong states.

Monarchy's multifaceted symbolism and ritual

Nations are necessarily marred by contradictions. They are imagined to be culturally homogeneous communities of members of equal standing. Yet, their culturally diverse populations are vastly unequal in economic and political power. National identity provides a sense of belonging and continuity. Yet, it has been long noted that it depends on reinterpretations and selective remembrance. Arguably, such contradictions are most glaring in periods of nation-building. These contradictions between the imagined and the real society cannot be solved. They can, however, be managed by symbolic politics and ritual.

Political symbols derive their power from their ambiguity. Different groups can interpret them differently at the same time or the same individuals can interpret them differently at different times. Nevertheless, because of their singular nature, they appear to offer a unified perspective.[14] This is also the case for monarchy. A case implicitly made in the famous discussion of the British monarchy by Walter Bagehot, here read together with an introduction and summary by Arthur J. Balfour, the First Earl of Balfour. In the texts, the monarchy is seen as instrumental in creating a sense of 'unity and continuity' as a necessary foundation for patriotic sentiment and for strengthening the government. As a reading of both texts shows, this capacity rests on the institution's multifaceted symbolism, which merges different, if not polar opposite, meanings in the royal body. The monarch symbolizes both a united and a diverse nation; a nation which is both ancient and modern.[15]

Ritual plays a very minor role for Bagehot and Balfour. For Bagehot, spectacle is simply a necessary distraction for his less-educated compatriots.[16] Balfour mentions 'great ceremonial occasions' but does not link them to his further discussions.[17] Here ritual is understood as central to the monarchy's ability to negotiate between its multifaceted meanings, for it is a quintessentially ritual institution. One becomes monarch through ritual and must subsequently maintain this status through its continuous performance.[18] Furthermore, kingship is a relational institution, and it is through ritual that relationships are formed, negotiated and maintained.[19]

Insights from the field of cognitive studies shed light on how ritual can reconcile different, if not opposite, meanings.[20] Over time, participation in repetitive yet low-intensity rituals, such as those performed on national holidays, are not remembered as specific episodes. Rather, participants remember general roles and ideas within repetitive performances. This allows strangers to identify as members of a common imagined community and fosters mutual trust and cooperation. At the same time, it also reduces the reflective engagement with the meaning of the rituals as well as associated doctrines.

The Meiji Restoration and the making of modern Japan

In early January 1868, over 250 years of rule by the Tokugawa clan came to an end in Japan. Members of the court nobility, supported by feudal lords from the western domains of Satsuma and Choshu as well as low-ranking samurai, had taken control of the young Emperor Meiji and had him declare the restoration of imperial rule.[21] There were several reasons why this palace coup could usher in the sociopolitical revolution, as the Meiji Restoration would become known. Tokugawa Japan had been a feudal polity. The lords of the approximately 200 feudal domains were vassals of the shogun, demonstrating their loyalty through rites of submission.[22] Since the twelfth century, the title of *shogun* was acquired through investiture by the emperor, but for the Tokugawa this was only one of several sources of legitimacy. It rested additionally on a combination of conceptions derived from the Chinese classics, Buddhism and indigenous ideas.[23] From the mid-seventeenth century onwards, however, an increasingly influential scholarly tradition had emerged, which merged Confucian political ideals with the *kokutai*-myth. According to this myth, Japan was unique and superior to all other countries because of the rule by an unbroken line of emperors, who descended from the sun goddess herself.[24] Against the background of a social and economic crisis, which worsened after the integration of Japan into the global economy through a series of unequal treaties from 1854 onwards, attacks on the Tokugawas' legitimacy increased with arguments derived from this discourse. In 1863, the penultimate Tokugawa *shogun* travelled himself to the emperor to petition him for support and thus publicly accepting the latter's higher authority, setting the stage for the coup six years later.[25]

By mid-1869, the new political elite had defeated the last Tokugawa forces and had gained international recognition.[26] In the following years, the modernizers within the restoration alliance quickly asserted themselves and embarked on an ambitious modernizing project. A general agreement existed among the restoration leaders regarding the need to 'capture the people's hearts' and provide legitimacy for the state for the success of their project.[27] There was also an agreement that only the emperor was available to serve in this function, because Buddhism had been discredited for its having been crucial in Tokugawa rule.[28] Furthermore, of course, the emperor had been the unifying symbol of the movement supporting the takeover.

In reality, however, in the mid-nineteenth century, the role and function of the emperor was not widely known or he was considered an otherworldly being.[29] At first, an attempt was made to create a state-religion around the veneration of the emperor and to convert the people to this new faith.[30] In this process, an often violent separation of the veneration of indigenous deities from Buddhism took place in the cultic centres on which Japanese religious life had concentrated and where indigenous deities had been interpreted as local manifestations of Bodhisattvas.[31] Buddhist rituals in the imperial palace were discontinued and new ones introduced.[32] Within a couple of years, however, it became obvious that this endeavour was fruitless. The missionaries, who had been sent out to teach the population about the new imperial cult, could not compete with experienced Buddhist preachers. Neither was there a consensus among shrine priests on their teachings.[33] Importantly, it was also realized that the renegotiation of the unequal treaties depended on the granting of the freedom of religion.[34]

What captured the 'people's hearts' and served as the state's legitimization in everyday life was a ritual system that had in essence been assembled around the year 1891 rather than a state religion. In this system, Emperor Meiji served as both a modern and constitutional monarch equal to his European peers as well as the embodiment of the *kokutai*-myth.[35] This ritual system thus included modern national pageantries comparable to those of the European modern monarchies, studied by high-ranking missions to Europe.[36] By the end of the reign of Emperor Meiji in 1912, the loosely integrated feudal polity of the Tokugawa had become an industrializing nation-state and constitutional monarchy at the centre of a colonial empire. New treaties negotiated with the colonial powers had confirmed the empire's equal standing with them.[37] As the feline narrator in one of the most famous novels of Meiji Japan recounted, the reign of Emperor Meiji was both an 'enlightened' one in which Japan was an ally of the British Empire and the health benefits of swimming in the sea were known, and a time in which 'traditional ways' were still observed.[38]

The revival of the Thai monarchy after World War II

Nearly simultaneously with Japan, the Kingdom of Siam signed the first of a series of unequal treaties, the 1855 Bowring Treaty, with Great Britain. The economic changes resulting from the integration into the global economy allowed King Chulalongkorn (1853–1910, r. since 1868) to embark on a project to build a modern state and an absolute monarchy from the 1870s onwards.[39] Traditional Siam had been a ritual polity, as is evident in the contents of the Palace Law that stipulated the working of the traditional power centre, the Royal Palace. Roughly a quarter of the law's stipulations cover the various ceremonies performed by the king over the year.[40] Through these ceremonies and the additional performance of roles derived from the Theravada-Buddhist tradition, kings demonstrated their royal status and legitimacy.[41] In the reign of King Chulalongkorn, the annual ceremonies, which he described in writing, were complemented by modern state pageantries similar to those performed by his European royal peers or Emperor Meiji in Japan as heads of modern nation-states.[42]

His sons and successors King Vajiravudh (1880–1925, r. since 1910) and King Prajadhipok (1893–1941, r.1925–35) continued the royal modernization project. Faced with a growing and increasingly critical urban bourgeoisie, they additionally attempted to shore up their legitimacy by introducing a royal nationalism rather than making political concessions. The state and nation-building project was still ongoing, when in June 1932 a group of young officers and bureaucrats, who called themselves the People's Party, overthrew the absolute monarchy through the country's first successful coup d'état.[43]

The new ruling elite embarked on their own nation and state-building project. For the first time, attempts were made to integrate the whole nation through roads and the offer of primary education to all. Once firmly in power, however, a struggle ensued between the civilian faction under Pridi Banomyong (1900–83) and the military factions under Phibun Songkhram (1897–1964), which was decided by the military wing in their favour.[44] Phibun launched a nation-building project that attempted to make the kingdom's population both culturally homogeneous and civilized according to western norms. Ethnic minorities had no space in this conception of the nation. At the same time, it attempted to reduce the role of the monarchy to a minimum.[45] This was supported by the fact that King Prajadhipok had abdicated in 1935 and the new king Ananda (1925–46, r. since 1935) was a minor residing in Switzerland with his family.[46]

During World War II, the Phibun government aligned themselves with imperial Japan. This alliance allowed for a rapprochement between the civilian wing of the People's Party and royalists in Thailand as well as abroad. Supported by Great Britain and the United States, this alliance pushed Phibun out of office – the summer of 1944.[47] The first free elections under universal suffrage revealed in 1946 that conservatives and royalists stood no chance against the progressives under Pridi, ending the war-time alliance. Following a campaign accusing the government of corruption as well as of being involved in the mysterious death by gunshot of King Ananda in his bedchamber in June 1946, a coup was conducted in 1947. Shortly afterwards, Phibun assumed the premiership once again.[48] Presenting himself as a staunch anti-Communist, he could gain recognition as well as material and political support from the United States.[49]

In 1951, King Bhumibol, King Ananda's younger brother, returned from his studies in Switzerland. Phibun continued to reduce the public role of the monarchy by restricting the king's movements, limiting palace funds and attempting to take over royal functions such as the sponsoring of temple renovations or officiating at the ceremonies for the 1957 Buddhist centennial.[50]

Nevertheless, during the 1950s, a new 'royalist hegemony' emerged through the publication of newspaper articles, historical works and novels by royalist intellectuals.[51] Phibun could not suppress these works, because the coup that had brought him back to power had cited the need to protect the monarchy. By this time, the monarchy had also gained the support of the US government, who had come to believe that its appeal was crucial to prevent a communist takeover of the country.[52]

Phibun was overthrown the way he had come to power, when in 1957 then army chief General Sarit Thanarat conducted a successful coup. The general knew that he was not widely supported beyond his narrow army base, and that he was viewed with suspicion by the United States due to his ownership of newspapers that had been critical of US policies in Southeast Asia.[53] Sarit thus needed a source of legitimacy that appealed to Thais as well as to the United States. By the late 1950s, it had become clear that only the monarchy could achieve this. The Sarit years and the years of his successor, Thanom Kittikachorn, saw massive efforts to 'develop' Thailand with the support of the United States and through the encouragement of foreign investment. Similar to Meiji Japan, during these years both modernity, as development, was pursued, and an ostensibly authentic national identity centred on the monarchy shaped.[54]

The imagined as ritual communities

The *English Constitution* with its discussion of the British monarchy's multifaceted symbolism was known in both Meiji Japan and post-war Thailand. The liberal writer, educator and entrepreneur Fukuzawa Yukichi's (1835–1901) *On the Imperial House* envisaged not only a role for the Japanese emperor, which was essentially similar to that described by Bagehot, but also quoted the work directly.[55] The Meiji leaders, however, would rely more on Prussia as a model.[56] This is not to say, however, that the nation and state-building elites in either case depended on foreign sources for understanding the efficiency of royal symbols and ritual for political integration and social cohesion. For Shimazono Susume, the ritual system of Meiji Japan was an adaptation of the 'unity of rites and rule', which had been propagated in the widely read *New Theses* (1825) of samurai-scholar Aizawa Seishisei (1781–1863).[57] This work was so widely read and influential that it is commonly referred to as the 'bible' of the restoration activists.[58]

The *New Theses* proposed a 'long-range policy' to create a harmonious Japanese society through the 'unity of rites and rule' and thus strengthen Japan against the colonial powers whose ships were increasingly coming to Japanese shores. The foreign 'barbarians' did not so much pose a threat due to their superior military technology, but due to Christianity's ability to subvert the 'stupid commoners'.[59] To prevent this, the people had to be united in spirit and in their veneration of the emperor. Looking for guidance to the golden ages of the ancestral deity of the imperial house, 'sage emperors' and also to the Chinese classics, Aizawa offered a blueprint for the building of a hierarchical yet harmonious community. The living symbol of the emperor and ritual are central to this work. *Shinron* stresses the importance of the emperor performing rites in public as a 'living exemplar', arguing that such a ritual system was vastly superior in creating social cohesion in comparison to 'explanation or exhortation'.[60]

The British-educated nobility of Thailand were also aware of Bagehot. The private letters as well as memorandum written to the young King Bhumibol in 1947 by Prince Subha Svasti (1900–67) reveal, through their choice of wording, that the *English Constitution* was well read in court circles.[61] One of the royalist intellectuals who resurrected the monarchy in post-war Thailand was Prince Dhani Nivat (hereafter, Prince Dhani, 1885–1974). As a nephew of King Chulalongkorn, he had lived in the palace as a child and gained an intimate knowledge of the royal ceremonies, before receiving an elite education in Britain.[62] Upon his return, the prince first entered the Ministry of the Interior and later became Minister of Education. He lived a private life after the revolution but rose to prominence after World War II when he became regent for King Bhumibol, and then a member and later president of the Privy Council. He also served as the tutor of King Bhumibol in cultural regards.[63] A lecture given by Prince Dhani on the 'Siamese conception of the Monarchy' in 1946 marked the beginning of the revival as well as Prince Dhani's influence in it.[64] This lecture read together with other writings by the prince offers insights into his conception of the Thai monarchy and nation, and thus of the underlying assumptions of the royalist revival.

Prince Dhani emphasized the performative and ritual nature of kingship. Its authority in the past had rested on being instinctively embraced rather than understood, as its ideals had been 'ever kept before the public eye in literature, in sermons, and in any other channel of publicity'.[65] For him the monarchy was the political, social and moral 'nucleus' of the Thai nation understood as a community of 'individuals bound together by their loyalty to the sovereign'.[66] One can argue that this conception of the Thai nation is a projection of the realm of the *cakkavatti*-king upon the national territory. This ideal Buddhist monarch ruling the whole world is described in detail in the thirteenth-century cosmology of the 'three worlds', which can be considered the 'foundation of Thai political thought'.[67] Pre-modern Thai kings directly claimed this status in chronicles, letters and through ritual performances. All the world's rulers submit to the *cakkavatti*, overawed by his virtue, but are reinstated subsequently.[68] Without doubt, conservatives, who revived the Thai monarchy in the 1950s, also knew the *Royal Rites of the Twelve Months*: the inventory of royal ceremonies written by King Chulalongkorn himself. The king stressed in the introduction that these rituals served to foster social cohesion among participants, but that they were also worthwhile to maintain as 'traditions of the country'.[69]

Taking possession of the realm

The Meiji leaders shared the post-war Thai royalists' performative view of kingship, as well as the conviction that for the monarchies to become foundation stones for national identities able to provide the states with legitimacy, first and foremost, the monarchs had to be seen reigning by their subjects. For this reason, the very month after the restoration of imperial rule, Okubo Toshimichi (1830–78), one of the new political leaders, advised that Emperor Meiji had to come out from the 'jewelled curtains'.[70] During the first two decades of his reign, the emperor traversed his realm inspecting it, but also showing himself to the local residents. For the sociologist Ozawa Masachi, it was precisely through the local receptions of the travelling emperor that Japanese could imagine the communities that they experienced in daily life were part of a larger national community.[71] From the late 1880s the imperial progresses were replaced by grand state ceremonies in Tokyo as the main form of imperial pageantry. By this time, however, a hierarchy of national shrines had been established at which rites were conducted at the same time as those undertaken at the palace sanctuary in Tokyo. National time was ordered by national holidays making the nation indeed a ritual community.[72] Furthermore, the country's schools became central ritual spaces for the imperial cult. In 1890, the Imperial Rescript on Education was issued demanding loyalty and filial devotion from all students. The Rescript was held to be sacrosanct and was ceremonially read on holidays. By 1897, all schools had an official imperial portrait.[73] At the same time, however, Article 28 of the 1889 constitution of imperial Japan granted the 'freedom of religious belief' as long as that was not 'antagonistic to their duties as subjects', such as participating in rites in schools and at state shrines not considered to be religious.

In post-war Thailand, royalists who wished to revive the monarchy also saw the need for King Bhumibol to travel beyond the vicinity of the capital to be seen by his subjects.[74] This became possible only through the support of the United States. By 1953, Washington had become convinced that to prevent communist subversion, the traditional institution of the monarchy had to be both relied upon and reinvigorated.[75] The area of most concern was the impoverished north-eastern region of Isan: the ethnic Lao inhabiting the region were known to have strongly supported the Pridi government and were generally treated with contempt by officials of the state and the Thais of Bangkok.[76] US pressure forced the Phibun government to allow the king to travel this region as a nation-building effort in 1955. This was the first time since the revolution that a king had travelled beyond the immediate vicinity of the capital and the first time that a king of the reigning dynasty had visited this region.[77] The visit proved that in the countryside the traditional prestige of the Buddhist monarchy had not diminished over the quarter century that had passed since the revolution. Local residents were willing to travel large distances to see the king themselves. This enthusiastic reception by the population quickly convinced the government, however, not to support any further journeys due to Phibun's fear of being overthrown.[78] Following Sarit's coup in 1957, however, the king travelled widely throughout Thailand visiting all of Thai provinces.[79] Also, from the mid-1950s onwards, the royal portrait was distributed nationally with the support of the United States Information Service.[80] It not only became a prominent feature of the Thai geobody but also featured prominently during ceremonies in the now rapidly expanding school system.[81] From 1966 onwards, King Bhumpol additionally began to bestow Buddha images consecrated by himself to all provinces.[82]

Virtue, authenticity and modernity

The ability of monarchs to bind together a nation's various social groups derives not from ritual performance alone, as Bagehot had already noted; but rather, they have to be embodiments of virtue. For Japan and Thailand, where modernization necessarily meant the adoption of western practices, this was closely related to the embodiment of national authenticity.

Aizawa had stressed the importance of public imperial ritual for the legitimacy of imperial rule and the people's embrace of the dual virtues of filial devotion and imperial loyalty.[83] In this vein, Emperor Meiji began shortly from the restoration onwards to embody the myth of his divine descent and demonstrate his virtue publicly. Travelling from the former imperial residence of Kyoto to the new capital of Tokyo in 1868, he thus visited the sun goddess's shrine in Ise.[84] During his later progresses through the realm, the emperor would – without fail – visit other important shrines and pay homage to his ancestors and imperial loyalists of the past. In Tokyo, he would discharge daily ritual duties in the palace sanctuary. Through schooling and newspaper reporting, the emperor's subjects were consistently made aware of this discharge of his ritual and state obligations and thus exhorted to do the same with their own. According to a biographer, Emperor Meiji did indeed embrace and discharge his duties faithfully.[85] This served not only to sanctify imperial rule but also provided the emerging national community as a whole with a unique and superior collective identity.

The Meiji leaders recognized that in addition to embodying an authentic Japan, Emperor Meiji also had to become a modern monarch for colonial powers to accept Japan as an equal. From 1872, the emperor would only appear in western uniform in public, and he would also discharge the duties of a modern head of state.[86] In rapidly modernizing Meiji Japan, the emperor as head of state became increasingly the embodiment of a modern nation.[87] The renegotiation of the unequal treaties in the 1890s, the Anglo Japanese Alliance between the two monarchies and the victories that the imperial army gained with Emperor Meiji as the nominal commander-in-chief, confirmed Japanese equality with the west. In an article published after the emperor's death in 1912, his lifetime was explicitly associated with the progress of 'western civilization' in his realm.[88]

Prince Dhani's 1946 lecture on Thai kingship had pointed out the importance of the embodiment of Buddhist virtues for the legitimacy of the monarchy.[89] However, Phibun government's restriction on royal activities initially hindered such a dual embodiment of virtue and authenticity by King Bhumibol. One activity shaping the public perception of King Bhumibol as a virtuous monarch from early on in his reign was charitable giving.[90] In particular, royal charities related to agricultural development are of interest due to their multifaceted symbolism. First, they were, of course, an expression of the Buddhist virtue of charity, but they also emphasized the king's mastery of 'food organization': a traditional field of royal knowledge.[91] Simultaneously, these agricultural development projects could be seen as modern adaptations of the traditional royal duty to promote the fertility of the realm, as one of the king's daughters has related.[92]

In 1956, the king entered the monkhood following the death of his grandmother, Queen Saovabha. The ordination was highly symbolic: his grandmother had been Queen to King Chulalongkorn and he stayed, as monk, in the very room his great-grandfather had resided in for twenty-seven years as a monk.[93] After 1957, the court was once again the centre of traditional and religious life through the restoration of royal pageantries of the past and the inventions of new traditions.[94] New holidays and the redefinition of existing ones cemented the function of the monarchy as the central temporal axis of national time into daily life.[95] A memorandum prepared for President Johnson prior to a meeting with King Bhumibol in 1967 explicitly pointed out that the 'King [was] deeply revered and as a person [was] highly admired for his exemplary personal life'.[96] The revival of the monarchy and its ceremonies was not aimed at resurrecting a golden past in its entirety. As Prince Dhani related in interviews, he not only considered his view of an authentic Thai culture to be reconcilable with modernity but also saw it as a necessary foundation for modernization.[97] As it has been with authenticity and virtue, modernity was also symbolized by the Thai monarchy from the 1950s onwards. Through weekly jazz concerts as well as through photos and movies of the royal family, the king was a symbol of a modern and cosmopolitan Thailand. The monarchy could thus connect to the very urban bourgeoisie who had supported the 1932 revolution.[98]

Recognition as an equal member of the international society had been a major goal of the kingdom's foreign policy since the nineteenth century. After 1957, King

Bhumibol travelled not only domestically but also received foreign heads of state in Bangkok. He also travelled internationally, where he was received with the full diplomatic honours of a foreign head of state. The positive press coverage of these trips not only presented the regime at home in a much better light than Sarit could have hoped to achieve but was also a source of much domestic pride.[99] As an observer noted in the early 1970s on this embodiment of both authenticity and modernity, 'neither the traditionalists can find argument against the constitutional monarch nor can the modernists complain about a lack of flexibility and openness to new ideas'.[100]

National and local identities

The royal nation-building projects were seen as necessary, precisely because the populations of Japan and Thailand were not viewed as homogeneous. Arguably, an important similarity between the two cases is that the royal symbolism and ritual allowed for a certain degree of negotiation between national and local identities rather than simply negating the latter.

Aizawa did not assume in his work that a homogeneous Japanese people had always existed. He recounted a history of conquests and subsequent integration of 'barbarians' into a centralized political structure through ritual.[101] Accordingly, the ritual system described is also not homogeneous. Political integration was achieved through the integration of rites for local ancestral and tutelary deities into the overall ritual system.[102] The same can be said for the ritual landscape that began to emerge after the Meiji restoration. Of course, national holidays were celebrated nation-wide in state-shrines; yet, each and every one of these shrines was unique. The enshrined imperial ancestors and loyalists had also local significance, and the festivals celebrated by their shrines proved the important role of the specific place and its people in the nation and thus confirmed both national and local identities.[103]

In Thailand, the realm of the *cakkavatti* had also been understood to be a diverse one, which was held together through submission to the virtuous ruler. Prince Dhani's view of the Thai nation reflects this understanding, as does King Chulalongkorn's description of royal ceremonies. Chinese immigrants had been a growing and economically important minority since the foundation of Bangkok. King Chulalongkorn included a Chinese New Year ceremony in his list of royal rites.[104] In a similar vein, links between the urban bourgeoisie, who were very often of Chinese descent or immigrants themselves, and the monarchy were created from early on in King Bhumibol's reign. Through their participation in royal charity through donations, they were symbolically integrated into the Thai nation, and the king also sponsored marriages and handed out diplomas for university graduates.[105] In a 1969 novel about a family of Chinese immigrants in Bangkok, becoming Thai means having a Thai education, being a Thai citizen and being a subject of the king of Thailand.[106]

The connections between the king and distinct geographic regions of the kingdom was symbolized though the construction of royal palaces in those regions from 1959 onwards. The royal couple rotated around these residences, travelling at least eight months per year outside of the capital working on development projects.[107] For the anthropologist Charles Keyes who has studied Isan since the 1960s, these bonds created between the king and the region's inhabitants proved to be crucial to its successful integration into the Thai nation-state. The people of Isan could think of themselves as ethnic Lao as well as Thai citizens by virtue of being subjects of a Thai king.[108]

Much less successful was the integration of the population of the southernmost provinces where ethnic ethnic Malay Muslims were a two-fold minority: a long-running insurgence has intensified since 2004. Yet, there is evidence that conceiving of oneself as a subject of a virtuous monarch and patron of Islam made it possible to engage with a state perceived as oppressive and despite rejecting a Thai national identity.[109]

Order and hierarchy

To be Japanese or Thai became to mean, first of all, to be equally a subject of the respective monarchs. Unsurprisingly, this did not mean that all subjects or social groups were equals among themselves.

During Emperor Meiji's progresses, it was first of all the local notables who had direct access to the visiting monarch, which in turn confirmed their status in their communities.[110] A new nobility was created in 1869 merging the previous distinct estates of the court nobility and feudal lords, but also permitting successful and loyal entrepreneurs and bureaucrats. This social hierarchy reflected in physical close-ness to the emperor was, due to the emperor's association with virtue, authenticity and modernity, not only a legitimate one but also a moral one.[111] The hierarchical conception of Thai society with the monarchy at its apex was similarly evident in ritual clearly marking status differences.[112] As such, to move up in the social hier-archy meant to move physically closer to the king and, therefore, closer to society's virtuous centre.[113] Certain groups developed closer ties to the monarchs. In both imperial Japan and post-war Thailand, to the present day, this has been the case for the military. The armed forces are first of all protectors of the monarchy sworn to defend the institution. This special relationship between monarch and military was expressed through royal/ imperial symbolism and ritual, and resulted practically in a lack of civilian control over the armed forces. Due to this visible special relation-ship, the militaries could claim to partake in the virtue embodied in the monarchies and claim a special political role – in the case of Thailand until the present day.[114]

Conclusion

Today, Japan and Thailand can be seen as royal nations par excellence, where the monarchies form the symbolic core of the respective dominant nationalist dis-courses. Yet, at the time of the Meiji Restoration in 1868, the emperor was little known in Japan. While in Thailand, when King Bhumibol returned in 1951, the kingdom had not had a resident king for nearly two decades, and the governments since the overthrow of the absolute monarchy had vastly reduced the public role of the institution. Therefore, rather than always having been unifying symbols, the roy-al-and-imperial hegemonies must be understood as the outcome of nation-building projects centred on the monarchies. In Meiji Japan and during the years of the Sarit and Thanom dictatorships in Thailand, simultaneously, modernity was pursued and what was perceived to be national authenticity revived. It has been argued here that the success of this royal nation-building was, in part, a result of the symbolic and ritual nature of monarchy.

As symbolic and ritual institutions, the monarchies proved to be uniquely well equipped to negotiate between the contradictions among the imagined communities and their social realities. It was through imperial/royal ceremonies that individuals could view themselves as members of both an observable local community and a much larger national community that could only be imagined. Through ritual the monarchs could build ties between the court and various social groups that were nevertheless all members of the royal/imperial nation. As embodiments of virtue, the social orders centred on them became sanctified by them. Moreover, through their performance of the dual roles of heads-of-states of modern nations and embodiments of national authenticity, the monarchs demonstrated that traditions and modernity were indeed reconcilable and that their nations were equal members of the international communities.

Notes

1 George L. Mosse, *Die Nationalisierung der Massen: Von den Befreiungskriegen bis zum Dritten Reich* (Frankfurt: Ullstein, 1976), 14–28.
2 Regarding the management of social complexity through ritual, see Adam B. Seligman et al., *Ritual and its Consequences: An Essay on the Limits of Sincerity* (New York: Oxford University Press, 2008), 10–14, 20.
3 For the terms 'royal nation' and 'modern monarchy', see Milinda Banerjee, Charlotte Backerra and Cathleen Sarti, eds., "Introduction," in *Transnational Histories of the 'Royal Nation'* (Basingstoke: Palgrave Macmillan, 2017). For examples of assumptions of cultural homogeneity centred on the monarchy in Japan and Thailand, see Stein Tønnesson and Hans Antlöv, eds., "Asia in Theories of Nationalism and National Identity," in *Asian Forms of the Nation* (Richmond: Curzon, 1996), 20; Anthony D. Smith, *Nationalism: Theory, Ideology, History* (Cambridge: Polity, 2001), 113.
4 Eric Nelson, *The Hebrew Republic: Jewish Sources and the Transformation of European Political Thought* (Cambridge: Harvard University Press, 2010), 3; Hans-Ulrich Wehler, *Nationalismus: Geschichte, Formen, Folgen* (Munich: C.H. Beck, 2007), 27–28.
5 David Cannadine, "The Context, Performance and Meaning of Ritual: The British Monarchy and the 'Invention of Tradition', c. 1820–1977," in *The Invention of Tradition*, eds. Eric Hobsbawm and Terrance Ranger (Cambridge: Cambridge University Press, 2010), 122; Prasenjit Duara, *Sovereignity and Authenticity: Manchukuo and the East Asian Modern* (Lanham: Rowman, 2004), 31.
6 Wehler, *Nationalism*, 45–47.
7 Constantine N. Vaporis, "Linking the Realm: The Gokaidô Highway Network in Early Modern Japan (1603–1868)," in *Highways, Byways, and Road Systems in the Pre-Modern World*, eds. Susan E. Alcock et al. (Chichester: John Wiley & Sons, 2012): 90–95, 100–101.
8 Osawa Masachi, *Kindai Nihon no nashonarizumu* (Tokyo: Kodansha, 2011), 62.
9 Roel Ramaer, *The Railways of Thailand* (Bangkok: White Lotus Press, 1994), 10.
10 Chris Dixon, *The Thai Economy: Uneven Development and Internationalisation* (London: Routledge, 1999), 36–37.
11 Saito Yasuo, "Shikiji noryoku, shikiji ritsu no rekishiteki suii: Nihon no keiken," in *Journal of International Cooperation in Education* 15, no. 1 (2012): 53–56.
12 Nigel J. Brailey, *Thailand and the Fall of Singapore: A Frustrated Asian Revolution* (Boulder: Westview Press, 1986), 72.
13 CIA Records Search Tool, CIA-RDP80R01731R000700450029-9, *Proposed Revision by Department of State PSB D–20*, 24 July 1953, 10.
14 Murray Edelman, *Politics as Symbolic Action: Mass Arousal and Quiescence* (New York: Academic Press, 1971), 6–7, 16.
15 Walter Bagehot, *The English Constitution* (London: Oxford University Press, 1928), 40–41, 47. Arthur J. Balfour, "Introduction," in *The English Constitution, Walter Bagehot* (London: Oxford University Press, 1928), xx, xxv–xxvi.
16 Bagehot, *Constitution*, 34–35, 41.

17 Balfour, *Introduction*, xiii.
18 Declan Quigley, "Introduction: The Character of Kingship," in *The Character of Kingship,* ed. Declan Quigley (New York: Berg, 2005), 3–6.
19 Lynette Mitchell and Charles Melville, eds., "Every Inch a King: Kings and Kingship in the Ancient and Medieval Worlds," in *Every Inch a King: Comparative Studies on Kings and Kingship in the Ancient and Medieval Worlds* (Leiden and Boston: Brill, 2013), 12; Catherine Bell, *Ritual: Perspectives and Dimensions* (New York: Oxford University Press, 1997), 82–83.
20 Harvey Whitehouse, "Ritual, Cognition, and Evolution," in *Grounding the Social Sciences in Cognitive Sciences,* ed. Ron Sun (Cambridge and London: MIT Press, 2012), 274–275.
21 Andrew Gordon, *A Modern History of Japan: From Tokugawa Times to the Present* (New York: Oxford University Press, 2003), 58.
22 ibid., 11–19. On the ritual aspects of the Tokugawa-polity, see Luke S. Roberts, *Performing the Great Peace: Political Space and Open Secrets in Tokugawa Japan* (Honolulu: Hawaii University Press, 2015).
23 Watanabe Hiroshi, *Nihon seiji-shisoshi: 17–19 seiki* (Tokyo: Tokyo Daigaku Shuppankai, 2010), 55–68.
24 Klaus Antoni, *Shintô und die Konzeption des japanischen Nationalwesens (Kokutai): Der religiöse Traditionalismus in Neuzeit und Moderne Japans* (Leiden: Brill, 1998), 131–173.
25 On the end of the Tokugawa polity, see Gordon, *History of Japan,* 46–59.
26 Gordon, *History of Japan,* 59.
27 Trent E. Maxey, *The "Greatest Problem": Religion and State Formation in Meiji Japan* (Cambridge: Harvard University Press, 2014), 10.
28 Joseph Pittau, *Political Thought in Early Meiji Japan 1868–1889* (Cambridge: Harvard University Press, 1967), 177–178.
29 Takashi Fujitani, Splendid Monarchy: Power and Pageantry in Modern Japan (Berkeley: University of California Press, 1998), 7–9.
30 Helen Hardacre, *Shintō and the State, 1868–1988* (Princeton: Princeton University Press, 1991), 42.
31 Allan G. Grapard, *The Protocol of the Gods: A Study of the Kasuga Cult in Japanese History* (Berkeley: University of California Press, 1992), 3–11, 248–251.
32 Fabio Rambelli, "The Emperor's New Robes: Processes of Resignification in Shingon Imperial Rituals," in *Cahiers d'Extrême Asie* 13, no. 1 (2002): 428.
33 Hardacare, *Shintō*, 45–51.
34 Hardacare, *Shintō*, 31.
35 John Breen, *Reigi to kenryoku: Tenno no Meiji Ishin* (Tokyo: Heibonsha, 2011), 34–39.
36 Ian Nish, "Introduction," in *Japan Rising: The Iwakura Embassy to the USA and Europe 1871– 1873, Kume Kunitake,* compiled by Kunitake Kume, eds. Chushichi Tsuzuki and R. Jules Young (Cambridge: Cambridge University Press, 2009), xxiv.
37 Gordon, *History of Japan,* 78, 94, 119–121.
38 Natsume Soseki, *I am a Cat* (Clarendon: Tuttle, 2002), 226, 309, 455.
39 Chris Baker and Pasuk Phongpaichit, *A History of Thailand* (Cambridge: Cambridge University Press, 2009), 45–58.
40 Chris Baker and Pasuk Phongpaichit, *The Palace Law of Ayutthaya and the Thammasat: Law and Kingship in Siam* (Ithaca: Southeast Asia Program, Cornell University, 2016), 51, 58.
41 Stanley J. Tambiah, *World Conqueror and World Renouncer* (Cambridge: Cambridge University Press, 1977), 73.
42 Maurizio Peleggi, *Lords of Things: The Fashioning of the Siamese Monarchy's Modern Image* (Honolulu: University of Hawaii Press, 2002), 113–114.
43 Baker and Phongpaichit, *History of Thailand,* 105–119.
44 Ibid., 121–125.
45 Ibid., 125–135.
46 Ibid., 121.
47 Sorasak Ngamcachonkulkid, *Free Thai: The New History of the Seri Thai Movement* (Bangkok: Institute of Asian Studies, Chulalongkorn University, 2010), 21–26.
48 Ngamcachonkulkid, *Free Thai,* 172–187.

49 Daniel Fineman, *A Special Relationship: The United States and Military Government in Thailand, 1947–1958* (Honolulu: University of Hawaii Press), 20–63.

50 Kobkua Suwannathat-Pian, *Thailand's Durable Premier: Phibun Through Three Decades 1932–1957* (Kuala Lumpur: Oxford University Press, 1995), 140–144.

51 Prin Tepnarin, "Kan kotua khong udomkan Racha-chatniyom 2490–2510," *Warasan Thammasat* 32, no. 1 (2013): 3–4.

52 Natthaphon Chaiching, *Kho fan fai nai fan an lueachuea khwamkhlueanwai khong khabuan-kan patipak patiwat Sayam* (Phoso 2475–2500) (Nothaburi: Fadiaokan, 2013), 315.

53 Fineman, *Relationship*, 233–257.

54 It is interesting to note that the Thai intellectual and politician Wichit Wathakan, who was an influential adviser of Sarit Thanarat, had seen imperial Japan has an exemplar for a constitutional Thai monarchy in the 1930s, see David M. Malitz, *Japanese-Siamese Relations: From the Meiji Restoration to the End of World War II* (Bochum: ProjektVerlag, 2016), 308–312.

55 Fukuzawa Yukichi, *Teishitsuron* (Tokyo: Maruzen, 1882), 64.

56 Gordon, *History of Japan*, 85.

57 Shimazono Susumu, *Kokka shinto to Nihonjin* (Iwanami: Tokyo, 2010), ii–iv, vii, 7–8; Aizawa Seishisai, "New Theses," in *Anti-Foreignism and Western Learning in Early-Modern Japan: The New Theses of 1825*, ed. Bob T. Wakabayashi (Harvard University Press: Cambridge, 1991).

58 For example, see Shimazono, *Kokka shinto*, 113.

59 Aizawa, *Shinron*, 202, 211–212, 245.

60 Aizawa, *Shinron*, 252–268.

61 Prince Subha Svasti, *1 satawat Supphasawat, 23 Singhakhom 2543* (Bangkok: Amarin, 2000), 495, 537, 558.

62 Prince Dhani Nivat, *Chet rop ayu Krommuen Phithayalap Pharuethiyakon* (Bangkok: Rongphim Phrachan, 1969), 4–5.

63 Sulak Sivaraksa, "'The Last of the Princes': A Centennial Reflection on the Life and Work of Prince Dhani-Nivat Kromamun Bidyalabh," *Journal of the Siam Society* 74 (1986): 158–163; Baker and Phongpaichit, *History of Thailand*, 105–119, 296–297.

64 This lecture was subsequently published, see Prince Dhani Nivat, "The Old Siamese Conception of the Monarchy," *Journal of the Siam Society*, 36 (1946): 91–106.

65 Prince Dhani, *Conception of the Monarchy*, 103.

66 Prince Dhani Nivat, "The Reconstruction of Rama I of the Chakri Dynasty," *Journal of the Siam Society* 43, no. 1 (1955): 22. See also Prince Dhani, *Chet rop ayu*, 85–91.

67 Chonthira Klatyu, *Traiphum Phraruang: Rakthan khong udomkan kanmueang Thai, Warasan Thammasat* 4, no. 1 (1974): 104, 109.

68 Frank E. and Mani B. Reynolds, *Three Worlds According to King Ruang: A Thai Buddhist Cosmology* (Berkeley: University of California Press, 1982), 135–172.

69 Robert W. Moore, "Thailand Bolsters its Freedom," *National Geographic Magazine* 119 (1961): 828; King Chulalongkorn, *Phraratchaphithi sipsong duean* (Bangkok: Sangdao, 2013), 31–32.

70 Fujitani, *Splendid Monarchy*, 42–43.

71 Osawa Masachi, *Kindai Nihon*, 60.

72 Fujitani, *Splendid Monarchy*, 13–18.

73 Shimazono, *Kokka shinto*, 30, 35–39; Fujitani, *Splendid Monarchy*, 84.

74 Chaiching, *Kho fan fai nai fan*, 330.

75 CIA Records Search Tool, *Proposed Revision by Department of State PSB D–20*, 12.

76 Keyes, *Isan* (Ithaca: Southeast Asia Program, Cornell University, 1967), 38–58.

77 Phiyonphan Photchanalawan, *Kamnoet "Prathet Thai" phaitai phadetkan* (Bangkok: Matichon, 2015), 221.

78 Chaiching, *Kho fan fai nai fan*, 332.

79 Nicholas Grossman, King Bhumibol Adulyadej, *A Life's Work: Thailand's Monarchy in Perspective* (Singapore: Editions Didier Millet, 2011), 104. Kobkua Suwannathat-Pian, *Kings, Country and Constitutions: Thailand's Political Development, 1932–2000* (London: Routledge Curzon, 2003), 156–157.

80 Chaiching, *Kho fan fai nai fan*, 328.

81 For a contemporary description, see Charles Keyes, *Field Notes, Thailand: 1963–06 (June 1963), Mahasarakham, Roi Et*, 14–15, https://digital.lib.washington.edu/researchworks/bitstream/

handle/1773/19294/1963_June_Keyes_Fieldnotes_Mahasarakham.pdf?sequence=1&is Allowed=y (accessed 17 July 2017).

82 Krom Sinlapakon, *Chotmaihet ngan somphot Krung Rattanakosin 200 pi* (Bangkok: Fine Arts Department, 2002), 454.

83 Aizawa, *Shinron*, 157–158, 253–254.

84 Breen, *Reigi to kenryoku*, 27–34.

85 Donal Keene, *Emperor of Japan Meiji and His World, 1852–1912* (New York: Columbia University Press, 2002), 175–176, 191, 301, 416, 444, 560, 702, 718, 722.

86 Julia Meech-Pekarik, *The World of the Meiji Print: Impressions of a New Civilization* (New York: Weatherhill, 1986), 105–107, 170–171, 229.

87 Carol Gluck, *Japan's Modern Myths: Ideology in the Late Meiji Period* (Princeton University Press, 1985), 101.

88 Tokyo Asahi Shinbun, *Meiji no hajime to tsui*, 2 August 1912, 1.

89 Prince Dhani, *Conception of Monarchy*, 94.

90 Grossman et al., *King Bhumibol Adulyadej*, 100–101.

91 Prince Dhani, *Conception of Monarchy*, 95.

92 Princess Maha Chakri Sirindhorn, *Khao Thai pai Yipun* (Bangkok: Amarin, 1995), 129–130.

93 Grossman et al., *King Bhumibol Adulyadej*, 103.

94 Grossman et al., *King Bhumibol Adulyadej*, 233; Suwannathat-Pian, *Kings, Country, and Constitution*, 156.

95 Baker and Phongpaichit, *History of Thailand*, 177.

96 347. Memorandum From Acting Secretary of State Katzenbach to President Johnson, in *Mainland Southeast Asia; Regional Affairs (Foreign Relations of the United States, 1964–1968, Volume XXVII)*. VitalBook file.

97 Robert W. Moore, "Thailand Bolsters its Freedom," *National* 828; Surendranath H.H., "Prince Tripathi, Dhaninivat Kormamun Bidyalabh," *Bangkok Magazine* 8 November 1970, 22.

98 Grossman et al., *King Bhumibol Adulyadej*, 101; Pasuk Phongpaichit and Chris Baker, *Thailand: Economy and Politics* (Kuala Lumpur: Oxford University Press, 1995), 282–283.

99 Nicholas Grossman et al., *King Bhumibol Adulyadej*, 108–113; That Chaloemtiarana, *Thailand: The Politics of Despotic Paternalism* (Ithaca: Southeast Asia Program, Cornell University, 2007), 206–207.

100 Ruth-Inge Heinze, *The Role of the Sangha in Modern Thailand* (Taipei: Orient Cultural Service, 1977), 109.

101 Aizawa, *Shinron*, 257.

102 Aizawa, *Shinron*, 254–255.

103 For example, see Naoko Gunji, "Redesigning the Death Rite and Redesigning the Tomb: The Separation of Kami and Buddhist Deities at the Mortuary Site for Emperor Antoku," *Japanese Journal of Religious Studies* 38, no. 1 (2011): 55–92.

104 King Chulalongkorn, *Phraratchaphithi*, 145–147.

105 Phongpaichit and Baker, *Thailand*, 282; Chaloemtiarana, *Politics*, 214–215.

106 Botan, *Letters from Thailand* (Chiang Mai: Silkworm Books, 2002), 379.

107 Phongpaichit and Baker, *Thailand*, 314–315.

108 Keyes, *Isan*, 59–61; Charles F. Keyes, *Finding Their Voice: Northeastern Villagers in the Thai State* (Chiang Mai: Silkworm Books, 2014), 10–11.

109 Anusorn Unno, "'Rao Rak Nay Luang': Crafting Malay Muslims' Subjectivity through the Sovereign Thai Monarch," *Thammasat Review* 19, no. 2 (2016): 58.

110 Kyu Hyun Kim, "The Mikado's August Body: 'Divinity' and 'Corporeality' of the Meiij Emperor and the Ideological Construction of Imperial Rule," in *Politics and Religion in Modern Japan: Red Sun, White Lotus*, ed. Roy Starrs (Basingstoke: Palgrave Macmillan, 2011), 74–75.

111 Gordon, *History*, 126; Fujitani, *Splendid Monarchy*, 184.

112 Charles F. Keyes, *Thailand: Buddhist Kingdom as Modern Nation-State* (Boulder: Westview Press, 1987), 2.

113 Keyes, *Isan*, 60.

114 Suwannathat-Pian, *Kings, Country, and Constitutions*, 157; Mikiso Hane, *Modern Japan* (Boulder: Westview, 2001), 140–141.

Key works (English only)

Chaloemtiarana, Thak, *Thailand: The Politics of Despotic Paternalism* (Ithaca: Southeast Asia Program, Cornell University, 2007).

Dhani Nivat, Prince, "The Old Siamese Conception of the Monarchy," *Journal of the Siam Society* 36, no. 2 (1946): 91–106.

Dhani Nivat, Prince, "The Reconstruction of Rama I of the Chakri Dynasty," *Journal of the Siam Society* 43, no. 1 (1955): 21–47.

Fujitani, Takashi, *Splendid Monarchy: Power and Pageantry in Modern Japan* (Berkeley: University of California Press, 1998).

Hardacre, Helen, *Shintō and the State: 1868–1988* (Princeton: Princeton University Press, 1989).

Suwannathat-Pian, Kobkua, *Kings, Country and Constitutions: Thailand's Political Development, 1932–2000* (London: Routledge Curzon, 2003).

11

THE NATIONALIZATION AND MEDIATIZATION OF EUROPEAN MONARCHIES IN TIMES OF SORROW

Royal deaths and funerals in the second half of the nineteenth century[1]

Christoph De Spiegeleer

European monarchies withstood the challenges of the French Revolution and the democratization of politics surprisingly well through a mixture of tradition and new techniques and ideas.[2] This chapter explores how two long-term tendencies – nationalization and mediatization of royal lives and rituals – manifested themselves during the second half of the nineteenth century in the responses to the deaths and the organization of the funerals of Leopold I of Belgium (1865), Vittorio Emanuele II of Italy (1878) and German emperor Wilhelm I (1888).

These funerals occurred during a period that witnessed a renewal of ceremonial splendour on a European scale. Growing international rivalry and developments in the media made it necessary to present monarchs as the heads of their nations in all the splendour of their rituals. This chapter will show that royal funerals in the second half of the nineteenth century can often be described as '(re)invented traditions'. Old ritual and symbolic practices were combined with new symbols and rituals in order to stimulate a feeling of national unity and (artificial) historical continuity.[3]

After its separation from the United Kingdom of the Netherlands in 1830, the newly formed Belgian state chose to offer the throne to a German prince of the House of Saxe-Coburg and Gotha. Leopold I became a major diplomatic factor in consolidating Belgium's independence. In Italy and Germany, state-building was the result of hegemonic unification where one regional monarchical power seized the initiative. The Kingdom of Piedmont-Sardinia took the lead in the struggle for Italian unification with Vittorio Emanuele II as the founder of the Kingdom of Italy in 1861. Vittorio Emmanuele's popularity was almost exclusively linked to his role as military leader during the Risorgimento and the wars of liberation.[4] In 1871, Wilhelm I of the House of Hohenzollern, king of Prussia, became the first German emperor with the successful unification of Germany in the Franco-Prussian war. Wilhelm I received the title of German Emperor, instead of Emperor of Germany, as federal statehood was the central fact of the existence of the newly founded Empire. In Italy, there was nothing comparable to the continuing dualism of Prussia and Empire. Piedmont-Sardinia was completely absorbed into the unitary Italian state.[5]

In the first section, this chapter identifies the use of funerals in royal theatres of power during the Ancien Régime and assesses the importance for nineteenth-century monarchs to represent their nation in all its glory and prestige. The second and third sections of this chapter explore this process of nationalization by analysing how the three deaths and funerals were used by journalists, politicians, architects and royal families to further the notion of a unified nation, and if these efforts were successful. The second section will analyse the three funerals as 'cultural performances', while the third section will look into the broader responses to the royal deaths in media accounts. Deaths of heads of state can create unique moments of emotional connection between nation and dynasty, but these great deaths can also expose the lack of shared values and serve to break whatever fragile consensus existed.[6] The fourth and final section of this chapter will assess the extent to which the royal deaths and funerals became 'mediatized'. In order to fully understand the meaning of these events within their historical context, it is necessary to know whether the media landscape in all three countries was able to describe these royal deathbeds and funeral ceremonies with emotional immediacy and vividness for a broad section of the public.[7]

Royal funerals in Europe

The desire to mark royal funerals with elaborate ritual and theatricality and international rivalry of funerary pomp were no new phenomena in the second half of the nineteenth century. The main components of royal burials – the lying-in-state, the funeral procession and the requiem service – were in place from the late Middle Ages onwards. During the late Middle Ages and the early modern period, royal funeral rites were often lavish manifestations of political power and authority. As royal succession was often contested, the royal body became subject to great ritual elaboration with, for example, the use of funeral effigies in order to deny the break in continuity.[8] Already during the eleventh and twelfth centuries, Holy Roman emperors received magnificent obsequies. By the early fourteenth century, the funerals of English and French sovereigns had become important and ceremonial occasions as well.[9] In the sixteenth century, the need to reaffirm the social and political hierarchy after the passing of a sovereign gave way to a 'royal theatre of death' throughout Europe. This encompassed an important political role for funeral processions, even without the presence of the mortal remains.[10] The commemorative funeral held in Brussels for Emperor Charles V in 1558 became an international example and inspiration for other courts. Philip II presented himself on this occasion as the sole and legitimate successor of his father and his famous Burgundian ancestors.[11]

Throughout the seventeenth and eighteenth centuries, this Renaissance theatre of power and death disappeared in various European kingdoms.[12] However, during the second half of the nineteenth century, a new efflorescence in ritual and tradition can be observed throughout Europe. Monarchs became visible figures through public representations and served as focal points of national unity.[13] A solid basis for the position of monarchs in almost all nation-states, except in multinational empires such as Russia and Austria-Hungary, lay in a theatrical support of the nation, using symbolic and ritual language to exalt royal influence or to conceal its weakness.[14]

Even more so than other ritual life-cycle events, such as births and marriages, royal funerals became, together with coronations and jubilees, ceremonies *par excellence* through which the nationalization of nineteenth-century western European monarchies could be carried out in the public sphere against the background of international competition in royal pageantry.[15] With the funerals of Queen Victoria and King Edward VII in the first decade of the twentieth century, the British monarchy rediscovered the Renaissance 'theatre of death'. When his mother died in 1901, Edward VII needed to present himself as the focal point of national and imperial unity, and in organizing Victoria's funeral he probably wanted to emulate the impressive funeral accorded to Alexander III of Russia in 1894.[16] In both royal and republican regimes the rise of theatricality in international politics also manifested itself in grand funerary and memorial rituals for non-royal political leaders who acquired iconic national significance.[17] For example, the funerals of US President Abraham Lincoln (1865), the Italian Risorgimento-hero Giuseppe Garibaldi (1882) and former British Prime Minister William Gladstone (1898) were arranged as public spectacles with wide popular participation.[18]

In all three countries analysed in this chapter the organizers consciously staged the royal lying-in-state as a public affair in order to bolster support for the monarchy. Leopold I, Vittorio Emanuele II and Wilhelm I lay in state for several days in the Royal Palace in Brussels, the Quirinal in Rome (Figure 11.1) and the Berlin Cathedral (the 'Dom') respectively.[19] Not only was the lying-in-state but also the burial of the remains of the head of state in or near the capital of the young nation-state an essential step to identify the monarch successfully with the nation. In December 1865, the Belgian royal heir, Leopold II, withheld the existence of a letter in which his father asked to be buried in Windsor next to his first wife Charlotte, Princess of Wales. In fact, Leopold's successor and Sylvain van de Weyer, Belgium's official representative in London, reasoned that it was in the nation's interest to bury Leopold I in the kingdom founded by him. Leopold I was eventually buried next to his second wife Louise, Queen of Belgium, in the crypt of the church of Laken, a suburb in north-west Brussels.[20]

After the unexpected death of Italy's first king in January 1878, the issue of where to bury Vittorio Emanuele II unleashed a more public discussion. The new Italian Minister of the Interior, Francesco Crispi, intervened within the council of ministers to bury the king in Rome and not in the basilica of Superga near Turin, where the Savoy dynasty had had its traditional resting place since the middle of the eighteenth century. His colleagues in the cabinet and Vittorio Emanuel's eldest son Umberto agreed, but the decision met with considerable resistance in Turin. By deciding to bury the king in Rome, the left-wing government tried to strengthen the young nation's bond with the monarchy and its capital.[21] Wilhelm I wished to be buried next to his parents in the royal mausoleum in Charlottenburg (near Berlin), built as a tomb for his mother, Queen Luise, in the early nineteenth century.[22] Wilhelm's appeal in the 1870s and 1880s was in fact linked to the popular image of his mother.[23]

Royal funerals as cultural performances: mise-en-scène and social power

Royal funerals can be analysed as cultural performances. According to Jeffrey C. Alexander, 'fused cultural performances' are symbolic activities where the audience emotionally connects with actors and where background symbols and cultural scripts,

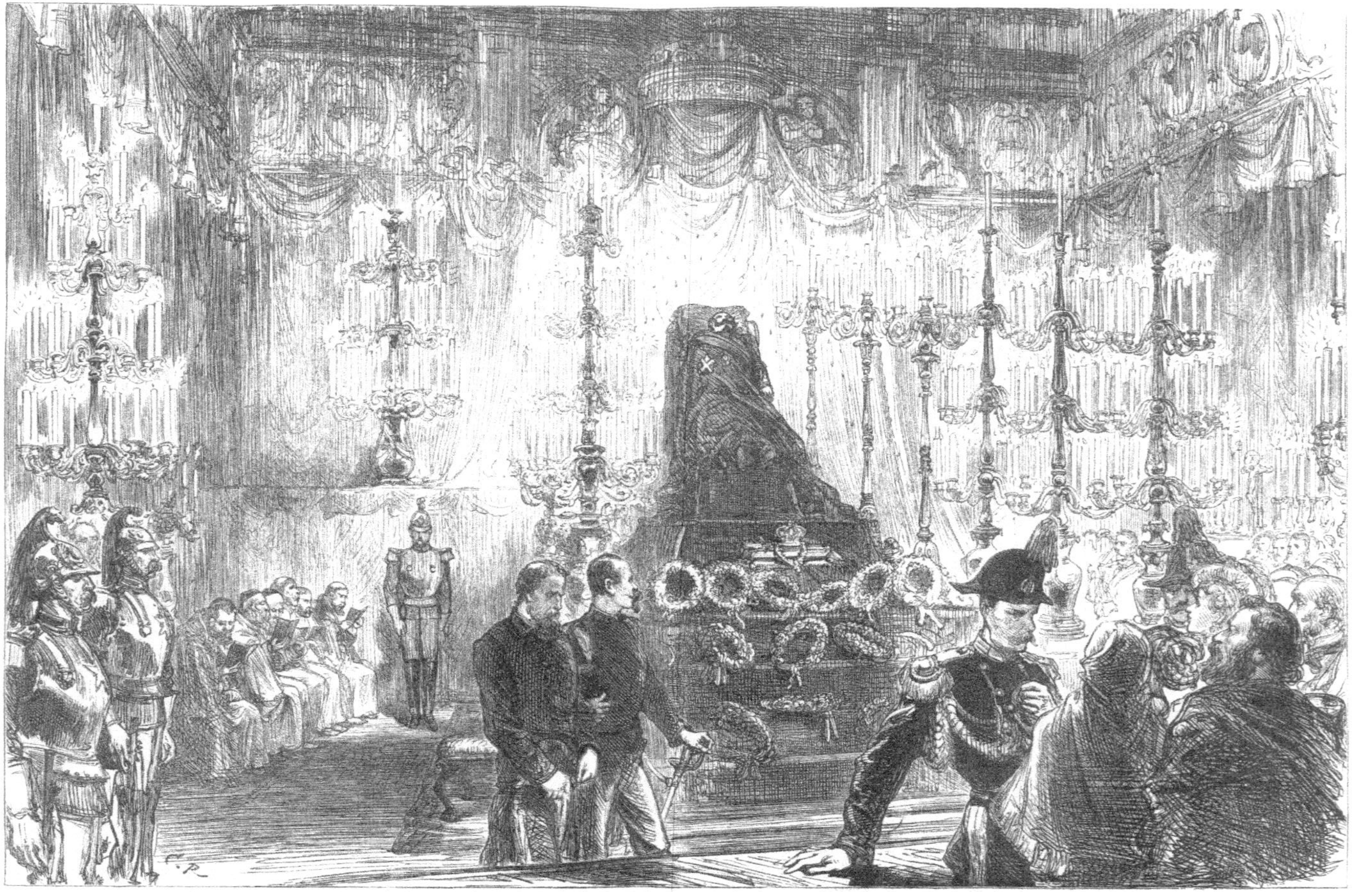

THE LATE KING VICTOR EMMANUEL LYING IN STATE AT THE QUIRINAL, ROME.

Figure 11.1 Lying-in-state, Vittorio Emanuele II, The Illustrated London News, 1878 (GUL, BIB.J.002999)

ranging from old traditions to 'invented traditions' created on the spot, achieve verisimilitude through effective mise-en-scène.[24]

Alexander mentions material means of symbolic production (objects, a physical place and clothing) and mise-en-scène (a spatial and chronological choreography) as important elements of cultural performances to assure the transmission of the performance to the crowds.[25] Even though Leopold I and Vittorio Emanuele II were never crowned, royal regalia that emphasized the continuity of the monarchy, such as the royal crown and sceptre, were laid on their coffins in 1865 and 1878.[26] The Belgian government charged prominent architects and entrepreneurs to construct a monumental hearse (Figure 11.2) to transport Leopold's remains to the church of Laken and to erect a temporary wooden chapel/temple in front of the church to perform the Protestant service before burial in the crypt on 16 December 1865. The decorations of the hearse combined national and dynastic symbols, with the Belgian coat of arms displayed on the front.[27] The heraldic design of this coat of arms, with the Belgian lion, was based on the coat of arms of the Dukes of Brabant, feudal rulers of the heart of the historic Low Countries since the twelfth century. The baldachin of the hearse used for Wilhelm's I funeral on 16 March 1888 was extensively decorated with the coat of arms of the German Empire in a similarly theatrical way. This imperial coat of arms had reintroduced the medieval single-headed black eagle of the Holy Roman emperors (Figure 11.3).[28]

When staging the funeral of the Italian kingdom's founder in 1878, Minister of the Interior Crispi was, like his Belgian colleagues before him, fully aware of the importance of a convincing mise-en-scène, material objects and '(re-)invented traditions' to stimulate a sense of historical continuity. Cesare Correnti, former Risorgimento revolutionary and ex-Minister of Education, advised Crispi to invent a new state ritual that would arouse patriotic sentiments.[29] Correnti proposed to carry the Iron Crown of Lombardy in front of the funeral car and to include flags of the most important cities in the funeral procession. The origins of the crown of Lombardy are shrouded in mystery. It has been used for the coronation of various kings of Italy, presumably since at least the eleventh century. This made it the perfect object to stress the historical continuity between the Italian kingdom and a remote past. Correnti eventually carried the Iron Crown on a cushion in the funeral cortege on 17 January 1878.[30] The Iron Crown became a typical example of an 'invented tradition' that tried to establish a (factitious) continuity with a historical past. A copy of the crown adorned the king's tomb in the Pantheon since 1885, and in 1890 the Iron Crown became part of the coat of arms of the Kingdom of Italy.[31]

Crispi chose the Pantheon in Rome to house the tomb of Vittorio Emanuele II. Originally dedicated to all the gods, this ancient temple had been converted into a consecrated church for centuries. The government attempted to augment the legitimacy of the Italian royal office by equating it with the traditions of Roman antiquity.[32] On 16 February 1878, one month after Vittorio Emanuele's funeral, a second funeral mass for the king was held in the Pantheon. A special committee of architects, art historians, sculptors and engineers turned the Pantheon into a temple that glorified the king and the house of Savoy by fusing national and monarchical symbols. A massive star of Italy decorated the central aperture. A large Savoy coat of arms appeared over the main altar and the arms of the most important cities of Italy hung around the walls. Inscriptions praised the king for his role in uniting the Italian people.[33]

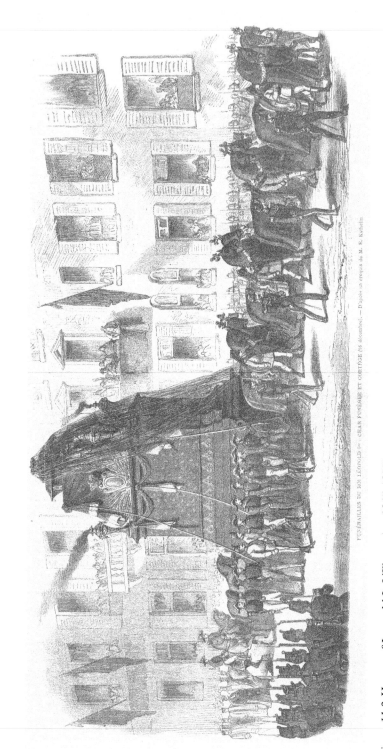

FUNÉRAILLES DU ROI LÉOPOLD Ier — CHAR FUNÈBRE ET CORTÉGE (16 décembre). — D'après un croquis de M. E. Kobelin.

Figure 11.2 Hearse of Leopold I, *L'Illustration*, 1865 (GUL, BIB.J.000016)

In Berlin, the temporary decoration produced for the funeral of Wilhelm I in March 1888 also created a theatrical air (Figure 11.3).[34] The German Empire did not have its own imperial insignia. In fact, the insignia displayed at the Berlin Dom during the lying-in-state presented Wilhelm as king of Prussia and not as German emperor. However, the architects who designed the street decoration for the funeral cortege between the Dom and the Brandenburg Gate privileged national German motifs, such as an inscription honouring 'the creator of the German Reich' and a statue of Germania.[35] The exterior decoration of the Dom focused on the imperial power of Wilhelm I. An imperial crown on top of a *castrum doloris*, which was erected on the crossing of the Unter den Linden-boulevard and the Friedrichstraße, symbolized the continuity of the German Empire.[36]

The decorators in Rome and Berlin tried to transform the funeral processions into triumphal marches by taking advantage of the symbolic associations of the Pantheon and the Brandenburg Gate with immortality and fame. The Berlin architects focused on the symbolic function of the Brandenburg Gate, a neo-classical monument built on the site of a former city gate, as a threshold between two worlds. 'Vale Senex Imperator' (Farewell, Old Emperor) was written in large letters across the black-draped monument.[37] On the other hand, the choice for the Pantheon as the tomb of Vittorio Emanuele II in Rome ten years earlier had to do with the Pantheon's resemblance to nearby ancient imperial mausoleums The use of this former temple could also exploit the modern concept of a 'Pantheon' as the place where a nation worships and immortalizes its heroes. For the second funeral mass in February 1878, the exterior of the Pantheon was decorated with allegories of fame and the inscription 'A Vittorio Emanuele II padre della Patria', a direct translation of 'Pater Patriae' – the epithet of Roman emperors including Augustus.[38]

Alexander identifies distribution of power in society – the nature of its political, economic and status hierarchies – as another element that profoundly affects cultural performances, as not everyone was allowed to participate.[39] In order to fulfil a royal funeral's central political purpose, to represent the continuity of the king's office and dignity, the presence of the heir in the funeral procession had become important. Yet, Umberto I did not accompany the remains of his father through the streets of Rome in 1878. He waited in the Pantheon.[40] Wilhelm I's son and successor Friedrich was too ill to attend the ceremonies in 1888. The prominent position of Crown Prince Wilhelm (future Wilhelm II) behind the hearse made it clear that a new generation was soon going to rule the German Empire. Friedrich had in fact only three months to live.[41]

Military units opened the funeral processions of all three monarchs in order to represent their connection to the military and to power.[42] Nevertheless, great care was taken in Brussels to underline that Leopold had been a constitutional monarch and the embodiment of the entire nation. The Presidents of the Belgian Chamber and the Senate symbolically flanked the coffin. The funeral cortege included all deputies and Senators and representatives of various sections of the state and civil society, such as judges, members of the city councils, academics from the universities and so on. The inclusion of some groups was highly symbolic due to their patriotic significance, like veterans of the Belgian revolution and old members of the National Congress of 1830 (the legislative assembly that had created the constitution of the new state).[43]

The funeral of Vittorio Emanuele II in Rome was carefully arranged as a combination of traditional, dynastic rituals of the House of Savoy, one of the oldest royal families in the world, and new elements that had to represent the young parliamentarian Italian state. The traditions of the House of Savoy were examined by looking at the funerals of the dukes of Savoy/kings of Sardinia Carlo Emanuele III and Carlo Felice in 1773 and 1831.[44] The lying-in-state with the mantle of the chivalric Order of Saints Maurice and Lazarus, the king's aide-de-camp on horseback bearing the monarch's sword, and the presence of the knights of the Savoy order of the Annonciade in the funeral procession referred to old Savoy traditions.

It was also important to stress that Vittorio Emanuele had been a constitutional monarch. For this reason, General Luigi Pelloux of the War Office examined the funeral procession of Belgium's first king twelve years earlier. In fact, the funeral of Leopold I in 1865 provided a useful precedent on how to underline the constitutional character of the monarchy by including all kinds of politicians and state officials in the procession.[45] On 17 January 1878, the Presidents of the Chamber and the Senate, the Minister of Interior Crispi and Prime Minister Depretis walked beside the hearse. Just like in Brussels, representatives of various sections of the state and civil society were included in the cortege, for instance town councillors, judges, students, workers and even Alpine guides.[46]

Deputies and Senators preceded the clergy and foreign representatives in the funeral processions in Brussels and Rome. The message behind this remained unclear in the Italian case. Compared with the members of Parliament, the clergy and foreign representatives were positioned far closer to the hearse.[47] In Berlin, the Court Marshal and the emperor's successor Friedrich III rejected the request of the legislators of the Reichstag and the Prussian House of Deputies to be included in the funeral service, though the presidents of the two Chambers were invited. The representatives of the legislative bodies of the German Empire and the Kingdom of Prussia who were allowed in the procession followed in the tail end, and they were not given very much attention in the press accounts. The royal court followed protocol regulations and gave priority to traditional elites, such as aristocrats, military officers and government officials. The people's elected representatives in the Reichstag were not considered eminent political citizens, and those of noble blood outranked commoners.[48] The dynasty clearly planned for the cortege to represent the nature and distribution of power in the German Empire and the national character of the imperial state was neglected.[49]

Taking all three funerals into account, the most impressive group of European royals gathered in Berlin in 1888, as the German Empire was undoubtedly the most powerful monarchy on the continent. The crowned heads of Saxony, Romania and Belgium and the heirs of Britain, Italy, Austria-Hungary and Russia accompanied Crown Prince Wilhelm in the streets of Berlin, followed by almost all the rulers of the German Empire's constituent states.[50]

Royal deaths and the unity of the nation

Catholic and Liberal Belgian newspapers went out of their way to emphasize the patriotic atmosphere and sincere mourning among Belgians of all classes and parties after Leopold's death in 1865.[51] In 1878 both left- and right-wing monarchist

Italian newspapers stressed the need to unify all Italians behind the Savoy throne in a similar way. Vittorio Emanuele was frequently referred to as 'Padre della patria' ('Father of the fatherland').[52] In 1888, newspapers from various parts of the German Empire also underlined the loyalty of all Germans ('das deutsche Volk'), and not only the Prussians, towards their Kaiser, and necrological articles mostly focused on the Kaiser as a symbol of national unity, reaffirming the pre-eminence of his role as the Empire's founder over his royal Prussian role.[53] When covering royal funerals, nineteenth-century newspapers were also eager to frame public displays of mourning rituals as shared by the entire nation.[54]

We should be careful not to solely rely on newspaper accounts. The freedom to publish often came with conditions to protect monarchs against press attacks.[55] Moreover, the distinction between mere curiosity and veneration for the deceased monarch was often thin among the mobilized crowds. In order to find out if royal deaths and funerals brought the nation together, it is necessary to take the specific cultural and political milieu within each country into account.[56]

Due to the tensions rife in the national and international political context, it was conceivable that a crisis would arise in Belgium after the death of the kingdom's founding monarch. A general atmosphere of anxiety about a possible annexation of Belgium to the Second Empire of Napoleon III persisted throughout the 1860s.[57] The death of Leopold I temporally effaced the political and social conflicts between Catholics and Liberals over the place of religious alliances in modern polity. This truce manifested itself at the level of the political discourse that was produced by Leopold's death and during the actual funeral ceremonies. The death and funeral of Belgium's first king produced national bonds of social solidarity among participants and commentators who lacked consensus on the cultural and ideological level.[58]

Despite Belgium being an overwhelmingly Catholic country, the Lutheran Leopold never converted to Catholicism and received a Protestant funeral. This made it impossible for Catholic priests and bishops to participate in the religious ceremonies and also caused difficulties for those organizing his burial in the Catholic royal crypt. The leaders of the Belgian Catholic Church were aware of the unpatriotic impression their absence from the funeral and a refusal to bury Leopold in the crypt would make. The Belgian archbishop eventually reached an agreement with the royal court. The Belgian bishops were given the opportunity to offer their condolences to Leopold's successor at the Palace before the start of the ceremonies, and the Catholic clergy of Brussels took part in the funeral procession. A Protestant service took place in a temporary wooden temple at the front of the Church of Laken with the royal crypt. It was agreed that the Protestant pastors would not enter the church for burial in the crypt. The royal crypt was 'neutralized' to allow the Protestant monarch to rest next to his Catholic wife.[59] This compromise averted a public conflict that risked overshadowing the succession.

A clear example of the existence of a truce of death was the conciliatory discourse used by organizations and sections in society that did not share or opposed Leopold's religious and political views. During the 1860s, the Protestant king publicly joined the Catholic opposition against emerging freethinkers' associations. Due to the royal policy of imposing fortifications around the port-city of Antwerp, Leopold was also confronted with strong anti-monarchist sentiments within the majority of the Antwerp city council.[60] Nonetheless, both the Brussels freethinkers' magazine

Le Libre Examen and the city council of Antwerp issued firm patriotic statements in which anti-clerical freethinkers and anti-militarist councillors proclaimed their loyalty to the constitutional monarchy. They were clearly motivated by a desire to stress the unity of Belgium against the lingering threat of annexation.[61]

Just as in Belgium, a peaceful transition in late nineteenth-century Italy was by no means guaranteed after the death of the kingdom's founder. Compared with the peaceful social and political atmosphere in Belgium after Leopold's death, it proved far more difficult to transcend the political sphere in Italy after Vittorio Emanuele's passing. During the weeks following the succession, several pamphlets expressed anxiety over the young Italian monarchy's capacity to survive the death of its first king.[62] In fact, except for the Catholic faith, hardly anything linked together Italians from Lombardy and Sicily. From 1848 onwards, the Church had been on a collision course with Italian nationalism as the unification of the country under the Savoia monarchy and the promotion of a national identity became inimical to the interests of the papacy.[63]

Despite the fact the Vittorio Emanuele's funeral was carefully politically and culturally orchestrated by the political establishment, the events in Rome failed to be completely socially integrative 'fused performances'. Italian society remained too regionally and politically divided.[64] The Vatican regretted the decision of the government to bury the king in Rome. The choice for Rome also went against the explicit wish of the majority of the municipal council of Turin. The Turin council wanted to bury the king in the basilica of Superga.[65] The presence of the papacy and the 'Roman question' made the church–state antagonism in Italy quite distinctive.[66] The capture of Rome in 1870 ended the centuries-long reign of the Papal States. Pius IX did not recognize the right of the government and the king to be in the eternal city. However, having a Catholic monarch's funeral in Rome without the participation of the clergy was unimaginable. The Vatican eventually allowed the priests of the local parish to take part in the funeral in Rome, but forbade bishops or confraternities from participating.[67]

For their part, intransigent Catholics and Church leaders rejected any compromise with the liberal Italian state. After the king's death, disrespectful articles towards the Italian monarchy appeared in papers such as *Veneto Cattolico*, *L'Osservatore Cattolico* and *La Civiltà Cattolica*. This was not to the liking of all Italian Catholics. Moderate Milanese priests, who believed the king had a firm claim to rule, criticized journalist–priest Davide Albertario for his harsh words and sarcastic comments in his paper *L'Osservatore Cattolica*, even though Albertario was backed by Pius IX himself.[68]

Violent encounters between angry demonstrators and prominent Catholics occurred in different cities in the Emilia-Romagna region, a traditional bastion of anti-clericalism. Anti-clericals clearly tried to make use of royalist sentiments to attack Church officials who found themselves in an uncomfortable position following Vittorio Emanuele's death. The Bishop of Piacenza had to be protected against angry demonstrators as he refused to use the cathedral for a funeral observance.[69] The most excessive violence occurred in Bologna when hundreds of men, mostly students, vandalized the residence of Archbishop Lucido Parocchi and other important buildings of the Catholic community after hearing the news that the Archbishop refused to allow funeral masses for the king.[70] No major incidents triggered by anti-Savoy movements seem to have occurred in the southern part of Italy. This is important to note because thousands had lost their lives in the civil war between southern rural anti-Savoy insurgents and the Italian authorities through the 1860s.[71] In Napoli, a group of monarchists even demonstrated against the republican journal *La Spira* for its critical stance towards the monarchy by publicly shredding copies of the journal into pieces.[72]

Despite the fact that internal resistance to national unification was not as great and violent in Germany as in Italy, the Hohenzollerns still faced the tremendous challenge of providing historical legitimacy for the founding of the Empire under their leadership after 1871. Wilhelm's military actions in 1866 and his acquiescence to the *Kulturkampf*, the struggle triggered by Bismarck's salvo of laws which intended to neutralize Catholicism as a political force in the Kingdom of Prussia, made it difficult for him to act as a figure of national and political integration.[73] During the last decades of his life the old Kaiser essentially remained a Prussian king. Nevertheless, after his death in 1888, there was a great need to publicly transform Wilhelm I into a national symbol as the father of the Second German Empire.[74]

In 1888, the relationship between throne and altar in the German Empire had become far less problematic than in Italy. The *Kulturkampf* in Prussia was over, with the last peace law of 1887 readmitting all religious orders, except the Jesuits. Wilhelm I was the conscientious 'Summus episcopus' (Supreme Governor) of the Protestant State Church of Prussia ('Evangelische Landeskirche der älteren Provinzen Preußens'). He instructed that his lying-in-state should take place in the Dom of Berlin, and he stipulated the hymns and texts for his Protestant funeral. The court preacher Rudolf Kögel, an important figure in the Prussian State Church, played a major role in the religious ceremonies surrounding Wilhelm's death and funeral.[75] The celebration and commemoration of Wilhelm I in death contributed to the advancement of the national idea across confessional and regional divisions. The popular response to Wilhelm's death in Bavaria, an overwhelming Catholic state in the southeast where Catholics had been vividly opposing the liberal project of German unification under Prussian leadership, shows that the imperial national cult already extended substantially to Catholic regions in the late 1880s. There was a clear willingness among both Protestants and Catholics in Bavaria to participate in local funerary ceremonies for Wilhelm I in 1888.[76]

The Catholic Church may have reached a *modus vivendi* with the German Empire, but the social and political tensions around the rise of the German Social-Democratic Party were still very much present. Shortly before Wilhelm's death, Bismarck's Anti-Socialist Laws of 1878, which banned all social-democratic associations, meetings and newspapers, had been renewed for the fourth time. In 1888, Social-Democrats were still seen as 'enemies of the Empire'.[77] The Social-Democratic exile press never forgave Wilhelm I for his bloody repression of revolts during the 1848 revolutions and described him as a mass murderer and an authoritarian ruler. *Der Sozialdemokrat*, the main press organ of German socialism (published in Zurich and illegally distributed in Germany), completely rejected the monarchical, authoritarian government and did not even bother to describe the Kaiser's funeral.[78] In other words, the responses to the deaths of Vittorio Emanuele II and Wilhelm I undoubtedly contributed to the nationalization of the Italian Savoy monarchy and the German Empire across regional and political allegiances. Be that as it may, not even after their deaths were both monarchs able to act as figures of national integration for all Italians and Germans.

The mediatization of royal deathbeds and funerals

Mediatization refers to an ongoing process whereby media increasingly change human relations and behaviour, becoming relevant for the social construction of society and culture.[79] In the early modern period, media was already important in publicizing royal deaths and funerals such as the ceremonies for Emperor Charles V in Brussels in 1558. The nineteenth century witnessed the growth of a mass print and visual culture with a tremendous expansion in the market for newspapers, books, periodicals, lithographic prints and engravings.[80] The nineteenth-century media transformation and graphic revolution was characterized by the attention given to the great personalities of the time, such as monarchs.[81] For example, nineteenth-century newspapers offering their readers romanticized descriptions of touching scenes of familial togetherness at royal deathbeds as the 'embourgeoisement of the monarchy' became an important strategy to legitimize royal regimes.[82]

Belgian and Italian newspapers turned the last hours of Leopold I and Vittorio Emanuele II into symbolic mediatized events with competing partisan representations. Belgian Catholic and Liberal high-brow journals publicly discussed whether the Protestant Leopold had shown signs of religiosity on his deathbed in December 1865.[83] In Italy, the didactic and symbolic resonance of the king's deathbed was even greater due to the Roman question. On his deathbed, Vittorio Emanuele II asked his chaplain to convey to the pope that he apologized for any displeasure he had caused the Holy Father and that he had never intended to cause any damage to religion. The Archbishop Giulio Lento, vice-regent of Rome, deemed this dubious confession sufficient to allow the administration of the Eucharist and Holy Unction.[84] The kingdom's official newspaper, the *Gazzetta Ufficiale del Regno d'Italia*, remained silent on the king's apology, whereas the Catholic papers *L'Osservatore Romano* and *La Civiltà Cattolica* focused on the king's supposed repentance.[85]

The news that the king had died a good Catholic who received the last rites was information that could be used for great profit by the Italian government, as it demonstrated that there was no conflict between loyalty to the Italian State and devotion to the Church.[86] This explains the attention to the administration of the last rites in the *Gazetta Ufficiale del Regno d'Italia* and various Roman newspapers. However, the suggestion spread by the Catholic press that the king had expressed regret on his deathbed for conquering the Papal States delegitimized the very existence of the Italian nation. Crispi did not hesitate to prepare a counterattack and stated through Italy's leading press agency that Vittorio Emanuele had not made any declaration that repudiated his glorious life as Italian king.[87]

Royal families were one of the principal beneficiaries of the expansion in the reproduction of the visual image that took place during the nineteenth century.[88] In the 1840s, a new generation of illustrated weekly newspapers appeared: *The Illustrated London News* (London, 1842), *L'Illustration* (Paris, 1843) and *Der Illustrirte Zeitung* (Leipzig, 1843).[89] These newsweeklies, aimed at a bourgeois readership, used the method of wood engraving for their detailed illustrations of current events in Europe. The monumental and heavily decorated funeral hearses were a popular subject of illustration in these periodicals. In contrast to early modern prints, which solely offered a macro-perspective on whole processions, the engravings of the hearses and funeral processions in illustrated nineteenth-century weeklies tried to give the readers a realistic image of the funeral cortege as seen from a particular, somewhat spatially manipulated point of view. Illustrators often highlighted some well-chosen architectural surroundings for theatrical effect or for the symbolic connection between a certain public space and the late monarch.[90]

The development and possibilities of the illustrated press varied between the three nation-states in the different decades analysed here. In 1865, Belgium still lacked a national equivalent of *The Illustrated London News* and *L'Illustration*. Nevertheless, one or two weeks after the events in Brussels, the most important illustrated bourgeois magazines of France and England already offered their readers wood engravings of the transport of Leopold's remains to the Palace in Brussels, the lying-in-state, the funeral procession and the burial service in Laken (Figure 11.2).[91]

While wealthy Belgian citizens had to buy foreign weeklies with illustrations of their king's funeral, Italians and Germans were able to purchase national illustrated periodicals with images of the funerals of Vittorio Emanuele II and Wilhelm I. The Milan-based *Illustrazione Italiana* (founded in 1873) was the leading illustrated bourgeois newsmagazine of its day in Italy.[92] Its readership was mostly an urban bourgeoisie that spanned much of the country. Public patriotic rituals and monuments were the magazine's favourite topic, as paraphernalia of the monarchy and the government were ideal to celebrate the unified Italian nation-state.[93] The magazine provided thorough coverage, with multiple images and detailed stories, of each phase in the ceremonies surrounding Vittorio Emanuele's death and funeral in 1878.[94] The editors of the periodical actively tried to reinforce the king's central position within Italian patriotic imagery through illustrations.[95]

In Germany, *Die Gartenlaube* (Leipzig, 1853) was the most popular magazine with a circulation of almost 380,000 in 1881.[96] Just like *Illustrazione Italiana*, *Die Gartenlaube* tried to stimulate national consciousness among its readers. As a family magazine, *Die Gartenlaube* did not focus on describing weekly news events. It nevertheless published a reportage of the Kaiser's funeral in 1888 with large illustrations of the cortege (Figure 11.3). In order to stress the popularity of Wilhelm I, the novelist Hermann Heiberg focused on the enormous crowds standing along the roads, eager to catch a glimpse of the spectacle in the freezing cold.[97]

Conclusion

The three royal deaths analysed here proved to be important occasions for cultural nation-building, albeit in a different manner. The organizers of Leopold I's and Vittorio Emanuele II's funerals consciously staged these events as public affirmations of patriotism and national unity. The ceremonies in Brussels and Rome combined old symbols and rituals – such as extravagant displays of coats of arms and orders of chivalry – with new elements, which represented the new parliamentary nation-state in order to stimulate a feeling of national unity and historical continuity. In Berlin, on the other hand, the royal family and Court Marshal regarded the traditional representation of the dynasty during Wilhelm I's funeral as much more important than the representation of the unified German nation. The latter was favoured by journalists and those responsible for the funerary decoration. The nationalization of the monarchy in Berlin was less straightforward due to the particular character of the German Empire being a confederation of sovereign principalities with Wilhelm I as

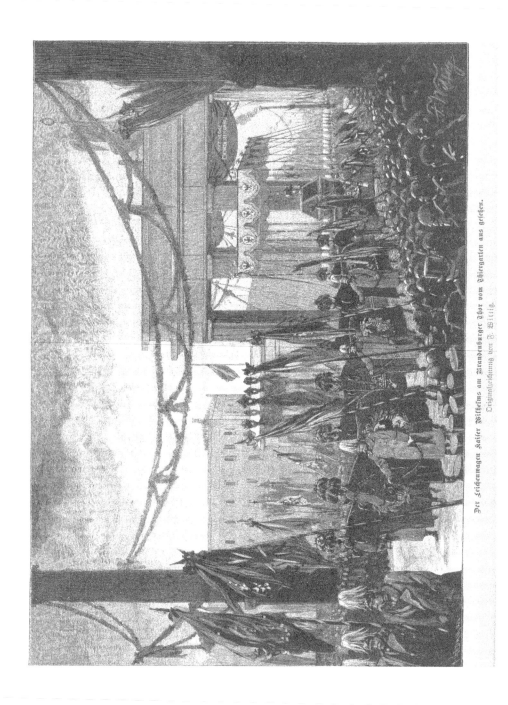

Der Leichenwagen Kaiser Wilhelms am Brandenburger Thor vom Thiergarten aus gesehen.
Originalzeichnung von F. Wittig.

Figure 11.3 Funeral procession, Wilhelm I, *Die Gartenlaube*, 1888 (Ghent University Library, BIB.P.006858)

primus inter pares among the German princes and kings. The ceremonies in Berlin had both a Prussian and imperial national dimension, and the composition of the funeral cortege symbolized the subordinate role of the Reichstag towards the Kaiser in the authoritarian political system of the German Empire.

Compared to the Italian and German cases, the responses to the death of Leopold I succeeded most in sustaining the coherence of the nation. Explicit dissent was absent. This had everything to do with the precarious geopolitical situation of the Kingdom of Belgium, though the discourse of consensus and solidarity certainly concealed a diversity of inward ideological attitudes. The responses to the deaths of Vittorio Emanuele II and Wilhelm I did not succeed in being fully integrative on a national level. Italian intransigent Catholics and German Social-Democrats repudiated everything the Italian king and German emperor stood for. The deaths of Vittorio Emanuele II and Wilhelm I deepened the divide between these political and social groups and the Kingdom of Italy and the German Empire even further. The death and funeral of Vittorio Emanuele II not only heightened tensions between Catholics and anti-clericals in different cities but also widened the gap between liberal and intransigent Catholics.

Descriptions and illustrations in the press played an increasingly important role in the process of stimulating national consciousness through royal events, with technical innovations and growing readership towards the end of the century. The deathbeds and funerals of all three monarchs became subject to mediatization processes, which influenced the construction of collective sentiments and solidarities. The emergent mass media did more than simply report or 'mediate' the royal deaths and ceremonies; daily newspapers and illustrated weeklies invoked public solidarities by framing public displays of mourning as shared by the whole nation or by focusing on specific symbolic acts on the deathbed.

Notes

1 I would like to thank Peter Laroy, director of Liberas for the institutional support to write this chapter, as well as the editors of this volume and the anonymous reviewers for their valuable comments.

2 Frank Lorenz Müller, "Stabilizing a 'Great Historic System' in the Nineteenth Century? Royal Heirs and Succession in an Age of Monarchy," in *Sons and Heirs: Succession and Political Culture in 19th-Century Europe*, eds. Frank Lorenz Müller and Heidi Mehrkens (New York: Palgrave Macmillan, 2016), 2–5.

3 David Cannadine, "The Context, Performance and Meaning of Ritual: The British Monarchy and the 'Invention of Tradition', c. 1820–1977," in *The Invention of Tradition*, eds. Eric Hobsbawm and Terrence Ranger (Cambridge: Cambridge University Press, 1983), 133, 161; Eric Hobsbawm, "Introduction: Inventing Traditions," in *The Invention of Tradition*, 1–2.

4 Alex Körner, *Politics of Culture in Liberal Italy: From Unification to Fascism* (London: Routledge, 2009), 200.

5 Jürgen Osterhammel, *The Transformation of the World. A Global History of the Nineteenth Century* (Princeton: Princeton University Press, 2014), 410–411.

6 John Wolffe, *Great Deaths: Grieving, Religion and Nationhood in Victorian and Edwardian England* (Oxford: Oxford University Press, 2000), 4–5. For the Belgian monarchy's ability to act as an integrative or polarizing force after the untimely deaths of three heirs during the nineteenth century and the accidental deaths of King Albert and Queen Astrid in 1934–5, see Christoph De Spiegeleer, "1834–1849–1891: The Untimely Deaths of Thee Heirs to the Belgian Throne," in *Sons and Heirs*, 79–196; and Christoph De Spiegeleer,

"Royal Losses, Symbolic Politics and Media Events in Interwar Europe: Responses to the Accidental Deaths of King Albert I and Queen Astrid of Belgium (1934–1935)," *Contemporary European History* 24, no. 2 (2015): 155–174.

7 Cannadine, "The Context," 123.

8 For a European perspective on the deaths, funerals and tombs of late medieval rulers, with a focus on Holy Roman Emperor Friedrich III, see *Der Tod des Mächtigen: Kult und Kultur des Todes spätmittelalterlicher Herrscher*, ed. Lothar Kolmer (Paderborn: Ferdinand Schöningh, 1997). For a European perspective on the early modern period, see *Les funérailles princières en Europe, XVIe–XVIIIe siècle. Volume 1. Le grand théâtre de la mort*, eds. Juliusz Chroscicki, Mark Hengerer and Gérard Sabatier (Paris: Éditions de la Maison des sciences de l'homme, 2012). For Renaissance France, see Ralph Giesey, *The Royal Funeral Ceremony in Renaissance France* (Geneva: Libraririe E. Droz, 1960). For a critique of Giesey's thesis on the political meaning of the use of effigies in royal funeral processions in Renaissance France, see Alain Boureau and Jacques Revel, "Le corps séparé des rois français," in *La mort du roi: Essai d'ethnographie politique comparée*, ed. Jacques Julliard (Paris: Gallimard, 1999), 113–133. For early modern England, see Jennifer Woodward, *The Theatre of Death: The Ritual Management of Royal Funerals in Renaissance England, 1570–1625* (Woodbridge: The Boydell Press, 1997); Sarah Tarlow, *Ritual, Belief and the Dead in Early Modern Britain and Ireland* (New York: Cambridge University Press, 2011), 112–115; and Clare Gittings, *Death, Burial and the Individual in Early Modern England* (London: Routledge, 1984), 216–234.

9 Elizabeth M. Hallam, "Royal Burial and the Cult of Kingship in France and England 1060–1330," *Journal of Medieval History* 8 (1982): 359–380; and Ralph Griffiths, "Succession and the Royal Dead in Later Medieval England," in *Making and Breaking the Rules: Succession in Medieval Europe, c. 1000–c.1600*, eds. Frédérique Lachaud and Michael Penman (Turnhout: Brepols Publishers, 2007), 97–107.

10 Gérard Sabatier and Mark Hengerer, "Le grand théâtre de la mort," in *Les funérailles princières*, 9.

11 Minou Schraven, *Festive Funerals in Early Modern Italy: The Art and Culture of Conspicuous Commemoration* (Farnham: Ashgate, 2014), 59.

12 Sabatier and Hengerer, "Le grand théâtre," 10.

13 Jaap Van Osta, "The Emperor's New Clothes: The Reappearance of the Performing Monarchy in Europe, c. 1870–1914," in *Mystifying the Monarch: Studies on Discourse, Power and History*, eds. Gita Deneckere and Jeroen Deploige (Amsterdam: Amsterdam University Press, 2006), 183; David Cannadine, "The Context," 128; Eva Giloi, *Monarchy, Myth, and Material Culture in Germany, 1750–1950* (Cambridge: Cambridge University Press, 2011), 335; Frank-Lothar Kroll, "Zwischen europäischen Bewußtsein und nationaler Identität. Legitimationsstrategien monarchischer Eliten im Europa des 19. und frühen 20. Jahrhunderts," in *Geschichte der Politik: Alte und neue Wege*, eds. Hans-Christof Kraus and Thomas Nicklas (Munich: Oldenbourg, 2007), 353; and Johannes Paulmann, *Pomp und Politik: Monarchenbegegnungen in Europa zwischen Ancien Régime und Erstem Weltkrieg* (Paderborn: Ferdinand Schöningh, 2000), 406.

14 Maria Grever, "Staging Modern Monarchs: Royalty at the World Exhibitions of 1851 and 1867," in *Mystifying the Monarch*, 163; Kroll, "Zwischen europäischen Bewußtsein und nationaler Identität," 364; Paulmann, *Pomp und Politik*, 17–172; and Alexis Schwarzenbach, *Königliche Träume: Eine Kulturgeschichte der Monarchie, 1789–1997* (Munich: Collection Rolf Heyne, 2012), 111.

15 Kroll, "Zwischen europäischen Bewußtsein und nationaler Identität," 361.

16 Wolffe, *Great Deaths*, 222, 237.

17 Cannadine, "The Context," 128–129.

18 Wolffe, *Great Deaths*, 181–191; Barry Schwartz, "Mourning and the Making of a Saced Symbol: Durkheim and the Lincoln Assassination," *Social Forces* 70, no. 2 (1991): 343–344; and Lucy Riall, *Garibaldi: Invention of a Hero* (New Haven: Yale University Press, 2007), 358–359.

19 Alberto Mario Banti, "The Remembrance of Heroes," in *The Risorgimento Revisited: Nationalism and Culture in Nineteenth-Century Italy*, eds. Silvana Patriarca and Lucy Riall (New York: Palgrave Macmillan, 2012), 173; Volker Ackermann, *Nationale Totenfeiern in*

Deutschland: Von Wilhelm I. bis Franz Josef Strauß. Eine Studie zur politischen Semiotik (Stuttgart: Klett-Cotta, 1990), 77; and Gita Deneckere, *Leopold I: De eerste koning van Europa* (Antwerp: De Bezige Bij, 2011), 665.

20 Deneckere, *Leopold I*, 666.

21 Umberto Levra, *Fare gli Italiani: Memoria e celebrazione del Risorgimento* (Turin: Comitato di Torino dell'Istituto per la storia del Risorgimento, 1992), 27–31; Pietro Pirri, *Pio IX e Vittorio Emanuele II dal loro carteggio privato. III. La Questione Romana, 1864-1870. Parte II. I documenti* (Rome: Pontificia Università Gregoriana, 1961), 444–447; Banti, "The Remembrance of Heroes," 181 and Körner, *Politics of Culture in Liberal Italy*, 198.

22 "Kaiser Wilhelm," *Berliner Börsen-Zeitung*, 119, 10 March 1888, 3; *Kaiser Wilhelm: Sein Leben und seine Zeit, 1797–1888* (Berlin, 1888), 204. For the Charlottenburg mausoleum, see chapter in Philipp Demandt, *Luisenkult: Die Unsterblichkeit der Königin von preußen* (Cologne: Böhlau Verlag Köln, 2003).

23 Giloi, *Monarchy*, 328.

24 Jeffrey C. Alexander, "Cultural Pragmatics: Social Performance between Ritual and Strategy," *Sociological Theory* 22, no. 4 (2004): 527–533.

25 Alexander, "Cultural Pragmatics," 532.

26 Banti, "The Remembrance of Heroes," 174.

27 *L'Indépendance Belge*, 15 December 1865, 1.

28 "Die Beisetzung Kaiser Wilhelms," *Allgemeine Zeitung* (Munich), 19 March 1888, 1155.

29 Levra, *Fare gli Italiani*, 18–19.

30 Catherine Brice, *Monarchie et identité nationale en Italie (1861–1900)* (Paris: Éditions de l'École des hautes études en sciences sociales, 2010), 184; Christopher Duggan, *Francesco Crispi, 1818–1901: From Nation to Nationalism* (Oxford: Oxford University Press, 2002), 379; Giacomo Martina, *Pio IX (1867–1878)* (Rome: Pontifica Università Gregoriana, 1990), 518; and Bruno Tobia, "Die Toten der Nation. Gedenkfeiern, Staatsbegräbnisse und Gefallenenkult im Liberalen Italien (1870–1921)," in *Inszenierung des Nationalstaats. Politische Feiern in Italien und Deutschland seit 1860/1871*, eds. Sabine Behrenbeck and Alexander Nützenadel (Cologne: SH-Verlag, 2000), 74–75.

31 Tobia, "Die Toten der Nation," 76.

32 "Perchè siasi prescelta la basilica di S. Maria ad Martyres per la tomba di Vittorio Emmanuele II," *La Civiltà Cattolica*, 11–25 January 1878, 376; Tobia, "Die Toten der Nation," 74; and Robin B. Williams, "Rome as State Image: The Architecture and Urbanism of the Royal Italian Government, 1870–1900" (PhD dissertation, University of Pennsylvania, 1993), 228.

33 Williams, "Rome as State Image," 230; Tobia, "Die Toten der Nation," 77; Brice, *Monarchie*, 192–193; and "L'esequie per Vittorio Emmanuele al Pantheon," *L'Illustrazione Italiana*, 3 March 1878, 139.

34 For the theatrical and monumental air of the architectural decoration, see "Berliner Briefe. II," *Beilage zur Allgemeine Zeitung* (Munich), 18 March 1888, 1145.

35 Michael L. Hughes, "Splendid Demonstrations: The Political Funerals of Kaiser Wilhelm I and Wilhelm Liebknecht," *Central European History* 41, no. 2 (2008): 234, 236; Ackermann, *Nationale Totenfeiern*, 244–245 and "Kaiser Wilhelm," *Berliner Börsen-Zeitung*, 16 March 1888, 130, 1–2.

36 Ackermann, *Nationale Totenfeiern*, 241–243; "Kaiser Wilhelm," 3.

37 Ackermann, *Nationale Totenfeiern*, 227, 243–244.

38 Williams, *Rome as State Image*, 231.

39 Alexander, "Cultural Pragmatics," 532.

40 Brice, *Monarchie*, 189.

41 Ackermann, *Nationale Totenfeiern*, 285–256; Hughes, "Splendid Demonstrations," 239–240, 242; "Berliner Briefe. II,"; "Kaiser Friedrich," *Berliner Börsen-Zeitung*, 120, 10 March 1888, 3; and Alexa Geisthövel, "Tote Monarchen: Die Beisetzungsfeierlichkeiten für Wilhelm I. und Friedrich III.," in *Das politische Zeremoniell im Deutschen Kaiserreich 1871–1918*, eds. Biefang Andreas, Epkenhans Michael and Tenfelde Klaus (Düsseldorf: Droste Verlag, 2008), 146–147.

42 "Funérailles du roi," *Le Journal de Bruxelles*, 17 December 1865, 1; Joachim Wendler, *Rituale des Abschieds. Eine Studie über das staatliche Begräbniszeremoniell in Deutschland* (Stuttgart:

Ibidem-Verlag, 2007), 52; "Ordine del convoglio funebre di SM il Re Vittorio Emanuele II," *Gazzetta Ufficiale del Regno d'Italia*, 16 January 1878, 194.

43 "Funérailles du roi," *Le Journal de Bruxelles*, 17 December 1865, 1; "Funérailles du roi Léopold," *L'Indépendance Belge*, 17 December 1865, 1.

44 Levra, *Fare gli Italiani*, 21–23; Brice, *Monarchie*, 188.

45 Levra, *Fare gli Italiani*, 21; Luigi Pelloux, *Quelques souvenirs de ma vie: A cura e con introduzione di Gastone Manacorda* (Rome: Instituto per la storia del Risorgimento Italiano, 1967), 102–103.

46 "Ordine del convoglio funebre,"; "I funerali del re," *L'Illustrazione Italiana*, 3 February 1878, 66.

47 "Funérailles du roi Léopold,"; Brice, *Monarchie*, 187; "Ordine del convoglio funebre,".

48 Hughes, "Splendid Demonstrations," 238–240; Ackermann, *Nationale Totenfeiern*, 286.

49 Ackermann, *Nationale Totenfeiern*, 285–286.

50 Ackermannn, *Nationale Totenfeiern*, 339; Geisthövel, "Tote Monarchen," 146.

51 "Mort du roi," *Le Journal de Bruxelles*, 11 December 1865, 1; "Mort du roi," *L'Écho du Parlement*, 11 December 1865, 1; "Mort du roi," *Le Journal de Liège*, 11 December 1865, 1

52 Levra, "Fare gli Italiani," 8–16.

53 Hughes, "Splendid Demonstrations," 235; Ackermann, *Nationale Totenfeiern*, 81, 85–86. For example, "Kaiser Wilhelm I," *Allgemeine Zeitung* (Munich), 10 March 1888, 1025–1027; "Der Kaiser, der Kaiser gestorben!" *Berliner Börsen-Zeitung*, 119, 10 March 1888, 1–2; Karl Biedermann, "Zum Gedächtniß Kaiser Wilhelms," *Die Gartenlaube*, 1888, 11, 166–168.

54 Hughes, "Splendid Demonstrations," 243. For example, "Funérailles du roi,"; "Funérailles du roi Léopold,"; "Funérailles de S.M. Léopold Ier," *L'Écho du Parlement*, 17 December 1865, 1; "Berliner Briefe. II"; and "Kaiser Wilhelm,".

55 The morning edition of the Roman, Mazzinian paper *Il Dovere* was confiscated on 10 January 1878 by order of the attorney general for an article that gave offence to the monarchy. "Cronaca Cittadina," *L'Osservatore Romano*, 12 January 1878, 2.

56 Cannadine, "The Context," 105.

57 Coenraad Arnold Tamse, *Nederland en België in Europa (1859–1871)* (The Hague: Martinus Nijhoff, 1973), 130–134.

58 For the difference between social solidarity and cultural consensus, see David I. Kertzer, *Ritual, Politics, and Power* (New Haven: Yale University Press, 1988), 67–69.

59 Deneckere, *Leopold I*, 665.

60 Jean Stengers, *De koningen der Belgen: Van Leopold I tot Albert II* (Leuven: Davidsfonds, 1997), 229; Deneckere, *Leopold I*, 579.

61 "Avènement du roi léopold II," *Le Libre Examen*, 20 December 1865, 1; "Conseil communal, séance du 14 décembre 1865," *Ville d'Anvers. Bulletin communal*, 75, 1865, 906–908.

62 Alex Körner, "Heirs and their Wives: Setting the Scene for Umbertian Italy," in *Sons and Heirs*, 49.

63 Martin Papenheim, "Roma o morte: Culture Wars in Italy," in *Culture Wars. Secular-Catholic Conflict in Nineteenth-Century Europe* (Cambridge: Cambridge University Press, 2003), 202.

64 Brice, *Monarchie*, 178.

65 Levra, *Fare gli Italiani*, 28–34; Banti, "The Remembrance," 181.

66 See Papenheim, "Roma o morte," 202–226.

67 Kertzer, *Prisoner*, 128, 131; Martina, *Pio IX*, 516; Brice, *Monarchie*, 176, 178; and Pirri, *Pio IX*, 447–452.

68 Martina, *Pio IX*, 521; Kertzer, *Prisoner*, 127; Brice, *Monarchie*, 206; "L'Osservatore Cattolico di Milano," *L'Osservatore Romano*, 22 January 1878, 3; and "Breve del Santo Padre in lode dell' Osservatore Cattolico di Milano," *La Civiltà Cattolica*, 26 January–8 February 1878, 492–493.

69 "Altre violenze," *L'Osservatore Romano*, 22 January 1878, 1–2.

70 "Ultime notizie," *L'Osservatore Romano*, 18 January 1878, 3; "I fatti di Bologna," *L'Osservatore Romano*, 19 January 1878, 1; "Altre violenze,"; "Violenza a Bologna ed in altre città pei funerali a Vittorio Emmanuele," *La Civiltà Cattolica*, 9–28 March 1878, 104; and Kertzer, *Politics*, 130.

71 Osterhammel, *The Transformation*, 412.

72 "Appunti sulla stampa Italiana," *L'Osservatore Romano*, 13 January 1878, 2; "Dimonstrazione a Napoli," *L'Osservatore Romano*, 15 January 1878, 2.

73 Giloi, *Monarchy*, 21, 181, 332.

74 Christopher Clark, *Iron Kingdom: The Rise and Downfall of Prussia, 1600–1947* (London: Penguin Books, 2007), 588–589; Eric Hobsbawm, "Mass-Producing Traditions: Europe, 1870–1914," in *The Invention of Tradition*, 264.

75 Hughes, "Splendid Demonstrations," 239; Ackermann, *Nationale Totenfeiern*, 88–89, 242; "Rede des Oberhofpredigers D. Kögel," *Berliner Börsen-Zeitung*, 16 March 1888, 3–4.

76 Erwin Fink, "Symbolic Representations of the Nation: Baden, Bavaria, and Saxony, c.1860–80," in *Different Paths to the Nation: Regional and National Identities in Central Europe and Italy, 1830–70*, ed. Laurence Cole (New York: Palgrave Macmillan, 2007), 212, 215; Werner K. Blessing, *Staat und Kirche in der Gesellschaft. Institutionelle Autorität und mentaler Wandel in Bayern während des 19. Jahrhunderts* (Göttingen: Vandenhoeck & Ruprecht, 1982), 179–180.

77 Ackermann, *Nationale Totenfeiern*, 83.

78 Hughes, "Splendid Demonstrations," 244.

79 Friedrich Krotz, "Mediatization: A Concept With Which to Grasp Media and Societal Change," in *Mediatization: Concept, Changes, Consequences*, ed. Knut Lundby (New York: Peter Lang, 2009), 24; Johanna Sumiala and Outi Hakola, "Introduction: Media and Death," *Thanatos* 2, no. 2 (2013): 1–5.

80 John Plunkett, *Queen Victoria: First Media Monarch* (Oxford: Oxford University Press, 2003), 1; Osterhammel, *The Transformation*, 29.

81 Gian Luca Fruci, "The Two Faces of Daniele Manin: French Republican Celebrity and Italian Monarchic Icon (1848–1880)," *Journal of Modern Italian Studies* 18, no. 2 (2013): 158.

82 For the adoption of middle-class cultural values such as hard work, modesty and a harmonious family life by sovereigns, see Heinz Dollinger, "Das Leitbild des 'Bügerkönigtums' in der europäischen Monarchie des 19. Jahrhunderts," in *Hof, Kultur und Politik im 19. Jahrhundert*, ed. Karl Ferdinand Werner (Bonn: Ludwig Röhrscheid Verlag, 1985), 325–362. For ideals of femininity in middle-class narratives around queens, see Regina Schulte, "The Queen: A Middle-Class Tragedy – The Writing of History and the Creation of Myths in Nineteenth-Century France and Germany," *Gender & History* 14, no. 2 (2002): 266–293.

83 "Mort du roi," *Le Journal de Bruxelles*, 12 December 1865, 1; *L'Indépendance Belge*, 12 December 1865, 1; "Circulaire maçonnique," *Le Bien Public*, 13 December 1865, 2.

84 For correspondence on the king's death, see Pirri, *Pio IX*, 427–453.

85 "La morte del Re Vittorio Emanuele II," *Gazzetta Ufficiale del Regno d'Italia*, 10 January 1878, 8, 113–114; "Roma 10 gennaio," *L'Osservatore Romano*, 11 January 1878, 1; "Roma 12 gennaio," *L'Osservatore Romano*, 13 January 1878, 1; "Una nota dell' Osservatore Romano," *La Civiltà Cattolica*, 29 December 1877–10 January 1878, 250–251; and "Appunti sulla stampa Italiana," *L'Osservatore Romano*, 23 January 1878, 2.

86 Kertzer, *Prisoner*, 127.

87 Pirri, *Pio IX*, 442; "Cronaca Cittadina," *L'Osservatore Romano*, 11 January 1878, 2; "Politica e religione del F: Crispi nella congiuntura della morte di Vittorio Emmanuele II," *La Civiltà Cattolica*, 11–25 January 1878, 363–364.

88 Plunkett, *Queen Victoria*, 5–6.

89 Bacot, *La presse illustrée au XIXe siècle : Une histoire oubliée* (Limoges: Presses Universitaires de Limoges, 2005), 13–14, 43–56.

90 Geisthövel, "Tote Monarchen", 155, 157–158. See, for example, "Funeral of the Late King of the Belgians: The Funeral Car Passing the Column in Place du Congès at Brussels," *The Illustrated London News*, 30 December 1865, 640; "Funeral of the Late King of Italy at Rome: The Procession in the Piazza di Spagna," *The Illustrated London News*, 2 February 1878, 101; "Roma: il funerale del re: 17 gennaio," *L'illustrazione Italiana*, 3 February 1878, 72–73; "Die Leichenbegägniß: Die Minister mit den Rechsinsignien und die Trauerpforte al Schneidungspunkt der Friederichsstraße," *Illustrirte Zeitung*, 24 March 1888, 299; and "Der Leichenwagen Kaiser Wilhelms am Brandenburger Thor vom Thiergarten aus gesehen," *Die Gartenlaube*, 1888, 13, 216.

91 *The Illustrated London News*, 30 December 1865, 639–641; *L'Illustration*, 23 December 1865, 404; *L'Illustration*, 30 December 1865, 420–421; *Le Monde Illustré*, 23 December 1865, 408–409.

92 Bacot, *La presse illustrée*, 87.

93 John Dickie, *Darkest Italy: The Nation and Stereotypes of the Mezzogiorno, 1860–1900* (New York: Saint Martin's Press, 1999), 84–86.

94 Robin B. Williams, "Popularizing Roma Capitale: Representations of a Royal Rome in the Pages of L'Illustrazione Italiana in the Late 19th Century," *Tahiti* 4 (2016), http://tahiti.fi/04-2016/tieteelliset-artikkelit/popularizing-roma-capitale-representations-of-a-royal-rome-in-the-pages-of-l%E2%80%99illustrazione-italiana-in-the-late-19th-century/ (accessed 23 March 2019).

95 *L'Illustrazione Italiana*, 27 January 1878, 55.

96 See Kirsten Belgum, *Popularizing the Nation: Audience, Representation, and the Production of Identity in Die Gartenlaube, 1853–1900* (Lincoln: University of Nebraska Press, 1998); Bacot, *La presse illustrée*, 55–56.

97 Hermann Heiberg, "Trauertage und des großen Kaisers Leichenbegängniß," *Die Gartenlaube*, 1888, 13, 209–211.

Key works

Ackermann, Volker, *Nationale Totenfeiern in Deutschland" Von Wilhelm I. bis Franz Josef Strauß – Eine Studie zur politischen Semiotik* (Stuttgart: Klett-Cotta, 1990).

Brice, Catherine, *Monarchie et identité nationale en Italie (1861–1900)* (Paris: Éditions de l'École des hautes études en sciences sociales, 2010).

Cannadine, David, "The Context, Performance and Meaning of Ritual: The British Monarchy and the 'Invention of Tradition', c. 1820–1977," in *The Invention of Tradition*, eds. Eric Hobsbawm and Terrence Ranger (Cambridge: Cambridge University Press, 1983), 101–164.

Deneckere, Gita, *Leopold I. De eerste koning van Europa* (Antwerp: De Bezige Bij, 2011).

Levra, Umberto, *Fare gli Italiani: Memoria e celebrazione del Risorgimento* (Turin: Comitato di Torino dell'Istituto per la storia del Risorgimento, 1992).

Williams, Robin, "Rome as State Image: The Architecture and Urbanism of the Royal Italian Government, 1870–1900" (PhD dissertation, University of Pennsylvania, 1993).

12

A USELESS CEREMONY OF SOME USE

A comparative study of attitudes to coronations in Norway and Sweden in the nineteenth and twentieth centuries

Trond Norén Isaksen

On the eve of King Charles X of France's coronation in the Cathedral of Reims in 1825, François de Chateaubriand asked himself if the king would recall seeing his eldest brother being anointed on the same spot. 'Will he believe that a coronation provides protection against misfortune? There is no longer any hand virtuous enough to heal the King's evil, no longer any holy phial salutary enough to make kings inviolable', he wrote.[1] While Louis XVI had touched 2,400 sufferers from 'the King's evil' at his coronation fifty years earlier, only 120–130 showed up to be 'healed' by Charles X.[2]

Critical voices had been heard already at the time of Louis XVI's coronation.[3] In the words of Jacques Le Goff, that occasion marked the 'end of belief in the coronation': 'From a liturgical officium it had during the sixteenth and seventeenth centuries transformed itself into a ceremony and in 1775 finally into a theatre performance. The mystery had become opera.'[4] Indeed, the ideas embodied by a coronation could hardly be reconciled with the ideas of the enlightenment and belief in the sovereignty of the people. Upon his accession in 1740, King Friedrich II of Prussia described a crown as nothing but a hat that let the rain in and told Voltaire that he would 'receive homage without benefit of the flask of holy oil and those other useless and empty ceremonies introduced because of ignorance'.[5]

By the end of the eighteenth and beginning of the nineteenth centuries coronations were on the wane in Europe. Russia retained the ritual until the last emperor's coronation in 1896, while the Habsburgs were crowned in Hungary until 1916, in Bohemia until 1836 and in Lombardy-Venetia in 1838, but never in Austria. In 1861 Wilhelm I became the first Prussian monarch to be crowned since 1701, but none of his successors followed suit.[6] Other European kingdoms had long let go of coronations. The only Portuguese coronations were in 1579 and 1641, while Spain did not hold coronations after its unification in the fifteenth century.[7] At his accession in 1830, King William IV of Britain wished to abstain from a coronation, but did not get his way. At the end of the turbulent seventeenth century the ritual had acquired new meaning at the coronation of the joint monarchs William III and Mary II in 1689, when the coronation oath was rewritten so that the monarchs clearly acknowledged their subordination to the law. In the words of Roy Strong, this made coronation 'one of the foundation stones of the modern state' and helps explain why the ritual has survived in Britain to the present day.[8]

Among the new or reborn kingdoms of the early nineteenth century, Bavaria, the Netherlands and Greece planned coronations, but various circumstances got in the way.[9] The new kingdoms of Württemberg, Saxony, Hanover and Belgium also did without coronations. Emperor Alexander I of Russia abstained from being crowned in the resurrected Kingdom of Poland, but his successors Nicholas I and Alexander II were crowned in Poland in 1829 and 1856 respectively. The odd one out among the new kingdoms was Norway, whose constitution of 17 May 1814 included article 12: 'The King's coronation and anointing is held, after he has reached his majority, in the Cathedral of Trondhjem at the time and with the ceremonial he himself decides upon'.[10] Coronations had been held in Norway from 1164 to 1514, but ceased when Norway was incorporated into Denmark at the time of the Lutheran Reformation in 1536. Thereafter the kings were crowned or – after the introduction of absolute monarchy in 1660 – anointed only in Denmark. Since the absolute monarchy's collapse in 1848–9, no Danish monarchs have been crowned or anointed, but when Norway became a constitutional monarchy the ritual was even codified.[11]

From 1807 Denmark–Norway was allied with France, while Crown Prince Carl Johan of Sweden forged an alliance with Britain and Russia in 1812 and was promised Norway as his reward. In January 1814, Carl Johan forced Frederik VI to cede Norway. However, the Norwegians rebelled and convened a constituent assembly, which proclaimed Norway's independence and passed a liberal constitution. The constitution was largely based on a draft by Johan Gunder Adler and Christian Magnus Falsen, but this version did not mention coronations. Coronation was however included in several other drafts.[12] The fact that coronation was not mentioned in Adler and Falsen's draft does not necessarily mean that they were opposed to it, as it was in fact unusual to codify coronations. One exception was the Danish *Lex Regia* of 1665, the fundamental law of the absolute monarchy, which stipulated that the kings should be anointed.[13] France offers a contemporaneous exception. A declaration of the *Senatus-consultus* of 17 February 1810 stated: 'After being crowned in the Church of Notre-Dame de Paris, the Emperors will be crowned in the Church of St. Peter [in Rome] before the completion of the tenth year of their reign.' Further to this, Louis XVIII's constitutional charter of 4 June 1814 stipulated that the kings should swear to uphold the charter at their coronations, thus implying that such a ceremony would take place.[14]

Interestingly, the founding fathers of modern Norway did not discuss whether their future kings should be crowned. Rather, the debate dealt almost exclusively with the ceremony's location. This is the more surprising given that coronations were no longer 'fashionable'. The idea of the sovereignty of the people appears to have been commonly accepted in the Dano-Norwegian realm in the second half of the eighteenth century and divine monarchy consequently viewed as outdated.[15] In 1757, the political scientist Jens Schjelderup Sneedorff called coronation and anointing 'unnecessary' and 'merely a ceremony'.[16] The sources do not explain why the Constituent Assembly went against the tide and insisted on perpetuating coronations. One possible explanation is that it was an attempt to underline Norway's status as an independent kingdom of its own should it again come to form a union with another state. Just a day after the constitution was passed, on 17 May 1814, the Constituent

Assembly elected the leader of the rebellion, Prince Christian Frederik, who was also heir presumptive to the Danish crown, king of Norway. Furthermore, Sweden was unlikely to abandon its claim on Norway. Another union thus seemed likely.[17]

In the summer of 1814 Sweden invaded Norway and, after a short war, the still uncrowned Christian Frederik renounced the crown. On 4 November, the Norwegian parliament passed a revised constitution whereby Norway entered into a union of crowns with Sweden, a very loose arrangement in which both countries remained independent and in which only the king and the foreign service were shared by the two states. The coronation article was retained unaltered, although renumbered as article 10. This created a discrepancy as the Swedish constitution had no similar requirement, although the preamble of the Act of Succession of 21 August 1810, which had transformed Marshal Bernadotte into Crown Prince Carl Johan, stated that after Carl XIII's death, Carl Johan should succeed him and 'be crowned and acclaimed as King of Sweden'. In the following, this chapter will explore how Swedish and Norwegian views on coronations came to diverge greatly in the decades that followed.

The coronations of Carl XIV Johan and Oscar I

Despite the constitutional requirement for a coronation, Carl XIII never made it to Norway before his death on 5 February 1818. On 11 May Carl XIV Johan was crowned king of Sweden in the Great Church (now the Cathedral) in Stockholm. The Norwegian parliament sent a deputation of twelve MPs, who expressed the hope soon to see 'the crown of Norway once more placed upon the head of a hero'.[18] The king replied in the affirmative and he was duly crowned in the Cathedral of Trondhjem on 7 September 1818.[19] Queen Desideria was still living in France at the time, but after she eventually came north she was crowned Queen of Sweden in Stockholm on 21 August 1829. Her Norwegian coronation was set for Christiania (now Oslo) in the late summer of 1830, but was cancelled when the outbreak of revolution in Paris threw Europe into turmoil and made the king fear a general European war might break out and that the Norwegians might rebel.[20]

After Carl Johan's death, his only son, Oscar I, was crowned together with Queen Josephine in Stockholm's Great Church on 28 September 1844. The event drew some criticism from members of the estates. One of them, Thore Petre, said that 'coronation cannot be seen as anything but an outdated ceremony, which our days' ever progressing enlightenment should abolish'. Some claimed that the tradition was rooted in a firm popular faith, but if so this faith was merely a sort of superstition, 'which the spirit of the times ought to defeat', Petre said.[21] In Norway, on the other hand, no objections were heard, probably because the king being crowned in Norway would highlight its independence and equality with Sweden. His representative in Norway, the Lieutenant of the Realm, Severin Løvenskiold, advised him not to delay longer than until the following year, as a longer delay would hurt the 'pious and loyal feelings' of the people.[22]

On 29 March 1845, the Speaker of Parliament proposed inviting the king to be crowned and received the support of all but twenty-one of the MPs.[23] The constitution said nothing of the queen's coronation, but on 9 April the Speaker proposed that Queen Josephine should also be invited to be crowned and won unanimous support.[24]

The king readily agreed on behalf of both of them.[25] However, as Trondhjem Cathedral was in urgent need of repairs, the king did not set a date for the ceremony.

Soon a heated debate about the queen's coronation broke out. The Bishop of Trondhjem, Hans Riddervold, wrote to the Church Ministry that the crowning of someone who was not to exercise royal power would be in contradiction to the meaning of the act of coronation and that to crown a queen consort would, therefore, weaken the significance of the king's coronation.[26] The official catalogue to the Norwegian crown jewels and many other books claim that Riddervold refused to crown Josephine as she remained Catholic, but this is a myth.[27] First, Riddervold never once mentioned Josephine's faith and argued only in terms of the queen's constitutional position – or rather lack thereof. Second, it was not the Bishop of Trondhjem but the Bishop of Christiania who was to perform the coronation. Third, Riddervold offered to renounce his bishopric so as not to stand in the way. Fourth, the primary sources show that preparations for the coronation went ahead regardless of Riddervold's intervention, which was hotly debated in the press.[28]

The king agreed to the government's recommendation to ignore Riddervold's objections and Riddervold was allowed to absent himself from the ceremony.[29] On 12 April 1847 Riddervold informed the Provost of Innherred that the king was expected to arrive in Trondhjem on 21 July ahead of his coronation, but on 13 May the king resolved to postpone the ceremony due to failing crops and the threat of food shortage.[30] The peasants were obliged to provide horses for transportation, and Queen Josephine later wrote that her husband 'partly could not enjoy himself while the people suffered and partly also feared that a Royal journey . . . with on such an occasion unavoidably large entourage would weigh heavily on the transporting populace – who were so dear to him'.[31] Later, a wealth of circumstances which included a disagreement with parliament over funds, the 1848 revolutions, a state of war in neighbouring Denmark and the Crimean war came in the way of Oscar I's coronation until he eventually seems to have lost interest and his health broke down, leading to his death in 1859 at the age of sixty.[32]

The coronations of Carl XV

In 1860 the Norwegian author and journalist Aasmund Olavsson Vinje observed that:

> Many a good king has lived and died in power and glory even though he was not anointed; while other kings have been both deposed and even executed by their people even though they in their days had been anointed so that they dripped of oil.

He added that coronations were becoming an increasingly rare sight 'as many people are becoming so unbelieving that they do not see any sanctity in this anointing with oil but on the contrary mock it'.[33] This scepticism was already evident when the Swedish estates met in the autumn of 1859. The first issue brought before them was a proposal to petition the new king, Carl XV, to be crowned during the meeting of the estates. The nobility, the priests and the burghers agreed, but among the peasants the motion met with such opposition that it was withdrawn.[34] The people's love for its king would be neither greater nor smaller through expensive ceremonies 'which only satisfy the curiosity of the spectators', said one member of the peasants' estate, Robert Fredrik Gross, while another, Sven Heurlin, expressed a desire to do 'away with all such prejudices in a constitutional country!'[35] Parts of the press also opposed the idea that Carl XV should be crowned.[36] *Illustrerad Tidning* called it an expensive, empty anachronism, while *Aftonbladet* reminded its readers that there was no constitutional requirement for a coronation and argued that Oscar I's position in Norway had not been weakened by his failure to be crowned. It also correctly predicted that if Europe's most powerful monarch, Napoléon III, were one day to fall it would not be because he had not been crowned and anointed. The idea that a prelate could give a free people's lawful monarch a higher consecration not only belonged to a time that was long past but contradicted 'our times' entire erudition and its idea of church and state'.[37]

Once again, the criticism was confined to Sweden. On 3 December 1859, the Speaker of the Norwegian parliament suggested inviting King Carl and Queen Louise to be crowned. Only three MPs voted against, one of whom explained that he did not oppose a coronation but merely thought it unnecessary to issue such an invitation.[38] The king replied that he intended to be crowned in the coming year and in January he set the dates as 3 May for Sweden and 5 August for Norway.[39]

A broken vow came to cast a shadow over the Norwegian coronation. As the king was primarily resident in Stockholm, three members of the Norwegian cabinet resided in the Swedish capital to be near him. In the monarch's absence, a Lieutenant of the Realm presided in the cabinet in Christiania. The Norwegians disapproved of this and considered the lieutenancy a colonial stigma unworthy of an independent kingdom. As Crown Prince, Carl XV had promised that he would consent to the lieutenancy's abolition when he became king.[40] However, when parliament voted to abolish it in December 1859, strong voices in the Swedish estates and press objected and demanded that the king should not assent without consulting the Swedish estates and without ensuring a revision of the terms of the union in Swedish favour.[41] To the fury of the Norwegians, who insisted that this was an exclusively Norwegian issue, King Carl allowed himself to be pressured by Swedish politicians into breaking his vow.[42] It thus seemed obvious that he was first and foremost king of Sweden and only secondly of Norway.

In the wake of this the coronation in Trondhjem would not be 'without political significance', Eugéne Forcade wrote in *Revue des deux Mondes*. However, the Norwegian people's love for the union and the dynasty was strong, Forcade thought, and he predicted that 'particularly at this moment' one would see the Norwegians 'far from receiving the coronation with coldness but greet the new king of Norway with jubilation'.[43] Similarly, a Danish newspaper reported that the inhabitants of Trondhjem were intent on 'forgetting the Swedish Parliament's and government's behaviour and regard the coronation as what it is: a demonstration to the whole world that Norway is an independent, free country'.[44] The newspaper *Christiania-Posten*'s correspondent also believed that everyone must rejoice that the king and queen had been crowned, for foreign nations, 'who so slowly learn to recognise our country as an independent kingdom', would have got the wrong idea if the royal couple had been crowned only in Sweden. Perhaps it was useful that the coronation took place at a time 'when our constitutional independence so recently has been the subject of discussion', he mused.[45]

Indeed, much of the explanation as to why coronations were viewed more favourably in Norway than in Sweden seems to have been that they were the most visible demonstrations possible of the fact that Norway, the junior partner of the union, was an independent kingdom of equal status with Sweden. In other words, what was increasingly derided in Sweden as a useless ceremony was of some use to the Norwegians.

Oscar II's coronations

Having lost his only son at an early age, Carl XV was succeeded by his younger brother when he died at the age of forty-six on 18 September 1872. Oscar II's reign began with a dispute over his Swedish coronation. The estates had now been replaced by a bicameral parliament, and on 25 January 1873, the vice-Speakers of the two chambers moved that they should ask the king whether he and Queen Sophie intended to allow themselves to be crowned. The vice-Speakers admitted that there was no constitutional requirement for a coronation, but stressed that the constitution of Norway 'explicitly says (Article 10) that [a] king must be crowned'. Previous generations of parliamentarians had listened to 'the call of the heart and the people's desire' every time a king had ascended the throne and had greeted him by requesting that he would 'let the crown be placed upon his head in the temple of the Lord'. The vice-Speakers assumed that the MPs would now follow 'old, time-honoured use and Swedish custom'.[46]

The liberal firebrand Adolf Hedin made a barn-storming speech when the issue reached the second chamber. He asked whether one thought Sweden's position in the union would suffer if the king were crowned only in Norway. Did one perhaps think that the degree of the king's obligations towards the people and country would increase through an 'unreasonable, for some tasteless, for others ridiculous ceremony'? Or was one perhaps so uncertain of one's feelings that it was necessary to 'undertake special theatrical measures to puff them up to a higher temperature'? Or was it still believed in 1873 that the awe for royal authority could be fortified 'through such public entertainments for children and old women?' Was one sure that one did not accomplish the opposite of one's intention if the public saw through the pomp and realized that the monarchy depended on nonsense and humbug, he wondered.[47]

Several other MPs also spoke against coronations in themselves or the idea that parliament should petition the king to be crowned.[48] 'The people no longer attach any value to the coronations of kings. They are only concerned with their king's personal qualities', said Carl Anders Larsson.[49] The vice-Speaker was alone in maintaining that the people in rural areas still thought it important that the king be crowned.[50] In the end, 124 members of the second chamber voted not to petition the king, while fifty-one supported a motion that parliament should invite the king to decide whether or not he intended to be crowned, but should not itself take any action in the matter.[51]

The liberal press also reacted strongly against the idea of a coronation. *Aftonbladet* opined that in 'our age, that of the bourgeois monarchy', the people's trust was a stronger foundation than 'some imposing emblems'.[52] *Dagens Nyheter* doubted that there was any popular desire for such a superfluous ceremony and pointed out that anointing did not give any protection, while it was 'the King's qualities and actions that make up his rightful and secure crown'.[53] The newspaper thought the debate was 'a sign of our times' which testified to 'how public opinion regarding "the royautée's imposing problems" has changed during the past decade'.[54]

Despite the opposition, Oscar II, who was known for his love of pomp and circumstance,[55] insisted on being crowned in Stockholm's Great Church on 12 May 1873.

Norwegian newspapers reported the Swedish debate in detail, particularly Hedin's speech, but once again there was no debate in Norway. Just a week after the Swedish parliament's second chamber had rejected the proposal to petition the king, the Norwegian parliament did the exact opposite and invited the king and queen to be crowned.[56] The king replied that he saw this as 'renewed proof of the Norwegian people's feelings for its royal house' and set the date for 18 July 1873.[57] The reason why there were no objections in Norway again seems to have been that a coronation would broadcast Norway's independence.

The newspaper *Dagbladet*, no friend of the monarchy, opined that the king's Swedish coronation made a Norwegian coronation 'a political necessity' and commended King Oscar for his presumed wish to assist in making things clear to those who imagine him to be a 'union king', the point being that, strictly speaking, in law there was no king of the union; the king of Sweden and the king of Norway just happened to be the same man. Perhaps the constitution's and the Act of Union's words about Norway being 'a free, independent, indivisible and inalienable realm, united with Sweden under one king' ought to be enough so that one did not have to illustrate them with 'an expensive medieval ceremony' that might muddle conceptions of the nature of a constitutional monarchy, the paper mused. Nevertheless, the paper had to agree with the king's supposed view that it was sometimes:

> [n]ecessary to use a language that speaks more directly to the senses when one wants a fact to be clearly perceived and retained by public opinion in those groups of states where it may be of the greatest interest that there is no lack of clarity about our state's independence.[58]

Oscar II contributed to making his and Queen Sophie's coronation a roaring success when he on 5 June agreed to the abolition of the lieutenancy, thus fulfilling his brother's broken vow. The king wrote in his memoirs:

> In Norway one was of course jubilant, and this jubilation followed me in increasing tones during the journey I soon thereafter undertook to the northernmost provinces of Norway, which had not been visited by any king since Christian IV [in 1599], and reached its crescendo when I received the crown in the choir of Trondhjem's ancient cathedral on the anniversary of Norway's millennium [the millennium of Norway's unification had been celebrated on 18 July 1872].[59]

There is a lot of braggadocio and misrepresentations in Oscar II's memoirs, but this statement is supported by the contemporary press coverage.

Before the coronation, King Oscar travelled through the vast northern half of Norway, all the way to the North Cape and the border with Russia, while Queen

Sophie made a similar tour of the southern part of the country. Already in 1818, Carl XIV Johan had basked in public gratitude when he travelled to Trondhjem for his coronation as he had personally helped relieve the people's hardships through gifts of grain and by lending money, thus presenting himself as the people's friend to a greater degree than their chosen representatives in parliament.[60] But King Oscar II and Queen Sophie were the first royal couple to make a nationwide coronation tour, which provided them with the opportunity to form a personal bond with the people all over the country.

Their example was followed by King Haakon VII and Queen Maud in connection with their coronation in 1906, and later by King Olav and his daughter, Princess Astrid, at the time of his solemn blessing in 1958 and then by King Harald V and Queen Sonja when they were solemnly blessed in 1991. Similar tours have been undertaken on a number of other occasions, most recently the king's silver jubilee in 2016, and are now considered more important than solemn ceremonies when it comes to connecting with the people and thereby strengthening the monarchy's standing.

The end of coronations

Oscar II's Norwegian coronation was a master class in how to win the people and marked the union's golden hour. For various reasons it would, nevertheless, fall apart in his lifetime. On 7 June 1905, he was deposed by the Norwegian parliament and the union consequently dissolved. Following negotiations between the two states, Oscar II formally renounced the crown of Norway and, after a referendum in which 78.9% voted in his favour, Prince Carl of Denmark was unanimously elected King Haakon VII by parliament on 18 November. Three days earlier, the cabinet had struck 'by the grace of God' from the royal title, which it had been part of since the reign of Magnus Erlingsson, who in 1164 was the first king of Norway to be crowned.[61]

When he was first offered the crown, Prince Carl had set certain conditions, including that he should be crowned. This may seem rather puzzling as he also stated his wish to live rather modestly with a small household, but the reason for his demand was apparently simply that he considered himself bound by the constitution's coronation article.[62] However, now that a coronation was no longer needed to remind the world of Norway's independence, the ritual had outlived its usefulness and for the first time it came in for heavy criticism.

Two weeks after the new royal family's arrival, four Labour MPs proposed abolishing the coronation article. As the coronation was inextricably linked to the idea of monarchy 'by the grace of God', its abolition was a necessary consequence of this having been struck from the royal title. The four MPs claimed that a coronation was really 'a debasement of the church and an abuse of the church service' and, as the king's swearing-in marked his accession, a coronation was merely 'a superfluous ceremony that causes great expenses for the state and the municipality'. Parliament may only vote over constitutional amendments after the next general election, and in the meantime the proposers expected that Haakon VII's coronation would be postponed.[63] This did not happen, but this time parliament did not invite the king to be crowned.

As they were cut off from debating the amendment, parliament instead engaged in a lengthy debate when voting over funds for the coronation on 6 April 1906. Alfred Eriksen, one of the MPs who had proposed the amendment, found it unbelievable that a parliamentary majority could possibly support spending NOK100,000 of taxpayers' money on an 'empty, meaningless, medieval custom' connected to a way of thought that had 'long passed away'.[64] Adam Egede-Nissen, another of the Labour MPs behind the amendment, warned that the people might both laugh and snarl at 'all this ridiculousness' that was staged at their expense.[65] Moreover, Liberal MP Wollert Konow thought that King Haakon would have become more loved if he had refrained from a coronation and would thus have 'built his dynasty on a more secure foundation', partly because of the nation's straightened financial circumstances, 'partly because it is an old, antiquated ceremony'.[66]

Not a single MP offered a principled defence of coronations. However, the leader of the Budget Committee, Peter Collett Solberg (Conservative), stated that the coronation would be 'the new royal family's true day of entry into the country' and thought that the general populace would want this to be marked in a proper way.[67] Finance Minister Edvard Hagerup Bull (Conservative) admitted that one could do without coronations, but did not find this the right moment to abolish them. He was convinced that many would regard 'the day when a fully independent Norwegian king is installed in his position by a Norwegian bishop for the first time in centuries a national day of celebration'.[68] Abraham Berge of the Liberal Party saw King Haakon's coronation as the very completion of Norway's revival. He thought it odd that some would deny that 'it is a festive moment, not for the sake of the coronation, not for the sake of the oil, but because the entire Norwegian people has found itself again after 600 years'.[69] This became the theme of the coronation on 22 June 1906. When the ritual no longer harmonized with the times, it was interpreted as an act that reconnected Norway with its past and marked the completion of its struggle to free itself of dependence on other countries.

Ahead of the coronation, Bishop Anton Christian Bang of Kristiania had publicly called for the ceremonial to undergo 'a thorough if not radical reworking, so that it may more or less correspond with our days' feelings and views in both political and ecclesiastical respect'. As it was not possible to scrap the act of anointing altogether, Bang felt that it ought to be toned down as much as possible and that the crown jewels ought to be presented not by prelates but by representatives of parliament, who were the real kingmakers.[70] In the end, the ceremonial was somewhat simplified but mostly followed the precedents of 1818, 1860 and 1873, including the anointing of both king and queen.

In his coronation sermon, Bang pointed out that the last man to be crowned king of Norway without simultaneously being king of another realm was Håkon V Magnusson in 1299. On this day it was as 'if old and new times reach out to each other, it is as if broken ties are bound together again'. Now 'the crown will be placed upon king and queen, and with that the crown shall be placed upon a completed work that connects past to present and present to past', he enthused.[71] Several newspapers echoed this view.[72] 'Today the work of 7 June [1905] is crowned', wrote *Aftenposten*, while *Fredriksstad Tilskuer*'s reporter called the crowning 'a wondrous, unforgettable moment' and thought he had seen tears in many eyes 'at the great historical moment when the crown of liberated Norway was placed on the descendant of the House of Harald [the earliest royal dynasty] and the ring around past, present and future was completed'.[73]

Stavanger Aftenblad's reporter was unimpressed, however. He thought the act 'did not really belong in our times. The coronation's bonds did not quite succeed in connecting old and new times'. He found it all too theatrical and thought that 'in the people's conscience the throne was erected and the crown fastened when Haakon was chosen as King of Norway by the Parliament of Norway'. However, on this day all Norway knew that this would be the last coronation, he went on:

> This time we wanted it. To demonstrate to the world that the work is completed. That Norway is a whole, independent kingdom, united with no one, ours, ours alone. For us a meaningless act, an attestation, a commercial, but a beautiful commercial.[74]

Bishop Bang agreed: 'Although without political significance it [the coronation] found its justification in the historical situation. It pointed back to 1319 [when the centuries of unions began] and symbolised the linking of the old and the new Norway'. Yet he realized that this was most likely the last coronation. 'In a modern state there is really no room for a ceremony that to such an extent as a royal coronation is based on medieval ideas and circumstances'.[75]

It also turned out to be the last coronation in all of Scandinavia. Two weeks after the death of Oscar II on 8 December 1907, King Gustaf V informed the Swedish cabinet that he would not be crowned 'as he held the opinion that a coronation, which is not required by the Constitution of the realm, was superfluous and did not correspond with the spirit of the age'. He added that the money might also be spent on something more useful.[76] The Marshal of the Realm (i.e. Lord Chamberlain) told the press that the new king was 'a man of action, who does not like unnecessary formalities . . . he wants to go forwards and he likes simplicity'.[77] *Aftonbladet* believed the decision would be welcomed throughout the country, while *Dagens Nyheter* observed:

> In our days the royal crown sits as securely on an un-anointed as on an anointed head; and Sweden's monarchs win nothing in popular respect through a priestly act of coronation . . . And the fact that democratic Norway has inaugurated its new era with a coronation festivity in the most outdated form need not diminish the Swedish pleasure over the fact that our royal house feel sufficiently deeply rooted in the country's soil to manage without this arguably meaningless ceremony.[78]

Meanwhile a general election had been held in Norway and parliament could thus vote over the constitutional amendment proposed in December 1905. When it did so on 29 February 1908, no one rose to speak and only two MPs voted against the abolition of the coronation article.[79] With the dissolution of the union and the re-establishment of a national monarchy, a coronation was no longer needed to remind the world of Norway's independence.

A replacement for coronations

Despite the removal of the coronation article from the Norwegian constitution, some voices occasionally suggested that there might be more coronations as no ban had come in its place.[80] The issue was raised in the summer of 1945, when the 73-year-old King Haakon VII returned to Norway in triumph at the end of the World War II. Arne Fjellbu, who became Bishop of Nidaros, as the bishopric of Trondheim had now been renamed, in the autumn observed that given the current standing of the royal family, who had been the foremost symbols of resistance and independence during the war, a coronation would 'surely be felt natural and self-evident'. However, Fjellbu himself opposed the idea and thought that only the English were sufficiently traditional to be able to stomach a coronation.[81]

About the same time, the Bishop of Oslo, Eivind Berggrav, told Crown Prince Olav that he found it wrong that there had been no replacement for the coronation article. Berggrav thought that most people were not aware of this and would consider it a void if there were no solemn event in Trondheim when the crown prince ascended the throne. He therefore suggested marking the event with a simpler ceremony in Nidaros Cathedral.[82] Berggrav brought the suggestion to the attention of King Haakon, who 'at once showed great interest', but who would later tell his son to insist on a coronation.[83] Prime Minister Einar Gerhardsen, the Speaker of Parliament and the Minister of Church and Education were also in favour of the idea and, according to Berggrav, they believed that 'the people would expect and desire such a solemn event'.[84]

When Haakon VII died in 1957, some newspapers and one MP publicly called for Olav V to be crowned, but several Social Democratic newspapers opposed the idea.[85] At the end of his life, King Olav admitted that he had wanted to be crowned.[86] He told one biographer that he felt it could only have been done if there had been a popular demand for it, but told another biographer that he would have wanted it if that option 'had not been abolished'.[87] The latter was a misinterpretation, and the Ministry of Justice had publicly confirmed that there were no constitutional or legal barriers to a coronation.[88]

However, had the new king insisted on a coronation he would probably have met fierce resistance from the cabinet. Although the government had initially been favourably disposed to the new ceremony proposed by Berggrav, Olav faced considerable opposition in the years that followed. There is no space to enter into the details of this byzantine process, but in short the Labour government favoured a much simpler ceremony.[89] In 1950, the Minister of Church and Education told Berggrav that the ceremony should not resemble a coronation and suggested that it could take place in Oslo's modest cathedral rather than in the Gothic splendours of Nidaros Cathedral. The new king and queen should sit in a prominent position in the choir, but there should be no laying on of hands when they were blessed.[90] Crown Prince Olav insisted that he should kneel and the Bishop lay his hand on his head as he blessed him. Shortly after returning from the coronation of Queen Elizabeth II in Britain, the land of his birth, in 1953, he told Bishop Fjellbu:

> When one is about to marry and set up a home it is a serious matter. Then one wants to kneel at the Lord's altar and be blessed by the laying on of hands and prayer. When one becomes king it is also a serious matter. Then I want to kneel at the Lord's altar and be blessed by the laying on of hands and prayer.[91]

In the end, the crown prince decided to let the matter rest until his accession and then succeeded in outmanoeuvring Gerhardsen completely. The result was a rather pompous affair in Nidaros Cathedral on 22 June 1958, in which the widowed king knelt in front of the high altar and was solemnly blessed by Fjellbu, who laid his hand on the king's head. Although it was really just a blessing in solemn forms, King Olav preferred the English translation 'consecration' with all its sacral connotations even though he was not anointed.[92] He later said that the ritual was 'very important to me'.[93] His relationship to the Church of Norway, whose head he was, would 'not have been the same without the consecration. I would not have felt the same right to authority'.[94] He explained that although he was not king *by* the grace of God, he wanted to be king *with* the grace of God.[95] King Olav considered the solemn blessing a marriage to his people, a bond that could only be broken by death, and told his family that abdication 'would be a betrayal of the consecration'.[96]

The ceremony was repeated with even greater splendour for King Harald V and Queen Sonja on 23 June 1991. By then it met with no political opposition whatsoever and only one critical voice was heard in the press. Twenty-five years later King Harald said: 'Receiving God's blessing of our task – and to kneel down where both my father and my grandfather [sic] had earlier received the same blessing, felt like a great strength'.[97] The accession of the current king of Sweden, Carl XVI Gustaf, was on the contrary marked solely by secular ceremonies. On 19 September 1973, four days after the death of his grandfather, he took the oath in a council of state and thereafter gave a speech from the throne in the Royal Palace's Hall of State.

At the close of the twentieth century, Norway was the only European kingdom besides Britain that marked the accession of a new monarch with a religious ritual. At the time of the next accession things may, however, be different. Since a constitutional amendment in 2012 the king is no longer head of the Church of Norway, which was made independent of the state in 2017. Nevertheless, the constitution still accords the Church of Norway a privileged position, and the requirement for the king to profess the Lutheran faith was retained on the personal request of King Harald.[98] In an interview in 2013 Crown Prince Haakon hinted that there may well be another solemn blessing, although it may be done in a somewhat different manner.[99]

Conclusion

The constitution which was passed when Norway won back its independence in 1814 stipulated that the king should be crowned in the Cathedral of Trondhjem. This created a discrepancy when Norway was forced into a personal union with Sweden later that year, as there was no such constitutional requirement for the king of Sweden.

By then, many European monarchies had done away with coronations, a ritual which was not easily compatible with the ideas of the enlightenment. Throughout the nineteenth century, opposition to coronations grew ever stronger in Sweden, to the extent that in 1873 Oscar II was crowned against parliament's wish.

In Norway, on the other hand, critical voices barely registered. The reason was clearly that the fact the king had two coronations demonstrated to the world Norway was an independent kingdom of equal status with Sweden and not merely a Swedish appendage.

This rationale for coronations disappeared when the union was dissolved in 1905. Against some opposition, Haakon VII was crowned king of Norway the following year, a ceremony which was widely considered the symbolical completion of Norway's national rebirth. Two years later, the coronation article was struck from the constitution.

In the meantime, Gustaf V had brought the Swedish coronation tradition to an end by refusing to be crowned when he came to the throne in 1907. While Sweden since then has marked a monarch's accession with secular ceremonies only, King Olav V of Norway devised a new religious ritual, the solemn blessing, which perpetuated some of the ideas associated with coronations.

Notes

1 François-René de Chateaubriand, *Memoirs from Beyond the Tomb*, trans. Robert Baldick (London: Penguin, 2014 [1849–50]), 332.
2 Marc Bloch, *The Royal Touch: Sacred Monarchy and Scrofula in England and France*, trans. J.E. Anderson (London: Routledge & Kegan Paul and Montreal: McGill-Queen's University Press, 1973 [1961]), 227.
3 Jacques Le Goff, *Reims: Krönungsstadt*, trans. Bernd Schwibs (Berlin: Verlag Klaus Wagenbach, 1997 [1986]), 84. All translations into English from sources in other languages than English are mine.
4 Le Goff, *Reims*, 87.
5 Quoted in Nicholas Henshall, *The Zenith of European Monarchy and Its Elies: The Politics of Culture, 1650–1750* (Basingstoke and New York: Palgrave Macmillan, 2010), 91; Friedrich Heer, *The Holy Roman Empire*, trans. Janet Sondheimer (London: Phoenix, 1995 [1967]), 248.
6 Lord Twining, *European Regalia* (London: B.T. Batsford, 1967), 81.
7 David Williamson, *Debrett's Guide to Heraldry and Regalia* (London: Headline Book, 1992), 152–153; Twining, *Regalia*, 78–79.
8 Roy Strong, *Coronation: A History of Kingship and the British Monarchy* (London: Harper Collins, 2005), 281.
9 Hans Ottomeyer, *Die Kroninsignien des Königreiches Bayern* (Munich: Schnell & Steiner, 1979), 28–29; "Sabine Heym, Prachtvolle Kroninsignien für Bayern – aber keine Krönung," in *Bayerns Krone 1806: 200 Jahre Königreich Bayern*, eds. Johannes Erichsen and Katharina Heinemann (Munich: Hirmer, 2006), 37, 47.
10 Eli Fure, *Eidsvoll 1814: Hvordan grunnloven ble til* (Oslo: Dreyer, 1989), 376; Mads T. Andenæs, *Grunnloven vår: 1814 til 2001* (Oslo: Universitetsforlaget, 2001 [1949]), 150.
11 See Trond Norén Isaksen, *Norges krone: Kroninger, signinger og maktkamper fra sagatid til nåtid* (Oslo: Historie & Kultur, 2015).
12 Yngvar Nielsen, *Bidrag til Norges Historie i 1814: Afhandlinger og Aktstykker*, vol. 1 (Kristiania: Den norske historiske Forening, 1882), 52, 233.
13 Christian Ejlers, ed., *Kongeloven: Thomæsons håndskrift* (Copenhagen: Jurist- og Økonomforbundets Forlag, 2012), 161 (§ XVI).
14 Quoted in Émile Dard, *Napoleon and Talleyrand* (London: Philip Allan, 1937), 354; Le Goff, *Reims*, 91.
15 Jens Arup Seip, "Teorien om det opinionsstyrte enevelde," *Historisk tidsskrift* 38 (1957–1958): 407.
16 Jens Schjelderup Sneedorff, *Om den borgerlige Regjering* (Copenhagen: Johann Benjamin Ackermann, 1774), 275, 277.
17 Among a vast literature on the events of 1814 one of the best books is Sverre Steen, *Det frie Norge*, vol. 1, 1814 (Oslo: J.W. Cappelen, 1951).
18 Stortingsforhandlinger 1818, vol. 2, part 2, 143–144.
19 Ibid, 203.
20 See Norén Isaksen, *Norges krone*, 259–263, 269–270.
21 Quoted in Posthumus [Johan Carl Hellberg], *Ur minnet och dagboken om mina samtida personer och händelser efter 1815 inom och utom fäderneslandet*, vol. 2 (Stockholm: Iwar Haggström, 1870), 22.

22 Letter from Severin Løvenskiold to Oscar I, 7 October 1844, The Bernadotte Archive: Oscar I's and Queen Josephina's archive, vol. 42.

23 Stortingsforhandlinger 1845, vol. 7, 106, 149.

24 Ibid., 171.

25 Stortingsforhandlinger 1845, vol. 9, 358.

26 Copy of letter from Hans Riddervold to the Church Ministry, 6 March 1846, State Archive of Trondheim: Trondhjems biskops kopibok, no. 31, 1844–1847.

27 See Norén Isaksen, *Norges krone*, 275–291.

28 Trygve Lysaker, *Domkirken i Trondheim*, vol. 3 (Oslo: Land og Kirke, 1973), 292–294; letters from Severin Løvenskiold to Oscar I, 15 November 1846, 31 December 1846, 4 and 18 March 1847, The Bernadotte Archive: Oscar I's and Josephina's archive, vol. 42; Stortingsforhandlinger 1848, vol. 2, 482; Stortingsforhandlinger 1851, vol. 7, 423; *Trondhjems borgerlige Realskoles alene privilegerede Adressecontoirs-Efterretninger*, 4 June 1847.

29 "Protocol ført i Statsraad for Hans Majestæt Kongen," Stockholm Palace, 11 April 1846, National Archives of Norway (hereafter NRA): Statssekretariatet, Kongelige resolusjoner, 1846, I, RA/S-1001/A/Ab/L0063); letter from Severin Løvenskiold to Oscar I, 18 March 1847, The Bernadotte Archive: Oscar I's and Josephina's archive, vol. 42.

30 Copy of letter from Hans Riddervold to Hans Sever Arentz, 12 April 1847, State Archive of Trondheim: Trondhjems Biskop, Kopibog nr. 32, 1846–1853; "Protocol ført i Statsraad for Hans Majestæt Kongen," 13 May 1847, NRA, Statssekretariatet, Kongelige resolusjoner, 1847, I, RA/S-1001/A/Ab/L0065.

31 Queen Josephine's notes on the life of King Oscar I, 1859, National Archives of Sweden: Katolska biskopsämbetet, Joseph Müllers samling om drottning Josephina, vol. 19, 1481: 05.

32 See Norén Isaksen, *Norges krone*, 291–296.

33 Aasmund Olavsson Vinje, *Ferdaminne fraa sumaren 1860* (Oslo: Gyldendal, 1996 [1861]), 131.

34 *Aftonbladet*, 2 November 1859.

35 Bondeståndets protokoll vid Riksdagen 1859–1860, vol. 1, 141–143.

36 Cecilia Bååth-Holmberg, *Carl XV: Som enskild man, konung och konstnär* (Stockholm: Fahlcrantz, 1891), 95.

37 *Illustrerad Tidning*, no. 19, 12 May 1860; *Aftonbladet*, 3 November 1859.

38 Stortingsforhandlinger 1859–1860, vol. 9, 34; *Drammens Tidende*, 6 December 1859.

39 Stortingsforhandlinger 1859–1860, vol. 9, 34, 47, 49.

40 Sven Eriksson, *Carl XV* (Stockholm: Wahlström & Widstrand, 1954), 301; Bo Stråth, *Union och demokrati: De Förenade rikena Sverige-Norge 1814–1905*, vol. 2 of *Sverige och Norge under 200 år* (Nora: Nya Doxa, 2005), 218; J. Ernst Sars, *Norges politiske historie, 1815–1885* (Kristiania, Oscar Andersen, 1904), 502.

41 Eriksson, *Carl XV*, 307; Stråth, *Union och demokrati*, 2005, 218–220; Sars, *Norges politiske historie*, 507–515.

42 Stortingsforhandlinger 1859–1860, vol. 9, 73–77; Eriksson, *Carl XV*, 314; Stråth, *Union och demokrati*, 2005, 220; Sars, *Norges politiske historie*, 515–516.

43 Quoted in *Morgenbladet*, 16 August 1860.

44 *Fædrelandet*, quoted in *Christiania-Posten*, 13 August 1860.

45 *Christiania-Posten*, 21 August 1860.

46 Riksdagens protokoll vid lagtima riksmötet år 1873: Andra kammaren, vol. 1, 26–27.

47 Ibid., 54–55.

48 Ibid., 55–54.

49 Ibid., 56.

50 Ibid., 58.

51 Ibid., 217–222.

52 *Aftonbladet*, 28 January 1873.

53 *Dagens Nyheter*, 27 January 1873.

54 Ibid., 28 January 1873.

55 See for instance Jakob Schøning's diary, 18 January 1905, printed in Jacob S. Worm-Müller (ed.), *Jakob Schønings dagbøker: Fra Stortinget 1895–97 og fra Regjeringen 1903–05* (Oslo: Tanum, 1950), 280.

56 *Stortingstidende*, no. 16, 1873.
57 Stortingsforhandlinger 1873, vol. 5, doc. no. 56.
58 *Dagbladet*, 18 July 1873.
59 Oscar II, *Mina memoarer*, vol. 2 (Stockholm: Norstedts, 1961), 19.
60 *Den Norske Rigstidende*, 5 September 1818; copy of Jacob De la Gardie'sdiary, 24 August 1818, National Library of Norway: Manuscript Collection, Ms. fol. 647; Sverre Steen, *Det frie Norge*, vol. 2 (Oslo: Cappelen, 1953), 265.
61 J.V. Heiberg, ed., *Unionens opløsning: Officielle aktstykker vedrørende unionskrisen og Norges gjenreisning som helt suveræn stat* (Kristiania: Stensersen, 1906), 977; Absalon Taranger, *Trondheimens forfatningshistorie* (Trondheim: Brun, 1929), 42.
62 Tim Greve, *Haakon VII: Menneske og monark* (Oslo: Gyldendal, 1980), 104; Trygve Ramberg, *Med folket: Historien om vårt kongehus* (Oslo: Gyldendal, 1987), 439.
63 Stortingsforhandlinger 1905–1906, vol. 5, 52.
64 Stortingsforhandlinger 1905–1906, vol. 7b, 1519–1522.
65 Ibid., 1525.
66 Ibid., 1537.
67 Ibid., 1523.
68 Ibid., 1527.
69 Ibid., 1533.
70 *Morgenbladet*, 8 April 1906, morning edition.
71 Anton Christian Bang, *Taler og foredrag ved særlige anledninger* (Kristiania: Cammermeyer, 1907), 165, 170–171.
72 *Morgenbladet*, 22 June 1906, evening edition; *Ørebladet*, 22 June 1906; *Hedemarkens Amtstidende*, 22 June 1906.
73 *Aftenposten*, 22 June 1906, morning edition; *Fredriksstad Tilskuer*, 22 June 1906.
74 *Stavanger Aftenblad*, 26 June 1906.
75 Anton Christian Bang, *Erindringer* (Kristiania and Copenhagen: Gyldendal, 1909), 449.
76 Quoted in Karl Hildebrand, *Gustaf V som människa och regent*, vol. 1 (Stockholm: Svensk Litteratur, 1945), 513; Per-Erik Lindorm, "I den sjätte Bernadottens tid," in *Gustaf VI Adolf: Hela folkets kung*, eds. Karl-Ragnar Gierow, Nils-Gustaf Holmquist and P. G. Peterson (Stockholm: Hemmets Journal, 1971), 174.
77 *Dagens Nyheter*, 24 December 1907.
78 *Aftonbladet*, 23 December 1907; *Dagens Nyheter*, 24 December 1907.
79 Stortingsforhandlinger 1908, vol. 7, 609.
80 Taranger, *Trondheimens forfatningshistorie*, 53–54; *Dagsposten*, 22 November 1938.
81 Arne Fjellbu, *En biskop ser tilbake* (Oslo: Gyldendal, 1960), 364–365.
82 Letter from Eivind Berggrav to Minister of Church and Education Lars Moen, 23 December 1949, cited in memorandum from Minister of Church and Education Birger Bergersen to other cabinet members, 19 February 1958, NRA, Kirke- og undervisningsdepartementet, Kirkeavdelingen A Kontoret for Kirke og geistlighet, Kongehuset 1818–1958, nr. 183, RA/S-1007/D/Dd/L0183/0001.
83 Ibid.; Eivind Berggrav's notes from a conversation with Haakon VII, 22 July 1947, NRA, Privatarkiv 320, arkivdel 1, eske 39, Andre saker knyttet til Berggravs virksomhet, Kongefamilien.
84 Letter from Eivind Berggrav to Minister of Church and Education Lars Moen, 23 December 1949, cited in memorandum from Minister of Church and Education Birger Bergersen to other cabinet members, 19 February 1958, NRA, Kirke- og undervisningsdepartementet, Kirkeavdelingen A Kontoret for Kirke og geistlighet, Kongehuset 1818–1958, nr. 183, RA/S-1007/D/Dd/L0183/0001.
85 *Adresseavisen*, 26 September and 12 October 1957; *Aftenposten*, 14 October 1957, morning edition; *VG*, 14 October 1957.
86 Jo Benkow, *Olav: Menneske og monark* (Oslo: Gyldendal, 1991), 264.
87 Lars Roar Langslet, *Kong Olav V av Norge: Monarkiet i en brytningstid* (Oslo: Cappelen, 1992), 339–340; Benkow, *Olav*, 264.
88 *VG*, 15 October 1957.

89 See Norén Isaksen, *Norges krone*, 370–378.
90 Letter from Minister of Church and Education Lars Moen to Eivind Berggrav, 9 November 1950, cited in memorandum from Minister of Church and Education Birger Bergersen to other cabinet members, 19 February 1958, NRA, Kirke- og undervisningsdepartementet, Kirkeavdelingen A Kontoret for Kirke og geistlighet, Kongehuset 1818–1958, nr. 183, RA/S-1007/D/Dd/L0183/0001.
91 Fjellbu, *En biskop*, 365.
92 Langslet, *Kong Olav*, 192.
93 Ibid., 340.
94 Ibid., 351.
95 Ibid., 340.
96 Ibid., 192.
97 https://royalcorrespondent.com/2016/12/31/video-a-new-years-message-from-his-majesty-king-harald-v-of-norway/ (last accessed 29 March 2019).
98 *Dagbladet*, 11 April 2008; Jens Stoltenberg, *Min historie* (Oslo: Gyldendal, 2016), 454.
99 "Kronprins Haakon: Veien til et kongerike," broadcast on NRK1, 20 July 2013, http://tv.nrk.no/program/MKTF40000013/kronprins-haakon-veien-til-et-kongerike# (last accessed 29 March 2019).

Key works

The Bernadotte Archive: Oscar I's and Josephina's archive, volume 42.

Bondeståndets protokoll vid Riksdagen 1859–1860, vol. 1.

"Memorandum from Minister of Church and Education Birger Bergersen to other cabinet members," 19 February 1958 (National Archives of Norway: Kirke- og undervisnings departementet, Kirkeavdelingen A Kontoret for Kirke og geistlighet, Kongehuset 1818–1958, nr. 183, RA/S-1007/D/Dd/L0183/0001).

Norén Isaksen, Trond, *Norges krone: Kroninger, signinger og maktkamper fra sagatid til nåtid* (Oslo: Forlaget Historie & Kultur, 2015).

Riksdagens protokoll vid lagtima riksmötet år 1873: Andra kammaren, vol. 1.

Stortingsforhandlinger 1818, vol. 2, part 1–2; 1845, vols.7, 9; 1848, vol. 2; 1851, vol. 7; 1859–1860, vol. 9; 1873, vol. 5; 1905–1906, vols. 5, 7b; 1908, vol. 7.

13

NEGOTIATING WITH THE NEIGHBOURS

Kingship and diplomacy in Munhumutapa

Eugénia Rodrigues[1]

This chapter analyses the diplomatic culture and practices of Munhumutapa, or Monomotapa,[2] focusing on relations with the Portuguese. It aims to shed light on the social and cultural dimensions of diplomacy between African and European polities in the early modern world. Munhumutapa was the most famous of the states created by the Karanga people (present-day Shona) in East Africa. Its mythical gold wealth attracted foreign merchants: this was the case for the Portuguese, who established a government in Mozambique Island in the sixteenth century in the framework of their Indian Ocean Empire.[3] The relationship between these sovereignties located in distant parts of the world involved distinct political, social, economic and cultural traditions. However, despite their differences, Portuguese and Karanga also shared some features and interests that enabled them to develop diplomatic interactions, that is 'a set of practices designed to establish mutual confidence between polities'.[4] Indeed, in a manner similar to the ongoing contemporary process in Europe, the rulers of Munhumutapa and other African states had established ritual diplomatic procedures that allowed them to conduct negotiations with Europeans.[5]

In recent years, early modern diplomacy has attracted increased academic interest, creating a significant body of research. This literature explores issues such as the symbolic aspects of the ceremonial, the meanings of gift giving, the cross-cultural exchanges and the actors involved in diplomatic practice.[6] In the framework of the first globalization, scholars have also examined the relationships between Europeans and polities in Asia, America and Africa. This work demonstrates that diplomacy was frequently a device of empire building and offered opportunities for cultural exchanges, even though it often took place in the context of violence.[7] Nonetheless, there has been little discussion of the practical functioning of diplomacy with African polities, principally in East Africa.[8] Despite cultural differences and violent conflicts, this chapter shows that mutual interests existed between the Karanga and the Portuguese during early modernity. Thus, besides war, they were involved in repeated negotiations and exchanges of envoys aimed at reaching agreements.

There are three aspects of recent scholarly developments on diplomacy that offer a framework for approaching these particular relations. First is the notion of diplomacy as a set of ritual practices of representation and political mediation carried out by an array of actors ranging from ambassadors, spies and missionaries to captains and interpreters.[9] This approach encourages the cross-examination of a wide variety of diplomatic activities and agents operating in the East African landscape. Second, in considering the symbolic dimensions of the ritual associated with negotiations, scholarship has identified how ceremonial interactions functioned as a means to shape hierarchies of power, rank and prestige among states and political actors.[10] Unlike their relations with other African rulers, the Portuguese kings did not receive Karanga embassies in Portugal; therefore, the symbolic meanings of diplomatic ritual emerged mainly within the Munhumutapa court and the settlements of the Portuguese colony in Mozambique. As such, by examining the embassies of the respective sovereigns, this chapter sheds light on the Karanga ways of formalizing rulers' power by rituals in a part of the world where 'ritual power and social networks appear to be at the core of the very notion of power'.[11] In both cases, ambassadorial ceremony was a tool to perform power and rank among Karanga leaders. Indeed, as scholars have argued for Europe, there was not a clear line between domestic and external issues.[12] Lastly, scholars have stressed how diplomacy constituted a space for cross-cultural interactions and exchanges between rulers and their communities.[13] Moreover, the material culture surrounding diplomatic contacts, such as gifts, could pose challenges to dissimilar polities making this a pertinent area of analysis for Karanga-Portuguese diplomacy.[14]

This chapter is divided into four sections. The first analyses the role of diplomacy in the negotiation of power relationships between Munhumutapa and the Portuguese, highlighting stages of cooperation between the two sides and Portuguese hegemony over the Karanga, in both cases using treaties. The second focuses on Karanga ceremonial protocol when receiving and sending embassies, emphasizing how this protocol, even though flexible, reinforced the power of the sovereigns. The third addresses the cultural exchanges associated with diplomacy, such as gift giving, and explores how the Karanga appropriated the material culture of European and Indian origin and integrated this into its political culture as a means of supporting rulers' power. The fourth examines the processes of legitimization of agreements, underlining how African devices prevailed in the negotiation of pacts, although the European pattern of establishing alliances existed in parallel.

Munhumutapa and its relations with the Portuguese: pathways of diplomacy and war

The interaction between the Munhumutapa and the Portuguese was developed in the framework of the European overseas expansion and the ongoing processes of empire building. The Munhumutapa emerged in the fifteenth century in the northeast of the plateau south of the Zambezi River. Also identified as Mukaranga, the Portuguese perceived this state as having tutelary authority over other powerful Karanga rulers. Therefore, translating local to European political categories, they referred to this state as an empire and its ruler, the mutapa, as an emperor.[15]

The Karanga expansion to the northern reaches of the plateau implied conquest as well as alliances with local chieftainships, which became their tributaries. The mutapa called these allies their 'wives', and allowed them a certain degree of autonomy, creating kinship ties which enabled their political incorporation into Mukaranga.[16] Owing to the large number of subjects and an increasingly complex state administration, a hierarchy of chiefs emerged and there was a growing demand for imported articles to reward them. Wares such as gold, copper and ivory were exchanged for textiles and beads from India, which became fundamental items to distinguish the status of the elite. This long-distance trade developed through Muslim and Portuguese merchants, first in coastal Sofala and later in the Zambezi valley.[17]

In the context of their empire building in the Indian Ocean, which was a crown-run enterprise called *Estado da Índia* governed by viceroys in Goa, the Portuguese considered the Munhumutapa to be a sufficiently wealthy and powerful empire to establish diplomatic relations with in order to trade and conduct missionary activities. By this time, the Portuguese had already accumulated a great deal of experience of diplomacy with rulers in Atlantic Africa, such as Kongo, and this served as a template for dealings with the Karanga.[18]

As in the case of Atlantic Africa and Asia alike, the fundamental divisions along the political, cultural, social and religious lines did not prevent a longstanding relationship between both polities, which went through several stages and encompassed different levels of assistance and conflict.[19] In an earlier phase, the mutapa took the initiative to send embassies to the Portuguese factory in Sofala (established in 1505), and these were reciprocated by Portuguese envoys to the zimbabwe, the designation of the capitals of Mukaranga.[20]

A stage of more closer relationships was opened around the mid-sixteenth century when Portuguese merchants – then a designation which encompassed individuals with roots in Europe and in India, as well as a rising number of local mixed-race persons – moved to the Zambezi valley. At this point the merchants, and then the captain of Mozambique, paid a tax known as *kuruva*, which was charged by the ruler for allowing trading activities in Mukaranga. The 'captain of the gates', who discharged fiscal and judicial duties at Massapa fair, delivered this rate in the name of the mutapa. This captain also acted as a resident Portuguese representative, since the 'Monomotapa ruler dealt with this captain for every matter concerning his subjects and the Portuguese and replies are sent through him'.[21] This commercial partnership paved the way for initiatives by the Portuguese monarchy. Subsequent to the assassination in 1561 of the Jesuit Dom Gonçalo da Silveira on the mutapa's orders, the Portuguese crown sent a large army to 'conquer' the Munhumutapa, which aimed to guarantee the freedom to trade, access to the mines and permission to preach Christianity. Yet, the mutapa accepted the conditions presented by the expedition's commander, Francisco Barreto (who died in the Zambezi valley), through the embassy that he dispatched to the zimbabwe in 1572, and the army left the country.[22]

While the balance of power did not change on the ground, the mutapa became increasingly dependent on alliances with Portuguese merchants to face the Maravi expansion towards the southern Zambezi, as well as for support in internal disputes. Against this backdrop, in 1607, mutapa Gatsi Rusere negotiated the donation of mining areas in exchange for military assistance from the Portuguese. The transfer of the mines to the Portuguese crown was the basis for successive military ventures and intense diplomatic exchanges to take effective possession of them with the hope of discovering silver wealth similar to that of the Spanish colonies in America.[23]

However, up to the 1620s, the political relationship between both parties remained essentially shaped by forms of negotiation rather than one-sided imposition.

The results of diplomacy ultimately created legal rights for the Portuguese crown over the Munhumutapa. In 1629, mutapa Mavhura established an alliance with the Portuguese crown in which he recognized himself as its vassal in exchange for military support. This new condition implied the end of the *kuruva*; instead, the mutapa was directed to pay a tribute according his vassal status. Yet the Portuguese king ordered that the tribute correspond to an equally substantial gift, called *saguate*, similarly to the embassies sent to powerful rulers in Persia, India, China and Japan.[24] For the Portuguese crown, dominance over this famous 'empire' emphasized its prestige, and this was increased further by the mutapa's baptism. This treaty did not predicate a Portuguese administration over Mukaranga, neither did the mutapa court adopt European institutions as occurred in Kongo.[25] Nevertheless, the treaty did usher in a phase of greater intervention by the Portuguese, including military hostilities and territorial appropriation.[26] To counter resistance by the Karanga elite and to ensure the mutapa's safety, Portuguese administration stationed a garrison at the zimbabwe and the captains acted as mediators in relationships with the rulers. Similarly, the Dominican missionaries who established a parish in Munhumutapa were particularly active in supporting one candidate against other. Moreover, during the seventeenth century, a Catholic baptism was integrated into the ritual of enthroning the mutapa, and the ceremony was preceded by an exchange of envoys.[27] All of these actors – captains and missionaries – were also resident ambassadors paralleling contemporary diplomatic trends in Europe.[28]

Portuguese dominion over Mukaranga was broken by the appearance of an important player in the southwestern plateau, the changamire of Butwa, who expelled the Portuguese from the Karanga highlands in 1693. This pivotal moment enforced a new equilibrium of power between the two parties. Karanga rulers ceased to acknowledge their vassalage in relation to the Portuguese crown, and, with the subsequent political fragmentation, the mutapa lost control of the plateau. Now focusing on the lowlands near the Zambezi, and becoming a smaller state, the Karanga pillaged the territory under the Portuguese crown and increased taxes on trade.[29]

The Portuguese continued to hold the mutapa garrison but, from the 1740s, they only travelled to the zimbabwe to conduct the annual *saguates*. Without the capacity to impose its rules, the Portuguese administration was compelled to accept the mutapa's demands, presented through frequent embassies, and enter into agreements to preserve trading links. Given the great political competition, some deposed mutapa and other chiefs struggling for power also sent emissaries to the Portuguese. Moreover, the sovereigns exchanged envoys with several merchants, which sometimes contravened the Portuguese crown's policies.[30] Thereafter, Portuguese and Karanga developed multi-layered relations that connected different actors beyond the delegates of the two sovereigns.

In brief, although entangled by phases of cooperation and opposition, there was a longstanding interaction between the Karanga and the Portuguese. Even without expression in formal pacts, many of the rules that regulated these interactions derived from practices and the capacity of each side to impose its goals on the other party.

Receiving and sending embassies

Portuguese descriptions of the mutapa's embassies reveal how a structured and refined diplomatic culture prevailed in Mukaranga which prescribed well-established norms for all actors. Roosen argues there existed an 'elaborated body of rules governing the behaviour of participants' for European courts, which 'greatly lessened the possibility of wrong messages being sent or perceived'.[31] The Karanga rules were aimed at manifesting and symbolically reinforcing the prestige and power of the mutapa, as well as delimiting the place of each actor. In effect, the setting arrangements, the motion of the actors in the scenario and all gestures codified the power of the mutapa vis-à-vis his subjects and the Portuguese to ensure he was recognized as the sovereign.

Portuguese reports indicate that by the sixteenth century an elaborate protocol already existed shaped by the mutapa's relations with other African rulers, which functioned as a template for diplomatic contacts with the Portuguese. An important moment in the construction of the power of the mutapa was the *chivabvu* annual festivities: a ceremonial renegotiation of the obedience of all dependent chiefs, using imported luxury items as rewards and symbolically formalizing the hierarchy of power among chiefs. According to their status, these chiefs would either appear personally or send representatives to the zimbabwe. Thus, the chiefs classified in lower ranks would attend in person, being received somewhere and immediately processed; while those who held a higher position sent ambassadors, who were received with diplomatic formalities extended to envoys from other states on the plateau, such as *changamire* or the emissaries of the Portuguese administration.[32] This representational differentiation corresponded to recognition of the power that each of these chiefs held in Munhumutapa's political context, while simultaneously affirming the sovereign's authority.

The embassies were usually slow and involved various audiences as negotiations unfolded. According to the hospitality rules in Africa, which were in force in Asian legations alike, the ambassadors were lodged in houses close to the zimbabwe, where they awaited their first audience.[33] At this stage, the mutapa received the gifts sent for him and formally took note of the subject of the embassy. A few days later the emissaries would be summoned for a new audience at which they would either be bid farewell or instructed to stay for new sessions.[34]

As stated in an early seventeenth-century description, the audiences took place on the great patio next to the residences of the mutapa. During the audiences, the ruler stayed inside his dwelling and the ambassadors could only access the external courtyard. The separation of actors in these spaces indicated a political hierarchy which was reinforced by the impeded visual contact with the sovereign. Ambassadors were also forced to carry out the *zumbaya* ritual, which was a formality associated with recognizing the status of the sovereign: it entailed entering the courtyard on their knees and prostrating themselves on the ground when they drew close to the mutapa. All the visitors would speak without looking in the direction of the mutapa and accompanied their speeches with clapping, a gesture which was considered to be very courteous. Moreover, the Portuguese had to present themselves barefoot, without hats and sans weapons, quite different from the way they would appear in European courts. Despite these prescriptive rules, the sovereign allowed some people the privilege of being able to speak with him while standing and looking at him. The singular honour of a face-to-face contact was conceded, for example, to the Jesuit Dom Gonçalo da Silveira.[35]

As the limited visibility of the mutapa acted as a device to affirm his power, the means of communication used in the audiences similarly underscored his political rank. The ambassadors submitted their proposals orally to the lowest dignitary, and it was repeated by different individuals until it reached the ruler, who would respond using the same chain of communication. Likewise, the gifts brought by the ambassadors were delivered through various officials in a hierarchical chain that ended at the mutapa.[36]

Even though the Europeans adjusted to these practices in order to be able to negotiate, as they did in embassies to the Asian courts,[37] they perceived Karanga rituals as particularly vexatious. The Jesuit Júlio César Vertua, who was part of an embassy in 1619, considered having to crawl on a floor finished with cow dung to be incompatible with the 'decorum of a priest'.[38] In this context, the Portuguese tried to negotiate the etiquette to align with European practices, at least for the audiences of individuals of a higher status. Thus, when the Jesuit Silveira visited the zimbabwe he entered the mutapa's residence and sat on a carpet, but his interpreter had to remain at the door.[39] Similarly, a Portuguese merchant was sent ahead of the envoy dispatched by Francisco Barreto in 1572 to discuss the reception of the ambassadors prior to their arrival. The mutapa accepted the European protocols on this occasion, most probably due to the European army transported to the Zambezi valley. In this manner, the Portuguese emissaries were able to present themselves wearing hats and shoes, and a European setting was recreated for their reception, with a carpet and a chair on which the ambassador sat.[40]

The treaty of 1629 allowed the Portuguese opportunities to impose further and more permanent changes in the protocol. Indeed, they demanded to appear before the mutapa, as they would have attended the Portuguese court, and refused to clap while speaking. Furthermore, they demanded chairs for the ambassadors, while accepting that merchants could sit on the ground.[41] This change in ceremonial protocol acquired a marked significance in the context of new political relations with the mutapa, who, while still viewed as an 'emperor', was transformed into a vassal of the Portuguese crown by the aforementioned treaty. By means of a specific ritual the envoys of the Portuguese authorities thus began to distinguish themselves not just from African ambassadors but, likewise, from Portuguese merchants. Nevertheless, the sources indicate that, despite the Portuguese efforts, the essence of the protocol remained Karanga and demonstrates that this was still a compromise on both sides. When Friar Simão de São Tomás arrived at the zimbabwe in 1735, the mutapa took his hand and led him to his residence and offered him a chair, while he himself sat on an Indian-style chaise longue (*cataló*). The clergyman was surprised by this welcome since he had been informed that the mutapa only offered seating – and only on cushions – to the captain of the garrison and to the vicar of the zimbabwe, while everyone else sat on the floor.[42]

Descriptions of embassies in the second half of the eighteenth century suggest further changes in the protocol, with fewer formalities and greater access to the mutapa. At this time, the rulers no longer remained within their residence but instead went out to the external courtyard, where all the dignitaries and ambassadors would gather. Here, the hierarchy of the space was now underscored by two parasols (*sombreiros*) provided by the Portuguese administration. The mutapa would sit under them on his *quite* (footstool or throne), or, occasionally, on the ground like all the other members of the court. The ambassadors, including the Portuguese envoys, would cross the courtyard clapping and would then sit on the floor, handing over their gifts and describing the matters concerning the respective embassy. The account of the Portuguese embassies sent to the mutapa Ganyambadzi in 1780–1, reveals how the ruler was visible in successive audiences and even participated in the *pemberações*, which was the war dance performed at such events.[43] The Karanga ceremonial was not, therefore, static but adapted and reshaped over time. The evolution of the rituals was probably due to both the waning power of the mutapa, whereby the ruler became less distinct from the smaller Karanga elite, and continuing interaction with European cultural models of officials and merchants at the Portuguese colony. Indeed, instead of the complexity of the ritual, the sovereigns increasingly used imported artefacts to distinguish themselves.

The embassies dispatched by the mutapa to the Portuguese were also correspondingly shaped by rules aimed at building the power of the sovereigns. According to S.I.G. Mudenge, there were various categories of envoys, and these depended on the importance and quality of the matter.[44] Nonetheless, Portuguese records do not make such distinctions: there were repeated references to the designation *mutume* until the seventeenth century and *manamucate* during the eighteenth, in parallel with the more comprehensive designation of ambassador. Indeed, it seems that, as in Europe, there was a certain degree of flexibility and it is impossible to find fixed categories of representatives.[45]

Friar João dos Santos described the embassies of the Karanga ruler of Kiteve, at the end of the sixteenth century, affirming them to be analogous to those who represented the mutapa. This clergyman mentioned the existence of four ambassadors: the first performed the person of the king; the second acted as his mouth, speaking in his name; the third represented his eyes; and the fourth his ears.[46] In a predominantly oral culture, multiple ambassadors helped to ensure that details were faithfully described to the sovereign. These ambassadors were high-ranking individuals, chosen from among the ruler's sons and officials of the court, and accompanied by a large entourage. One of the embassies sent to Sofala consisted of 100 individuals, including porters, musicians, dancers and the ambassadors, who were in the rear guard of this retinue.[47] In 1572 the embassy the mutapa dispatched to Tete in the Zambezi valley, counted more than 200 individuals, comprising 10 or 12 dignitaries.[48] These ambassadors carried royal staffs, as a passport, which gave them immunity, a privilege that Europeans also acknowledged to diplomats. Indeed, as in Europe and most African polities, the Munhumutapa had a set of rules to protect the envoys it sent and received.[49] It was clear that through these embassies the Karanga sovereigns intended to demonstrate their authority and wealth, not just to the receiving party but also to those rulers whose territories they travelled through en route.

By the last decades of the eighteenth century, the embassies generally included five or six ambassadors.[50] At this time, the role of envoy was also performed by the *vanyiai*, the soldiers of the Karanga chiefs, a category that emerged in the late seventeenth century, probably to fight the armies of *achikunda* (African slaves) of the Portuguese lords.[51] The Portuguese considered this number excessive, arguing that in the preceding period embassies had consisted of only two *manamucates.* It is unknown whether any agreement existed on the composition of the embassies in the past. Likely, the Portuguese argument reflected the ongoing process in Europe where embassies, while preserving the complexity of the ceremonial, tended to be smaller.[52] However, by sending constant embassies and various ambassadors, the mutapa clearly tried to increase the tributes paid by the Portuguese to trade, demanding that they 'provide clothing' for their envoys. Actually, ambassadors, in accordance with African and European practices, had also to be honoured with gifts. The Portuguese often had no option other than to satisfy the Karanga demands.[53]

In terms of the composition of the embassies, the main novelty by 1780 was the inclusion of women. In a society where women held considerable authority, up until the early seventeenth century some of the mutapa's wives played a role as brokers in relations with Muslim and Portuguese merchants. The women held the titles of *nehanda,* the ruler's sister, and *mazvarira,* his father's sister, and they served important diplomatic functions at the zimbabwe: the former was the interlocutor of the Muslim, while the latter interceded for the Portuguese.[54] In the eighteenth century, women referred to as the mutapa's 'daughters', his 'empress' or his 'elder sister', or only as *mukaranga* (woman), figured among the embassies of the sovereign sent to the Portuguese authorities. At a time of great conflicts, when communication was essential, the mutapa probably preferred to send his female relatives as his representatives. This could also have been a method to obtain luxury items for these women who, as ambassadors, were recompensed by the Portuguese. Thus, for example, the mutapa Ganyambadzi complained that princess Vamuturo was not given the carpet and the cushion on which she sat in Tete.[55] These women gained a political role and became protagonists of diplomatic exchanges. Altogether, these envoys, whether made up of women and/or men, do not seem to have had much autonomy vis-à-vis the mutapa and their counsellors. The accounts of the embassies received in Portuguese settlements record the voices of the ambassadors and the answers given to them. However, envoys returned to the zimbabwe to transmit those responses, with the final decisions taken by the mutapa and their counsellors.

Diplomacy and gift exchange

Any negotiations among the Karanga entailed offering gifts, creating a chain of reciprocity over time. In fact, as in other societies, a gift meant an obligation to correspond with another present, introducing cohesion via social ties.[56] This exchange had two important and immediate purposes in a diplomatic context. On the one hand, it had a political significance, reflecting the confidence and mutual recognition between parties that enabled negotiations. On the other, it had a material purpose translating into the redistribution of goods in which each of the parties had an interest. It is also important to note that these practices also encompassed the ambassadors as mediators for the respective sovereigns.

In Karanga diplomacy, there were various categories of gifts according to the phase of the negotiations and the status of the recipients. For example, a gift called *boca* (mouth), which was viewed as a request to speak, accompanied the opening of talks and the main gift was only handed over later. In this context, until 1629, before paying the *kuruva,* the tax due to the mutapa for engaging in trade, the Portuguese would send a preliminary embassy to the zimbabwe with the *boca*. These envoys would then return to Tete accompanied by the mutapa's ambassadors to escort a new embassy, which was to present the *kuruva*. In the eighteenth century, the *saguates* the Portuguese gifted to the mutapa consisted of an annual present, which continued to be called *boca*, and, every three years, a gift of a higher value known as *estado* (state), which substituted for the erstwhile *kuruva* and complied with the same ceremonial. Moreover, the mutapa would send other embassies with *boca* presents. In 1780, mutapa Changara offered a *boca* of two slaves.[57] Furthermore, apart from the gifts designed for their rulers, the ambassadors themselves received 'clothing' gifts, the *bairações*. These ambassadors acted according to legal conventions and had common expectations in relation to the benefits the post afforded. The fact that, at least since the 1780s, the Portuguese authorities tried to reduce or eliminate these gifts in light of innumerable embassies and ambassadors, gave rise to friction and more protracted negotiations.[58]

From both the Karanga and the Portuguese perspective the exchange of gifts was to observe the principle of reciprocity, which also regulated diplomatic contacts in Europe.[59] In 1572, Francisco Barreto sent the mutapa innumerable textiles and 'rich items', very similar to the gifts the Portuguese State of India forwarded to powerful kings in Asia.[60] The African ruler expressed himself very pleased and responded with eight gold bracelets, a present of exceptional honour, since, allegedly, these were only used by the sovereign. However, the Portuguese felt that, as the bangles were very slim, the value of the present fell short of the gift they had sent and hence the 'honour and benefits were not equal'.[61] On another occasion, in 1780, an embassy sent by mutapa Changara reduced the gift for a Portuguese commander as the reciprocal present was deemed of inferior importance. As these exchanges were meant to be symmetrical and of equivalent substance, breaking this rule could generate conflicts and misunderstandings.[62]

Karanga gifts generally consisted of gold, livestock and, by the late 1700s, slaves, all of them valued by the Portuguese. The gifts offered by Portuguese embassies included high prestigious imported goods, with an emphasis on cotton and silk textiles and beads. Depending on cross-cultural exchanges, the type of articles earmarked for the mutapa varied, embracing European and Indian goods, mainly due to Karanga demands. After the 1607 pact, for example, mutapa Gatsi Rusere demanded two horses that the Portuguese had transported to the Zambezi valley, stating that he had long yearned to possess them. He later requested a battlefield banner made of coloured silk, a golden *ndoro* (a conus shell and a royal insignia) studded with gems, and silk fabrics, mirrors, pins, needles, knives, scissors, lamps, pepper, soap, porcelain and Portuguese saffron.[63] In the eighteenth century, Portuguese gifts continued to comprise a vast array of goods, such as weapons, gunpowder, drinks, spices, coral, tin or stitched clothes, at the request of the Karanga. A Portuguese official explained the need to include these items, 'as he [the mutapa] has repeatedly insisted upon this with me . . . and because if we do not give them the said goods, which they prize and are currently in their possession, it could have serious consequences for the State'.[64] In effect, with the dissemination of textiles and imported beads, some articles took on the role of differentiating the mutapa among the Karanga elite and, as such, the deposed mutapa wanted them too.

The imported goods changed the material culture of the Karanga elite, mainly in the case of the mutapa and his family who received the most exclusive products.

The Karanga incorporated foreign elements into their decoration, such as parasols, carpets, chairs, cushions and chaise longues, which became a characteristic feature of royal quarters. Intercultural contact also influenced the garments worn by the mutapa, who mixed European and Asian styles. Several mutapa used *quimões* (a sort of kimono), *cabaias* (a long tunic), coats, shirts and caps, in addition to their usual fabrics.[65] Thus, it is not surprising that chiefs struggling for power and seeking recognition settled at strategic sites in an attempt to control trade routes so as to acquire the material culture that these merchants could supply. For example, in 1781, the deposed mutapa Changara complained to a Portuguese captain that:

> [t]he *cabaia* he had sent him was too small and did not fit him and thus he should send him a larger and better one, and since he had sent him a pair of stockings he should also send him shoes, breeches, shirt, coatee [a short coat], and dress coat, to complement the stockings, which on its own was no use without the other items.

In addition to the habitual textiles and beads, he also asked for a parasol, cushion, carpet, gunpowder and a pig 'which he wished to eat'.[66] In effect, the Karanga adopted aspects of Asian and European culture, and Portuguese and Indian merchants ensured the flow of the respective wares. However, the selection of the imported items depended substantially on the mutapa's choice and the significance of the articles to the Karanga.

Legitimizing external relations

External relations raised the question of how to formalize and legitimize the agreements between the mutapa and the neighbouring polities. Karanga diplomacy was based on orality and unwritten contracts and was represented by objects that served as a 'signature'. However, by the early modern period, texts were the dominant source of legitimacy for agreements in Europe. As such, relations between the Karanga and Portuguese entailed a combination of mechanisms of legitimization: treaties and other arrangements between the polities were based on dual practices – unwritten and written. As Benton argues for Atlantic Africa: 'Despite the emphasis among Europeans on written sources in European law, Portuguese traders learned that Africans recognized unwritten contracts, sanctified by oaths or other unwritten practices.'[67]

In Karanga culture orality was the most common form of diplomatic communication. In 1572, the Jesuit Francisco Monclaro described how verbal communication was an essential tool for diplomacy: 'They receive and send embassies by means of words and they describe everything that happened to them to the king, from the time they leave until they return, in meticulous detail, and they spend many hours in these narrations'.[68] The description of eighteenth-century agreements underscore how, two centuries later, each clause was still discussed and repeated orally. After the close of negotiations, the agreement entailed handing over an artefact, 'a trifle for personal use . . . which by its ritual is the sign of registering a contract'.[69] The ceding of personal goods reflected the possessor's acquiescence with the pact concluded. These objects became *ressambo* (a signature or receipt) and acquired symbolic value in the system of relations between rulers, who would undoubtedly have maintained a repository for such objects.

The Portuguese were obliged to recognize the legitimacy of African practices. Just like other ambassadors in diverse parts of the world, they faced 'a whole universe of entirely unfamiliar artefacts and artefact-related practices'.[70] The Portuguese strove to obtain these objects to validate their pacts, after which they could confront Karanga chiefs with their commitments. The Portuguese administration in Mozambique kept an archive of these 'signs' associated with concluded negotiations.[71] Portuguese sources record innumerable examples of the Karanga way of regulating external conventions. For instance, the Portuguese and the mutapa Ganyambadzi authenticated the treaty accorded in 1781 by handing over a box, which ensured that merchants could freely travel to the Zumbo fair.[72] Some of the objects used in pacts were related to particular meanings. For example, handing over offensive weapons, such as arrows and spears, generally implied that the owner allowed the bearer to wage a given war or to kill a certain individual. Thus, in the 1781 treaty, the Portuguese administration tried, unsuccessfully, to obtain one of these weapons from the mutapa as permission to attack individuals who pillaged the lands under the Portuguese crown. The Portuguese also appropriated this legal language and handed over weapons to Karanga chiefs to allow them to execute Portuguese subjects.[73] In order to operate in a society that did not use writing, the Portuguese had to manipulate local mechanisms of legitimization using a complex set of symbolic materials.

In a scenario in which each interlocutor tried to affirm their legal order, the Portuguese also sought to impose their norms, namely written communications. Unlike the case of Kongo and Angola, where various chiefs adopted writing as a means of communication and archiving, few members of the Karanga elite learnt Portuguese, and written correspondence entailed Portuguese intermediaries.[74] During the seventeenth century, some Dominican clergymen mediated such interactions. Friar Manuel da Purificação, for example, wrote the letters for the mutapa Mavhura, who also appointed him as his delegate to Goa in 1645.[75] However, the Portuguese administration soon appointed clerks and interpreters for the mutapa's court, trying to ensure a channel for political communication. These men were chosen from among the residents of the Portuguese colony, so they understood the Karanga language and culture. From the mid-eighteenth century onward, their role in diplomatic relations became especially important since these clerks were the only Portuguese personnel to stay at the zimbabwe for long periods, albeit not permanently. As was the case for their diplomatic predecessors in the zimbabwe, they were to spy on what was happening there and persuade the mutapa to favour Portuguese affairs.[76] Their functions were to envoys in Europe, where spying and information gathering also featured among diplomatic activities.[77]

Even though European practices of written agreements did not dominate, the Karanga accommodated their use in diplomacy. Treaties from 1607 and letters prepared in the name of the mutapa from 1619 onward became instruments of communication and tools to regulate relations with the Portuguese. Their importance varied according to the context. Written communication also became a device of power for the Karanga sovereigns, as illustrated by the case of Changara, the mutapa deposed in 1780, who demanded that a merchant go to his zimbabwe to write a letter to the Portuguese governor.[78] Treaties and letters were validated, mainly during the 1600s, by the sovereign's signature – marked as a cross, as was usual in Portugal for individuals who did not know how to write – and, sometimes, these bore his seal in red lacquer.[79] This symbol depicted a lion whose front paws rested on a bow and arrow. The lion was associated with the sovereign's power, it being believed that after dying the mutapa's spirit would live on in this animal, while the Portuguese understood the bow and arrow to be symbols of his power. The Portuguese likely encouraged the adoption of seals, as this was a practice associated with European royalty. Nonetheless, the incorporation of Karanga symbols reflected Portuguese perceptions of the political importance of these emblems and, possibly, was the result of negotiations with the mutapa. Similarly, the letters exchanged between the Portuguese administration and the mutapa reproduced European forms of address – 'Your Highness', 'Your Very Faithful Majesty' – which expressed Portuguese recognition of the mutapa's ranking.[80] Indeed, written communications were instruments of diplomacy that could encompass embassies, or replace them, in some stages of negotiations.

Oral and written communication also constituted a field of dispute where both sides and their intermediaries clashed. Each actor had their own interests and could manipulate information in their favour. For example, mutapa Ganyambadzi had his own interpreter. In 1781, the Portuguese governor demanded that only the Portuguese clerk was to read out the letters he sent to the mutapa and that the sovereign was to personally dictate his letters to the Portuguese clerk, so as to 'avoid fraud and intrigues'.[81] In effect, Karanga and Portuguese perceptions of given issues could generate misunderstandings and mistrust. Forms of legitimating agreements were a core aspect of diplomatic relationships between the two societies with very different cultural backgrounds. Albeit accommodating European written devices, Karanga successfully imposed on the Portuguese their own prevailing standard as the rule.

Conclusion

This chapter analysed the dynamics of the diplomatic contacts and underlying cultural exchanges between two polities – one African, the Munhumutapa, and the other European, Portugal – which the first globalization brought into contact. These two early modern polities were located in distant geographical settings with different cultural backgrounds, although shared interests existed. Both were monarchies in the process of consolidation and expansion of the sovereign's power. The mutapa had built their power by extending their dominion over the northeast of the plateau. They depended on the Portuguese for access to imported luxury goods, and to confront internal and external opponents. For the Karanga, the alliance with the Europeans was a flexible device to support mutapaship and ensure the continuity of trade routes. The Portuguese monarchy, in its turn, was engaged in an ongoing process of overseas expansion in the Indian Ocean and looked for allies to support it. For the Portuguese this partnership was pivotal to access to the gold and ivory of the plateau, as well as to Christianize the Karanga, even if this last objective became less important over time. Accordingly, the association between the mutapa and the European kings was rooted in related interests, although this did not prevent conflict and the Portuguese hegemony over Mukaranga (1629–93). However, diplomacy, as war, functioned as a tool to negotiate power relations between the Karanga and the Portuguese in a number of ways.

276

First, Africans and Europeans acknowledged formal agreements as a legitimate means of engaging in diplomacy even if they were sealed in different ways. The practice of drawing up treaties was prominent until the early seventeenth century and during the eighteenth century, which were periods witnessing a greater balance of power between the Karanga and the Portuguese. These treaties encompassed military assistance, trading and mining conditions, security aspects and even diplomatic protocols, but they also promoted, in the 1629 pact, the transfer of sovereign rights to the Portuguese crown. Nevertheless, some negotiations on agreements reveal how the mutapa could reject Portuguese proposals. Second, African and European political cultures accepted the role of ambassadors as mediators between rulers. The set of envoys encompassed a range of actors, recruited usually among high-ranking individuals. While in Europe women were not formal diplomats, the Portuguese recognized their role among the envoys of the mutapa. Furthermore, both polities acknowledged the diplomatic immunity and hospitality owed to ambassadors in order to ensure their safety. This allowed Karanga and Portuguese ambassadors to act in distinct cultural contexts, trying to negotiate mutual norms even in contexts of intense dispute.

Third, African and European polities shared the notion of the symbolic dimensions of diplomatic rituals as well as its relevance in the affirmation of the power and prestige of the rulers. The etiquette associated with diplomacy reveals how the Karanga created an elaborate set of rules for all interactions with the mutapa with a significant symbolic value. The reception of ambassadors was a staged moment, affirming the ranking and power of the mutapa, regarding their subjects as well as other African rulers and the Europeans. Finally, for Karanga and Europeans, the exchange of gifts was a key tool of diplomacy. To both cultures, the structure of gift exchange confirms the status of both sides by reciprocity. Conversely, due to distinct cultural contexts, both parties had to accommodate the practices of the other party; it was clear that, even in times of hegemony, the Portuguese could not fully impose their European standard. This was evident, with some concessions, in the embassies' ceremonial as well as regarding the tools of legitimizing agreements. Indeed, while treaties were sometimes written and sealed, they were often struck in the Karanga fashion, by means of symbolic artefacts. Diplomacy also reveals cross-cultural exchanges. While maintaining the core of the Karanga diplomatic culture, the mutapa's court appropriated some aspects of Portuguese and Indo-Portuguese culture, and especially material culture. The kind of gifts requested by Karanga, and their subsequent uses, shed some light on intercultural dynamics. These gifts were mainly specific luxury objects from Portugal and India, which illustrate changing consumption patterns among the Karanga, and defined social and political hierarchies in order to strengthen the sovereign's status and power vis-à-vis his subjects and neighbouring polities. However, cross-cultural exchanges were never as strong as in the case of some polities in the Atlantic Africa, such as Kongo.[82]

In the context of intercultural diplomacy, it is important to stress that early modern polities in Europe and Africa were able to accommodate the values and practices of the other party in order to achieve their aims. Hence, despite distinct political, social, cultural and religious backgrounds, the fact that they shared some institutions and interests was essential to the establishment of long-standing diplomatic relationships.

Notes

1 This work was funded by national funds by FCT – Foundation for Science and Technology, Portugal, under the project UID/HIS/04311/2013.
2 I follow the designation Munhumutapa, according to S.I.G. Mudenge, *A Political History of Munhumutapa c. 1400–1902* (Harare: Zimbabwe Publishing House, 1988).
3 From the 1530s Mozambique Island, where the Portuguese had built a fort and a factory in 1507, gradually replaced Sofala as the seat of government of the captaincy of Sofala and Mozambique.
4 Eric Hinderaker, "Diplomacy between Britons and Native Americans, *c.* 1600–1830," in *Britain's Oceanic Empire: British expansion in the Atlantic and Indian Ocean worlds, c. 1550–1850*, eds. H.V. Bowen, Elizabeth Mancke and John G. Reid (Cambridge: Cambridge University Press, 2012), 220.
5 On Atlantic Africa, see Lauren Benton, *Law and Colonial Cultures: Legal Regimes in World History, 1400–1900* (Cambridge: Cambridge University Press, 2002), 31–79. I use 'external' instead of 'international' relations, considering the criticism that surrounds the idea of nations in the early modern world. See Daniela Frigo, ed., *Politics and Diplomacy in Early Modern Italy: The Structure of Diplomatic Practice, 1450–1800* (Cambridge: Cambridge University Press, 2000), 8.
6 For example, see Christopher Storrs, *War, Diplomacy and the Rise of Savoy, 1690–1720* (Cambridge: Cambridge University Press, 2004); Robyn Adams and Rosanna Cox, eds., *Diplomacy and Early Modern Culture* (New York: Palgrave Macmillan, 2011); Catherine Fletcher, *Diplomacy in Renaissance Rome: The Rise of the Resident Ambassador* (Cambridge: Cambridge University Press, 2015); Tracey A. Sowerby and Jan Hennings, eds., *Practices of Diplomacy in the Early Modern World c. 1410–1800* (New York: Routledge, 2017).
7 See, for example, Saliha Belmessous, ed., *Empire by Treaty: Negotiating European Expansion, 1600–1900* (New York: Oxford University Press, 2015); Shogo Suzuki, Yongjin Zhang and Joel Quirk, eds., *International Orders in the Early Modern World before the rise of the West* (London: Routledge, 2014); Christian Windler, "Diplomatic History as a Field for Cultural Analysis: Muslim-Cultural Relations in Runis, 1700–1840," *Historical Journal*, 44 (2001), 79–106.
8 On Atlantic Africa, see Robert S. Smith, *Warfare and Diplomacy in Pre-Colonial West Africa* (Madison: University of Wisconsin Press, 1976); Toyin Falola and Robyn Law, eds., *Warfare and Diplomacy in Precolonial Nigeria* (Madison: University of Wisconsin Press, 1992); Joel Quirk and David Richardson, "Europeans, Africans and the Atlantic World, 1450–1850," in Suzuki, Zhang and Quirk, *International*, 138–158.
9 Frigo, *Politics*; Adams and Cox, *Diplomacy*; Sowerby and Hennings, *Practices*.
10 Frigo, *Politics*.
11 Peter de Maret, "From Kinship to Kingship: an African Journey into Complexity," *Azania* 47, no. 3 (2012): 314–326.
12 Storrs, *War*; Fletcher, *Diplomacy*.
13 Adams and Cox, *Diplomacy*; Sowerby and Hennings, *Practices*.
14 Fletcher, *Diplomacy*; Harriet Rudolph, ed., *Material Culture in Modern Diplomacy from the 15th to the 20th Century* (Berlin: Walter de Gruyter, 2016).
15 David Beach, *The Shona and the Zimbabwe 900–1850* (London: Heineman, 1980); Mudenge, *Political*; Innocent Pikirayi, *The Zimbabwe Culture. Origins and Decline of Southern Zambezian States* (Walnut Creek: Altamira Press, 2001).
16 Gai Roufe, "Local Perceptions of the Political Systems of the Southern Bank of the Zambesi Valley in the Sixteenth and Early Seventeenth Century," *The International Journal of African Historical Studies* 49, no. 1 (2016): 53–75.
17 Pikirayi, *Zimbabwe*, 157–194; G. Pwiti, "Peasants, Chiefs and Kings: A Model of Development of Cultural Complexity in Northern Zimbabwe," *Zambezia* 33, no. 1 (1996): 31–52; Mudenge, *Political*, 77–160; Beach, *Shona*, 113–121.
18 Ivana Elbl, "Cross-Cultural Trade and Diplomacy: Portuguese Relations with West Africa, 1441–1521," *Journal of World History* 3, no. 2 (1992): 165–204.
19 For Atlantic Africa, see Quirk and Richardson, "Europeans." On Kongo, see John K. Thornton, *The Kingdom of Kongo: Civil War and Transition 1641–1718* (Madison: The

University of Wisconsin Press, 1983); Linda Heywood and John Thornton "Central African Leadership and the Appropriation of European Culture," in *The Atlantic World and Virginia, 1550–1624*, ed. Peter C. Mancall (Chapel Hill: The University of North Carolina Press, 2007), 194–224. On Asia, see Stefan Halikowski-Smith, "'The Friendship of Kings was in the Ambassadors': Portuguese Diplomatic Embassies in Asia and Africa during the Sixteenth and Seventeenth Centuries," *Portuguese Studies* 22, no. 1 (2006): 101–134.

20 Eugénia Rodrigues, "Embaixadas portuguesas à corte dos mutapa," in *D. João III e o Império*, eds. Roberto Carneiro and Artur Teodoro de Matos (Lisbon: CHAM/CEPCEP, 2004), 753–779. The capitals of the Karanga states were called 'zimbabwe', literally 'houses of stone'. Pikiraiy, *Zimbabwe*, 123–139, 163–176.

21 Bocarro, *Década*, 536.

22 Mudenge, *Political*, 203–221; Malyn Newitt, *A History of Mozambique* (London: Hurst & Company, 1995), 56–60; Eugénia Rodrigues, *Portugueses e Africanos nos Rios de Sena: Os Prazos da Coroa em Moçambique nos Séculos XVII e XVIII* (Lisbon: Imprensa Nacional-Casa da Moeda, 2013), 81–104.

23 Mudenge, *Political*, 224–262; Newitt, *History*, 83–92. Contemporary geological research proved the existence of some silver north of Tete, but far away from being a Potosi. Rodrigues, *Portugueses*, 117–164.

24 Mudenge, *Political*, 258–259; Newitt, *History*, 90–92; Rodrigues, *Portugueses*, 141–146. For Asia, see Halikowski-Smith, "Friendship."

25 On Kongo, see Thornton, *Kingdom*; Heywood and Thornton "Central African."

26 Pikirayi, *Zimbabwe*, 222–230; Rodrigues, *Portugueses*, 173–206.

27 Newitt, *History*, 92–93.

28 Ibid., 193–207. On Europe, see Frigo, *Politics*. In the Karanga state Barue, the ruler makombe could only be enthroned after receiving the baptism water from the Portuguese ambassadors. Allen Isaacman, "Madzi-manga, Mhondoro and the Use of Oral Traditions: A Chapter in Barue Religious and Political History," *Journal of African History* 14, no. 3 (1973): 395–409.

29 Beach, *Shona*, 145–147; Pikiraiy, *Zimbabwe*, 192–193; Rodrigues, *Portugueses*, 239–254.

30 Rodrigues, *Portugueses*, 264–334; Mudenge, *Political*, 285–347; Newitt, *History*. For European examples, see Frigo, *Politics*, 7.

31 William Roosen, "Early Modern Diplomatic Ceremonial: A Systems Approach," *The Journal of Modern History* 52, no. 3 (1980): 466.

32 António Bocarro, *Década 13* (Lisbon: Academia das Sciencias de Lisboa, 1876), 541–542; António da Conceição, "Tratado dos Rios de Cuama," (1696) *O Chronista de Tissuary* 15 (1867): 67; António Pinto Miranda, "Memória sobre a Costa de África," *c.* 1766, in *Relações de Moçambique Setecentista*, ed. António Banha de Andrade (Lisbon: AGU, 1955), 306–307. See, also Mudenge, *Political*, 85–86.

33 On Asia, see Halikowski-Smith, "Friendship."

34 Miranda, "Memória," 306–307.

35 Bocarro, *Década*, 538; João de Barros, *Ásia* (Lisbon: AGU, 1944 [1552]), 396; Diogo do Couto, "Capítulos XX a XXV da Década IX da Ásia," (post. 1573) in *Documentos sobre os Portugueses em Moçambique e na África Central* (Lisbon: National Archives of Rhodesia and Centro de Estudos Históricos Ultramarinos, 1962–89), vol. VIII, 274; Francisco Monclaro, "Relação (cópia), feita pelo padre Francisco Monclaro [post 1573]," in *Documentos*, vol. VIII, 376; João dos Santos, *Etiópia Oriental e Vária História de Cousas Notáveis do Oriente* (Lisbon: CNPCD, 1999 [1609]), 94; Conceição, "Tratado," 67.

36 Monclaro, "Relação," 380; Miranda, "Memória," 306–307; Mudenge, *Political*, 147–148.

37 Halikowski-Smith, "Friendship."

38 Archivum Romanum Societatis Iesu, *Goa*, 9, I, fls.56–7v (3.10.1623). See also António Gomes, "Viagem que fez o Padre Antº Gomes da Comp.ª de Jesus, ao Imperio de de (sic) Manomotapa; e assistência que fez nas ditas terras de Alg'us annos," (1648) ed. E. Axelson, *STVDIA* 3 (1959): 239–240.

39 "Carta (copia) do padre jesuíta Luís Fróis," (15.12.1561), in *Documentos*, vol. VIII, 34–58.

40 Monclaro, "Relação," 396, 416–418; Couto, "Capítulos," 274–282.

41 "Treslado das capitulações que fizeram os Portugueses com ElRy de Monomotapa," (24.05.1629) in *Records of South-Eastern Africa collected in various libraries and archive departments in Europe*, ed. George McCall Theal (Cape Town, 1898–1903), vol. 5, 287–288.

42 Biblioteca Nacional de Portugal (hereinafter, BNP), Reservados, *Fundo Geral*, cód.866, fls.2–7 (10.06.1735).

43 Miranda, "Memória," 306–307; Arquivo Histórico Ultramarino (hereinafter, AHU), *Moçambique* cx.34, doc.84. (1780–81).

44 Mudenge, *Political*, 143–144.

45 On Europe, see Frigo, *Politics*, 8.

46 Santos, *Etiópia*, 133.

47 Ibid., 133–134.

48 Monclaro, "Relação," 416–418.

49 On Africa, see Smith, *Warfare*.

50 AHU, *Moçambique*, cx.33, doc.81 (12.05.1780); cx.38, doc.7 (7.01.1782).

51 AHU, Moç. cx.34, doc.84 (1780–81). On the *vanyiai*, see Beach, *Shona*, 149–151; Newitt, *History*, 220–221. For an approach arguing that the *vanyiai* were only envoys, see Mudenge, *Political*, 135, 144–145.

52 Pedro Cardim, "A prática diplomática na Europa do Antigo Regime," in *História e Relações Internacionais*, eds. Luís Nuno Rodrigues and Fernando Martins (Évora: CIDHEUS, 2004).

53 AHU, *Moçambique*, cx.33, doc.95 (1781); cx.42, doc.70 (1783).

54 Bocarro, *Década*, 539; Santos, *Etiópia*, 220–223. On these women, see Mudenge, *Political*, 104–110; Eugénia Rodrigues, "Rainhas, princesas e donas: formas de poder político das mulheres na África Oriental nos séculos XVI a XVIII," *Cadernos Pagu* 49 (2017). For a perspective arguing that these women were men, see Roufe, "Local."

55 AHU, *Moçambique*, cx.34, doc.84 (1780–81); cx.35, doc.5 (10.01.1781); cx.38, doc.5 (5.01.1782). See, also Rodrigues, "Rainhas."

56 There is an extensive literature on the meanings of gift giving. For an overview, see Ilana Krausman Ben-Amos, *The Culture of Giving: Informal Support and Gift-Exchange in Early Modern England* (New York: Cambridge University Press, 2008); Fletcher, *Diplomacy*, 145–167.

57 AHU, *Moçambique*, cx.33, doc.77 (6.05.1780).

58 Santos, *Etiópia*, 134; Miranda, "Memória," 306–307; AHU, *Moçambique*, cx.33, doc.95 (1781); cx.42, doc.70 (1783).

59 On Europe, see Fletcher, *Diplomacy*, 161.

60 For more on Portuguese and European gifts in Asia, see Halikowski-Smith, "Friendship"; Zoltán Biedermann, Giorgio Riello and Anne Gerritsen, eds., *Global Gifts: The Material Culture of Diplomacy in Early Modern Eurasia* (Cambridge: Cambridge University Press, 2018).

61 Monclaro, "Relação," 410–418.

62 AHU, *Moçambique*, cx.41, doc.14. (28.12.1780).

63 Rodrigues, "Embaixadas," 772–723.

64 AHU, cód.2127, fl.157–7v (1.10.1774).

65 Miranda, "Memória," 308–309.

66 AHU, *Moçambique*, cx.35, doc.28 (14.02.1781).

67 Benton, *Law*, 55–56.

68 Monclaro, "Relação," 380.

69 AHU, *Moçambique*, cx.71, doc.58 (28.11.1794). See also A.C.P. Gamito, *O Muata Cazembe e os Povos Maraves, Chevas, Muizas, Muembas, Lundas e outros da África Austral* (Lisbon: AGC, 1937), vol. I, 63–64.

70 Harriet Rudolph, "Entangled Objects and Hybrid Practices? Material Culture as a New Approach to the History of Diplomacy," in Rudolph, *Material*, 20.

71 Arquivo Histórico de Moçambique, *Quelimane*, cx.858, M2(10), (30.12.1811); AHU, *Moçambique*, cx.71, doc.58 (29.12.1795).

72 AHU, *Moçambique*, cx.33, doc.66 (6.04.1781); AHU, Moç. cx.34, doc.84 (1780–81).

73 AHU, *Moçambique*, cx.35, doc.46 (6.03.1781).

74 Missionaries educated some mutapas' sons. However, writing never expanded in Munhumutapa. Mudenge, *Political*. On Kongo, see Heywood and Thornton "Central African"; on Angola, see Ana Paula Tavares and Catarina Madeira Santos, eds., *Africæ Monumenta: A apropriação da escrita pelos Africanos* (Lisbon: IICT, 2002).

75 ANTT, LM 60, fls.233–4v (12.04.1645). See also AHU, *Moçambique*, cx.2, doc.119 (20.04.1663).
76 Rodrigues, "Embaixadas," 763–766.
77 Frigo, *Politics*, 9.
78 AHU, *Moçambique*, cx.35, doc.5 (14.02.1781).
79 BNP, Reservados, *Fundo Geral*, Mss.71, n.1 (1.05.1735); ANTT, LM60, fls.233–4v (12.04.1645).
80 AHU, *Moçambique*, cx.34, doc.84 (1780–81).
81 Ibid.
82 Thornton, *Kingdom*; Heywood and Thornton "Central African."

Key works

Beach, David, *The Shona and the Zimbabwe 900–1850* (London: Heineman, 1980).

Frigo, Daniela, *Politics and Diplomacy in Early Modern Italy: The Structure of Diplomatic Practice, 1450–1800* (Cambridge: Cambridge University Press, 2000).

Mudenge, S.I.G., *A Political History of Munhumutapa c. 1400–1902* (Harare: Zimbabwe Publishing House, 1988).

Newitt, Malyn, *A History of Mozambique* (London: Hurst & Company, 1995).

Rodrigues, Eugénia, *Portugueses e Africanos nos Rios de Sena: Os Prazos da Coroa em Moçambique nos Séculos XVII e XVIII* (Lisbon: Imprensa Nacional-Casa da Moeda, 2013).

14

EARLY MODERN MONARCHY AND FOREIGN TRAVEL

Philippa Woodcock

In 2007 the newly elected French President, Nicolas Sarkozy, declared 'François Mitterrand travelled for his own amusement . . . Not me. I've been President for four months. There's no time to lose. I must meet, with all haste, as many leaders as possible.'[1] Travel was essential to his perception of the exercise of power, where he would personally represent his country and its diplomatic aims. Like a monarch, he was trailed by an impressive entourage and a throng of reporting journalists. In the *Ancien Régime*, travel, or its notable absence, was equally important in the exercise of French royal power. This was as true for Merovingian kings who 'ritually journeyed' around their realm, as for the Capetians.[2] By the medieval period, travel by rulers became necessary for international relations where frontier meetings sealed alliances. However, as Colette Beaune and Albert Babeau have shown, political murders hindered travel: indeed, Louis XI (r.1461–83) and Edward IV of England (r.1461–83) were forced to embrace through a primitive security grill at Pecquigny in 1475.[3] As such, the early modern period saw ambassadors more commonly take the place and the risks of travelling royals. For Lucien Bély, they were the 'travellers for the prince'.[4] Given that it was dangerous to travel, this chapter will consider the foreign journeys undertaken by sixteenth-century Valois monarchs, exploring how they generated change, ideas and images which extended royal authority, rather than threatening its survival. Of course, travel for conquest extended dynastic power, whether by upholding inherited claims to territories or meeting relatives, but this chapter will also demonstrate that it indirectly strengthened the state and shaped royal identity.

Considering the modern age, Philip Long identifies that royal travel continues to 'attract considerable attention both at home and abroad'.[5] In the sixteenth century this public interest was manifest in records of royal entries, often held as kings set off or returned from their travels.[6] The occasion consolidated royal power for, as part of these parades, set tableaux made colourful reference to episodes of royal travel and conquest. For example, in the entry organized by the city of Lyon on 12 July 1515, François I's preparations to invade Italy were celebrated in a scene where the ship of state or *nef de France* was shown being steered towards success by the king's military commanders, Gian Giacomo Trivulzio and the Constable of Bourbon, both soon to take part in the invasion (Figure 14.1).[7]

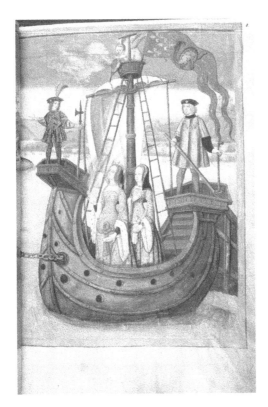

Figure 14.1 The Constable of Bourbon (in feathered cap) and Gian Giaomo Trivulzio (in
yellow and green), steering the ship of state. The entry of François I to Lyon,
1515, Cod. Guelf. 86.4 Extrav, fol. 8r. Courtesy of Herzog August Bibliothek,
Wolfenbuttel

Monarchs also ensured that their own glory and prowess as travellers was
recorded, for like those journalists following Sarkozy, Louis XII (r.1498–1515)
commissioned poets Jean d'Auton (*c.*1466–1528) and Jean Marot (*c.*1463–1526)
to laud his voyages to Italy in 1499, 1507 and 1509.[8] D'Auton's strictly chronological accounts hint at wider advantages to the country from the 'beneficial acts and
commendable deeds of the victorious French, carried out during the conquest of
the duchy of Milan'.[9] Marot's praise is more fulsome and explicit, with travels presented as of undoubted value and felicity for Louis XII who was the 'Most Christian
Virtuous King of France/ Bearing the Heaven born Lily. Anointed with Heavenly
Oil/ Mighty Hercules, of invincible strength'.[10] Of course, as Cynthia Jane Brown
argues, such works also combined 'rhetorical and historical tendencies' and were
used as propaganda to win public support for the Italian wars.[11] The importance
of travel was also expressed materially in the royal commissions of tombs in the
basilica of St Denis, which depicted Louis XII and François I (r.1515–47) on their
respective Italian travels for posterity.

Ideas about the connection between French royal travel and power also resonated
beyond the kingdom in the sixteenth century. For the foreign perspective, we can

look to the 1588 *Cronica breve dei fatti illustri de re di Francia*, published in the Republic of Venice and dedicated to the French ambassador in the Republic. This presents annotated portraits of all the kings of France, ending with the last Valois, Henri III (r.1574–89).[12] The text mentions travel among the first, defining achievements of each monarch from Charles VIII (r.1483–98) onwards (Table 14.1). However, there is an inconsistent visual association between the kings who went abroad with armies, and the idea that the French king also possessed imperial power. For example, François I and Henri II (r.1547–59) are adorned with imperial laurels and Roman-style armour (see Figure 14.2), but Charles VIII and Louis XII are not, perhaps because they had occasionally been opposed to Venice.

Table 14.1 Illustrations and texts from the *Cronica breve de i fatti illustri de' re di Francia, con le loro effigie dal naturale*, Venice: Bernardo Giunti: 1588

King	Main travel undertaken	Text	Image
Charles VIII	1494–5 Conquest of Naples	fece l'impresa del Regno di Napoli. . .senza quasi mai sfodrar la spada, scorse tutta l'Italia.	Non-military dress and collar of Saint Michel (* it was forbidden to wear the collar with armour)
Louis XII 1498–1515	1499 Conquest of Milan 1500 Final victory in Milan 1507 Conquest of Genoa 1509 Presence in Italy after Agnadello	Passo in Italia e prese Milano . . . dette una gra[n] rotta a Venetiani	Non-military dress and collar of St Michel
François I 1515–47	1515 Conquest of Milan 1524 Reconquest of Milan 1525–6 Spanish imprisonment	Passo con esercito in Italia et rotti Svizari prese Milano . . . menato in Spagna	Imperial laurels and armour
Henri II 1547–59	1551 Chévauchée in Imperial lands – Metz and 3 bishoprics	Fu bellicoso . . . passo in Alemagna, e prese alcuni luochi dell'Imperator Carlo Quinto	Imperial laurels and armour
François II 1559–60		Hebbe etiandio il Regno di Scotia	Royal regalia
Charles IX 1560–74	(1564–6 Undertook journey in France with his mother)	–	Court dress
Henri III 1574–89	1573–4 Travel from France to Krakow as elected king of Poland June-July 1574 Return from Krakow via Vienna, Venice, Padua, Mantua, Turin and Marseille	Fu in vita del fratello, eletto da i poloni lor Re, e coronato in Cracovia . . . ritorno con prestezza in Francia	Court dress

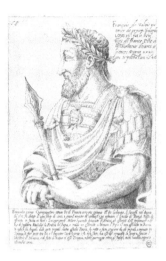

Figure 14.2 Francois I, Cronica breve dei fatti illustri de re' di Francia p. 58, courtesy of the BNF

In this instance, contemporaries saw French claims to imperial power corre-lated with travel for conquest, whether in Italy or Germany. Isabelle Haquet argues that this is characteristic of Valois representations from the reign of Charles VIII onwards, where the French kings' challenge to Habsburg power harnessed images of Roman emperors.[13] If the Holy Roman emperors were the heirs to Rome, French monarchs were not averse either to claiming this inheritance and its universal authority. As this chapter will show, travel allowed this claim to be exercised in diverse ways. However, not all French monarchs travelled as conquerors, and some were invited voyagers and guests.

This exploration of travel by rulers contributes to a key debate in early modern French history. Travel history is an expanding area of scholarship, yet when histori-ans' gaze has fallen on royal travellers, it has most notably been on non-French cases. For example, the ever-peripatetic Holy Roman Emperor, Charles V (r.1519–56), was forced by the problems of governing an empire of geographically disparate territo-ries to spend much of his life in the saddle.[14] More outlandishly, Peter the Great, tsar of Russia (r.1682–1725), undertook tours to the west for his own education, pleasure and political goals.[15] Other case studies have focused on extremes, such as the young Cosimo III de'Medici (r.1670–1723), who before his accession was sent to the Spanish Low Countries to allow time for marital hatred to abate.[16] Table 14.1 has shown the significance of travel for perceptions of the Valois. Thus, study of French foreign royal travel is an important addition to the field.

Moreover, it further nuances discussion of royal power, where the connection between a displaced court and authority is particularly key for early modern France. For a long time, Valois power was characterized as increasingly absolutist and cen-tralized around royal institutions and the king's person, whether in Paris or at the monarch's residences in the Île de France, especially from the reign of François I onwards. What is more, after 1600 it was increasingly sedentary. While over even twenty years ago, Robert Knecht was able to summarize new historiography refuting such ideas about the Valois, little attention has been paid to the real impact of a court which continued to be itinerant, and the kings' forays beyond France.[17] Instead, where travel is considered as a means to rule, it is as a domestic phenomenon, for example, in Charles IX and Catherine de Medici's 'grand tour' of France in 1564–6, as explored by Jean Boutier et al. and most recently by Linda Briggs.[18] However, rather than the reigns of the first Bourbon monarchs ushering in something quite different to the Valois, some historians have challenged the idea of a sedentary Bourbon court. For example, Jean-Claude Cuignet has shown how the first Bourbon king, the ever-peripatetic Henri IV (r.1589–1610), spent the majority of his life on the road in war torn France.[19] More significantly, Marc W.S. Jaffré has overturned assumptions about Louis XIII's style of rule, to argue that even if the king did not leave France, he was often on the move. Moreover, an itinerant court was a key part of the king's politics, rather than any sign of weakness or inability to attract nobles to a fixed court.[20] Hence, travel really is a key part of the understanding of early modern French monarchy.

Nonetheless, the idea justifiably persists that the later Bourbon dynasty based their authority on sedentary rule. For example, 2004's *Dictionnaire de l'Ancien Régime* describes a situation after 1660 where 'a settled court at Versailles became the key space for daily ceremonies'.[21] Rather than foreign adventures, Christophe Levantal's plotting of Louis XIV's whereabouts during his rule shows an ever less itinerant court, which when it moved only did so in a small circumference between Versailles and its satellite châteaux.[22] This is confirmed in the archival dossiers for *Voyages Royales*, which add the occasional sortie to the front in Flanders and the journey to Spain of Philip V.[23] The world simply came to Versailles to be near to the king. Thus travel, or rather the lack of it, was key to later Bourbon royal authority. The most damning mark of the risks of royal travel came in June 1791. The royal family's flight to escape France ending ignominiously at Varennes, brought an end to the constitutional monarchy and precipitated charges of treason against Louis XVI (r.1774–92) and Marie-Antoinette. Thus, it is important to know what the Valois gained by travel when the later Bourbons were increasingly disinclined towards it.

In order to make effective comparison, the chapter will principally contrast the experience of Louis XII with that of Henri, duc d'Anjou, later Henri III (hereafter referred to as Henri III). These cases help reflect on two of the lesser studied Valois monarchs in a century dominated by the reign of François I, who famously travelled as a conqueror to Italy, as a prisoner to Spain and received his great rivals, the Holy Roman Emperor Charles V and Henry VIII, as guests in his own realm. However, it was Louis XII and his army who first successfully crossed the Alps several times to conquer Milan in 1499 and 1500, and to subdue Genoa (1507). Louis, rather than François, consolidated the Orléans dynastic claim to Milan, inherited from Valentina Visconti, and it was Louis and his courtiers who really fostered the import of Italian artists to France, as well as Italian delicacies.[24] In contrast, the prelude to Henri III's reign was a period of intense non-military travel, allowing for discussion of the gains of travel when not at the head of an army. Henri III went reluctantly to Poland in 1573 as its elected monarch, but much more willingly from Warsaw to Italy in 1574, before returning to France to become the king of a nation divided by religious and political hatred. While his journey, and in particular his stay in Venice, has attracted scholarly discussion focused on its extravagant festivals, relatively little has been said about the impact of non-military travel on a king's domestic power.[25] This chapter will now use these two case studies to explore some of the methods of travel available to, and preferred by, the Valois monarchs. It shows how the physical act of travel – its speed and difficulty – consolidated their power beyond the acquisition of land and titles.

Entourage and anonymity

Once on the road, monarchs usually travelled with vast retinues and households, their journey assured by passports and safe conducts. Such entourages were an established way for kings to display their power to their people and to other rulers. This relationship is evident in contemporary imagery, from illuminations of Louis XII followed by his entourage in d'Auton's *Chroniques* (*c*.1501–8), to the 'travel' episode of the Valois Tapestries (*c*.1580–9), where courtiers follow Henri III and his siblings, royal carriages, baggage trains and mounted guards. This shows that one impact of royal travel was to force the great magnates to leave home, dislocating them from their own power bases and placing them under royal supervision. It thus achieved through movement what Versailles later guaranteed by stasis, and shows how travel could contribute directly to royal management of the nobility.

While the Spanish ambassador in France, Diego de Cuniga, told Philip II that Henri III would travel to Poland with 500 companions and 800 cavaliers, Henri III's correspondence gives us evidence of a king carefully selecting a small number of gentlemen for his close entourage during his journey to Poland.[26] Thus, to the duc de Daimville, Henri wrote that 'I love you so much that the King, my said lord and brother, could not allow anyone to accompany me whose company I would find more agreeable.'[27] Indeed, in one print Henri is shown travelling to Poland with just a few gentlemen (Figure 14.3). These represent the core of his favourites, rather than the full extent of his followers.[28]

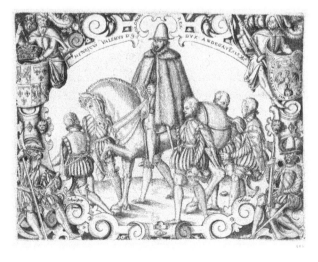

Figure 14.3 Henri, duc d'Anjou, leaving for Poland, FRBNF41499892, courtesy of the BNF

This illustrates how travel offered the crown another means to control the nobility, with the exercise of preference keeping certain nobles near and in competition for proximity.

Numbers, hierarchy and overwhelming power characterized martial expeditions. In his *Chroniques*, d'Auton suggested Louis XII's army in 1499 numbered at least 16,000 men, while at his entry to Milan he was 'so well accompanied that my quill (pen) buckles under the weight of the description'.[29] Similarly, Didier Le Fur, Robert Knecht and Pierre Brasme have quantified the French armies of Louis XII, François I and Henri II as numbering between 16,000 and 40,000 men.[30] Knowing how many were in the 'close' entourage is harder. It is possible to follow the titled knights who processed behind Louis XII in his Milanese entries, but we do not know total numbers for combined households, as each noble might travel with his own sizeable personal entourage.[31] The Milanese duchy records only provide information on the permanent garrison, rather than the invading force.[32] Neither was this precision a concern for the official chroniclers, with d'Auton 'fearing, that if the account is too long, to weary the listeners'.[33]

This lack of detail speaks of the equivocal benefits of entourage. Although weight of numbers demonstrated loyalty to the king and the kingdom's noble might, if d'Auton or Marot gave it too much attention, it could distract from the focus on the royal achievement of crossing the mountains. Thus, in 1507 Marot referred in greater detail to the components of Louis' artillery than to his companions' identities:

> The King .../ Crossed the mountains to avenge this defiance/ More promptly than ever was King ... Fire arms, Serpentines, Canons, / And other arms for which I do not know the name, Thus the king [went], with all his baronage, and the greatest of his royal lineage.[34]

In contrast, Henri III's return to France shows just how sparsely a king could travel. Having learnt of his brother's death and his own accession to the French crown in June 1574, Henri decided on a hasty departure from Krakow. Fearing that the Poles would detain him if recognized, he 'secretly [And to the disappointment of the senate and Polish lords] withdrew with only eight or nine horses . . . to return to France to take possession of the French kingdom'.[35] Thus, when in some circumstances a vast entourage was part of the performance of power, when Henri did not wish to be recognized as a king, and travelled illicitly, a small retinue was adopted for safety. This mechanism was once again reversed when he set foot on friendly territory on his return journey to France. Here, numbers confirmed his legitimacy as king. Equally, the distance that welcoming parties travelled towards him was a mark of his authority. For example, in Venice on 18 July 1574, quite unusually, the Doge, Alvise Mocenigo, travelled to the Lido and offered Henri the seat of honour on the ducal barge, the *Bucintoro*. In France, Henri's younger brother, François, duke of Alençon (1555–84) and his brother-in-law, Navarre (the future Henri IV) were dispatched to the frontier to acknowledge his power.[36] Henri III even wrote to his mother to 'Command the nobility to come to meet me on the road to Lyon', showing once again a king's power to impose travel upon his court.[37]

As Henri III's flight from Poland proves, monarchs also perceived advantages to travelling incognito, correlating with moments where royal status was rejected in return for some other benefit. Such journeys were undertaken from personal caprice, economy or security. Peter the Great provides the most famous early modern example of an anonymous royal traveller, touring western Europe to improve his knowledge of shipbuilding under the guise of Peter Mikhailov. Likewise, Ulrich Langen, although arguing that this aspect of royal travel has been neglected, has explored different incognito journeys by seventeenth- and eighteenth-century Danish kings, who used courtesy princely titles to divert attention from their higher status when travelling.[38] However, these attempts at anonymity largely failed. The young Cosimo III, wishing to travel incognito, was frustrated to be greeted by civic largesse and gun salutes at each town he visited in the Spanish Netherlands.[39] Rather than the problems of divorcing oneself from entourage and command, Langen suggests that, at least for seventeenth- or eighteenth-century royal travellers, incognito travel was understood differently from anonymity. Instead, it was more the opportunity to 'cut back on formal and ceremonial duties', and to make savings, rather than the 'complete obscuring of a person's identity'.[40] Indeed, dictionaries of early modern French qualify incognito royal travellers as those still enjoying high status activities, but without their full 'ordinary retinue, or the other marks which distinguish them'.[41]

The Valois also attempted to travel incognito, but rarely managed to fully shrug off their royal identity. Louis XII is said to have gone incognito to the Berry to visit the tomb of his first wife, Jeanne de France.[42] In this instance, he did so to avoid further censure of his repudiation of Jeanne in 1498, after twenty-two years of marriage. When Henri III slipped out of his temporary Venetian palace, the Ca' Foscari, to melt into the Venetian crowds, it was as a private citizen, Henri de Valois, ready to visit Venice's best addresses and follow something of the established tourist route for gentlemanly visitors.[43] This signified his putting off of his royal role to visit the city without moral scrutiny and with no obligation to enter into formal ceremonial or ritual at all moments of his stay. He was not anonymous though; he was followed by crowds, and Venetian jewellers sought to charge him the highest price for their wares.[44] The correlation between incognito royal travel and real anonymity was perhaps only achieved when disguise was used, for example when Henri III fled from Poland dressed as a servant, stabling his own horse at a roadside inn. Thus, entourage was an essential accessory to making royal power visible but was a hindrance when speed and anonymity were of the essence. Safety could be found in numbers, yet while entourages literally moved the nobility in tandem with the crown, they also had to be used carefully in relation to stressing the virtues of kings as individuals, for fear of their accomplishments being overwhelmed by the collective magnificence.

Transport

In contrast to modern luxury jet or royal yacht, the preferred methods of early modern royal travel, if varied, were rarely the most luxurious. Nonetheless, all methods were turned to message-bearing advantage, and in this period the horse remained the supreme mark of status, conveying both the wealth and the virility of the rider. In Figure 14.3, Henri III's social superiority is marked by his being the sole rider, around whom all the other figures cluster on foot. The majority of journeys considered here were on horseback, as this was the speediest available transport and the animals were far easier to manoeuvre than a lumbering coach.[45] However, even this had limits, as François I wrote to his mother in 1515 during his crossing of the Alps, 'We are finding it irksome to wear armour in these mountains, most of the time we have to go on foot, leading our horses by the bridle.'[46]

Images of the Valois monarchs on horseback continued the loaded connection between royalty and the authority of the Roman emperors, while extending the symbolic Valois challenge to the Holy Roman emperors.[47] Titian's equestrian portrait of the emperor Charles V, commemorating the battle of Mühlberg (1547), spoke of the emperor's control over many disparate and unruly peoples, as well as his military ability.[48] As such, it directly referenced equestrian images of the Roman emperors. Similar ideas are present in the even earlier illuminations in d'Auton and Marot, which show Louis XII on a war horse entering conquered Italian cities.[49] It was not only the power of the horse but also its heraldic caparison and harnessing which bore messages of royal authority, down to mottos embossed on the stirrups.[50] For example, Louis XII's horse in his 'Journey from Alexandria' (Marot) wears a caparison decorated with beehives and bees, symbolizing the king's ability to both punish and be clement.[51]

The slowest mode of royal transport was horse-drawn travel. This did not have the positive connotations associated with the highly ornate court coaches of the seventeenth century, which according to John M. Hunt had the ability, when suitably decorated and accompanied, to become 'a prince's ceremonial face'.[52] The luxury coach was rare beyond the urban setting in sixteenth-century France, and was barely more comfortable than the farm carts from which they had developed.[53] They were associated with female royals and their physical weaknesses.[54] For example, Queen Claude was conducted to Guines in June 1520 by coach because of her pregnancy with Princess Madeleine. On her 1564–5 progress, Catherine de' Medici used a coach or litter due to her expanding girth, while her daughter Marguerite and small son Charles were simultaneously showcased and protected in a smaller, 'gilded cage' of a coach.[55] Thus, if the coach symbolized royalty, it also represented the constraints and dangers of the position.

The easiest way to travel was by water. It also had great symbolic potential. Henri III's travel by water transport in Italy was part of his successful visit to the Republic of Venice, and would resonate in later royal interests. For example, when the Doge met Henri in the ducal barge, the *Bucintoro*, the king was offered the Doge's seat, representing the alliance between France and Venice, and indeed, the honour done to this uncrowned king.[56] When he returned to France in late August and made his entry into Lyon, crossing the Saône to the archbishop's palace, the city offered him 'a boat which reminded him of the *Bucintoro*', recalling the diplomatic success of his Venetian stay.[57] Equally, Henri III's reception in Venice was accompanied by waterborne parties, and he was the first French king to travel by gondola. He had experienced the new and unusual, adding to the idea of royal connoisseurship and extraordinary knowledge. A century later, the ongoing friendship between France and Venice was emphasized in a gift of 1674 to Louis XIV of several gondolas and gondoliers for the canal at Versailles.[58] While the exchange of valuable horses was an established diplomatic gift, here the use and gifting of exotic travel methods could symbolize new and strengthening alliances.[59]

While Henri III crossed the Alps by litter, kings at the head of their armies made their return journeys to France by sea.[60] It was quicker, safer and reinforced royal power by allowing for the exercise of royal command. Landing at Marseille or a nearby port, the king could review his naval capability. Travelling by water to another realm was also a means to bring royal power into the view of another ruler. Thus, the last illumination to d'Auton's *Chroniques* shows Louis XII bidding farewell to his brother monarch, Ferdinand of Aragon (who was by now married to Louis' niece, Germaine de Foix).[61] All Ferdinand's teeming fleet of ships bear sails in his colours, Or/Geules, emphasizing to the French court his naval power, his mobility, and ability to attack and defend.

From a wider perspective, royal travel – whether in peace or for war – had a secondary impact on transport, technology and logistics. For example, the development of coaches owed something to contact with Italy during Louis XII and François I's Italian campaigns (1499–1529). Coach travel was fashionable in the peninsula's many urban centres before it spread to France, and the kings and their commanders who travelled to Italy may have promoted coach travel on their return to France.[62] Manuscript illuminations show Louis XII in both fixed-axle ceremonial chariots and canopied coaches: contemporaries who travelled to Italy also commissioned similar images.[63] While the chariot echoed Rome adding to messages about Louis XII's imperial power, the comfort and manoeuvrability of coaches were helped by new military technology, such as the inclusion of the 'pivoting front end, no doubt inspired by the new artillery carriages tested during the Italian wars'.[64] Furthermore, the kings' occasional need to travel to certain parts of their kingdom to conduct war led to an improved national infrastructure. For example, Daniel Nordman has shown that 'the presence of paths (or even tracks) is linked to military concerns, [the] Italian wars'.[65] Likewise, royal movement led to developments in cartography, and such maps may have contributed to economic growth by 'focusing interest (political, commercial)' on linking markets and infrastructure, and indirectly strengthening the kingdom.[66] This surely echoes d'Auton's comment, noted earlier, on the 'beneficial' elements of foreign travel and conquest.

Royal travel, therefore, was symbolic of imperium and power. Military technology had the potential to speed up the development and forms of civilian transport, which potentially encouraged economic growth. The routes trodden by royal armies and entourages consolidated domestic royal authority by improving knowledge of the realm and its infrastructure, as well as awareness of the extent of the king's powers, contested lands and fluid borders. Ultimately, each man's identity was reinforced by their choice of transport, which demonstrated their command and experience, whether travelling on horseback like Roman emperors, or in extreme leisure and comfort.

Speed and difficulty

In an age when travel was difficult, the very fact that foreign campaigns or extended trips were safely undertaken demonstrated power and character. For example, Louis XII's success was underlined both by the speed of his journeys and the difficult nature of the mountainous landscape that he traversed. This was in sharp contrast to Henri III's travels, which were designed to be as easy as possible and avoid all potential confrontation. However, the political fallout of his flight from Poland involved Henri deploying ingenuity and guile, and then, once in safety, using his charm to convey France's magnificence.[67]

In royal iconography and legend, as well as the estimation of their contemporaries, going beyond France's mountain borders was also testimony to authority. For Louis XII, as for François I, the Alps were 'conquered' as much as any Italian rival. While enemies were only human, the mountains were timeless, and their crossing was proof of the king's power and success. Interestingly, Louis XII did not physically accompany his army on its first conquest of Milan, only arriving there when the duchy had been secured, but did travel with them on later journeys. Nonetheless, the king's role in the fall of Milan is central to his iconography: a panel from Louis XII's tomb (commissioned by his successor, François I) shows the king entering the duchy of Milan as its conqueror, the mountains providing a backdrop of 'trophies'. Similarly, François I's tomb shows cannons being hauled over the mountains, symbolizing the physical barrier crushed by Valois might. Inevitably, for both kings, comparisons were made to Hannibal and Caesar, and a Venetian observer stated: 'nothing comparable had happened since Hannibal's crossing of the Alps'.[68]

For d'Auton and Marot, the ability of Louis XII's army to haul his equipment to Genoa from France was 'a near marvellous thing that so many and so large artillery pieces, were driven so carefully over the knoll of the mountains'.[69] In such official histories, the speed at which this difficult passage was achieved was proof of the king's ability. Thus in 1499, 'the journey was so brief that in less than 15 days [the road] from Lyon to Asti was armed, with all its array', while in 1507 Louis XII 'crossed the mountains without stopping for a single day'.[70] He then swiftly reconquered Genoa. This sense of ease and speed is a reflection of the king's mastery of a hostile landscape, as well as his enemies.

Visual representations of Louis XII's successful travels depict him with imperium over further geographical, as well as political landscapes. Indeed, for Le Fur, Louis' power was linked to his ability to travel and restrict others' travel, for he was 'king of the sea and lord of the land'.[71] Control over Naples, Genoa and the Duchy of Milan gave him influence in the Mediterranean basin, with the keys to Africa and Asia. He was well placed to travel further, using his base in Naples to uphold the Angevin claim to Jerusalem and be a truly 'Holy Roman Emperor'. Even if this remained an unrealized dream, the potential was presaged in the frontispiece to Giovanni Michele Nagonio's *c.*1500 *De laudibus galliae*, which shows the soldier-emperor Aurelian, who had reunited the Gallic provinces with Rome, handing the king a globe, and hence dominion over France and Italy, if not beyond (Figure 14.4).[72]

Likewise, Louis' control over Italy was further developed in first-hand knowledge of it. He had travelled in the peninsula since 1492 and, with successive victories, seemed to hold Italy in his hand. This is encapsulated in the surviving fragment of one of the three statues of Louis XII from Cardinal d'Amboise's château at Gaillon, near Rouen. Defaced in 1793, the remaining *all'antica* armoured torso is identified with the king by its collar of St Michel and a map of Italy clasped in its left hand.[73] This shows the peninsula's main cities, all within Louis XII's grasp, as well as features of its landscape – which he had mastered – just like a Roman emperor.

In contrast, speed and power had a different relationship in Henri III's journeys. Indeed, he largely took his time when travelling, allowing him to be seen, to learn and to enjoy himself. For example, although elected king of Poland on 11 May 1573, he only left French sovereign territory in late November, and seemed to take all possible chances to delay his final arrival in Poland on 24 January.[74] This characterized

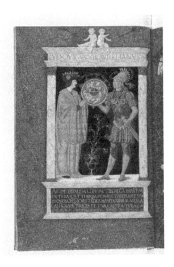

Figure 14.4 BN MS Latin 8132, frontispiece, Giovanni Michele Nagonio, *De Laudibus Galliae* (1500), courtesy of the BNF

a man loathe to agree to all of Poland's terms for his rule and fearful that his future domestic power would be challenged by his younger brother, Alençon. In contrast, his letters use a politic discourse of haste. For example, on 17 July 1573, he wrote to 'a palatin . . . with the promise to arrive in Poland as soon as possible'.[75] Three days later he told the duc de Daimville: 'I am in a great hurry to take to the road and it seems that I will never be able to get there fast enough according to my subjects.'[76] This prevarication also took the form of manner of travel. Having decided on 14 August that he would travel through Germany *sans armes*, it took a further ten days to return a boat lent to him by the baron de la Garde, when it had been envisaged that he might travel to Poland by sea. Yet, when he wanted to travel, Henri was capable of great speed, but it reflected his ability to evade the grasp of a foreign power – Poland – rather than anything akin to Louis' swift domination of northern Italy. The *Cronica breve* states that upon learning of Charles IX's death, Henri hastened to France and *ritorno con prestezza*.[77] This is only partially true. In his flight from Krakow to Vienna, and thence to Venice, which took less than three weeks, Henri paused to write to his mother on 22 June from Wisternitz (Vestonice, Czech Republic) that 'If I had the time and means from where I am to write to you at length as I desire, I would tell you in detail the story of my happy departure from Poland.' He would return swiftly, but on his own terms, for 'Having seen Germany, I shall go to Italy, and I will go to Venice.'[78] This was at his own leisure. Indeed, after his trip to Venice, he took a leisurely Italian meander. Having been formally recognized by the Venetian Republic and the emperor in Vienna on 25 June, he also met the dukes of Ferrara and Mantua – using 'slow' travel to make personal diplomatic bonds, like earlier medieval princes. He then took a 'water coach' to Turin where he 'arrived on 11 August and was there received with great joy and magnificence by the duke and duchess of Savoy, his aunt'.[79] Thus, a king who controlled his own trajectory was master of his own destiny and could manipulate travel to his own purposes. If Louis XII could swiftly subdue landscapes and subjects, Henri III's authority was manifest when he made his subjects and allies – in Poland, France and Italy – wait for his presence.

Beyond comment on the pleasurable evenings of his stay in Venice, the political significance of his visit to the Republic, the first paid by a French monarch, has drawn attention.[80] Unusually, this was an occasion for a monarch, who had not yet been crowned, to meet another head of state. It could have been an uneasy encounter, and indeed, Philippe de Commines, Charles VIII of France's travelling companion and counsellor, argued that: 'Great princes should never meet, if they want to remain friends.'[81] In Henri's case the visit was positive, and Marie Viallon argues his entry and visit was 'a twofold approach of seduction by the inviting power as by the guest'.[82] It profited his international and domestic position, as he gained recognition as king by powerful friends, underlining his legitimacy in the face of any potential challenge by Alençon.[83]

Such political gains were derived from Henri's manipulation of honours paid to him and pleasurable *divertissements*, for in effect the king was his own ambassador to Venice and observing diplomats. Although he sat in the *Bucintoro* and visited the Senate, Henri was also under public scrutiny from shopkeepers and soldiers.[84] Here, the importance of personal contact in royal travel is evident. The king engaged in the ritual of gift giving, judging his participation and the level of gift in a largely appropriate style. Images of his reception suggest he was also careful to show his difference from Venetian regalia and opulence. Vicentino's depiction of the event, painted for the ducal palace twenty years after Henri's visit, suggests that despite his Italian mother, he incarnated France: his black velvet *tenue*, cut in the modern French style, and sober goffered ruff distinguishes him from the rich red archaic costume of the Venetian senators, confirming the different characters and statuses of the two states. It emphasized that he alone was France, while Venice was a corporate government, rejecting individualism.

Once returned to France and crowned as king, ideas associated with physical travel did not have an obvious impact on Henri's power, as his reign became bogged down in the latter stages of the French Wars of Religion.[85] However, the fact that he had travelled to Poland – whatever the distance, speed and domestic political difficulties – and been crowned its king was clearly remarkable, as shown by the foregrounded comment in the *Cronica breve*. It was also later instrumental in France in his challenge to noble rivals for his throne and was used to underline his divinely appointed power. For example, he continued to maintain his claim to the Polish crown, albeit wrongly, and this crown was represented alongside that of France in his developing iconography. Haquet has shown how, as early as 1575, Henri's motto of 'MANET VLTIMA COELO' (the kingdom of heaven is above all others) was coupled with French and Polish closed imperial crowns and encircled by earthly laurels and palm leaves, which referred to a third, 'last' kingdom – heaven.[86] This endowed Henri with a huge geographical and unimaginably large spiritual domain, in comparison to Louis XII's earthly dominion *au-delà des monts*. In this context, the fact that he had travelled to Poland to perform his duty to the electors and been crowned Polish king, as well as being a divinely appointed French monarch, was used as propaganda as he strove to consolidate his domestic power against challenges from the Catholic League and the Huguenots.

As difficult as royal travel might be, Louis XII and Henri III successfully traversed perilous landscapes and hostile states. Physical and political challenges, speed – and the control thereof – was turned to political advantage by emphasizing resulting Herculean feats, political accomplishments and deft handling of circumstances and imagery.

Conclusion

Travel shaped early modern royal identities, whether as conqueror for Louis XII, or for Henri III as a new king, who used his experience of travel, rule and public acclaim beyond France to silence domestic rivals. Successful travel communicated power, resilience and statesmanship, and was keenly watched by followers, propagandists and diplomats in order to judge the calibre of a king. It was a public act and could not be otherwise, no matter how hard some rulers strove for anonymity.

Royal travel beyond France's borders in the sixteenth century could never be as frequent or wide-ranging as the modern-day presidential experience. Where Sarkozy sought friendships and economic partnerships, the Valois' journeys were equally fruitful. Although Champdor scornfully states that: 'Charles VIII brought back a melon from his Italian campaign, and this was, in the final analysis, the only benefit to France from the expedition to Naples,' the European experiences of Louis XII and Henri III did more than just expand French culinary horizons.[87] The passage of Louis XII's armies and developments in military technology may have hastened transport developments, and were linked to improved infrastructure. Ideas about French power transformed as Italy fell to Valois armies, with Louis XII presented as a Roman emperor in his control of territory and method of transport. Where ambassadors had begun to replace kings as travellers, Henri III's visit to Venice showed how valuable personal contact remained. He also met in person with his Italian kinsmen, reinforcing alliances between certain Italian states and France.

This chapter demonstrates that during the sixteenth century, royal travel remained an important part of the exercise of domestic power. While there has not been room to explore how regional noble ambitions were disrupted when they were obliged to follow the king and court, it has shown the importance of the entourage. The opportunity to accompany a king on his travels was a similar mark of favour to an invite to remain with the king at Versailles a century later. Ultimately, the symbolic potential of travel, as a conqueror and guest, as world emperor or heavenly ruler, allowed the Valois monarchs to sustain a challenge to their main rivals: the image of travel was used to underline personal power, whether against Habsburg emperors, ambitious younger brothers, or factional leaders.

Notes

1 Bruno Dive, *Air Sarko. Chroniques des Voyages Présidentielle* (Paris: Jacob-Duverent, 2008), 16, 'François Mitterrand voyageait pour son bon plaisir . . . Moi pas. Je suis président depuis quatre mois. Je n'ai pas de temps à perdre. Il faut que je rencontre, très vite, le plus possible de dirigeants.'

2 Janet L. Nelson, "Carolingian Royal Ritual," in *Rituals of Royalty*, eds. David Cannadine and Simon Price (Cambridge: Cambridge University Press, 1987), 140.

3 Albert Babeau, "Les souverains étrangers en France du Xe au XVIIIe siècle," *Revue des questions historiques* (1903), 5; Colette Beaune, "Preface," in *Fastes de Cour. Les enjeux d'un voyage princier à Blois en 1501* eds. Monique Chatenet and Pierre-Gilles Girault (Rennes: Presses Universitaires de Rennes, 2010), 7.

4 Lucien Bély, *Espions et ambassadeurs au temps de Louis XIV* (Paris: Fayard, 1990), 351: voyageurs du prince.

5 Philip Long, "Introduction," in *Royal Tourism Excursions around Monarchy*, eds. Philip Long and Nicola J. Palmer (Clevedon: Channel View Publications, 2008), 1.

6 Cynthia Jane Brown, *The Shaping of History and Poetry in Late Medieval France: Propaganda and Artistic Expression in the Works of the Rhetoriqueurs* (Birmingham, AL: Summa, 1985), 37–42 explores Gringore's poetry for the return triumphs; Albert Champdor, *Les Rois de France à Lyon* (Lyon: Albert Guillot, 1986), 23–29, 32–34.

7 For recent scholarship on entries see Tania Levy, "La fête imprévue: entrées royales et solennelles à Lyon (1460–1530)," *Questes* 31 (2015): 33–44.

8 The main works produced are Jean d'Auton, *Chroniques de Louis XII*, Bibliothèque Nationale de France (BN) MS Fr 5081, 5082, 5083; Jean d'Auton, *Les alarmes de Mars sur le voyage de Millan, avecques la conqueste et entrée d'icelle , par le roi Louis XII, le 6 octobre 1499*, BN MS Fr 5089; Jean Marot, *Sur les deux heureux voyages de Gênes et Venise victorieusement mys à fin par le très chrestien roy Loys douziesme de ce nom, père du peuple , et véritablement escriptz par iceluy Jan Marot, alors poete & escriuain de la tresmagnanime Royne Anne, Duchesse de Bretaigne, & depuys, Valet de chambre du treschrestien Roy Francoys, premier du nom* (Paris : Pierre Roffet, 1533), reprinted as Jean Marot, *Sur les deux heureux voyages de Gênes et Venise victorieusement mys à fin* (Edn. 1532) (Paris: Hachette BNF, n.d.).

9 Jean d'Auton, *Chroniques de Louis XII*, ed. René de Maulde la Clavière (Paris: Renouard, 1889–1895), 4 vols, vol. 1 (1899), 3: 'actes florissans et oeuvres recomandables des victorieux Françoiz, par eux faictes en la conquest de la duché de Milan'.

10 Marot, *Sur les deux heureux voyages*, xxxiiii: 'Treschrestien verueulx Roy de France/Portant le Lys qui de Ciel print naissance. Sacre de Lhuille aux Saictz Cieux embasmee/ Fort Hercules dinvincible puissance.'

11 For stylistic analysis see Brown, *The Shaping of History*, 37, 40.

12 This edition is held in the British Library. The digitized copy in the Bibliothèque Nationale de France (BN) is incomplete for Louis XII, with no written commentary to the portrait.

13 Isabelle Haquet, *L'énigme Henri III. Ce que nous révèlent les images* (Paris: Presses Universitaires de Paris Ouest, 2011), 40.

14 Historiography includes Henri Lapeyre, "Les voyages de Charles Quint," *L'Histoire* 30 (1981): 58–65; Hugo O'Donnell and Duque de Estrada, "La travesia maritima de Carlos V para su coronacion imperial en 1520," *Revista de Historia Naval* 19, no. 72 (2001): 49–64; José I. Uriol, "Viajes de Carlos V por España," *Historia y Vida* 19, no. 219 (1986): 36–49; José Miguel Morales Folguera, "El viaje triunfal de Carlos V por Sicilia tras la victoria de Túnez," *Imago: revista de emblemática y cultura visual* 7 (2015): 97–111. Thanks are due to Rocío Martinez for her knowledge of this literature.

15 Recent literature includes Jacob Abbott, *Peter the Great* (New York: Seven Treasures, 2009); Gwenola Firmin, Francine-Dominique Liechtenhan and Thierry Sarmant, eds., *Peter the Great: A Tsar in France–1717* (Versailles: Lienart, 2017).

16 Joseph Cuvetier, "Un Voyage princier en Belgique au XVIIe siècle," *Extract of the Bulletin Officiel du Touring Club de Belgique* (Brussels: F van Buggenhoudt, 1923).

17 Robert Knecht, *Renaissance Warrior and Patron: The Reign of Francis I* (Cambridge: Cambridge University Press, 1994), xviii–xix.

18 Jean, Boutier, Alain Dewerpe and Daniel Nordman, *Un tour de France royal: Le voyage de Charles IX 1564–66* (Paris: Aubier, 1984); Linda Briggs, "'Concernant le service de leurs dictes Majestez et auctorite de leur justice': Perceptions of Royal Power in the Entries of Charles IX and Catherine de Medicis (1564–1566)," in *Ceremonial Entries in Early Modern Europe: The Iconography of Power*, eds. J.R. Mulryne, Maria Ines Aliverti and Anna Maria Testaverde (Farnham: Ashgate, 2015), 37–52.

19 Jean-Claude Cuignet, *L'Itinéraire d'Henri IV: Les 20597 jours de sa vie* (Bizanos: Héraclès, 1997).

20 Marc W.S. Jaffré, "The Early Bourbon Courts" (unpublished PhD thesis, St Andrews University, 2017), 163–165.

21 Anne Conchon, Bruno Maes, Isabelle Paresys, ed. Robert Muchembled, *Dictionnaire de l'Ancien Régime* (Paris: Armand-Colin, 2004), 52: 'une cour sédentarisée à Versailles devient l'espace essentielle des cérémonies quotidiennes.'

22 Christophe Levantal, *Louis XIV chronographie d'un règne: ou biographie chronologique du Roi-Soleil établie d'après la "Gazette" de Théophraste Renaudot – les 28121 journées du Roi entre le 5 septembre 1638 et le 1er septembre 1715* (2 vols. Gollion: Paris, 2009).

23 Voyages des Grands Valets de Pied, Archives Nationales de France (AN), O/1/904.

24 D'Auton, *Chroniques*, vol. 1, 320–321 mentions a number of objects transported to France from Italy under Louis XII's command. This includes *fromaiges de Milan*.

25 Recent literature includes Evelyn Korsch, "Renaissance Venice and the Sacred-Political Connotations of Waterborne Pageants," in *Waterborne Pageants and Festivities in the Renaissance. Essays in honour of J.R. Mulryne*, eds. Margaret Shewring and Linda Briggs (Farnham: Ashgate, 2013), 79–97; Evelyn Korsch, "Diplomatic Gifts on Henri III's visit to Venice in 1574," *Studies in the Decorative Arts* 15 (2007): 83–113; Marie Viallon, "Les honneurs de Venise à Henri de Valois, roi de France et de Pologne: Etude du séjour vénitien du roi Henri III en 1574." Congrès annuel de la RSA, April 2010, Venice. https://halshs.archives-ouvertes.fr/halshs-00550971/document (last accessed 23 March 2019), 1–13.

26 "Diego de Cuniga to Philip II," n.d., AN K/1532/b.35.

27 Pierre Champion, ed., *Lettres de Henri III, roi de France* (Paris: Klinksieck, 1959), vol. 1, 294: 'je vous ayme tant que le Roy mondict seigneur et frere ne pourroit permettre a personne venir avecques moy duquel la compaignie me fust plus agreable.'

28 Georges Bordenove, *Henri III* (Paris: Pygmalion, 1988), 138, lists his gentlemen.

29 D'Auton, *Chroniques*, vol. 1, 14, 95: 'si bien accompagné que le pouhoir de ma plume plye soubz la description de ce'.

30 Didier Le Fur, *Louis XII* (Paris: Perrin, 2010), 63; Knecht, *Renaissance Warrior*, 69–70; Pierre Brasme, *Quand Metz reçoit la France: souverains et chefs d'État français dans la cité messine* (Metz: Paraiges, 2011), 30–31.

31 For the entourage in 1499 see d'Auton, *Chroniques*, vol. 1, 100; for entourage in Milan, see Philippa Woodcock, "Living Like a King? The Entourage of Odet de Foix, Vicomte de Lautrec, Governor of Milan," *Royal Studies Journal* 2, no. 2 (2015): 10–11.

32 Estats de Millan AN J/910/1–6 partially preserves the duchy's financial records; for their transcripts see *Stati di guerra. I bilanci della Lombardia francese del primo Cinquecento* eds. Matteo di Tullio and Luca Fois (Rome: Ecole Francaise de Rome, 2014), 107–314.

33 D'Auton, *Chroniques*, 14: 'doubtant, par trop eslargie le compte, les oyans a ennui provoquer'.

34 Marot, *Sur les deux heureux voyages* (reprint), 13r-v: 'Le Roy voyant le grant crisme & forfaict/ Que genevoys envoys luy auroient faict . . . Passe les montz pour venger de defroy/ Plus promptement que jamais ne fist Roy . . . Pieces a Feu, Serpentines, Canons,/ Et aultres mainctz dont je ne scay les noms . . . Ainsi le Roy, avecques tout son bernaige/ Et des plus grans de son royal lignaige.'

35 "Journal de Pierre Lestoile," in *Nouvelle Collection des Mémoires pour servir à l'Histoire de France depuis le XIIIe siecle jusqu'à la fin du XVIIIe*, second series, vol 1, part 1 (Paris: Edouard Proux, 1837), 40: 's'estoit secrettement [et au desceu du senat et seigneurs polonnois] retire avec huict ou neuf chevaux seulement . . . pour revenir en France prendre possession du roiaume francois'.

36 Hector de la Ferrière-Percy, Gustave Baguenault de Puchesse, André Lesort eds., *Lettres de Catherine de Médicis*, 11 vols. (Paris: Imprimerie nationale, 1880–1943), vol. 5 (1895), xxxiii.

37 *Lettres de Henri III*, vol. 1, 358: 'Ordonnez le chemin de Lyon de la noblesse pour me venir trouver.'

38 Ulrich Langen, "The Meaning of Incognito," *The Court Historian* 7, no. 2 (2002): 145–155.

39 Cuvetier, "Un voyage," 3.

40 Langen, "The Meaning of Incognito," 155.

41 *Le Dictionnaire de l'Académie française 1694*, vol. 1 [1694], 'Incognito: . . . train ordinaire, ni les autres marques qui les distinguent', https://artfl-project.uchicago.edu/content/dictionnaires-dautrefois (accessed 1 July 2017).

42 Philippe-Jacques de Bengy de Puyvallée, *Mémoire historique sur le Berry : et particulièrement sur quelques châteaux du département de Cher* (Bourges: Vermeil, 1842), 14.

43 Viallon. "Les honneurs," 8–9, suggests that Henri III spent the night of 21/22 July away from his temporary palace, the Ca'Foscari, entertaining himself elsewhere. A similar night was spent on 22/23 July; for gentleman tourists to Venice, see the permissions granted to visit the Doge's palace in Archivio di Stato di Venezia (ASV), Consiglio di Dieci, Deliberazioni, Comuni, Filze 264, e.g. 7 February 1607.

44 Viallon, "Les honneurs," 9.

45 For speeds see Cuignet, *L'itineraire*, 16–17.

46 Knecht, *Renaissance Warrior*, 72. The original letter is in "François I to Louise of Savoy," August 1515, BNF Ms Fr 3012, f. 2.

47 For imperial imagery in Valois iconography see Nicole Hochner, *Louis XII: Les dérèglements de l'image royale* (Seyssel: Champ Vallon, 2006); Nicole Hochner "Le Trône vacant du roi Louis XII: Significations politiques de la mise en scène royale en Milanais," in *Louis XII en Milanais*, eds. Philippe Contamine and Jean Guillaume (Paris: Librairie Honoré Champion, 2003), 227–244; Robert W. Scheller, "Ensigns of Authority: French Royal Symbolism in the Age of Louis XII," *Simiolus* 13 (1983): 75–141; Robert W. Scheller, "Gallia cisalpine: Louis XII and Italy 1499–1508," *Simiolus* 15 (1985): 5–60; Michael Sherman, "Pomp and Circumstances: Pageantry, Politics and Propaganda in France during the Reign of Louis XII, 1498–1515," *Sixteenth Century Journal* 9 (1978): 13–32.

48 Titian, *The Emperor Charles V at Mühlberg*, oil on canvas, 1548. Museo del Prado, Madrid; Jerry Brotton, *The Renaissance Bazaar* (Oxford: Oxford University Press, 2002), 117.

49 BN Ms Fr 5082, f.104r; BN MS Fr 5083, f.44v; BN MS Fr 5089, frontispiece.

50 For example, François I's pre-1525 golden stirrups, Musée de la Renaissance, Ecouen E. Cl 21108 A and B.

51 Juan Antonio Ramirez, *The Beehive Metaphor: From Gaudi to Le Corbusier* (London: Reaktion, 2000), 18.

52 John M. Hunt, "The Ceremonial Possession of a City: Ambassadors and their Carriages in Early Modern Rome," *Royal Studies Journal* 3, no. 2 (2016): 69–89, at 70.

53 Hélène Delalex, *La galerie des Carrosses Château de Versailles* (Paris: Editions Artlys, 2016), 18–25 for the seventeenth century development and construction of royal coaches; Daniel Roche, "Introduction," in *Voitures, chevaux et attelages, du XVIe au XIXe siècle*, ed. Daniel Reytier (Paris: Art équestre de Versailles, 2000), 8.

54 Julian Munby, "Les Origines du Coche," in ed. Reytier, *Voitures*, 76.

55 Peter Edwards, "Une forme d'étalage ostentatoire: la mode des carrosses et l'aristocratie anglaise du XVIIe siècle," in ed. Reytier, *Voitures*, 41.

56 Korsch, "Diplomatic Gifts," 86–87; Viallon. "Les honneurs," 5.

57 *Lettres de Catherine de Médicis*, vol. 5, xxxiii: 'un bateau qui lui rappeller le Bucentaure'.

58 Jerôme de la Gorce, Béatrix Saule and Elisabeth Caudé, eds., *Fêtes et divertissements à la cour, exhibition catalogue, Château de Versailles, 29 November 2016–26 March 2017* (Paris: Galimard, 2016) 194–198.

59 Brotton, *The Renaissance Bazaar*, 2.

60 *Lettres de Catherine de Médicis*, vol. 5, xxxiii.

61 BN MS Fr 5083, f.124r.

62 For coach travel in Rome see John M. Hunt, "Carriages, Violence, and Masculinity in Early Modern Rome," in *I Tatti Studies in the Italian Renaissance* 17 (2014): 175–196.

63 For example, the illumination of 'Portrait allégorique de Louis de Chandio conduit par la Magnanimité et la Force', Illumination in *Le Fort Chandio*, BNF MS Fr 1194, ff.6v–7.

64 Daniel Roche, "Introduction," in *Voitures*, 9: 'l'avant train pivotant, sans doute inspiré par les trains de l'artillerie nouvelle expérimentée pendant les guerres d'Italie'. For such illuminations see: BN MS Fr 5089, frontispiece, and Giovanni Michele Nagonio, *De laudibus Galliae*, BN MS Latin 8132, inner frontispiece.

65 Jean Boutier, Alain Dewerpe and Daniel Nordman, *Un tour de France royal: Le voyage de Charles IX 1564–66* (Paris: Aubier, 1984), 47: 'la presence de chemins (ou seulement de passages) est liée à des préoccupations militaires, guerres d'Italie.'

66 Boutier, Dewerpe and Nordman, *Un tour*, 44–45; Daniel Nordman, "La connaissance géographique de l'état (XIVe-XVIIe siècles)," in *L'état moderne, le droit, l'espace: actes du colloque tenu à la Baume Les Aix, 11–12 octobre 1984*, ed. Noel Coulet (Paris: CNRS, 1990), 181: 'focaliser l'interêt (politique, commercial)'.

67 Champion, *Henri III*, 7–42 for his crossing of Germany.

68 Marot, *Sur les deux heureux voyages* (reprint), 5r; Knecht, *Renaissance Warrior*, 72.

69 D'Auton, *Chroniques*, 16: 'une chose prochaine de merveilles le charoy de tant et si grosses pieces d'artillerie, qui par-dessus la cruppe des montagnes si sainement fut conduyt.'

70 Ibid., 16: 'Le voyage fut si brief qu'en moings de quinze jours de Lyon en Ast fut armee, avecques tout son arroy'; Marot, *Sur les deux heureux voyages* (reprint), 13v: 'Passe les mons sans sejourner un jour.'

71 Le Fur, *Louis XII*, 235: 'roy de la mer et seigneur de la terre'.

72 BN MS Latin 8132, frontispiece. This is dated between 1499 and 1500. This is discussed in Le Fur, *Louis XII*, 229–231.

73 Pascale Thibault, ed., *Louis XII : Images d'un Roi de l'imperateur au père du peuple, exhibition catalogue, Château de Blois, 18 December 1987–14 February 1988* (Blois: Ville de Blois, Conservation du château et des musées, 1987), 63–64.

74 Viallon, "Les honneurs," 2; Champion, *Henri III*, 7–42; Champion, *Lettres de Henri III*, 307 and 294–310.

75 *Lettres de Henri III*, 292: 'avec promesse de gagner aussi rapidement que possible la Pologne'.

76 Ibid., 294: 'je suis fort pressé de m'acheminer et semble que je n'arriveray jamais assez tost par dela au gré de mes subgetcz'.

77 Bernardo Giunti, *Cronica breve di i fatti illustri de' re di Francia, con le loro effigie dal naturale* (Venice: Bernardo Giunti: 1588), 62.

78 *Lettres de Henri III*, 358: 'ayant veu l'Allemagne, je iray en Italie, et iray a Venise'.

79 Lestoile, "Journal," 41: 'il arriva l'onziesme d'aoust, et y fust à grande joie et magnificence reçue par le duc et par la duchesse de Savoie, sa tante.'

80 See note 26.

81 Commines, *Mémoires*, cited in Babeau, "Les souverains étrangers," 8: 'Les grands princes ne se doivent jamais voir, s'ils veulent demeurer amis.'

82 Viallon, "Les honneurs," 1: 'une double démarche de séduction de la puissance invitante comme de l'invité.'

83 Ibid.

84 Ibid., 4, 6–7.

85 For the later French Wars of Religion see Stuart Carroll, *Martryrs and Murderers: The Guise Family and the Making of Europe* (Oxford: Oxford University Press, 2009), 221–280; R.J. Knecht, *The Rise and Fall of Renaissance France* (London: Fontana, 1996), 512–541; R.J. Knecht, *The French Wars of Religion, 1559–1598* (Abingdon: Routledge, 2014), 62–73.

86 Haquet, *L'énigme Henri III*, 42–43.

87 Albert Champdor, *Les Rois*, 29: 'Charles VIII rapporta un melon de sa campagne d'Italie. Ce fut un trophée comme un autre, et ce fut, même, en fin de compte, le seul bénéfice que valut à la France l'expédition de Naples.'

Key works

Knecht, R.J., *The Rise and Fall of Renaissance France* (London: Fontana, 1996).

Le Fur, Didier, *Louis XII* (Paris: Perrin, 2010).

Mulryne, J.R., Maria Ines Aliverti and Anna Maria Testaverde, eds., *Ceremonial Entries in Early Modern Europe: The Iconography of Power* (Farnham: Ashgate, 2015).

Reytier, Daniel, ed., *Voitures, chevaux et attelages, du XVIe au XIXe siècle* (Paris: Art équestre de Versailles, 2000).

Sherman, Michael, "Pomp and Circumstances: Pageantry, Politics and Propaganda in France during the Reign of Louis XII, 1498–1515," *Sixteenth Century Journal* 9 (1978): 13–32.

Shewring, Margaret and Linda Briggs, eds., *Waterborne Pageants and Festivities in the Renaissance. Essays in honour of J.R. Mulryne* (Farnham: Ashgate, 2013).

15

KINGSHIP AND MASCULINITY IN RENAISSANCE PORTUGAL (FIFTEENTH AND SIXTEENTH CENTURIES)

Hélder Carvalhal[1]

This chapter seeks to examine the relationship between gender – more specifically, masculinity – and the upholding of both the power of the king and the monarchy in Renaissance Portugal, more specifically during the last generations of the House of Avis. It will be argued that, along with other variables, gender seems to have been relevant to maintaining political stability and dynastic power through a set of practices that may or may not have been in accordance with established models of expressing masculinity.

The study of masculinities has been a growing field for historians since the late 1990s, influenced greatly by the theoretical framework developed by R. Connell, particularly the hegemonic masculinity concept. To put this in simple terms, hegemonic masculinity defines the dominance of a group of men towards women and other groups of men, the latter appearing here, at least temporarily, as subordinated. The concept itself has generated several critiques in the past decades as well as developments in several areas. Differences among gender models are now debated as one of the results of hierarchical societies and their political order.[2] Similarly, both historians of royal courts and political historians have reflected on the way in which perceptions and expressions of masculinity could affect a ruler's performance and, by extension, the dynastic and political balance.[3] Scholars such as Marc Baer and Mats Hallenberg, have stressed the importance of masculinity and 'manly' behaviour to statecraft as part of royal performance, in regions such as northern Europe and the Near East.[4]

Despite these examples of historical studies on masculinity in terms of the monarchy, historians have not particularly discussed how Connell's theory affects the specific case of the premodern royal court. Part of this gap is perhaps due to the context in which masculinity studies was conceived: a modern world where political, religious, cultural and sexual paradigms, in theory, differ substantially from their medieval and early modern counterparts. Thus, application of the hegemonic masculinity model in an institution such as the royal court offers rich potential for additional research in this area, especially taking into account the diversity of the Renaissance court, where one can find distinct social hierarchies. Other issues regard the inherent transformation of the concept of masculinity during the period analysed here. It is not guaranteed that royal men conform themselves to the hegemonic model; neither is it certain that other groups would not attempt to enact this model. Moreover, such a model might not pervade in the long duration, given the need for adjustment according to political, social and cultural contexts. Despite the issues prevalent with this model, male monarchs and other members of the royal family analysed in this chapter will be considered an integral part of the hegemonic masculinity model, along with other members of the high nobility and also the upper strata of the clergy. Therefore, other groups of men and women visible in the daily workings of the court – such as low-ranking servants or slaves –will be considered as belonging to subordinate strata. Masculine models designed to influence the behaviour of royal men, balanced out with their respective practices, would come to influence not only subaltern groups of men and women but also other dominant men, regardless of their political position.

The following analysis will encompass two different subjects and will cover a period between the mid-fifteenth and the late-sixteenth centuries, more specifically the reigns of João II (r.1481–95), Manuel I (r.1495–1521) and João III (r.1521–57), with reference also to the reigns of Afonso V (r.1448–81) and Sebastião (r.1568–78).[5] One area of examination will be events held by the court, where gender order is present to disseminate a political message. Thus, a number of royal festivities will be examined in the analysis, including jousts, tournaments and weddings. In parallel, the evolution of didactic literature, or 'mirrors for princes', will be studied in order to identify changes in the expression of manhood, especially given the transformation observed in royal courts during the late medieval and early modern periods. In comparing the two areas, it will be verified if theory meets practice or if there are differences between what the models propose and that which royal persons – and, by extension, the court – perpetrated through their actions. These models and respective practices will be compared with those of the first generation of Avis princes to evaluate continuity and change within the period, while bearing in mind the political context of the time.

Moreover, in addition to demonstrating the verification of continuities within the Avis dynasty, this debate will also show the similarities with other European political units and, should it be the case, pinpoint any evidence of exceptions. Works written about the subject, such as the seminal study of Werner Paravicini about the Burgundian model, have already provided glimpses of northern European influence on Iberian court performances.[6] Such influences have produced echoes in the way masculinity is staged. The opposite, however, has not been fully acknowledged, which is interesting if one regards, for instance, the primacy in overseas expansion and the possible repercussions on masculinity models. Hence, southern influences on other European regions regarding the relationship between power, authority and masculinity will also be explored.

Context

At the beginning of the fifteenth century, the new Avis dynasty on the throne of Portugal felt that it needed to legitimize itself in the eyes of other European realms. After the rule of King João I (r.1385–1433), who was himself an illegitimate child, and the political action of his descendants – King Duarte (r.1433–8) and the *infantes* (princes) Pedro (1392–1449), Henrique (1394–1460) and Fernando (1402–43) – royal chroniclers idealized an image of dynastic identity where the expression of manhood in several forms was a key component. The monarch was described as a good ruler, good father and good warrior.[7] While there were additional features attributed to certain royal family members, such as chastity, and even sainthood in the case of *Infante* Fernando (1402–43),[8] many of them shared the same characteristics as the ruler himself. In short, apart from being a model of sainthood, male royal persons displayed a strong component of masculinity, which was based on two ideas. First, that the figure of the *pater familias* was responsible not only for family honour and reputation but also for the running of the household and the court – themes also examined in Estelle Paranque's chapter in this collection, which focuses on how early modern European monarchs used the father and warrior figures to assert their royal authority over their subjects. Fatherhood was also favoured at that time due to the availability and influence of works by authors such as Aristotle and Thomas Aquinas.[9] Second, there was the potent ideal of a chivalric *ethos*, which these men, as a social group, embodied by following a number of symbolic codes and correlative practices, with their paradoxes and contradictions.[10]

During the late fifteenth and the sixteenth centuries, the monarchs of the Avis dynasty generally tried to impose dynastic continuity. Yet this was sometimes challenged by the political context of the time, such as the unusual circumstance by which Manuel I (r.1495–1521) came to the throne. At the time of his birth, there were six men standing between him and the throne. Ironically, events of his predecessor's reign, such as the nobles' conspiracy against King João II (1483–4) and its outcomes, contributed indirectly to the later promotion of Manuel I as the heir to the throne, as João II lacked legitimate progeny after the death of *Infante* Afonso (1475–91).[11] This uncommon succession process left its mark on the higher echelons of nobility, forcing the new monarch to act in order to prevent political instability. Thus, considering the prominent reliance upon masculine dynastic identity by earlier Avis rulers, it should be addressed how expressions of manhood helped to shape the sixteenth-century monarchs' rule as an answer to political challenges.

The pervading influence of late medieval chivalric values in Iberia is something readily acknowledged. In terms of the situation in Portugal, for instance, it is known that Arthurian novels served as an inspiration for evening gatherings in noble and aristocratic palaces during the early modern period.[12] Other variables can explain this persistence, such as the relationship between Christian and Moorish populations. Research stresses that this scenario was marked by an attraction/repulsion dichotomy in late medieval and early modern Iberia. Moreover, forced conversions both in Spain and Portugal during the second half of the fifteenth century neither stopped cultural interaction nor prevented Moorish culture from being one of the factors on which a common identity was built.[13] Analysing this issue through a gender lens, one must stress the attempts of domination of the Moorish by Christian chroniclers. By juxtaposing the valour, courage, prowess and strength of the Christian warrior with the alleged delicate manners of their enemies of faith, they were establishing the border between the hegemonic model and a type of subservient masculinity.[14]

Despite this theoretical model, the practice differed substantially as Moorish people (until their forced conversion in 1497) were present in everyday court and city life. Court festivities in the late fifteenth century would have included Moorish and Jewish people parading and singing within the royal procession. To a certain extent, this involvement also helped to establish a dominant stance, separate from the evident hierarchies in court society.[15] Furthermore, it is reasonable to enquire to what extent this cultural basis influenced the continuing crusader spirit among sixteenth-century members of the House of Avis and, more importantly, how it became visible in their expression of manhood. It is certain that aspects such as the overseas expansion in North Africa and Southern Asia, or the occasional recreation of these environments in court, provided an appropriate context for these practices.

Regarding this late medieval to early modern transition period, one has to mention the progressive change of the expression of knightly masculinity, which was usually connected with the king and any male siblings.[16] Despite the continuous presence of sporadic episodes of violence in daily life at court (visible along with the occurrence of violence episodes in court games), the late fifteenth and early sixteenth centuries saw shifting models of the courtier that moved away from the medieval martial archetype, which had an effect on expressions of manhood.[17] Obviously, the transformation of the models of masculinity was not immediately all-embracing, and these shifting models definitely did not exclude former martial traditions of expressing manhood. Instead, they served the purpose of balancing gender practices and ways to represent dominance over other groups. As such, the warrior-like type of courtier – where legitimating practices were based on both physical imposition and aggressive speech – changed, in a slow and irregular way, to result in a courtier model more markedly defined by etiquette.

Such a process was more clearly demarcated further into the early modern period, as one can still verify evidence of the aforementioned warrior-like type courtier in the late fifteenth century. Good examples can be found, for instance, in the court poetry *corpus* gathered by Garcia de Resende (1470–1536), called the *Cancioneiro Geral* (1516). Within these pages, and among poetry written for other purposes, one can find many cases of misogyny and aggressive behaviour. For example, the case of the courtier, Rui Moniz, who decided to forcefully verbalize his opposition towards the attention a court damsel gave to another man, or even the advice given by a nobleman to his nephew, a recent courtier; advice that included, among other disrespectful actions, never to turn down a brawl.[18] Hence, the question remains: was the slight shift in the royal and princely models enough to affect significant change in the expression of manhood?

Portuguese Renaissance royal and princely models

Royal and princely models in the late fifteenth century and throughout the first half of the sixteenth century were generally influenced by two confluent variables. On the one hand, they continued to focus on the way the monarch should rule. Thus, treatises like *De Republica Gubernada per Regem* [*De Republica*] (1496), dedicated by Diogo Lopes Rebelo to King Manuel I, or the *Breve Doutrina e Ensinança de Príncipes* [*Breve Doutrina*] (1525), presented to King João III by Frei António de Beja, put emphasis on *topoi* like being a good ruler, having the ethos of a wise king, being a pious and merciful monarch, and being a good warrior, especially against enemies of faith.[19] It is also possible to trace continuity through older models at the court of the first Avis. Lopes Rebelo, when disserting in *De Republica* about the role of the monarch as a father to all his subjects, recalls the translation of Marcus Tullius Cicero's

De Officiis by *Infante* Pedro, son of João I and regent of the kingdom until his demise at the battle of Alfarrobeira (1449).[20] Likewise, works dedicated to other members of the royal family suggested similar ideas. *Doutrina*, dedicated by Lourenço de Cáceres to *Infante* Luís (1506–1555), the second son of King Manuel I and Queen Maria of Castile and Aragon, and one of the most influential court personalities of the time, is a perfect example. The *infante*'s teacher, Cáceres, encouraged his student to be a wise prince, while also praising military action against the enemies of Christianity.[21] All of these mirrors of princes highlighted how important it was to be a good patron (in the treatises, represented by the term *liberalidade*). Together with the concepts of love and political friendship, this doctrine emphasized the generosity of the monarch not only to his family members but also to other courtiers and, to a certain extent, all his subjects. These threads of discourse, so prominent in the advice to the early members of the dynasty, are also visible in the mirrors of the sixteenth century.[22]

The second variable, connected with the former, concerns the type of behaviour and/or attitudes which the ruler should avoid. Regarding this issue, the consensus among several works is to avoid greed and vices such as gambling and excessive recreational hunting.[23] Another interesting detail, which is especially noteworthy in mirrors from the sixteenth century dedicated to either young kings or royal heirs, is the condemnation of the deceitful character of late medieval chivalry novels. Frei António de Beja, in *Breve Doutrina*, suggested that João III should avoid paying too much attention to novels' characters, like Amadis (of Gaul) and Esplandião, both favourites for noble evening gatherings in halls and castles. In the same vein, while introducing *Libro Primero del Espejo del Príncipe* (1544) to the son of João III and heir, Prince João Manuel (1537–54), Francisco de Monçón (d.1575) pointed out the lack of realism in *Amadis* and expressed his opposition to such influences being given to a future ruler.[24] Lastly, there are also warnings against the hazard of over-relying on certain courtiers. In his *Tractado Moral de Louvores e Perigos Dalguns Estados Seculares* (1549), dedicated to Prince João Manuel, son and heir of King João III, Sancho de Noronha advised against the inherent danger of an adviser who wished to please his king more than his people.[25]

These tendencies present considerable similarities to the most important European coeval models. Despite Machiavelli's *The Prince* (1532) clearly preferring a strong, military sovereign to a more pious, friendly one, mentions of avoiding corrupt courtiers and secretaries are also present as a benefit to the people. Also identifiable is the neglect of, and even contempt for, the tradition provided by chivalric novels in works such as the *Relox de Príncipes* (1529), dedicated to the Holy Roman Emperor Charles V (1500–58) by the influential Fr. Antonio de Guevara (1480–1545). In fact, this tendency pervaded throughout the long sixteenth century in the Iberian peninsula, from the works of humanist Juan Luis Vives (1493–1540) to the renowned *Quijote* by Miguel de Cervantes (1547–1616).[26]

All homologous European mirrors of princes of the period stressed the virtues that a monarch should have. Among them, one still finds continuity with regard to late medieval works, namely the good patron, good father and wise king *topoi*.[27] The courtier renaissance model had its impact on models of masculinity. For instance, both Castiglione's model – *The Book of the Courtier*, published in Iberia in 1534 – and a good portion of Erasmus' work, such as *Institutio Principis Christiani* (1516), enforce the need to moderate one's masculinity.[28] In summary, one can point to differences between the mirrors of princes dedicated to Portuguese royal family members and the majority of their European counterparts, although these are of little (if any) significance for Portugal. Therefore, one can easily identify similarities within some general features expected of the monarch. Most of them, in fact, attempt to format the expression of manhood of the monarch and other court members into less violent and more gentle performances, although this does not necessarily mean that the recommendations given were followed, as an analysis of the practice of manhood will show.

Practices of masculinity and manhood in Renaissance Portugal

Just as their early fifteenth-century counterparts, the monarchs Afonso V, João II and Manuel I and their respective descendants also developed a particular taste for hunting, bullfights, jousts and tournaments. Before any analysis of the ceremonial performances of these monarchs, one has to stress an important detail. Out of all of them, only Afonso V, João II and Sebastião actually engaged in battle, all against the Moorish in North Africa and, in the case of the first two, against Castile and Leon (1475–9). Equally, not all of them participated in performative events in the same way, and their respective roles must be differentiated. Regarding jousts, it should be noted that João II and Sebastião had a very active role, while Manuel I and João III preferred an observant role from a privileged vantage point and, thus, to emphasize their role as patrons rather than participants. According to royal chronicles, João II had a preference for tournaments, bullfights and jousts. During the marriage celebrations of Crown Prince Afonso (d.1491) with Princess Isabel of Castile and Aragon (1490), King João II could be found either participating actively in the jousts or chairing the event from a privileged position.[29] In contrast, Manuel I, for instance, would lend vestments to his courtiers when it was time to joust, thus displaying the same type of behaviour that one identifies in Henry VII of England, who often preferred not to joust himself.[30] Apart from his prominence as a patron, Manuel I also geared his rule towards overseas expansion, keeping in mind the crusader ethos. In this way, he could meet the expectations of a portion of the Portuguese nobility who were eager to acquire additional income and honour from fighting enemies of faith.[31]

João III, however, found a different political context. He faced other challenges in terms of politics inside and outside the kingdom, with consequences that affected his expression of masculinity. Out of all of the case studies mentioned, this monarch seems to have been the only one who chose not to be depicted in military attire. His overseas priorities lay in the South Atlantic and Asia, which meant that he relegated commonly held interests in North Africa and the Mediterranean to the background, despite these geographic areas being perceived as the standard destination for the crusaders. These choices in terms of representation and overseas foci meant that the king faced a substantial degree of opposition, not only in terms of his decision-making but also in terms of political representation.

Ironically, another of King Manuel I's descendants, *Infante* Luís (1506–55), was the main ideological heir of the dynastic crusader ideology. Along with João III's other brother – *Infante* Duarte (1515–40) – and a considerable part of the nobility, Luís was an avid promoter of jousts, games of canes (an Iberian game where two teams – Christian versus Moorish – of six horse riders each throw canes at each other) and tournaments. King João III authorised these events as the majority of them took place within court festivities and celebrations, where he was part of the audience so as to represent the monarch's role as a patron.

One important episode regarding these political differences took place during a joust organized by *Infante* Luís when a set of gifts, of sumptuous horse attire, given by Emperor Charles V (1500–58) arrived in Portugal. The gifts themselves had strong symbolic connotations relating to the recent participation of the *Infante* in the conquest of Tunis (1535). Seizing upon the arrival of such meaningful gifts, Luís quickly organized a festivity, not only to display the attire but also to reinforce the crusader ethos by staging a confrontation between Christian knights and Moorish warriors.[32]

The embodiment of masculinity in the chivalric figure of a Christian knight is a recurring feature, both in terms of the influence of Arthurian novels during the period and later, and when looking at other evidence, such as material culture.[33] Descendants of King Manuel I, especially the *Infantes* Luís, Fernando (1507–34) and Duarte were very active in this area. Also, it is known that embodying the role of the knight errant was something inherent to the performances mentioned. A good example is found in the royal jousts that took place in Rossio Square (Lisbon) on the Sunday after Christmas in 1522. *Infante* Luís appeared, disguised and unrecognizable before the marshals of the joust, wearing a shield that depicted a woman with a fan covering half of her face (one of the chivalric *leitmotivs*), along with the rest of his uncommon attire. Not recognizing Luís, referees asked him to introduce himself, something he promptly refused to do, saying only that he was a noble who wanted to joust. And so he did, breaking two of his opponents' spears. Later, he revealed his identity and felt the general amusement of the audience, which included the monarch, other members of the royal court and foreign ambassadors.[34] However, none of this pattern of behaviour is found exclusively in Portugal. For instance, several monarchs observed similar patterns in medieval and early modern England, especially in relation to nobles hiding their identities during performances. Henry VIII of England, a contemporary of Luís, used masks during tournaments as a tool with which to enact a particular type of knightly masculinity, which had political outcomes.[35]

Lastly, there is the interesting case of King Sebastião. Just as other Avis royal men, the young king had an extremely pious profile combined with a strong crusader ethos. To a certain extent, his behaviour reflected the image and representation of his two great influences, the *Infante* Luís and Emperor Charles V.[36] Nevertheless, some of his features did not match the characteristics of either. One of these characteristics, clearly the most problematic for a king, was the inability to surround himself with women. Note that all of the monarchs in this study had descendants from one or several wives (as in the case of Manuel I, who married three times and had more than a dozen children), sometimes even children outside of marriage (examples can be found in Duarte [1523–43], son of João III and Ana Moniz, a court damsel, or Jorge [1481–1550], governor of the military orders of Avis and Santiago, son of João II and Ana de Mendonça, also a court damsel). Since Sebastião's early days at court, both high strata courtiers (who were close to him) and foreign ambassadors noticed how this inability could be an issue to the survival of his direct dynastic line and, therefore, the dynasty more broadly, as few descendants of Manuel I were still alive by the 1560s and 1570s and the king showed no interest in marriage proposals.[37] Apart from the consequences to the dynasty, a gender implication could also be observed. According to the chivalric tradition, men used women and their attention to excel in their respective position, thus diminishing the status and hierarchy of possible competitors.[38] Sebastião, an enthusiast of spectacles such as bullfights and horse riding, asked Pope Pius V (1566–72) to suspend the excommunication penalty for participants in this activity as he was not particularly interested in competing for the attention of ladies. Chronicles tell of the king's introversion when his horse walked past the female section of the audience; he did not even look at them, neither did he perform any type of salute.[39] This, along with other attitudes such as his aversion to certain lavish clothes or the tendency to take refuge in convents and/or peripheral royal residences, makes it reasonable to argue that he lacked the ability to impose his knightly masculinity during public events.

Given the specific characteristics of this king, one must evaluate other coeval examples in order to launch possible points of comparison. A case study worthy of note is the French monarch Henri III (r.1575–89). Like Sebastião, doubts about Henri's sexual orientation and/or alleged inaptitude to entertain himself with women had a negative impact on his reputation as a king. Just like the Portuguese monarch, Henri III had considerably more interest in religion than in government, and also paid an overwhelming amount of attention to his close male courtiers, *les mignons*.[40] While Sebastião did not suffer considerable internal opposition, political opponents of Henri III seized on his flaws and used them to disrupt his rule.

The relevance of manliness in the level described becomes larger still when one compares Henri III to his father, Henri II (r.1547–59). Works written about the latter described him as a kind father, a loyal friend and a good ruler, despite his heavy reliance on advisers. One must emphasize his penchant for riding and jousting, which ultimately took his life.[41] Nonetheless, this tragic episode could be argued to epitomize the way Henri II enacted his masculinity in a manner very appropriate to his office; so much so that even his widow, Catherine of Médici (1519–89), urged her son Henri III to act in a more 'manly fashion', imitating, for instance, his father's taste for courtly sports.[42] Despite the French king's lack of interest for jousting, Paranque's chapter offers another approach to Henri III's masculinity and argues that he used the warrior figure in his speeches to project a strong royal authority into the public sphere. As such, this argument demonstrates that there were other forms of enacting masculinity, apart from the performances involving physical attainment, to obtain political advantages, but challenges were more likely to be lodged against those who did not conform to expected manly roles.

The ability of the monarch to express a certain type of masculinity was important for his ruling, as it contributed to political stability across social groups, with particular gains in the dominant group of the nobility. Less clear, perhaps, is the representation of the dominant role of the hegemonic knightly masculinity model over a subordinated group of men and women in everyday court life.

Hegemonic vs. subaltern masculinities

This is perhaps the dimension of gender studies in the Renaissance and early modern court which remains more obscure even today: how individuals embodying the hegemonic model performed towards other groups, including individuals who enacted subaltern non-dominant forms of masculinity, and women. A good example to debate this point is related to the Moorish presence in the Iberian territory, mentioned earlier. From a general perspective, there are countless episodes where the late medieval tradition of chronicles was used to diminish the masculinity of Moorish men, which served as a vehicle for the domination of the Christian warrior. Portuguese court festivities were replete with these episodes. Parades and court games, such as tournaments (for instance, the improvised scene organized by *Infante* Luís shortly after the conquest of Tunis) and the game of canes were not the only times that symbolic domination could be noted. The monarchy itself promoted such displays by providing either Christian or Moorish vestments to knights to replicate the idea of confronting the infidel on the battlefield (as seen in King Manuel I's case, see earlier). Similarities can be found with festivities in the Holy Roman Empire. Following the great example of his grandfather, Maximilian I (1459–1519), as a promoter of tournaments within the imperial court, Ferdinand I (1503–64) was renowned for including a clear political message in his 'Hungarian tournaments', in which elite imperial troops – Hungarian hussars – faced a team made up of Moorish and Turkish soldiers.[43]

Additional features of Moorish material culture were used to set gender differences, even among members of the same upper echelons of society. In the early sixteenth century, for example, there were notable differences between seating to identify certain individuals as dominant: women and children were seated on cushions, whereas the monarch and other male elites would be seated on chairs to place them in a physically higher position and promote dominance. As such, dominance could be promoted by associating such gendered objects with individuals who were considered of subaltern.[44] While the connotation of the Moorish warrior with effeminate manners had implications on their expression of manhood, other subtle examples existed during the late medieval and Renaissance periods. One case to explore involves the political representation of 'savages', who were considered to hold the same subaltern position as the Moorish in Iberia (or the Ottoman in central Europe during the early modern period), elsewhere in Europe. These glimpses have remote origins in land expansion and in the image of the monarch as conqueror. The representation of savages was not an early modern innovation, as early representations can be seen, for instance, in the late medieval Danish coat of arms of Christian I (r.1450–81). Many interpretations have arisen of the significance of such iconography, although it is reasonable to assume that royal power and domination over other subjects – in this case, savages from other Baltic areas – were at stake.[45]

An alternative and noteworthy representation of 'savages', in this case from the South Atlantic, was also present in early Portuguese court festivities.[46] A good case study can be found in the matrimonial festivities held for Emperor Frederick III and Princess Leonor (1434–67), sister of King Afonso V of Portugal. A foreign observer, the ambassador Niklas Lankmann von Falkenstein, described an early scene where a group of 'savages', who introduced themselves as being from the Canary Islands, under dispute by the Portuguese crown at that time, were sent by their local tribe leaders to pay homage to Afonso V, thus showing subordination to the alleged new conqueror.[47] Additional research into Portuguese court festivities during the mid-sixteenth century shows a similar pattern. The tournament of Xabregas (1550) staged a similar scene, where a group of four 'savages' with long hair and vestments made of bear fur was taken before Prince João Manuel and Queen Catherine of Austria (d.1578), delivering a manuscript with the rules agreed by each of the competitors.[48] Such an act contained an important symbolic dimension. It was Prince João Manuel's first tournament – he was thirteen years old at the time. Being in possession of the aforementioned manuscript elevated him in terms of authority and made him the patron of the festivities. These symbolic actions, together with being the sponsor of one of the participating teams, mediated his frail physical condition, which was probably one of the reasons why he did not join the team as captain. Thus, in terms of masculinity, João Manuel took a step towards coming of age and, ultimately, emancipation.

Once again, points of comparison can be made with other monarchies. Court events in early modern Scotland used 'savages', sometimes together with Moors and Highland men, emphasizing their 'wild' origins to serve political purposes. James IV (r.1488–1513), a tournament adept, included wild men and Moors within festivities, sometimes with great prominence.[49] In the same vein, Mary, Queen of Scots (r.1542–67) also adopted this ceremonial usage of the 'savage', with a particularly potent episode at the baptism celebrations (1566) of her son, the future James VI (r.1567–1625), with the participation of wild men in a mocking tournament influenced by the Valois model.[50] The French case also provides a useful comparison. Henri II, for instance, was known for using 'savages' during his royal entries. In the case of the entry into Rouen in 1550, in which the young Mary, Queen of Scots, participated as the dauphine, the French monarch had an evidently political purpose: to stage a South American conflict between the Portuguese, the French and their respective indigenous allies. Also noteworthy was the attempt to represent Henri II as both a civilized and chivalric king, which was further extended to the 'humanistic' savages he allied himself with. By adding a modified representation of the Greek mythological character Hercules – at this time not only displaying brute force but also eloquence – the scene legitimized Henri II as the bringer of a new era.[51] Apart from the overseas dispute, there is a side of domination that involves gender that should not be overlooked. The differences in this case, when compared to the Portuguese example, lie in the type of masculinity displayed by the French king. This was a paradoxical combination of a monarch embodying new court practices with a former model recovered by Henri II, who relied on knightly masculinity by being enthusiastic in court games where a display of physical prowess was key to the expression of manhood.

Conclusions

Gender – in this case, masculinity and the expression of manhood – contributed to the political stability of a dynasty that had reasonably visible flaws. It was not just a matter of keeping the monarchy's power and authority. The sixteenth-century Avisians recovered and reused masculinity models that belonged to their fifteenth-century counterparts, regardless of the rise of new courtier models that were more polite, more refined in their manners and, from a contemporary perspective, even more effeminate. Apart from models of fatherhood and sainthood, the crusader dynamics fuelled by a chivalric ethos were taken on by all Avis monarchs, apart from João III.

All of them cultivated, to a greater or lesser extent, a taste for court games, where physical display was an important part of a political spectacle. The knightly masculinity model pervaded throughout the period studied here, which may as well be the main mark of gender identity that affected the course of this dynasty until its extinction at the end of the sixteenth century (1595).[52] The best example to understand this dynamic can be found in the fatal tragedy of King Sebastião, whose demise in 1578 resulted from an open battle in northern Morocco, an act inspired by the first Avis kings, which illustrates that the survival and potency of the crusader ethos was still alive.

Regarding the model and practices of masculinity enacted by these men, the context in which each sovereign was created has to be stressed as one of the most relevant factors to their later performance. Still, some of the recommendations were carefully followed and their gender expression allowed the king and his kin to keep and/or increase political power. Perhaps the most followed advice focused on the role of the king as a patron and the role of the king in the war against the enemies of faith. Note also that, in the absence of these, internal conflict could emerge. Generally speaking, Portuguese monarchs of the period ruled in order to avoid political intrigue and upheaval. However, it is fair to mention that some research is still to be done on several aspects that could have a possible influence on the expression of manhood. One of them is to evaluate implications of the Roman Catholic Counter Reformation on these models of masculinity.

It is also useful to project these conclusions within the European framework, where the knightly masculinity model can generally be seen to continue into the sixteenth century and beyond. Political and religious circumstances surely stimulated this. Whether the monarch had a more active role in the expression of manhood, going off to war and/or taking part in court games – for example Charles V, Henry VIII, François I, Henri II, Gustav Vasa (r.1523–60) – or distinguished himself more on the representative side, associations with war, violence and military prowess were effectively present. One can also argue that this was a fading model, at a time when the most notable European warrior-kings had given way, slowly and gradually, to a different type of monarch. The Renaissance courtier model had an impact and moderated the way in which manhood was displayed by the king and his subjects. An example can be found in Philip II of Spain (r.1556–98), who despite his early participation in tournaments (especially between 1540 and 1560) and his will to fight every enemy of Spain, was mostly recognized as a bureaucratic king. If this is true, there are coeval examples to show how representations of the martial 'medieval' warrior archetype were still relevant, especially concerning the high levels of animosity experienced at the time, with conflicts among several European powers.[53]

Lastly, there are considerations to be made regarding the possibility of masculinity models converging between southern and northern Europe. While there is no substantial comparative work allowing for a full assessment, one can definitely see evidence of considerable cultural exchange of models and ways of displaying manhood among all European courts. Although this is straight forward among the dominant group – the monarch, his kin and the high nobility – doubts still remain about whether this took place regarding domination over subjects. The examples previously debated imply that this type of cultural exchange existed, especially in the use of symbolic 'savages'. The Moorish case is, however, unique given the Iberian late Christian *Reconquista* and its aftermath in the form of the advent of overseas expansion during the fifteenth and sixteenth centuries. This point requires further research in order to evaluate possible models and discussions of manly domination for legitimizing a new reality.

Notes

1 CIDEHUS, University of Évora (UID/HIS/00057/2019). The author would like to thank Estelle Paranque, Isabel dos Guimarães Sá and Lucinda Dean for valuable comments to an early version of this chapter and also to Ana Maria Rodrigues, Jonathan Spangler and Marta Manuel dos Santos for additional bibliographic suggestions.

2 R.W. Connell, *Masculinities*, second ed. (Berkeley: University of California Press, 2005), 76–81; Raewyn Connell and James W. Messerschmidt, "Hegemonic Masculinity: Rethinking the Concept," *Gender & Society* 19, no. 6 (2005): 829–859; see also John Tosh, "Hegemonic Masculinity and the History of Gender," in *Masculinities in Politics and War. Gendering Modern History*, eds. Stefan Dudink, Karen Hagemann and John Tosh (Manchester: Manchester University Press, 2004), 41–58.

3 For examples, see Katherine J. Lewis, *Kingship and Masculinity in Late Medieval England* (New York: Routledge, 2013); Christopher Fletcher, "Manhood, Kingship and the Public in Late Medieval England," *Edad Media. Revista de Historia*, 13 (2012): 123–142.

4 Marc Baer, "Manliness, Male Virtue and History Writing at the Seventeenth-Century Ottoman Court," *Gender & History* 20, no. 1 (2008): 128–148; Mats Hallenberg, "The Golden Age of the Agressive Male? Violence, Masculinity and the State in Sixteenth-Century Sweden," *Gender & History* 25, no. 1 (2013): 132–149.

5 The gap between 1557 and 1568 it is due to a period of regency of Queen Catherine of Austria (d.1578) and Cardinal Henrique (1512–80), in the minority of King Sebastião, who was only three years old when enthroned.

6 Werner Paravicini, "The Court of the Dukes of Burgundy: A Model for Europe?" in *Princes, Patronage, and the Nobility: The Court at the Beginning of the Modern Age, c.1450–1650*, eds. Ronald G. Asch and Adolf M. Birke (London and New York: German Historical Institute and Oxford University Press, 1991), 69–102; on the circulation of courtier models, see also Sydney Anglo, "The Courtier: the Renaissance and Changing Ideals," in *The Courts of Europe: Politics, Patronage and Royalty, 1400–1800*, ed. A G. Dickens (London: Thames & Hudson, 1997), 33–53.

7 Duarte I, *Leal Conselheiro*, ed. João Morais Barbosa (Lisbon: IN-CM, 1982), 416, 427–428; Ana Maria Rodrigues, "Gender and Legitimacy in the First Generations of the Avis Dynasty" (paper presented at the congress Kings & Queens IV: Dynastic Changes and Legitimacy, Lisbon, 23–27 June 2015); see also Mariana Bonat Trevisan, "A Primeira Geração de Avis: uma Família 'Exemplar' (Portugal -século XV)" (PhD dissertation, Universidade Federal Fluminense, 2016).

8 João Luís Inglês Fontes, *Percursos e memória: do Infante D. Fernando ao Infante Santo* (Cascais: Patrimonia, 2000).

9 Daniela Frigo, *Il padre di famiglia: Governo della casa e governo civile nella tradizione dell'economica' tra cinque e seicento* (Rome: Bulzoni, 1985); António M. Hespanha, "Carne de uma só carne: para uma compreensão dos fundamentos histórico-antropológicos da família na época moderna," *Análise Social* 28, nos 123–124 (1993): 951–973.

10 Maurice Keen, *Chivalry* (New Haven: Yale University Press, 2005), 1–17; Jesus D. Rodríguez-Velasco, *Order and Chivalry: Knighthood and Citizenship in Late Medieval Castile* (Philadelphia: University of Pennsylvania Press, 2010), 17–45.

11 Garcia de Resende, *Crónica*, 80; Jean Aubin, *Le Latin et l'Astrolabe. Études inédites sur le règne de D. Manuel, 1495–1521* (Paris: Centre Culturel Calouste Gulbenkian, 2006), vol. III, 3–12. Note that Manuel was both João II's cousin and brother-in-law (as the youngest brother of Queen Leonor [1458–1525]).

12 José Hermano Saraiva, ed., *Ditos Portugueses Dignos de Memória* (Mem Martins: Europa-América, 1997), 479.

13 Regarding this idea, see Barbara Fuchs, *Exotic Nation: Maurophilia and the Construction of Early Modern Spain* (Philadelphia: University of Pennsylvania Press, 2011).

14 Louise Mirrer, "Representing 'Other' Men: Muslims, Jews, and Masculine Ideals in Medieval Castilian Epic and Ballad," in *Medieval Masculinities: Regarding Men in the Middle Ages*, ed. Claire Lees (Minneapolis: University of Minnesota Press, 1994), 169–186.

15 Garcia de Resende, *Crónica de D. João II e Miscelânea*, ed. and pref. Joaquim Veríssimo Serrão (Lisbon: Imprensa Nacional-Casa da Moeda, 1973), 170 [chapter CXXIII].

16 See, for instance, Hélder Carvalhal and Isabel dos Guimarães Sá, "Knightly Masculinity, Court Games and Material Culture in Late-Medieval Portugal: The Case of Constable Afonso (*c.*1480–1504)," *Gender & History* 28, no. 2 (2016): 387–400.

17 For these shifts, the seminal work of Elias is still indispensable. See Norbert Elias, *The Civilizing Process: Sociogenetic and Psychogenetic Investigations*, trans. Edmund Jephcott (London: Blackwell, 2000 [1939]), vol. II, 387–396.

18 Garcia de Resende, *Cancioneiro Geral*, ed. Aida Fernandes Dias (Lisbon: Imprensa Nacional-Casa da Moeda, 1990–2003), vol. I, 172–179, vol. II, 7–8.

19 Diogo Lopes Rebelo, *Do Governo da República pelo Rei*, ed. Manuel Cadafaz de Matos (Lisbon: Távola Redonda/C.E.H.L.E., 2000), 139–147; Frei António de Beja, *Breve Doutrina e Ensinança de Príncipes*, ed. Mário Tavares Dias (Lisbon: Instituto de Alta Cultura, 1965), 115–131.

20 Rebelo, *Do Governo*, 155–157.

21 Lourenço de Cáceres, "Doutrina ao Infante D. Luís," in *Antologia do Pensamento Político Português*, ed. António Alberto de Andrade (Lisbon: ISCSPU: 1965), vol. I, 29–87, at 34–35.

22 Ana Isabel Buescu, *Imagens do Príncipe. Discurso Normativo e Representação (1525–49)* (Lisbon: Cosmos, 1996), 69.

23 *Doutrina*, 50–53, 55–57; *De Republica*, 101–111, 121–125.

24 Nuno J. Espinosa Gomes da Silva, *Humanismo e direito em Portugal no século XVI* (Lisbon: E.N.P., 1964), 26.

25 Buescu, *Imagens*, 161.

26 Buescu, *Imagens*, 174–175.

27 About the wise king topos in medieval Europe, see Manuel Alejandro Rodriguez de la Peña, "The 'wise king' topos in context", 38–53.

28 Todd W. Reeser, *Moderating Masculinity in Early Modern Culture* (Chapel Hill: University of North Carolina, Department of Romance Languages, 2006), 11–48.

29 Garcia de Resende, *Crónica*, 177–187 [chapters CXXVI–CXXVIII].

30 Steven Gunn, "Chivalry and the Politics of the Early Tudor Court," in *Chivalry in the Renaissance*, ed. Sydney Anglo (Woodbridge: The Boydell Press, 1990), 107–128, at 122.

31 Luís Filipe Thomaz, "L´idée impériale manueline," in *La Découverte, le Portugal et l'Europe*, ed. Jean Aubin (Paris: Fondation Calouste Gulbenkian, 1990), 35–103.

32 Archivo General de Simancas [AGS], *Estado*, leg. 371, nº 85. Published in Sylvie Deswarte-Rosa, "Espoirs et désespoir de l'infant D. Luís," *Mare Liberum* 3 (1991): 234–298, at 285.

33 Glenn Richardson, "Boys and Their Toys: Kingship, Masculinity and Material Culture in the Sixteenth Century," in *The Image and Perception of Monarchy in Medieval and Early Modern Europe*, eds. Sean McGlynn and Elena Woodacre (London: Cambridge Scholars Publishing, 2014), 183–206; Isabel dos Guimarães Sá, "The Uses of Luxury: Some Examples from the Portuguese Courts from 1480 to 1580," *Análise Social* 44, no. 192 (2009): 589–604.

34 Lisbon Academy of Sciences [ACL], Série Vermelha, nº 159, fls. 124–124v. Published in Pedro Pinto, "Apêndice. Resumos e transcrições de documentos relativos à Rua Nova," in *The Global City: Lisbon in Renaissance. Exhibition Catalogue*, eds. Annemarie Jordan and Kate Lowe (Lisbon: MNAA/IN-CM, 2017), 365–381, at 376.

35 On this topic, see Meg Twyncross and Sarah Carpenter, *Masks and Masking in Medieval and Early Tudor England* (Aldershot: Ashgate, 2002). Regarding tournaments in early Tudor period, see Emma Levitt, "Woodville versus the Bastard," *History Today* November (2016): 6.

36 Regarding Charles V's image, see Fernando Checa Cremades, "Héroes, guerreros y batallas en la imagen artística de la Monarquía española: De los Reyes Católicos a Carlos II," in *Historia Militar de España. III, Edad Moderna. II*, eds. Hugo O'Donnell, Duque de Estrada and Luís Ribot (Madrid: R.A.H./Ministerio de Defensa, 2014), 471–517, at 479–499.

37 Maria Augusta da Lima Cruz, *D. Sebastião* (Mem Martins: Temas e Debates, 2009), 94–104.

38 Ruth Mazo Karras, *From Boys to Men: Formations of Masculinity in Late Medieval Europe* (Philadelphia: University of Pennsylvania Press, 2003), 47–57.

39 Cruz, *D. Sebastião*, 101–104.

40 Nicolas Le Roux, *La faveur du roi: mignons et courtisans au temps des derniers Valois (vers 1547-vers 1589)* (Seyssel: Éditions Champ-Vallon, 2002), 660–670.

41 R.J. Knecht, *Catherine de Medici* (New York and London: Routledge, 1997), 37–39; Ivan Cloulas, *Henri II* (Paris: Fayard, 1985), 388.

42 Anita M. Walker and Edmund H. Dickerman, "The King Who Would Be a Man: Henri III, Gender Identity and the Murders at Blois, 1588," *Historical Reflections/Réflexions Historiques* 24, no. 2 (Summer 1998): 253–281, at 270.

43 Veronika Sandbichler, "Torneos y Fiestas de Corte de los Habsburgo en los Siglos XV y XVI," in *El Legado de Borgoña: Fiesta y Ceremonia Cortesana en la Europa de los Austrias (1454–1648)*, eds. Krista De Jonge, Bernardo J. García García and Alicia Esteban Estríngana (Madrid: Fundación Carlos de Amberes/Marcial Pons, 2010), 607–624, at 612–615.

44 Sá, "The Uses," 596.

45 Nils G. Bartholdy, "De danske kongers skjoldholdere," *Heraldisk Tidsskrift* 98 (2008): 345–357.

46 For example, see Fernando António Baptista Pereira, "Notas sobre a representação do Homem Silvestre na Arte Portuguesa dos séculos XV e XVI," *História e Crítica* 9 (1982): 57–66.

47 Aires Augusto Nascimento, ed., *Leonor de Portugal, Imperatriz da Alemanha: diário de viagem do embaixador Nicolau Lanckmen de Valckenstein* (Lisboa: Cosmos, 1992), 35.

48 António Dias Miguel, "Carta que Francisco de Morais enviou a Raynha de França em que lhe escreve os Torneos, e Festa que se fes em Xabregas Era / de 155," *Arquivos do Centro Cultural* XXXVII (1998): 132.

49 Louise Fradenburg, *City, Marriage, Tournament: Arts of Rule in Late Medieval Scotland* (Madison: University of Wisconsin Press, 1991), 235–236.

50 Michael Lynch, "Queen Mary's Triumph: The Baptismal Celebrations at Stirling in December 1566," *The Scottish Historical Review* 69/1, no. 187 (1990): 1–21, at 6–9.

51 Michael Wintroub, "Civilizing the Savage and Making a King: The Royal Entry Festival of Henri II (Rouen, 1550)," *The Sixteenth Century Journal* 29, no. 2 (1998): 165–191.

52 It is taken as 1595 instead of 1580 as the end of the dynasty because this was the year that Antonio, Prior do Crato, passed away in France. This option, still debatable today within academia, is justified by the pretension to the Portuguese throne that Antonio maintained until his demise, claiming he belonged to the dynasty of Avis as a natural son of *Infante* Luís and grandson of King Manuel I.

53 For example, see Estelle Paranque, "Royal representation through the father and warrior figures", 314–329 in this volume.

Key works

Connell, R.W., *Masculinities*, second ed. (Berkeley: University of California Press, 2005).

Hallenberg, Mats, "The Golden Age of the Agressive Male? Violence, Masculinity and the State in Sixteenth-Century Sweden," *Gender & History* 25, no. 1 (2013): 132–149.

Karras, Ruth Mazo, *From Boys to Men: Formations of Masculinity in Late Medieval Europe* (Philadelphia: University of Pennsylvania Press, 2003).

Lewis, Katherine J., *Kingship and Masculinity in Late Medieval England* (New York: Routledge, 2013).

Reeser, Todd W., *Moderating Masculinity in Early Modern Culture* (Chapel Hill: University of North Carolina, Department of Romance Languages, 2006).

Tosh, John, "Hegemonic Masculinity and the History of Gender," in *Masculinities in Politics and War: Gendering Modern History*, eds. Stefan Dudink, Karen Hagemann and John Tosh (Manchester: Manchester University Press, 2004), 41–58.

16

ROYAL REPRESENTATIONS THROUGH THE FATHER AND WARRIOR FIGURES IN EARLY MODERN EUROPE

Estelle Paranque

'I know I have the body but of a weak and feeble woman; but I have the heart and stomach of a king.'[1] Powerful rhetoric has the ability to resonate through history. The opening quote, spoken by Elizabeth I over 400 years ago, is a prime example of the way well-chosen words can reverberate through the centuries. Monarchs were expected to protect the borders of their realm, demonstrate their power at court and beyond, and forge bonds with the people over whom they reigned. Rhetoric was an essential weapon in the arsenal of a monarch in order to project their strength, real or imagined, into the public sphere. This chapter pays special attention to two dominant tropes – that of the father and that of the warrior – and how these were utilized in royal rhetoric in particular. The image of a warrior and father were often intertwined, as they both implied the necessity of protecting a realm and its people.[2] That these images were shared by early modern European monarchs, bypassing their religious beliefs or political ambitions, can be demonstrated by drawing parallels between the uses of rhetoric to govern by different rulers. While focusing on how many times rulers won battles can help to examine their military prowess, this would not indicate the importance of projecting martial authority into the public sphere and what tools they used to do so.

Scholars have expressed an increasing interest in kingship, queenship and how royal authority was asserted.[3] The importance of being able to project a strong royal image into a public sphere has also led historians to explore how monarchs were represented and how these representations were a crucial component of their rulership. For example, in France, Henry III (r. 1574–89) and Louis XVI (r. 1774–91) have particularly been demonized throughout history, impacting their reputation as strong monarchs for centuries and showing the importance of representations when shaping royal authority.[4] Other scholars, such as Yann Lignereux and Kevin Sharpe, offer a more visual and well-rounded representation of the French and English monarchies.[5] Lignereux argues that royal self-representation and representations by others needed one another. For Sharpe all these representations, both shaped by a monarch and by others, were necessary for preserving royal authority. Therefore, an analysis of both royal letters and proclamations in parallel with how the subjects received these royal images is fundamental to understanding the significance of certain images projected in the public sphere.

Furthermore, utilizing pamphlets, drawings and paintings, studies of queenship have demonstrated that strong and stable leadership produced effective representations in a variety of forms and medium.[6] The importance of material culture, iconography, paintings and architecture have also been examined in relation to these interrogations.[7] This chapter aims to further these discussions by addressing two crucial aspects of the kingly image, that of a father and that of a warrior, through the medium of rhetoric of monarchs and subjects.[8]

During the medieval and early modern period, it is not surprising that authority was intertwined with the image of a warrior king. Rulers were expected to go to war and demonstrate strength and courage.[9] Glenn Richardson has drawn comparisons between the reigns of Henry VIII of England, Francis I of France and Charles V of Spain. Richardson insists that although kings could not wage war in perpetuity, it was nonetheless crucial for them to fashion a warlike authority and image if they wanted to be respected domestically and abroad.[10] Yet, this warlike image was used differently by monarchs.

The warrior king is enmeshed with ideas of hegemonic masculinity, and the relationship between kingship and masculinity has become a new focus of interest among historians. This is illustrated in Hélder Carvalhal's chapter on hegemonic masculinity in Renaissance Portugal in this volume, a complementary study to this chapter. Here, however, wider questions of gender are explored. Anna Whitelock has paid particular attention to the limitations that a martial identity posed to queenship. She explained that Mary I of England and Elizabeth I of England, as queens regnant, often had to rely on their army officers 'to do the military business for them' yet that to some extent they could still be perceived as warrior queens.[11] Whitelock is right to make this difference.

Yet, this chapter goes further and also explores how rulers used the father figure to assert their royal authority. Kevin Sharpe explains the importance for monarchs to develop such an image, in order to bond with their people.[12] Perhaps more importantly, a father figure allows rulers to defend and protect their royal authority.[13] Interestingly, one can wonder at how this impacted a queen regnant's rulership. A concrete example will be the case of Elizabeth I of England who, in remaining single, ruled as both king and queen of England, and as result was both father and mother to her country.

The aims of this current chapter are threefold. First, it will reveal the significance of the father and warrior figures in rhetorical representations. Second, this chapter examines how such representations were intertwined with religion and humanist ideas, as well as being used during times of war or times of peace to achieve different outcomes. Finally, the comparative approach exposes the complexities and fragilities behind rhetorical representations used in speeches to provide a more comprehensive understanding of what it meant to be a monarch in early modern Europe.

This will be achieved by looking at two themes in the round before drilling down into representative case studies undertaking close analysis of the speeches and writings of early modern monarchs. The first section centres on the father figure, demonstrating ways in which the image was used by different kings and how it was associated with the ideal of a Christian figure, with a case study on Elizabeth I of England (r.1558–1603), who was also engaged with the father figure, though she was obliged to bypass masculine ideals. Following this will be a definition of the warrior figure and what this entailed during the early modern period. Rulers were not always at war, meaning that the warrior representation depended on other martial activities such as tournaments, hunting and chivalric expectations. Finally, the chapter offers a case study on Henry III of France (r.1574–89), a king reputed to be weak, but who also employed the image of a warrior in his writings. This chapter analyses the use of the father and warrior figures by early modern European monarchs in their own speeches and other forms of writing, as well as how their subjects responded to them. The two case studies help to re-evaluate the significance of fashioning such images to assert a strong and indisputable royal authority both within and outside the border of one's realm.

Monarchs as fathers to their country: divine rights and the defence of Christianity

In 1680, Robert Filmer, an English political theorist who advocated the divine right of kings, wrote:

> If we compare the natural rights of a father with those of a King, we find them all one, without any differences at all, but only in the latitude or extent of them: as the father over one family, so the King as father over many families extends his care to preserve, feed, clothe, instruct and defend the Commonwealth.[14]

Filmer's intention was to defend the divine right of rulers through the everyday contemporary expectation of a father who was in charge of his family. It is not surprising that this father figure was commonly found in monarchs' speeches long before Filmer's defence of the king's natural rights as most early modern rulers were influenced by humanists, such as Desiderius Erasmus. In 1516, Erasmus wrote and dedicated *The Education of a Christian Prince* to the future king of Spain and Holy Roman Emperor Charles V, later father of Philip II of Spain. He explained 'it is the spirit that is right for a prince: being like a father to the state'.[15] Erasmus claimed that a king needed to care for 'the advantage of all his subjects', and strongly differentiated a prince from a tyrant, affirming that 'there is the same difference between a prince and a tyrant as there is between a benevolent father and a cruel master'.[16] In France, the humanist Guillaume Budé wrote *L'Institution du Prince* and dedicated it to Francis I of France in 1519. His work was later published in 1547. Budé insisted on the importance of good qualities for a king to be successful – qualities similar to those described by Erasmus in order to fashion a fatherly image.[17]

These works and ideas had shaped princes' and princesses' education for hundreds of years. Therefore, kings had used the paternalistic image to reinforce their divine rights and to shield themselves from accusations of tyranny by representing themselves as true Christian patriarchs. Embodying the image of a father to his people was notably used by a king to govern in times of conflict or discord among the people – a rhetorical device which was not always successful but which remained necessary to preserve one's authority.[18] Furthermore, these thinkers who were also subjects of rulers also demonstrate that the people also used fatherly images in order to bond with their monarchs and remind them of their duties to their subjects.

During the eighth war of the French Wars of Religion, Beauvais and Amiens were major strongholds that had to be protected from the Spanish army. Since the conversion to Catholicism by Henry IV of France (r.1589–1610) on 25 July 1593, the Protestant majority in Beauvais had felt betrayed and abandoned by their prince.[19] In 1594, the king decided to revive their faith in him by gathering the nobles and gentry of neighbouring Amiens. There, Leonard Driot, a lawyer, began his speech explaining why the king had lost the support of Beauvais's inhabitants by reminding him of his divine rights and therefore his duties as father to his people:

> The Prince is the image of God; he is the father of his people and of his subjects. . . . a father loves his child with an extreme love which overcomes any other kind of affections . . . If the child separates himself from his father, abandons his house for riot and disobedience, and then after he comes back in his father's house, his father kisses him and greets him in good graces.[20]

Shrewdly, Driot made strong comparisons between the images of king and father, and more importantly, he aimed to use this father figure ideal to defend the abandoned inhabitants of Beauvais.[21] His reference to the father figure also helped him to make a political move and ensure that the king would forgive the inhabitants of Beauvais for their disloyalty to him – reminding him that they were his children. Therefore, the father figure seems to have been employed as a rhetorical tool by the people as well as the monarch in order to gain forgiveness.

In a private audience, the Bourbon king agreed with Driot's statement on the image of God as a benevolent figure who did not seek revenge.[22] Yet, throughout his own speech in Beauvais, Henry expressed discontent with the people who had betrayed him by supporting Philip II of Spain's war against France. Although he never used the word 'father', Henry insisted that he was a clement king who would pardon his disloyal subjects as long as they recognized him as the legitimate king of France.[23] He continued his speech, stating 'I forbid anyone to practise this supposed reformed religion . . . and promise with my God that . . . you all, and everyone else in my realms, will live under one and only Catholic, apostolic and roman Church.'[24] Henry's words and general tone were harsh and firm, but he counterbalanced their severity by reminding his audience that he had been the Huguenot king of Navarre who had ruled as 'their leader for twenty-two years and with softness I will bring them under the true Church'. Henry continued by expressing his ideal of France:

> I have in my realm of Bearn, two provinces next to each other, separated only by a river, in which there never was a riot under my reign, some were living under the Roman Catholic and Apostolic Church and others never went to Mass, yet no dispute ever arose among them.[25]

In this speech, Henry's desire to unify his country and provide peace for his people was indisputable. Despite his audience being primarily Protestant, he proved his sincerity regarding his conversion as well as showing the example to be followed in order to maintain peace in France. As he stressed in his speech, 'our Holy Father the Pope gave me absolution . . . you can be assured that I am part of his prayers and benedictions, as it is supposed to be for his elder son that I am'.[26] If the Pope – the

Father on earth – was able to welcome Henry into the Catholic faith as his son, he could welcome all Henry's subjects or 'children' who might decide to convert as well. Politically it was the only way he could unify the realm, but arguably Henry also converted at least in part to play this role of a spiritual father in France and to ward off any criticism, enabling him to unify the two religions and the two factions of the realm under a single sovereign, their anointed father and projecting a stronger royal authority into the public sphere.

While Henry's conversion helped to legitimize his authority and reduce resistance to his rule from the Catholic League, it was not sufficient to bring peace among all the factions in his realm. In April 1598 he issued the Edict of Nantes, a statement of tolerance and a peace treaty that granted a level of freedom of religion to the Huguenots. On 25 February 1599, after many contestations following the ratification of the edict, the Bourbon king gave another speech in which he reminded his audience of the role he meant to play for France:

> [y]ou are seeing me in my private office, where I come to speak to you, not dressed in royal gowns, nor with the sword and the cape, like my predecessors, nor like a prince who greets ambassadors, but dressed with a robe like a father to speak frankly to his children . . . I beg you to ratify the Edict that I granted to all regarding religion.[27]

Strikingly, Henry was not wearing a royal garb but instead chose to present himself in a 'robe' – a garment showing closeness but more importantly reminding his audience of Henry's pure Christianity. Indeed, as Erasmus explained:

> Admittedly, the prince is not a priest . . . he has not made his profession in the order of St Benedict, and therefore does not wear the cowl. But, more than all this, he is a Christian. The order in which he has made his profession is not that of Francis but of Christ himself, and he has received the white robe from him.[28]

Thus, in the French context and supported by principles of religious tolerance, Henry IV's conversion to Catholicism helped him not only to propagate the image of a spiritual father to all his people but also to unify the realm under one authority that could not be questioned.

Another example of a monarchical effort to resolve conflicts through the father figure ideal can be seen in the case of Philip II of Spain (r.1556–98). Sylvène Edouard's study of the Spanish king partly examines the challenges that the inhabitants of the Spanish Netherlands posed to his royal authority.[29] During a failed uprising in 1570, Philip II gave a speech to pardon his Dutch people using the image of a loving father to emphasize his sincerity towards them and remind them of their duty towards him.[30] However, Edouard argues that this fatherly love could only be bestowed upon good Catholics – thus associating the father figure with that of defender of the faith.[31] This distinction was very much used by the people in times of conflict with their king.

In 1573, during a conflict between the army of Philip II of Spain, led by the Duke of Alva, and William of Orange, leader of the Dutch rebels, the latter wrote to Philip appealing to his 'natural affection and fatherly inclination' and demanding that measures be taken against the Duke of Alva's tyrannical attitude.[32] In his open letter to the Spanish king, Orange positioned himself and the Dutch as Philip's subjects, in need of his love and protection. Through this bond, he made strong demands regarding quality of life and their rights, assuring the king of 'the fidelitie & obedience of your subiectes, which were accused to your Maiestie as rebels and traytours'.[33] Through the prism of a father-child relationship, William of Orange denounced the harsh treatment of the Protestants in Spanish dominions. However, for Philip, his role as a father was intertwined with the image of the defender of the Catholic faith, and therefore he rejected the rebels' demands.[34] In a speech given in 1590 in Madrid later translated into French, Philip stated that he was devoted to:

> [o]ur mother the Holy Catholic Apostolic and Roman Church, for the rest of good Catholics, under the obedience of their legitimate princes, for the extirpation of all forms of heresy, peace and concord of Christian Princes, for which to achieve, we are ready not only to employ any means but also our own life.[35]

Princes were devoted to the care of souls and often the line between a priestly and paternal role is blurred. Yet, in humanist ideas, such as the ones demonstrated in Erasmus's work, these two roles were intertwined to present the image of a good Christian father to the people. For both Henry and Philip, their fatherly image was connected to a priestly one. Yet, Henry chose to rally all his people around him, Protestants and Catholics, while Philip ended up antagonizing his Dutch Protestant subjects.

As previously demonstrated, this image of the father figure was often triggered during periods of conflict between the people and their sovereign, and the Protestant Charles I of England (r.1625–49) was no exception to the rule. During the British Civil Wars, his royal authority was not only challenged but actively undermined by parliament and the different court factions seeking power. In 1647 a letter written in Charles' own hand was published, revealing the importance of preserving the paternal representation.[36] The declaration began by explaining the predicament the English monarch was facing:

> [f]or I shall earnestly and incessantly endeavour the setting of a safe and well-grounded peace, where ever I am, or shall be; And that (as much as may be) without the effusion of more Christian blood, for which how many times have I desired, prest to be heard, and yet no eare given to me.[37]

At the end of his speech, Charles insisted on reminding his people of his role as a father to his country, proclaiming, 'let me be heard with freedome, honour, and safety, and I shall (instantly) breake through this cloud of retirement, and shew my selfe really to be *Pater Patriae*'.[38] In this difficult and dangerous situation, by associating 'freedome, honour, and safety' with paternalistic images, Charles strove to distance himself from the widespread portrayals of him as a tyrant by reminding the people of his role as a father to them. He reminded his audience that a fatherly king had to ensure freedom and stability to his people and, therefore, positioned himself at the top of his realm and family.

While his detractors portrayed him as a tyrant who did not care for the wellbeing of his people, the father figure helped Charles to counterbalance this negative image and enhance his benevolent image that would be at the root of efforts to raise him as a martyr after his death. Furthermore, in using the father figure, he implied that he should not be disobeyed and that if he was it would end all order in the commonwealth. In doing so, he was therefore appealing to the fear of inversion that was part of the shared culture of early modern England.[39]

As the image of father figure often embodied the idea of protection, it often proved to be an inevitable and powerful tool for monarchs in times of crisis. Equally, this same rhetoric allowed the subjects to appeal to their monarch in a manner that chimed with tropes used in royal representation, if to varying effect in different contexts. Despite this mode of rhetoric not always being a success, through protection rulers asserted their royal authority over their subjects. In other cases, it also allowed them to find compromises and stability within their realm.

Queen Elizabeth I of England: a father to her country?

The virgin queen, Deborah, mother of her country, and the equal of a king, are all images of the last Tudor queen that have been thoroughly studied by scholars, yet this chapter offers a challenge to the image of Elizabeth as mother to her country.[40] As Carole Levin explains, by remaining single, Elizabeth ruled as both king and queen of England, and as a result served as both father and mother to her country.[41] Erasmus himself insisted that the main difference between a tyrant and a king was love: 'the tyrant strives to be feared, the king to be loved' and added, 'a king has the one interest of fostering harmony'.[42] According to Ilona Bell, 'the rhetoric of love was also traditional political discourse, regularly used by male monarchs to win the support of their subjects'.[43] This theme was similarly employed by Elizabeth in order to assert her own strength and royal authority. She used the rhetoric of love combined with that of protection to project and fashion the image of a father to her country.

During the early modern period, a mother's love was associated with the care she provided to young children. As Cissie Fairchilds explains they 'bore almost total responsibility for the care of children under six' while fathers were expected to love their young children as well 'but at a distance'.[44] To some extent, a motherly love involved more devotion and selflessness than one of a father, but more importantly, a motherly love is often connected to the protection of a younger person.[45] Furthermore, Sara Mendelson and Patricia Crawford reveal that 'maternity followed soon after marriage'.[46] Therefore, a maternal love could only be provided by a wife. By remaining single, Elizabeth could not be the mother of her country, she had to care for all her subjects, the young ones as well as the elders. She was not physically caring for them. Instead, she was protecting and ensuring their well-being from afar: as a father.

In 1593, while England was still at war with Spain, Elizabeth stated in a speech in front of her parliament: 'Many wiser princes than myself you have had, but one only excepted, none more careful over you'. She continued:

I may truly say none whose love and care can be greater or whose desire can be more to fathom deeper for prevention of danger to come or resisting of dangers, if attempted towards you, shall ever be found to exceed myself in love towards you and care over you.[47]

The expressions of love for her people, coupled with the discussion of herself in comparison with other 'princes', emphasized Elizabeth's desire to be seen as a clement and caring father to her country. As Erasmus acclaimed, the first characteristic of a king is being a father.[48] Thus by using the rhetoric of love mostly used by men in the public sphere, Elizabeth bonded with her people and represented herself as a king through the father figure.

In her Golden Speech of 1601, Elizabeth again insisted on her love for her people, declaring that: 'There will never [a] queen sit in my seat with more zeal to my country, care to my subjects, and that will sooner with willingness venture her life for your good and safety, than myself'.[49] To some extent, by denying herself the opportunity to marry and have her own children, Elizabeth sacrificed her maternal instincts to be a father to her people. The queen's desire to appear as both benevolent and able to protect her country was striking.

As with many other monarchs of the era, Elizabeth's father figure image was also based on the ideal of the Defender of the Faith. As Bell points out, 'because Elizabeth was not only a monarch but also a queen, the ambassadors judged her words and actions according to the assumptions about women that dominated their world. Misogyny pervades early modern discourse'.[50] After she was crowned Queen of England on 15 January 1559, Parliament passed two important acts: the Act of Uniformity and the Act of Supremacy. She could not be named the controversial 'Supreme Head of the Church of England', a term that referred to the patriarchal hierarchy, so instead settled for 'Supreme Governor of the Church of England'.[51] Yet, in practice, she was indeed the 'head' and her speeches consciously use the word 'head' to assert her sovereignty and, to some extent, her paternal authority. As the de facto head of her Church, Elizabeth was effectively the father of the Church of England, a title that allowed her to defend her hegemonic legitimacy as well as unite the country under her rule. During a speech given in 1566, as a response to the Parliament's pressure on her to marry, she declared firmly, 'I will deal therein for your safety and offer it unto you as your prince and head, without request. For it is monstrous that the feet should direct the head'.[52] By using the words 'safety' and 'your prince and head', Elizabeth was insisting on a prevailing concept of fatherhood: protection. The word 'prince', which could be applied to both female and male monarchs, did not in this case refer to her gender. However, it was nevertheless associated with the term 'head', which emphasized the 'male' royal identity of Elizabeth. Moreover, the last sentence of this quotation referred directly to the well-known declaration of John Knox that 'the head shuld not folowe the feet', wherein 'the head' represented men and 'the feet' symbolized women.[53] Elizabeth no longer positioned herself as a woman but as the only monarch of England, the only governor of the Church of England, and consequently the only father of her country. Therefore, 'the feet' became a reference to all men, while the 'head' became the queen. Through this reference to the 'head', Elizabeth once more bypassed the same misogynistic preconceptions that she had to overcome in order to assert her warrior figure.[54]

Monarchs as warriors: military prowess and public demonstrations of power

Erasmus stated in 1516 that 'The good prince will never start a war at all unless, after everything else has been tried, it cannot by any means be avoided'.[55] In warning of the dangers and the disasters that wars could bring to a realm, Erasmus thoroughly explained how a Christian prince needed to seek peace at all costs to avoid the risk of losing his country.[56] This wise advice was widely adhered to, at least in theory, by early modern European rulers. Addressing his son in *Basilikon Doron*, for example, James VI of Scotland (r.1568–1625) and future James I of England (r.1603–25) explained:

> And as I haue counselled you to be slow in taking on a warre, so aduise you to be slow in peace-making. Before ye agree, looke that the ground of your warres be satisfied in your peace; and that ye see a good suretie for you and your people; otherwaies a honourable and iust warre is more tollerable, than a dishonourable and disaduantageous peace.[57]

The balance between being a just king and a warrior was often perceived by monarchs as difficult to identify and achieve.[58] As previously stated, despite the numerous wars that had ravaged Europe from 1500 to 1800, widespread conflict was not the perpetual state of affairs. However, even in peacetime, being a warrior remained a quality that needed to be pursued and demonstrated in order to assert one's royal authority. Historians have discussed the links between military prowess and fame in tournaments, chivalric orders, pageantry and hunting.[59] The latter activity particularly needs to be further analysed in terms of how it was utilized by monarchs to demonstrate their power.

During his reign, Charles IX of France (r.1560–74) authored *La Chasse Royale* (the Royal Hunt), which was published posthumously in 1625 and dedicated to Louis XIII of France (r.1610–43). In 1807, the book was reprinted with the original dedication to Louis by Mr Gervais Alliot, a printer in Paris, along with responses to Charles's work by contemporaries such as François d'Amboise and Pierre de Ronsard. In the introduction by Henri Chevreuil, it was noted that Charles IX was barely remembered a mere half century after his death, and was primarily associated with the St Bartholomew's Day Massacre in 1572.[60] However, Chevreuil insisted that there was more glory to Charles's reign than his critics had credited, praising his military prowess by reminding the reader that Charles had won major battles, and that he had fought against the Huguenots 'riding a horse' at seventeen years old.[61] In his dedication to Louis, Alliot explained that *La Chasse Royale* was meant to 'entertain' the king, as hunting was an exercise that had helped his predecessor to 'endure the fatigue from war'.[62] While Charles's *La Chasse Royale* does not offer any advice in terms of hunting strategy and focuses more on imparting knowledge of stags and the training of hunting dogs, Alliot's allusion to the links between hunting and war is noteworthy.

References to hunting as a demonstration of power were also found in correspondence concerning Elizabeth I of England from the French ambassador, La Mothe Fénélon, to the French royal family. Extensive and thorough analyses have been made of the descriptions of Elizabeth's hunting skills and physical strength as revealed by La Mothe Fénélon's letters.[63] The ideal of the warrior figure was based on qualities of strength and power making martial skill a significant part of how monarchs were represented, remembered and chose to represent themselves.

Edouard has explored in detail how Philip II of Spain based his royal authority on the image of a warrior. She argues that through invocation of King Solomon, Philip II managed to impose the impression of 'strength, temperance, and prudence', with representations of the Spanish king as a warrior thus closely associated with his religious zeal.[64] The 'stomach of King Philip' was mentioned in a French propagation pamphlet regarding the Franco-Spanish war in the 1590s.[65] While Henry IV's victory was noted, Philip II nonetheless appeared as a strong warrior king who threatened France's prosperity. On the other hand, in 1595, amid the eighth religious civil war ravaging France, a tribute to Henry IV was printed that praised his victories and military prowess against Spain.[66] Its author, the Bishop of Evreux proclaimed:

> After so many fights worthy of so many stories
> All covered with glory, full of victories
> Come to see Ô Great King the high walls of Paris
> And you who for honour no danger no refuses
> Comes back full of honour after so many dangers
> To collect the fruits of Mars in the Muses's fields
> Paris, for the love of God, letters of the journey
> Pallas's Temple is awaiting for you in this beautiful day.[67]

References to Mars and Pallas, important warrior figures in classical mythology, reinforced the image of Henry IV as a successful warrior king who had saved Paris from a Spanish invasion. His glory was infused with an almost godly power, and Paris represented the child that needed to be protected by the invaders. Such references to Mars were not unusual, for they allowed contemporary writers to draw strong parallels between a royal power and a martial one. At his death, Charles IX of France was also remembered for his 'strength from Mars'.[68]

In contrast with the previous examples, which include a mixture of self-fashioning and the fashioning by others, Charles II of the British Isles offers a prime example of how a monarch could shape his own military reputation. After the destruction of the War of the Three Kingdoms (1639–51), the British people needed stability again. Charles II declared:

> [w]herein is expressed the late cruel, Tyrannical and perfidious practises and proceedings of a pack'd piece of a Parliament or Juncto, who have assumed a Power to themselves far beyond what ever hath been acted or done by any of Our Predecessors, contrary to Law, Reason and the just Rights and Priviledges of all Our good Subjects . . . To which end and purpose, We have already provided shipping, and embarqued a considerable part of Our Army

to be landed at one of the places therein mentioned; resolving with Our Self to appear in Our own Royall Person at the head of those Forces.[69]

It was as a strong warrior figure that Charles projected himself into the public sphere in order to appear as a legitimate ruler worthy of the title: one prepared to bring stability to his country and fight for his birth rights. After his exile and his father's execution, Charles understood the necessity of imposing his authority and legitimacy as the true ruler of the British Isles over the parliament. He became the 'head' of his country again and, as such, was in control of it. Interestingly, in differentiating himself from the image of tyrant, Charles in turn accused parliament of having been tyrannical with his 'loving subjects'. This distinction between the warrior leader of a rescuing force and a tyrant lay at the centre of early modern monarchical representations. As monarchs used the warrior figure to rule effectively, they had to be aware of the correlations between a tyrant and a warrior monarch. Hence, the warrior figure was rarely used on its own, and as previously mentioned, was often combined with the father figure.

King Henry III of France: a warrior king?

Henry III of France has long suffered a bad reputation due to his inability to put an end to the religious civil wars that ravaged France in the second part of the sixteenth century. In trying to find compromises with the Huguenots, Henry was seen by his contemporaries and later by most historians as too mild and too tolerant. Annie Duprat and Jean-Marie Constant offer an explanation as to how his religious tolerance was misinterpreted and denounced by the king's contemporaries.[70] Representations of Henry III both during and after his reign were largely monopolized by Catholic League propaganda, and his failures to impose catholicism over his subjects caused Henry III to be considered as insufficiently Catholic, or even worse, according to Keith Cameron, 'as the enemy of both of the true Catholic faith and of the Huguenots'.[71] Yet, this perspective on Henry III is greatly criticized by historians like Nicolas Le Roux, who recognize Henry as a fervent defender of the Catholic faith, while Jacqueline Boucher goes even further to claim that he was 'indisputably the most fervent in his Catholic faith'.[72]

The bond between Henry III and catholicism appears to have been central in terms of how he represented himself. However, a crucial component of his royal representation that has often been overlooked is that of a warrior king. By devoting closer attention to his speeches, which were often printed and distributed throughout the country, one can realize that Henry III strove to project a warlike royal authority over his subjects using rhetorical means. The warrior figure as striven towards by Henry III has been analysed through such quotations as 'I want my people to know that I have a heart and stomach as big as any of my predecessors'.[73] These words, stated by Henry in May 1588, obviously recall the opening quote to this paper and are immortalized by Elizabeth I of England at Tilbury in 1588: 'I know I have the body but of a weak and feeble woman but I have the heart and stomach of a king, and of a king of England too.'[74] Though long connected to Elizabeth for this particular statement and its particular resonance, references to 'the heart and stomach', and to the military prowess of their predecessors, helped many monarchs to be respected and rule effectively.

At the death of Henry III's younger brother, Francis duke of Anjou, in 1584, the next heir presumptive to the throne was Henry of Navarre, the future Henry IV. Yet, the Guises declared that they could not bear to have a Protestant as a king, and swore to defend the French crown at any cost – with or without Henry III's support and approval.[75] Various Catholic factions were created, and the eighth religious civil war in France erupted in 1585.[76] During that period, Henry III's desire to appear as a strong warrior king was paramount. In 1587, the last Valois king gave a speech that was printed and spread among his people. The title of this speech evoked a warlike image: 'The Copy of the Speech given by the King to Messieurs of Paris in front of them riding a horse, to go to war'. Henry stated that he was:

> [w]ell-resolved to ride a horse and gather the biggest army possible in order to protect our people from the misery and calamity into which it has been sucked through this wet nurse mother of this disease that we name civil war generated by this new religion.[77]

He continued his speech with the claim that he would sacrifice his life for the commonwealth of his people.[78] This rhetoric of sacrifice, which demonstrated a monarch's devotion to their people, was also used by other monarchs, including Elizabeth I of England and Charles I of England, when they fashioned their warrior figures.[79] Henry ended his discourse by affirming that he 'would always be ready to save you and meet your needs'.[80] A year later, in an address to his General States, he reiterated that he cared more about his people than 'the conservation of his own life' in his calls for unity.[81] The rhetoric of a sacrificial saviour was an expression of Henry's efforts to represent himself as a protector to his people, undoubtedly linked to the father figure.

Despite his widespread and enduring reputation as a tyrannical figure, his own words are crucial when analysing the shaping of Henry's royal authority, and some evidence suggests that such rhetoric was at least partly successful. At his death, most of the printed pamphlets denounced his tyrannical behaviour rather than emphasizing his efforts to preserve French unity.[82] Yet, one publication praised Henry's bravery with echoes of the same rhetoric alluding to Mars and Pallas that had been used for his older brother, Charles IX.[83] This illustrates that Henry's reputation among the French had not been entirely tarnished and that this prominent rhetoric had cut through the vitriolic criticism in some quarters.

Conclusion

The hereditary nature of early modern monarchies meant that there were those who succeeded despite being unsuited to the role and thus struggled to maintain authority, or – in the case of Elizabeth – were perfectly capable but hindered by contemporary opinion. Monarchs were expected to unify their country, protect borders and care for their people. Through two significant royal representations, this chapter has shown how early modern European leaders engaged with a paternal and warlike rhetoric in order to assert their royal authority and confront challenges to their reign. The two case studies have highlighted ways in which Elizabeth I of England and Henry III of France used rhetoric commonly employed by early modern European rulers to fashion a strong monarchical authority. Scholars have too often overlooked these images in monarchs' speeches, missing interesting parallels between rulers who ended up with different fates and reputations. By comparing the use of rhetoric as exercised by various rulers to fashion their powerful royal representations, this chapter has further demonstrated the complexities of monarchical reigns during the early modern period. Monarchs had to negotiate their royal identities with their subjects. Through speeches, declarations and pamphlets, this chapter has revealed the complexities behind the warrior and father figures and what such representations actually entailed for rulers, It also revealed the importance of such verbalized representations to maintaining good relations between rulers and their people. As such these ideals played a crucial role in the success of their rulership. Appearing as a benevolent and protective father was used as a political rhetoric in order to control public opinion and mediate the very necessary, but often potentially challenging, representation of warrior monarch.

Notes

1 "Queen Elizabeth's Armada Speech to the troops at Tilbury, 9 August 1588," in *Elizabeth I: Collected Works*, eds. Leah Marcus, Janel Mueller and Mary Beth Rose (Chicago: Chicago University Press 2000), 326.
2 David Carpenter, *The Minority of Henry III* (Los Angeles: University of California Press, 1990); Jean Flory, *Richard Cœur de Lion: Le Roi Chevalier* (Paris: Payot, 1999); Gérard Sivéry, *Louis VIII le Lion* (Paris: Fayard, 1995); Georges Minois, *Charles VII: un roi shakespearien* (Paris: Le Grand livre du mois, 2005); John Gillingham, *Richard Cœur de Lion: Kingship, Chivalry and War in The Twelfth Century* (London: Hambledon Continuum, 1994).
3 Glenn Richardson, *Renaissance Monarchy: The Reigns of Henry VIII, Francis I and Charles V* (London: Hodder Education, 2002); Jacqueline Boucher, *La cour de Henri III* (Rennes: Persée, 1986); Louis Montrose, *The Subject of Elizabeth I: Authority, Gender and Representation* (Chicago: Chicago University Press, 2006); John Adamson, ed., *The Princely Courts of Europe, 1500–1750* (London: Weidenfield and Nicolson, 2000).
4 Annie Duprat, *Les rois de papier, la caricature de Henri III à Louis XVI* (Paris: Belin, 2002).
5 Yann Lignereux, *Les Rois Imaginaires: Une Histoire Visuelle de la Monarchie de Charles VIII à Louis XIV* (Rennes: Presses Universitaires de Rennes, 2016) and Kevin Sharpe, *Selling the Tudor Monarchy: Authority and Image in Sixteenth Century England* (New Haven: Yale University Press, 2009).
6 Carole Levin and Christine Stewart-Munez, eds., *Scholars and Poets Talk About Queens* (New York: Palgrave Macmillan, 2015); Zita Eva Rohr and Lisa Benz, eds., *Queenship, Gender, and Reputation in the Medieval and Early Modern West, 1060–1600* (New York: Palgrave Macmillan, 2016); and Debra Barrett-Graves, ed., *The Emblematic Queen: Extra-Literary Representations of Early Modern Queenship* (New York: Palgrave Macmillan, 2013).
7 Kate Buchanan, Lucinda H. S. Dean, Michael Penman, eds., *Medieval and Early Modern Representations of Authority in Scotland and the British Isles* (Abingdon: Routledge, 2016); Malcom Vale, *The Princely Court: Medieval Courts and Culture in Northwest Europe, 1270–1380* (Oxford: Oxford University Press, 2001); Sean MacGlynn and Elena Woodacre, eds., *The Image and Perception of Monarchy in Medieval and Early Modern Europe* (Newcastle: Cambridge Scholar Publishing, 2014).
8 Kevin Sharpe, "The King's Writ: Royal Authors and Royal Authority in Early Modern England," *Culture and Politics in Early Stuart England*, eds. Kevin Sharpe and Peter Lake (Stanford: Stanford University Press, 1993), 117–138 ; Carole Levin and Patricia A. Sullivan, *Political Rhetoric, Power, and Renaissance Women* (New York: SUNY Press, 1995).
9 Marie-Claude Canova-Green, "Warrior King or King of War? Louis XIII's Entries into his *Bonnes Villes* (1620–1629)," *Ceremonial Entries in Early Modern Europe: The Iconography of Power*, eds. J.R. Mulryne, Maria Ines Aliverti and Anna Maria Testaverde (Farnham: Ashgate, 2015), 77–98.
10 Richardson, *Renaissance Monarchy*, 36–37.

11 Anna Whitelock, "Woman, Warrior, Queen? Rethinking Mary and Elizabeth," *Tudor Queenship: the Reigns of Mary and Elizabeth*, eds. Alice Hunt and Anna Whitelock (New York: Palgrave Macmillan, 2010), 173–189.

12 Kevin Sharpe, *Reading Authority and Representing Rule in Early Modern England* (London: Bloomsbury Academic, 2013), 160.

13 Mark Fortier, "Equity and Ideas: Coke, Ellesmere, and James VI and I," in *Royal Subjects: Essays on the Writings of James VI and I*, eds. Daniel Fischlin and Mark Fortier (Detroit: Wayne State University Press, 2002), 276.

14 Robert Filmer, *Patriarcha, or, the Natural Power of Kings* (London, 1680), 23–24.

15 Desiderius Erasmus, *The Education of a Christian Prince*, 1516, ed. Lisa Jardine (Cambridge: Cambridge University Press, 1997), 17.

16 Ibid., 27–28 and 25.

17 Guillaume Budé, *L'Institution du Prince* (Paris, 1547), 13–15.

18 For a discussion on Henry III of France's father figure see Estelle Paranque, "Catherine of Medici: Henry III's Inspiration to be a Father to His People," in *Royal Mothers and their Ruling Children: Wielding Political Authority from Antiquity to the Early Modern Era*, eds. Elena Woodacre and Carey Fleiner (New York: Palgrave Macmillan, 2015), 225–240.

19 Michal Wolfe, *The Conversion of Henri IV: Politics, Power, and Religious Belief in Early Modern France* (Cambridge: Cambridge University Press, 1993).

20 Discours fait au Roi Henri IV, à Amiens, le 21 Aout 1594 (Paris, 1787), 14–15.

21 Ibid., 15.

22 Henry IV of France, *Le Roy devant les Desputes, le dimanche 21 Aout 1594* (Paris, 1787), 16.

23 Ibid., 17–23.

24 Ibid., 19–20.

25 Ibid., 21.

26 Ibid., 23.

27 *Collection Complète des Mémoires Relatifs à l'Histoire de France par M. Petitot, Mémoire Journaux par Pierre de L'Estoile*, Tome XLVII (Paris, 1825), 244–245.

28 Erasmus, *The Education of a Christian Prince*, 19.

29 Sylvène Edouard, *L'Empire imaginaire de Philippe II, pouvoir des images et discours du pouvoir sous les Habsbourg d'Espagne au XVIe siècle* (Paris: Honoré Champion, 2005).

30 Philip II of Spain, *Grâce et pardon général donné par la Majesté du roy catholique [Philippe II] à cause des troubles et séditions survenues en Flandres et pays circonvoisins*, printed by Benoist Rigaud (Lyon, 1570).

31 Edouard, *L'Empire imaginaire de Philippe II*, 166.

32 William I of Orange, *A supplication to the Kings Maiestie of Spayne, made by the Prince of Orange, the states of Holland and Zeland, with all other his faithfull subiectes of the low Countreys, presently suppressed by the tyranny of the Duke of Alba and Spaniards. By which is declared the originall beginning of al the commotions [and] troubles happened in the sayd low Countrie: to the relief wherof, they require his Maiesties speedy redresse and remedie. Faithfully translated out of Duytsch into English, by T.W.* (1573), 2–3.

33 Ibid., 7–9.

34 Philip II of Spain, *Grâce et pardon général donné par la Majesté du roy catholique*, 3.

35 Philip II of Spain, *Declaration du Roy d'Espaigne sur les troubles miseres, & calamitez qui affligent la Chrestienté, & notamment le Royaume de France (8 mars 1590)* (Lyon, 1590), 8.

36 Charles I of England, A declaration by the Kings Majestie concerning His Majesties going away from Hampton-Court written by his own hand and left upon the table in His Majesties bed-chamber, dated at Hampton-Court Novemb. 11, 1647: presented to the Parliament . . . Friday Nov. 12, 1647, with His Majesties propositions for satisfying of the Presbyterians and Independents, the Army, and all His Majesties subjects of England and Scotland, (Hampton Court, 12 November 1647).

37 Ibid., 2–3.

38 Ibid., 5.

39 Susan D. Amussen and David E. Underdown, *Gender, Culture and Politics in England, 1560–1640: Turning the World Upside Down* (London: Bloomsbury Academic, 2017), 3–4.

40 On works on Elizabeth's representations, see Carole Levin, *The Heart and Stomach of a King: Elizabeth I and the Politics of Sex and Power* (Philadelphia: Pennsylvania University Press,

1994, second edition 2013); Susan Doran, "An Old Testament King," in *Tudor Queenship, the Reigns of Mary and Elizabeth*, eds. Alice Hunt and Anna Whitelock (New York: Palgrave Macmillan, 2010), 95–110; Alexandra Walsham, "'A Very Deborah?' The Myth of Elizabeth I as a Providential Monarch," in *The Myth of Elizabeth*, eds. Susan Doran and Thomas S. Freeman (New York: Palgrave Macmillan, 2003), 143–170; Helen Hackett, *Virgin Mother, Maiden Queen: Elizabeth I and the Cult of the Virgin Mary* (London, 1994) and Roy Strong, *The Cult of Elizabeth: Elizabethan Portraiture and Pageantry* (London, 1999). On the mother figure, see Christine Coch, "'Mother of my Contreye': Elizabeth I and Tudor Constructions of Motherhood," *English Literary Renaissance* 26, no. 3 (1996): 423–450.

41 Levin, *The Heart and Stomach of a King*, 148.

42 Erasmus, *The Education of a Christian Prince*, 28.

43 Ilona Bell, *Elizabeth I: The Voice of a Monarch* (New York: Palgrave Macmillan, 2010), xiii.

44 Cissie C. Fairchilds, *Women in Early Modern Europe, 1500–1700* (Harlow: Longman 2007), 96.

45 Ibid., 97.

46 Sara Mendelson and Patricia Crawford, *Women in Early Modern England*, second edition (Oxford: Oxford University Press, 2003), 49.

47 "Queen Elizabeth's Speech at the Closing of Parliament, April 10, 1593," in *Elizabeth I: Collected Works*, eds. Leah Marcus, Janel Mueller and Mary Beth Rose (Chicago: Chicago University Press, 2000), 328–330.

48 Erasmus, *The Education of a Christian Prince*, 35.

49 "Elizabeth's Golden Speech, November 30, 1601," in *Collected Works*, 339.

50 Bell, *Elizabeth I: The Voice of a Monarch*, 86.

51 For a discussion on Elizabeth's title, see Carole Levin, *The Reign of Elizabeth* (New York: Palgrave Macmillan, 2002), 22–24.

52 "Queen Elizabeth's Speech to a Joint Delegation of Lords and Commons, November 5, 1566," in *Collected Works*, 98.

53 John Knox, *The First Blast of the Trumpet Against the Monstruous Regiment of Women* (Geneva, 1558), STC 15070, 7.

54 See Estelle Paranque, "The Representations and Ambiguities of the Warlike Female Kingship of Elizabeth I of England," in *Medieval and Early Modern Representations of Authority*, 163–176.

55 Erasmus, *The Education of a Christian Prince*, 103.

56 Ibid., 102–104.

57 King James VI & I, *Basilikon Doron Or His Maiesties Instructions to his Dearest Sonne, Henry the Prince* (1599, reprint 1603), in *Political Writings*, ed. Johann P. Sommerville (Cambridge: Cambridge University Press, 1994), 33.

58 Paranque, "Representations and Ambiguities," 165–168. See also Whitelock, "Woman, Warrior, Queen," 173–189; Ben Spiller, "Warlike Mates? Queen Elizabeth and Joan La Pucelle in 1 Henri VI," in *Goddesses and Queens: The Iconography of Elizabeth I*, eds. Annaliese Connolly and Lisa Hopkins (Manchester: Manchester University Press, 2007), 34–44.

59 Richardson, *Renaissance Monarchy*, 36. Also see, Glenn Richardson, *The Fields of Cloth of Gold* (New Haven: Yale University Press, 2013); Jan Frans Verbruggen, *The Art of Warfare in Western Europe during the Middle Ages, from the Eighth Century to 1340*, second edition (Woodbridge: Boydell Press, 1997); Kylie Murray, "'Out of My Contree': Visions of Royal Authority in the Courts of James I and James II," in *Medieval and Early Modern Representations of Authority*, 214–234.

60 *La Chasse Royale Composée par le Roi Charles IX et dédiée au roi très-chrétien de France et de Navarre, Louis XIII*, Nouvelle édition précédée d'une introduction par Henri Chevreuil (Paris, 1807), i–ii.

61 Ibid., iv.

62 Ibid., 3.

63 Estelle Paranque, "Queen Elizabeth and the Elizabethan Court in the French Ambassador's Eyes," in *Queens Matter in Early Modern Studies*, ed. Anna Bertolet Riehl (New York: Palgrave Macmillan, 2017), 267–284. On Elizabeth's hunting, see Dustin Neighbors, "'With My Rulinge': Agency, Queenship and Political Culture through Royal Progresses in the Reign of Elizabeth I" (PhD thesis, York University, forthcoming).

64 Edouard, *L'Empire imaginaire de Philippe II*, 177, 244, 255.

65 Alexandre de Pontaymeri, *Discours d'Estats, Où la necessité et les moyens de faire la guerre en Espagne mesme, sont richement exposez* (Lyon, 1595), 15.

66 Monsieur du Perron, Bishop of Evreux, *Stances sur les Victoires du Roy et son advement à la Coronne* (Lyon, 1595).

67 Ibid., 3.

68 Pierre de Ronsard, *Le Tombeau du Feu Roy Tres-Chrétien Charles Neufvieme, Prince Tres Débonnaire, Tres vertueux et Tres eloquent* (Lyon, 1574), 2.

69 Charles II of England, *By the Kings Most Excellent Majestie a Declaration to All His Maiesties Loving Subiects in his Kingdoms [sic] of England, Scotland, and Ireland, &c.*, (Antwerp, 1659), 1.

70 Annie Duprat, *Les rois de papier, la caricature de Henri III à Louis XVI* (Paris: Belin 2002), 23 and Jean-Marie Constant, *Les Guise* (Paris: Hachette, 1984), 137.

71 Keith Cameron, "Introduction," in Keith Cameron, ed., *From Valois to Bourbon: Dynasty, State and Society in Early Modern France* (Exeter: Exeter University Press, 1989), 2.

72 Nicolas Le Roux, *Un régicide au nom de Dieu* (Paris: Gallimard, 2006), 39 and Jacqueline Boucher, *La cour de Henri III*, 179.

73 "Propos que le Roi a tenu à Chartres aux Députés de la Cour de Parlement, imprimé à Paris, chez Lhuillier May 1588," *Mémoires de la Ligue*, Tome II (Amsterdam: Arkstee & Merkus, 1758), 364. For an analysis of this speech, see Estelle Paranque, "Another Spare to the French Crown: Henry III's Self-Representation and Royal Authority," in *Unexpected Heirs in Early Modern Europe: Potential Kings and Queens*, ed. Valerie Schutte (New York: Palgrave Macmillan, 2017), 139–158.

74 "Queen Elizabeth's Armada Speech to the Troops at Tilbury, August 9, 1588," in *Collected Works*, 326.

75 "Déclaration des causes qui ont mu monseigneur le cardinal de bourbon et les pairs, princes, seigneurs, villes et communautés catholiques de ce royaume de France, de s'opposer à ceux qui par tous moyens s'efforcent de subvertir la religion catholique et l'Etat. March 31, 1585," *Mémoires de la Ligue*, Tome I (Amsterdam: Arkstee &Merkus, 1758), 55–56.

76 Robert J. Knecht, *Hero or Tyrant: Henry III, King of France, 1574–1589* (Farnham: Ashgate, 2014), 244–248.

77 Henry III of France, *La Coppie de la Harangue qu'a faict le Roy, à Messieurs de Paris devant que monter à cheval, pour aller à la guerre* (Lyon, 1587), 3–4.

78 Ibid., 4–5.

79 Paranque, "Representations and Ambiguities," 170–174; Edouard, *L'Empire imaginaire de Philippe II*, 177–178.

80 *La Coppie de la Harangue qu'a faict le Roy*, 6.

81 Henry III of France, *La Harangue faite par le Roy Henry Troisième de France et de Pologne, à l'ouverture de l'assemblee des Trois Estats generaux de son Royaume, en la ville de Blois, le seizième jour d'Octobre, 1588* (Lyon, 1588), 3.

82 Two of them are particularly striking in their rhetoric, see *Le Discours au Vray sur la Mort et Trepas de Henry de Valois* (Paris, 1589), 3–15; and *Discours de Préparations faictes par frere Iacques Clement, religieux de l'ordre de S. Dominicque, pour delivrer la France de Henry de Valois, lequel fust tue à S. Cloud à Paris, le premier iour d'Aoust, 1589* (Lyon, 1589), 3–15.

83 *Discours de la Guerre Civile et Mort Tres-Regrettee de Henry III, Roy de France et de Polongne* (Tours, 1590), 9.

Key works

Boucher, Jacqueline, *La cour de Henri III* (Rennes: Persée, 1986).

Knecht, Robert, J., *Hero or Tyrant: Henry III, King of France, 1574–1589* (Farnham: Ashgate, 2014).

Le Roux, Nicolas, *Un régicide au nom de Dieu* (Paris: Gallimard, 2006).

Levin, Carole, *The Heart and Stomach of a King: Elizabeth I and the Politics of Sex and Power* (Philadelphia: Pennsylvania University Press, 1994, second edition 2013).

Strong, Roy, *The Cult of Elizabeth: Elizabethan Portraiture and Pageantry* (London: Pimlico, 1999).

17

CHASING ST LOUIS

The English monarchy's pursuit of sainthood

Anna M. Duch

During the High Middle Ages, the concept of *beata stirps* (holy stock or roots) came to prominence in royal and noble families throughout Europe. It was believed that a tendency towards sanctity could be transmitted through bloodlines, much like royal power. Being of *beata stirps*, preferably with papally authorized canonizations, was desirable, as it enhanced the reputation of one's family. Perhaps the best-known example of this in effect was the later reign of Philippe IV of France (r.1285–1314). After the canonization of Louis IX (r.1226–70) in 1297 by Pope Boniface VIII (r.1295–1303), Philippe's power escalated over both Church and State within France, climaxing with the Templar trials and having the long-term effect of creating an increasingly conciliatory Papacy.[1]

At first glance, the French influence on the papacy could explain why there were no medieval English royal saints created after Edward the Confessor (r.1046–66, canonized 1161), despite several campaigns during the thirteenth, fourteenth and fifteenth centuries. Indeed, as André Vauchez observes, the Papacy created only one English saint during its time in Avignon (1309–78): Bishop Thomas Cantilupe in 1320.[2] However, this is an oversimplification of a more complicated world. In order to address some of the complexities of dynastic sanctity, this chapter will first argue that the desirable features of a royal saint and the purview of papal authority had changed between the canonizations of Edward the Confessor and of St Louis and also after the canonization of St Louis. Second, the candidates for English sainthood and their respective failures will be assessed in their English context. Third, it will be argued that, although prior historiography is correct that political strife within England was detrimental in achieving papal canonization, other features of English culture also affected the viability of saintly causes, especially when compared to continental use of saints and *beata stirps*.

Certain parameters must be applied to this study. First, the saints considered here are limited to those who were officially canonized by the Papacy, their cult recognized as legitimate. Papal reforms of the twelfth and thirteenth centuries resulted in a more rigorous and critical process in determining sanctity, which also made receiving such recognition a particularly enviable prize. Second, this chapter will address only saints that were canonized prior to the English Reformation. While this may seem obvious, some medieval saints were not canonized until after the Reformation or even the twentieth century. Considering their papal canonization as a medieval achievement would be an anachronism.

Who and what made a medieval royal saint?

Gábor Klaniczay has identified the two major archetypes of a royal saint during the twelfth century: either 'an intrepid, victorious knight' or 'a chaste, ascetic prince, striving for moral perfection and committed to the service of the Church'.[3] Both types of ruler would have undermined common images of a good secular king. The fighting knight may have had a shortened lifespan or destabilized kingdom, while the chaste prince may have been disinclined towards producing dynastic heirs. The *vitae* of Edward the Confessor, the last Anglo-Saxon king of England, state that he maintained his virginity for the sake of the kingdom and its well-being.[4] Upon his death in 1066, however, the kingdom of England was the subject of multiple attempted conquests. At the time, it was common for bishops to declare local saints independently and only seek Church-wide recognition through formal canonization by the pope later – such was the case for Edward.[5]

Pope Gregory VII (r.1073–85) had delineated royal power from sacred power, arguing that being of noble blood did not grant sanctity by default.[6] Pope Alexander III's (r.1159–81) canonization of royal saints, including the chaste Edward the Confessor of England and the warrior-saints Olaf of Norway in 1164 and Canute Lavard of Denmark in 1170, may suggest a reversal in policy.[7] However, Vauchez frames the events in the assertion of the papal privilege to actively control the cult of saints.[8] The processes of centralizing papal power and carefully moulding the shape of royal sainthood continued during the thirteenth century. Through reforms by Pope Innocent III (r.1198–1216), the process of canonization was to be under the direct supervision of the Holy See and required the *verbatim* testimonies of witnesses, information pertaining to the life, miracles, character and overall reputation of the candidate.[9] The number of submitted causes for sainthood dramatically declined.

The composition of a royal saint changed due to these reforms. In general, male saints represent a vast majority of saints papally canonized.[10] Rodney Stark has suggested that this was due to the lack of female access to church offices and to education.[11] Upon removing popes, academics and post-medieval figures from his list of saints, Stark found that 30.2% of the remaining saints were female, of which 42.5% were from royal families. In contrast, only 13.1% of male saints were from royal families.[12] Prior to the thirteenth century, most saintly ruling men fit into either the mould of chivalrous warrior or chaste prince. However, with the more demanding requirements for forming a cause for canonization, a death in battle or childlessness could not be entered as *prima facie* evidence.

The proliferation of female royal saints came mostly from central Europe and Scandinavia and centred on women who practised asceticism, an outright rejection of their intended role in the world.[13] While some of these women had been mothers prior to joining an order (and thus contributors to a dynasty), the cloistered and virginal were still able to grant their families some prestige by expressing – proving – that sanctity was present in the family line. Klaniczay considers the rise of the holy princesses as catering to both popular religious sentiments and diplomatic and dynastic needs, but observes that this phenomenon 'was less likely to subordinate the cult of saints . . . to political goals'.[14] By the thirteenth century, it was more prudent to canonize women than their active, ruling male counterparts.

Thus, in the context of papal authority and the changing face of a royal saint, the canonization of Louis IX in 1297 was an aberration. As noted by Klaniczay, St Louis' canonization was a twenty-seven-year struggle. Though he arguably fit both the chaste prince (faithful to his queen) and the chivalric warrior (a crusader) paradigms of the eleventh and twelfth centuries, the Papacy's preferred traits had changed during the thirteenth century to favour non-regnant and religious members of a dynasty.[15] Once it was achieved, the canonization was a turning point in the feud between Philippe IV of France and Pope Boniface VIII.[16]

A brief summary of the dispute follows. Boniface VIII issued the papal bull *Clericis Laicos* on 24 February 1296, which threatened the French and English crowns with excommunication for taxing clergy without consultation or papal permission.[17] Philippe IV's response to the bull was to stop sending money to Rome altogether.[18] Boniface angrily responded in the further papal bull *Inefabilis Amoris* on 20 September 1296.[19] M.C. Gaposchkin has argued that with this bull, Boniface VIII began a campaign of critique against Philippe IV by contrasting him with his grandfather, Louis IX.[20] By this stage, the process for Louis' canonization had stalled several times due to the deaths of the popes and investigators involved with the cause.[21] The invocation of Louis can be viewed as a veiled threat against the completion of the process.

However, in 1297, Boniface VIII and Philippe IV were reconciled, cemented by the issuance of two bulls, *Etsi De Statu* (which provided an exception to *Clericis Laicos* to Philippe and his line) and the canonization bull for Louis IX.[22] Unsurprisingly, Philippe seized upon the political advantage immediately, ignoring any sort of criticism from Boniface.[23] The dispute between Philippe and Boniface would resume after a brief respite, and this culminated in Boniface's assault at Anagni in 1303 and his death five weeks thereafter.[24] The significance of Boniface's death to the medieval public may have been built up in retrospect.[25] However, the intimidation factor probably was not lost on the Curia nor on Boniface's successors. In his measured assessment, P.N.R. Zutshi states that there was a beneficial, reciprocal relationship between the Avignon papacy and the French crown, but the Papacy was, in general, more willing to appease secular powers than in prior times.[26]

In terms of saintly causes from royal houses, the impact of Louis IX's canonization was significant. After 1297, only the French or one of their affiliates, the Angevins of Sicily and the Hungarians, were successful in attaining a canonization, none of them regnant kings.[27] The more politically safe choices of non-regnant or religious family members were preferred. Before hastily concluding that a successful royal English cause for sainthood was impossible, each of the potential candidates must be assessed based upon his own merits and his own shortcomings and placed in an English context before extending into the wider, western European world.

The English candidates

The first candidate for sainthood was Henry III (r.1216–72), Louis IX's contemporary and brother-in-law. Whether Henry III was ever formally proposed for sainthood has always been questionable. There is no evidence that there was a unified, conscious effort of having him canonized. The minimal chronicle references to Henry's supposed sanctity suggest some clerical enthusiasm, but there was no overt action by Edward I (r.1272–1307), Henry's son and successor, to push the cause forward.

Within the first ten years of his death, miracles seemed to happen at Henry's tomb, following the pattern of reports after Louis IX's interment. Two chronicle reports are brief and undetailed, the nature of the miracles unmentioned.[28] In 1281, a man claimed to have had his sight restored by visiting Henry III's tomb, and he approached Henry's widow, Eleanor of Provence. Edward I, their son, quickly intervened and angrily drove out the intruder, believing this to be an attempt to defraud his mother.[29] In 1290, Henry III's body was moved from its temporary resting place in the former tomb of Edward the Confessor in Westminster Abbey to a permanent tomb to the north of the Confessor's Shrine. The Bury St Edmunds Chronicler simply reports that Edward I moved Henry in the dead of night.[30] D.A. Carpenter and W.C. Jordan accept that the cult was promoted but failed.[31] Carpenter has noted that seven bishops between 1276 and 1287 had issued indulgences for those who visited Henry's tomb, but there seems to have been little to no royal support or popular support.[32] The lack of other documentary evidence and Edward I's reactions suggest that any motion to promote Henry's cause was primarily in the ecclesiastical realm.

In 1328 or 1329, John de Stratford, bishop of Winchester, issued an indulgence for those visiting Westminster Abbey, specifically if they made an offering or prayed at the tomb of Henry III.[33] The indulgence is actually about Edward II (r.1307–27) or, more accurately, the effort to stunt his cult. Edward II had been deposed in January 1327, and his son, Edward III (r.1327–77) was crowned. In September 1327, Edward II died at Berkeley Castle and was interred at Gloucester in December 1327. Regents Queen Isabella and Roger Mortimer had deliberately chosen the site and paid for the body's transport to keep it far from London and the political scene.[34] However, as their regime faltered, Edward II became the focus of a political cult.[35]

A two-pronged effort was employed to thwart the cult's popularity. First, it is suggested that Bishop Stratford, who had been part of the committee that persuaded Edward II to abdicate, issued the abovementioned indulgence to draw pilgrims away from Gloucester and bring them to Westminster. Second, Isabella and Mortimer attempted to manipulate the local cult of Thomas of Lancaster, personal and political rival of his first cousin, Edward II.[36] Edward II had executed Thomas in 1322, and stories began to circulate that miracles happened at Thomas' grave. These stories were resurrected, and the regency wrote to the pope in support of Thomas' official canonization at least three times.[37] Edward II's cult arose partly in pity for him and partly in dissatisfaction with Isabella and Mortimer.[38] Contemporary attitudes expressed in the chronicle at Melsa and in the *Polychronicon* acknowledge these motivations, and despite *in vulgo* rumours, no specific miracles were linked to Edward II.[39] Popularity of both cults died down once the kingdom stabilized.

Richard II (r.1377–99), grandson of Edward III, became interested in the cult of Edward II early on in his reign. This was not out of character, due to his devout religious observances as well as his assertion of the royal prerogative, and he petitioned Urban VI for Edward's canonization in 1385.[40] In 1389, Boniface IX requested an investigation of Edward II's miracles, in order for the canonization to proceed.[41] This suggests that in the wake of the Merciless Parliament, which compromised the king's personal authority and prestige, Richard had renewed the 1385 request.

The Westminster Chronicler reports that Richard II met with Archbishop William Courtenay of Canterbury and Bishop Robert Braybrooke at Gloucester to discuss 'whether the miracles [were] genuine or fictitious'.[42] Having decided that the cause was legitimate, a book of miracles was compiled and sent off to Rome. Richard would pursue this cause for the rest of his life. Unfortunately, the book has been lost, the content unknown.[43]

The pursuit of sainthood for Edward II would become increasingly political as Richard II's reign progressed. Chris Given-Wilson has rightly argued that after 1397, the desire for canonization was fuelled by both vindication for Edward II and the desire to acquire Lancastrian lands by reversing the return of Thomas of Lancaster's inheritance to his heirs in 1326–7.[44] The current duke of Lancaster, John of Gaunt, was among the richest men in England, and rumours had swirled around his ambitions and the royal succession.[45] At Gaunt's death in February 1399, Richard II disinherited Gaunt's son, Henry, which led to Henry's invasion in September 1399 and ultimately to Richard's deposition and the end of Edward II's cause for sainthood.[46] The new regime promoted the cult of Thomas of Lancaster but with no formal success.[47]

Henry VI (r.1422–61, 1470–1) represented the best – possibly the only – chance of the medieval English monarchy attaining a saint. Becoming king of England and France before he was a year old, Henry VI was necessarily promoted as a promised child, the pinnacle of both England and France, as he descended from St Louis from both parents (through his father Henry V via Isabella of France, Edward III's mother, and through his mother Catherine of Valois, Princess of France).[48] His coronation at Westminster in 1429 reflected this, right down to the 'subtleties', or heavily decorated pastries. The first course's selection depicted him as supported by Edward the Confessor and St Louis.[49] Henry VI's own psalter depicted his presentations to the Madonna by St Louis and by St Catherine of Alexandria, who was supposedly a princess (Figures 17.1 and 17.2).[50]

Public perception of Henry VI as a potential saint did not manifest until his death and funeral in 1471. The deceased Henry was paraded with an open visage, and according to *Warkworth's Chronicle*, the coffin leaked blood on the ground once at St Paul's and once at Blackfriars.[51] Bleeding after death was considered a sign of a martyr, and Henry VI quickly acquired a religious following.[52] Henry VI's exequies also were thought to be pitiful by contemporaries.[53] Events that suggested piety and inspired pity were potent ingredients for an anti-Yorkist political cult. Within a year, shrines appeared in honour of Holy King Henry at Ripon, Durham and York. On 12 July 1473, Edward IV (r.1461–70, 1471–83) issued a proclamation stating that anyone going on pilgrimage needed to have letters of permission with an itinerary sealed with the Great Seal.[54] Brian Spencer believes the main cause for the letter may have been the meteoric rise of the Henry VI cult and the flow of pilgrims to Chertsey.[55] During the reign of Edward IV, Holy King Henry's cult had low chances of long-term success due to its political overtones.

Unlike Edward IV, Richard III (r.1483–5) did not implement any laws or discourage the cult of Henry VI. Rather, he seemed to hope it would die out on its own, and it appears that he tried to help this along by erecting a tomb fit for a king, not a shrine. British Library Additional MS 6298, f. 148, depicts a tomb box with a recumbent tomb effigy, all made of alabaster (see Figure 17.3).

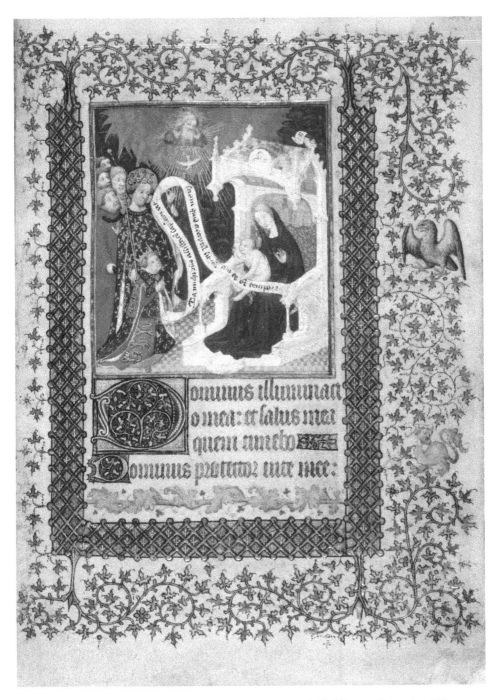

Figure 17.1 St Louis presenting Henry VI to the Virgin, British Library, Cottonian MS
Domitian A xvii, f.50

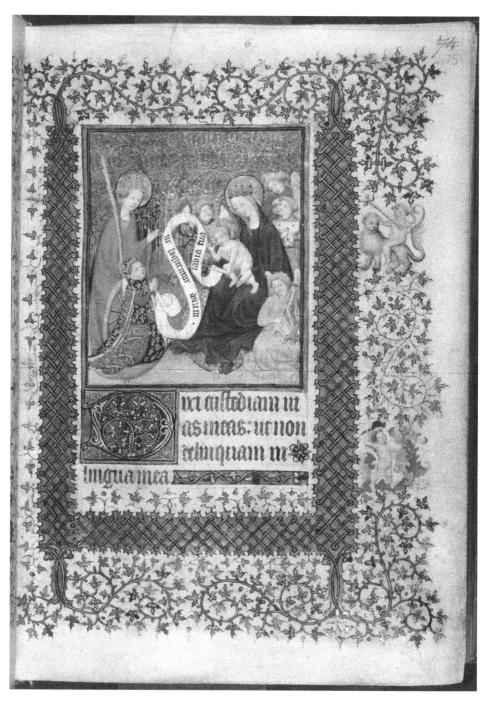

Figure 17.2 St Catherine presenting Henry VI to the Virgin, British Library, Cottonian MS
Domitian A xvii, f. 75r

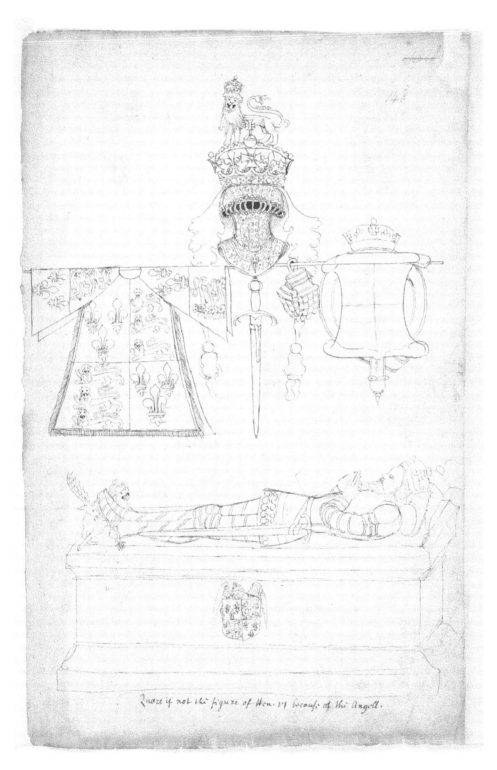

Figure 17.3 Presumed to be design for Henry VI's tomb at Windsor, British Library, Additional MS 6298, f. 148,

The tomb shows a bearded king surrounded by various symbols of monarchy, such as his various coats of arms, lions at his feet and angels about his crowned head. Based upon the labelling in the manuscript and the tomb's appearance, this was likely a depiction of Henry VI's tomb in Windsor, as erected by Richard III after he moved the royal body in 1484.[56] By representing Henry VI as a king of England, the Yorkist king Richard III had attempted to reconcile with remaining Lancastrian partisans and to draw attention away from the spectre of Holy King Henry. It was better to have Henry as a dead political rival than as a martyr at the hands of Edward IV.

Regardless of what stood in Windsor, people still claimed that miracles occurred, the most effective fuel for any saint's cult. Unlike Henry III and Edward II, specific accounts of the miracles of Henry VI survive. John Blacman, Henry's sometime confessor, completed his hagiographic *Henry the Sixth* prior to the victory of Henry VII at Bosworth in 1485.[57] How much circulation it had prior to Henry VII's canonization campaign in the 1490s is uncertain.[58] A four-volume collection of *miracula*, BL Royal MS 13 C VIII, survived the Reformation.[59] The miracles include a variety of interventions, but Henry appears to have had a specialization in healing or rescuing those in immediate, unexpected danger.[60] In the wake of a civil war, this was a powerful, useful, and comforting saintly attribute. Leigh Ann Craig has argued that Henry VI's devotees were more than political creatures. They were sincere and diverse because of Henry's range as a saintly helper.[61]

Because of this popular and ecclesiastical support, the aspirations of Henry VII (r.1485–1509) for his uncle's canonization were not necessarily in vain. As noted by Bertram Wolffe, the problem remained as to whether Henry VI's virtues outweighed his shortcomings.[62] Henry was popularly claimed to have been good-natured in life, had a sorrowful death and performed charitable miracles. However, it was questionable whether this all could counterbalance his bad rule and his known mental health issues. Even Louis IX's cause foundered at times, despite fitting into multiple earlier paradigms of sainthood with no notable problems.

Work began in 1498 to move Henry VI from Windsor to Westminster Abbey, where he would lie in Henry VII's Lady Chapel in a shrine, not far from the intended tomb site of Henry VII and Elizabeth of York.[63] Though Henry VII attested to these continued desires in his 1509 will, his son did not share such sentiments.[64] Several times, Henry VIII altered his father's plans for the Chapel, and ultimately, rather than placing the elaborate Torrigiano tomb in front of the high altar of the new Lady Chapel, it was positioned where the shrine to Henry VI should have been, behind the high altar.[65] The eastern-most area of the church was commonly reserved for saints' shrines, as seen with the Confessor's Chapel in the main body of Westminster Abbey, the former shrine site of Becket at Canterbury Cathedral, and St Margaret's tomb before the Reformation and after post-Reformation alterations at Dunfermline.[66] As such, one can assume that Henry VIII had no interest in moving Henry VI from Windsor after 1512. The cult of Henry VI continued to flourish through the sixteenth century, and the cause was still being examined in Rome when the English Reformation occurred.[67] The time for a medieval English royal saint had passed, as England then had a church with the monarch as the Supreme Head. What need was there for a saintly relative? By 1611, Henry VI's tomb at Windsor, though not built as a saint's shrine, was dismantled, and his resting place lost for over 300 years.[68]

J.M. Theilmann has persuasively argued that saintly royal and baronial figures were raised in England as a means of establishing legitimacy on the political scene from the twelfth through to the fourteenth century, particularly during the reign of Richard II. In some ways, these saints represented efforts to compensate for a lack of actual power.[69] This concept was first discussed by J.C. Russell in his essay 'The Canonisation of Opposition to the King in Angevin England'. Popular saints such as Thomas Becket (d.1174), Simon de Montfort (d.1264) and Thomas of Lancaster appeared in opposition to the king's perceived injustice.[70] The saints were popular precisely because they resisted the Crown's authority. Both the cults of Edward II and Henry VI fit this template early on, as the royal 'St' Edward II and Holy King Henry had been raised in opposition to bad new royal governments. Edward II's cult dissipated once the situation had been resolved. While still alive, both Henry III and Edward II had opposition political cults raised against them, which likely compromised their own causes. Although Henry VI's cult persisted after the political conflict, it was eventually royal neglect and the English Reformation that rendered the issue null.

The English problems: the international front

The arguments of Theilmann and Russell, while well grounded, tend towards being insular, with the external influences of the continent not addressed. As stated in the first section, the establishment of papal privilege and the criteria for saints changed the process and qualities of saint-making. However, closer examination of each English cause in an international context, including that of Edward the Confessor, reveals that English culture had significant differences in mentality towards royal sainthood compared to the continent and the Papacy itself.

The first problem was the matter of producing relics. First-class relics are the divided body parts of saints or items directly affiliated with Jesus Christ or his mother Mary, which were believed, as early as the sixth century, to radiate holy power that could offer healing to eager pilgrims. Second-class relics include physical items that came into direct contact with the saint – not as potent or valuable. Much like the cult of saints, by the thirteenth century, relics needed to be regulated due to their popularity and the tendency to declare any found bone a saintly by-product.[71] Saints' shrines in churches attracted pilgrims' devotion and their money.[72] The disarticulation of saints' bodies presented a problem to English royal funerary practices. By the fourteenth century, the process for preparing an English king's body for burial was committed to parchment, appearing in the *Liber Regalis* (*c.*1380) at Westminster Abbey, the *Liber Regie Capelle* (*c.*1449) and other later royal regulatory texts, and its application was extended to the nobility at the time of Henry VII. This written description, titled *De Exequiis Regalibus*, indicates that the viscera be removed and the brain somehow dealt with. Then, the person of status was to be dressed and presented as he would have appeared in life, right down to the footwear.[73] Full-body preservation was required, and as far as the records suggest, all post-Conquest English kings were interred in their entirety, save for the viscera.[74]

This is consistent with the treatment of Edward the Confessor's remains, as recorded by Osbert of Clare. In 1102, the Confessor's tomb was opened, and his body was found to be incorrupt. The preservation of a body during the Middle Ages, particularly years after its demise, tended to be viewed as a sign of sanctity.[75] The bishop of Rochester attempted to pluck out a hair from the Confessor's beard. He was severely upbraided for such a transgression. Instead, Edward's crown and sceptre were removed.[76] In 1163, only a ring and cloth were taken from the Confessor's tomb.[77] Similarly, when Henry III was moved to his current tomb in 1290, a London chronicler made it a point to mention that Henry was well preserved, and his beard was intact.[78] While incorruptibility was considered a sign of sanctity, no potential relics were reported to be taken from the king's coffin, which argues against a religious cult. The dearth of relics would have severely reduced the appeal of a cult and challenged its long-term viability.

In contrast, other European monarchies and courts did not demand an intact body post-mortem. The French were particularly enthusiastic about distributing their body parts across multiple churches. Due to his death abroad, Louis IX had been excarnated, the flesh interred in Tunis, the innards taken by his brother Charles of Anjou for burial in Sicily, and the bones forwarded to Saint-Denis for burial.[79] The head was later separated and taken to the Sainte-Chapelle.[80] In Hungary, there were no qualms about splitting up a royal saintly body. During the conquest of Croatia, the Hungarians installed the head reliquary of St Stephen in Zagreb.[81] When her remains were moved in 1236, the head of St Elizabeth of Hungary (princess and Landgravine of Thuringia, 1207–31) was crowned in its own reliquary.[82] This raises the point that more presentable body parts (bones, fingers, toes, heads, etc.) were desirable for display as venerable relics. The English royal house, though it removed internal organs, had a set tradition of preserving and maintaining the integrity of the external aspect of the king's body, even that of the Confessor.

A second problem is tied to the political tendency of popular English saints: support tended to be situational or temporary. D.A Carpenter once summed up the differences between Louis IX of France and his brother-in-law, Henry III of England: 'Above all, Louis was far more successful as a king.' However, the following sentence provides an inaccurate qualifier: 'He was made a saint, and Henry was not.'[83] Sainthood can only be attained after death, so judging Henry III's success as a king by whether he was made a saint puts an unfair burden on his corpse. He had no control over the process of canonization or the activities of his successors to procure this. This also ignores the extensive efforts of the living to attain canonization, as well as the tangible benefits to their descendants. The cause for Louis' canonization was sustained over the course of nearly thirty years. No English royal candidate received such consistent support. There were also potential disadvantages for claiming good kingship as a qualifying factor for sainthood. As discussed by Gaposchkin, not only did Philippe IV use St Louis to promote his political agenda, but Boniface VIII weaponized Louis' good rulership to criticize Philippe's shortcomings.[84] The investment of time and money and potential risks may have been discouraging factors for the English crown, especially considering the domestic situation.

Out of the English political 'saints' described by Russell and Theilmann, only Becket was papally canonized, and he was a churchman. Saints with ecclesiastical backgrounds were always beneficial to the prestige of the Church itself, even in awkward situations. Thomas Cantilupe, bishop of Hereford, was canonized in 1320 despite, at one point, being excommunicated by the Archbishop of Canterbury, John Pecham.[85] However, Cantilupe had universal support from the populace, his ecclesiastical successors at Hereford, and both Edward I and Edward II. This perfect storm of endorsements rarely manifested for any figure in England. Popular political saints opposed the government, and no amount of ecclesiastical support could induce the Papacy to risk being on the wrong side of the conflict. The Church could risk a little internal conflict, as seen in the case of Cantilupe, but breeding enmity between the ecclesiastical and temporal or the popular and royal was wholly imprudent.[86]

That said, the very canonization of Edward the Confessor was a political manoeuvre: it was an expression of gratitude by a pope under threat. Alexander III's election in 1159 had been contested by Emperor Frederick Barbarossa of the Holy Roman Empire. At the same time, Henry II of England (r.1154–89) desired further consolidation of his claim to the English throne, as he had become king after a lengthy succession crisis. By supporting Alexander III's election, Henry received the Church's support in return through two papal bulls, issued on 7 February 1161, which canonized Edward the Confessor and added him to the Calendar of Saints.[87] B.W Scholz concludes that Henry II had lent himself to the cause for the canonization of Edward the Confessor in order to provide his line of inheritance with 'the halo of an inherent sanctity'.[88]

The canonization of the Confessor was not the only route to this assertion of legitimacy. Henry's mother, Matilda, was a descendant of Margaret of Scotland, great-granddaughter of Edmund Ironside, half-brother to Edward Confessor. In her own lifetime, Margaret's holiness was recognized, partly by relation to the Confessor, and her canonization in 1250 remarked upon this.[89] However, Henry II made the choice to rely primarily upon the alleged political nomination rather than the transmitted holiness through Edward and Margaret. By the legitimacy and sanctity of Edward the Confessor, his chosen successors, William the Conqueror and his descendants, were incontestable kings.

This was perhaps the greatest detractor to English royal causes, as it emphasized political choice over the transmission of holiness and saintly characteristics. St Louis, on the other hand, gave political legitimacy, but he transmitted a certain standard of behaviour to worthy kings, as demonstrated by Boniface VIII's criticism of Philippe IV.[90] English kings could not imitate Edward the Confessor as holistically as the French kings could St Louis. The Confessor was a king of chastity and peace, not a man with heirs who went on a crusade.[91]

The continental powers also built up their *beata stirps* by having multiple, lower ranking members of the family canonized, not just kings regnant or queens consort. The diverse portfolio of saints in the royal families of France, Hungary and Angevin Sicily was a long-term investment, as it made their causes more plausible to the Papacy. Charles Robert, king of Hungary (r.1301/8–42) was able to claim his throne through an appeal to his *beata stirps*. On his paternal side, Charles Robert was the grandson of Charles II of Naples and the great-nephew of St Louis of Toulouse (bishop of Toulouse, canonized 1317). The uncle to both Charles II and St Louis of Toulouse was St Louis of France. Through Charles Robert's paternal grandmother, Maria of Hungary, his great-great-grandfather was the brother of St Elizabeth of Hungary (mentioned above and canonized 1235), and St Elizabeth's maternal aunt was St Hedwig of Andechs (canonized 1267). It was through this network of canonized saints that Charles Robert gained support (see Figure 17.4).[92]

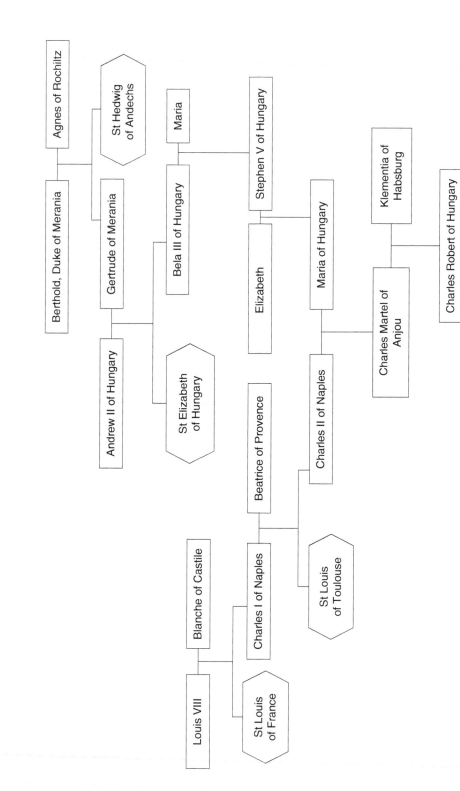

Figure 17.4 Genealogy of Charles Robert

The English royal house did not attempt to create a familial network of saints. Rather, in the fourteenth century, it turned its attention to St George, a Greek soldier-saint whose popularity had spiked during the Crusades.[93] As D.A.L. Morgan and W.M. Ormrod identify, this was partly due to the upbringing of Edward III. He was taught to appreciate both his Plantagenet and Capetian heritages and their devotions to various saints, including St George.[94] His mother's Hungarian cousin, the aforementioned Charles Robert, founded the Order of St George *c.*1326–7. After Edward III's triumphant return from France in 1347, he began a programme that promoted St George's support of England and the protection of the royal family, culminating in the foundation of the Order of the Garter.[95] The use of St George during the Hundred Years' War by both Edward III and Henry V offered a devotional focus for military achievement and chivalric practice that Edward the Confessor could not provide.[96] The lack of bloodline connection or any attempt to make such a connection suggests that the English royal house had different values and uses for their saints compared to the continent.

The early dialogue of the Hundred Years' War reflects these cultural differences. After the deaths of all of Philippe IV's son, the French crown passed to Philippe VI in 1328, a nephew of Philippe IV, due to the Salic law; this passed over Edward III of England, who was a grandson of Philippe IV through his mother, Isabella of France. Edward III argued against this, citing his political authority as a descendant of St Louis in 1340 and swearing to uphold St Louis' laws.[97] This apparently earned him the mocking nickname 'Edward Louis' on the continent, as seen in *The Vows of the Heron*, a French satirical poem.[98] What is most striking is that Edward III appealed to political authority, not his own *beata stirps*. Instead of affiliating himself with saintly characteristics of St Louis, he attempted to use Louis IX as his English progenitors had used Edward the Confessor: the claim to the throne was all about political legitimacy. In contrast, from the beginning of his reign, Philippe VI had made sure to emulate St Louis' behaviour and emphasize his connections to him by the wording of his legislation, minting coins like St Louis had, and attempting to go on crusade in 1336.[99] Though Edward owned relics of the Confessor and other Anglo-Saxon saints, he did not refer to Edward the Confessor or signal he would follow a saintly role model.[100] One may suggest that Edward's formulation of his claim to the French throne failed to appeal to French audiences because of how he couched his relationship with St Louis.

Although Edward III had pursued the French crown along traditional, English lines of political legitimacy, his grandson, Richard II, showed some awareness of the continent's appreciation of *beata stirps*. Richard first petitioned Urban VI for Edward II's canonization in 1385. His wife, Anne of Bohemia, was a descendant of Ludmilla the protomartyr of Bohemia and Good King Wenceslas, and she had dynastic connections to the blessed Agnes of Bohemia, who had died in 1282. Thanks to Agnes' parentage, Agnes was first cousin to St Elizabeth of Hungary (and thus connected to St. Hedwig). The popular Abbess Kunigunde (d.1321, never papally canonized) was Agnes' great niece and the sister of Anne's great grandfather.[101] Richard would have been well aware of his wife's heritage, and it would have been fitting for his to somehow match (see see Figure 17.5). A letter from Anne to her brother Wenceslas in 1384 indicates the couple were trying to conceive.[102] If Richard had been successful in having Edward II canonized, the resulting child would have come from *beata stirps* on both sides, a highly desirable feature on the continent. If we must ascribe some of Richard's actions to French influence, then the model of Capetian sanctity and legitimacy via saintly networks would be appropriate here. However, Richard II never had children by his wife Anne nor by his second wife, Isabella of France, another princess coming from an established saintly line.

Edward the Confessor was still needed by the king of England. On 8 May 1389, Richard II issued letters patent for the creation of vestments for Westminster Abbey for use on the Feast of St Edward the Confessor, as the Confessor was to be honoured as Richard's predecessor from thereon.[103] The immediate context of this order pertains to the compromise of Richard's power and dignity during the Merciless Parliament. Richard needed the Confessor's historical legitimacy, first utilized by Henry II, in order to stabilize his kingship. The fact that Richard wished to be a king of peace, as well as his lack of children, only amplified his relationship with the Confessor.[104] Likewise, Anne's father, Charles IV, Holy Roman Emperor and king of Bohemia, had actively pursued connections to the image of the Bohemian royal saint, Wenceslas, as his claim to the Bohemian crown came through the female line. The royal saint was used to bolster his legitimacy to the end of his life in 1378, but Charles IV also found Wenceslas to be appealing due to their familial connections.[105] Richard was both traditional and innovative by maintaining the political legitimacy of the Confessor, yet also pursuing *beata stirps* through Edward II and through his marriages, though these efforts failed.

In an international context, the cause of Henry VI was still viable. Although he had been buried intact, there were second-class relics, such as his hat, a pillow and even several different weapons proclaimed to be instruments of his martyrdom. As mentioned earlier, he was of Louis IX's bloodline, though proclaiming this king a saint did not have the same downsides as the canonization of Louis IX. Henry VI had no direct descendants, as Henry VII was a nephew through a half-brother, Edmund Tudor. The Papacy's canonization of Henry VI would have resulted in a somewhat 'safe' status of *beata stirps* for Henry VII, providing some defence for his legitimacy while not threatening papal power over the new English king. Yet, aside from the inclusion of St Louis in a commissioned dynastic stained glass window at Greenwich and his will's mention of Catherine of Valois's final resting place within Westminster Abbey, there are no signs that Henry VII gave significant thought to using the argument of *beata stirps*, both for the cause of Henry VI or as a rallying point for his own legitimacy.[106] In the broader family, although the English monarchy did have princesses and widowed queens in convents and half-siblings of the king as bishops, there is no evidence that any of them were considered to be saintly by the clergy or by their natal families.[107] Because the English monarchy so valued the political appointment by the Confessor, they did not work with the concept of *beata stirps*, which was a critical, favourable factor in considering continental causes. Without counterweight, royal English causes were not as likely to succeed.

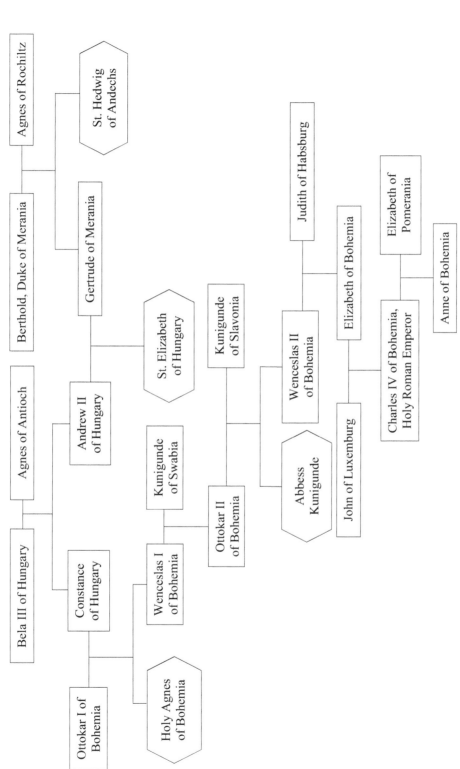

Figure 17.5 Genealogy of Anne of Bohemia

Conclusions

As established by Russell and Theilmann, problems within England detracted from the kingdom's saintly causes, particularly since the English people tended to support saints that died in opposition to the crown. This chapter has shown that there were other internal and external factors that were detrimental to the success of causes in Rome. Continental powers cultivated saintly networks through these family members, substantiating claims of *beata stirps*. However, being of *beata stirps* was not critical evidence of political legitimacy in England. Rather, being a successor of the Confessor was most relevant. While the Hungarian monarchy could draw upon their saintly cousins in France and the Angevins could draw upon the holy women of Hungary, the English monarchy did not assert these connections, possibly to the impairment of their saintly causes. What mattered in Rome did not necessarily matter in England. The Confessor was used as a political reference, not a template, for a pious English king. The popular desire for relics ran against the tradition of maintaining the English royal corpse *in toto*. The lack of unanimity among the royal house, the ecclesiastics and the populace made canonization a political risk to the Papacy, which already was subject to heavy pressure from the French monarchy during the fourteenth century. After the fall-out from Louis IX's canonization, the Papacy had every right to be cautious of canonizing a leader within living memory or to cater to the desires of a direct, bloodline descendant. Two kings, Edward III by his parentage and Richard II by his marriages, were positioned to access the continental saintly network to enhance their statuses, but this was ultimately untapped. In the case of Henry VI, although identified from the beginning of his nominal reign as a descendant of St Louis through both his parents and the political heir of Edward the Confessor, his troubled life and reign caused hesitation in Rome, and Henry VII did not pursue the *beata stirps* line of argument. After the death of Henry VII, Henry VIII tacitly declined to exert effort in the matter, and Henry VI's cause was never concluded due to the English church breaking away from Rome in 1532. Once again, the consistent support of consecutive kings did not materialize. The medieval causes for the papal canonization of English royal saints failed because of these varied and vital cultural factors. The English crown would only gain a saint in 1660, when the Convocations of Canterbury and York elevated Charles I as 'Blessed King Charles the Martyr' in the Church of England.[108] The pope, however, was not consulted.

Notes

1 J. Théry, "A Heresy of State: Philip the Fair, the Trial of the 'Perfidious Templars,' and the Pontificalization of the French Monarchy," *Journal of Medieval Religious Cultures* 39, no. 2 (2013): 117–148. While the proposed level of absolute power achieved is debatable, the article does capture the aspirations and logical conclusions.

2 A. Vauchez, *Sainthood in the Later Middle Ages*, trans. J. Birrell (New York: Cambridge University Press, 1997), 78.

3 G. Klaniczay, *Holy Rulers and Blessed Princesses: Dynastic Cults in Medieval Central Europe*, trans. E. Palmai (New York: Cambridge University Press, 2000), 295.

4 P. Cullum, "'Give Me Chastity': Masculinity and Attitudes to Chastity and Celibacy in the Middle Ages," *Gender and History* 25, no. 3 (November 2013): 626–627.

5 Vauchez, *Sainthood in the Later Middle Ages*, 22–30.

6 Ibid., 165–166.

7 J. Lindow, "St Olaf and the Skalds," in *Sanctity in North: Saints, Lives, and Cults in Medieval Scandinavia*, ed. T. DuBois (Toronto: University of Toronto Press, 2008), 105–106.

8 Vauchez, *Sainthood in the Later Middle Ages*, 24–25.

9 Ibid., 38.

10 A. Vauchez, "Between Virginity and Spiritual Espousals: Models of Feminine Sainthood in the Christian West in the Middle Ages," *The Medieval History Journal* 2, no. 2 (1999): 349–350, places this number at less than 10%, while Stark (see note below) places it at closer to 17.5%.

11 R. Stark, "Upper Class Asceticism Social Origins of Ascetic Movements and Medieval Saints," *Review of Religious Research* 45, no. 1 (September 2003): 13.

12 Ibid., 14.

13 Vauchez, "Between Virginity and Spiritual Espousals," 355–356.

14 Klaniczay, *Holy Rulers, Blessed Princesses*, 295.

15 Ibid., 297.

16 B. Tierney, *The Crisis of Church and State with Selected Documents* (Englewood: Prentice Hall, Inc., 1980) 172–192. E.A.R. Brown, "Death and the Human Body in the Later Middle Ages: The Legislation of Boniface VIII on the Division of the Corpse," *Viator* 12 (1981): 221–270; E.A.R. Brown, "Authority, the Family, and the Dead in Late Medieval France," *French Historical Studies* 16, no. 4 (Autumn 1990): 803–832; M.C. Gaposchkin, "Boniface VIII, Philip the Fair, and the Sanctity of Louis IX," *Journal of Medieval History* 29, no. 1 (2003): 1–26; J.H. Denton, "Taxation and the Conflict between Philip the Fair and Boniface VIII," *French History* 11, no. 3 (1997): 241–244; and others.

17 G. Digard, M. Faucon and A. Thomas, eds., *Les Registres de Boniface VIII: Recueil Des Bulles de Ce Pape*, i (Paris: Librairie Des Écoles Française D'Athènes & De Rome, 1885), 583, no. 1567.

18 M.C. Gaposchkin, *The Making of St Louis: Kingship, Sanctity, and Crusade in the Later Middle Ages* (Ithaca: Cornell University Press, 2008), 50.

19 *Les Registres de Boniface VIII*, i, 614–619, no. 1653.

20 Gaposchkin, *The Making of St Louis*, 57–59.

21 Vauchez, *Sainthood in the Later Middle Ages*, 63, n. 7.

22 *Les Registres de Boniface VIII*, i, 941–942, no. 2354; 788, no. 2047.

23 Gaposchkin, *The Making of St Louis*, 63.

24 G. Martin, "Did Pope Boniface Die of a Subdural?" *Journal of Clinical Neuroscience* 8, no. 1 (2001): 8–9. A subdural haematoma is a more plausible cause of death than dying of shame.

25 T.F. Ruiz, "Reaction to Anagni," *The Catholic Historical Review* 65, no. 3 (July 1979): 385–401.

26 P.N.R. Zutshi, "The Avignon Papacy," in *The New Cambridge Medieval History*, vi, ed. M. Jones (Cambridge: Cambridge University Press, 2000), 658–659.

27 I. McCleery, "Isabel of Aragon (d.1336): Model Queen or Model Saint?" *The Journal of Ecclesiastical History* 57, no. 4 (October 2006): 677.

28 *Flores Historiarum*, iii, ed. H.R. Luard. RS 95 (London: 1890), 28; "A Continuation of William of Newburgh's History to AD 1298," in *Chronicles of the Reigns of Stephen, Henry II, and Richard I*, ii, ed. R. Howlett. RS 82 (London, 1885), 571.

29 W. Rishanger, "Chronica," in *Chronica Monasterii Sancti Albani*, ii, ed. H.T. Riley. RS 28 (London, 1865), 98.

30 *The Chronicle of Bury St Edmunds, 1212–1301*, ed. A. Gransden (London: Nelson, 1964), 94.

31 W.C. Jordan, *A Tale of Two Monasteries* (Princeton: Princeton University Press, 2009), 203–204; Carpenter, "Meetings," 28–29.

32 D.A. Carpenter, "King Henry III and the Cosmati Work at Westminster Abbey," in *The Cloister and the World: Essays in Medieval History in Honour of Barbara Harvey*, eds. J. Blair and B. Golding (Oxford: Clarendon Press, 1996), 194.

33 Westminster Abbey Muniments (WAM) 6672.

34 The National Archives (hereafter TNA), E 368/100, m. 8; TNA, E 101/383/1. See also S. Phillips, *Edward II* (New Haven: Yale University Press, 2010), 551–554 for details of the treatment of the body and its burial at Gloucester.

35 *Historia et cartularium Monasterii Sancti Petri Gloucestriae*, i, ed. W.H. Hart (London: Longman, Green, Longman, Roberts, and Green, 1863), 46. The cult may have been the spur for the great building project at Gloucester during the 1330s.

36 See J.R. Bray, "Concepts of Sainthood in Fourteenth Century England," *Bulletin of the John Rylands Library* 66 (1984): 51–55, for a summary of their enmity.

37 Phillips, *Edward II*, 600–601; J.M. Theilmann, "Political Canonization and Political Symbolism in Medieval England," *Journal of British Studies* 29, no. 3 (July 1990): 252.

38 Vauchez, *Sainthood in the Late Middle Ages*, 160; Bray, "Concepts of Sainthood," 60–61.

39 W.M. Ormrod, "The Personal Religion of Edward III," *Speculum* 64, no. 4 (October 1989): 870.

40 N. Saul, *Richard II* (New Haven: Yale University Press, 1997), 323.

41 Phillips, *Edward II*, 604.

42 *The Westminster Chronicle, 1381–1394*, eds. L.C. Hector and B.F. Harvey (Oxford: Clarendon Press, 1982), 436–439.

43 Phillips, *Edward II*, 605, n. 141.

44 C. Given-Wilson, "Richard II, Edward II, and the Lancastrian Inheritance," *English Historical Review* 109, no. 432 (June 1994): 570.

45 Saul, *Richard II*, 396–397, for the immediate context of this; see also M. Bennett, "Edward III's Entail and the Succession to the Crown, 1376–1471," *English Historical Review* 113, no. 452 (June 1998): 580–609 for further discussion of this.

46 Saul, *Richard II*, 403–404.

47 Phillips, *Edward II*, 605.

48 J.W. McKenna, "Henry VI of England the Dual Monarchy: Aspects of Royal Political Propaganda, 1422–1432," *Journal of the Warburg and Courtauld Institutes* 28 (1965): 151–155, with illustrations.

49 B. Wolffe, *Henry VI* (London: Eyre Methuen, 1981), 51–52.

50 British Library (hereafter BL), Cotton MS Domitian A VII, f. 50r., 75r.

51 *The Great Chronicle of London*, ed. A.H. Thomas and I.D. Thornley (London: George W. Jones at the Sign of the Dolphin, 1938), 220; T. Warkworth, "Warkworth's Chronicle: A Chronicle of the First Thirteen Years of the Reign of King Edward the Fourth," ed. J.O. Halliwell, in *Three Chronicles of the Reign of Edward IV* (Gloucester: Alan Sutton Publishing, 1988), 43.

52 E. Duffy, *Stripping the Altars: Traditional Religion of England, 1400–1580* (New Haven: Yale University Press, 1992), 161.

53 *The Great Chronicle of London*, 220; R. Fabyan, *The New Chronicles of England and France*, ed. Henry Ellis (London: F.C. and J. Rivington, et al., 1811), 662, express such sentiments.

54 *Calendar of Close Rolls, 1468–1476*, eds. W.H.B. Bird and K.H. Ledward (London: Her Majesty's Stationery Office, 1953), 299.

55 B. Spencer, "King Henry of Windsor and the London Pilgrim," in *Collectanea Londiniensia: Studies Presented to Ralph Merrifield*, eds. J. Bird, H. Chapman and J. Clark (London: London and Middlesex Archaeological Society, 1978), 240.

56 P. Lindley, "'The singular mediacions and prayers of the holie companie of Heven': Sculptural Functions and Forms in Henry VII's Chapel," in *Westminster Abbey: The Lady Chapel of Henry VII*, eds. T. Tatton-Brown and R. Mortimer (Woodbridge: Boydell Press, 2003), 266; C.R. Beard, "The Tomb and Achievements of King Henry VI at Windsor," in *Fragmenta Armamentaria, Volume II, Part 1*, ed. F.H.C. Day (Frome: Butler and Tanner, 1936), 17.

57 J. Blacman, *Henry the Sixth: A Reprint of John Blacman's Memoir with Translation and Notes*, ed. M.R. James (Cambridge: Cambridge: University Press, 1919).

58 Wolffe, *Henry VI*, 355–357.

59 *Henrici VI Angliae Regis Miracula Postuma: Ex Codice Musei Britannici Regio 13 C VIII*, ed. P. Grosjean (Brussels: Société des Bollandistes, 1935), 39, 45.

60 These included rescuing people from sudden accidents (falling 'devilish' weights of sand, housefires), stemming the flow of a broken wine cask, and resurrecting small children.

61 L.A. Craig, "Royalty, Virtue, and Adversity: The Cult of King Henry VI," *Albion* 35, no. 2 (Summer 2003): 208–209.

62 Wolffe, *Henry VI*, 4–7.

63 R. Griffiths, "Succession and the Royal Dead in Later Medieval England," in *Making and Breaking the Rules: Succession in Medieval Europe, c. 1000–c. 1600*, eds. F. Lachaud and M. Penman (Turnhout: Brepols, 2008), 108–109. See also *Calendar of Close Rolls 1500–1509*, ed. R.A. Latham (London: Her Majesty's Stationery, 1963), 138, no. 389, for Henry VII's extensive commemoration of his relatives and the planned removal of Henry VI from Windsor to Westminster Abbey, dated 1504.

64 TNA E 23/3.

65 M. Condon, "God Save the King! Piety, Propaganda and the Perpetual Memorial," in *Westminster Abbey: The Lady Chapel of Henry VII*, eds. T. Tatton-Brown and R. Mortimer (Woodbridge: Boydell Press, 2003), 60.

66 R. Bartlett, *Why Can the Dead Do Such Great Things?: Saints and Worshippers from the Martyrs to the Reformation* (Princeton: Princeton University Press, 2013), 253.

67 For the survival of the cult of Henry VI, see Spencer, "King Henry of Windsor and the London Pilgrim," 235–264.

68 Lindley "'The singular mediacions'," 266.

69 Theilmann, "Political Canonization and Political Symbolism," 241–266.

70 J.C. Russell, "The Canonization of Opposition to the King in Angevin England," in *Anniversary Essays in Mediaeval History by Students of Charles Homer Haskins*, ed. C.H. Taylor (Boston and New York: Houghton Mifflin, 1929), 280–285.

71 R.C. Finucane, *Miracles and Pilgrims: Popular Beliefs in Medieval England* (Totowa: Rowman and Littlefield, 1977), 26–31. Innocent III and council explicitly ruled about the verification, regulation and sale of relics in Canon 62 of the Fourth Lateran Council.

72 A.R. Bell and R.S. Dale, "The Medieval Pilgrimage Business," *Enterprise and Society* 12, no. 3 (2011): 601–627.

73 *Missale ad Usum Ecclesie Westmonasteriensis*, ii, ed. J.W. Legg. Henry Bradshaw Society 5 (Woodbridge: Boydell Press, 1999), col. 735; *Liber Regie Capelle*, ed. W. Ullman. Henry Bradshaw Society 92 (Woodbridge: Boydell Press, 2010), 112; *A Collection of Ordinances and Regulations for the Government of the Royal Household, Made in Diverse Reigns*, ed. J. Nichols (London: J. Nichols, 1790), 129–133.

74 P.D. Mitchell, H. Yeh, J. Appleby and R. Buckley, "The Intestinal Parasites of King Richard III," *The Lancet*, 382 (4 September 2013): 888. The presence of roundworms in the sacral area of Richard III's remains indicates that he was not eviscerated, a key element of embalming. The embalming process is extensively discussed in A.M. Duch, "The Royal Funerary and Burial Ceremonies of Medieval English Kings, 1216–1509" (PhD dissertation, University of York, 2016), chapter III.

75 P. Camporesi, *The Incorruptible Flesh: Bodily Mutilation and Mortification in Religion and Folklore* (New York: Cambridge University Press, 1983), 75, 155.

76 Frank Barlow, *Edward the Confessor* (Berkeley: University of California Press, 1984), 267–269.

77 Ibid., 282. It is worthwhile to consider that the high medieval English opposition to the post-mortem division of royal bodies springs from the shame that the action carried in the Anglo-Saxon period; see N .Marafioti, *The King's Body* (Toronto: University of Toronto Press, 2015).

78 "Annales Londoniensis," in *Chronicles of the Reigns of Edward I and Edward II*, i, ed. W. Stubbs. RS 76 (London: 1882), 98.

79 Brown, "Death and the Human Body," 231–232.

80 E.A.R. Brown, "Philippe le Bel and the Remains of Saint Louis," *Gazette Des Beaux-Arts* 95 (May–June 1980): 175–182.

81 Klaniczay, *Holy Rulers, Blessed Princesses*, 147.

82 Ibid., 210.

83 D.A. Carpenter, "The Meetings of Kings Henry III and Louis IX," in *Thirteenth Century England X: Proceedings of the Durham Conference, 2003*, eds. M. Prestwich, R.H. Britnell, and R. Frame (Woodbridge: Boydell Press, 2005), 1.

84 Gaposchkin, *The Making of St Louis*, 64–66.

85 R.C. Finucane, "Cantilupe, Thomas de [St Thomas of Hereford] (c.1220–1282)," *Oxford Dictionary of National Biography*, doi: 10.1093/ref:odnb/4570 (accessed 20 May 2018). This was deemed to not have been an excommunication at all in 1307.

86 Bray, "Concepts of Sainthood," 42–43.

87 E.W. Kemp, "Pope Alexander III and the Canonization of Saints: The Alexander Prize Essay," *Transactions of the Royal Historical Society* 27 (1945): 17.

88 B.W. Scholz, "The Canonization of Edward the Confessor," *Speculum* 36, no. 1 (January 1961): 49, 59.

89 J. Huntington, "St Margaret of Scotland: Conspicuous Consumption, Genealogical Inheritance, and Post-Conquest Authority," *Journal of Scottish Historical Studies* 33, no. 2 (2013): 156–160.

90 Gaposchkin, *The Making of St Louis*, 237.

91 Paul Binski, *Westminster Abbey and the Plantagenets* (New Haven: Yale University Press, 1995), 523, suggests that Edward I may have actively abandoned the Confessor as a role model, despite Henry III's utter devotion.

92 Klaniczay, *Holy Rulers and Blessed Princesses*, 324–326.

93 D.A.L. Morgan, "The Banner Bearer of Christ and Our Lady's Knight: How God became an Englishman revisited," in *St George's Chapel, Windsor, in the Fourteenth Century*, ed. N. Saul (Woodbridge: Boydell, 2005), 57; W.M. Ormrod, *Edward III* (New Haven: Yale University Press, 2011), 15.

94 Morgan, "The Banner Bearer," 58–59.

95 J. Hillson, "Edward III and the Art of Authority," in *Medieval and Early Modern Representations of Authority in Scotland and the British Isles*, eds. K. Buchanan and L.H.S. Dean (London: Routledge, 2016), 116–117.

96 Morgan, "The Banner Bearer," 60–61; W.M. Ormrod, "For Arthur and St George: Edward III, Windsor Castle and the Order of the Garter," in *St George's Chapel, Windsor, in the Fourteenth Century*, ed. N. Saul (Woodbridge: Boydell, 2005), 19–21.

97 *Foedera*, ii, part 2, ed. Records Commission (London: 1821), 1108.

98 Ormrod, *Edward III*, 4.

99 Gaposchkin, *The Making of St Louis*, 233; C. Tyerman, "Philip VI and the Recovery of the Holy Land," *English Historical Review* 100, no. 394 (January 1985): 25–52.

100 Ormrod, *Edward III*, 101.

101 A. Thomas, *Reading Women in Medieval Europe: Anne of Bohemia and Chaucer's Female Audience* (New York: Palgrave MacMillan, 2015), 27–28.

102 K. Geaman, "A Letter Written by Anne of Bohemia," *English Historical Review* 128, no 534 (October 2013): 1089.

103 E. Scheifele, "Richard II and the Visual Arts," in *Richard II: The Art of Kingship*, eds. A. Goodman and J. Gillespie (Oxford: Clarendon Press, 2003), 259.

104 Saul, *Richard II*, 312, 456–457.

105 I. Rosario, *Art and Propaganda: Charles IV of Bohemia, 1346–1378* (Woodbridge: Boydell, 2000), 51.

106 Condon, "Piety, Propaganda, and the Perpetual Memorial," 63. The order for the window is found in BL Egerton MS 2341AB. Henry's will, TNA E 23/3, gave some importance to Catherine, but not enough to re-inter or even seal her coffin after it was disturbed during the construction of the Lady Chapel.

107 Among these are Eleanor of Provence, Mary daughter of Edward I, and Cardinal Henry Beaufort.

108 Charles I was added to the calendar of saints in the Book of Common Prayer and his feast day was a 'red letter day' until 1859 with a prayer referring to him as saint and martyr read on his feast.

Key works

Gaposchkin, M.C., *The Making of St Louis: Kingship, Sanctity, and Crusade in the Later Middle Ages* (Ithaca: Cornell University Press, 2008).

Klaniczay, G., *Holy Rulers and Blessed Princesses: Dynastic Cults in Medieval Central Europe*, trans. E. Palmai (New York: Cambridge University Press, 2000).

Russell, J.C., "The Canonization of Opposition to the King in Angevin England," in *Anniversary Essays in Mediaeval History by Students of Charles Homer Haskins*, ed., C.H. Taylor (Boston and New York: Houghton Mifflin, 1929), 279–290.

Theilmann, J.M., "Political Canonization and Political Symbolism in Medieval England," *Journal of British Studies* 29, no. 3 (July 1990): 241–266.

Vauchez, A., *Sainthood in the Later Middle Ages*, trans. J. Birrell (New York: Cambridge University Press, 1997).

18

RAISING ROYAL BODIES

Stuart authority and the monumental image

Catriona Murray

Throughout early modern Europe, the royal body was elevated and sacralized. While the reclusive hidden monarchy of Philip II of Spain was intended to mystify the king's person, the idealized and ever-youthful visual image of Elizabeth I of England was meant to immortalize her increasingly fragile frame.[1] In turn, the conspicuous display of Louis XIV's *levers* and *couchers* served to regulate and ritualize the bodily functions of the French sovereign.[2] At its most elemental, the royal body was the physical site of monarchical power, a living, breathing centre from which divinely appointed authority originated. Through representations of the princely figure, the body became a stage on which the sanctification of kingship was repeatedly performed. The treatment of the royal body not only reflected sovereignty but also sustained it.

Nevertheless, when James VI & I acceded to the English throne in 1603, the Stuart monarchy also inherited the effects of a slow but steady shift towards a publicized royal body. Under Henry VIII and the Tudors, representation had been increasingly performed through a rapidly expanding print culture, exposing royal mystique to the public sphere.[3] This development was to prompt critical changes in the relationships between rulers and subjects. A tension emerged between royal mystique and exposure – between the private and the public body.[4] As the printed word and image brought audiences closer to the monarchy, layers of majesty were uncovered and the monarch's person was rendered ever more profane.[5] Of course, the ultimate act in stripping the Stuart royal body of its sacred power was the execution of Charles I in 1649. From this moment on, the monarch's body as both site and image of authority was fractured. Although, after the Restoration of Charles II, significant attempts were made to re-mystify kingship, the nature of princely power had been irretrievably remodelled.[6] Later, Stuart and Hanoverian rulers would return to the representation of sanctified monarchy, but the royal body was now a contested icon.

Monumental sculpture was naturally implicated in this process. Monuments literally recreated the royal body; they were carved or cast stand-ins for, or extensions of, the monarch. As such, they too were endowed with a symbolic power. Indeed, by reforming and refiguring the sovereign, some of the sacred aura of kingship was conferred upon their effigies. Early modern Europe saw a gradual but significant shift in approaches to princely monuments, as public statuary supplemented and, in Britain's case, supplanted funerary sculpture. Royal sculpted images emerged from spiritual spaces into secular environments. The physicality, tangibility and immediacy of statues, as well as their very public display in strategically selected urban locations, again served to familiarize the people with their princes. Thus, paradoxically, monuments served both to solidify and to dissolve the mystique surrounding the royal body. This complex and apparently contradictory political performance could provoke mixed reactions. The coalition of the sanctified and the earthly, which Stuart statuary embodied, prompted popular wonder and suspicion. In moments of political tension, this potent combination could incite physical acts of devotion and destruction. As substitutes for the royal body, monuments were both venerated and attacked. They became a public stage upon which the relationships between sovereign and subject were symbolically played out. From the ancient Romans to the French Revolutionaries, audiences have recognized and resisted the monumental body's power. Scholars though have consistently neglected the origins and development of public monuments as an art of political communication in early modern Britain.[7] By focusing on the Stuart sculpted image at moments of dynastic change, political transition and representational development, this chapter aims, in part, to remedy this oversight, while teasing out far-reaching issues surrounding the representation and perception of monarchy in monumental form.

Sacred bodies

Under the Stuarts, the focus of royal monuments shifted from religious to secular commemoration.[8] Nevertheless, within a year of the accession to the English throne of James VI & I, a significant programme of tomb erection was initiated.[9] Peter Sherlock has argued that the dearth of post-medieval English royal funeral monuments marks those actually realized as 'memorials to discontinuity', intended to convey definite, calculated messages that highlighted change, while asserting providential succession and political legitimacy.[10] Certainly, in commissioning a series of tombs, James was breaking with recent English tradition. His homeland, however, offered more recent precedents. Following his death in 1542, a monument had been erected to James V of Scots at Holyrood Abbey, although it was subsequently destroyed by Henry VIII's troops during the Rough Wooing.[11] South of the border, royal funerary sculpture had thrived under the Plantagenet dynasty, but with the accession of the Tudors, this commemorative drive had faltered. James' initiative then produced the first royal memorials installed at Westminster Abbey since the completion of Henry VII's funerary chapel and tomb almost a century earlier.[12] Although Henry's impressive monument was only erected after his death, it is clear that the monarch's posthumous representation had been a major concern during his lifetime. His will left detailed and explicit instructions for the decoration of his chapel and the execution of his monument:

> [t]hat for the said Sepulture of us and our derest late wif the Quene, whose soule God p'donne, be made a Towmbe of Stone called Touche [black marble], sufficient in largieur for us booth. And upon the same, oon Ymage of our figure, and another of hers, either of them of Copure and gilte of such faction [sic], and in suche maner, as shal be thought moost convenient by the discretion of our Executours.[13]

Pietro Torrigiano's executed scheme, completed in 1519, largely fulfils the late king's wishes. The gilt-bronze effigies of Henry and his queen recline upon a black marble tomb chest, eyes open and hands clasped in prayer. Aside from its Italianate flair, with classicizing roundels and fleshy *putti* ornamenting the basic structure, the arrangement is conservative, even archaic – the regal figures recall medieval sculptural precedents. In establishing a monumental presence at Westminster, the Tudor dynasty looked back to its forbears. The visual traditions of the Plantagenet tombs, scattered throughout the Abbey, were adopted in order to present the new line as the latest stage in England's royal succession.[14]

By embarking upon a scheme of monumental commissions, James was following in the footsteps of his Tudor great-great-grandfather. However, unlike Henry, who had planned to aggrandize the new dynasty through his own tomb, James instead chose to memorialize those familial connections that had secured his new throne. Both kings sought to establish their line at the royal sepulchre but, in commemorating his ancestors, James incorporated complex messages into this monumental integration. He exploited associations and manipulated memories to revise historical narratives and re-present his monarchy. At the heart of James' scheme were two women: Mary, Queen of Scots, who, in life, chose marriage and motherhood to strengthen Stuart claims to the English crown; and Elizabeth I, who, in a childless death had ensured that those claims were realized. According to Ernst Kantorowicz's theory of the 'King's Two Bodies', a monarch had both a natural body, which was personal, corporeal and mortal, and a political body, which was public, abstract and incorruptible.[15] The political body was a social institution which survived the death of the natural body. The treatment of each queen's monumental likeness had significant implications for both their natural and political bodies. Royal remains, representations and reputations were repositioned to align with the new sovereign's preferred versions of the past.

From the outset, the king's hand had been forced. It would appear that Robert Cecil, Secretary of State to both Elizabeth and James, initiated the tomb project of his former mistress, settling a contract without royal approval.[16] In March 1605, Sir Thomas Lake reported the king's reluctance to endorse Cecil's preparations, indicating that his consent was not without caveat: 'So he passed it but with this addition, that he hoped when there was more store of money others should be remembered, which you may guess whom he meant.'[17] James' retort implies that any honour due to his Tudor predecessor would also be accorded to his Stuart mother. Of course, this plan was further complicated by the tangled histories of these two women, the former having ordered the latter to be executed as a traitor. It is not surprising then that James was partisan. Julia Walker has argued that he actively marginalized the English queen.[18] Rather, in revising and rehabilitating the posthumous image of his mother, he fashioned a pointed contrast between the two monuments and their subjects, in which Elizabeth inevitably lost out.

Elizabeth left no instructions for her funeral, no directions for her burial and no orders for a monument.[19] Indeed, she may have believed that to have done so would have compromised her public image, which had attempted for so long to deny her mortality. Nevertheless, when the time came, she was accorded a great state funeral, in line with regal precedents, and interred in the same vault as her grandfather, Henry VII.[20] This was not to be her final resting place, however.

In 1606, her corpse was removed from its original position and placed in a crypt in the north aisle of Henry VII's Chapel, resting on top of the coffin of her half-sister, Mary I, and beneath the spot where Elizabeth's monument now stands.[21] The irony of placing her with her elder half-sister and predecessor, whose own memory Elizabeth had done little to honour, may not have been lost on James.[22] In fact, the turbulent relationship between the two women was diminished in one of the inscriptions that designated the tomb's inhabitants 'partners both in throne and grave'. In a reflection of James' conciliatory religious policy, the Protestant Elizabeth's mortal remains were placed in a symbolic embrace with those of her Catholic sister.[23]

Elizabeth's monument comprises a recumbent marble effigy, resting upon a shallow chest. Corinthian columns extend from the base, bearing two entablatures, which meet in an arched canopy. Her figure lies crowned, holding sceptre and orb and cloaked in ermine (Figure 18.1).

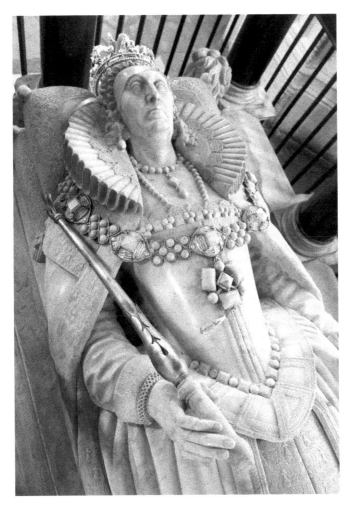

Figure 18.1 Maximillian Colt, *Tomb Effigy of Elizabeth I*, 1606, Henry VII Chapel, Westminster Abbey, Country Life Picture Library.

In correspondence with accounts of her appearance towards the end of her reign, her likeness wears a curled wig, high fanned-out ruff, low-cut bodice and a quantity of jewels.[24] The effect was rendered more striking by 'radiant colours', resembling enamels, which the royal limner, Nicholas Hilliard, applied.[25] In fact, his involvement in the project highlights the striking incongruity of one aspect of Elizabeth's appearance: her physiognomy. It is, after all, Hilliard who is credited with creating the portrait face pattern known as the 'mask of youth' that idealized and rejuvenated her visage, rejecting the ravages of time. Instead, in a gesture of visual realism, which Elizabeth would surely have rejected, her effigy's face was likely modelled on the queen's death mask. The hooded eyes, high receding hairline, sunken cheeks and sagging jowls reflect an aging queen. This is not the iconic Gloriana, but an elderly woman. Certainly, efforts to refashion Elizabeth's body image were supported by the accompanying Latin inscriptions. Contrary to her celebrated statement that she wished her epitaph to memorialize her virginity – 'pure untill her Death' – no mention is made of her lifelong chastity.[26] Rather, the text casts her, somewhat conventionally, as a conquering ruler, praised for her 'regal Vertues beyond her Sex'.[27] James, in turn, is positioned not only as heir to her throne but as heir to those virtues too.[28] Glossing over Elizabeth's sexual denial and prolonged maidenhood, she is instead characterized as a happy septuagenarian, 'quietly by death departed'.[29] Thus, Elizabeth's body politic – pure, ageless and divine – was posthumously brought into alignment with her natural one. Her monumental likeness, resting over her mortal remains, accentuated her humanity and lifted the veil on the Virgin Queen's mystique.

Work on the monument to Mary, Queen of Scots, began in 1606 but was not completed until 1612. The spot selected for her memorial was in the south aisle of the Henry VII Chapel, corresponding to that of Elizabeth in the north aisle. Placed between the tombs of two royal matriarchs, Margaret Beaufort, mother of Henry VII, and Margaret Douglas, mother of Henry, Lord Darnley, and grandmother of James, the situation of Mary's tomb made a marked distinction. While the north aisle accommodated the tombs of childless Tudor women, the south became representative of maternity, fruitfulness and lineal continuity.[30] This was entirely consistent with the rhetoric of family and succession, which James employed to justify his prerogative. The interment of Mary's corpse in the vault beneath her tomb was a more complicated affair than the transferal of Elizabeth's body had been. Executed some twenty-five years earlier, the Scots queen's remains had originally been buried at Peterborough Cathedral. Mary's memorial was to be a tomb not a cenotaph, however, and the union of her natural and monumental bodies was symbolically important. In a letter to the Dean of Peterborough ordering the translation of her remains, the king explains: 'wee think it app'aynes to the Justice wee owe to our deerest mother that like honour should be done to hair bodye and like Monument to be extant to her as to others.'[31] The treatment of Mary's body was particularly significant given the indignities that she had suffered at her execution. Of course, the ultimate act of desecration had been the removal of the Queen's head, which had taken three attempts, but there had been other affronts too. Before the axe was swung, Mary had publicly undressed to her petticoats; as the executioner held up her head to the audience, her wig fell and her tightly cut grey hair was revealed; finally, her corpse was stripped by the headsmen, who pocketed garments as intimate as her garters.[32] In light of these insults, the sanctity of the royal body needed to be restored.

Mary's second funeral was held on 11 October 1612, when she was interred with great solemnity at Westminster Abbey.[33] This ritual elevation of the queen's body was reflected in her monument and effigy. The violence of her death was replaced with the serenity of her final rest. In form, Mary's monument resembles that of Elizabeth, with effigy and sarcophagus surmounted by an arched canopy. In a patent display of the king's sympathies, his mother's tomb is, however, grander both in terms of scale and embellishment. The queen's effigy is derived from a portrait type dating from the late 1570s, during her time in captivity, which proliferated after her death (Figure 18.2).[34]

She wears a lace-trimmed widow's cap, her frizzed hair rolled on either side of her head. An intricate ruff adorns her neck, a chemise covers her chest and shoulders, and an ermine-lined cloak encloses her bodice and skirts. In contrast with Elizabeth, the only flesh Mary reveals is that of her face and hands. Her countenance is peaceful; her palms meet together in prayer. In fact, the delicate sensitivity with which Mary's effigy has been carved also differs from the more direct monumentality of the English queen's form. An even more striking distinction, however, would have been the finish of the two figures; where Elizabeth's dazzled with vibrant colour, Mary's gleamed in plain white marble. As such, artifice was countered with purity. The process of rewriting Mary's body was extended by the tomb inscriptions. Emphasizing the violent nature of her death, which she accepted 'piously, patiently and courageously', Mary's 'murder' was recast as a noble sacrifice for the promotion of her son.[35] She was simultaneously cast as martyr and mother. While Elizabeth had exceeded the merits of her sex, Mary's praise was couched in her gendered female roles: 'Great in marriage, greater still in lineage, greatest of all in her progeny, here lies buried the daughter, the bride and mother of kings.'[36]

By refashioning the natural and political bodies of both queens, James refigured memory on his own terms. Elizabeth's monumental body was represented in concord with the mortal one that rested beneath it, while Mary's monumental body repaired and remedied the damage done to her remains lying below. Revised family histories converged on James, with the new king presented alternately as the political son of one monarch and the natural son of the other. In effect, he is the fruition of their achievements. James had both complicated and elaborated the implications of the royal sculpted image. As monumental bodies entered secular spaces, the combination of location, imagery, materiality and text would continue to create new meanings.

Public bodies

The public monument tradition was reborn in fifteenth-century Italy, where sculptors – such as Donatello and Andrea del Verrocchio – embraced classical precedents and initiated a trend that would leave its indelible mark upon the cities of early modern Europe. It was not until the seventeenth century, however, that the power of public sculpture was fully realized and exploited in Britain. The monumental body, which for centuries had reclined resplendent on marble tomb chests, became animated: positioned upon sandstone plinths and within limestone niches. From the reign of Charles I, the vertical statue succeeded the horizontal effigy as the principal form of

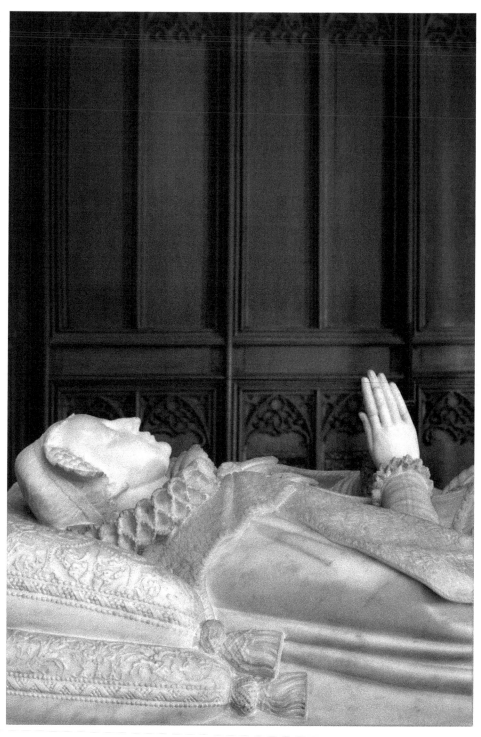

Figure 18.2 Cornelius Cure, *Tomb Effigy of Mary, Queen of Scots*, 1612, Henry VII Chapel, Westminster Abbey, UK/Bridgeman Images.

sculptural commemoration. The relocation and reformation of princely monuments was an exercise in persuasion and control. Public statues acted as agents of Stuart authority, creating a royal presence beyond court and capital. Predominantly commissioned and erected during a monarch's lifetime, these monuments, in a sense, amalgamated the 'King's Two Bodies' by 'incorporating the mystique of kingship into the figurative bodies of real but largely invisible kings'.[37] More than that though, they allowed monarchs to present a multiplicity of political bodies to their subjects. New monumental iconographies developed to display different aspects of a monarch's public image. Kings and queens were portrayed in coronation robes, classical drapery and contemporary armour: they held books, globes and handkerchiefs. Their likenesses were executed in stone, bronze and lead, erected in public squares, college quads and aristocratic estates, with both English and Latin inscriptions. As statues began to populate the British landscape, therefore, new meanings and, indeed, new readings, were conferred upon the royal body. It was at once both openly displayed and publicly exposed.

With a keen eye on monumental developments in France and Italy, Charles I and his courtiers commissioned busts, and both freestanding and equestrian statues. Charles was a connoisseur king, with his finger on the pulse of artistic trends on the continent, and his aesthetic interests allied closely with his political beliefs. Indeed, among the state papers of his reign are copies of the inscriptions that accompanied the statues of Henry IV at the Pont Neuf and of Louis XIII at the Place Royale in Paris, suggesting that, for Charles, art and politics were intimately connected.[38] The King endeavoured to recruit to his court sculptors of international standing. Indeed, in 1639, based on reputation alone and without first-hand knowledge of the artist's work, Charles requested that the master of Baroque sculpture, Gian Lorenzo Bernini, execute his portrait:

> The fame of your sublime genius and of the illustrious works that you have so felicitously brought to fruition has extended beyond the frontiers of Italy and, indeed, nigh beyond those of Europe itself, and brought to our England your glorious name, exalted above those of all men of talent who have exercised your profession to this day.[39]

The infamous bust was lost in the Whitehall fire of 1698, but its commission speaks of the artistic ambitions and expansive outlook of its patron.[40] Charles succeeded in wooing two accomplished sculptors to his court in the 1630s: the Italian, Francesco Fanelli, and the Fleming, François Dieussart. It was the French-born, Hubert Le Sueur, however, who dominated royal monument production, from his arrival in London in 1625 until his departure, around 1642, as England's political climate worsened. Le Sueur had been a sculptor-in-ordinary to the French crown, an artist of marked, but not remarkable, talent.[41] Nevertheless, it was his robust and stately effigies of the king, in a variety of guises, which would inhabit England's public spaces. Indeed, a pair of sculptural schemes commissioned from Le Sueur by two of Charles' leading courtiers, William Laud, Archbishop of Canterbury, and Richard Weston, Earl of Portland, demonstrates the diversity of representational strategies employed. Each corresponds to an aspect of the king's public image, articulating related but distinct messages about his rule through a combination of sculptural devices.

Caroline court culture celebrated the marriage of Charles and his queen, Henrietta Maria, as a harmonious and balanced union. Husband and wife were complementary halves of a perfect whole. Their mutual love reflected that of the sovereign and his people and offered a rich metaphor for the unity of their kingdom.[42] In 1633, Laud commissioned Le Sueur to cast two bronze statues of the king and queen as part of a coordinated programme of display within Canterbury Quad of St. John's College, Oxford (Figures 18.3 and 18.4).[43] The Archbishop, a former President of the College, had been elected Chancellor of the university in 1630. Facing each other, positioned respectively above the east and west gateways of the square, the scheme extends the representation of marital equilibrium and concord, rendering the spirit of CARLOMARIA in sculptural form.

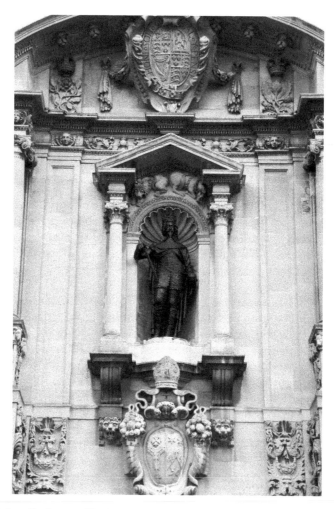

Figure 18.3 Hubert Le Sueur, *Charles I*, 1636, Canterbury Quad, St. John's College, Oxford, by permission of the President and Fellows of St. John's College, Oxford.

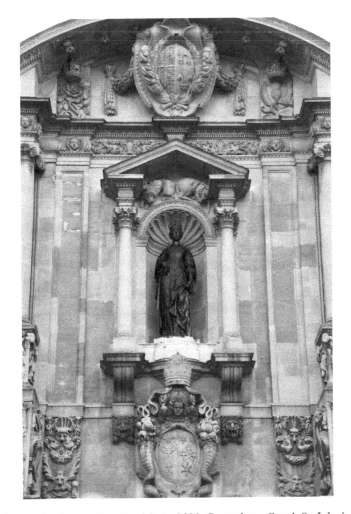

Figure 18.4 Hubert Le Sueur, *Henrietta Maria*, 1636, Canterbury Quad, St. John's College, Oxford, by permission of the President and Fellows of St. John's College, Oxford.

Full-length statues of queens consort are rare, and it is possible that Laud took inspiration for his royal pairing from the statues of Henrietta Maria's parents, Henry IV and Marie de Medici, now lost, which stood in the entrance pavilion to the Luxembourg Palace in Paris.[44] Even in posture, the figures represent a balancing act, with Charles assuming a *contrapposto* stance, leaning slightly to the right, and Henrietta Maria's posture bearing slightly to the left. Both are crowned. Charles wears an embellished suit of armour, under a mantle, with a baton of command in his right hand and the orb in his other. His queen wears a jewelled high-waisted bodice, her floral-embroidered skirt falling in heavy folds, contouring her legs beneath. She grasps her cloak with her left hand and grips a handkerchief between the fingers of her right. There is a hint of the medieval in the attire of both, something of the noble knight and the fair princess, in sympathy with Rubens' painting, *Landscape with St. George and the Dragon* (1630–5), in which the figures of the hero and his maiden allude to Charles and Henrietta Maria.[45] Certainly, in Thomas Carew's masque, *Coelum Britannicum* (1634), which coined the phrase CARLOMARIA as an expression of the unifying bonds of the royal marriage, the king was presented to the queen as 'St George himselfe'.[46] Henrietta Maria's handkerchief in particular – an intimate and romantic token of feminine affection – indicates that the statues were intended to be read within the chivalric context of courtly love.[47] Graham Parry has argued that the Caroline masques generally presented the king as the embodiment of heroic virtue and Henrietta Maria as the incarnation of divine beauty or love.[48] Le Sueur's statues then represent a sculptural extension of this rhetoric.

If the royal couple are presented as the reciprocal royal pairing valorized by the court masque, then how is their harmonious influence here represented? Most noticeably, carved into the stone pediment above each statue's niche, are the docile, languid figures of lion and unicorn, the heraldic supporters of the royal Stuart arms, which in their meek and subdued state signify the peaceful Union of the British Isles. Overhead, the Anglo-Scottish Union is again represented, this time by a crowned rose and thistle, while rosebuds, blossoms, fruit and foliage abound, symbolizing the fertility of the royal match, which had produced four surviving children by the time the Quad was completed in 1636. The imagery of fecundity also points to the bountiful reign of king and queen. Below the bronze figures, the carved arms of Laud himself are flanked by a pair of cornucopia, brimming with peaches, pears and pomegranates. The patron's heraldry, therefore, is contained within his rulers' imagery, associating Laud with their beneficent reign. Thus, the surrounding iconographic programme corresponds to, and enhances, the characterization of king and queen, portraying their union as serene, benevolent and fruitful. Walking through the quadrangle, the viewer is contained within a microcosm of Caroline rule. Architectural space, decorative masonry and bronze statues combine in a harmonious arrangement, which promotes the unity of husband and wife. When Charles and his queen visited the University of Oxford in 1636, their reception at St John's played upon this conceit. As the monarchs ascended the library stairs within the eastern range of the Quad, a bass sang 'Carlo Maria', answered by a treble who sang 'Maria Carlo', before a young scholar beseeched the pair, 'May you feast and frolicke heer with Love.'[49] Clearly, Laud was well versed in Caroline matrimonial imagery and shrewdly sought to align himself with its ideals. The figuratively conjoined royal bodies of king and queen reflected the inseparable relationship between ruler and nation.

Three years before Laud's commission, Richard Weston, Earl of Portland and Lord Treasurer, had chosen to commemorate a different aspect of Charles' *persona*. In 1630, a contract was drafted between Weston and Le Sueur for an equestrian statue of the king to be displayed in the Earl's gardens at his Roehampton estate. Significantly, the sculptor was also charged with executing a 'perfect modell of the said Worcke', which would be subject to the 'approbation of his Maj[esty] and content of his Lord[shi]p' before work on the monument proper began.[50] The statue portrays Charles larger than life, in contemporary armour, gripping a baton of command and mounted upon a great charger (Figure 18.5).

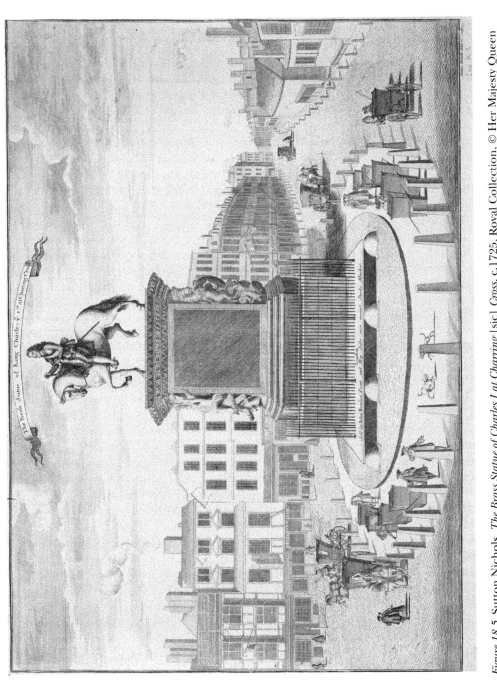

Figure 18.5 Sutton Nichols, *The Brass Statue of Charles I at Charring* [sic] *Cross*, c.1725, Royal Collection, © Her Majesty Queen Elizabeth II 2018.

As such, it draws upon a long tradition of equestrian monuments as signifiers of secular authority: from the ancient Roman sculpture of Emperor Marcus Aurelius on the Capitoline Hill in Rome, to Giambologna's statue of Cosimo I, Grand Duke of Tuscany, in Florence's Piazza della Signoria. The most immediate influences, however, were Pietro Tacca's monuments to Henry IV of France, erected at the Pont Neuf in 1614, and to Philip III of Spain, raised in the gardens of the Casa de Campo in 1616. Le Sueur would have been acquainted with the statue to Henry IV, which was set up during his employment for the French crown.[51] It is also possible that the king himself saw both sculptures during his abortive journey to secure a Spanish match with Philip IV's sister, the Infanta Maria. Charles passed through Paris in February 1623 and was in Madrid the following month. John Moffitt has proclaimed the equestrian image the 'predominant leit-motif' of Charles I's reign.[52] It is worth noting then that Le Sueur's sculptural attempt at this type precedes, in conception at least, Anthony van Dyck's painted renditions.[53] Charles' statue drew upon associations with ancient and modern rulers – it was the climax of an imperial sculptural succession.

In its treatment, however, parallels with Henry IV's statue are particularly striking. The afterlives of both Stuart and Bourbon sculptures mirror the shifting fortunes of the royal families they represented. Good King Henry's monument, for instance, stood at Pont Neuf for 178 years before it became a victim of the French Revolution, suffering demolition in 1792, only to be recreated and reinstated in 1818, following the return of the monarchy and the restoration of Louis XVIII.[54] Discussing the statue's treatment, Victoria Thompson has argued that public sculptures act as repositories of collective memory, over time assuming meanings which are 'multiple, fluid and overlapping'.[55] Certainly, the fate of Charles I's statue evidences how monuments could be read and re-read in response to altering situations. Portland and his estate at Roehampton were not to enjoy their bronze effigy for long. When the Earl died in 1635, his statue was sequestered and eventually ended up as the property of a small group of Covent Garden residents. With the political situation deteriorating, Le Sueur's figure languished in Covent Garden Churchyard until, in the early 1650s, it came into the hands of John Revett, a brazier. He was ordered by the Protectorate government to break up the statue, but instead he buried it.[56] The authorities' aim had been to ensure that 'nothing might Remaine in memorie of his said Majestie'.[57] In an entrepreneurial feat of ingenuity, however, Revett fabricated large numbers of brass handles for forks and knives, which he sold as remnants and relics of the supposedly lost statue.[58] Thus, while the Protectorate sought to obliterate the royal body, Revett's actions served, in a way, to proliferate it. In its pretended destruction, its mystique was both undermined and enhanced. Following the restoration of Charles II, on hearing of the monument's survival, the second Earl of Portland demanded its return. Finally, in 1675, his widow sold it to the king and it was erected upon a new stone pedestal at Charing Cross, facing towards Whitehall. The location was significant, standing close to the spot where the regicides had been executed, while, in turn, overlooking the Banqueting House and the site of Charles I's beheading.[59] The resurrected statue therefore symbolized the triumph of monarchy over unlawful rebellion – the Stuart dynasty lived on and legitimate authority had been restored. Of course, the statue also stood upon an ancient royal memorial site: that of the Eleanor Cross at Charing. The medieval monument, which had been destroyed in 1647, was the grandest of a series of crosses marking the points at which the funeral cortege of Edward I's consort, Eleanor of Castile, paused on its way from Lincoln to Westminster in 1290.[60] By locating Le Sueur's statue on the site of a Plantagenet royal cenotaph, it was raised to the same status. It served as a public commemoration of grief and loss, while also signifying the durability of monarchy. The newly commissioned pedestal also advanced this re-presentation of the monument. Executed by Joshua Marshall to Christopher Wren's design, it was carved with two sets of the royal Stuart arms. On the side facing towards Whitehall, instead of the traditional supporters of lion and unicorn, the arms are borne by two *putti*, holding palms, traditional symbols of martyrdom and the victory of life over death. Charles had made the ultimate sacrifice in the name of royal prerogative. Progressively then, multiple meanings became embedded in the equestrian statue of Charles I. Its original significance was supplemented, as it became both a symbol of the termination of Stuart power and then of its resurgence.

Public statuary promoted and promulgated the Stuart body. Under Charles, monuments came to serve as royal proxies, enabling the king to present altering aspects of his image to his subjects. This heterogeneity, however, opened up new meanings and interpretations, as his political bodies were increasingly shaped outside of his control. Whether loyal or subversive, complex issues of authorship and ownership were now at play. Monumental bodies had become contested and the afterlives of Stuart statues charged with evolving perceptions and recollections of political power. More and more, fashioning the sculpted royal body would become a participatory process.

Monumental interventions

Sculptures have long been physical sites for public interventions, which both support and contest authority. Whether laying a wreath at the Tomb of the Unknown Soldier, or adorning an equestrian statue with the ubiquitous traffic cone, monumental mediations contribute further meaning. Even passing, fleeting actions can impose deferential or derogatory readings, shifting authorial power. Indeed, as early as 1623, a copy of a libel was placed in the hand of Elizabeth I's tomb effigy, lamenting the end of her golden age and the corruption of the regime of James I.[61] Offered to 'the blessed St. Eliza: of most famous memory', the petition advocated for 'hir now most wretched and most Contemptible the Commons of poor distressed England'.[62] This documentary addition to the monument recast the scheme, presenting James' rule as undermining, rather than upholding, the queen's policy. It also served to activate Elizabeth's reclining figure, addressing her political body as a surrogate for her spiritual one – an intermediary between the earthly and heavenly. Over a century later, in 1736, a statue of the last Stuart monarch, Queen Anne, erected in Gloucester, was dressed in black mourning dress.[63] Nostalgic for the heyday of Tory rule, local opponents of Robert Walpole's Whig administration, under George II, thereby transformed the statue's significance, presenting the queen as grieving for the end of her own political legacy. In both instances, these momentary, ephemeral interventions served to elevate the memory of a past sovereign at the expense of the current one, temporarily rewriting the royal body. As stand-ins for the monarch's person, monuments too were subject to more enduring acts of veneration and contempt. At moments of real political tension, the toppling of a statue could symbolize the toppling of a regime. The desecration of the monumental body, therefore, reflected the dismantling of a ruler's personal authority. Yet, acts of iconoclasm likewise point to the perceived power of the royal sculpted form. In attacking the monumental body, the mob also acknowledged its authority.

Despite the brevity of his reign – less than four years – James II & VII was the subject of seven statues, of which only two now survive.[64] The rapid rise and fall, following the Revolution of 1688, of his monumental representations demonstrates how respect could quickly descend into disdain. James' statue at University College, Oxford, was inaugurated with great ceremony in February 1687. The installation of the king's likeness, in Roman dress and crowned with a laurel wreath, above the western gateway in the college quadrangle, was greeted with several rounds of small shot, accompanied by cries from the assembled spectators. Feasting, music and speeches followed. Edward Hales, the orator and a student of the college, recited James' virtues and achievements, commending the ancient practice of erecting statues to heroes and worthies as exemplars for imitation, before concluding with thanks to the donor who had bestowed 'this durable representation of our prince'.[65] With the solemnities over, lit candles were placed to illuminate the windows surrounding the quadrangle, those facing the street and those in the Chapel.[66] The king's stone figure was bathed in light, while the college appeared brilliant against the night sky. In not only erecting but also celebrating the king's monumental body, therefore, the college performed its loyalty to the crown. Through an elaborate spectacle focused upon the statue, the installation festivities attached additional layers of meaning, directing how it was received and understood.

Oxford's enduring Jacobite sympathies and the monument's position, high up in a niche above a gateway, probably contributed to its survival after the king's deposition. His equestrian statue in Newcastle was not so fortunate, however. Commissioned from William Larson in 1686 by the Common Council, the monument portrayed the king in contemporary riding dress upon a free-standing rearing horse: a considerable technical feat. Indeed, there were only two antecedents, in the bronze equestrian statues to Leopold V at Innsbruck and Philip IV at Madrid.[67] Erected in the market place at Sandhill, the king's cast likeness stood for less than a year before his deposition dictated its demise. On the evening of 11 May 1689, goaded on by the local soldiery, the statue was attacked by the 'common people'.[68] Again, this was a performative act, with speeches and displays of largesse centring on the statue. The order was given by a Colonel Hayford, who publicized the deed with an announcement at Hedlam's coffee house. Meanwhile, Captain Killigrew delivered a speech from the mountebank's stage at the market, throwing money among the rabble. His few recorded words are informative. Pointing to the monument, he declared: 'Our laws, liberties and properties were taken away and all by that picture.'[69] For Killigrew then, the ousted ruler and his statue were synonymous. His speech recognized the power residing within the monumental body, while seeking to overthrow it. Next, a soldier threw a rope round the statue's head and pulled 'the man' from the horse, before the throng beat it with stones.[70] The royal body was violated in effigy, and the statue's fall signified that of the king. Yet, such behaviour constituted a threat, even to the new post-Revolution regime. Within a fortnight, the recently installed mayor, Nicholas Ridley, held a formal inquiry into the attack.[71] Whether royal loser or victor, the challenge to authority that this desecration represented was a very real concern.

Of course, politically motivated assaults on images were nothing new. Sculpted representations of Roman and Byzantine elites who became subject to what would later be dubbed *damnatio memoriae* – a legally sanctioned act of conscious forgetting or erasure of memory – were frequently dismantled and destroyed.[72] Bente Kiilerich has also pointed to the related practice of refashioning and replacing images, whereby statues or reliefs of deposed Roman or Byzantine rulers were reworked into the likenesses of their successors.[73] This process of revision has some relevance for James' monument. In 1695, All Saints' Parish petitioned for the 'metal of the statue' to be recast for their bells.[74] There is some irony in the appropriation of a Catholic king's bronze figure to ring out the Protestant calendar. Interest in the monument persisted well beyond its material transformation, however. In 1742, Joseph Barber, a Newcastle stationer, advertised a print of the lost statue, published by subscription (Figure 18.6).

The engraving on 'two large sheets of genoa paper' and originally 'illustrated with near 200 coats of arms' representing the subscribers, is a largely imaginary concoction.[75] Certainly, the king's mount and figure are derived from a seventeenth-century Dutch print of James II on the battlefield.[76] Underneath, the caption relates the sad fate of the town's 'very great Ornam[en]t'. It is worth noting here that Stuart monuments inspired a rich subsidiary culture of prints, medals and texts, which publicized the monumental body beyond its immediate public location. Indeed, in this state, Barber's print constitutes a retrospective record of what should have been an enduring expression of civic pride and regal loyalty. There is, however, another state of this print, published by William Herbert 'at the Golden Globe on London Bridge'.

With a new inscription and some slight alterations to the face, the engraving has been transformed into a representation of James' royal challenger and successor, William III (Figure 18.7). These two images, therefore, secondary fragments of a lost sculptural form, pictorially exemplify the fall and rise of Stuart power during the Glorious Revolution. The process of refashioning and replacing has been imposed on the visual culture generated from the statue. The prints serve as an epilogue to its complex object biography. The monumental body has been revived and reshaped in ephemeral form.

Once the royal body became public, it also became contested. This chapter has explored public sculpture's role in this process, probing issues of display, reception and control. Early modern monuments were sites for a series of exchanges between the monarchy and its subjects, which both sustained and undermined regal power. Under the early Stuarts, tomb sculpture refashioned the relationships between the natural and political bodies. A rich combination of setting, materiality, iconography and inscriptions was employed in an effort to revise history and to control memory. This process was extended once monuments emerged into secular surroundings. The imposition of a royal sculptural presence in civic and institutional spaces, as well as noble estates, visually articulated the reach of royal authority and of public allegiance. What is more, the monumental body was no longer confined to a solitary tomb effigy but to a host of statues, assuming different forms and significances. Rulers projected a range of *personae*, adapting their representations to their settings. Yet, with this plasticity of approach came a fluidity of meaning, which was progressively shaped outside regal influence. The afterlives of Stuart statues demonstrate how these authoritarian images became vulnerable to public mediations. Both shifting contexts and direct interventions could distort their original messages or contribute new ones, so that multiple meanings co-existed within a single

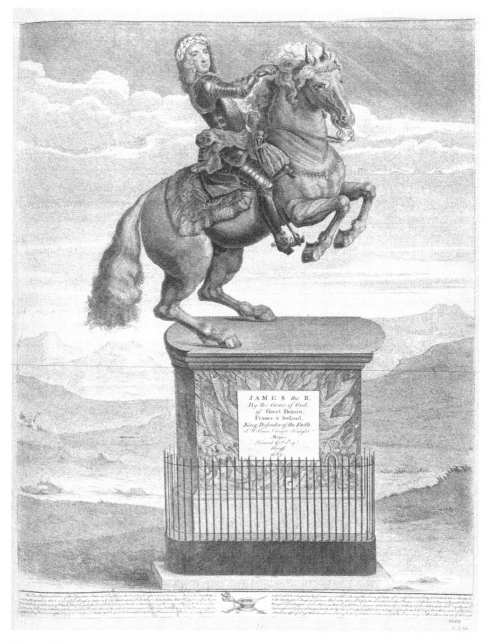

Figure 18.6 Anonymous (published by Joseph Barber), *James II's Statue at Sandhill, Newcastle,* 1742, Royal Collection, © Her Majesty Queen Elizabeth II 2018.

monument. Even attempts to obliterate the monumental body could not halt this progression. In their erasure, the mystical aura and special power of Stuart statues was both acknowledged and undercut. Finally, lost sculptures might live on through textual and visual spin-offs, where meanings were further revised. The royal body,

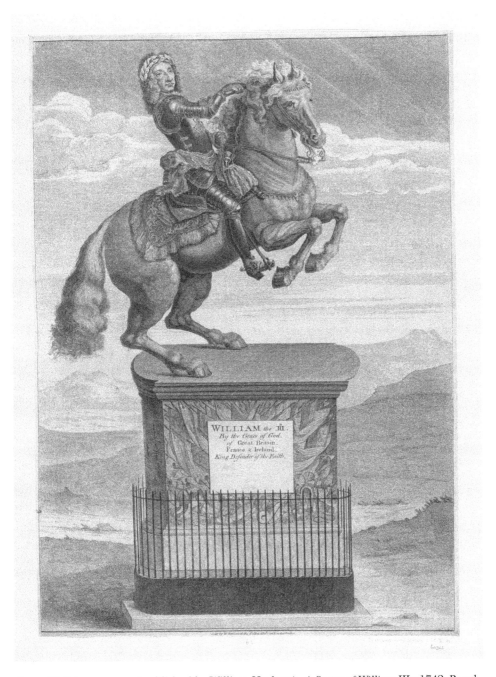

Figure 18.7 Anonymous (published by William Herbert), *A Statue of William III* c.1742, Royal Collection, © Her Majesty Queen Elizabeth II 2018.

therefore, was increasingly exposed and subject to popular forces. Monumental bodies became registers of public opinion, inscribed by the altering relationships between monarch and realm.

Notes

1 J.H. Elliot, "The Court of the Spanish Habsburgs: A Peculiar Institution?" in *Politics and Culture in Early Modern Europe, Essays in Honor of H.G. Koenigsberger*, eds. Phyllis Mack and Margaret C. Jacob (Cambridge: Cambridge University Press, 1987), 17; Kevin Sharpe, *Selling the Tudor Monarchy: Authority and Image in Sixteenth-Century England* (New Haven: Yale University Press, 2009), 387–388.

2 Jeffrey Merrick, "The Body Politics of French Absolutism," in *From the Royal to the Republican Body: Incorporating the Physical in Seventeenth- and Eighteenth-Century France*, eds. Sara E. Melzer and Kathryn Norberg (Berkeley: University of California Press, 1998), 16–17.

3 Kevin Sharpe, "Sacralisation and Demystification: The Publicization of Monarchy in Early Modern England," in *Mystifying the Monarch: Studies on Discourse, Power and History*, eds. Jeroen Deploige and Gita Deneckere (Amsterdam: Amsterdam University Press, 2006), 106.

4 Sharpe, "Sacralisation and Demystification," 112.

5 Sharpe, "Sacralistation and Demystification," 101.

6 Paul Hammond, "The King's Two Bodies: Representations of Charles II," in *Culture, Politics and Society in Britain, 1660–1800*, eds. Jeremy Black and Jeremy Gregory (Manchester: Manchester University Press, 1991), 13.

7 Important scholarship has been published on sixteenth- and seventeenth-century English tomb monuments, most notably Nigel Llewellyn's *Funeral Monuments in Post-Reformation England* (Cambridge: Cambridge University Press, 2000) and Peter Sherlock's *Monuments and Memory in Early Modern England* (Aldershot: Ashgate, 2008). A comprehensive analysis of public sculpture as a potent political language in early modern Britain has yet to be written, however.

8 With the exception of James II, no Stuart monarch ruling after 1603 was commemorated with a funeral monument. Monuments to James were erected in the Church of St Louis at St.-Germain-en-Laye, and in the chapels of the Scots College and the English Benedictine Monastery in Paris. For proposed but unrealized monuments, see Sir Christopher Wren's drawings for a *Mausoleum to Charles I* (Oxford: All Souls College, 1678); Grinling Gibbons' drawings for a *Monument to William III and Mary II* (London: British Museum, 1702); and Nicholas Hawksmoor's drawings for an *Equestrian Monument to William III* (*c.*1702, Oxford: All Souls College and the Victoria and Albert Museum, London).

9 As well as commissioning monuments to Elizabeth I and Mary, Queen of Scots, James also ordered tombs for his infant daughters, Sophia and Mary, in 1606 and 1607 respectively.

10 Peter Sherlock, "The Monuments of Elizabeth Tudor and Mary Stuart: King James and the Manipulation of Memory," *Journal of British Studies*, 46, no. 2 (April 2007): 265.

11 Michael Penman, "A Programme for Royal Tombs in Scotland?" in *Monuments and Monumentality across Medieval and Early Modern Europe*, ed. Michael Penman (Donington: Shaun Tyas, 2013), 253; George MacKenzie, *The Lives and Characters of the Most Eminent Writers of the Scottish Nation* (Edinburgh, 1711), 2:594.

12 Plans for a magnificent monument to Henry VIII went through several permutations but were never completed. For the tomb projects to Henry VII and Henry VIII, see Michael Wyatt, *The Italian Encounter with Tudor England* (Cambridge: Cambridge University Press, 2005) and Nigel Llewellyn, "The Royal Body: Monuments to the Dead for the Living," in *Renaissance Bodies: The Human Figure in English Culture c. 1540–1660*, eds. Lucy Gent and Nigel Llewellyn (London: Reaktion Books, 1995).

13 Thomas Astle, ed., *The Will of King Henry VII* (London, 1775), 4.

14 David Howarth, *Images of Rule: Art and Politics in the English Renaissance, 1485–1649* (Berkeley: University of California Press, 1997), 158.

15 Ernst Kantorowicz, *The King's Two Bodies: A Study in Medieval Political Theology* (Princeton: University of Princeton Press, 1957).

16 Sherlock, "The Monuments of Elizabeth Tudor and Mary Stuart," 269.

17 M.S. Giuseppi, ed., *Calendar of the Cecil Papers in Hatfield House: Volume 17, 1605* (London: His Majesty's Stationery Office, 1938), 79.

18 Julia M. Walker, "Reading the Tombs of Elizabeth I," *English Literary Renaissance* 26, no. 3 (Autumn 1996): 515.

19 Sherlock, "The Monuments of Elizabeth Tudor and Mary Stuart," 266.
20 Walker, "Reading the Tombs of Elizabeth I," 515. For Elizabeth's funeral, see Jennifer Woodward, *The Theatre of Death: The Ritual Management of Royal Funerals in Renaissance England, 1570–1625* (Woodbridge: The Boydell Press, 1997), 87–115.
21 Sherlock, "The Monuments of Elizabeth Tudor and Mary Stuart," 283; Walker, "Reading the Tombs of Elizabeth I," 522.
22 Judith Richards, "Examples and Admonitions: What Mary Demonstrated for Elizabeth," in *Tudor Queenship: The Reigns of Mary and Elizabeth*, eds. Alice Hunt and Anna Whitelock (New York: Palgrave Macmillan, 2010), 41.
23 For James' religious policies, see W.B. Patterson, *King James VI and I and the Reunion of Christendom* (Cambridge: Cambridge University Press, 1997), and Malcolm Smuts, "The Making of Rex Pacificus: James VI and I and the Problem of Peace in an Age of Religious War," in *Royal Subjects: Essays on the Writings of James VI and I*, eds. Daniel Fischlin and Mark Fortier (Detroit: Wayne State University Press, 2002), 371–387.
24 Louis Montrose, *The Subject of Elizabeth: Authority, Gender and Representation* (Chicago: University of Chicago Press, 2006), 231–232.
25 M.S. Giuseppi, ed., *Calendar of Cecil Papers in Hatfield House: Volume 18, 1606* (London: His Majesty's Stationery Office, 1940), 409; June Schlueter, "Three Early Seventeenth-Century Watercolours of the Tombs of Henry VII and Elizabeth I in Westminster Abbey," *The Burlington Magazine* 151, no. 1281 (December 2009): 820. All trace of the effigy's colouring has now disappeared.
26 Elizabeth's statement concludes the speech she made to Parliament on 10 February 1559, in response to a petition from the House of Commons urging her to marry. William Camden, *Annales the True and Royall Historie of the Famous Empresse Elizabeth, Queene of Englande France and Ireland* (London, 1625), 29.
27 Quoted from a translation of the inscriptions in Francis Sandford, *A Genealogical History of the Kings and Queens of England, and Monarchs of Great Britain, from the Conquest, Anno 1066 to the year 1707* (London, 1707), 520.
28 Sandford, *A Genealogical History*, 521.
29 Ibid.
30 Sherlock, "The Monuments of Elizabeth Tudor and Mary Stuart," 271; Walker, "Reading the Tombs of Elizabeth I," 524.
31 "James VI and I to the Dean and Chapter of Peterborough Cathedral, 28 September 1612," quoted in Woodward, *The Theatre of Death*, 138.
32 Maria Hayward, "'We Should Dress Us Fairly For Our End': The Significance of the Clothing Worn at Elite Executions in England in the Long Sixteenth Century," *History* 101, no. 345 (April 2016): 240, 237, 241.
33 For Mary's second funeral, see Woodward, *The Theatre of Death*, 138–140.
34 See, for example, Anon., *Mary, Queen of Scots* (Hardwick Hall, Derbyshire, 1578); and Nicholas Hilliard, *Mary, Queen of Scots*, c.1592, Royal Collection, London.
35 Margaret Stephenson's translation of the Latin epitaph is available at www.westminster-abbey.org/our-history/royals/mary-queen-of-scots (last accessed 30 March 2019).
36 "Mary Queen of Scots," *Westminster Abbey*, www.westminster-abbey.org/our-history/royals/mary-queen-of-scots (last accessed 30 March 2019).
37 Jeffrey Merrick, *Order and Disorder under the Ancien Regime* (Cambridge: Cambridge Scholars Publishing, 2007), 50.
38 The National Archives, SP 78/100, f. 102; SP 78/108, f. 246.
39 "Charles I to Gian Lorenzo Bernini, 17 March 1636," quoted in Domenico Bernini, *The Life of Gian Lorenzo Bernini*, ed. and trans. Franco Mormando (University Park: Pennsylvania State University Press, 2011), 142.
40 For Charles I's sculpture collections, see David Howarth, "Charles I, Sculpture and Sculptors," in *The Late King's Goods: Collections, Possessions and Patronage of Charles I in the Light of the Commonwealth Sale Inventories*, ed. Arthur MacGregor (London: Alistair McAlpine and Oxford: Oxford University Press, 1989), 73–113.
41 Charles Avery, "Hubert Le Sueur, the 'Unworthy Praxiteles' of King Charles I," *The Volume of the Walpole Society* 48 (1980–2): 138.

42 Su Fang Ng, *Literature and the Politics of Family in Seventeenth-Century England* (Cambridge: Cambridge University Press, 2007), 42; Graham Parry, *The Golden Age Restor'd: The Culture of the Stuart Court, 1603–42* (Manchester: Manchester University Press, 1981), 184.

43 For the contract, see The National Archives, SP 16/238, f. 21.

44 Géraldine A. Johnson, "Imagining Images of Powerful Women: Maria de' Medici's Patronage of Art and Architecture," in *Women and Art in Early Modern Europe: Patrons, Collectors and Connoisseurs*, ed. Cynthia Lawrence (University Park: Pennsylvania State University Press, 1999), 141.

45 Howarth, *Images of Rule*, 72. See Peter Paul Rubens, *Landscape with St. George and the Dragon* (*c.*1630, Royal Collection, London).

46 J.S.A. Adamson, "Chivalry and Political Culture in Caroline England," in *Culture and Politics in Early Stuart England*, eds. Kevin Sharpe and Peter Lake (Stanford: Stanford University Press, 1993), 174.

47 Will Fisher, *Materializing Gender in Early Modern English Literature and Culture* (Cambridge: Cambridge University Press, 2006), 58.

48 Parry, *The Golden Age Restor'd*, 184.

49 "Verses Spoken in St Johns Library at the Entertainment of the K[in]g and Queen anno 1636," Bodleian Library, MS Malone 21, ff. 52v-53.

50 "Balthazar Gerbier to Lord Treasurer Weston, 16 January 1630," quoted in William Hookham Carpenter, *Pictorial Notices: Consisting of a Memoir of Sir Anthony Van Dyck* (London, 1844), 190.

51 Avery, "Hubert Le Sueur, the 'Unworthy Praxiteles' of King Charles I," 140.

52 John F. Moffitt, "'Le Roi á la ciasse'? Kings, Christian Knights, and Van Dyck's Singular Dismounted Equestrian Portrait of Charles I," *Artibus et Historiae* 4, no. 7 (1983): 80.

53 Van Dyck's first equestrian portrait of the king is *Charles I with M. de St. Antoine* (1633, Royal Collection, London).

54 Victoria Thompson, "The Creation, Destruction and Recreation of Henry IV: Seeing Popular Sovereignty in the Statue of a King," *History and Memory*, 24, no. 2 (Fall/Winter 2012): 6.

55 Thompson, "The Creation, Destruction and Recreation of Henry IV," 6.

56 Nicola Smith, *The Royal Image and the English People* (Aldershot: Ashgate, 2001), 75.

57 "The Answer of John Revet Gentleman Defendant to the Informacion of Geoffrey Palmer Knight, 14 November 1662," quoted in Smith, *The Royal Image and the English People*, 75.

58 Edward Gleichen, *London's Open-Air Statuary* (Bath: Cedric Chivers, 1973), 3. The story of Revett's entrepreneurship is first recounted by the historian, Johann Wilhelm von Archenholz, in *A Picture of England: Containing a Description of the Laws, Customs and Manners of England* (Dublin, 1791), 229.

59 G.H. Gater and E.P. Wheeler, eds., *Survey of London, St Martin-in-the-Fields I: Charing Cross* (London: London County Council, 1935), 16:262.

60 Smith, *The Royal Image and the English People*, 59.

61 "The Coppie of a Libell put into the hand of Queen Elizabeths statue in Westminster by an unknowne person Anno d[omi]ni 1621," Bodleian Library, MS Malone 23, fol. 41.

62 Bodleian Library, MS Malone 23, fol. 41.

63 Matthew Craske, *The Silent Rhetoric of the Body, A History of Monumental Sculpture and Commemorative Art in England 1720–1770* (New Haven: Yale University Press, 2007), 233. John Rickett's statue was set up in 1712 at Gloucester's Southgate and now stands in Gloucester Park.

64 Statues to James were installed in the Privy Garden at Whitehall, outside Gloucester's Holy Trinity Church and at The Royal Exchange; University College, Oxford; Southwark Old Town Hall; King's Lynn market place; and Newcastle's Sandhill.

65 Andrew Clark, ed., *The Life and Times of Anthony Wood, Antiquary of Oxford, 1632–1695* (Oxford, 1891), 210–212.

66 Clark, *The Life and Times of Anthony Wood*, 210.

67 Smith, *The Royal Image and the English People*, 130.

68 *Calendar of State Papers Domestic: William and Mary, 1689–90* (London, 1895), 111. Hereafter *CSPD: W&M*.

69 *CSPD: W&M, 1689–90*, 115.

70 *CSPD: W&M, 1689–90*, 115.
71 *CSPD: W&M, 1689–90*, 115.
72 Bente Kiilerich, "Defacement and Replacement as Political Strategies in Ancient and Byzantine Ruler Images," in *Iconoclasm from Antiquity to Modernity*, eds. Kristine Kolrud and Marina Prusac (London: Routledge, 2016), 58.
73 Kiilerich, "Defacement and Replacement," 68.
74 E. MacKenzie, *A Descriptive and Historical Account of the Town and County of Newcastle Upon Tyne* (Newcastle, 1827), 162.
75 M. A. Richardson, *The Local Historian's Table Book, Of Remarkable Occurrences* (Newcastle, 1841), 1:321.
76 See an anonymous engraving, *Jacobus II by de Gratie Godts Koningh van Engelant, Schotlant, Vrancryck en Irlant* (*c.*1685), Royal Collection, London.

Key works

Howarth, David, *Images of Rule: Art and Politics in the English Renaissance, 1485–1649* (Berkeley: University of California Press, 1997).
Kiilerich, Bente, "Defacement and Replacement as Political Strategies in Ancient and Byzantine Ruler Images." in *Iconoclasm from Antiquity to Modernity*, eds. Kristine Kolrud and Marina Prusac (London: Routledge, 2016), 57–73.
Llewellyn, Nigel, "The Royal Body: Monuments to the Dead for the Living," in *Renaissance Bodies: The Human Figure in English Culture c.1540-1660*, eds. Lucy Gent and Nigel Llewellyn (London: Reaktion Books, 1995), 218–240.
Sharpe, Kevin, "Sacralisation and Demystification: The Publicization of Monarchy in Early Modern England," in *Mystifying the Monarch: Studies on Discourse, Power and History*, eds. Jeroen Deploige and Gita Deneckere (Amsterdam: Amsterdam University Press, 2006), 99–116.
Sherlock, Peter, "The Monuments of Elizabeth Tudor and Mary Stuart: King James and the Manipulation of Memory," *Journal of British Studies* 46, no. 2 (April 2007): 263–289.
Thompson, Victoria, "The Creation, Destruction and Recreation of Henry IV: Seeing Popular Sovereignty in the Statue of a King," *History and Memory* 24, no. 2 (Fall/Winter 2012): 5–46.

19

IN PURSUIT OF SOCIAL ALLIES

Royal residences and political legitimacy in post-revolutionary Europe, 1804–30[1]

Mikolaj Getka-Kenig

The outbreak of the French Revolution in 1789 transformed the monarchy from an absolutist style to a constitutional one. The new status of the Bourbon king Louis XVI as a national leader, rather than God's plenipotentiary, required such symbolic measures as the forced abandonment of a century-long royal isolation at Versailles. The court was moved to Paris, where the monarch was expected to live among his people; installed in the previously neglected palace of the Tuileries, situated in the heart of the bustling city. Although the palace had a long history behind it, it was not a return to an earlier form of monarchy but rather a first step in the process of the modern change of royal representation. However, the question of where and how an absolutist-turned-constitutional king should live was not definitely settled. Even a few months before the final abolition of the monarchy in 1791, the National Constituent Assembly still discussed the problem of royal representation in the constitutional state, and even then deputy Bertrand Barère suggested extending the royal palace and transforming it into a new *Palais National*.[2] For Barère, such an extension would provide the legislative and executive bodies of the new state with duly magnificent headquarters, while also sharing the space with the royal family and their court. Barère hoped that such a palace would have served as a true representation of national sovereignty, contrasting with antidemocratic 'superstitions surrounding the throne' that were a traditional driving force behind royal architectural undertakings, and that 'so often corrupted the hearts of kings and subjugated the minds of the people'.[3]

It is notable that the changes, both those effective such as the court's movement to Paris, and those merely speculative such as Barère's project, did not come from the monarch himself. Ambrogio A. Caiani has recently argued that Louis's unwillingness to adapt his monarchical representation to the expectations of new political elites and popular opinion 'played an active role in stoking the fires of radicalism during the Revolution' and eventually contributed to the constitutional monarchy's ephemeral existence.[4] This reflection supports a more general and already well-established argument in the social and political historiography, that monarchical pageantry is by no means an empty show but a key element of political culture in monarchical regimes, as it serves as an instrument of their legitimacy. It is, as Richard Wortman put it, 'a simulacrum of a state directed by the ruler's will'.[5] It influences the way in which monarchs are seen by their subjects, and thus it has a direct impact on their obedience and commitment to the throne, serving to reinvigorate or bolster such positive feelings. However, if it is misdirected and out of touch with prevailing popular views, it can do harm to monarchical prestige and undermine the crown's political authority both in the residential setting and beyond.

Residences play a crucial role in the royal representation mainly because, as symbols of monarchical legitimacy, they are not only attention drawing but also permanent. It makes them distinct from spectacular instruments of self-fashioning, such as ceremonies and festivals. Any decision concerning their exterior, public internal parts or surroundings can be interpreted as a political move that is intended to fashion the royal image. Building on this idea, this chapter deals with the political role of royal residences in monarchical propaganda and self-fashioning, not only in France but also in other parts of Europe in the period that directly followed the French Revolution in the first half of the nineteenth century. It is the 'age' of monarchical revival in Europe that started with the return of monarchy in Napoleonic France in 1804 and declined in the aftermath of the July Revolution in 1830 and the deposition of the restored French kings of the Bourbon dynasty. The revival of monarchy in post-Revolutionary Europe was contingent on the readiness of the reaffirmed monarchical regimes to confront the rise of the political ambitions of commoners, and especially those who belonged to the expanding, largely urbanized middle class who had means and determination (as well as self-respect) to engage in public life. In the course of the Revolution and the consequent Napoleonic Wars, they progressed in the development of their modern self-identification, not only as subjects but also as agents of political community. Therefore, as William Doyle once observed, this revolutionary experience made the post-1789 European monarchs 'learn that they needed social allies' if they wanted to be strong and long-lived.[6]

This chapter argues that in those circumstances, the Old Regime pan-European idea of royal residence, which focused on the glorification of monarchs and emphasized their utmost superiority over the people, was an ambiguous legacy for their post-Revolutionary successors. As a matter of course, palatial edifices, already characteristic for pre-absolutist monarchies, but much developed in terms of magnificence throughout the seventeenth and eighteenth centuries, were a well-established expression of royal standing. They helped the post-Revolutionary crowned heads to stress their prestige and, furthermore, symbolized the stability and firmness of the social and political order that a monarchical regime entailed. However, they also contributed to the symbolic distance between royal majesty and their subjects (in this case, the middle-class public) that was problematic in the post-Revolutionary time when, according to Wortman, the symbolic discourse of political legitimacy started to be inclined towards 'demonstration[s] of affinity between government and governed' that have been 'marking European political systems as legitimate' ever since.[7] Therefore, in contrast to the reluctant and consequently unhappy Louis XVI, those European monarchs who found themselves in need of supporting their legitimacy and looked for 'social allies' in the aftermath of the Revolution, provided their publicly seen seats with notable signs of their close proximity to the common but politically aspiring people who needed to be reckoned with.

There are three distinct stages of this phenomenon's gradual development on an international scale, which this chapter discusses in separate sections, providing the reader with a selection of residences that underwent most notable modifications in the period in question. The first section of the chapter concerns post-Revolutionary France, where Napoleon Bonaparte revived a monarchical regime in 1804. It was there where the ambiguity of the traditional architectural representation of monarchy was first experienced and dealt with. The second section of the chapter is focused on Napoleonic satellite monarchies in other parts of Europe. There, the problem became evident as a result of both the French conquest as well as the French-style sociopolitical modernization that was imposed on dependant territories. Finally, the third section of the chapter offers a survey of characteristic cases to show that residences also played a role in courting 'social allies' for monarchs in the period of the post-Napoleonic restoration.

Legitimizing a return

The return of the monarchy in Napoleonic France in 1804 was intended to entrench the political stability of the Consulate (1799–1804) that followed the atrocities of the Revolutionary Terror (1793–4) and the chronic disorder of the Directory (1795–9). Quite paradoxically, General Napoleon Bonaparte presented monarchy to the public as the only solution to save the republican legacy of the Revolution, and won their support that found its expression in a popular plebiscite in which the French opted in favour of Bonaparte's enthronement. The imperial election in itself was a propaganda technique that served to express the republican meritocratic values, which would motivate the way in which the emperor would form the imperial elite, tending to base it on personal achievements rather than lineage and inheritance.[8] The political credit that Napoleon's co-citizens-turned-subjects gave him was a consequence of spectacular military victories that the French army achieved under his guidance. Owing to them, the sociopolitical ambitions of the French Revolution were provided with a truly universal scope. Therefore, the French domination in Europe that followed Napoleon's election and coronation was the principle upon which the popular authority and legitimacy of the Napoleonic monarchy was founded.

The emperor as the successor of the former kings of France meant he had many former royal residences at his disposal. He paid regular visits to the Grand Trianon, Saint Cloud and Fontainebleau outside Paris. Towards the end of his reign, he was in possession of forty-four seats in France proper as well as in other parts of his pan-European empire, and most of them had a long tradition of monarchical ownership and use.[9] However, it was the abovementioned Tuileries in Paris, already used by him during the Consulate, where the imperial court was ordinarily based and seen in public. This choice addressed the popular expectation of having the monarch close to the people.[10]

The First Consul, and subsequently emperor, was much absorbed with redecorating the interiors of the palace of the Tuileries in his preferred idiom of neoclassicism, known to art-historians as the *Empire* style. It was characterized by rich ornamental decoration and the predominance of the Corinthian over the other classical architectural orders. It brought back the pre-Revolutionary opulence of royalty but subjected it to the strictness of the classical regime. It disciplined this absolutist legacy in accordance with the rules of natural and rational harmony, which could be expressive of the idea of the Napoleonic empire as a natural and rational form of exercising monarchical power. It did this in a much more direct and pure (anti-Baroque) way than the Bourbon kings had previously embraced in their own architectural and artistic undertakings that were also expressive of the classical taste, and intended to express the classical ideas of order and naturalness as the principles of their rule.[11] The *Empire* style was also a direct reference to the idealized political legacy of the Roman empire. It was a successful method tried and tested by many monarchs around Europe in the early modern period. However, it was specifically this monarchical precedent of the Augustan and post-Augustan Roman empire, invented in order to preserve the legacy of the old Republic, which sanctioned the propriety of Napoleon's aspirations and induced him to use those historical associations in his propaganda. What is more, it was this specific idea of monarchical rule that grounded its popular legitimacy on successful military leadership, which accounted for its relevance to the modern situation of the French.[12]

However, the most public part of the Tuileries palace – its magnificent Renaissance exterior with a 266-metre façade – was left virtually intact. It is possible that the huge cost of redecoration was a discouraging factor, as well as the duration of any works that would have left Napoleon without an appropriate place of representation in the capital for an extended period of time. Nevertheless, the enormous scale and classically inspired architecture of the royal palace's exterior, described by contemporary arbiters of taste as being 'of elegant and delicate style', seemed to satisfy his ambitions.[13] Moreover, its preservation was an expression of Napoleon's intention to maintain direct links with the tradition of French monarchy and its apparently still valid social prestige. In popular opinion, the Tuileries was still the 'palais des Henris' and thus acted as a memento of two well-loved kings of early modern France, Henry II and Henry IV, who contributed much to the history of the palace.[14] The latter, in particular, was an esteemed figure; he managed to rebuild the national economy that had been in a dire state after a long-standing period of internal upheavals. Therefore, the emperor had a vested interest in maintaining direct associations with him in his propaganda, even if privately he was not entirely appreciative about Henry IV's regal achievements (although he reportedly expressed his criticism only after his abdication).[15]

However, Napoleon found it essential to enrich this great architectural symbol with a specific element that could distinguish him from his pre-Revolutionary predecessors. This addition was a new gateway that took the form of a triumphal arch. Charles Percier and Pierre Francois Leonard Fontaine, who are credited with the invention of the *Empire* style, designed it. The structure's richly decorated architecture was praised for being 'perfectly in accord' with the Tuileries' façade.[16] It was more than a mere point of spectacular entry that had been a customary element of royal residences in Europe for ages as an instrument of monarchical glorification. It was a monument to the glory of the French army and as such it was Napoleon's homage to the nation-in-arms: the nation of citizen-soldiers for whom the idea of mass military service in the age of the Revolutionary and Napoleonic Wars was a source of respect and political significance. The arch, known as the *Arc de Triomphe du Carrousel* ('Carrousel' is the name of the adjacent square), specifically commemorated the campaign against the Third Anti-French Coalition. It culminated with the victory at Austerlitz in 1805 and was the first great military achievement of the empire after its establishment. That military success consolidated the empire's powerful position in Europe and validated the French nation's pretensions to be seen as the modern

successor of the Roman imperial glory.[17] The Roman connection was also emphasized by the Horses of Saint Mark at its top.[18] This set of ancient bronze horses was
brought to Paris as booty from Venice, and they were thought to originally adorn
a triumphal arch in the Roman Forum.[19] Reportedly, some French officials also
wanted to place Napoleon's statue on the top of the arch, but the emperor declined,
stressing that it would be 'very inconvenient' to give him the honour of 'apotheosis'
while he dedicated this monument to 'the glory of the army he had the honour
to command'.[20] Each of the arch's columns was crowned with a statue of a soldier
representing a specific army formation. With such focus on the soldiers themselves,
the arch used traditional architectural language for honouring a monarch or leader
but did not glorify him alone. It was a monument to a collective national effort, and
its erection in front of the emperor's palace served the official propaganda of the
republican and meritocratic foundations of the Napoleonic regime.

The *Arc du Carrousel* linked the monarchical majesty, represented by the palace,
with the imperial identity of the nation-in-arms that had elected Napoleon as their
leader and could then praise itself for this apparently felicitous choice. The responsibility of the emperor for the military excellence of the nation as a requirement for
his monarchical legitimacy was additionally stressed by the military use of the square
in front of the palace, serving as a parade and review ground that was open to the
public. Moreover, the square's perspective was closed by the Louvre complex. Unlike
the Tuileries, this former royal residence was not restored to its original use, but
due to its associations with artistic exhibitions – dating from the pre-Revolutionary
period – it was chosen to house the *Musée Napoléon*. There, the precious spoils of
Republican and Imperial successful wars were exhibited to the public, being the ultimate symbols of national greatness under the guidance of the emperor who resided
on the other side of the square.[21]

The only major royal palace that Napoleon was unable to decide how to make
ideological use of in the post-Revolutionary political circumstances was Versailles.
After a long period of intentional neglect during the Revolution, this monument
of French monarchy needed renovation after its re-establishment, but it appears
that Napoleon did not know how to adapt it to the specific needs of imperial representation. According to Fontaine, Napoleon regretted that Louis XVI 'left him his
splendour to use' and 'the Revolution its excesses to mend'.[22] He started to repair
some minor and most dilapidated parts of the structure, musing about the possibility
of its comprehensive rebuilding. He was even presented with designs regarding this
project, but none of them got any further than paper.

He eventually lost his original interest in Versailles after the birth of his son, the
king of Rome, in 1811, which confronted him with the problem of secure dynasti-
cal succession. For many, the birth of the king of Rome was, according to Adolphe
Thiers, a 'pledge of the perpetuity of the Napoleon dynasty granted by Providence'
that finally secured the permanence of the empire.[23] However, it did not discharge
the emperor from obligation to clarify to the post-Revolutionary generation of the
French why the hereditary regime was advantageous for them.[24] It seems to explain
why Napoleon decided to renounce the idea of rebuilding Versailles, which apart
from its problematic connotations with the legacy of the absolutist political order
could hardly support his claims for being more independent from the past and worthy of establishing a new dynasty. Last, but not least, such an expensive enterprise

was bound to prevent him from investing in any other spectacular architectural project that could benefit him more in his new situation. He therefore focused his attention on building a new residence for his closest family that, even if clearly inspired by the grandeur of the suburban seat of the Bourbons, would be an independent enterprise manifesting his ambition to establish a new dynasty for the new post-Revolutionary order.[25]

This palace, designed by Percier and Fontaine in 1811 but ultimately unbuilt, fell prey to the political upheavals of 1812–14 and the subsequent downfall of the empire. It was called the *Palais du Roi de Rome*, and this name was apparently a reference to the promise of Napoleonic France's great future under his successor. The palace was expected to be built on the immediate outskirts of the capital, namely Chaillot Hill, as an integral part of a grand architectural ensemble. The harmonious complex was designed to house military barracks and a military hospital, as well as public institutions of other kinds. These included the Imperial University, the School of Fine Arts, the state archive and a building intended to provide grace-and-favour accommodation for 'retired professors, intellectuals and men of distinction who due to their outstanding services, or their talents, merited respect and national recognition'.[26] All these structures were to be centred around the field of exercise (*Champ de Mars*) for the pupils of the *Ecole militaire*, whose mid-eighteenth-century building stands in front of the hill. The merger of the new Versailles-scale palace with those public institutions expressed the idea of this new hereditary rule. The latter was to be based not on self-aggrandizement, but rather on the championship of national excellence and greatness, patronized by the crown and administered by the state-sponsored institutions of knowledge management that were responsible for the meritocratic development of the nation and the formation of its knowledge-based new elite.[27] In combining monarchical splendour with the meritocratic vision of the (nonetheless hierarchical) society, it was a Versailles of the modern era. The prominence given to a military school was a salient feature of the design. This symbolic juxtaposition of imperial authority with the army was building on those ideas that were originally embodied in the developments undertaken at the Tuileries.

Legitimizing conquest

The French model of using residences as an instrument of bridging the symbolic gap between monarchical majesty and the people set an example for those monarchies established by Napoleon in the occupied part of Europe, and ruled by his relatives. This policy served to support the legitimacy of the conquerors who needed to convince their new subjects (and especially those on whose support they intended to base their power) that their regimes were better than the preceding ones. From the French point of view, it was Napoleonic France that served as a model society, combining Revolutionary ideals with monarchical tradition. However, this paradigm was not universally applicable and needed to be modified with respect to local history and sociopolitical traditions. This situation influenced the character and extent of changes that those crowned conquerors decided to implement in their residences.

One of those new monarchs, Napoleon's brother-in-law, Joachim Murat, was made king of Naples, a country that had an established tradition of absolutist rule under a side branch of the Bourbons. Murat did not want to repudiate the existing symbols of monarchical power that could add to his popular prestige. He therefore moved into the old palace in the Parthenopean capital. He did not change the building a great deal, except for the *Empire* redecoration of the interiors.[28] He preferred to focus his attention on the public area that unfolded immediately in front of the main façade. He launched a competition, and eventually decided to commission Leopoldo Laperuta to replace a chaotic and rather claustrophobic mass of unassuming structures (including two Catholic churches and adjoining monasteries) with the classical dignity and order of a porticoed semi-circle.[29] Laperuta wanted to crown this monumental structure with a pavilion, situated exactly vis-à-vis the entrance gate of the palace. It was not a gloriette or a gazebo, which were typical elements of pre-Revolutionary royal residential ensembles, but a public assembly hall that served for such gatherings as exhibitions of industry and fine arts. Those state-patronized events promoted the progress of national creative output, which in turn could be a source of national prosperity;[30] they were addressed to the Napolitan middle class that gained significance in the course of the French-style anti-feudal reforms and were the natural social basis of the new regime.[31] Renata de Lorenzo noted that: 'the symmetrical, balanced and classically inspired square . . . is mirroring the new union between social forces and powers of the state'.[32] This ensemble – the structure closing the perspective of the palace's outer and publicly accessible courtyard – expressed in its form and use the idea of economic and cultural growth of the kingdom's modernized society that the new ruler intended to champion. It was also an emblematic act of ideological separation from the Bourbon past, counterbalancing the signs of Murat's apparent traditionalism expressed by his inhabitancy of the little-changed palace.[33] However, it was Napoleon's, and not Murat's, effigy that was planned to be placed in the centre of the square. The equestrian statue by Antonio Canova would not have been only a symbol of political dependence. It could also indicate the official model of civilizational development under Murat's rule. This ambitious enterprise was, nevertheless, unfinished before the empire's eventual collapse and the consequent deposition of the crowned usurper. Murat was therefore unable to see whether his original idea would prove to be an ideological asset.

The Kingdom of Westphalia represented a different model of a Napoleonic monarchical state. Being previously composed of separate territories such as the landgraviate of Hesse-Kassel, it had no precedent.[34] The fact that the kingdom was an artificial creation motivated Napoleon to make it a model monarchy of Napoleonic Europe. There, it was seemingly easier to effectively implement political, economic and social innovations of the Revolutionary pedigree, such as the abolition of the feudal stratification of society and the consequent introduction of bureaucratic administration as well as parliamentarian representation that was open not only to noble landowners but also urbanized intellectuals and tradespeople.[35] As a result, a political life in Westphalia became more democratic than it had been in the pre-Napoleonic era (although still most inhabitants of the kingdom had no political rights). In the emperor's view, the 'liberty', 'equality' and 'degree of well-being unknown to the people of Germany', resulting from the reforms, were secure foundations of the French hegemony in this part of Europe.[36]

Napoleon chose his youngest brother, Jérôme, to execute this ambitious plan. The source of the new king's legitimacy resided in his sibling's supremacy over Europe. It is then no surprise that the name of the country seat of one of this territory's former rulers at *Wilhelmshöhe* (Wilhelm's Heights), outside Kassel, was changed to *Napoleonshöhe*.[37] This palatial structure, built in the last two decades of the previous century, satisfied the requirements of the official classical taste of the empire. However, the apparent problem was the insufficient ideological impact such a palace might have on the politically engaged public.

Even though the suburban grounds of *Napoleonshöhe* were accessible to the subjects of the 'model' monarchy, the king also paid attention to his representation in the capital proper, where the kingdom's parliament had its seat.[38] The fact that noble landowners opposed the French-style reforms and the Napoleonic ideas of liberty and equality (although the king did his best to curry favour with them), also could be a driving factor behind Jérôme's special interest in the kingdom's rapidly developing metropolis, where the rising, politically emancipated middle class could be his ally.[39] The comprehensive rebuilding of the former castle of the Hessian landgraves in the inner city was not taken into account. All the works that concerned the castle were limited to the superficial classicization of its façades and interiors.[40] Much like his brother in Paris and his brother-in-law in Naples, Jérôme focused his efforts on the reorganization of the area around the building. One of the principal features of August-Henri-Victor Grandjean de Montigny's conception of the castle's new spatial environment was a four-and-a-half-metre-high memorial to the king himself, with his statue standing on a plinth, decorated with bas-reliefs featuring Jérôme's glorious deeds.[41] The design explicitly stated that the king was to be portrayed 'en pied' and in marble, but lacks further details. However, it seems probable that it was the only known standing marble statue of the king by François Joseph Bosio that Montigny had in mind as a model. The nearly two-metre-high sculpture, placed on a circular pedestal, and corresponding with what Montigny drew in his design, depicts the monarch in a moment of taking an oath. It was a very unusual pose for a monarchical monument that had traditionally depicted rulers as military leaders or law-givers. It was a novel invention in the history of royal iconography, representing the king of Westphalia ('by the grace of God and the constitution') as a constitutional monarch by focusing on the solemn public declaration of obeying the kingdom's fundamental law.[42] If the statue was intended for public display in front of the royal palace, it would be a most spectacular sign of recognition of the public acceptance as a source of legitimacy. However, the very fact of planning a royal statue in this place is noteworthy in itself. By representing the monarch as a man of merit (through the representation of his achievements), it provided his residence with a public visual expression of meritocratic values on which the Napoleonic idea of monarchy was founded. Much like in Napoleon's case, the people's obedience to Jérôme was not only a question of metaphysical order but was apparently also expected to result from a rational appreciation of all the benefits the Westphalians gained from his rule. The statue was intended to occupy a specific point of the castle's grandiose forecourt, namely a square where the axis leading from the castle's entrance façade would be crossed with the axis of another square, where the building of parliament was standing. The visual connection between both squares, and thus both politically important structures, was linked by the statue of the king. It even more profoundly manifested the idea of integral connection between the royal authority and the political agency of the subjects (at least, some part of them).

Yet another of Napoleon's brothers, Louis, was positioned as the ruler of Holland. In contrast to Naples and the patchwork state of Westphalia, this newly established Napoleonic kingdom replaced not an absolutist monarchy but a centuries-old republic. However, the material legacy of the republican system apparently suited the needs of Napoleonic monarchical propaganda. After spending some time looking for a suitable royal seat and a centre of state administration (the Republic of the Netherlands had been a federation of self-governing entities, and the Dutch had no former capital), Louis settled in Amsterdam, which was the biggest city of the country and its commercial hub.[43] There, he chose to reside in a former city hall, the traditional headquarters of the city's self-government and the centre of the republican commune's political life. The building was not confiscated but – in a propagandist move – granted to the king by the city as a token of the citizens of Amsterdam's will to 'see Your Majesty among us as well as respect and cherish him as a king who after his elevation to the throne, has not ceased to love and protect us'.[44] In his response, Louis prudently remarked that 'A country where the king would be entirely isolated from his people, would soon perish.'[45] He was evidently determined to use the former city hall as an instrument of his royal self-fashioning – he moved to it despite being discouraged by some courtiers who found this place humid and cold, and thus inappropriate to live in.[46] The evocations of the ancient Roman Republic in the seventeenth-century building's classical architecture, that had originally served to promote the image of Amsterdam as a new Rome, proved ideally suited to the requirements of the Napoleonic royal court. Nevertheless, the city hall's interior decoration needed some changes to make it dignified enough to express its new status as a royal palace. This work was entrusted to the French architect Jean Thomas Thibault and his Dutch collaborator, Bartholomeus Ziesenis.[47] The main assembly room of the building, the Citizens' Hall, provided a spectacular venue for ceremonies, receptions and other displays of royal pomp. What is more, the original universalistic programme of its decoration, glorifying the global colonial influence of the city and making references to Rome as its predecessor, corresponded with the ambitions of the empire with which Louis's kingdom was integrally associated.

The transformation of the city hall into a royal residence brought natural restrictions of access to the former public building, guided by etiquette. It was the reason why a balcony was added to the front façade. It was there where the monarch could make public appearances before his subjects, who had free space to gather in front of the palace after some 'gothic' buildings that adjoined it had been demolished.[48] As argued earlier, the rearrangements of squares that played the role of the palaces' public forecourts was a common preoccupation of Napoleonic monarchs. They may appear to be acts of paternalistic civic appropriation, but there is no evidence that they were seen as such in the period under discussion. It was the monarchs' privilege to shape the public space of their residential cities, and they did it according to the narrative they favoured and found advantageous for their image. However, the king of Holland did not content himself with only this innovation. The royal palace still had its public part to which admission was not an exclusive privilege of the guest of the court, and this area housed an art gallery. It identified the prestige of the royal office with the protection of the internationally famous patrimony of the Dutch that had been the pride of Amsterdam's citizens in the previous century, when the city's magistrates provided accommodation for an 'art chamber' in the city hall.[49] It also could be a reference to the Parisian example of joining the monarchical palace (the Tuileries) with the public museum (the Louvre).

Legitimizing restoration

For Napoleonic rulers, the pre-Revolutionary tradition of monarchical representation was not an easy legacy to deal with, but neither was it for the Restoration monarchs who ruled their people after the Congress of Vienna in 1815. In order to survive without risking new disorders, the Restoration was marked by efforts to adjust monarchical rule to the post-Revolutionary world that witnessed the rise of new social forces and, above all, the political ambition of the urbanized middle class that was nurtured by the Napoleonic regime. It is true that Restoration regimes excelled in applying the Napoleonic model of administrative control of society, rather than in satisfying their subjects' expectations and aspirations for active participation and subjectivity in political life. It was a main source of revolutionary upheavals that Europe faced after the Congress of Vienna, which was convoked with an intention to secure the stability of the 'restored' order in post-Napoleonic Europe.[50] Still, many of those monarchs who were confronted with a need for a *modus vivendi* wanted to address sociopolitical anxieties, at least symbolically. Many residences, as it is evidenced in the following survey, proved to be an operative instrument of marrying the traditional majesty with the Revolutionary legacy, both in those monarchies that were directly affected by Napoleonic reforms and in those in which this influence was indirect and did not result in revolutionary changes regarding government systems and divisions of political power.

Prussia and Austria, two absolutist states that played a significant role in the destruction of the Napoleonic empire, are good examples of the second group. While the Royal Castle in downtown Berlin, where the court's ceremonial life was centred, remained largely unchanged in the aftermath of the Congress of Vienna, its environs were metamorphosed to a meaningful degree.[51] In the 1820s, the king's private pleasure garden (*Lustgarten*), which had provided the military with exercise grounds throughout the eighteenth century, was redesigned by Peter Joseph Lenné into a green area for the public. As such, it became the main public park in the city. At its far end, directly opposite the castle, Friedrich Wilhelm III (r.1797–1840) built the magnificent edifice of the Royal Museum, designed by Karl Friedrich Schinkel, which made the king's private collection of art (mainly ancient classical) accessible to his subjects.[52] The Austrian emperor, Francis I (r.1804–35; previously Francis II as the Holy Roman Emperor, 1792–1806), followed a similar path. A 'people's garden' (*Volksgarten*) was opened next to the Hofburg Castle in Vienna, in the area that was originally occupied by its fortifications.[53] There, the court architect Peter Nobile designed a Doric temple-like pavilion. It served as a place of public exhibition for the monumental neoclassical sculpture of *Theseus and the Centaur* by Antonio Canova. Originally commissioned in 1805 by Napoleon as his victory monument, it was subsequently acquired by the Habsburgs after 1815. It gave the Viennese public an opportunity to see an example of artistic excellence that had a political meaning in itself. According to Charlotte Stokes, 'the classical rules that once gave a sense of order to the Revolution [and the Napoleonic empire] were appropriated by a conservative government in order to set strict standards that precluded any revolution in style' and thus in Austrian society as well.[54] The association of Austria with classical tradition was made even more convincing by the display of Roman archaeological findings from the Habsburg lands in the catacombs of the Temple.[55] Both in Berlin and Vienna, monarchical residential precincts turned into open spaces that were generally accessible not only to nobility and guests of the court but also to the middle classes. This served the pro-monarchical ideology by showing regard for the latter and recognizing their social significance, while simultaneously being a sign of the monarchs' anxiety about this new sociopolitical situation in which the absolutist Hohenzollerns and Habsburgs found themselves after the Napoleonic Wars, in the so-called *Vormärz* period that ended with the outbreak of the bourgeois revolutions of 1848.

In Russia, it was not an underdeveloped middle-class public, but members of the noble elite – the class of civil and military servicemen – who put political pressure on the monarch and were determined to obtain their share in the government. Tsar Alexander I (r.1801–25) himself added fuel to their ambitions because of his ambiguous suggestions about the possibility of granting the Russians a constitution. However, there was strong opposition by many conservative nobles for whom the autocracy was an instrument of social control. From their point of view, liberal changes could have a negative impact on their relations with peasant serfs they owned in their estates.[56] Oscillating between both sides of this conflict, Alexander I came up with an idea of a monument to the glory of the Russian victory over Napoleon that contributed to the rise of liberal views in Russia. His intention was to build a commemorative gallery in the Winter Palace, the main seat of the tsars in St Petersburg, which would feature effigies of all the Russian generals of the successful 'patriotic' war against Napoleon. He commissioned the English painter George Dawe to make almost 350 portraits of the war heroes.[57] However, due to the dictates of political exigency, the gallery was inaugurated in 1826 (before the painter finished his long-standing work) by Alexander's successor Nicholas I (r.1825–55), who ascended the throne in the aftermath of the quenched pro-constitution Decembrist revolt.[58] The suppression of this aristocratic uprising solidified the political position of the young tsar who was an ardent proponent of traditional autocracy. On the other hand, it also prompted him to reinvigorate the cult of the 'patriotic war' that could appease the decimated elite that had recently suffered detention, conviction, forced displacement or execution of many members of their social circle. The gallery, designed by Carlo Rossi and displaying rows of portraits that culminated with the large-size likeness of Alexander I on horseback, was situated next to the throne room as its immediate antechamber. The prestigious placement of the gallery pointed to the idea of collective contribution to the common good that was contingent on nobles' faithful service to the emperor.[59] A gigantic column in the palace square nevertheless emphasized the utmost prominence of the latter visually linking the imperial residence with the building of the Russian general staff. Nicholas erected that monument to the memory of his late brother as the one who was responsible for the victory, but it was officially dedicated by the Russian nation. It was consequently a spectacular symbol of national gratitude that contributed to the image of the emperor as father of the nation and shield against enemies.

Monarchies that experienced a Napoleonic rule did not need remarkable modifications of royal residences but tried to accommodate those ones with which they were left after 1815. In Naples, for example, King Ferdinand I (r.1816–25, previously Ferdinand IV of Naples and Ferdinand III of Sicily, 1759–1816) upheld the Napoleonic concept of the forum in front of the palace, harnessing the progressivist ideology of Murat's transformation to support the legitimacy of his restoration. However, the central pavilion was no longer a secular assembly room, but a church. By this modification, the Bourbon king restored the original sacral character of the palace's forecourt and simultaneously undermined – in a symbolic but also very destructive way – the conceptual foundations of the previous intervention by Murat.[60] It was a powerful reaction against Napoleonic desecration and the relegation of monarchical legitimacy to the sphere of social relations rather than divine intervention. Another modification concerned the equestrian statue. Ferdinand himself occupied the plinth that was previously intended for Napoleon. However, the king was not left without a companion since a correspondent statue was unveiled nearby, that of his father, Charles VII. Thus, the natural right of succession, undermined by the meritocratic ideology of the Napoleonic regime, found its expression in this discourse of legitimacy that manifested itself in the precincts of the royal palace. The church was inaugurated only by his grandson, Ferdinand II (r.1830–59), in 1836, but this elapse of generations only added fuel to the dynastic connotation of this building that served the royal propaganda. It was evidenced by an official commemorative medal that featured the effigy of the current monarch beside that of his father and grandfather.[61]

While the Napolitan monarch could feel free to redirect the meaning of the invading regime's symbolic enterprises that were nevertheless retained and developed, his French cousins, Louis XVIII (r.1814–24) and Charles X (r.1824–30), needed to accept the Napoleonic heritage unconditionally because they returned to rule the people who had previously toppled their family from the throne. Therefore, they prudently established their court at the Tuileries, following the tradition of the constitutional monarchy that they willingly espoused. They preserved the *Arc de Triomphe du Carousel* in front of the palace and did not redecorate the interiors. The etiquette in their Parisian palace also took inspiration from the Napoleonic heritage, shortening the distance between a monarch and his subjects that was so characteristic of the Versailles court.[62] However, both Louis and Charles were clearly eager to use the Versailles palace as a seat, at least in summer time. It was not only a symbol of the old French monarchy but also the place where they were born and brought up. Ultimately, they did not have enough courage to put this idea into practice, but simultaneously did not leave their family home without due care, financing its upkeep and repair.[63] The Versailles question was eventually solved only after the July Revolution of 1830, which resulted in the deposition of the 'legitimate' line of the ruling family and their replacement with the head of the distant Orleanist branch, known for his liberal viewpoint and fondness of the Revolutionary and Napoleonic past. The new king 'of the French' (instead of France), Louis Philippe (r. 1830–48), made decisive steps to sever the symbolic connections of the current French monarchy with the tradition of absolutism. This policy included the restoration of the Versailles complex's former role as a public museum that it had previously played during the Republican period.[64]

Conclusion

The Revolutionary experiences of 1789–91 had a profound impact on the way that European monarchs represented themselves to their subjects through residences. At first glance, it may seem that the change was not drastic and merely superficial, but the examples analysed here demonstrate that even minor modifications could serve to refashion the image of monarchy as a political phenomenon that had much in common with their (at least those better off) people and was absorbed with their development, excellence and prestige. In the period between 1804 and 1830, the precincts of royal palaces in France, Naples, Prussia and Austria started to be linked with museums, assembly rooms, common green spaces and national memorials. In some cases, their interiors also had such public functions, such as in Russia, where the political participation of the society was limited to the noble elite, or in the Netherlands, where the republican traditions apparently deprived the monarch of the ability to prevent the people from accessing at least some part of his palace. Such modifications apparently became essential to win popularity. The symbolic integration of royal residences with society intensified throughout subsequent generations in response to the growing power of the middle class in the second half of the nineteenth century. In the Habsburg empire, this phenomenon was exemplified by the 'Emperor's Forum' (*Kaiserforum*) that formed part of the Hofburg complex (1870s). In Russia, it was the transformation of the Hermitage wing of the Winter Palace into a public museum (1852). In Naples, it was a series of the statues of Napolitan crowned heroes that were added to the entrance façade of the palace by the new king of the unified Italian state (1888). In the twentieth century, the process of 'democratization' of royal palaces entered a completely new phase of its history. Being a reflection of the further social democratization of the public life, it was motivated by the progress of media coverage of royal public and private life and consequent demand for the further reduction of distance that monarchical majesty was traditionally generating. It was only then that a truly mass public started to witness and virtually participate in state ceremonies taking place there, as well as directly experience the internal opulence that became accessible to commoners through guided tours and open days. No more a source of isolation, but constantly a symbol of royal dignity, palaces are still apparently able to adapt to new social circumstances, supporting their royal inhabitants in their incessant endeavours to retain popularity and public legitimacy.

Notes

1 I would like to thank De Brzezie Lanckoronski Foundation and the Polish Academy of Learning for the award of a research grant in 2016 that enabled me to consult a number of secondary sources that are not available in Poland. This chapter was written while I was a National Science Centre (Poland) post-doctoral researcher at the Jagiellonian University in Cracow (2016/20/S/HS2/00053).

2 The National Assembly was already the king's neighbour, but it resided in an adjacent riding hall rather than in the palace proper. C.J. Mitchel, *The French Legislative Assembly of 1791* (Leiden: E.J. Brill, 1988), 9–10.

3 A fragment of Bertrand Barère's speech is included in Ambrogio A. Caiani, *Louis XVI and the French Revolution, 1789–1792* (Cambridge: Cambridge University Press, 2012), 69. The idea was not originally his, because it had already attracted the attention of architects: Richard Etlin, *Symbolic Space: French Enlightenment Architecture and its Legacy* (Chicago:

The University of Chicago Press, 1996), 31; Jean-Claude Daufresne, *Louvre & Tuileries: Architectures de papier* (Liège-Bruxelles: Pierre Mardaga, 1987), 122–134.

4 Caiani, *Louis XVI*, 8, 21.

5 Richard S. Wortman, *Scenarios of Power: Myth and Ceremony in Russian Monarchy from Peter the Great to the Abdication of Nicholas II* (Princeton: Princeton University Press, 2006), 3–4.

6 William Doyle, *France and the Age of Revolution* (New York: I.B. Tauris, 2013), 126.

7 Wortman, *Scenarios of Power*, 10.

8 For more on the idea and practice of Napoleon's monarchy, see Alan Forrest, "Napoleon as Monarch: A Political Evolution," in *The Bee and the Eagle: Napoleonic France and the End of the Holy Roman Empire, 1806*, eds. Alan Forrest and Peter H. Wilson (New York: Palgrave Macmillan, 2009), 112–130; and William Doyle, "The Political Culture of the Napoleonic Empire," in *The Bee and the Eagle: Napoleonic France and the End of the Holy Roman Empire, 1806*, eds. Alan Forrest and Peter H. Wilson (New York: Palgrave Macmillan, 2009), 83–93. On the Napoleonic elite, see Alexander Grab, *Napoleon and the Transformation of Europe* (New York, Palgrave Macmillan: 2003), 41–43.

9 Philip Mansel, *The Court of France 1789–1830* (Cambridge, Cambridge University Press, 1988), 70. See also Philip Mansel, *The Eagle in Splendour: Inside the Court of Napoleon* (London: I.B. Tauris, 2015), 67–80.

10 On Napoleon's court in general, see Mansel, *The Eagle*, passim.

11 See: Mitchell Schwarzer, "The Sources of Architectural Nationalism," in *Nationalism and Architecture*, eds. Raymond Quek, Darren Deane and Sarah Butler (London: Routledge, 2012), 21.

12 On the problem of Roman references in Napoleonic propaganda see Valerie Huet, "Napoleon I: A New Augustus?" in *Roman Presences: Receptions of Rome in European Culture, 1789–1945*, ed. Catherine Edwards (Cambridge: Cambridge University Press, 1999), 53–69; Matthew D Zarzeczny, *Meteors that Enlighten the Earth: Napoleon and the Cult of Great Men* (Newcastle-upon-Tyne: Cambridge Scholars Publishing, 2013), 128–140.

13 *Rapport du jury institué par S. M. L'Empereur et Roi pour le jugement des prix décennaux* (Paris: Imprimerie Imperiale, 1810), 164.

14 Aubry, *Le guide des étrangers aux monumens publics de Paris* (Paris: Aubry, 1808), 75; Anne-Adrien-Firmin Pillon-Duchemin, *Numa-Pompilius au palais des Tuileries: Hommage a l'occasion de la naissance de S.M. le Roi de Rome* (Paris: J.B. Hautecoeur, 1811), 8. The palace was built during the reign of the first and rebuilt by the second.

15 Susan Conner, *The Age of Napoleon* (Westport: Greenwood Press, 2004), 75; Zarzeczny, *Meteors*, 109; Lord Rosebery, *Napoleon: The Last Phase* (London: Humphreys, 1900), 179.

16 *Rapports et discussions de toutes les classes de l'Institut de France sur les ouvrages admis au concours pour les prix décennaux* (Paris: Baudouin et cie., 1810), 52.

17 Diana Rowell, *Paris: The 'New Rome' of Napoleon* (London: Bloomsbury, 2014), 47–48.

18 Rowell, *The "New Rome"*, 52–53.

19 A. Person de Teyssèdre, *Conducteur général de l'étranger dans Paris* (Paris: Garnier, 1837), 72.

20 Charles Percier and Pierre-François-Léonard Fontaine, *Résidences de souverains: Parallèle entre plusierus résidences de souverains de France, d'Allemagne, de Suède, de Russie, d'Espagne, et d'Italie* (Paris: n.p., 1833), 23.

21 Rowell, *The "New Rome"*, 8, 48–49.

22 *Palais de Versailles: Domaine de la couronne* (Paris: Imprimerie de Pihan Delaforest, 1836), 14.

23 Adolphe Thiers, *History of the Consulate and the Empire of France under Napoleon*, trans. D. Forbes Campbell and H.W. Herbert (Philadelphia: J.B. Lipincott & Co., 1864), 4–9.

24 Jean Tulard, *Napoléon II* (Paris: Fayard, 1992), 54–62.

25 Hans-Joachim Haassengier, *Das Palais du Roi de Rome auf dem Hügel von Chaillot* (Frankfurt am Main: Peter Lang, 1983), 18.

26 Percier and Fontaine, *Résidences*, 11.

27 See Rafe Blaufarb, *The French Army 1750–1820: Careers, Talent, Merit* (Manchester: Manchester University Press, 2002), 170.

28 Felice de Filippis, *Il Palazzo Reale di Napoli* (Naples: Montanino, 1960), 57–60.

29 Arnoldo Venditti, *Architettura neoclassica a Napoli* (Naples: Edizioni scientifiche italiane, 1961), 159–168; John A. Davis, *Naples and Napoleon: Southern Italy and the European Revolutions, 1780–1860* (Oxford: Oxford University Press, 2006), 206.

30 Pasquale Villani, *Italia napoleonica* (Napoli: Guida, 1978), 144.

31 Renata de Lorenzo, *Murat* (Rome: Salerno Editrice, 2011), 209–213.

32 De Lorenzo, *Murat*, 232.

33 See: Paolo Mascilli Migliorini, "Valori civili dell'architettura," in *A passo di carica: Murat re di Napoli*, ed. Luigi Mascilli Migliorini (Napoli: Arte'm, 2015), 39–40.

34 Georg Hassel, *Das Königreich Westphalen von seiner Organisation Statistisch dargestellt* (Braunschweig: F. Vieweg, 1807), 4.

35 Ewald Grothe, "Model or Myth? The Constitution of Westphalia of 1807 and Early German Constitutionalism," *German Studies Review* 28, no. 1 (2005): 1–19; Grab, *Napoleon*, 101–103.

36 Napoleon's letter to his brother Jérôme, November 1807, quoted in Grab, *Napoleon*, 99.

37 Thorsten Smidt, "Residenzen," in *König lustik!? Jerome Bonaparte und der Modellstaat Konigreich Westphalen*, eds. Michael Eisenhauer, Arnulf Siebeneicker and Thorsten Smidt (Munich: Hirmer, 2008), 314; Arnulf Siebeneicker, "Repräsentanten der ganzen westphälischen Nation: Das Parlament im politischen System des Königreichs Westphalen," in *König lustik!? Jerome Bonaparte und der Modellstaat Konigreich Westphalen*, eds. Michael Eisenhauer, Arnulf Siebeneicker and Thorsten Smidt (Munich: Hirmer, 2008), 117. For more on Jerome's connection with this palace, see Guillaume Nicoud, "Napoléonshöhe, joyau de la couronne de Westphalie," in *Jérôme Napoléon, roi de Westphalie*, ed. Aube Lebel (Paris: Éditions de la Réunion des musées nationaux, 2008), 93–101.

38 Smidt, "Residenzen," 314.

39 Grab, *Napoleon*, 99.

40 Dorothea Heppe, *Das Schloß der Landgrafen von Hessen in Kassel von 1557 bis 1811* (Marburg: Jonas, 1995), 283–285; Gerd Fenner, "Das kleine teutsche Paris? Zum Bauwesen in der Hauptstadt des Königreichs Westphalen," in *König lustik!? Jerome Bonaparte und der Modellstaat Konigreich Westphalen*, eds. Michael Eisenhauer, Arnulf Siebeneicker and Thorsten Smidt (Munich: Hirmer, 2008), 85.

41 Heppe, *Das Schloß*, 289. The plan by Montigny is in Hessisches Staatsarchiv, Marburg, Karten P II 9578/2. Fenner, "Das kleine teutsche Paris," 85.

42 *König Lustik!? Jerome Bonaparte und der Modellstaat Konigreich Westphalen*, eds. Michael Eisenhauer, Arnulf Siebeneicker and Thorsten Smidt (Munich: Hirmer, 2008), 180–181.

43 Dominique Labarre de Raillicourt, *Louis Bonaparte, 1778–1846, roi de Hollande, frère et père d'empereurs* (Paris: Peyronnet, 1963), 230–231, 235; Frans Grijzenhout, "King of Empire," in *King Louis Napoleon and His Palace in Dam Square* (Amsterdam: Koninklijk Paleis Amsterdam, 2012), 19–20; Annie Jourdan, "La Hollande en tant 'qu'objet de désir' et le roi Louis, fondateur d'une monarchie nationale," in *Louis Bonaparte, Roi de Hollande*, ed. Annie Jourdan (Paris: Nouveau Mondé éditions, 2010), 11.

44 Raillicourt, *Louis Bonaparte*, 236.

45 Raillicourt, *Louis Bonaparte*, 237.

46 Thomas Dunk von der, "Le roi Louis et l'architecture: une politique nationale," in *Louis Bonaparte, Roi de Hollande*, ed. Annie Jourdan (Paris: Nouveau Mondé éditions, 2010), 289.

47 On the architectural and artistic development of the palace in this period, see Paul Rem, "Les palais de Louis Napoléon, leur aménagement et leur mobilier," in *Louis Napoléon Premier Roi de Hollande (1806–1810)*, eds. Paul Rem and George Sanders (Zutphen: Walburg Pers, 2007), 30–32, 38–39; Renske Cohen Tervaert and Aagje Gosliga, "A Royal Transformation: The Empire Style at the Royal Palace in Amsterdam," in *King Louis Napoleon and His Palace in Dam Square*, ed. Marianna van der Zwaag (Amsterdam: Amsterdam Royal Palace, 2012), 53–86.

48 Grijzenhout, "King," 24, 29; Raillicourt, *Louis Bonaparte*, 237.

49 Grijzenhout, "King," 29–30. See also Bergvelt, "Louis Bonaparte," 328.

50 David Laven and Lucy Riall, "Restoration Government and the Legacy of Napoleon," in *Napoleon's Legacy: Problems of Government in Restoration Europe*, eds. David Laven and Lucy Riall (Oxford: Berg, 2000), 19.

51 On the ceremonial role of the Royal Castle, see Wolfgang Neugebauer, *Residenz-Verwaltung-Repräsentation: Das Berliner Schloss und seine historischen Funktionen vom 15. bis 20. Jahrhundert* (Potsdam: Verlag für Berlin-Brandenburg, 1999), 52–57.

52 See: Markus Jager, *Der Berliner Lustgarten. Gardenkunst und Stadgestalt in Preussens Mitte* (Munich: Deutscher Kunst Verlag, 2005), 133–167.

53 Richard Perger, *Straßen, Türme und Basteien: Das Straßennetz der Wiener City in seiner Entwicklung und seinen Namen* (Vienna: Franz Deuticke, 1991), 149.
54 Charlotte Stokes, "Taming the Eagles: The Habsburg Monarchy's Political Use of the 'Revolutionary' Neoclassical Style," in *Austria in the Age of the French Revolution 1789–1815*, eds. Kinley Brauer and William E. Wright (Minneapolis: Center for Austrian Studies, University of Minnesota, 1990), 80.
55 Franz Tschischka, *Der Gefährte auf Reisen in dem österreichischen Kaiserstaate* (Vienna: F. Beck, 1834), 497.
56 Janet M. Hartley, *Alexander I* (London: Longman, 1994), 166–168.
57 Galina Andreeva, *Geniuses of War, Weal and Beauty: George Dawe, RA Pinx* (Moscow: ICOM Russia, 2012), 146.
58 Andreeva, *Geniuses of War*, 196.
59 Andreeva argues that the mode of hanging those portraits was inspired by iconostases: the relationship between the tsar and his generals would then reflect the relationship between God and saints. Andreeva, *Geniuses of War*, 197.
60 On this transformation, see Arnoldo Venditti, *Architettura neoclassica a Napoli* (Naples: Edizioni scientifiche italiane, 1961), 168–172.
61 Massimo Carafa Jacobini, Susanna Marra and Francesco Petrucci, eds., *Dall' Aspromonte a Porta Pisa. I Borbone, Pio IX e Garibaldi* (Rome: Gangemi Editore, 2011), 46.
62 Mansel, *The Court*, 126–128.
63 Hélène Himelfarb, "Versailles: Functions and Legends," in *Rethinking France: Les Lieux de Mémoire, Volume I: The State*, eds. Pierre Nora and David P. Jordan, trans. Mary Trouille (Chicago: University of Chicago Press, 2001), 317.
64 Himelfarb, "Versailles," 310.

Key works

Benoît, Jérémie, *Napoléon et Versailles* (Paris: Réunion des Musées nationaux, 2005).
Featherstone, Michael, Jean-Michel Spieser, Gülru Tanman and Ulrike Wulf-Rheidt, eds., *The Emperor's House: Palaces from Augustus to the Age of Absolutism* (Berlin: De Gruyter, 2015).
Möckl, Karl ed., *Hof und Hofgesselschaft in den deutschen Staaten im 19. und 20. Jahrhundert* (Boppard am Rhein: Harald Boldt Verlag, 1990).
Telesko, Werner, Richard Kurdiovsky and Andreas Nierhaus, eds., *Die Wiener Hofburg und der Residenzbau in Mitteleuropa im 19. Jahrhundert: Monarchische Repräsentation zwischen Ideal und Wirklichkeit* (Vienna: Böhlau, 2010).
Werner, Karl Ferdinand, ed., *Hof, Kultur und Politik im 19. Jahrhundert* (Bonn: Ludwig Röhrscheid Verlag, 1985).
Zieseniss, Charles Otto, *Napoléon et la cour impériale* (Paris: Tallandier, 1980).

20

CLOTHING ROYAL BODIES

Changing attitudes to royal dress and appearance from the Middle Ages to modernity

Benjamin Wild[1]

In 2016, Queen Elizabeth II of the United Kingdom is said to have remarked, 'I have to be seen to be believed.'[2] Her maxim is apt for describing royals throughout history, whose appearance has been paramount in the projection, maintenance and diminution of their authority. The issue of what royalty wears has long been a source of popular comment. Sustained scholarly interest in royal clothing, however, is more recent. Much of the academic writing about royal dress has been in conjunction with museums. Exhibition catalogues have provided in-depth analysis of the clothing and dress accessories worn by royalty between the fourth and twentieth centuries.[3] Books on Chinese imperial dress and European ceremonial clothing, which follow a recognizable catalogue format, have also been published.[4] The work of specialist curators, these volumes are valuable for their visual and technical insights, but they can be difficult to incorporate into wider historical studies because they provide limited contextualization. A singular focus on rulers' wardrobes, which emphasize the role of garments in defining social and political hierarchies, is also out of step with recent clothing studies that emphasize multiple motivations and different methodologies for the creation and consumption of dress.[5] This chapter re-engages with the topic of what rulers wore by considering changing attitudes to royal dress and appearance between the Middle Ages and modernity in western Europe.

Historians have tended to engage with royal clothing only in larger studies that consider the public presentation of monarchy,[6] although there are some exceptions.[7] Medieval and early modern historians have also been successful in combining studies of royal clothing with political commentary, which is probably because the main sources for royal clothing from these periods are textual, thus diminishing the need for specialized clothing or curatorial knowledge.[8] Scholars of the pre-early modern period have certainly led the way in transcribing and translating sources that document royal clothes and jewellery.[9] Work on royal dress has not occurred in isolation, however, and attempts to place the topic in a wider cultural frame have been made, notably by Philip Mansel, Robert Ross, and Dominique Gaulme and François Gaulme.[10] Additionally, and underlining the important point that commentary on royal dress remains popular, in the *London Review of Books*, author Hilary Mantel has considered the appearance of royal bodies in a polemic about the objectification of modern monarchy.[11] While these authors pursue different lines of enquiry, they emphasize the difficulty of writing a history of royal dress and appearance, which is never quite the sum of its parts.

Arguably, royal dress has become a more critical means of defining royal status: where royal dress had long been important for reflecting the power of monarchy, it is now important for refracting its relative powerlessness. If this appears counterintuitive, it reveals the ambivalence of modern monarchy in the face of increasing public scrutiny, which has followed the establishment of representative institutions and the continuation of globalization. As rulers and their families have increasingly been required to justify their positions, their clothing choices have become subject to a larger range of interpretations as they try to satisfy conflicting demands to remain distinct and regal, while also becoming approachable and relevant. As Hilary Mantel argues of royals who now fulfil a largely symbolic role, it is as though they have become 'things'. Deprived of executive authority and now politically neutral, they are somewhere between 'gods and beasts'.[12] David Cannadine has made a similar, if more measured, point, remarking that the public perception of Britain's monarchy changed from 'impotence to aloofness to veneration to grandeur' between *c.*1820 and 1977.[13] By taking the *longue durée* approach to encompass the medieval to the modern, this chapter will suggest the 200 years between *c.*1640 and *c.*1840 were an important transitional period in changing attitudes to royal dress and appearance. This transition was largely due to the period's witnessing of the decisive curtailment of the executive and spiritual authority of royalty, even if the institution of monarchy in Europe continued to be widespread until the first half of the twentieth century.

The demonstration of royal authority: royal dress and appearance before *c.*1640

To comprehend the changes that occurred to alter attitudes towards royal dress and appearance between *c.*1640 and *c.*1840, it is necessary to understand how royal bodies were clothed before this point. Between the ninth and sixteenth centuries, royal bodies were visually distinct. Clothing styles, fabrics and decoration were enforced by sumptuary legislation that demarcated people's social position. Despite, or perhaps due to, the potent socialized belief, informed by Christian teaching, that clothing conveyed character, such laws were difficult to enforce as the desire to emulate was ever present.[14] Colour associations were particularly important in determining the appearance of royalty, who ruled by God's grace. Blue, which represented heaven and the clothing of the Virgin Mary, denoted loyalty in northwest Europe; red was associated with faith and charity. Yellow signified the fire and brimstone of hell.[15] Blue and red were popular colours in the heraldry of northwest Europe and, because of their positive meaning, became the colours of the royal houses of France and England, respectively. Yellow, which was conventionally linked with disorder, is uncommon in European heraldry. The colour was typically worn by jesters and associated with people who defied royal authority. In the seventeenth century, when yellow became controversially popular at court, notably in Britain, it was linked to those who critiqued royal authority.[16] In the east, where similar sartorial injunctions existed, different faiths invested colours with different values.[17] Wearing yellow was a prerogative of China's emperor. The colour is associated with the Qing dynasty

(1644–1911), who adopted it to distinguish themselves from the Ming dynasty (1368–1644), whose official colour had been red.[18] In an interesting parallel to its European usage, the colour was adopted by rebels who wore yellow turbans to symbolize their protest.[19] As sartorial vogues and values were disseminated from the royal courts, they reinforced the rigid hierarchies that first produced them.

The importance of clothing and colour in conveying a ruler's authority is exemplified by fifteenth-century Burgundy, even though its head was not an anointed monarch. Philip the Good (r.1419–67) popularized the wearing of black, which he wore frequently after the assassination of his father by the French. Black clothing could represent mourning, but Till-Hoger Borchert argues it sent a strident message that the French treachery would not be forgotten.[20] Difficult to achieve through dyeing, pure black was also commensurately expensive and desirable.[21] The miniature of Philip on the dedication page of the *Chroniques de Hainault* – he is dressed in his polyvalent and pricey black – demonstrates how he embraced the latest fashions (pointed shoes, pinched waist and padded fur-trimmed sleeves) to exalt his authority through signs of taste, power and wealth.[22]

In the early modern period, images of royals dressed in elaborate and expensive clothing were particularly important in clarifying their singular authority, as concepts of royal magnificence and splendour could be projected through dress. The commission of royal portraits that could be viewed beyond the court, albeit largely in elite circles, was useful at a time when the establishment of representative institutions increased the number of politically active subjects.[23] England's Elizabeth I (r.1558–1603) used portraiture to assert her political status and to deflect prejudices connected to her womanhood and age.[24] *The Rainbow Portrait* of the queen, executed by Marcus Gheeraerts the Younger around 1600, which now hangs in Hatfield House, shows Elizabeth wearing a dress and cloak embroidered with allegorical symbols (Figure 20.1).

The eyes and ears on the cloak reference the story of Astraea, Greek goddess of innocence, and suggest that the queen sees and hears all; the jewelled serpent on her left sleeve represents wisdom. The long strings of pearls that hang from Elizabeth's hair, neck and wrist represent purity.[25] The rich decoration highlights the queen's sartorial distinction, but in recasting her as Astraea, it does more than this. The painting's motto *Non sine sole iris* ('no rainbow without sun') indicates that Elizabeth's qualities, intact despite her advanced age, would continue to ensure peace in England.[26] To make this connection explicit, the queen achieves the impossible and holds a rainbow in her right hand.

The idea that a monarch's dress could be 'read' as a barometer of their nation's political fortunes became clear during the sixteenth and seventeenth centuries, which saw the expansion of the state to unprecedented proportions. As royal authority affected more people, rulers' role as national figurehead and lodestar became commensurately important. Long before the seventeenth century, however, a ruler's appearance was equated with their ideals and style of politics, at least for those subjects who saw them frequently. When Henry I (r.1100–35) became king of England, he ordered his male courtiers to cut their hair and to forgo ostentatious dress, to make a public statement that he would rule prudently, in contrast to his brother William II (r.1087–1100), whose court had been criticized for licentiousness.[27] A similar gesture had been made by Charlemagne, king of the Franks (r.768–814), who

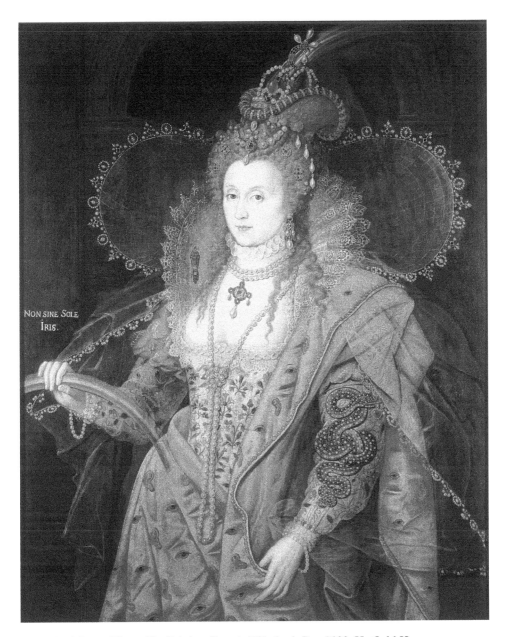

NON SINE SOLE
IRIS.

Figure 20.1 Isaac Oliver, *The Rainbow Portrait* (Elizabeth I), *c.*1600. Hatfield House, Hertfordshire, UK/Bridgeman Images

changed his hairstyle after his accession, to cauterize the break from the Merovingian rulers he replaced.[28]

Propaganda can be a problematic word for use in the pre-modern world, but people were aware that their rulers' clothing choices communicated more than personal tastes, and they were critical judges of what their overlords wore. For example, when the army of Henry III of England (r.1216–72) laid siege to Kenilworth Castle in 1266 – which had been occupied by a rebel garrison following a period of civil disturbance – the king wore a gambeson. This military tunic afforded protection, but its use of contrasting colours and decoration with gold embroidery suggests it was worn for its visual impact. This conclusion is plausible because Henry was probably more visible to a larger group of his subjects during the siege, and for a longer period of time than at any previous point in his reign.[29] The king's military clothing presumably sought to demonstrate his commitment to the campaign. Whatever the intended message, the rebels, who held out until Henry agreed to negotiate over their confiscated lands, presumably interpreted the gambeson as a sign of royal anger and bellicosity.[30] This example demonstrates a broader point about royal dress and appearance in the medieval and early modern periods: namely, that even the principle of strict sartorial hierarchy could not guarantee the successful reception of messages conveyed through dress. Clothes could reflect the wearer's status, but they did not necessarily convincingly reconstitute it.

The defence of royal authority: royal dress and appearance between *c.*1640 and *c.*1840

An example of how rulers found it increasingly difficult to use dress to demonstrate their authority during the later early modern period may be provided by the reign of Peter the Great of Russia (r.1682–1721). To exalt his authority, as much to demonstrate the political and economic transformation that was occurring under his rule, Peter used dress in two contrasting ways. First, he reclothed the monarchy, aristocracy and bourgeoisie by promoting 'German dress' and banning some traditional garments and beards to project the modernity of his nation. On 4 January 1700, the government printed a list of acceptable clothing that could be worn; on 16 January 1705, beards were prohibited across all social levels, unless a permit had been purchased.[31] By defining what could be worn, and using his court as a model of appropriate dress and comportment, Peter was demonstrating the reach of his authority and his apparent ability to shape his subjects' outlook. His method was similar to that of other European monarchs before him. For example, Peter's monarchical fiat is analogous to that displayed by Henry VIII of England (r.1509–47) in May 1535. Apparently, the king had his hair and beard cut short, perhaps to maintain a youthful appearance as he continued to gain weight, and 'commanded all about his court to poll their heads'.[32] A closer parallel to Peter's reforms is that of Louis XIV of France (r.1643–1715), who used his court 'as a showcase for the French cloth and dress industry'.[33] In a dramatic demonstration of Louis' support for his kingdom's clothing industry, and to ensure that his family's dress reflected this, Philip Mansel refers to an occasion when Louis ordered one of his son's coats to be burned because it was cut from imported cloth.[34]

Alongside these conventional clothing strictures, however, Peter's second sartorial strategy encouraged carnivalesque entertainments, largely based on western traditions, which inverted political and ecclesiastical positions through raucous behaviour and fancy dress. For the New Year, festivities within the tsar's court were celebrated with the 'All-Mad, All-Jesting, All-Drunken Assembly'. Costumes worn by members of the Assembly included monk's habits and animals' tails; on one occasion in 1698, Peter dressed as a Freisian peasant.[35] Lindsey Hughes suggests the tsar's comedic reversal of order reinforced his singular authority: Peter's rule in this fantasy placed in sharp relief his rule in reality.[36] Peter's actions in this example are intriguing because they suggest the tsar acknowledged that a change of dress and appearance did not fundamentally alter the character of its wearer. His position with regards to dress therefore seems contradictory. On the one hand, he inaugurated clothing reforms, which followed long-standing sartorial strategies used by other European monarchs and implied that he did believe his subjects' outlook could be affected by altering their clothing. On the other, through the Assembly, Peter's use of dress suggests he recognized that clothing merely reflected its wearer's character and did not change it; carnivalesque dress enabled individuals to take on the guise of things they were not. It is possible the tension between Peter's clothing reforms reflect, in microcosm, the challenges that were facing the institution of monarchy throughout Europe with the rise of the professionally trained officials and the increasing powers of representative parliaments.[37]

The acceleration of the growth of royal administrations across Europe that occurred between c.1640 and c.1840 was a double-edged sword for rulers' authority. On the one hand, royals gained greater knowledge of their kingdom's resources and new methods to exploit them, but on the other, the encroachment of royal offices and officials created a more litigious, demanding and often critical public. The expansion of the state, which deprived people of interpersonal bonds, could also engender feelings of loneliness that alienated them from their nation, to the point of creating an antagonistic relationship between the rulers and ruled.[38] Responding to Max Weber's remarks on the pronounced secularization or 'disenchantment' (*Entzauberung der Welt*) of this period, historians have charted the severance of personal bonds and the obfuscation of traditional beliefs.[39] New modes of courtly consumption, driven by commercial expansion and the wiles of monarchs who wanted to emasculate their leading subjects by encouraging penurious status expenditure, increased the social and cultural distance between the rulers and the ruled.[40] These developments were most apparent in western Europe, and in Britain and France in particular, where monarchical authority was more firmly established, and where, not coincidentally, the calls for representative institutions and restraint in royal dress were heard early and vociferously. The advent of Protestantism during the sixteenth and seventeenth centuries was also important in changing attitudes towards statecraft and matters sartorial. The re-establishment of a Protestant monarchy in England after the Glorious Revolution of 1688 strengthened the socialized notion that clothing conveyed character because indicators of luxury and effeminacy, which had been popular hallmarks of Catholic and royalist sympathisers, were denounced.[41] In this context, the dress of Charles I (r.1625–49) and his court, evocatively immortalized in Van Dyck portraits, was rebuked for its perceived opulence and decadence.[42]

Concerns about clothing and comportment were, of course, not confined to male members of the royal family and their court. During the seventeenth and eighteenth centuries, the dress of royal women was increasingly subject to comment. In their respective countries, Mary of Modena, wife of James II of England (r.1685–8), and Marie Antoinette, wife of Louis XVI of France (r.1774–93), popularized the wearing of male riding habits, which had been worn at least since the reign of Charles II of England (r.1660–85).[43] The fashion is illustrated in a portrait of Mary of Modena by Simon Verelst of *c.*1675, which forms part of the Royal Collection.[44] Diarist Samuel Pepys disapproved, remarking that 'Nobody could take [Mary and her female attendants] for women in any point whatever; which was an odd sight, and a sight [that] did not please me.'[45] In France, Marie Antoinette's dress, called *justaucorps* ('just on the body') because of its close-fitting silhouette, was also considered unladylike.[46] Central to these concerns was a belief that male attire would encourage women to transgress their gendered roles.[47] This specific anxiety reflected the opinions of privileged conservatives, but debates about the meaning of dress became urgent during the seventeenth and eighteenth centuries. People began to question the 'transnaturing' capacity of clothing – the ability of garments to alter the behaviour of their wearer – at a time when political and religious upheaval was 'turning the world upside down', to paraphrase a contemporary aphorism.[48]

In the face of sustained criticism and suspicion about their policies and their apparel, monarchs between *c.*1640 and *c.*1840 attempted to reclothe and reconstitute their social and political authority. After his return to England as king, Charles II introduced plainer court dress for men. This embryonic three-piece suit was an attempt, analogous to Henry I's in the twelfth century, to demonstrate that England's monarchy had a new moral compass and a more prudent style of governance.[49] Three years before the king's edict, in 1663, privy councillor Samuel Fortrey had advised the monarch that, 'it seems to be more honourable for a King of England, rather to become a pattern to his own people, than to conform to the humors and fancies of other nations'.[50] The reform faltered initially, and there were continued tensions between the simplicity of dress and the royal encouragement to wear fine clothing and lavish jewellery at court events, but the adoption of an aesthetics of restraint in the style of dress persisted among England's royalty. When the Protestant William III (r.1689–1702) replaced his Catholic father-in-law James II, it was noted that he 'probably wore a simple cinnamon-colored suit [for his coronation] and presented a rather modest, certainly civilian, surely benign picture' of kingship.[51] England's rulers were not alone in adopting ascetic attire in response to crisis. Mariana of Austria (r.1649–96), who acted as regent following the death of her husband Philip IV of Spain (r.1621–65), wore a mourning habit for the remainder of her life. The mourning habit had been worn by Habsburg widows and regents for over a century, but Mariana stands out for asserting its political meaning. Her dress demonstrated her piety and moral probity as the realm's ruler.[52] In a series of portraits, Mariana is shown seated at a desk, wearing her clothes of mourning and attending to matters of state. The queen's dress and demeanour is deliberately used to proclaim Mariana's 'vicarious authority' and to reassure courtiers and officials of her capacity to govern.[53]

During the eighteenth and nineteenth centuries, the tendency of European royals to wear spartan attire increased, and many wore variations of military dress, in itself a highly regulated mode of dress. There are several reasons for this. Martial clothing reflected the fact that Europe's leading powers were engaged in almost continuous conflict between the War of Spanish Succession (1702–15) and the Franco-Prussian War (1870–1).[54] Wearing uniforms can, in some instances, be elided with the period's pronounced growth of nationalism and the emergence of new states. Perhaps more importantly, the vogue for uniforms followed a period when the institution of monarchy in Europe had been severely weakened by rebellion and revolution. The rulers that remained needed to defend royal prerogatives clearly, and military dress facilitated this. As Robert Ross observes, uniforms are unambiguous in their depiction and promotion of rank.[55] Worn at a time when royal authority was being physically and theoretically challenged, uniforms also reminded subjects of the ruler's role as protector. Philip Mansel suggests that Frederick II of Prussia (r.1740–86) wore shabby uniforms to emphasize his successful leadership of his kingdom's army and to provide an unusual and striking sign of his singular authority.[56]

A particular advocate of military and national dress in the eighteenth century was Gustav III of Sweden (r.1771–92).[57] In contrast to Frederick II, Lena Rangström suggests Gustav used colourful military dress and insignia to give his unprepossessing physical stature greater authority.[58] In France, Napoleon I (r.1804–15) reminded his subjects of his right to rule by wearing military clothing. While he did wear aristocratic breeches and enforced court dress as conceived by artist Jacques-Louis David, Napoleon's frequent portrayals in uniform visually distanced him from the *ancien régime* he had deposed. In a portrait by David of 1812, now in Washington's National Gallery of Art, Napoleon wears the uniform of a Colonel in the Imperial Guard Foot Grenadiers (Figure 20.2). The emperor is both impressive and dishevelled. The clue as to why he is depicted so is provided by the time on the clock behind him – which shows thirteen minutes past four – and a nearly burned-out candle to his right, which indicates that this is early morning. Furniture is stacked with documents, which the viewer is to assume he has been reviewing. The presentation of the emperor as a 'flesh-and-blood politician working overtime' is significant considering changing attitudes to royal rule and dress.[59]

The working portrait of Napoleon, while similar in purpose to those of Mariana of Austria in seventeenth-century Spain, reflects, perhaps, a broader shift in attitudes to royal authority because it was not the only means of depicting him. In other of his portraits, David presented Napoleon as an all-powerful ruler, notably his coronation scene of 1806–7, now in the Musée du Louvre.[60] The emphasis on relevance, or what might be termed the 'humanizing' of monarchy, can be traced through changes in the depiction of other monarchs. For example, Frederick II, who was frequently painted in martial attire during his lifetime, was depicted, six decades after his death, in civilian clothing playing a flute in Adolph Menzel's 'Flute-concert of Frederick the Great at Sanssouci' of 1850–2, now in Berlin's Alte Nationalgalerie.[61] The adoption of such contrasting methods to portray Napoleon and Frederick suggests that royal authority could not be taken for granted, as it had been in Gheeraerts's seventeenth-century portrait of Elizabeth I. In the nineteenth century, it had to be cognisant of subjects' expectations and demonstrated. Two centuries apart, the depictions of Elizabeth and Napoleon indicate how the clothing of royal bodies was changing as attitudes to rulers' executive authority became censorious.

The tendency of eighteenth- and nineteenth-century royal dress, and depictions of it, to allude to the day-to-day work of ruling reflected the fact that its wearers no longer provided the sole steer for their realms, politically or socially. Exact turning points are difficult to establish. However, the beheading of Charles I in 1649 by English Parliamentarians, the assassination of Gustav III by a subject in 1792 and Louis XVI's guillotining by his subjects in 1793 demonstrates that attitudes to the royal body had shifted a long way from those espoused by Scottish king James VI in

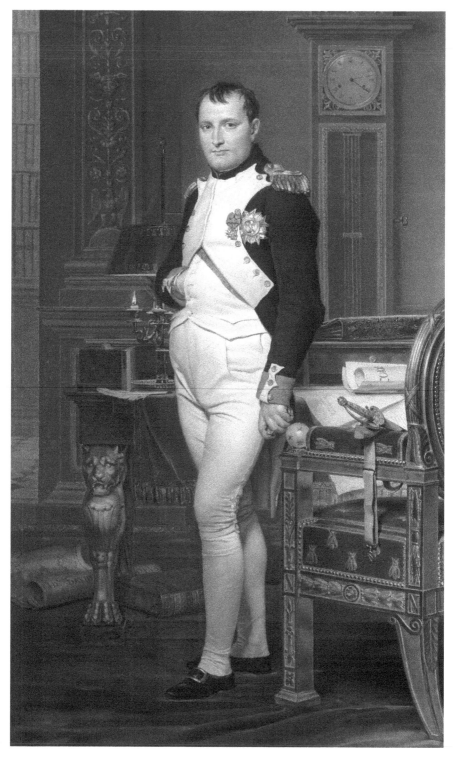

Figure 20.2 Jacques-Louis David, *The Emperor Napoleon in His Study at the Tuileries*, 1812, Courtesy of the National Gallery of Art, Washington

his *Basilikon Doron* (1599), which argued that monarchs were divine.[62] The Glorious Revolution of 1688, the French Revolution of 1789 and the revolutions that occurred across Europe in 1848, highlighted that the institution of monarchy was in flux and in a critical state. Industrial and technological developments of the eighteenth and nineteenth centuries provided further clarification of the challenges monarchy faced. In part, this was because emerging multinational companies diluted royal authority, even if they were nominally controlled by crown officials. To offer one example that pertains to clothing, during the late seventeenth century, the East India Company had tried its hand at market manipulation by flooding London with ready-made cotton shirting to encourage the moderately affluent to change their habits of consumption.[63] The scheme faltered, but it showed well enough that a monarch's ability to influence clothing preferences beyond their court was waning in direct proportion to their political prominence, which happened to be negatively correlated to the waxing of a globalized fashion industry. Instead of shaping clothing habits, royals now did their best to reflect them. The fate of the coronation, the grandest occasion for royal sartorial display, was an early casualty of this evolving state of mind because of its conspicuous emphasis on heavenly ordained distinction. In Britain, a turning point is apparent: the coronation of George IV (r.1820–30) on 19 July 1821.

The cost of George IV's coronation is reckoned to have been £238,000, although a maximum expenditure of £400,000 is feasible.[64] The outlay dwarfed George's annual income when he had been Prince Regent and the £70,000 spent on his father's coronation in 1761.[65] The unusual robes worn by George IV and his privy councillors were the chief reason for the expense. Confections of the king's aesthetic mind, the garments of the royal train were inspired by Elizabethan and Jacobean vogues and constructed from cloth of gold, satin, crimson and navy velvet.[66] In part, the theatrical nature of George IV's coronation was reflective of what Cannadine calls the 'revived ceremonial' of this period, which was apparent across Europe and America, but it was also more than this.[67] The pageantry was conceived to heighten George's singular position at a time when royal prerogatives were being curtailed and assumed by elected officials. For example, the symbols of the British territories that he ruled (such as the rose, thistle and shamrock, representing England, Scotland and Ireland respectively) were embroidered on his robe. It is tempting to contend that the atypical grandeur of George's coronation was also conceived to compete with Napoleon I's imperial coronation of 1804; after all, 'indemnities from France as a consequence of her defeat in the Napoleonic Wars' had partly covered the ceremony's costs.[68] If George's coronation appeared 'beyond measure magnificent' to some observers, the gulf between the actual powers of monarchy and those which the king appeared to be claiming caused others to react critically; the royal brothers were said to have made a 'deplorable spectacle'.[69] Changing attitudes to royal dress and appearance can thus be gauged by responses to the coronation more generally, which became more personal and public as its emphasis shifted, albeit by degrees, to demonstrate a ruler's responsibility to their subjects.

The coronation of George IV reveals much about the king's personal tastes, but it is also important for highlighting how, by the nineteenth century, the dress and appearance of all royals was interpreted more critically. Social, political, religious and technological developments over at least the past century had reduced monarchical authority. Royals remained politically and morally powerful, but they were no longer, like Henry VIII, Gustav III and Louis XIV, the lodestar of their realms or the uncontested national figurehead. Peter the Great's seemingly paradoxical clothing strategies, and George IV's coronation robe that unambiguously proclaimed his rule over England, Scotland, Wales and Ireland, indicate that royal bodies were becoming increasingly polyvalent to demonstrate the continued necessity of a role that was, perhaps, less clear as traditional social structures and mores were being challenged by their subjects and changed.

The display of royal authority: royal dress and appearance after *c*.1840

A turning point in the ceremonial appearance and dress of Britain's royals is perhaps easier to identify than for other European countries where the institution of monarchy has not survived. Nevertheless, during the nineteenth century, Philip Mansel has suggested that royals suffered 'clothes mania', characterized by a fastidious adherence to sartorial detail and etiquette, as they used dress to bolster their position.[70] In Austria, Germany and Russia, in particular, he notes there was a continued emphasis on military attire.[71] In Britain, anxiety about royal dress is apparent in the letters of Queen Victoria. For example, when she criticized the dress and hair of her eldest son (later, Edward VII, r.1901–10), which she did not like to see parted in the middle because it looked 'effeminate and girlish', she (inadvertently) acknowledged the need to project a powerful image of royalty.[72] Her admonishment is interesting for its suggestion that a potent appearance was achieved by conforming to contemporary tastes.

The reduced sartorial influence of royalty was entrenched by World Wars I and II. As an indication of how influential the global fashion industry had become at the start of the twentieth century, the major combatants used dress to galvanize morale. For Germany and Austria, the war provided an opportunity to create a national clothing industry to rival that in France. Kaiser Wilhelm II's youngest son, Prince Joachim of Prussia, appeared on the cover of *Elegante Welt* in 1914 wearing his battle fatigues in a patriotic demonstration of Germany's fighting and fashion force.[73] However, markets, rather than monarchs, were responsible for the alteration in wartime silhouettes. In 1916, a comic sketch by Thomas Theodor, *Die enttäuschte Pariserin* ('The disappointed Parisian'), was published in the satirical magazine *Simplicissimus*. In the first panel of the cartoon, a fashionable Parisian lady ponders how her opposite number in Germany will dress without the benefit of French models. In the panels that follow, the Parisian speculates on the German's appearance: *Brünhilde*, 'militaristic', 'Turkish' (a nod to Germany's ally), or perhaps she will give up and cover her nakedness with oak leaves. At the end of the conflict, the Parisian is dismayed that the fashionable German *Frau* looks identical to her.[74] The cartoon illustrates that fashion was too unwieldy a force to be controlled by national governments, let alone hereditary heads of state whose courts were closed for much of the war, some never to reopen.

In one sense, the impact of the twentieth century's global conflicts on royal authority and dress was predictable; no longer did they alone set the fashions in their respective countries. The popularity of democracy and democratic figureheads in the wake of global conflict, which had been waged against the ascendant political forces of fascism and communism, conspired to make the notion of ordained rulers seem anachronistic, even errant. Adolf Hitler, one of the period's most abhorrently capti-vating demagogic leaders, considered hereditary monarchy a 'biological blunder'.[75] The arbiters of peace were elected officials and these men (and women) increasingly surpassed royals as the representatives of their nation's values and vogues thereafter. After World War II, figures in Britain's labour government denounced Christian Dior's New Look, which they thought frivolous; the chancellor of the exchequer said it should be outlawed.[76] In America, presidential candidate John F. Kennedy alarmed his nation's hatters in the late 1950s by eschewing headwear.[77] Already regarded as a fashionable trendsetter, along with his wife Jackie, Kennedy apparently sparked fears that sales of men's hats would plummet, to the extent that he was sent multiple versions to wear on the campaign trail. The fears were not without consequence, for he was the last president to wear a top hat at the inauguration.[78]

If the political powerlessness of European royalty became more apparent after 1945, the social and political upheavals that followed the conflict provided it with a new function as an 'embodiment of consensus, stability and community'.[79] In this symbolic or talismanic role, which was sustained on memories of royal power from the past and by political neutrality in the present, the position of royalty became fossilized and, as Cannadine has argued, almost impervious to contemporary criti-cism.[80] This ambivalent position affected the role of royal dress considerably. First, royal regalia, now wholly symbolic, became a potent reminder of royalty's former power. Correlatively, it was an important source of imitation, particularly for auto-cratic rulers who sought legitimacy. In Iran, for example, the last shah, Mohammad Reza Pahlavi (r.1941–79) synthesized imperial Persian motifs through western royal military dress. The shah's coronation of 1967 muddled medievalism and modern-ism, and included royal garb made on London's Savile Row, which had long dressed European royalty.[81] Cultural juxtapositions were no less apparent in one of the most opulent royal festivities of the first half of the twentieth century: Haile Selassie of Ethopia's coronation in November 1930. The vestments worn by the emperor and empress appeared traditional, but the ceremony was punctuated by western ref-erences.[82] Selassie's coronation coach had belonged to Wilhelm II, its coachmen had served Franz Josef I, and police and members of Selassie's bodyguard were issued with khaki uniforms imported from Belgium.[83] Second, the ambivalent sta-tus of royalty – typified in Hilary Mantel's 'Gods and Beasts' description – meant that non-ceremonial dress became more important as one of the few indicators to express a royal's personal choice. Consequently, critics and celebrants of monarchy came to scrutinize rulers' wardrobes to gauge the abiding moral authority that its wearers, as national figureheads, were obliged to assert.

In the twenty-first century, with the advent of social media, interest in royal dress has become commonplace. Commentary on contemporary royal clothing is gener-ally approving, for as Cannadine opines for the period 1820 to 1977, how could it be otherwise for 'an institution that combine[s] political neutrality with personal integrity?'[84] A similar point is made by Jaap van Osta, who suggests that European royals between c.1870 and 1914 constituted a 'People's Monarchy' in the sense that they endeavoured to appear proximate to their subjects and to 'elicit emotional and affectionate feelings'.[85] Social media is an unconventional source for academic study, but it does much to demonstrate contemporary engagement and understanding of royal dress. The inclusion of social media in this discussion is an attempt to respond to van Osta's observation that a 'personal and bibliographical approach' is more appropriate in the study of twenty-first-century monarchies.[86]

The clothing of rulers from around the world has become a source of visual inspiration on Instagram, with accounts from Kurdistan to Brazil documenting the dress of the Duchess of Cambridge, formerly Catherine Middleton.[87] The appeal and influence of royal dress is also demonstrable in the global fashion industry. In 2016, to mark the sixty-third anniversary of the coronation of Elizabeth II, Italian fashion brand Gucci staged a fashion show in the cloister of Westminster Abbey. Creative director Alessandro Michele said of Britain's monarch, 'The Queen is one of the most quirky people in the world . . . She is very inspiring. It is clear that she loves color.'[88] British royals are not alone in providing sartorial stimulus. In an interview for *Esquire* magazine in 2016, Jeremy Langmead, brand and content director for online menswear retailer Mr Porter, claimed inspiration from Haile Selassie: 'At school, I used to sketch outfits for him in the back of my maths book.'[89]

The positive interest in, and commentary on, royal dress is predicated on its equivalence to clothing worn by everybody else. A recent exhibition at Bath's Fashion Museum, 'Royal Women', is noteworthy in this context for looking at 'wives and daughters, sisters and mothers; none of the Royal women featured in the exhibition was monarch, yet each played a key role in British monarchy'.[90] The similitude between ruler and ruled is necessary because it enables royals, possessing a limited and perhaps poorly understood constitutional role, to appear relevant.[91] Where royal dress of the eleventh century had proclaimed the power of its wearers, royal clothing in the present reflects a more ambivalent role because its wearers are politically powerless and symbolically polyvalent, as they represent the diverse values of their subjects.

The critical function that contemporary royal clothing performs is apparent from media coverage. For example, in April 2013, one of the Duchess of Cambridge's outfits was itemized by the *The Daily Mail* under the headline: 'Kate's £1,000 dress is not such a common touch.'[92] The Duchess's ensemble – a '£1,065 Erdem dress, £350 blue Prada heels and a £2,800 diamond Asprey button pendant' – was criticized for its insensitivity because her destination, Wythenshawe, was said to be the 'second biggest [housing] estate of its kind in Europe' and 'a notorious area of Manchester'.[93] By contrast, when *Vogue* featured the Duchess on the cover of its centenary issue in July 2016, her clothing was deemed too ordinary.[94] In these scenarios there is a tension between the expectation that the royal body appear both distinct and demure. In a similar way, the appearance of Elizabeth II in a bright green outfit during her ninetieth birthday celebrations in 2016 divided opinion. Surprised by the monarch's atypical choice of colour, many people used mocking hashtags on social media and compared the green to the digital screens used in film-making.[95]

If Elizabeth II's green dress indicates that royal bodies continue to use clothing to define their status akin to their medieval predecessors, it demonstrates how the context in which they appear has fundamentally changed. The political, economic and religious transformations that occurred between *c.*1640 and *c.*1840 permanently deprived rulers of their spiritual and executive authority, and fundamentally changed how they were perceived. Before 1640, green would have been an unusual royal colour, because it symbolized youth and chaos in Christian thought, but against Elizabeth no such concerns were raised: the green dress was criticized at face value because of its hue, and not for any apparent symbolism.[96] Moreover, few subjects would have critiqued their monarch's dress publicly. Rulers' circumscribed position was confirmed by 1945, when their role became almost wholly symbolic and their non-ceremonial dress became equivalent to that of their subjects, if still carrying a royal price tag, produced by the finest designers and worn as a performer might don a costume. Borne of this experience, Elizabeth II's remark that a monarch needs to be seen to be believed is true indeed.

Notes

1 I am grateful to Giles Reynolds for his comments on this chapter.
2 Charlotte Lytton, "'I Have to Be Seen to Be Believed': The Hidden Significance of the Queen's Colourful Wardrobe," *The Telegraph*, 20 April 2016, www.telegraph.co.uk/fashion/people/i-have-to-be-seen-to-be-believed-the-hidden-significance-of-the/.
3 For example, Robin Cormack and Maria Vassilaki, eds., *Byzantium, 330–1453* (London: Royal Academy of Arts, 2008); Svetlana A. Amelekhina and Alexey K. Levykin, *Magnificence of the Tsars: Ceremonial Men's Dress of the Russian Imperial Court, 1721–1917* (London: V&A Publishing, 2008); Susan Marti, Till-Holger Borchert and Gabrielle Keck, eds., *Charles the Bold (1433–1477): Splendour of Burgundy* (Brussels: Mercatorfonds, 2009); Joaquín Yarza Luaces, ed., *Vestiduras Ricas: El Monasterio de Las Huelgas Y Su Época 1170–1430* (Madrid: Patrimonio Nacional, 2005); and Anna Reynolds, *In Fine Style: The Art of Tudor and Stuart Fashion* (London: Royal Collection Trust, 2013).
4 John E. Vollmer, *Ruling from the Dragon Throne: Costume of the Qing Dynasty (1644–1911)* (Berkeley: Ten Speed Press, 2002); Gary Dickinson and Linda Wrigglesworth, *Imperial Wardrobe* (Berkeley: Ten Speed Press, 2000); Tessa Rose, *The Coronation Ceremony of the Kings and Queens of England and the Crown Jewels* (London: Her Majesty's Stationery Office, 1992); Zillah Halls, *Coronation Costume and Accessories 1685–1953* (London: Her Majesty's Stationery Office, 1973).
5 The contemporary approach to clothing studies has been challenged. For different views, see Fred Davis, *Fashion, Culture, and Identity* (Chicago: The University of Chicago Press, 1992), 9; and Benjamin L. Wild, "The Civilizing Process and Sartorial Studies," *Clothing Cultures* 1, no. 3 (2014): 213–224.
6 For example, Peter Burke, *The Fabrication of Louis XIV* (New Haven: Yale University Press, 1992); Larry Silver, *Marketing Maximilian: The Visual Ideology of a Holy Roman Emperor* (Princeton: Princeton University Press, 2008); and Barbara Stollberg-Rilinger, Matthias Puhle, Jutta Götzmann and Gerd Althoff, eds., *Spektakel der Macht: Rituale im Alten Europa 800–1800* (Darmstadt: Wissenschaftliche Buchgellschaft, 2008).
7 For example, Lena Rangström, *Kläder för tid och evighet: Gustaf III sedd genom sina dräkter* (Helsingborg: AB Boktryck, 1997); Kay Staniland, *In Royal Fashion: The Clothes of Princess Charlotte of Wales and Queen Victoria 1760–1901* (London: Museum of London, 1997); and Kate Strasdin, *Inside the Royal Wardrobe: A Dress History of Queen Alexandra* (London: Bloomsbury, 2017).
8 For example, Malcolm Vale, *The Princely Court: Medieval Courts and Culture in North-West Europe, 1270–1380* (Oxford: Oxford University Press, 2001); John Gillingham, "Wirtschaftlichkeit oder Ehre? Die Ausgaben der Englischen Könige im 12. bis zum 18. Jahrhundert," in *Luxus und Integration: Materielle Hofkultur Westeuropas vom 12. bis zum 18. Jahrhundert*, ed. W. Paravicini (Munich: Oldenbourg Wissenschaftsverlag, 2010), 151–167.
9 For example, see Robert Fawtier, ed., *Comptes du Trésor (1296, 1316, 1384, 1477)* (Paris: Imprimerie nationale, 1830); Maria Hayward, ed., *Dress at the Court of King Henry VIII: The Wardrobe Book of the Wardrobe of Robes prepared by James Worsley in December 1516, edited from Harley MS 2284, and his Inventory prepared on 17 January 1521, edited from Harley MS 4127, both in the British Library* (Leeds: Maney Publishing, 2007); and Benjamin L. Wild, ed., *The Wardrobe Accounts of Henry III* (London: Pipe Roll Society, 2012).

10 Philip Mansel, *Dressed to Rule: Royal and Court Costume from Louis XIV to Elizabeth II* (New Haven: Yale University Press, 2005); Robert Ross, *Clothing: A Global History. Or, The Imperialists' New Clothes* (Cambridge: Polity Press, 2008); and Dominique Gaulme and François Gaulme, *Power and Style: A World History of Politics and Dress* (Paris: Flammarion S.A., 2012).

11 Hilary Mantel, "Royal Bodies," *London Review of Books*, 35, no. 4 (21 February 2013), www.lrb.co.uk/v35/n04/hilary-mantel/royal-bodies (accessed 30 March 2019).

12 Ibid.

13 David Cannadine, "The Context, Performance and Meaning of Ritual: The British Monarchy and the 'Invention of Tradition', *c*.1820–1977," in *The Invention of Tradition*, eds. Eric Hobsbawm and Terence Ranger (Cambridge: Cambridge University Press, 2016), 139.

14 Michel Pastoureau, ed., *Le Vêtement: Histoire, archéologie et symbolique vestimentaires au Moyen Age* (Paris: Cahiers du Léopard d'Or, 1989); Frédérique Lachaud, "Dress and Social Status in England before the Sumptuary Laws," in *Heraldry, Pageantry and Social Display in Medieval England*, eds. Peter Coss and Maurice Keen (Woodbridge: Boydell Press, 2002), 105–124; and Ross, *Clothing: A Global History*, 13–22.

15 Michel Pastoureau, *Figures et Couleurs: Études sur le symbolique et la sensibilité médiévales* (Paris: Le Léopard d'Or, 1986), 40.

16 A.G. Hassall and W.O. Hassall, *The Douce Apocalypse* (London: Faber and Faber Limited, 1961), 22–23; and Ann Rosalind Jones and Peter Stallybrass, *Renaissance Clothing and the Materials of Memory* (Cambridge: Cambridge University Press, 2000), 59–86.

17 Wolfram Eberhard, *A History of China* (London: Routledge and Kegan Paul, 1977), 218–219.

18 Vollmer, *Ruling from the Dragon Throne*, 82–84.

19 Ibid., 100, 161–162.

20 Till-Holger Borchert, "Philip the Good," in *Charles the Bold (1433–1477)*, 174.

21 John Harvey, "From Black in Spain to Black in Shakespeare," in *The Men's Fashion Reader*, eds. Peter McNeil and Vicki Karaminas (Oxford, Berg, 2009), 19–43.

22 *Chroniques de Hainaut*, Brussels, Bibliothèque royale de Belgique, MS. 9242, f. 1r.

23 Tatiana C. String, *Art and Communication in the Reign of Henry VIII* (Aldershot: Ashgate, 2008), 45–47.

24 Roy Strong, *Gloriana: The Portraits of Queen Elizabeth I* (London: Thames and Hudson, 1987).

25 Catherine L. Howey, "Dressing a Virgin Queen: Dress, and Fashioning the Image of England's Queen Elizabeth I," *Early Modern Women* 4 (Fall 2009): 201–208.

26 Frances A. Yates, "Queen Elizabeth as Astraea," *Journal of the Warburg and Courtauld Institutes* 10 (1947): 27–82.

27 C. Warren Hollister, *Henry I* (New Haven: Yale University Press, 2001), 331.

28 Paul E. Dutton, *Charlemagne's Mustache and Other Cultural Clusters of a Dark Age* (New York: Palgrave Macmillan, 2004), 3–42.

29 Wild, *The Wardrobe Accounts of Henry III*, clxxv, 136.

30 Benjamin L. Wild, "Reasserting Medieval Kingship: King Henry III and the Dictum of Kenilworth," in *Baronial Reform and Rebellion in England 1258–1267*, ed. Adrian Jobson (Woodbridge: Boydell Press, 2016), 241–242.

31 Lindsey Hughes, *Russia in the Age of Peter the Great* (New Haven: Yale University Press, 1998), 282.

32 Quoted in Alison Weir, *Henry VIII: King and Court* (London: Jonathan Cape, 2001), 366.

33 Mansel, *Dressed to Rule*, 8.

34 Ibid.

35 Hughes, *Peter the Great*, 250–255. For possible Russian precursors to the Assembly, see William Willeford, *The Fool and His Scepter: A Study in Clowns and Jesters and Their Appearance* (London: Edward Arnold Ltd., 1969), 159–161.

36 Ibid., 255–257.

37 Wild, "Reasserting Medieval Kingship," 237–238; John Keane, *The Life and Death of Democracy* (London: Simon & Schuster Ltd, 2009), 235–272.

38 These observations have been made by historians and sociologists. They are central to Norbert Elias' work. See Norbert Elias, *The Civilizing Process: Sociogenetic and Pscyhogenetic Investigations*, rev. ed., trans. Edmund Jephcott, eds. Eric Dunning, Johan Goudsblom

and Stephen Mennell (London: Basil Blackwell, 1939); and Norbert Elias, *The Society of Individuals*, trans. Edmund Jephcott, ed. Micahel Schröter (London: Basil Blackwell, 1991). For consideration of Elias' work in relation to dress, see Benjamin L. Wild, "The Civilizing Process and Sartorial Studies," *Clothing Cultures* 1, no. 3 (2014): 213–224.

39 Burke, *The Fabrication of Louis XIV*, 128–129; Peter Burke, *Popular Culture in Early Modern Europe*, third edition (Farnham: Ashgate, 2009), 366–380.

40 Grant McCracken, *Culture and Consumption: New Approaches to the Symbolic Character of Consumer Goods and Activities* (Bloomington: Indiana University Press, 1990), 11–16; David Kuchta, *The Three-Piece Suit and Modern Masculinity: England, 1550–1850* (Berkeley: University of California Press, 2002), 39–40.

41 Kuchta, *The Three-Piece Suit*, 93–102.

42 Reynolds, *In Fine Style*, 87–99.

43 Caroline Weber, *Queen of Fashion: What Marie Antoinette Wore to the Revolution* (London: Aurum Press Ltd, 2006), 81–83.

44 RCIN 404920. The painting can be viewed via the Royal Collection's website: www.royal collection.org.uk/collection/404920/mary-of-modena-1658–1718-when-duchess-of-york (accessed 30 March 2019).

45 Mynors Bright, ed., *The Diary of Samuel Pepys* (London: J.M. Dent and Sons Ltd, 1959), 2:272.

46 Weber, *Queen of Fashion*, 81–82.

47 Reynolds, *In Fine Style*, 261–263.

48 Ann Rosalind Jones and Peter Stallybrass, *Renaissance Clothing and the Materials of Memory*, 4; Christopher Hill, *The World Turned Upside Down: Radical Ideas during the English Revolution* (London: Penguin Books, 1975); and David Underdown, *Revel, Riot and Rebellion: Popular Politics and Culture in England 1603–1660* (Oxford: Oxford University Press, 1985).

49 Kuchta, *The Three-Piece Suit*, 78–90.

50 Quoted in Kuchta, *The Three-Piece Suit*, 77–78.

51 Quoted in Kuchta, *The Three-Piece Suit*, 93.

52 Mercedes Llorente, "Mariana of Austria's Portraits as Ruler-Governor and Curadora by Juan Carreño de Miranda and Claudio Coello," in *Early Modern Habsburg Women: Transnational Contexts, Cultural Conflicts, Dynastic Continuities*, eds. Anne J. Cruz and Maria Galli Stampino (Farnham: Ashgate, 2013), 200–205.

53 Ibid., 197–198.

54 Mansel, *Dressed to Rule*, 111–129.

55 Ross, *Clothing: A Global History*, 103–104.

56 Mansel, *Dressed to Rule*, 23–24.

57 Ibid., 51–54.

58 Rangström, *Kläder för tid och evighet*, 243.

59 Robert Rosenblum, "Portraiture: Facts versus Fiction," in *Citizens and Kings: Portraits in the Age of Revolution 1760–1830*, eds. David Breuer and Robert Rosenblum (London: Royal Academy of Arts, 2007), 17.

60 "The Consecration of the Emperor Napoleon and the Coronation of Empress Joséphine on December 2, 1804," inv. 3699. An image of the painting can be viewed on the Louvre's website, www.louvre.fr/en/oeuvre-notices/consecration-emperor-napoleon-and-coronation-empress-josephine-december-2-1804 (accessed 30 March 2019).

61 Alte Nationalgalerie, inv. A I 206. The painting has been digitized by Google, https://artsandculture.google.com/asset/flute-concert-with-frederick-the-great-in-sanssouci/WAFEF2zy8Ym8vQ (accessed 30 March 2019).

62 S. J. Houston, *James I* (Harlow: Longman Group, 1973), 37–38.

63 John Styles, *The Dress of the People: Everyday Fashion in Eighteenth-Century England* (New Haven: Yale University Press, 2007), 128–129.

64 Rose, *The Coronation Ceremony*, 85.

65 E.A. Smith, *George IV* (New Haven: Yale University Press, 1999), 88–92, 186.

66 Ibid., 84–85; Halls, *Coronation Costume*, 47–49.

67 Cannadine, "The British Monarchy," 138.

68 Rose, *The Coronation Ceremony*, 85.

69 Smith, *George IV*, 188, 190.

70 Mansel, *Dressed to Rule*, 138.
71 Ibid., 111–129.
72 Jane Ridley, *Bertie: A Life of Edward VII* (London: Vintage Books, 2012), 44.
73 Adelheid Rasche, "New Fashion Trends during the First World War," in *Wardrobes in Wartime: Fashion and Fashion Images during the First World War, 1914–1918*, ed. Adeleide Rasche (Berlin: Staatliche Museen zu Berlin, 2015), 74.
74 Ibid., 19.
75 Hugh R. Trevor-Roper, *Hitler's Table Talk, 1941–1945: His Private Conversations* (London: Phoenix, 2000), 385.
76 Ross, *Clothing: A Global History*, 141–142.
77 Alan Mansfield, *Ceremonial Costume: Court, Civil and Civic Costume from 1660 to the Present Day* (London: Adam and Charles Black, 1980), 158–164.
78 Ted Lewis and Jerry Greene, "John F. Kennedy is Sworn in as the 35th President of the United States in 1961," *Daily News*, 21 January 1961, www.nydailynews.com/news/national/jfk-sworn-35th-president-u-s-1961-article-1.2479922.
79 Cannadine, "The British Monarchy," 140.
80 Ibid., 141.
81 Gaulme and Gaulme, *Power and Style*, 240–241; James Sherwood, *Savile Row: The Master Tailors of British Bespoke* (London: Thames and Hudson, 2010), 32–71; Peter Tilley, "By Royal Appointment: Outfitters to the Empire," in *One Savile Row: The Invention of the English Gentleman, Gieves & Hawkes*, ed. Sarah Rozelle (Paris: Flammarion S.A., 2014), 57–132.
82 Asfa-Wossen Asserate, *King of Kings: The Triumph and Tragedy of Emperor Haile Selassie I of Ethiopia* (London: Haus Publishing Ltd, 2015), 82–88.
83 Ibid., 76, 77.
84 Cannadine, "The British Monarchy," 141.
85 Jaap van Osta, "The Emperor's New Clothes: The Reappearance of the Performing Monarchy in Europe, c.1870–1914," *Mystifying the Monarch: Studies on Discourse, Power, and History*, eds. Jeroen Deploige and Gita Deneckere (Amsterdam: Amsterdam University Press, 2006), 182.
86 Ibid., 192.
87 For example, @Katemiddleton-kurdistan and @Katemiddletonbr.
88 Rebeca Mead, "Costume Drama," *The New Yorker* (19 September 2006): 52.
89 Michael Bracewell, "Just So," *Esquire: The Big Black Book A/W 2016* 8 (2016): 156.
90 "Royal Women," *Fashion Museum Bath*, www.fashionmuseum.co.uk/events/royal-women (accessed 30 March 2019).
91 Cannadine, "The British Monarchy," 155.
92 Rebecca English, "Kate's £1,000 Dress is Not Such a Common Touch," *The Daily Mail* (24 April 2013): 5.
93 Ibid.
94 Liz Jones, "Is Kate Auditioning to be the Catalogue Queen," *The Daily Mail*, 30 April 2016, www.dailymail.co.uk/femail/article-3567529/Duchess-Vogue-cover-star-LIZ-JONES-dares-say-s-bit-Boden.html#ixzz49fRp9qzd.
95 Michael Safi, "Queen's 'Green Screen' Outfit Ensures She Stands out From the Crowd," *The Guardian* (12 June 2016), www.theguardian.com/uk-news/2016/jun/12/queens-green-screen-outfit-ensures-she-stands-out-from-the-crowd.
96 Pastoureau, *Figures et Couleurs*, 23–34. Henry VIII probably wanted to emphasize his youth by wearing green at the start of his reign. Hayward, *King Henry VIII*, 98.

Key works

Cannadine, David, "The Context, Performance and Meaning of Ritual: The British Monarchy and the 'Invention of Tradition', c.1820–1977," in *The Invention of Tradition*, eds. Eric Hobsbawm and Terence Ranger (Cambridge: Cambridge University Press, 2016), 101–164.
Gaulme, Dominique and François Gaulme, *Power and Style: A World History of Politics and Dress* (Paris: Flammarion S.A., 2012).

Mansel, Philip, *Dressed to Rule: Royal and Court Costume from Louis XIV to Elizabeth II* (New Haven: Yale University Press, 2005).

Mantel, Hilary, "Royal Bodies," *London Review of Books* 35, no. 4 (21 February 2013): 3–7.

Rose, Tessa, *The Coronation Ceremony of the Kings and Queens of England and the Crown Jewels* (London: Her Majesty's Stationery Office, 1992).

Ross, Robert, *Clothing: A Global History. Or, The Imperialists' New Clothes.* (Cambridge: Polity Press, 2008).

PART III

DYNASTY AND SUCCESSION

INTRODUCTION

Russell E. Martin

As he lay dying of the Plague, Grand Prince Simeon Ivanovich of Moscow (b.1316, r.1340–1353) was thinking about the future. He was the third member of his branch of the Rjurikovich dynasty to rule as grand prince of Vladimir – the highest sovereign title in what we today call Russia – having followed his father (Ivan I Kalita, d.1340) and uncle (Iurii Daniilovich, d.1325), with some interruptions, onto that throne. He fretted that he would be the last of his line, having watched his two sons and direct heirs, Ivan and Simeon, die of the same deadly disease that was about to shorten his own life. All that stood between him and the extinction of his branch of the family, the Daniilovichi, were his two younger brothers and their young sons – slender threads of hope in times of rampant pestilence. Simeon naturally enough turned at that moment of bracing reality to the writing of his will, in which he laid out all his bequests and made provisions for his widow. Towards the end of the text, in a unique and affecting passage, he wrote, 'And lo, I write this to you so that the memory of our parents and of us may not die, and so that the candle may not go out.'[1] Here, Grand Prince Simeon looks back to his parents, to the family to which he belonged, and forward to the ruling house that needed to continue, even if not in his direct line. Here we see an awareness that, as the Muscovite historian Edward Keenan put it, 'in the culture of the Muscovite court there was simply no responsibility of the monarch more important than the generation of viable male issue'.[2]

Grand Prince Simeon's will displays not only his awareness of his responsibility to produce 'viable male issue' but his consciousness of dynasty, as well; a recognition that he was part of a larger familial structure, which included his siblings, nephews and nieces. These kin could remember their common ancestors and pray for the commemoration of their souls (no small thing in an Orthodox culture) and assume the responsibility of keeping alight the candle of dynastic continuity (no small thing in a hereditary monarchy). But how common was that consciousness of dynasty? In places that were ruled by acknowledged dynasties, how were the relationships among relatives in them regulated? What place did women – mothers, wives, daughters, sisters, aunts – play in the running of the royal household, marriage of its members, or succession from one generation of monarchs to the next? Did women have rights of succession to the throne, and how were those rights represented and legitimized? How significant in all these matters were the monarchy's closest servitors – the 'magnates', 'nobles', or 'boyars' – who often ruled in degrees of collaboration with the monarch, even when the political myths and rituals suggested that power was vested in the ruler alone?

These questions have been asked by generations of modern historians, and the answers to them have evolved as new methods and sources have been brought to bear on the general *Problematik* of monarchy. One prominent model, perhaps, for thinking about these questions has been the early Capetians, whose history is comparatively well documented compared to most parts of western Europe and whose history has been written very closely to that of the general history of medieval France. One need turn only to the classic works of Robert Fawtier, Jean-François Lemarignier, Charles Wood, or Joseph Strayer, among others, to see the patterned alignment between the formation of France and the history of its *troisième race*.[3] The dynasty, it has been argued, laboured with almost divinely inspired prescience generation after generation to assert its legitimacy, control the succession, regulate its collaterals and accumulate the kingdom into its own hands. It is a model of dynasty and state that has been so handy and compelling that it has been searched for, and confidently found, in the histories of other kingdoms and other dynasties.[4]

This model for the study of state and dynasty has been reinvigorated – one might put it better, 'revised' – with new methods and emphases, and this recent work has thrust some of that traditional historiography into doubt. One need go no further than, for example, the work of Andrew W. Lewis, and those who have more recently followed in Lewis's footsteps (not always agreeing, of course, with all his ideas),[5] or to survey the on-going study today of the Jagiellonians, which has amply shown how the history of dynasties can and should be thought of independently of the history of the spaces they ruled.[6] The dynasty-and-state model is, therefore, ripe for revision. Gilbert Dagron, for example, has urged us to ignore the dynastic tables that sprinkle the pages of so many older histories of the Byzantine empire, and instead argues for the absence of any useful notion of dynasty in the Byzantine context. 'A dynasty', he writes, 'was never, in Byzantium, more than the unpredictable pursuit of an individual destiny, an extension to the family of a personal adventure.'[7] Even in the case of early East-Slavic history, the notion of a ruling dynasty among the ancestors of Grand Prince Simeon – descended, as was claimed, from the Varangian Rjurik and continuing in direct succession down to the collapse of Kyivan Rus' by the Mongols in the thirteenth century – has also been recently challenged.[8] There has emerged, then, among those studying royal courts, monarchical systems, dynastic families, royal women and succession a new set of vital questions. What constitutes a dynasty? How do dynasties compare over different times and spaces, and how important are they for understanding politics, power, families, and ideas in world history? The history of monarchy has been liberated from the constraining hold of national histories and has become, again and more seriously than before, a discrete topic of historical investigation.

The liberation has already had an effect. If Dagron and others have reminded us that we must be careful about the appearances of dynasty when there was, in fact, none, Jeroen Duindam has offered the most convincing and nuanced definition, if not defence, of the dynasty as a useful category for historical research.[9] As Duindam described it, dynasties are 'cultural constructs, based on a series of conventions regarding reproduction and eligibility for the throne'.[10] They may come in many forms and operate according to varied principles, but dynasties do offer us ways of understanding culture, religion, public space, political elites, and rituals and representations of power. Historians like Duindam have been aided considerably by the work of anthropologists (and historians influenced by them), who have helped us understand monarchical societies with much greater precision than before;[11] and the dynasty in the ancient world has again become a subject of some interest, as the recent work of Olivier Hekster has shown.[12] We have today reopened the inquiry again into the history and role of dynasties in pre-modern cultures, and this 'restoration' is of a size and scale that it by now constitutes, once again, a vibrant field in world history. Indeed, the field of royal studies has emerged as one of the most energized and active avenues of research today, finding outlets both in print and the Internet.[13] These are happy times for serious historians interested in kings and queens.

As this volume itself shows, there are many ways this new vibrant field is being approached, but one of the oldest and most fundamental questions in the history of dynasties remains succession. The highest royal rank (however it is called) can pass by primogeniture (or any systematic form of preference for an heir by birth order, such as ultimogeniture), agnatic succession (any male offspring of the ruler), collateral succession (passing to brothers then to the nephews in birth order or by age), and a host of variations of these forms. Succession can also exist outside of a dynastic framework, of course, as in the numerous cases of elective or appointive monarchy demonstrate. And law – either as written code or oral custom – invariably becomes a vital factor in determining the succession in many cultures around the globe. But in every place where monarchy reigns, the problem of how to regulate the succession is a fundamentally important matter. And a deadly serious one. The Ottoman succession was pockmarked, until surprisingly late in its run, by the massacres of all the successor's surviving brothers.[14] And in Russia, it was during acute moments in a dynasty's history – like royal betrothals and marriages, but also when a new ruler ascended to power – that, quoting Keenan again, 'one heard the thud of limp bodies in the Kremlin'.[15]

Understanding those 'thuds' requires thinking about how power pools and flows through dynasties. Dynasties are, after all, families, and any approach to grasping the political forms and structures of dynasties requires an investigation of familial order in the dynasty. The chapters in this part do just that: they investigate dynasties in various spaces and eras, they focus on the various members of these dynasties (fathers, mothers, siblings, children) and they explore how these forms and structures determine and maintain a system of succession to the highest title in the realm. These chapters are thus both a continuation of this new, discrete investigation of the history of monarchy and a venturesome new step forward in our understanding of the comparative history of succession and dynasty.

The part begins with Grand Prince Simeon's family, whose candle of dynastic continuity was flickering so precariously as he approached death in the year 1353. In 'Anticipatory association of the heir in early modern Russia: primogeniture and succession in Russia's ruling dynasties', I explore the development of primogenitural succession in Muscovy between the early fourteenth and late seventeenth centuries. Collateral succession had prevailed in Kyivan Rus' in the tenth through to the thirteenth century, and it continued in many of the successor states that survived its fall to the Mongols in 1240. Only in Moscow did the princely line adopt father-son succession – first as a bio-statistical accident, then as a conscious policy. But vertical succession did not come easy to Moscow, especially once collateral lines of the Moscow branch of the Rjurikovych began to flourish and insist on its customary rights to the succession. Different princes of Moscow tried different strategies to direct the succession to their lineal heirs, including anticipatory association – the crowning or by other means designating of the eldest son as co-ruler (and therefore successor) during the lifetime of the father. This chapter examines the strategies for installing primogeniture in Muscovy and situates the Muscovite practice of anticipatory association in and among other monarchical systems that employed the custom.

The customs of succession from one ruler to the next is also the focus of Derek Whaley's 'From *a* Salic Law to *the* Salic Law: the creation and re-creation of the royal succession system of medieval France'. The insistence by the French that their throne pass not to Edward III of England (r.1327–77) but to Philippe VI of Valois (r.1328–50) launched the Hundred Years' War (1337–1453), but even before the *arrière-ban* – the feudal call to war – was issued in April 1337, there were dynastic troubles in France. The infant Jean I (1316) had died without, of course, direct heirs – the first occasion a Capetian king had not provided an heir by the time of his death. The great lords of France handed the throne to Jean I's uncle, Philippe V (r.1316–22), rather than his sister (Jeanne, the eventual queen of Navarre, r.1328–49), amending the unwritten rules of succession with the provision that only males could inherit the throne. When Philippe V also failed to produce a male heir, the throne again passed to a collateral, his younger brother Charles IV (r.1322–28). But having run out of brothers, the French magnates were in quite the quandary when Charles IV died without male heirs. What the magnates did have, however, as Whaley shows, is the now established custom of strict male primogeniture. What they still needed was a written law code to back it up, thus they appropriated the ancient 'Salic Law' which originally had no relation to royal succession and applied it retroactively to justify the exclusion of women and female line claimants. Whaley's chapter explores the way the Salic Law came to be transformed and appropriated by the French magnates and the Valois branch of the Capetian dynasty to keep the English off the French throne. This chapter also casts new light on the legal thinking that went into this appropriation. 'The result' writes Whaley, 'was the Salic Law, a legal code based entirely on precedent and convenience.'

Jonathan Spangler's 'A family affair: cultural anxiety and political debate concerning the nature of monarchy in seventeenth-century France and Britain' pulls us forward into early modern Europe and broadens our study of succession to include the younger brothers and other agnatic relatives of the kings of France and England, whose position in the dynasty and in the kingdom was in flux following the Middle Ages. While younger royal siblings were essential to any dynastic system, they were also a tremendous danger to it, especially in systems that were in the process of adopting primogeniture and other forms of a vertical familial structure. These 'spares' had to be provided for, or else they could (and often did) object to the lesser role relegated to them as a function of their birth order. The French especially were cursed with fecundity, which quickly expanded the ranks of the Capetian-Valois dynasty and prompted the creation of *appanages* for the maintenance of royal collaterals. But as

Spangler shows, even in England where these dynasties posed fewer bio-statistical threats to the king, the royal family had to be accommodated. What Spangler gives us in this chapter is an important reminder and set of case studies of the importance of inter-dynastic relations in monarchies. Smooth successions from one generation of the dynasty to the next recommended and required that the 'question of the exercise of power by someone sitting so close to, though not on, the throne' be tackled. What Spangler shows is that, while the general trend in France and England (as elsewhere) leaned towards a general quelling of enmity between eldest son and younger brothers, the strains that were produced by the intersection of power and family never fully went away. At the end of the day, these conflicts and tensions were hardwired into the monarchy, and no custom, religious tenant, or legal code would ever be able to do more than mute the Cain-and-Abel rivalries that characterize rule by dynasty.

Our focus remains on dynasty in the next chapter, 'What's in a name? Dynasty, succession and England's queens regnant (1553–2016)', by Sarah Betts. Here, however, the focus shifts slightly to considering the ways female succession in England (where it was allowed, unlike France) affected dynastic identity and continuity. What is the effect on dynastic identity when the succession passes through the female line? Using a range of sources, Betts isolates the six English and British regnant queens since the early modern era, beginning with Mary I (r.1553–8) and proceeding to the current sovereign, Queen Elizabeth II (since 1952), and explores their attitudes and notional alliances to the previous dynasty or dynasties from which they derived their own claims to the throne. Betts grapples with the underlying definition of dynasty as a patrilineage and helps us understand the boundaries – sometimes firm and at other times elastic – that determined the definition of dynasty. In doing so, Betts raises important questions about periodization – the span of time and rulers that view themselves as belonging to the same dynasty – and concludes that 'dynastic periodization is still a "natural" and valuable way in which to analyse the history of the monarchy'. This is an important reminder and something of a revival and rehabilitation of a concept once considered outmoded: that dynasties (and reigns) represent discrete epochs in a nation's history. Betts' argument compels us, then, to look at periodization again, though with the admonition that the traditional boundaries between these epochs might not be so neatly delineated by the reign or lifespan of a man or woman.

We turn to royal women in the dynasties of the ancient Near East in Aidan Norrie's 'Female pharaohs in ancient Egypt'. Here the focus is on 'the way that female pharaohs reigned, and how they presented themselves and their reign'. Pharaonic dynasties, like all others, have lapsed or died out. In at least four cases, a dynasty was continued for a time by the elevation of a woman to the throne. Norrie looks at these four cases to explore how ancient Egyptians understood their own kingship. The chapter reveals that 'Egyptians understood that the office of *pharaoh* was distinct from the *person* of the pharaoh.' Since the most important role a pharaoh filled was maintaining *maat* (the 'divine order'), it mattered less who was pharaoh than that there *was* a pharaoh: 'an elderly, infant, disabled, or female pharaoh was not an issue, as long as there was a pharaoh on the throne'. Even so, the norm was to have a male on the throne: 'a man who was the son of the preceding pharaoh, who could sire future pharaohs, and who could successfully lead Egypt's armies'. Norrie shows how, despite the overriding role of *maat* as the underlying purpose of the ancient Egyptian monarchy – a quality a woman could possess as much as a man – the instances of female pharaohs nonetheless required adjustments to the way that the pharaoh were portrayed and represented as a political and religious figure. Gender played in two directions: female pharaohs appear to have gone to greater lengths to emphasize their legitimacy, downplaying, as it were, potential obstacles to the rarity of a female ruler; and at the same time they made the most of their uniquely female qualities and depicted themselves as pharaohs in their own right. All four were successful as rulers, and even more importantly (then and now), had reigns that are etched in stone (literally) and remembered.

The next several chapters situate our study of the role of women in dynasties in comparative perspective. In their 'Neither heir nor spare: childless queens and the practice of monarchy in pre-modern Europe', Kristen Geaman and Theresa Earenfight explore what they term the 'non-reproductive aspects of queenship'. Childlessness was something of a dynastic catastrophe in many cases, and royal couples, but especially queens, pulled out all the stops to remedy it. They tapped into the medical knowledge available to them at the time, went on pilgrimages to holy sites, or venerated holy relics to cure their condition. But barren couples also often found ways to turn what in most cases would be seen as a blemish on their reigns – their inability to produce an heir – into political and religious assets. Childlessness could be explained away and even exploited. Royal couples could be eschewing parenthood as an expression of Christian chastity; childless queens could be portrayed as holy or dutiful mothers of the whole realm. Geaman and Earenfight show how childless queens sometimes served as intercessors before the king for pardon and favour, they became cultural patrons of the arts and culture, and sometimes assumed vital and powerful political roles, especially when their husbands were absent. 'The evidence reveals', conclude Geaman and Earenfight, 'that pre-modern queenship was a complex cultural and political institution and that it was never just about having heirs, that maternity clearly is not the sole determinant of a queen's 'success.'

Lloyd Llewellyn-Jones takes our investigation into royal women back to the ancient Near East and into the harems of rulers spanning more than a thousand years in his 'Harem politics: royal women and succession crises in the ancient Near East (*c.*1400–300 BCE)'. Llewellyn-Jones seeks to corral 'evidence from across Near Eastern antiquity' in order to 'normalize harem participation in dynastic life'. Rejecting the common view of the harem 'as a brothel-like pleasure-palace', this chapter argues for the 'central role in the political milieu of a royal court or, indeed, of empires at large'. Harems in ancient Persia, Israel, pharaonic Egypt and, leaping forward, the Ottoman empire (as well as elsewhere) together present consistent evidence of the vital role the women inhabiting them played in the dynastic politics of these realms, especially in the way succession worked. Not only did the mothers of potential heirs insinuate themselves into the high politics of the ruler's court, they also became markers of power transfer and legitimacy when new rulers and dynasties came to power – possessing the harems of their predecessors legitimized more than one ancient Near Eastern usurper. This broadly comparative treatment understands the harem as a normative element of 'absolutist forms of dynastic government' and reveals the women inhabiting it as understanding 'that their family bloodline and their potential fecundity made them political agents in a world in which women were otherwise without direct power'.

What was the power of a mother when her young child became the monarch? This is the question posed by Emily Joan Ward in 'Child kings and guardianship in north-western Europe, *c.*1050–*c.*1250'. Regencies for kings who were minors developed fully only after the late fourteenth century. Before then, the role and powers that later would be associated with a regent would be understood in the Middle Ages in terms of guardianship. What Ward does is provide us a fleshed out and comparative history of the development of the regency by looking at guardianship in Germany, France and England in the eleventh through to the thirteenth century. Ward reveals that the power of a guardian evolved over time, and that 'new legal and martial influences on kingship, as well as changing concepts of lordship, meant that queen mothers in the thirteenth century had to become more creative to secure and maintain a place as guardian alongside the child king'. Ward also explores the vital question of the role of the 'magnates' in both securing a royal mother's guardianship powers and helping her exercise those powers in this changing environment. This study, then, has important implications not just for the history of royal women and queen mothers but also for the evolving nature of medieval kingship and dynastic rule. In many ways, magnates and royal mothers had much in common and were natural allies in times of a king's minority. They occupied both customary and ill-defined positions at court. While not always allies, royal mothers did at times find ways to make use of their circumstances to shore up their positions in the royal family and at court, which, as Ward suggests, turns on its head some of our preconceived notions about gender roles and the exercise of power in these realms and times.

Queen mothers are again the focus in Beverly J. Stoeltje's 'Creating chiefs and queen mothers in Ghana: obstacles and opportunities'. Here our attention shifts to the modern day and to the role of queen mothers (*Ohemaa*) in the succession to the chieftaincy, particularly among the Asante. The *Ohemaa* is more 'the mother of the clan' than necessarily the biological mother of the successor to the throne, but she played a political and dynastic role not unlike what we have seen elsewhere in other periods. Both metaphorically and functionally, the *Ohemaa* 'suckles' the dynasty and the heir, serving as a repository of knowledge about the ruling clan, especially (and importantly) genealogical knowledge. Much in this political world is vested in this maternal knowledge. The *Ohemaa* knows the characters of members of the clan, understands the current political trends and selects which of her kinsmen will rule next – that person often not being her own son but another relative with qualities appropriate for the post. In this respect, the *Ohemaa* can be compared and contrasted with the queen mothers of medieval Europe or the mothers in ancient Near Eastern harems, both in their notions of kinship and dynasty but also in their selfless dedication to good rulership. It is no wonder, as Stoeltje points out, that the government of Ghana takes so seriously and respectfully the role of monarchy in society today.

Finally, Cathleen Sarti reminds us that not all kings and queens died in their beds at a ripe old age. In her 'Depositions of monarchs in northern European kingdoms, 1300–1700', Sarti examines the 'removal of a monarch from their throne against their wishes' in Scotland, England, Denmark, Norway and Sweden, and makes the case for the key role played by a kingdom's 'political' elite – and later, 'the majority of the kingdom's inhabitants' – in the stability and continuance of any given reign. This approach is rich in connections, leading to insights on a range of related topics – such as the right to revolt, good and bad kingship, and the nature of power in these monarchies and monarchies in general. Particularly important is the suggestion here that kings rule with, not over, the great lords of their court. Good kingship is collaborative and rooted in consensus. Depositions and collaborative government were a productive and positive combination in these realms, says Sarti, as 'depositions formed states by forcing the negotiation of a new consensus of royal rule'. She is right to imply that depositions ought to be seen as just one more way one king succeeded another. What Sarti shows is the clear connections between dynasty, succession and the elite in the context of state-building. Sarti's chapter, then, brings us full circle in the cycle of kingship: from the rules and conventions (even laws) of succession to the throne, to how monarchs ruled with their wives and mothers, to how they lost their thrones when the times required.

These chapters illustrate a general observation that Duindam made about monarchy: that 'almost all peoples across the globe until very recently accepted dynastic rule as a god-given and desirable form of power', with 'divergent practices' that 'can be seen as part of the same pattern'.[16] When it comes to dynasty and succession, the practices are enormously divergent, but the pattern does appear to be the same. The striking feature of all these studies, despite the range of cultures and periods represented in them, is that the transfer of power from one ruler to the next was both the most important and the most dangerous moment in the life of the political system. These dangers were navigated variously, and these chapters demonstrate powerfully how important women were to the success of dynasties and monarchical systems in every corner of Afro-Eurasia, regardless of the underlying religious and political culture of a given space. But all these solutions were aimed at a single goal, to avoid the interregnum – what Ambrose Bierce called the 'period during which a monarchical country is governed by a warm spot on the cushion of the throne'.[17]

Notes

1 Translation from *The Testaments of The Grand Princes of Moscow*, trans. and ed., and with commentary, by Robert Craig Howes (Ithaca: Cornell University Press, 1967), 192.

2 Edward Keenan, "Ivan IV and the 'King's Evil': Ni Maka Li To Budet?" *Russian History* 20, nos. 1–4 (1993): 5–13, quote at 6.

3 See Robert Fawtier, *Les Capétiens et la France: Leur rôle dans sa construction* (Paris: Presses universitaires de France, 1942), published in English as *The Capetian Kings of France: Monarchy and Nation, 987–1328* (London: Macmillan; New York: St. Martin's, 1960); Jean-François Lemarignier, *Le gouvernement royal aux premiers temps capétiens (987–1108)* (Paris: Editions A. and J. Picard et Cie, 1965); Charles T. Wood, *The French Appanages and the Capetian Monarchy, 1224–1328* (Cambridge, MA: Harvard University Press, 1966); Joseph R. Strayer, *On the Medieval Origins of the Modern State* (Princeton: Princeton University Press, 1970). See also William Chester Jordan and Jenna Rebecca Phillips, eds., *The Capetian Century, 1214–1314*, in the series Cultural Encounters in Late Antiquity and the Middle Ages, 22 (Turnhout: Brepols Publishers, 2017).

4 See, for example, the Hohenzollerns and the formation of Germany, Daniel Schönpflug, *Die Heiraten der Hohenzollern: Verwandtschaft, Politik und Ritual in Europa 1640–1918* (Göttingen: Vandenhoeck & Ruprecht, 2013); Henry Bogdan, *Les Hohenzollern: La dynastie qui a fait l'Allemagne (1061–1918)* (Paris: Perrin, 2010); Christopher Clark, *Iron Kingdom: The Rise and Downfall of Prussia, 1600–1947* (Cambridge, MA: Belknap Press of Harvard University Press, 2006).

5 See Andrew W. Lewis, *Royal Succession in Capetian France: Studies on Familial Order and the State* (Cambridge, MA: Harvard University Press, 1982); Elizabeth A.R. Brown, *The Monarchy of Capetian France and Royal Ceremonial* (Aldershot: Variorum; and Brookfield: Gower, 1991); and Jim Bradbury, *The Capetians: Kings of France, 987–1328* (London: Hambledon Continuum, 2007).

6 On the Jagiellonians, see the extensive research project "The Jagiellonians: Dynasty, Memory and Identity in Central Europe," www.jagiellonians.com/ (accessed 25 March 2019); and one of the first of its resulting publications, Giedrė Mickūnaitė, "United in Blood, Divided by Faith: Elena Ivanovna and Aleksander Jagiellon," in *Frictions and Failures. Cultural Encounters in Crisis*, ed. Almut Bues, in the series Deutsches Historisches Institut Warschau. Quellen und Studien 34 (Wiesbaden: Harrassowitz, 2017), 181–200.

7 Gilbert Dagron, *Emperor and Priest: The Imperial Office in Byzantium*, trans. Jean Birrell (Cambridge: Cambridge University Press, 2003), 23.

8 Donald Ostrowski, "Was There a Riurikid Dynasty in Early Rus'," *Canadian-American Slavic Studies* 51, no. 1 (2017): 1–20.

9 Jeroen Duindam, *Dynasties: A Global History of Power, 1300–1800* (Cambridge, UK: Cambridge University Press, 2016). See also Jeroen Duindam, Tülay Artan and Metin Kunt, eds., *Royal Courts in Dynastic States and Empires: A Global Perspective* (Leiden: Brill, 2011).

10 Duindam, *Dynasties*, 88.

11 Edward Muir, *Ritual in Early Modern Europe*, second edition (Cambridge: Cambridge University Press, 2005); David I. Kertzer, *Ritual, Politics, and Power* (New Haven: Yale University Press, 1988); Catherine Bell, *Ritual: Perspectives and Dimensions* (Oxford: Oxford University Press, 1997).

12 Olivier Hekster, *Emperors and Ancestors: Roman Rulers and the Constrains of Tradition* (Oxford: Oxford University Press, 2015).

13 See, for example, the Royal Studies Network, https://www.royalstudiesnetwork.org/ (accessed 25 March 2019), and its new and highly respected online journal *Royal Studies Journal* at www. rsj.winchester.ac.uk/ (accessed 25 March 2019). See also the journal *The Court Historian*, which was launched in 1996 and which treats many of the themes raised in this volume.

14 Donald Quataert, *The Ottoman Empire, 1700–1922*, second edition, in the series New Approaches to European History, 34 (Cambridge: Cambridge University Press, 2005), 90–92; Colin Imber, *The Ottoman Empire, 1300–1659: The Structure of Power*, second edition (Basingstoke: Macmillan, 2009), 84–102.

15 Keenan, "Muscovite Political Folkways," *Russian Review* 45 (1986): 115–181, quote at 144.

16 Duindam, *Dynasties*, 2, 14.

17 Ambrose Bierce, *The Unabridged Devil's Dictionary*, eds. David E. Schultz and S. T. Joshi (Athens: University of Georgia Press, 2000), 135.

Key works

Bogdan, Henry, *Les Hohenzollern: La dynastie qui a fait l'Allemagne (1061–1918)* (Paris: Perrin, 2010).

Dagron, Gilbert, *Emperor and Priest: The Imperial Office in Byzantium*, trans. Jean Birrell (Cambridge: Cambridge University Press, 2003).

Duindam, Jeroen, *Dynasties: A Global History of Power, 1300–1800* (Cambridge: Cambridge University Press, 2016).

Hekster, Olivier, *Emperors and Ancestors: Roman Rulers and the Constrains of Tradition* (Oxford: Oxford University Press, 2015).

Imber, Colin, *The Ottoman Empire, 1300–1659: The Structure of Power*, second edition (Basingstoke: Palgrave Macmillan, 2009).

Lewis, Andrew W., *Royal Succession in Capetian France: Studies on Familial Order and the State* (Cambridge, MA: Harvard University Press, 1982).

21

ANTICIPATORY ASSOCIATION OF THE HEIR IN EARLY MODERN RUSSIA

Primogeniture and succession in Russia's ruling dynasties

Russell E. Martin

Residents and foreign visitors to Moscow since 1600 cannot help but notice the bell tower stretching skyward in the Kremlin, which was the tallest structure in Moscow until 1883. If they have good enough eyesight they might make out the inscription that wraps three times around the top of the tower, some 81 metres aloft, which reads:

> By the will of the Holy Trinity, [and] by order of the Great Sovereign, Tsar and Grand Prince Boris Fedorovich / of All Russia, Autocrat, and of his son the pious Great Sovereign, Tsarevich and Grand Prince / Fedor Borisovich, this Church was built and gilded in the second year of their reign in the year 1600.[1]

The inscription has been the source of some confusion, however – even among native Muscovites. First, there's the name of the bell tower: the Ivan the Great Bell Tower. It is popularly named after Ivan III (r.1462–1505), not Boris Godunov (r.1598–1605), because it was originally built in 1505–8 by the former and only refurbished and made two levels taller by the latter. But the bell tower takes its name not from Ivan III but from the church over which it rises, the Church of St John Climacus, which itself was originally built in 1329 by Grand Prince Ivan I Kalita (r.1325–40), in honour of the birth of his son, Ivan (the future Ivan II).[2] But the real confusion might lie in the possessive pronoun 'their' in the last line of the inscription at the very top of the tower: 'in the second year of *their* reign'. The text makes it clear that both father and son – Boris and Fedor – were the rulers of Russia: both are called 'Great Sovereign' (*velikii gosudar*), and 'Grand Prince' (*velikii kniaz*), though the father is 'tsar' and 'autocrat' (*samoderzhets*) while the son is 'tsarevich', the son of a tsar. It was 'their reign' together that is celebrated in the inscription, counted in years without distinction: as if father and son – sovereign and heir – ruled side by side.

Associating the heir – crowning or otherwise designating the heir as co-ruler for the purpose of clarifying the succession – is a custom found in many polities across the west Eurasian space. It was a regular feature of the Roman and Byzantine empires from the time of the earliest Caesars and was known in medieval western Europe, particularly in early Capetian France.[3] The several episodes of anticipatory association in Muscovy are well known too, but the practice has yet to receive much scholarly attention as a discrete topic; neither has a list of the instances of it been documented and discussed. In the literature on this topic, the practice is seen either in the narrow context of isolated dynastic struggles or as a device in the development of the centralized Muscovite state.[4] As a result, we still know very little about the custom: when it originated, why it died out and how it fitted together with other strategies for determining and controlling the succession. The relationship between association of the heir and primogeniture has also largely been unexplored in the Muscovite context, though historians have had much to say about the development of father-to-son succession in the fifteenth through to the seventeenth century and how primogeniturial succession contested with and eventually supplanted collateral succession.[5]

This chapter explores the relationship between anticipatory association and other means of indicating heirs and promoting primogeniture in Muscovy. I argue that several strategies – the use of testaments, treaties, surety oaths, public nomination ceremonies and the association of the heir – were employed at different times by different rulers, alone or in combination, with the single purpose of establishing succession by primogeniture in the line of the descendants of Ivan I Kalita. The struggle to convert the collateral system of succession that largely prevailed in Kyivan times (tenth to the thirteenth century), called agnatic seniority, into a vertical, father-to-son system in Muscovite times (fourteenth to the seventeenth century), called agnatic primogeniture, was significantly assisted by the adoption of the custom of anticipatory association, especially at times when there were multiple possible candidates for the succession.[6] The extinction in 1598 of the Muscovite house, the Daniilovichi (the name given to the line by later historians after the common ancestor, Prince Daniil of Moscow), brought new families to the throne and new concerns about securing the succession of the heir. Anticipatory association would be briefly trotted out by the first of these would-be new dynasties – Boris Godunov and his son, Fedor – but the Romanovs would demur. Examining the Muscovite system of succession in these centuries and through the rise and fall of multiple dynasties reveals how anticipatory association worked in Muscovy and how it and other strategies combined to clarify who the next ruler was supposed to be.

Testaments and primogeniture

The line that ruled the principality of Moscow had a successful ten-generation run.[7] Eleven grand princes (and later, tsars) of Vladimir (and later, Vladimir and Moscow) ruled with their seat in Moscow from 1319 to 1598. The line started with Prince Daniil Alexandrovich, the youngest son of Grand Prince Alexander Nevskii (see Figure 21.1).

Nevskii was himself a member of the sprawling Rjurikovych dynasty, nominally descended from the Varangian Rjurik, but probably only from Prince St Volodimer (ruled in Kyiv 978–1015), who is purported to have been a great-grandson of Rjurik (but almost certainly was not).[8] Nevskii died in 1263, and the grand princely throne passed to his next younger brother, Yaroslav Yaroslavich (r.1264–71), both in accordance with the lateral succession system practised then among the Rjurikovychi, and by appointment of the khan of the Ulus of Jochi (i.e. the Golden Horde), who gave

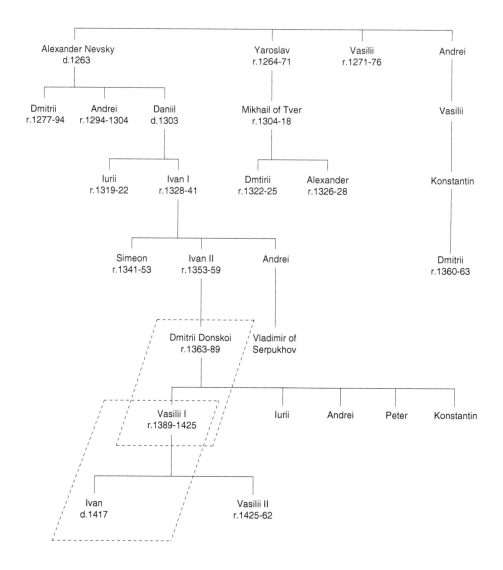

Key: Dotted boxes indicate possible cases of anticipatory association.

Figure 21.1 The Daniilovich dynasty and its competitors, 1263–1462, showing incidences of anticipatory association

out the *iarlyk*, or patent, to whomever he chose, though often (but not always) to the prince most senior in the succession system. Those customs favoured collateral heirs over lineal ones: younger brothers over sons and nephews. After Yaroslav Yaroslavich came his next oldest brother, Vasilii (r.1272–6); then the succession spiralled back to Nevskii's two sons in turn: Dmitrii Alexandrovich (r.1277–94) and Andrei Alexandrovich (r.1294–1304), each of whom had to receive the *iarlyk* from the khan to rule legitimately as grand prince of Vladimir.

Prince Daniil – the youngest of Alexander Nevskii's three sons – was only two years old when his father died. As a result, he got the leftover scraps of his father's patrimony: the outpost town of Moscow. Moscow was a latecomer to princely politics in Rus'. It is mentioned for the first time in the chronicles only in 1147, as one of the many towns founded by Grand Prince Iurii Dolgorukii of Kyiv.[9] Daniil's dynastic bad luck continued in that his own death in 1303, a year before his elder brother died, left his progeny ineligible to succeed to the title of grand prince of Vladimir (named after the town of Vladimir in northeast Rus', the nominal seat of the Rjurikovych dynasty after the fall of Kiev to the Mongols). Daniil's offspring were, in the terminology of this system, *izgoi* ('orphaned') – excluded from the subset of Rjurikovych princes who could succeed to the throne.[10] The succession and the *iarlyk* passed over Prince Daniil to his cousin, Prince Michael of Tver (r.1304–19), which launched a contest for the *iarlyk* and the title of Grand Prince of Vladimir between the houses of Moscow and Tver that lasted the next two decades: through the reigns of Iurii Daniilovich (r.1319–22), the first grand prince of the house of Moscow, and his second cousins Dmitrii Mikhailovich of Tver (r.1322–5) and Alexander Mikhailovich of Tver (r.1326–8).[11] In 1328, the khan handed the *iarlyk* to Moscow again, with Ivan I Kalita (r.1328–41), another son of Daniil Alexandrovich, as grand prince, and there it stayed, except for the brief reign of Grand Prince Dmitrii Konstantinovich of Suzdal (r.1360–3), who was placed briefly on the grand princely throne by the khan during the minority of Dmitrii Donskoi of Moscow (r.1363–89).[12]

Whatever the informal customs may have been about *izgoi* lines, the final arbiter of the succession was always the khan, and here Daniil's 'orphaned' offspring proved themselves to be very lucky. The descendants of Daniil Alexandrovich of Moscow did succeed to the grand princely throne thanks to their reliable collaboration with the Tatar overlords of northeastern Rus'. They then proceeded generation after generation to subdue the rest of the principalities of northeast Rus' such that, by 1521, Moscow was the only remaining principality in this space – uniting all the former territories of Kyivan Rus' except for those to the south and west that had fallen under the control of the Rzeczpospolita.[13]

That succession was collateral – moving across a generation, then, at the death of the last brother, moving to the eldest by birth order in the next generation (minus the males excluded by the *izgoi* rule) – was a tried and true custom in this space. Kyivan rulers largely followed it, as did other dynasties that ruled polities on the Pontic Steppe.[14] After Ivan I Kalita's reign, a combination of bio-statistical chance and dutifulness in the service of the khans in Sarai produced a rightening of the path of the succession: Ivan I Kalita had no brothers that outlived him and so was succeeded by his eldest son, Simeon (r.1341–53). Simeon had no surviving sons – he and his sons all fell victim to an outbreak of the Plague – and so was succeeded by his oldest sibling, Ivan II (r.1353–9).[15] Ivan II had only one son that survived him, Dmitrii (1363–89), called Donskoi for his victory over Mamai at the Battle of Kulikovo Field in 1380. Thus, the succession of the first three grand princes after Ivan I Kalita worked in a perfectly primogeniturial way, though only because of bio-statistical accident and the acquiescence of the khans.

The first deliberate move towards primogeniture appears in relation to Grand Prince Dmitrii Ivanovich Donskoi (1363–89) and his eldest son, Vasilii Dmitreevich (the future Vasilii I). Donskoi was the first in his line for four generations to have a brood of healthy sons survive him. In addition to Vasilii, Donskoi was survived by four other sons: Iurii, Andrei, Petr and Konstantin.[16] In the spring of 1389, Donskoi attempted to guarantee that his eldest son, Vasilii, and not his first cousin, Vladimir Andreevich, prince of Serpukhov and Borovsk, would succeed him. His method for providing that guarantee was through a treaty between himself and Prince Vladimir Andreevich, signed on 25 March 1389.[17] In it, Donskoi fixed the relative relationships between him and his eldest son, Vasilii, his other sons, and Vladimir Andreevich through kinship rankings. According to the treaty, Vladimir agreed to recognize Donskoi as occupying the position of his father, Donskoi's eldest son Vasilii as Vladimir's older brother, Donskoi's next son Iurii as equal to him, and Donskoi's other sons (Andrei, Petr and Konstantin) as younger than him – a kinship hierarchy that would assure that the throne passed from Donskoi to Vasilii upon Donskoi's death, then to Iurii, who was next in line according to agnatic primogeniture.

Donskoi's resolve in this treaty to have his son Vasilii succeed him is on even fuller display in his second last will and testament, which was signed by him perhaps only one month later (between 13 April and 16 May 1389) – only days before his death.[18] In the will, Donskoi 'bless[es] his son, Prince Vasilii, with his patrimony [*otchina*], the grand principality'.[19] This clear and unprecedented statement in the will of a grand prince was an important innovation. As Robert Crummey put it, this line in the will is a 'startling phrase' that assumed that the 'office [of grand prince] was his personal possession, to be passed on to his eldest son!'[20] The treaty and will together were indicators, as Nikolai Kazamzin put it, of 'a new order of succession to the grand princely succession, abolishing the ancient practice by which a nephew conceded the succession to his uncle'.[21] Donskoi was attempting to assure the succession of his son over a potential collateral heir. He used a treaty and a testament to impose this will on his relatives and to assert greater control over the succession at the expense of the khan's traditional prerogatives. But was there more than just nomination by treaty and testament going on?

For Vladislav Nazarov, the evidence from the treaty and testament provide proof, albeit indirectly, of the first instance of anticipatory association of the heir in Muscovy – the 'prototype', as he put it – for all subsequent instances of the custom.[22] Nazarov argued that the 1389 treaty displayed the new 'equal status' of father and son – Donskoi and Vasilii – vis-à-vis Vladimir Andreevich, and therefore signals anticipatory association, which Nazarov speculates was inaugurated 'in the spring of 1389, or perhaps even a little earlier'.[23] Nazarov points to a number of chronicle entries which indicate that 'the son fulfilled many of the functions of the father' in the years 1383–9. To be sure, Vasilii certainly did have an active and responsible role during his father's reign, including once even standing in for Donskoi (*v svoe mesto*) in a vital mission to Sarai to dispute Prince Michael Alexandrovich of Tver's claims to the grand princely title.[24] Other roles given Vasilii by his father likewise look like the things rulers, not heirs, do.[25] For Nazarov, the role played by Vasilii in these years compellingly 'demonstrates the feasibility of the hypothesis of co-rulership [*sopravitel'stvo*] of the heir with the grand prince' – in other words, the anticipatory association of the heir.[26]

Perhaps, but the evidence is not indisputable, the title given to Vasilii in both the treaty and the will is 'prince', not grand prince, though Nazarov explains this fact away by pointing to the 'political and legal realities of relations at that time with the Horde'. In other words, 'grand prince' was a title still bestowed only by the khan, regardless of one's position in fact in the Daniilovich dynasty. Nazarov goes on to assert that the 'motives' for associating Vasilii with his father are clear: 'to provide an additional guarantee – to the extent possible – of the transfer of power from Dmtirii Ivanovich to his eldest son'.[27] But this conclusion conflates two very different phenomena: primogeniture and anticipatory association. While the evidence is persuasive that Donskoi sought to pass his title to his eldest son, and failing that, to his next eldest son, rather than to his cousins, it is hard to prove anticipatory association by the treaty and testament alone. Given the continuing (though weakening) role of the khans in the succession, even after the Mongol-Tatar defeat at Kulikovo Field in 1380, it is hard to imagine that association would have even occurred as an option to Donskoi. But it is easy to imagine Donskoi wanting to resist against the claims of collateral heirs, especially those of Moscow's old nemesis Tver; and at this moment in time the best instrument for resisting collateral succession was through his last will and testament. Thus this episode is quite good evidence of an early push to institute primogeniture through testaments and treaties, bolstered by the decreasingly important but still essential imprimatur provided by the khan's *iarlyk*. It may not, however, have been an early instance of anticipatory association.

Nazarov also suggests that when Vasilii Dmitreevich himself took the throne in accordance with the provisions of his father's will – as Vasilii I – he likewise associated his own eldest son Ivan Vasil'evich in 1416. He concludes this because Ivan Vasil'evich is called the 'grand prince of Nizhnii Novgorod' in some chronicle references, though the usage is inconsistent.[28] It is a tempting speculation, to be sure. In one chronicle entry, he is called the 'officially designated grand prince' (*narechennyi kniaz' velikii*), suggesting not only that the title was more than honorary but that it had been bestowed upon him formally – through some undescribed rite of initiation.[29] Nazarov speculates that the title – and the co-rulership that it connoted – was granted to him at the time of his marriage in January 1416 (though in the chronicle entry for his marriage he is referred to only as 'prince').[30] This 'experiment' with anticipatory association, as Nazarov called it, was short-lived, however. Ivan Vasil'evich died in July 1417;[31] and if Ivan Vasil'evich was his father's co-ruler, the father for some reason did not choose to transfer the title and role to his next eldest son (and eventual successor), Vasilii Vasil'evich (the future Vasilii II). He did, however, nominate him as his successor – which by now had become a typical element of Daniilovich wills.[32] The first lines of the will after the obligatory preamble clearly indicates the heir: 'And I pass to [*blagosloviaiu*] my son, Vasilii, my patrimony, which my father passed [*blagoslovil*] to me.'[33]

The way to attack the old habits of mind that preferred collateral heirs to lineal ones was to put down in writing the name of your son as heir – to specify the succession in a text that received the seal of the grand prince, was produced in his chancellery by learned secretaries and that had the force of law. As Muscovy emerged from the years of Tatar domination, succession by *iarlyk* gradually gave way in part to succession by testamentary designation. The wills of the grand princes, which had been written at least since Ivan I Kalita's time, became the instruments of succession and an instrument for imposing primogeniture in the Daniilovich branch of the Rjurikovych dynasty.

Vasilii II and the Muscovite Civil War

The first clear instance of anticipatory association of the heir occurred by the summer of 1449, when Vasilii II the Blind (1425–62) declared his son, Ivan (the future Ivan III), 'grand prince' (see Figure 21.2). The date of this declaration is uncertain, however. A later source, a letter of Russian bishops dated 13 December 1459, describes the consecration of Metropolitan Iona of Moscow on 15 December 1448, and seems to indicate that the title of grand prince had by that date already been granted to the young Ivan: 'Grand Prince Vasilii Vasil'evich [Vasilii II] and his son Grand Prince Ivan Vasil'evich [the future Ivan III] having gathered us together, their intercessors, . . . consecrated our lord Iona, Metropolitan of Kiev and all Rus'.'[34] A treaty between Vasilii II and Prince Ivan Vasil'evich of Suzdal, seems to confirm the approximate date. Dated between December 1448 and July 1449, Ivan Vasil'evich is regularly referred to in it as 'Grand Prince Ivan Vasil'evich'.[35] As A.A. Zimin concluded:

> If this evidence [meaning the letter and the treaty] can be interpreted variously (in particular, that the title of grand prince could have been 'retrospectively' attributed to Ivan Vasil'evich in the letter), then another fact is indisputable: Prince Ivan was named grand prince in the treaty between Vasilii II and the Suzdal prince Ivan Vasil'evich.[36]

Nazarov rightly points out, however, that the usage of the title in a range of sources is inconsistent until 1452, after which it became the uniform and standard way to refer to the heir.[37] He concludes that the title was consistently used only after Ivan Vasil'evich had reached his majority – age twelve – in January 1452.[38] The fact that Ivan Vasil'evich married in June 1452 – he at the age of twelve, his bride, Mariia Borisovna of Tver, at the tender age of ten – only solidified his position as the heir of the dynasty and co-ruler with his father.[39]

Whether in 1448 or 1452, the decision to associate Ivan Vasil'evich with his father, Vasilii II the Blind, came at an opportune moment. It was precisely then that the feud between the two branches of the Daniilovich house – the main trunk, represented by Vasilii II, and a collateral branch, represented by Vasilii II's uncle, Iurii of Zvenigorod and Galich, and then, after Iurii's death in 1434, by his sons, Vasilii Kosoi and Dmitrii Shemiaka – was coming finally to a close.[40] The Muscovite Civil War, as it is called by later historians, lasted from 1433 to 1453 and was, as Edward Keenan put it, 'prolonged, bitter, and destructive'.[41]

It will be remembered that in his second will, Dmitrii Donskoi had nominated his son, Vasilii Dmitreevich (Vasilii I) to be his successor, but he also in this will stated that, should Vasilii die, the throne would go instead to the next eldest surviving son.[42] It will also be remembered that in the treaty between Donskoi and his cousin Prince Vladimir of Serpukhov, the next older brother, Iurii Dmitreevich, was treated as second in line to the throne. Iurii thus had good reason to think that the throne was his after Vasilii I's death. But Vasilii I had a son born to him in 1415, and as we have seen, he provided in his will that the throne should pass to this son, not his brother – which is what happened in 1425. Thus the Muscovite Civil War had its start in two different readings of Donskoi's will: one that saw the line of succession spelled out in it as fundamentally altered by the birth of a son (a reading that favoured Vasilii II), the other that relied rigidly on the text of the will

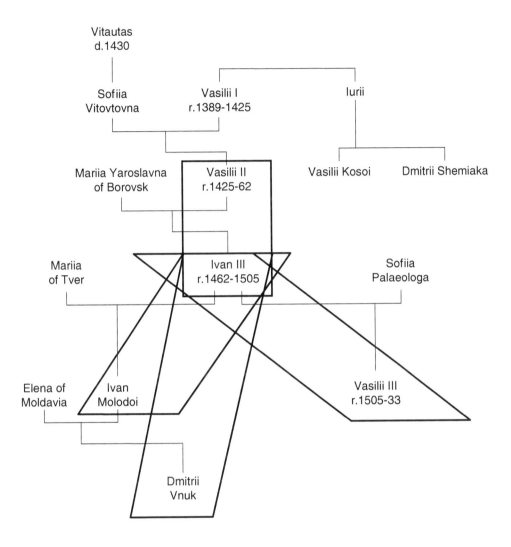

Key: Solid boxes indicate anticipatory association.

Figure 21.2 The Daniilovich dynasty, 1389–1533, showing incidences of anticipatory association

as originally signed (a reading that favoured Iurii). The Muscovite Civil War had its start as a hermeneutical dispute.

At first, Iurii Dmitreevich rejected the succession of his nephew, who was only ten years old at time, but he eventually relented, knowing that Vasilii II's claim was supported by his maternal grandfather, Grand Prince Vytautas the Great of Lithuania (r.1392–1430) and by Metropolitan Fotii. Iurii's position did not improve after Vytautas' death in 1430 or Fotii's in 1431, however. When, later that year, both Vasilii II and Iurii travelled to Sarai to make their cases before Khan Ulu-Muhammed, the *iarlyk* was handed to Vasilii II, though it took the khan nearly a year to make up his mind. There things stayed until the 1433 wedding of Vasilii II and Mariia Iaroslavna of Borovsk, where Vasilii II's mother, Sofiia Vitovtovna (Grand Duke Vytautas' daughter), got into a fierce row with Iurii's son, Vasilii Kosoi, over the rightful ownership of a golden belt Kosoi had worn to the wedding.[43] Iurii and his kin stormed out and shortly took up arms against his young nephew. War raged intermittently – with the grand princely title passing back and forth between the heads of the two feuding branches of the dynasty, with other members of the dynasty taking and then changing sides in the feud, and with each claimant to the throne taking turns blinding each other. Eventually, Vasilii II prevailed against his rivals, and, quoting Keenan again:

> [t]he winning coalition (Vasilii II and his allies) confirmed forever a new dynastic principle, whereby only the eldest son of only one family – that of Vasilii – was clearly designated as successor, his brothers and uncles being effectively excluded from political life, typically by means of imprisonment or exile in the so-called 'appanage' centers.[44]

It was with victory nearly in hand that Vasilii II sealed this 'new dynastic principle' by associating his son Ivan with him on the throne at the first opportunity: in 1448 (when Vasilii Kosoi died) or 1452 (when Ivan turned twelve). By then, Vasilii II was either certain of the khan's acquiescence or felt bold enough to ignore his opposition. Either way, the 'catastrophe' of the civil war prompted a bold solution to the question of the succession. That solution may well have been inspired by the Byzantine experience with co-rulership. The custom was common in Byzantium, and in the last Byzantine dynasty, the Palaeologi, every ruler but two was associated with his predecessor.[45]

Despite the regularity of associating heirs during the Palaeologus dynasty, the last association of a Byzantine co-ruler was in 1421, when Manuel II crowned his eldest son, John VIII, some three decades before the first instance of it in Muscovy.[46] Were the Muscovites aware of the Byzantine custom of co-rulership and, if so, did they deliberately adopt it? The custom is unreported in the *Letopisets Ellinskii i Rimskii* and the *Russkii Khronograf*, the chief written sources of Byzantine history and culture in Muscovy,[47] or in the description of Manuel II's coronation by the monk Ignatius of Smolensk in his 'Journey to Constantinople'.[48] Even so, the written sources hardly indicate the extent of Muscovite knowledge of court rituals, as even the later diplomatic correspondence with the 'Greek world' demonstrates.[49] That the future John VIII married Anna, the daughter of Vasilii I of Moscow, in 1411, certainly placed Muscovite diplomats, churchmen and courtiers close to the late Byzantine court.[50] That other Byzantine court customs that had long ago fallen into desuetude at home were picked up by the Muscovites, such as the bride-show, demonstrates both familiarity with Byzantine rites and a willingness to borrow them.[51] But as probable as it may be to see the Byzantine experience as the model for the association of Ivan Vasil'evich (Ivan III), we can do little more than suggest it until more conclusive evidence is unearthed.

Ivan III and the dynastic crisis of 1498–1502

The civil war won and the collateral lines of the dynasty duly chastised, the succession passed without challenge to Ivan III in 1462 on his father's death. But the possibility for trouble still loomed. Four of Ivan III's younger brothers were still alive and living on their distant apanages. It was an unhappy life, however, for most. Two of them were never permitted to marry and form collateral lines, and the other two married only in their twenties – rather late for a Muscovite dynast.[52] Ivan III would himself marry twice and have ten known children, including a son, Ivan Molodoi (the Younger) from his first wife, Mariia of Tver, and four sons and three daughters from his second wife, Sofiia Palaeologa, niece of both John VIII and Constantine XI. The threats to the succession posed by uncles and nephews may have been fainter than in 1425 because of the 'new dynastic principle' of primogeniture that came out of the civil war, but Ivan III nonetheless saw the need to associate his heir to make sure that the deal struck in 1453 at the conclusion of the civil war stuck.

Zimin believed that Ivan Ivanovich Molodoi was named his co-ruler with his father in 1477,[53] but Nancy Shields Kollmann and John Fennell are probably right that it was as early as 1471, when some chronicle entries and other sources begin consistently to refer to him as 'grand prince'.[54] Nazarov agrees that Ivan Ivanovich Molodoi took the title of 'grand prince' in 1471, and he connected the date with his father's campaign in that year against Novgorod, when the young heir (he was thirteen years old at the time) was left in Moscow as co-ruler.[55] Molodoi's position only solidified as his father's co-ruler in 1480 when he married Elena, the daughter of the Moldavian voevoda Stefan III the Great (r.1457–1504),[56] and had a son in 1483 – Dmitrii Vnuk (the grandson).[57] In 1485, Molodoi was handed the principality of Tver, which had just been conquered by his father, Ivan III.[58]

All the plans for the succession came crashing down, however, on 7 March 1490, with the death of the designated heir and co-ruler. Ivan Molodoi died of gout and from the inexpert treatment he received for it from a foreign doctor (who was, of course, later executed).[59] Afterwards, 'nominal control', in Fennell's words, of the principality of Tver transferred to Molodoi's half-brother, Vasilii – the eldest of Ivan III's children from his second marriage – who was just a few days short of his eleventh birthday.[60] Between March 1490 and February 1498, the succession remained in limbo: both potential heirs – Dmitrii Vnuk and Vasilii – are called 'princes' in the sources and neither was favoured in such a way as to suggest that Ivan III was leaning in one direction or another, much less had chosen a new heir and co-ruler. Then an apparent conspiracy in the summer of 1497 against Dmitrii by supporters of Vasilii was discovered and foiled. The heads of the conspirators rolled (literally) in December 1497, and Vasilii was placed under house arrest while his mother was officially 'disgraced' (*v opale*).[61] The conspiracy broke the tie between uncle and nephew: Ivan III decided to declare his grandson, Dmitrii Vnuk, his heir and co-ruler in a grand coronation on 4 February 1498, in the Dormition Cathedral in the Kremlin, modelled, in selective ways, after Byzantine coronations.[62]

Less than a year later, however, the pendulum swung in the other direction. Members and allies of the great Patrikeev boyar clan, related to the grand princely house by marriage, were arrested and condemned to death in January 1499. While only a few allies actually lost their heads, the patriarchs of the Patrikeev clan were forcibly tonsured monks – the political equivalent of a beheading – and sent away.[63] While historians have debated the connection between this attack on the Patrikeevs and the succession dispute between Dmitrii Vnuk and Vasilii, Kollmann's analysis of the interplay between the leading boyar clans at court and the dynasty is probably correct: 'The ambiguity in succession [between 1490 and 1498] coincided with rising tension at court, when the Patrikeevy's narrow faction was claiming more power and more privileges than other boyars would tolerate.'[64] Given the support of the Patrikeevs for Dmitrii Vnuk's candidacy, this attack on them was, according to Kollmann, an unmistakable harbinger of his downfall.[65] On 21 March 1499, Ivan formally 'forgave' Vasilii his earlier involvement in the conspiracy against Dmitrii and bestowed upon him the title 'grand prince' of Novgorod and Pskov – a title which, in part at least (Novgorod), had formally been held by Dmitrii.[66]

Back in his father's good graces, Vasilii was evidently still unsatisfied. Sometime after 1 September 1499, he conspired again against his father and nephew, fleeing to the border with Lithuania, threatening, not so implicitly, to side with them against his own father in the war for which both sides were prepping.[67] Unable or unwilling to take on his son and the Lithuanians at the same time, Ivan III relented. He received his prodigal son back in Moscow with rewards. In March 1501 he received the principality of Beloozero to add to his other titles.[68] But Vasilii's victory was only complete on 11 April 1502, when Dmitrii Vnuk and his mother were arrested.[69] The inevitable followed three days later:

> In the year 7010 [1502], on April 14, a Thursday, the feast day of our Father among the saints St. Martin, Pope of Rome, Grand Prince Ivan Vasil'evich of All Russia showed favor upon [*pozhaloval*] his son Vasilii, and blessed him and seated him on the grand princely throne [*na velikoe kniazhenie*] of Vladimir and Moscow and of all Russia, Autocrat.[70]

The final stage of the succession crisis of 1498–1502 raises one final problem for our study of anticipatory association. When did Dmtrii Vnuk cease to be his father's co-ruler? Put another way, how many co-rulers were there between 21 March 1499 (when Ivan III 'forgave' Vasilii and bestowed titles and territories upon him), and 14 April 1502 (when he formally 'seated' Vasilii on the grand princely throne)?

For Fennell, there remained during this interval only two co-rulers: Ivan III and his grandson, Dmitrii Vnuk. The appointment of Vasilii to the title 'grand prince' and to the principalities of Novgorod and Pskov on 21 March 1499, or of Beloozero in March 1501 'in no way lessened [Dmitrii's] authority as "grand prince of All Russia", co-ruler and heir to the throne'.[71] These titles and related income merely compensated for the clear favour shown the more senior heir, Dmitrii Vnuk. They did not signal a return to the ambiguous situation that prevailed between the two potential heirs in the years between 1490 and 1498. Nazarov, however, argues that there were 'three co-rulers in the period 1499–1502': Ivan III, Dmitrii Vnuk and Vasilii (the future Vasilii III).[72] But Nazarov's argument relies entirely on the use of the title 'grand prince': that both heirs are attested with it in these years. Fennell's view that the coronation of 1498 was still in effect and that Dmitrii Vnuk was still the lone co-ruler and heir seems most plausible. Not until Dmtrii Vnuk's arrest in 1502 does the pendulum make its full and final swing towards Vasilii. That is probably why the chronicle entry for the declaration of Vasilii (the future Vasilii III) on 14 April 1502 is so powerfully worded. The text was announcing not just the elevation of a son to the co-rulership with his father; it was declaring the demotion and ruination of a grandson and his mother.[73]

Heirs and successors in the new dynasties

The association of Vasilii III with his father in 1502 was the last time the custom was employed for nearly a century – until Boris Godunov associated his son, Fedor Borisovich, in 1598, as the bell tower of Ivan the Great testifies. This is not for lack of opportunities (see Figure 21.3).

Vasilii III's own two sons – Ivan Vasil'evich (the future Ivan IV) and Iurii Vasil'evich – were toddlers when he died in 1533, and so the opportunity to associate one or the

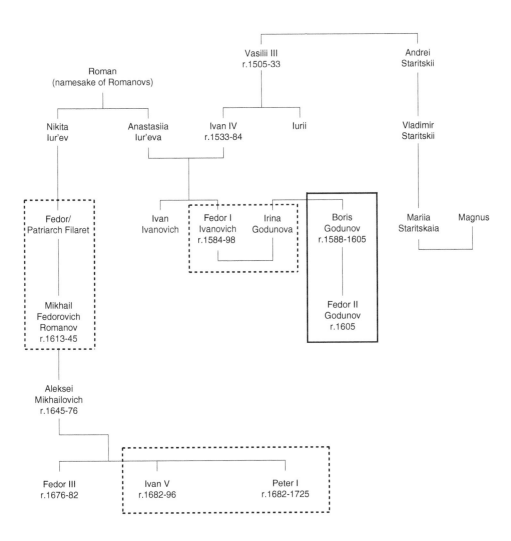

Key: Solid boxes indicate anticipatory association; dotted boxes indicate other forms of co-rulership.

Figure 21.3 The Daniilovich, Godunov and Romanov dynasties, 1533–1725, showing incidences of anticipatory association

other of them did not present itself. However, two of Ivan IV's sons – Ivan Ivanovich and Fedor Ivanovich (the future Fedor I) – did reach adulthood, but neither was ever associated with their father. In fact, Ivan IV's reign (r.1533–84) was in this respect, like in so many others, quite the contradiction. On the one hand, he married seven times (and planned other matches besides these) with the determined purpose of producing an heir of his body.[74] On the other hand, he rarely treated his sons as if they were heirs to his throne, much less co-rulers. In fact, he seemed to have had other plans at times: he divided the realm into two parts during the infamous 'Oprichnina' years (1565–72), giving control of one half to the boyars and keeping the other half as a 'privy domain'.[75] In 1573, he arranged the marriage of his cousin's daughter, Mariia Staritskaia, to Magnus, the son of King Christian III of Denmark, and declared at the time to a Danish diplomat that Magnus, not one of his sons, would succeed him after his death.[76] He also abdicated for about a year in favour of Simeon Bekbulatovich, a converted Chinggisid, who was 'grand prince of Moscow' from 1574 to 1575.[77] Ivan's sons must have spent their entire lives wondering if either of them would ever rule. As it turned out, the eldest surviving son, Ivan Ivanovich, predeceased his father, and the second son, Fedor Ivanovich, succeeded his father as tsar but died without heirs in 1598.[78]

Whatever Ivan IV's plans were for his sons, he had clearer ideas about his agnatic cousins, the Staritskii princes. The first Staritskii prince, Andrei Ivanovich, was the youngest brother of Vasilii III, who permitted Andrei to marry only in February 1533 at the advanced age, for the time, of forty-two – after an heir (the future Ivan IV) had been born in 1530.[79] Andrei's son Vladimir, born towards the end of 1533, would grow up with Ivan IV and come eventually to be regarded as a threat to Ivan IV's own line. In March 1553, when Ivan IV lay gravely ill, the court's loyalties waivered for a moment between swearing loyalty to Ivan's infant son, Dmitrii, or to Vladimir.[80] Ivan recovered but never forgot the incident. Vladimir was compelled immediately to sign a surety oath (*krestotseloval'naia zapis'*)[81] to assure his loyalty to Dmitrii, and then again the following year, after Dmitrii's death, and again the year after that.[82] Vladimir pledged to be loyal, should Ivan IV die, to the tsar's wife and offspring by her:

> Lo, I Prince Vladimir Andreevich pledge [literally, kiss the cross] to my Tsar and Grand Prince Ivan Vasil'evich of all Russia, and to his son, Tsarevich Dmitrii; and I shall give support (*khoteti mne dobra*) to my Tsar and Grand Prince Ivan Vasil'evich, and his Tsaritsa, Grand Princess Anastasiia, and their son Tsarevich Ivan, and to their children, whom God shall in the future give them.[83]

The use of a surety oath to guarantee loyalty was an old custom. Surety oaths appeared in the fourteenth century and became increasingly common in the reigns of Ivan III, Vasilii III and Ivan IV, but they were mostly employed to assure the loyalty of princes and boyars (and other servitors) who might flee Muscovy for greener pastures in Poland, Lithuania or elsewhere.[84] Surety oaths were adapted to assure the acquiescence of collaterals members of the ruling dynasty to vertical succession starting, perhaps, in 1531, when Vasilii III's younger brother, Iurii of Dmitrov, confirmed a surety oath to his older brother and to his older brother's son (the newborn Ivan, the future Ivan IV).[85] Andrei Staritskii did likewise, 'kissing the cross' in 1537 to the young Ivan IV (who was now on the throne): the forty-seven-year-old Andrei pledged himself 'to my senior [*svoemu stareishemu*], to Grand Prince Ivan Vasil'evich of all Russia, and to your mother, Grand Princess Elena, and to your children' – which, as a seven-year-old, Ivan did not yet have.[86] The adaptation of the surety oath to secure the succession clearly stood in for the custom of anticipatory association, which itself seems to have replaced the prior custom of using treaties and testaments. Why the custom of anticipatory association fell into disuse in the sixteenth century is harder to explain, but it may be that it was too strong a measure given the relative security of the succession in the direct line of Ivan III. Anticipatory association appeared when collaterals abounded and before the custom of vertical succession had become a firm habit of mind. The custom disappeared when Vasilii III reinforced the consensus that his lineage was firmly on the throne.

Boris Fedorovich Godunov was the founder of a new dynasty. He was the brother-in-law of Ivan IV's son and successor, Tsar Fedor Ivanovich (r.1584–98). Boris had been a steward (*kravchii*) and boyar in the later years of Ivan IV's reign and had become the principal figure at court in Fedor Ivanovich's reign. The death of the last Daniilovich tsar was a crisis of a system of succession that had come to rest on the firm posts and beams of primogeniture, now firmly enough established not to need confirmation by testament, treaty, or the association of the heir. The extinction of the dynasty in 1598, however, threw the entire system of succession into chaos. Fedor I was, after all, merely the last of one line of descent from Alexander Nevsky, which itself was merely one line of the larger Rjurikovych lineage. While contemporary courtiers in France had no trouble identifying who was next in line after Henri III (d.1589) – though they were horrified to contemplate that that heir, Henri de Navarre, was a Protestant – no one in Muscovy thought to scroll back through the generations of agnatic collaterals to find the next in line agnatic heir to Fedor I, though the sources for such an investigation were available. Instead, they turned to Fedor I's widow, Irina Fedorovna (née Godunova), who was for nine days after Fedor I's death nominally regnant tsaritsa, then to her brother, Boris. Some historians, such as Chester Dunning, have suggested that Irina was co-ruler with her husband, pointing principally to the fact that her name begins to appear next to his on various edicts after 1587, and because she came to be recognized by foreigners and courtiers as the tsar's closest adviser.[87] The evidence does point to an unusually expanded role for Irina in Fedor I's court, but it may be a venturesome speculation to call her Fedor I's co-ruler.[88] There is little doubt, however, that Irina, like her brother and nephew, was an able and bold personality: one of the extraordinary figures that made up the would-be House of Godunov.

So strong was the primogeniturial habit among the boyar kingmakers in the Kremlin in 1598 that they conceived of the dynasty as a single man – Fedor I – rather than as a vast lineage with many collateral lines still healthy and reproducing. Thus, what may look to the eye as a collateral shift in the succession – even to the point of moving the throne to a different, cognatic family – is actually an echo of the strong impulse towards primogeniture.

When an Assembly of the Land (*Zemskii sobor*) – a gathering of nobles, clergy and leading merchants from Moscow and other towns – was held in 1598 to decide the succession, they acted on that impulse and selected Godunov. After the requisite (and no doubt formulaic) number of refusals, Boris agreed and accepted the oaths of loyalty of his people, an oath made not only to him but to his entire family and line, including Godunov's wife, son and daughter. The assembly pledged their loyalty, or, in the words of the text, 'kissed the cross', to:

> [o]ur pious Tsar, Sovereign [*gosudar'*] and Grand Prince Boris Fedorovich of all Russia, and to his pious and Christ-loving Tsaritsa and Grand Princess Mariia, and to their royal [*tsarskim*] children, the Sovereign Tsarevich and Grand Prince Fedor Borisovich, and Sovereigness [*gosudarynia*] Tsarevna and Grand Princess [*velikoi kniazhne*] Ksen'e Borisovne, and to those children they, the Tsar and Tsaritsa, may yet have.[89]

The oath was to the entire family, because it had to be. A boyar clan was being remade into a royal house. And just as a Muscovite marriage transformed a commoner into a tsaritsa, this election and oath transformed a boyar into a tsar, a *boiarynia* into a tsaritsa, and their son and daughter into a tsarevich and tsarevna. To have this new identity extend in the oath a generation down – to Fedor Borisovich and Kseniia Borisovna – helped create the illusion of dynastic continuity and kept sacrosanct, fictively but no less meaningfully, the notions of dynastic continuity and primogeniturial succession.

That the son was co-ruler with the father is well documented. Even as early as 1594–5, when he was just five or six, Fedor Borisovich began to appear next to his father in diplomatic audiences and other court happenings. When his father was crowned in 1598, he showered the new tsar with gold coins, a high honour usually reserved for the most senior of courtiers. He bore the title 'great sovereign', and his name appears next to his father's on decrees and charters. And there is the bell tower inscription, plus many other signals from the sources that Fedor was more than the designated heir; he was co-ruler.[90] On Boris's death in April 1605, the sixteen-year-old son became tsar, but not for long. He was murdered by boyar conspirators on 10 June and replaced by the First False Dmitrii, who claimed to have been Ivan IV's son by his seventh wife, who escaped an assassination attempt back in 1591, hid out with the Poles in the intervening years, and had now returned to claim his throne, which he asserted was his by right of agnatic primogeniture.[91]

While it might look familiar, Godunov's use of anticipatory association was, in several respects, unlike the cases we have described during the reigns of Vasilii II and Ivan III. In these earlier cases, Muscovite rulers exploited the custom in specific instances to resolve specific disputes over the succession. In the sixteenth century, there were no similar crises of succession after Vasilii III had finally succeeded his father, except those engineered by the fickle and capricious Ivan IV. Godunov revived the custom not only to indicate his heir and thus assure the continuation of his dynasty – a concern of all rulers – but to bolster the legitimacy of the dynasty overall, something no Daniilovich ruler had to worry about. The trick about establishing the legitimacy of new dynasties was not only, or even principally, in nominating the second ruler of the new house. It was in getting the people that mattered at court and in the church to agree that the new house ought to supply the second ruler. Anticipatory association, then, had to do double duty for the Godunovs, and the weight of that responsibility overwhelmed the custom and helped undermine the would-be dynasty.

The Godunovs' successors learned the lesson. Vasilii Shuiskii (r.1606–10) frequently inserted his genealogical descent from the Rjurikovych dynasty in his decrees and charters during his brief and tumultuous reign, laying claim to the throne both by the election at a hastily convened Assembly of the Land and his descent from Prince Andrei Yaroslavich of Suzdal' (d.1264), Alexander Nevskii's younger brother.[92] Shuiskii never fathered a male heir (and his two daughters died in infancy). The description of Vasilii Shuiskii's coronation contains the homily of Metropolitan Isidor of Novgorod, in which he proclaims that 'It has been deemed good that you should occupy the throne of your ancestors and to be crowned according to your ancient royal customs.'[93] The loyalty oath that circulated shortly after Shuiskii's ascension likewise looks to his Rjurikovych ancestry – 'from the lineage [*ot koreni*] of . . . Alexander Yaroslavich Nevskii' – and ahead to a future dynasty, pledging loyalty to 'the sovereign, his tsaritsa and grand princess, and their royal children, as God may grant them'.[94] The hope was that a new dynasty was being founded; but like his two immediate predecessors on the throne, Shuiskii was deposed. He was forcibly tonsured a monk, captured by allies of the Poles and withered away in a Polish prison.[95]

The first tsar of the Romanov dynasty, the sixteen-year-old Mikhail Fedorovich (r.1613–45), also came to the throne through election at an Assembly of the Land in February 1613. The Confirmation Charter of 1613, like Shuiskii's, pledges loyalty to 'the sovereign, his pious tsaritsa, and their royal children, as God may grant him'.[96] That this oath was prospective is borne out by the simple fact that the new tsar not only had no children, but he had no wife yet. But he eventually would have both: Mikhail Fedorovich would live out his life on the throne and father ten children (three sons and seven daughters). When he died in 1645, he had one son to inherit the throne (and four daughters).[97] The *New Chronicle*, a post-1613 source and therefore written with a bias towards the new Romanov regime, nicely summarizes the content of the oaths on the succession of the new dynasty. After quoting the psalmist ('His seed shall be mighty upon earth: the generation of the upright shall be blessed' – Ps 112:2), the text entreats: 'Bless then, O God, and glorify the royal clan and kin [*plemia i srodstvo*].'[98]

Mikhail Fedorovich did not associate any of his sons with him on the throne, neither did he write a will designating an heir. But he and his Romanov supporters in the court did invent a new way to secure primogeniturial succession in the dynasty. In 1642, the long-standing ritual of the tsar wishing 'years of good health' to the members of his court on the first day of the church year (September 1) was modified to include a presentation of his eldest son, Aleksei Mikhailovich. The tsarevich stood with his father as the entire court exchanged New Year's congratulations with the tsar and his heir, and as prayers and incantations echoed across Palace Square in the Kremlin.[99] The first appearance of this new ritual is telling: the young Tsarevich had just turned thirteen, which, as we have seen, was the age of majority for male dynasts even in the Old Dynasty. The ritual of presenting the eldest son and heir would continue into the next two reigns, though sources for the ritual are spotty. Tsar Aleksei Mikhailovich (r.1645–76) presented his eldest son and heir, Tsarevich Aleksei Alekseevich, in 1667, 1668 and 1669 (he died, however, in 1670), and in 1674, he presented his next eldest son, Fedor, at the ritual, who had himself just turned thirteen.[100] In each of these cases, the heir presented was the eldest son.[101]

Wills and anticipatory association had passed out of fashion as tools of dynasticism, but primogeniture remained alive and well in Romanov Russia.

If the Romanovs no longer needed to associate the heir to provide for dynastic continuity, it is nonetheless only in Romanov times that we have perhaps the best examples of co-rulership in Russian history. But in both cases, the purpose was not succession as much as stability of rule. When Mikhail Fedorovich Romanov was elected tsar in 1613, his father, Fedor Nikitich Romanov – first a powerful boyar who had been forcibly tonsured by Boris Godunov, then metropolitan of Rostov, then patriarch-designate of the Second False Dmitrii – was being held prisoner in Poland. On his return to Moscow in 1619, he was quickly promoted to fill the vacant patriarchal throne and became, in a very real sense, the co-ruler of Russia, bearing even the title 'great sovereign' (*velikii gosudar*). Father and son – patriarch and tsar – ruled together until Filaret's death in October 1633, in perhaps the most remarkable example of Orthodox church-state collaboration since Byzantine times.[102]

Mikhail Fedorovich's grandsons, Ivan V and Peter I, provide the second example of co-rulership in Romanov Russia. Tsar Aleksei Mikhailovich was first succeeded by his son, Fedor III, who was bright but infirm and died without heirs in 1682, just short of his twenty-first birthday. The next oldest brother, Ivan, who was born of his father's first marriage, was physically and mentally handicapped, and so the boyars at court deemed him unfit to rule. They supported instead Peter, who was just ten years old and the son of his father's second marriage. A crisis ensued, as the families of the boys' mothers – the Miloslavskiis and the Naryshkins – clashed over which of Tsar Aleksei's Mikhailovich's sons would rule. A compromise was shortly reached: Ivan and Peter would rule together, with Ivan's full sister, Sofiia, as regent. The co-rulership of these two half-brothers ended only with Ivan V's death in 1696.[103]

All of the strategies employed in these centuries to regulate the succession in Muscovy – testaments, treaties, public presentations of heirs and anticipatory association – solved a set of related problems. First, the strategies helped variously to install a system of agnatic primogeniturial succession to the Muscovite throne in place of the former system of agnatic seniority. As Jeroen Duindam closely put it, 'male primogeniture, granting most rights and possessions to the first-born son, emerged in many European as well as in Han Chinese dynasties as the preferred solution' to what he called 'succession strife'. While it did work better than other systems, Duindam continues, primogeniture 'hardly removed conflict'.[104] Still, the moments when anticipatory association does appear in Muscovy – in the civil war, the succession crisis of 1496–1502 and at the opening of the Time of Troubles – are precisely those when primogeniture was most at risk. As imperfect as it was, primogeniture boasted obvious advantages to monarchical power in Muscovy, as it did elsewhere. The pursuit of it prompted the civil war in the mid-fifteenth century, and the victory in that war all but institutionalized it going forward.

The second problem addressed by these strategies was assuring that that heir actually succeeded to the throne as planned. Here, the rulers of Muscovy turned first to testaments and treaties, and then to anticipatory association, then to presentation rituals as the best method to try to control the future. When lines died out or the winds of fortune in the Kremlin changed, the elite in the Church, court and society at large stepped in to right the ship through election by the Assembly of the Land, with the hope that primogenitural succession would resume afterward. The ship would founder again, when Peter I the Great (r.1682–1725) issued his law of succession in 1722, which handed the succession over to the (capricious) will of the sovereign him- or herself. The emperor after Peter could name his own successor, whether a royal relative, a court favourite or his common-born wife. As it turned out, the succession remained among the Romanovs, bouncing back and forth over the course of the eighteenth century between the two branches of the dynasty.[105] But it was only when Paul I (r.1796–1801) enacted a new law of succession in 1797 (in which first-born males were preferred over junior males, and females succeeded in the absence of male heirs) that Russia finally got a system of succession that was both stable and clear.[106] These motives are even outlined in the text of the law: 'That the State should never be without an heir. That the heir should be determined by the law itself. That there should never be the least doubt as to who is to succeed.'[107] Much of the dynastic troubles in Russia before 1797 were for want of these words.

Notes

1 G. Istomin, *Ivanovskaia kolokol'nia v Moskve*, second edition (Moscow: Tipografiia Obshchestva rasprostraneniia poleznykh knig, 1893), 4.

2 On the bell tower, see A.I. Mikhailov, *Kolokol'nia Ivana Velikogo v Moskovskom Kremle* (Moscow: Iskusstvo, 1963); I.A. Bondarenko, "K voprosu o 'lestvichnom' postroenii tserkvi Ioanna Lestvichnika v Moskovskom kremle," *Restavratsiia i arkhitekturnaia arkheologia. Novye materialy i issledovaniia* 2 (1995), 109–116; V.V. Kavel'makher, "Bol'shie blagovestniki Moskvy 16 – pervoi poloviny 17-go veka," in *Kolokola. Istoriia i sovremennost'. 1990* (Moscow: Nauka, 1993), 75–118.

3 Olivier Hekster, *Emperors and Ancestors: Roman Rulers and the Constraints of Tradition* (Oxford: Oxford University Press, 2015), 2–19, 44, 70, 187–191, 314 and elsewhere; Gilbert Dagron, *Emperor and Priest: The Imperial Office in Byzantium*, trans. Jean Birrell (Cambridge: Cambridge University Press, 2003), 30, 79; Andrew W. Lewis, "Anticipatory Association of the Heir in Early Capetian France," *American Historical Review* 83, no. 4 (1978): 906–927.

4 La.G. Solodkin, "Sushchestvoval li institut sopravitel'stva v Moskovskom gosudarstve na rubezhe XVI – XVII vv.?" *Vestnik 'Al'ians-Arkheo'* 6 (2014): 8–15; V.D. Nazarov, "O sopravitel'stve v Moskovskom velikom kniazhestve (konets XIV – nachalo XVI veka)," in *Verkhovnaia vlast', elita i obshchestvo v Rossii XIV–pervoi poloviny XIX veka. Rossiiskaia monarkhiia v kontekste evropeiskikh i aziatskikh monarkhii i imperii*, ed., I.O. Mel'nikova (Moscow: Moscow Kremlin Museum, 2009), 112–115; S.A. Mel'nikov, *Pravovoi rezhim nasledovaniia prestola v drevnei Rusi IX – nachala XVI vv. Istoriko-pravovoe issledovanie* (Moscow: 'Inform-Znanie,' 2009); idem, "Nasledovanie prestola na Rusi i printsip sopravitel'stva kak faktory tsentralizatsii," *Voprosy istorii* 11–12 (2001): 102–108; Peter Nitsche, *Grossfürst und Thronfolger: Die Nachfolgepolitik der Moskauer Herrscher biz zum Ende des Rjurikidenhauses* (Köln: Böhlau Verlag, 1972).

5 See S.L. Kinev, "Printsipy nasledovaniia vlasti na Rusi XIV–XVI vv. v otechestvennoi istoriografii," *Vestnik Tomskogo gosudarstvennogo universiteta* 353 (2011): 85–92.

6 On these terms, see Donald Ostrowski, "Systems of Succession in Rus' and Steppe Polities," *Ruthenica* 11 (2012): 37–39.

7 On the genealogy of the Daniilovich dynasty, see V.A. Kuchkin, "Moskovskie Riurikovichi (genealogiia i demografiia)," *Istoricheskii vestnik* 14, no. 151 (June 2013): 6–73; Julius Forssman, *Die Bezeihungen altrussischer Fürstengeschlecter zu Westeuropa* (Bern: Verlag Herbert Lang & Cie AG, 1970), Tafeln I–X; Włodzimierz Dworzaczek, *Genealogia* (Warsaw: Państwowe wydawnictwo naukowe, 1959), Tablice 21–32; N. de Baumgarten, "Généalogies des branches régnantes de Rurikides du XIIIe au XVIe siècle," *Orientalia Christiana* 35, no. 94 (June 1934): 1–152.

8 Christian Raffensperger, *Ties of Kinship: Genealogy and Dynastic Marriage in Kyivan Rus'* (Cambridge, MA: Harvard Ukrainian Research Institute, 2016), 3, 9, 15.

9 *Polnoe sobranie russkikh letopisei* (hereafter *PSRL*), 43 vols. to date (St. Petersburg-Petrograd-Leningrad-Moscow: various publishers, 1841–2004), 2:339 (fol. 125).

10 Ostrowski, "Systems of Succession in Rus'," 41; Janet Martin, *Medieval Russia, 980–1584* (Cambridge: Cambridge University Press, 1995), 29; Nancy Shields Kollmann, "Collateral Succession in Kievan Rus'," *Harvard Ukrainian Studies* 14, no. 3/4 (1990): 377–387; A.D. Stokes, "The System of Succession to the Thrones of Russia, 1054–1113," in *Gorski Vijenats: A Garland of Essays Offered to Professor Elizabeth Mary Hill*, eds. R. Auty, L.R. Lewitter and A.P. Vlasto (Cambridge: Modern Humanities Research Association, 1970): 268–275.

11 Janet Martin, *Medieval Russia*, 199–248.

12 Janet Martin, *Medieval Russia*, 245–248.

13 Janet Martin, *Medieval Russia*, chapters 7 and 8; Robert O. Crummey, *The Formation of Muscovy, 1304–1613* (London and New York: Longman, 1987), chapters 2 and 3; A.A. Zimin, *Rossiia na poroge novogo vremeni* (Moscow: Mysl', 1972), 208–209.

14 Donald Ostrowski, "Systems of Succession in Rus'," 29–58; Janet Martin, "Calculating Seniority and the Contests for Succession in Kievan Rus'," *Russian History* 33, nos. 2–4 (2006): 267–281; Kollmann, "Collateral Succession in Kievan Rus'"; Stokes, "The System of Succession to the Thrones of Russia"; Peter Benjamin Golden, "Ascent by Scales: The System of Succession in Kievan Rus'," in *Eurasian Context, States, Societies, Cultures: East and West. Essays in Honor of Jaroslaw Pelenski*, eds., Janusz Duzinkiewicz, Myroslav Popovych, Vladyslav Verstiuk and Natalia Yakovenko (New York: Ross, 2004): 229–258. See also Janet Martin, *Medieval Russia*, 22–23, 25–29, 31–37, 50, 104–115, 118, 122–124 and elsewhere.

15 *Dukhovnye i dogovornye gramoty velikikh i udel'nykh kniazei XIV – XVI vv.*, ed. L. V. Cherepnin (Moscow-Leningrad: Izdatel'stvo Akademii nauk SSSR, 1950) (hereafter *DDG*), 14, no. 3. See also V.O. Kliuchevskii, *Kurs russkoi istorii*, vols. 1–5 of *Sochinenie v deviate tomakh*, 9 vols. (Moscow: Mysl', 1987–1990), 2:49.

16 Baumgarten, "Généalogies," 13, 16–17, table II.

17 *DDG*, 30–33 (no. 11).

18 *DDG*, 33–37 (no. 12). Donskoi's first will was prepared perhaps in 1475. See *DDG*, 24–25 (no. 8).

19 *DDG*, 34 (no. 12).

20 Crummey, *The Formation of Muscovy*, 51. For an alternative view of the will, see S.L. Kinev, "Dukhovnaia gramota velikogo kniazia Dmitriia Ivanovicha i poriadok nasledovaniia velikogo kniazheniia v severo-vostochnoi Rusi v XV v.," *Vestnik Tomskogo gosudarstvennogo universiteta* 363 (2012): 99–102.

21 Nikolai Mikhailovich Karamzin, *Istoriia gosudarstva Rossiiskogo*, fifth edition (Moscow, 1842–1843; reprint, 12 vols. in four books, Moscow: Kniga, 1988), book II (vol. 5), col. 59.

22 Nazarov, "O spravitel'stve," 113.

23 Nazarov, "O spravitel'stve," 113.

24 *PSRL*, 4:90, 5:238, 8:48.

25 See *Ukazatal' k pervym os'mi tomam Polnogo sobraniia russkikh letopisei*, 3 vols. (St. Petersburg: Tipografiia Edvarda Pratsa, 1868–1875), 1:87–91.

26 Nazarov, "O spravitel'stve," 113.

27 Nazarov, "O spravitel'stve," 113

28 Nazarov, "O spravitel'stve," 113. Ivan Vasil'evich is called 'grand prince of Nizhnii Novgorod' in *PSRL* 8:88, 35:161. Other chronicles refer to him only as 'prince'. *PSRL* 4:202, 5:260, 15:487. See also *Ukazatel' k pervym os'mi tomam*, 3:386–387.

29 *PSRL* 6:141, 8:88; Karamzin, *Istoriia Rossiiskogo gosudarstva*, Book II (vol. 5), 63 (notes to volume V), n. 146.

30 On the marriage, *PSRL* 15:487.

31 On his death, *PSRL* 4:202, 5:260, 6:141, 15:88.

32 *DDG*, 55–57 (no. 20); 57–60 (no. 21); 60–62 (no. 22). On these wills, see L.V. Cherepnin, *Russkie feodal'nye arkhivy XIV–XV vekov*, 2 vols. (Moscow and Leningrad: Izdatel'stvo Akademii nauk, 1948–1951), 1: 86–92.

33 Compare *DDG*, 55 (no. 20; Prince Ivan); 58 (no. 21; Prince Vasilii); and 61 (no. 22; Prince Vasilii). Quote at 58.

34 *Russkaia Istoricheskaia Biblioteka*, 39 vols. (St. Petersburg, Petrograd, Leningrad: various publishers, 1872–1927), 6:631–634 (no. 84) (quote at 6:633–634).

35 *DDG*, 155–160 (no. 52), at 158 and 159.

36 Zimin, *Vitiaz' na rasput'e: feodal'naia voina v XV v.* (Moscow: Mysl', 1991), 133.

37 Nazarov, "O sopravitel'stve," 114. See *DDG*, 126–140, 142–148, 150–155, 164–168, 179–186 (nos. 44, 45, 47, 48, 51, 55, 58); also compare *PSRL* 25: 269 and 271–276; *Gramoty Velikogo Novgoroda i Pskova*, ed. S.N. Valka (Moscow and Leningrad: Izdatel'stvo Akademii nauk SSSR, 1949), 39–43 (nos. 22 and 23).

38 See *DDG*, 150–155 (no. 51), at 153.

39 *PSRL*, 5:269, 5:271, 12:77, 15:495, 20:261, 23:158, 26:205. See also *The Monastic Rule of Iosif Volotsky*, ed. and trans. David M. Goldfrank, new revised edition (Kalamazoo, MI and Spencer, MA: Cistercian Publications, 2000), 96–97, 235–236.

40 See Zimin, *Vitiaz' na rasput'e*; Gustav Alef, "The Crisis of the Muscovite Aristocracy: A Factor in the Growth of Monarchical Power," *Forschungen zur Osteuropaischen Geschichte* 15 (1970): 15–58; and idem, "A History of the Muscovite Civil War: The Reign of Vasilii II (1425–62)," (PhD dissertation, Princeton University, 1956); Edward L. Keenan, "Muscovite Political Folkways," *Russian Review* 45 (1986): 115–181; and Nancy Shields Kollmann, *Kinship and Politics: The Making of the Muscovite Political System, 1346–1547* (Stanford: Stanford University Press, 1987), 108, 133–136, 153–159.

41 Keenan, "Muscovite Political Folkways," 129.

42 *DDG*, 35 (no. 12). The translation here is from *The Testaments of the Grand Princes of Moscow*, trans. and ed. Robert Craig Howes (Ithaca: Cornell University Press, 1967), 215.

43 *PSRL*, 26:189. See Cherie K. Woodworth, "Sophia and the Golden Belt: What Caused Moscow's 'Civil Wars' of 1425–1450," *Russian Review* 68, no. 2 (April 2009): 187–198.

44 Keenan, "Muscovite Political Folkways," 141.

45 Warren Treadgold, *A History of the Byzantine State and Society* (Stanford: Stanford University Press, 1997), 735–846; Donald M. Nicol, *The Last Centuries of Byzantium 1261–1453*, second edtion (Cambridge: Cambridge University Press, 1993); A.A. Vasiliev, *History of the Byzantine Empire*, 2 vols. (Madison: University of Wisconsin Press, 1952), 2:583–590.

46 Nicol, *The Last Centuries of Byzantium*, 330, 331.

47 *Letopisets Ellinskii i Rimskii*, vol. 1: *Tekst*, ed. O.V. Tvorogov (St. Petersburg: Dmitrii Bulanin, 1999); *PSRL* 22 (part 1): 419, 422, 428–430, 435.

48 George P. Majeska, ed., *Russian Travelers to Constantinople in the Fourteenth and Fifteenth Centuries*, Dumbarton Oaks Studies 19 (Washington, DC: Dumbarton Oaks Research Library and Collection, 1984), 48–113, 416–436.

49 See S.M. Kashtanov, ed., *Rossiia i grecheskii mir v XVI veke*, vol. 1 (Moscow: Nauka, 2004).

50 On the marriage, *PSRL* 4:113, 5:258, 6:139, 8:86, 11:217–218, 23:144. See also Zimin, *Vitiaz' na rasput'e*, 86. The *Khronograf* mistakenly reports that Anna married Manuel II, not John VIII. See *PSRL* 22:422.

51 Russell E. Martin, *A Bride for the Tsar: Bride-Shows and Marriage Politics in Early Modern Russia* (DeKalb: Northern Illinois University Press, 2012), 23–31.

52 Russell E. Martin, *A Bride for the Tsar*, 107–112.

53 Zimin, *Rossiia na rubezhe XV–XVI stoletii* (Moscow: Mysl', 1982), 66.

54 Nancy Shields Kollmann, "Consensus Politics: The Dynastic Crisis of the 1490s Reconsidered," *Russian Review* 45 (1986): 235, n. 2; J.L.I. Fennell, "The Dynastic Crisis 1497–1502," *Slavonic and East European Review* 39, no. 92 (December 1960), 1. Fennell does not cite his chronicle sources, but he likely meant the following two: *PSRL* 25:326 and 26:36. Ivan Molodoi appears with the title 'grand prince' in treaties as early as 1573. See *DDG*, 225–290 (nos. 69–76), and 293–328 (nos. 78–82).

55 Nazarov, "O sopravitel'stve," 114–115.

56 *PSRL* 4:134, 4:155, 6:36, 6:234–235, 8:214, 12:214, 18:270, 23:183; Kollmann, *Kinship and Politics*, 137. Fennell has the date of the marriage as 1483: J.L.I. Fennell, *Ivan the Great of Moscow* (London: Macmillan, 1961), 109, 324. Baumgarten has 1482: "Généalogies," 18, table III, no. 18.

57 On Dmitrii Vnuk's birth, *PSRL* 4:155, 6:235, 12:215.

58 *PSRL* 20:351, 23:184–185, 26:278; Kollmann, *Kinship and Politics*, 138; Fennell, *Ivan the Great*, 60–65.

59 Fennell, "Dynastic Crisis," 1–2; idem, *Ivan the Great*, 333–334.

60 Fennell, "Dynastic Crisis," 3, n. 5. See also *Akty sotsial'no-ikonomicheskoi istorii severo-vostochnoi Rusi* [hereafter *ASEI*], 3 vols. (Moscow: Izdatel'stvo Akademii nauk SSSR, 1958), 2:181–182 (no. 271).

61 *PSRL* 6:43, 8:234, 12:246.

62 George Majeska, "The Moscow Coronation of 1498 Reconsidered," *Jahrbücher für Geschichte Osteuropas*, Neue Folge, Bd. 26, H. 3 (1978): 353–361.

63 Kollmann, *Kinship and Politics*, 133–145. Iurii Patrikeev married Vasilii I's daughter, Anna, in 1418. See *PSRL* 24:232; Kollmann, *Kinship and Politics*, 131; and Karamzin, *Istoriia Rossiiskogo gosudarstva*, Book II (vol. 5), 109 (notes to volume V), n. 252.

64 Kollmann, "Dynastic Crisis," 260.

65 Kollmann, "Dynastic Crisis," 245. For an alternative view, see Fennell, "Dynastic Crisis," 9–12.

66 *PSRL* 12:264.

67 Fennell, "Dynastic Crisis," 7–8.

68 *ASEI*, 2:260–261 (no. 305); Fennell, "Dynastic Crisis," 8.

69 *PSRL* 8:242.

70 *PSRL* 8:242.

71 Fennell, "Dynastic Crisis," 6.

72 Nazarov, "O spravitel'stve," 115.

73 Dmitrii Vnuk's death in 1509, *PSRL* 5:261, 6:249, 8:250. For the death of his mother Elena in 1505, *PSRL* 6:50, 6:244, 8:244.

74 Russell E. Martin, *A Bride for the Tsar*, 112–166.

75 Edward L. Keenan, "The Privy Domain of Ivan Vasil'evich," in *The Rude and Barbarous Kingdom Revisited: Essays in Russian History and Culture in Honor of Robert O. Crummey*, eds. Chester S.L. Dunning, Russell E. Martin and Daniel Rowland (Columbus, Ohio: Slavica, 2008), 73–88.

76 Russell E. Martin, *A Bride for the Tsar*, 142–144.

77 Donald Ostrowski, "Simeon Bekbulatovich's Remarkable Career as Tatar Khan, Grand Prince of Rus', and Monastic Elder," *Russian History* 39 (2012): 269–299.

78 Paul Bushkovitch makes a compelling case that Ivan IV had nothing to do with his eldest surviving son's death: "Possevino and the Death of Ivan Ivanovich," *Cahiers du monde Russe* 55, nos. 1–2 (2014): 119–134. On Ivan IV's younger son and eventual heir, Dmitrii Volodikhin, *Tsar Fedor Ivanovich* (Moscow: Molodaia gvardiia, 2011).

79 Russell E. Martin, "Royal Weddings and Crimean Diplomacy: New Sources on Muscovite Chancery Practice During the Reign of Vasilii III," *Harvard Ukrainian Studies* 19, nos. 1–4 (1995): 389–427.

80 See Ruslan G. Skrynnikov, *Reign of Terror: Ivan IV*, trans. Paul Williams (Leiden: Brill, 2016), 59–72.

81 On the term, see I.G. Ponomareva, "O proiskhozhdenii moskovskikh 'ukreplennykh' gramot," *Arkheograficheskii ezhegodnik za 2012* (Moscow: Universitet Dmitriia Pozharskogo, 2016), 64–75.

82 *Sobranie gosudarstvennykh gramot i dogovorov, khraniashchikhsia v gosudarstvennoi kollegii inostrannykh del* [hereafter *SGGD*], 5 vols. (Moscow: Tipografiia N. S. Vsevolozhskogo, 1813–1894), 1:460–461 (no. 167); 462–464 (no. 168); 465–468 (no. 169). See also Mikhail Krom, *'Vdovstvuiushchee tsarstvo': Politicheskii krizis v Rossii 30–40-kh veka* (Moscow: Novoe literaturnoe obozrenie, 2010), 175–221; I.I. Smirnov, *Ocherki politicheskoi istorii russkogo gosudarstva 30–50-kh godov XVI veka* (Moscow-Leningrad: Izdatel'stvo Akademii nauk SSSR, 1958), 278–283.

83 *SGGD*, 1:460. The same formula is used for Tsarevich Ivan, Ivan IV's second son, after Dmitrii's death in 1533 (*SGGD*, 1:462, 1:465). On the Staritskiis, see Ann Kleimola, "Ivan IV and the Staritskie: Post-Modern Narratives from a Pre-Modern State," in *The Book of Royal Degrees and the Genesis of Russian Historical Consciousness / 'Stepennaia kniga tsarskogo*

rodosloviia' i genesis russkogo istoricheskogo soznaniia, eds. Gail Lenhoff and Ann Kleimola (Bloomington, IN: Slavica, 2011), 231–47.

84 See Peter F. Stefanovich, "Otnosheniia pravitelia i znati v severo-vostochnoi Rusi v XIV– nach. XVI v.: Krestotselovanie kak kliatva vernosti?" *Cahiers du monde russe* 46, nos. 1–2 (2005): 277–284; and Ponomareva, "O proiskhozhdenii moskovskikh 'ukreplennykh' gramot," 64–68.

85 *SGGD*, 1:443–448 (nos. 160 and 161)

86 *SGGD*, 1: 451–452 (no. 163), quote at 451.

87 Chester S.L. Dunning, *Russia's First Civil War: The Time of Troubles and the Founding of the Romanov Dynasty* (University Park, PA: Pennsylvania State University Press, 2001), 92. See also Isaiah Gruber, *Orthodox Russia in Crisis: Church and Nation in the Time of Troubles* (DeKalb: Northern Illinois University Press, 2012), 82; and Isolde Thyrêt, *Between God and the Tsar: Religious Symbolism and the Royal Women of Muscovite Russia* (DeKalb: Northern Illinois University Press, 2001), 80–81, 102–103, 117.

88 Zimin, *V kanun groznykh potriasenii* (Moscow: Mysl', 1986), 173–174; R.G. Skrynnikov, *Rossiia nakanune 'smutnogo vremeni,'* second edition (Moscow: Mysl', 1985), 36; S.F. Platonov, *Ocherki po istorii smuty v Moskovskom gosudarstve XVI–XVII vv.* (Moscow: Gosudarstvennoe sotsial'no-ekonomicheskoe izdatel'stvo, 1937), 153, 170–171; and Solodkin, "Sushchestvoval li institute sopravitel'stva," 8–11.

89 *Akty, sobrannye v bibliotekakh i arkhivakh Rossiiskoi imperii Arkheograficheskoiu ekspedit- sieiu Imperatorskoi Akademii nauk* [hereafter *AAE*], 4 vols. (St. Petersburg: Tipografiia II Otdeleniia Sobstvennoi E.I.V. Kantselarii, 1836), 2:36, 2:38–40 (quote at 40).

90 Solodkin inventories all the evidence for association of Fedor Borisovich with his father, but then abruptly dismisses it: "Sushchestvoval li institute sopravitel'stva," 11–14.

91 Maureen Perrie, *Pretenders and Popular Monarchism in Early Modern Russia* (Cambridge: Cambridge University Press, 1995), 33–106.

92 Gruber, *Orthodox Russia in Crisis*, 128–139; Platonov, *Ocherki*, 228. See also Baumgarten, "Généalogies," 10, 36–37, 45 (tables I, VII, and VIIa).

93 *AAE*, 2:105 (no. 47).

94 *Sobranie gosudarstvennykh gramot i dogovorov, khraniashchikhsia v gosudarstvennoi kollegii inostran- nykh del*, 5 vols. (Moscow: Tipografiia N. S. Vsevolozhskogo, 1813–1894), 2:300–301 (no. 142).

95 G.V. Abramovich, *Kniaz'ia Shuiskie i Rossiiskii tron* (Leningrad: Izdatel'stvo Leningradskogo universiteta, 1991), 134–168; Platonov, *Ocherki*, 333–340, 363.

96 S.A. Belokurov, ed., *Utverzhdennaia gramota ob izbranii na Moskovskoe gosudarstvo Mikhaila Fedorovicha Romanova*, second edition (Moscow: Izdatel'stvo Imperatorskogo Obshchestva istorii i drevnostei rossiiskikh pri Moskovskom universitete, 1906), 70. For other oaths, *Dopolneniia k Aktam istoricheskim, sobrannye i izdannye Arkheografeskoi kommissiei*, 12 vols. (St. Petersburg: Arkheograficheskaia kommissiia, 1846–1872), 2:1–3 (no. 1); *Drevniaia Rossiiskaia Vivliofika*, second edition, 20 vols. (Moscow: V tipografii Kompanii tipografich- eskoi, 1788–1791), 8:60–67, 8:67–83; L.E. Morozova, *Rossiia na puti iz Smuty: Izbranie na tsarstvo Mikhaila Fedorovicha* (Moscow: Nauka, 2005), 321–323, 325–329, 341–344, 385–386, 390–391, 405–407 (nos. 8, 9, 12–15, 19, 20, 36, 40, 54).

97 On the Romanov genealogy, G.I. Studenkin, "Romanovy, tsarstvuiushchii dom Rossiiskoi imperii s 1613 g.," *Russkaia Starina* 9 (April 1878): i–xxxii (at viii–ix).

98 *PSRL* 14:129.

99 *Vykhody gosudarei tsarei i velikikh kniazei, Mikhaila Fedorovicha, Alekseia Mikhailovicha, Fedora Alekseevicha vseia Rusi samoderzhtsev s 1632 po 1682 god*, ed. P.M. Stroev (Moscow: Tipografiia Avgusta Semena, 1844), 106. For a description of the ritual, Ivan Zabelin, *Domashnii byt russkikh tsarei v XVI i XVII stoletiiakh*, pt. 1 (Moscow: Iazyki russkoi kul'tury, 2000), 397–401; Philip Longworth, *Alexis: Tsar of All the Russias* (New York: Franklin Watts, 1984), 185–187.

100 *Vykhody gosudarei*, 480, 502, 581–582; S.A. Belokurov, ed., "Dneval'nye zapiski prikaza tainykh del 7165–7183 gg.," in *Chteniia v Imperatorskom obshchestve istorii i drevnostei Rossiiskikh pri Moskovskom universitete* (Moscow: Universitetskaia tipografiia, 1846–1918), vol. 225 (1908, no. 2): 252–253 (I. Materialy istoricheskie); *Dvortsovye razriady, po vysochaishemu poveleniiu, izdannye II-m otdeleniem sobstvennoi Ego Imperatorskogo Velikchestva kantserliarii*, 4

vols. (St. Petersburg: Tipografiia II otdeleniia Sobstvennoi E.I.V. kantseliarii, 1850–1855), 3:659–660, 3:973–981.

101 The custom disappeared during the turbulent times in the dynasty after Peter the Great's promulgation of a new law of succession in 1722, but was revived under Nicholas I as a cere-mony marking the coming of age of the heir and his taking the oath to the Pauline Law of Succession. See Richard S. Wortman, *Scenarios of Power: Myth and Ceremony in Russian Monarchy*, 2 vols. (Princeton: Princeton University Press, 1995–2000) 1:351, 1:354–362, 1:378, 2:170, 2:316–18.

102 J.H.L. Keep, "The Regime of Filaret 1619–1633," *Slavonic and European Review* 38 (1960): 334–360; Georg Michels, "Power, Patronage, and Repression in the Church Regime of Patriarch Filaret (1619–1633)," in *Religion und Integration im Moskauer Russland: Konzepte und Praktiken, Potentiale und Grenzen 14.–17. Jahrhundert*, ed., Ludwig Steindorff (Weisbaden: Harrassowitz Verlag, 2010; = *Forschungen zur Osteuropäischen Geschichte* 76), 81–96.

103 Paul Bushkovitch, *Peter the Great: The Struggle for Power, 1671–1725* (Cambridge: Cambridge University Press, 2001), 80–169; and Lindsey Hughes, *Sophia: Regent of Russia, 1657–1704* (New Haven: Yale University Press, 1990).

104 Jeroen Duindam, *Dynasties: A Global History of Power, 1300–1800* (Cambridge: Cambridge University Press, 2016), 88.

105 Russell E. Martin, "Law, Succession, and the Eighteenth-Century Refounding of the Romanov Dynasty," in *Dubitando: Studies in History and Culture in Honor of Donald Ostrowski*, eds. Brian Boeck, Russell E. Martin and Daniel Rowland (Bloomington: Slavica Press, 2012), 225–242.

106 O.A. Omel'chenko, "Stanovlenie zakonodatel'nogo regulirovaniia prestolonaslediia v Rossiiskoi imperii," *Themis: Yearbook of the History of Law and Jurisprudence* 7 (2006): 15–54; idem, "K problem pravovykh form russkogo absoliutizma vtoroi poloviny XVIII veka," in *Problemy istorii absoliutizma*, ed., K.I. Batyr (Moscow: Ministerstvo vysshego i srednego spet-sial'nogo obrazovaniia SSSR, Vsesoiuznyi iuridicheskii zaochnyi institute, 1983), 43–61; Richard S. Wortman, "Russian Monarchy and the Rule of Law: New Considerations of the Court Reform of 1864," *Kritika* 6, no. 1 (Winter 2005): 145–170; idem, "The Russian Imperial Family as Symbol," in *Imperial Russia: New Histories for the Empire*, eds. Jane Burbank and David L. Ransel (Bloomington: Indiana University Press, 1998), 60–86; and Russell E. Martin, "'For the Firm Maintenance of the Dignity and Tranquility of the Imperial Family': Law and Familial Order in the Romanov Dynasty," *Russian History* 37, no. 4 (2010): 389–411.

107 *Polnoe sobranie zakonov Rossiiskoi Imperii*, series 1: 1649–1825, 45 vols., with 3 vols. of plates (St. Petersburg: Tipografiia II Otdeleniia Sobstvennoi Ego Imperatorskogo Velicheskogo Kantseliarii, 1830), 6:588, no. 17.910 (5 April 1797).

Key works

Kollmann, Nancy Shields, "Collateral Succession in Kievan Rus'," *Harvard Ukrainian Studies* 14, nos. 3/4 (1990): 377–387.

Mel'nikov, S.A., "Nasledovanie prestola na Rusi i printsip sopravitel'stva kak faktory tsentrali-zatsii," *Voprosy istorii* 11–12 (2001): 102–108.

Nitsche, Peter, *Grossfürst und Thronfolger: Die Nachfolgepolitik der Moskauer Herrscher biz zum Ende des Rjurikidenhauses* (Cologne: Böhlau Verlag, 1972).

Omel'chenko, O.A., "Stanovlenie zakonodatel'nogo regulirovaniia prestolonaslediia v Rossiiskoi imperii," *Themis: Yearbook of the History of Law and Jurisprudence* 7 (2006): 15–54.

La. G. Solodkin, "Sushchestvoval li institut sopravitel'stva v Moskovskom gosudarstve na rubezhe XVI – XVII vv.?" *Vestnik 'Al'ians-Arkheo'* 6 (2014): 8–15.

Wortman, Richard S., "The Russian Imperial Family as Symbol," in *Imperial Russia: New Histories for the Empire*, eds. Jane Burbank and David L. Ransel (Bloomington: Indiana University Press, 1998), 160–186.

22

FROM *A* SALIC LAW TO *THE* SALIC LAW

The creation and re-creation of the royal succession system of France[1]

Derek Whaley

William Shakespeare's *Henry V*, the dramatic conclusion to the bard's Henriad tetralogy, begins with an explicit reference to the succession practices of France, specifically the Salic Law:

> Then hear me, gracious sovereign and you peers
> That owe yourselves, your lives, and services
> To this imperial throne. There is no bar
> To make against your highness' claim to France
> But this, which they produce from Pharamond:
> 'In terram Salicam mulieres ne succedant'–
> 'No woman shall succeed in Salic land'–
> Which 'Salic land' the French unjustly gloss
> To be the realm of France, and Pharamond
> The founder of this law and female bar.[2]

But what Shakespeare did not realize when he penned these verses was just how anachronistic they truly were. For although the Salic Law had achieved near-universal acceptance in France by the sixteenth century, it had no impact whatsoever on the English claim to the French throne. Shakespeare can be forgiven, however, for his confusion. These verses are evidence of a successful centuries-long campaign to justify the French royal succession system of male-only inheritance – agnatic succession. It was a movement that dredged out of the earliest years of the Middle Ages a legal code so neglected that none in the fourteenth century could adequately interpret it. Yet interpret it they did, first with miscomprehension and ultimately through juristic wand-waving, until a sixth-century legal clause in the Frankish *Pactus Legis Salicæ* ballooned into the first fundamental law of the French kingdom: the Salic Law. But the full history of this evolution and a survey of the French royal succession system in general have been largely neglected by historians despite a perennial interest in the development of the fifteenth-century iteration of the law.

Pactus Legis Salicæ

The immigration by the Salian Franks into Roman Gaul in Late Antiquity marked a turning point in European history.[3] No more were the Romans to rule the lands of the Loire and Seine – now that duty fell upon these Germanic wanderers whose dominions soon ranged from the Bay of Biscay to beyond the Rhine.[4] These nomads took with them a great wealth of laws, passed down orally from their ancestors, and, after settling in Gaul, these laws intermixed with the local customs of the indigenous inhabitants, the Gallo–Romans, Burgundians and Visigoths.[5] Indeed, it seems the *Pactus Legis Salicæ* was originally intended to clarify the differences between Roman and Salian law in northern Gaul, and Roman legal traditions certainly influenced and even precipitated the creation of this code.[6] The initial compilers of the laws of the Salian Franks are unknown, but the prologues to later versions of the code attribute authorship to four wise men who lived in the Rhineland.[7]

The law was first recorded in Latin between 507 and 511 during the reign of Clovis I, the first Christian king of the Salian Franks.[8] The earliest extant copies of the law date to the eighth century, after which versions become more widespread.[9] For the first hundred years of its existence, the *Pactus Legis Salicæ* was the only written code of law for the Franks, and it was expanded and updated as necessary by the Salian kings. However, the conquest and amalgamation in 613 of the Ripuarian Franks in Austrasia (modern-day western Germany) caused a legal crisis.[10] The Salians of Neustria (the Low Countries) had become increasingly Latinized by their interactions with the local Gallo–Roman population, while the Austrasians maintained their Germanic language and culture.[11] Although the *Pactus Legis Salicæ* reflected similar laws used in Austrasia, the Ripuarians felt that they needed their own king and their own written legal code. King Chlothar I relented and gave them his eldest son, Dagobert, as their king, who afterwards codified the Ripuarian laws into Latin as the *Lex Ripuaria* around 630.[12] From this point forward, there were two Frankish laws that held dominance over two autonomous kingdoms. While the *Lex Ripuaria* became a primary reference point for most later Germanic legal codes, the *Pactus Legis Salicæ* remained the primary code of law for what would eventually become northern France.[13]

Judicial reforms undertaken by Charlemagne in 798 led to a heavy revision of the *Pactus* in the form of the *Lex Salica Emendata*, which would later serve as the primary source for the fifteenth-century Salic Law. This revised *Pactus* was distributed widely across northern France and the Low Countries throughout the ninth century before merging into local customary laws and disappearing from regular usage.[14] It is from this redaction of the code that Shakespeare drew the Latin quotation included in the verse above. The full text of chapter 62, clause 6, reads:

> *De terra uero Salica nulla portio hered-* Regarding Salic land, no portion of the
> *itatis mulieri ueniat sed ad uirilem* inheritance in fact comes to the female,
> *sexum tota terræ hereditas perueniat.*[15] but all of the inheritance passes to the
> masculine (*virile*) sex.

Chapter 62, entitled 'De Alode', is essentially a short section of the *Emendata* focusing on the matter of female inheritance and how it differs from Roman Law.[16]

Specifically, it deals with how female succession works regarding *alodes* – autonomous, inheritable holdings.[17] Clause 6 basically states that, although women can inherit moveable goods and recently acquired lands, alodial holdings are treated differently.[18]

Changes to the *Pactus* under Charlemagne altered the original wording of clause 6 and made its original intent difficult to assess. However, the earliest known redaction of the *Pactus* makes the intention of 'De Alode' clearer. This version – found in chapter 59, clause 5 – reads:

> *De terra uero nulla in muliere hereditas non pertinebit, sed ad uirilem secum* [sic] *qui fratres fuerint tota terra perteneunt.*[19]

> Regarding land, none in fact belongs to a female, but all of the land should go to the masculine sex, who were (her) brothers.

Although it appears to be only a minor difference between these two versions of the clause, the fact that there is no mention of 'terra Salica' in the earlier version proves to be an important omission. Why was this term changed between the sixth and eighth centuries?

When Dagobert promulgated the *Lex Ripuaria*, it became necessary to clarify that the lands referenced in the *Pactus Legis Salicæ* only applied to Salian Franks. This change only appeared in redactions dated to the late eighth century, after Austrasia had been assimilated into the Frankish kingdom. The *Lex Ripuaria* replicated the clause (as chapter 57, clause 4) in clearer terms and never altered it, and an earlier proviso (chapter 35, clause 3) stipulated that people were to be judged by their own laws regardless of where they resided, a clarification absent from the *Pactus*.[20] Later French jurists spent countless hours discussing the true meaning of the term 'terra Salica', but in reality it was simply an ethnographic adjective to differentiate the land of a Salian from that of another people.[21]

A more fundamental, though less discussed, change between the versions is the disappearance of the qualifier 'qui fratres fuerint'. The original code specified that the inheritable land should be divided between a woman's brothers, while the later code simply says that it should go to males, not specifying whom.[22] While both versions make clear that women should not inherit ancestral land, this specific proviso included only in earlier redactions suggests that women could inherit if they had no brothers, since no alternative option is given.[23] Indeed, the *Lex Ripuaria* implies this and a later amendment to the *Pactus* states it precisely.[24] In contrast, the vagaries of the version in the *Emendata* make it easier for males of any degree to inherit, thus making female inheritance less likely.

Many writers since the sixteenth century have taken the position that the *Pactus Legis Salicæ* was intended specifically for private laws and had no impact on royal succession. François Hotman was the first to assert this in his *Francogallia* (1573), but others soon took the position as well and it was held by many historians and jurists well into the twentieth century.[25] Modern historians, however, such as Herbert Rowen and Édouard Perroy, have counterargued that the early Frankish kings would have found no difference between public and private law.[26] François Olivier-Martin states further that the Frankish kings treated their kingdoms as private lands, beholden to nobody but themselves and their laws, emphasizing that the stipulations in the *Pactus* dictated the royal succession.[27] Evidence of this can be found in the manner in which they succeeded to the throne.

Although the system invariably broke down due to sibling and cousinly disputes, the Frankish kings in general practised a form of succession known as agnatic pariage.[28] Ideally, before a king's death, a monarch would partition his realm between his sons in relatively equal parts – Ian Wood suggests that these portions were based more on parity in income than on strict territorial size.[29] Each king would technically reign co-regnant with his relatives, who ruled over other portions of the kingdom. In the case of the Merovingians – the first Salian ruling dynasty – a high mortality rate and frequent kinstrife kept the number of agnates relatively small, but on two separate occasions their domains were divided between four brothers who ruled separate portions of the realm.[30] Nevertheless, the dynasty gradually shrank until by the eighth century, only one king of the Franks ruled, more out of necessity than out of any desire to undermine the principles of pariage.[31] Notably, no women or maternal grandsons ever succeeded to a Frankish throne, which gives at least some credit to later historians who used this as evidence that a female had never reigned over the Franks.

The Carolingians, who replaced the Merovingians in 751, also used agnatic pariage initially – Charlemagne and his brother, Carloman, succeeded jointly in 768, and the former arranged for a similar division between his sons in 806.[32] However, under Charlemagne and with the support of local magnates, a new mode of succession became vogue: associative kingship. By this principle, the monarch, before dying, would crown his sons as client kings over various portions of the empire, thereby associating them with the domains over which they would one day rule. For example, Charlemagne appointed his second son, Pepin, king of Italy in 780 and his third son, Louis, king of Aquitaine in 781.[33] Practically, this was anticipative pariage – a pre-emptive, rather than testamentary, division of the kingdom. Like the Merovingians, though, the Carolingians never entirely embraced strict agnatic pariage or associative kingship simply because they were prone to the same sort of internecine wars. By 885, both forms of royal succession broke down entirely and the legacy of the *Pactus Legis Salicæ* on the royal succession faded into memory.

The Carolingian–Capetian transition

When Charlemagne's son, Louis the Pious, died in 840, his sons were supposed to divide the kingdom between them according to the tenets of agnatic pariage, but instead civil war erupted and three independent kingdoms emerged.[34] Middle Francia – the patrimony of the eldest son – collapsed between 869 and 875, after which its lands were fought over by the remaining Carolingian kings.[35] In West Francia, Louis II died in 879 leaving behind two teenage sons as well as a posthumous son.[36] The elder sons became co-kings according to agnatic pariage – the last time this system would be used by the Carolingians – but both were dead by 884, leaving the succession open.[37] In their stead, the magnates of West Francia allowed the East Frankish ruler, Charles the Fat, to reunite the entire Carolingian empire, but this decision quickly proved unpopular to all and revolts saw to his deposition in 887.[38] Charles' reign, however, highlights the sudden increase in power wielded by the Frankish elite over the throne. Prior to 884, the ideas presented in the *Pactus*

Legis Salicæ remained relevant, if often ignored. But after that date, all semblance of agnatic pariage within the Carolingian dynasty fell to the wayside.

In East Francia, Arnulf, an illegitimate son of an earlier king, was elected by the barons. He and his son would rule the East Franks until 911, when an election permanently took the kingdom out of the hands of the Carolingians.[39] Over time, electoral monarchy became the defining trait of the successor to the East Frankish realm: the Holy Roman Empire.[40] In West Francia, a series of kings were elected, beginning with the Robertine count Odo.[41] Louis II's youngest son, Charles the Simple, finally claimed his birth-right upon Odo's death in 898 but was deposed in a popular revolt in 922 headed by Odo's brother, Robert I.[42] Although Robert was defeated the next year by Charles' forces, the Carolingian claimant could not muster enough support to regain his throne, and so it passed to Robert's son-in-law, Rudolf of Burgundy.[43] The Carolingians were invited back to the West Francian throne in 936 – ostensibly through another election by the baronage – and they retained their position until 987.[44]

Fearing the loss and alienation of more territory, the last West Francian Carolingians abandoned agnatic pariage and instead adopted a policy of agnatic primogeniture to maintain the integrity of their kingdom.[45] Previously, agnatic pariage had caused siblings to quarrel over lands, titles and rights, but a half-century of civil war and elective monarchy had sapped them of their vast domains and power. Agnatic primogeniture – by which a single son succeeds to all his father's titles and lands – was considered to be the only option to avoid further diminution.[46] To reinforce the principle, the penultimate king, Lothaire, resumed the practice of associative kingship with his only son, Louis, installing him as king of Aquitaine in 982.[47] At the same time, he declined to give his brother, Charles, any portion of the inheritance. The fact that Charles continued to claim both a portion of West Francia and the whole kingdom after Louis's death in 987 suggests that he still recognized the lingering authority of the *Pactus Legis Salicæ* in Frankish royal succession law. Nonetheless, agnatic pariage would never again control the fate of the Franks.

Louis's death also prompted a brief revival of elective monarchy, a concept that had so crippled West Francia a century earlier. Since Louis died without an obvious heir, the Duke of the Franks and grandson of Robert I, Hugues Capet, assembled the magnates and was proclaimed king despite petitions by Charles of Lorraine.[48] Hugues' Carolingian ancestry was minimal, his personal domain tiny and his practical authority over West Francia non-existent.[49] There was every sign that West Francia had returned to full elective monarchy, as had already occurred in East Francia. The only thing that set Hugues apart from his Robertine forbears was the fact that he had an adult son in 987. This proved all the difference. Within months of his election, Hugues crowned his eldest son co-king, thereby resuming the practice of associative kingship.[50] Not only did it serve as a continuity marker, it ensured the stable transmission of royal authority from father to eldest son. Indeed, under the first seven Capetian kings, associative kingship and agnatic primogeniture walked hand-in-hand. Each king, from Hugues in 987 to Louis VII in 1179, continued this practice, with some kings even crowning multiple sons in succession when elder sons predeceased their fathers.[51] The system ensured an undisputed succession and also set a firm precedent for agnatic primogeniture in West Francia, and it endured even after associative kingship was abandoned by Philippe II Auguste.[52]

The fourteenth-century crises

The question as to whether a woman could inherit the French throne did not arise until Louis X died in 1316, leaving behind a pregnant wife who bore a short-lived son.[53] These deaths marked a watershed in the development of the French succession system. For the first time since 987, there was no obvious heir to the throne, although Louis did leave behind a young daughter, Jeanne, who, according to male-preference primogeniture, should have succeeded him.[54] Indeed, the viability of female rulers had already been confirmed in the Byzantine empire, Aragón, Castile, Jerusalem, Navarre, and Sicily, but there was no precedent for female succession in France. To complicate matters further, Jeanne had an ambitious uncle, Philippe, who already had eager sycophants willing to support his claim.[55] Nonetheless, circumstances were initially in favour of her receiving the throne. An agreement made between Jeanne's guardians and Philippe allowed for her to eventually succeed if her unborn sibling proved to be a girl.[56] However, no provisions were made if a boy was born and subsequently died, which is precisely what happened.[57] Philippe took advantage of this loophole to proclaim himself king, depriving his niece of her presumed rights.[58] At an assembly of barons held in February 1317 – notably a month *after* Philippe's coronation – it was declared that 'a woman does not succeed to the kingdom of France'.[59] This was not some spontaneous statement; rather it was an acceptance of the fact that, despite the *Pactus Legis Salicæ* ostensibly supporting female succession to inheritable rights and properties in lieu of males, no Merovingian or Carolingian princess had ever inherited any Frankish throne, suggesting that women were excluded from the very beginning. Few contemporary chroniclers disputed this point, but most noted some opposition to Philippe's election.[60] The precedent was repeated when Philippe died in 1322 and the throne passed uncontested to his brother Charles rather than to his eldest daughter.[61] Thus, it became an accepted fact that women were excluded from the French throne (Figure 22.1).

One might expect, therefore, that when Charles died without a son in 1328, the throne would pass to the next agnatic heir, Philippe de Valois. However, the precedents of 1316 and 1322 only confirmed male rule – the issue of whether the throne passed exclusively via strict agnatic primogeniture remained untested. Some lawyers, searching through civil and canon law, ruled that the nephew of the king should succeed, even if his claim came from his mother. Using this logic, they argued that Edward III, king of England and eldest son of Charles's sister, Isabelle, should become king of France.[62] Other lawyers argued against this, citing Roman law in saying that a man should not succeed to a title that his mother is incapable of holding herself.[63] This returned the debate to the issue of female regnants, to which the lawyers declared that, like the Roman emperorship, the French Crown was 'a dignity too eminent, a power too great, to devolve upon a mere woman'.[64] None at the time referenced the *Pactus Legis Salicæ*, which had either been forgotten by the early fourteenth century or simply considered inconsequential to the debates.[65] Although Edward later publicly proclaimed himself king in 1340 and his descendants maintained that claim until 1801, Philippe won the day and became the first king of the House of Valois, thereby establishing strict agnatic primogeniture as the official royal succession law for France.[66]

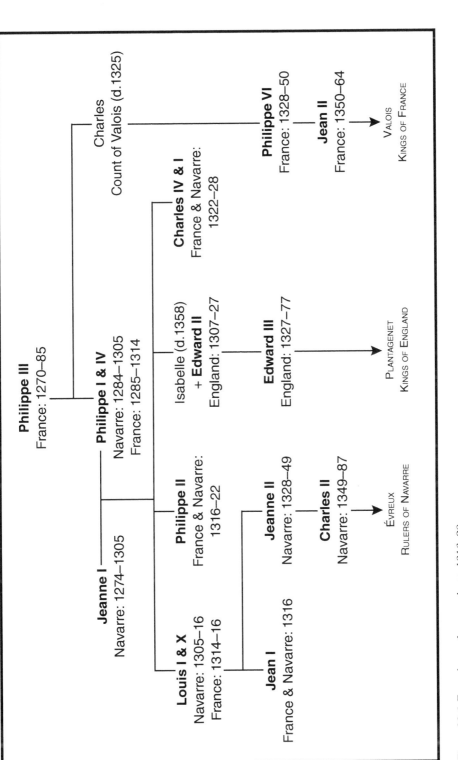

Figure 22.1 French royal successions, 1316–28

It cannot be ignored that election, or at least baronial input, was a key element in these successions. Most contemporary laws of inheritance in France, including Roman law, canon law and Parisian customary law, favoured Jeanne in 1316, and it was only with the support of important lords and prelates that Philippe V undermined her right to the throne. Similarly, the law was such that Edward III was undoubtedly a more proper successor than Philippe de Valois in 1328. He possessed all of the correct credentials – he was a French peer and territorial lord, had a Capetian mother and wife, and was fluent in the French language – and the University favoured him, but, as Paul Viollet writes, 'If the French heir had been a relative through women, and the English claimant a relative through males, [his opponents] would not have failed to proclaim the rights of women.'[67] Perhaps it was a xenophobic fear of an English king ruling over France, or the fact that Edward was still under the guardianship of his mother, but it is undeniable that baronial input handed the crown to Philippe. Contemporary authors downplayed the electoral nature of these successions, but it is nonetheless clear that royal election made a brief return to France in the early fourteenth century, if only to confirm strict agnatic succession in perpetuity.

Creating the Salic Law

Although these events reinforced agnatic primogeniture as the mode of royal succession, the precedent remained uncodified and undefined, and many still questioned whether they truly ended the debate or whether other more distantly related agnates could claim the crown. King Charles II of Navarre, maternal grandson of Louis X and heir to Jeanne, entered the scene in 1358 to address that question.[68] At this time, France's king sat in comfortable imprisonment in England after being captured at the Battle of Poitiers in 1356.[69] In his stead, the young Dauphin Charles tried desperately to suppress numerous rebellions and peasant uprisings while simultaneously fighting the English and ruling the kingdom.[70] With his strong claim to the French throne, his vast territories in Normandy and on the Spanish march, and his endless charismatic ambition, Charles II represented an existential threat to the Valois kingship.

It was within this context that the revival of the *Pactus Legis Salicæ* began. The Benedictine monk Richard Lescot, working out of the royal Abbey of Saint-Denis outside of Paris, rediscovered a manuscript of the *Lex Salica Emendata* while searching for justifications for the Valois succession to use against the claims of Charles II.[71] The monk soon referenced the law when scribing a short genealogy of the kings of France dating back to Clovis.[72] The copy of the *Emendata* Lescot used was included in a tome that collected some Merovingian genealogies, multiple Carolingian prologues and the law itself.[73] The monk assumed incorrectly that the genealogies represented a direct manifestation of the contents of the law, so when he penned his own genealogy, he placed the Merovingians, Carolingians and Capetians first, and then explained that all these successions were in accordance with the Salic Law, although he did not explain precisely how.[74] This work never reached a wide distribution, and its primary legacy is that it reintroduced the *Emendata* into French juristic culture.[75] Not long afterwards, Lescot wrote a now-lost treatise against English claims to the French throne, which likely included a transcription of clause 6 from 'De Alode', as it was written in the *Emendata*.[76] As stated earlier, this version of the clause lacked the clarification that a woman's male heirs should be her brothers and it included the adjective 'Salica'. At the time, none of this mattered since the moment of crisis had passed, but 'De Alode' had now decisively re-entered academic, diplomatic, and juristic discussions and quickly became a topic of debate that persists even to this day.

Discussions regarding the creation of the fifteenth-century Salic Law have always been highly politicized and remain so today. For a thoroughly academic look at the development of the law under the Capetians, no work compares to Ralph Giesey's *Le rôle méconnu de la Loi Salique*.[77] Meanwhile, Éliane Viennot takes a more focused approach when she discusses the development of French succession law in the context of women's history in *La France, les femmes et le pouvoir*.[78] However, neither of these works fully engage in the cultural debate that has raged since the mid-1990s over the intentions of the jurists who created the law. The major positions are held by Craig Taylor, Daisy Delogu and Tracy Adams, who generally assert that the political situation of the early fifteenth century guided events rather than overt sexism on the part of the jurists, and Sarah Hanley, who argues that the Salic Law was created explicitly to deprive women of their right to the French throne.[79] Indeed, almost any historical, political, or cultural study of the period 1300 to 1450 attempts to engage in the debate. Thus, for the purposes of this work, it is only necessary to provide a summary of the key moments that allowed an obscure clause in a Frankish legal code to become the first fundamental law of France.

The dual challenges of civil war and English invasion brought the archaic law to the forefront of French politics. In 1392, Charles VI of France became mentally unstable and his condition progressively worsened for the remainder of his life.[80] As a result, war erupted over who would rule as regent over the kingdom, fought between two agnatic lines, the Orléanists (later Armagnacs) and the Burgundians.[81] Both sides solicited the help of the English and, in 1413, Henry V invaded France and eventually came to occupy half of the kingdom.[82] Through the Treaty of Troyes (1420), Henry became Charles VI's heir, and the previous heir was disinherited and fled to the relative safety of central France, where he established his own counter-court and took the name Charles VII when his father died in 1422.[83] It was in this political morass that jurists definitively resurrected 'De Alode'. Between 1413 and 1463, dozens of polemical treatises were produced by Capetian lawyers and prelates proclaiming the inalienability of the realm, denouncing the English claim to the throne, and defending the hereditary rights of Charles VII. From the very beginning, they put the 'De alode' clause to work, using it in progressively abstract ways to justify not only the royal succession but the entire framework of French law as well.

There are three key treatises that represent attempts by the Capetian court to convert 'De Alode' into a functional justification for the Valois succession, although none of these treatises emphasized the clause as the sole – or even strongest – support for that succession.[84] *A toute la chevalerie* by Jean de Montreuil, written around 1413, was the earliest such polemic put into circulation.[85] Although it focuses very little on 'De Alode', its inclusion of a transcription of the clause made it important for later jurists who used the clause to argue in favour of the Valois against the claims of Henry V. The transcription was altered by Montreuil, however, to further support this political purpose, and the English occupation of Saint-Denis shortly afterwards, which deprived the treatise-writers of their access to the *Emendata* manuscript, allowed this altered version to survive well into the 1430s. In 1446, Jean Juvénal des Ursins reintroduced to juristic circles a proper transcription of the clause in his *Tres crestien, tres hault, tres puissant roy*.[86] This was the first polemic to discuss the Valois succession at length and the first to directly attribute the decision in 1328 to 'De Alode'.[87] *Tres crestien* quickly became the standard diplomatic text used when explaining the Valois right to the throne. One unexpected problem arose, however, out of the fact that it also attempted to undermine Lancastrian claims to the French throne by implicitly supporting the claims of the House of York, a tactic that backfired in 1461 when the Yorkists deposed the Lancastrians.[88] To remedy this situation, Louis XI commissioned Guillaume Cousinot to write an updated treatise, *Pour ce que plusieurs*, which was made available to diplomats in 1464 and became the definitive text that converted 'De Alode' into *the* Salic Law.[89] To bolster his argument, Cousinot inserted into the clause a detailed gloss that explained precisely how the law functioned, and, since it was written in Latin, the gloss became indistinct from the original clause, thereby blurring the lines between the two.[90]

The adoption of 'De Alode' to justify the royal succession was not a straightforward process, however. At its core, the clause supported male-preference pariage and only explicitly dealt with inherited property, not the kingdom as a whole. Montreuil approached the latter issue in *A toute la chevalerie* by equating 'Salic land' to the kingdom by simply adding the Latin words *in regno* (in the kingdom) directly into the clause.[91] Montreuil used a more accurate transcription in later treatises, adding after it a less ambiguous French gloss that explained how the law functioned in practice, but the earlier treatise remained his most widely read tract.[92] Thirty years later, Juvénal des Ursins stated outright in *Tres crestien* that 'Now the kingdom was governed by the said Salic Law, and it could be called Salic land.'[93] By the time Cousinot inserted his Latin gloss into the clause, the idea that Salic land equalled France was already firmly established in French diplomatic circles.[94] To overcome the former issue – male-preference pariage – the jurists relied on recent precedents and simple logic. Due to the widespread misinterpretation of 'De Alode' and the precedents of 1316–1328, women and their heirs were barred from the succession. This idea was further developed by jurists such as Jean de Terre Rouge and Noël de Fribois, who adopted Aristotelian logic to argue that only men have the ability to pass on the regenerative seed of kingship.[95] Primogeniture, meanwhile, was accepted on the basis that there was precedent supporting it in France dating back to 936 and that it followed natural law.[96] To undermine the concept of pariage, jurists argued for the inalienability of the realm.[97] Stated simply, if the realm could not be divided, then it must only fall to one person, who can only be the senior-most male member of the Capetian dynasty. Terre Rouge built upon this concept by arguing that it was impossible for an heir to be passed over by testament, treaty, or even personal desire because the dignity passed to him through transmission of royal authority, which was a fixed law.[98] By the end of the fifteenth century, the inalienability of the realm would sit beside the Salic Law as a fundamental law of France.[99] By interpreting 'De Alode' through this framework, the jurists argued that there could only ever be one heir to the French throne and that the English claim contravened the basic tenets of the fundamental laws of France.

All this new fundamental law needed was an auspicious origin story. From the time of Lescot, it was known that the *Pactus Legis Salicæ* owed its creation to Clovis and its final revision to Charlemagne and Louis the Pious.[100] This much was said in the prologues and epilogues of most copies of the law, and most jurists in the fifteenth century adopted it without hesitation.[101] The problem with this backstory, however, was that Clovis and Charlemagne already represented ideas in French royal mythology. Clovis was associated with the coronation ritual and Christian kingship, while Charlemagne represented the French imperial past and crusading glory.[102] Eager mythologists, therefore, looked elsewhere and settled upon the quasi-mythical Frankish king Pharamond, who was supposedly descended from the Trojans and purportedly became the first Frankish king in the fifth century. Conveniently, an eighth-century Frankish chronicle, the *Liber Historiae Francorum*, had already attributed the creation of the Salic Law to Pharamond, merging his story with that which appears in the *Pactus* prologues.[103] It was a concurrence the jurists could not ignore and they adopted this version wholesale by the late-fifteenth century.[104] By so doing, they placed Pharamond at the front of a series of historical kings upon whom a royal mythology had already been firmly developed. Pharamond's chronological placement in pre-Christian Gaul gave credit to the idea that the Salic Law was the first fundamental law of France, since it predated Christianity and placed the creation of the law concurrently with the foundation of the realm itself.[105] Only a century earlier, virtually nothing was known about this Late Antique legal code – now it was held aloft as the supreme embodiment of dynastic authority in France with a story carefully crafted to emphasize its illustrious past.

The Salic Law in France

This newly minted mythology paired with Cousinot's treatise, printed and mass-produced in the late fifteenth and early sixteenth centuries under the name *La Loy Salicque, premiere loy des françois*, spread the authority and legend of the Salic Law throughout France despite the fact that it was never formally codified.[106] The first evidence that the law had gained acceptance in the Valois court came in 1484 during the coronation procession of Charles VIII. Staged beside a re-enactment of Clovis receiving the royal anointing oil from Saint Remigius was a new dramatization showcasing Pharamond receiving the Salic Law from four councillors.[107] Although Pharamond had been recognized as a founder of the French kingdom for centuries, he was now elevated to near-equal status with Clovis, the great Christianizer of the Franks.[108] Yet the law itself remained only an idea. When Charles died without a son in 1498, the Salic Law was tested for the first time. Prior to his death, Charles acknowledged his cousin Duke Louis II of Orléans as his heir and the latter acceded to the throne as Louis XII without controversy, despite the fact that over a dozen relatives of maternal ancestry were bypassed in the process, including his own wife.[109] A second succession in 1515 of François, count of Angoulême, gave further credit to the Salic Law's validity, although only two females were debarred in this instance, the elder being the new king's spouse.[110] The Angoulême kings perpetuated the myths of the Salic Law wholesale: in three meetings of the Parlement of Paris between 1526 and 1537, François asserted the fundamentality of the Salic Law and the inalienability of the realm.[111] It came to speak for all royal lands in order to counter the

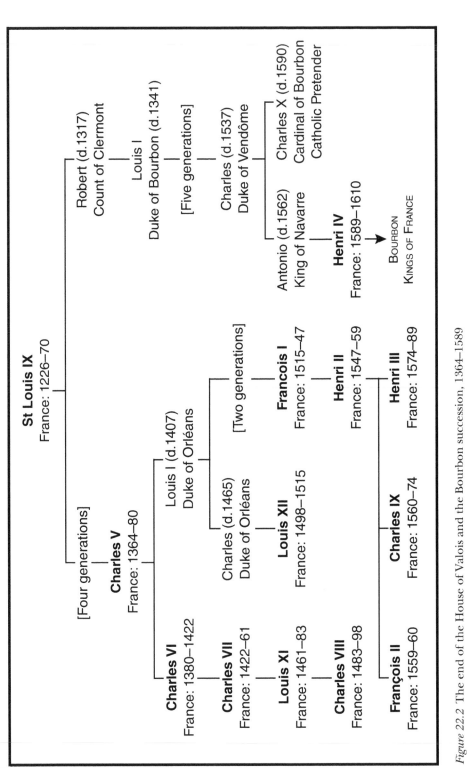

Figure 22.2 The end of the House of Valois and the Bourbon succession, 1364–1589

possibility that an heiress might alienate a portion of the realm through marriage.[112] When Holy Roman Emperor Karl V asserted his ancestral claim to the Duchy of Burgundy and County of Flanders, François countered that the Salic Law forbids the lands from inheritance via a maternal line, prompting a series of Franco–Imperial wars that dominated the mid-sixteenth century.[113] By 1584, the tenets of the law were firmly enmeshed within French political ideology, but the fluidity of the 1498 and 1515 successions left the law's limits undefined.

The inevitable crisis over the durability of the Salic Law finally came in the 1580s, when the senior-most Capetian prince after the French monarch became the Protestant warrior-king Henri of Navarre (Enrique III).[114] Henri was an extremely distant agnatic cousin of the last Angoulême king, Henri III, and no previous succession – agnatic or otherwise – had granted the throne to such distant kin. Despite fundamental laws advocating agnatic primogeniture, the inheritability of the senior male, and the indivisibility of the realm, a new question arose over whether the king had to be Catholic. Was Catholicism a fundamental requirement of kingship? Naturally, the Protestant supporters of Henri advocated the primacy of Salic Law above all other fundamental laws, and many jurists accepted the idea.[115] But others argued that Catholicism was also a fundamental law and, therefore, championed the claim of Cardinal Charles de Bourbon, Henri's uncle and the next male in the line of succession.[116] Despite his misgivings, Henri III had maintained support for Henri of Navarre as his successor, and when the former was assassinated in 1589, the Navarrese ruler ascended the French throne, the first king of the House of Bourbon.[117] To quell the ongoing resistance from those who challenged his claim, Henri publicly converted to Catholicism in 1593, in effect confirming adherence to the church as a fundamental law.[118] Others continued to resist him, culminating with his assassination in 1610, but the matter of the Bourbon succession became irrefutable under his Catholic descendants.[119] The Salic Law had triumphed and proved itself more authoritative than any other fundamental law.

It was in this political climate that Shakespeare penned his memorable monologue against the Salic Law in *Henry V*, drawing largely from Raphael Holinshed's recent history of Britain, which extolled the virtues of the English claim to France.[120] But Holinshed, drawing from arguments made by fifteenth-century English diplomats and jurists, misunderstood when and how the late medieval version of the law arose. He had inadvertently been drawn into the political rhetoric of the period and accepted their conclusions without further investigation. In fact, when *Henry V* was first performed in 1599, the Salic Law was fading in importance. It would not be called upon again for two centuries, and never truly be used to determine a royal succession. Over the course of the seventeenth and eighteenth centuries, most of the mythology behind the law was categorically debunked by humanist scholars, while the need for such legitimization had disappeared since the precedents alone justified the system.[121] It was only in 1791 that the French Revolutionary government enacted agnatic primogeniture for the first time into the legal code of France, including it as the standard mode of succession for the king.[122] But Louis XVI was beheaded in 1793, ending the brief constitutional monarchy, and his son died in prison two years later.[123] Salic Law determined that Louis' brother Louis Stanislas, rather than his daughter, gained the titular crown in 1795 as Louis XVIII, but that act was done outside French law since there no longer was a monarchy in France.[124] His status was only confirmed in 1814, when the victorious Allies restored the Bourbons to the throne.[125] His brother Charles X succeeded him, and his descendants continued to assert their right to the French throne as Legitimists until his line went extinct in 1883.[126] However, the Revolution of 1830 removed Charles from power, replacing him with the constitutional monarch Louis-Philippe, the head of the junior House of Bourbon–Orléans.[127] To justify the Orléans succession, French lawyers established the principle that the king must adhere to the tenets of constitutionalism and espouse popular nationalism, ideals Charles was unwilling to uphold.[128] Although this decision allowed for a popular monarchy built on a constitutional framework that overlooked the agnatic legacy of the recent past, the allure of Republicanism ended this experiment prematurely.[129] Louis-Philippe was forced off the throne in 1848, although his descendants continue to claim the French crown today as Orléanists, asserting their pretentions against the senior Bourbons (now the Spanish Bourbons), as well as the Bonapartists, for a title that has not existed for nearly two centuries and never entirely belonged to them.[130]

Out of France, into Europe

Outside of France, the Salic Law was given a second life. When the Peace of Utrecht in 1714 ended the War of the Spanish Succession, the grandson of Louis XIV of France was given the Spanish throne with a proviso that he would renounce the French throne for himself and his heirs and, rather contradictorily, adopt the Salic Law in order to avoid an eventual merger with the French crown.[131] In 1830, however, Fernando VII, who favoured his daughter Isabel over his brother Carlos, promulgated a pragmatic sanction that abolished the Salic Law in Spain to allow his daughter to succeed him.[132] Carlos, the dispossessed heir, refused to recognize the rights of his niece and proclaimed himself king, sparking the first of a series of Carlist Wars that punctuated Spanish politics well into the twentieth century.[133] To complicate matters further, upon the death of the last senior Bourbon in France, the Carlists also represented the senior agnates of the Capetian dynasty and claimed the French throne as the Legitimists, challenging the pretensions of the more junior Orléanists.[134] The Carlist line went extinct in 1936, but by that point the Spanish monarchy itself had been dissolved by the Second Republic.[135] The eldest son of the deposed Alfonso XIII renounced his right to the throne – although his descendants continue their French pretensions according to Salic Law – and a younger son and his descendants claimed, and eventually regained in 1975, the Spanish throne.[136]

The Spanish Bourbons also spread Salic Law into their other possessions. In 1734, Felipe V's son Carlos conquered Naples and Sicily from the Austrians and was proclaimed king of the two Sicilies.[137] Once in power, he introduced agnatic primogeniture into his new realms and it became the succession law used by the descendants of his second son and successor in southern Italy, Ferdinando I.[138] When Filippo, Carlos' brother, inherited the Duchy of Parma in 1748 from his mother, he imposed agnatic primogeniture upon his new Italian possession.[139] Thus, by the mid-eighteenth century, the royal succession in all of the Bourbon dynastic

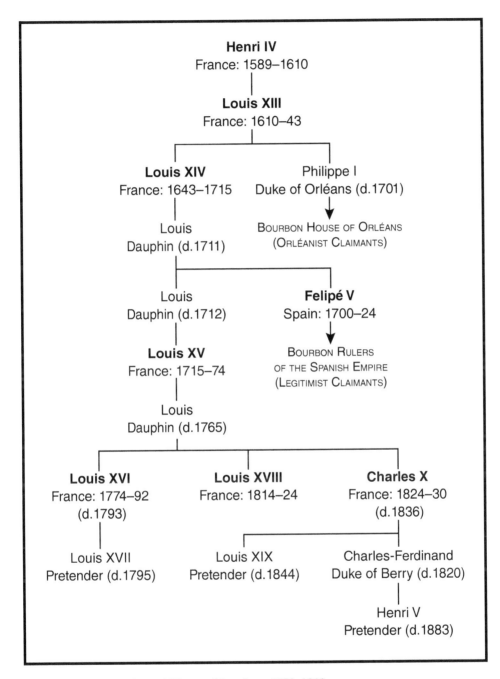

Figure 22.3 The French royal House of Bourbon, 1589–1830

possessions was regulated by agnatic primogeniture, although the term Salic Law was rarely used outside of France due to its specifically French origins.

The end of the Bourbons in France during the French Revolution, however, did not end the impact of the Salic Law on French politics. Indeed, the law owes much of its lasting legacy not to the Capetians, but to Napoléon Bonaparte. In 1804, only months after overseeing the creation of the Napoleonic Code, the emperor dictated the rules of imperial succession, adopting agnatic succession as the key tenet, with elective monarchy reserved for whether the Bonaparte line went extinct.[140] His great-nephew Napoléon III later re-enacted the same code in 1852.[141] The first Bonaparte emperor took agnatic primogeniture with him throughout Europe on his campaigns of conquest between 1796 and 1814.[142] Prior to 1650, most of Germany practised some form of agnatic pariage, a relic of the myriad legal codes promulgated by Charlemagne around 804 that all descended from the *Lex Ripuaria*, itself a scion of the *Pactus Legis Salicæ*.[143] Yet even as late as the early nineteenth century, the region was a kaleidoscope of hundreds of territories that nominally formed parts of larger duchies but in reality were entirely independent of each other.[144] Napoléon destroyed this system entirely and oversaw the reorganization of Germany, in the process encouraging or forcibly imposing the adoption of the Napoleonic Code by many of the newly formed states.[145] Other European countries such as Sweden also adopted agnatic primogeniture in imitation of France.[146] Long after Napoléon's defeat, the legacy of his Napoleonic Code survived and agnatic primogeniture became the primary royal succession law of central Europe.

More recently, the precepts of Salic Law have been viewed as increasingly counter to European ideals of gender equality and equal rights. The collapse of all dynastic monarchies in Germany and Italy after the World Wars led to the end of all royal succession laws in those regions, although pretenders continue to claim their lost thrones using them to the present.[147] Belgium was the last remaining monarchy to adhere to Salic Law, abandoning the practice in 1991.[148] Luxembourg, a former German state, was forced to abandon Salic Law when the House of Nassau went extinct in the male line in 1912, leading to the succession of two grand duchesses; Salic Law was legally abandoned there in 2010.[149] Although dozens of princes claim ancestral thrones by right of agnatic primogeniture, none currently holds a title by such right. As of 2016, nearly every monarchy remaining in Europe has adopted or promised to adopt absolute equal primogeniture, meaning that the eldest child, regardless of gender, becomes heir to the throne.[150] Liechtenstein is the only state to adhere to strict agnatic primogeniture, but its law traces its origin to other Germanic laws.[151]

Forged by the earliest Frankish kings and expanded and updated by the great Frankish emperor Charlemagne, the *Pactus Legis Salicæ* dictated and controlled the succession to the Frankish crown for nearly 400 years. But shifting perspectives and changing political situations allowed for the legal code to fall by the wayside. The Capetians embraced more pragmatic solutions to maintain the integrity of the French kingdom, adopting primogeniture and associative kingship. When a series of crises over the succession did finally occur between 1316 and 1328, the Capetian dynasty acted accordingly, protecting their interests and their dynasty's hold over the kingdom by embracing agnatic primogeniture as the law of the land. Yet rivals questioned the legality of this decision, prompting French jurists to develop complex explanations that resurrected the *Pactus* and put it to new use. The result was the Salic Law, a legal code based entirely on precedent and convenience. From 1498 until 1830, it decided all dynastic successions in France and quickly expanded into

Spain, Italy, Germany, and elsewhere, due to dynastic inheritances and Napoleonic might. Throughout the nineteenth century, most European nations were governed by variants of this law, but eventually it was eclipsed by modernity. In an age where democracy and gender equality is of paramount importance to Europeans, the Salic Law has no place.

Notes

1 Portions of this research were presented at the 11th Biennial Conference of the Australian & New Zealand Association for Medieval and Early Modern Studies (7–10 February 2017). Special thanks to Elisabeth Rolston, Matt Firth, George & Carol Blessing, and Anna Thomas for examining different potential angles to approach the Latin quotations. Thanks also to fellow ANZAMEMS panellists Jessica Hudepohl and Martin Laidlaw for moral and academic support, and Daniel Anderson and Tyler Farrington for providing outside opinions on the topic. Additional thanks to my doctoral supervisor, Dr. Chris Jones, who first advocated my research into Salic Law. And finally, endless love to my partner Kara, who continues to support my research despite my onerous ramblings.
2 William Shakespeare, *Henry V*, ed. Gary Taylor (Oxford: University Press, 1982), I.i.33–42.
3 Edward James, *The Franks* (Oxford: Basil Blackwell, 1988), 51, 57–58. See also J.B. Bury, *The Invasion of Europe by the Barbarians*, new edition (New York: W.W. Norton, 2000).
4 James, *Franks*, 78–108.
5 Colette Beaune, *The Birth of an Ideology: Myths and Symbols of Nation in Late-Medieval France*, trans. Susan Ross Huston and ed. Frederic L. Cheyette (Berkeley: University of California Press, 1991), 245; Craig Taylor, introduction to *Debating the Hundred Years War: Pour ce que plusieurs (La Loy Salique) and A declaration of the trew and dewe title of Henrie VIII*, Camden Fifth Series 29 (Cambridge: University Press, 2006), 18.
6 Katherine Fischer Drew, "Introduction," in *The Laws of the Salian Franks* (Philadelphia: University of Pennsylvania Press, 1991), 30; Patrick J. Geary, *Before France and Germany: The Creation and Transformation of the Merovingian World* (Oxford: University Press, 1988), 90–92.
7 Geneviève Bührer-Thierry and Charles Mériaux, *La France avant la France, 481–888* (Paris: Belin, 2010), 575–576; Ian Wood, *The Merovingian Kingdoms, 450–751* (London: Longman, 1994), 109.
8 Theodore John Rivers, "Introduction," in *Laws of the Salian and Ripuarian Franks* (New York: Ams Press, 1986), 2–3.
9 Drew, "Introduction," 52.
10 James, *Franks*, 88–89.
11 James, *Franks*, 233.
12 Rivers, "Introduction," 8.
13 Edward James, *The Origins of France: From Clovis to the Capetians, 500–1000* (Houndmills: Macmillan Education, 1987), 31.
14 Drew, "Introduction," 53.
15 Karl August Eckhardt, ed., *Pactus Legis Salicæ*, MGH LL nat. Germ. 4:1 (Hanover: Library of Hanover, 1962), 223. Translation mine.
16 Alexander C. Murray, *Germanic Kinship Structure: Studies in Law and Society in Antiquity and the Early Middle Ages*, Studies and Texts 65 (Toronto: Pontifical Institute of Medieval Studies, 1983), 212.
17 Murray, *Germanic*, 202; Susan Reynolds, *Fiefs and Vassals: The Medieval Evidence Reinterpreted*, second edition (Oxford: University Press, 1994), 75.
18 James, *Origins*, 85–86.
19 *Pactus Legis Salicæ*, 222. Translation mine.
20 James, *Origins*, 39; Rivers, *Laws*, 182, 192.
21 Beaune, *Birth*, 259–260.
22 Murray, *Germanic*, 208.

23 Murray, *Germanic*, 210.
24 The *Lex Ripuaria* reads:

> | | |
> |---|---|
> | *De terra uero Salica nulla portio hereditatis mulieri ueniat sed ad uirilem sexum tota terræ hereditas perueniat.* | Regarding Salic land, no portion of the inheritance in fact comes to the female, but all of the inheritance passes to the masculine (*virile*) sex. |

Karl August Eckhardt, ed., *Lex Ribuaria*, MGH LL nat. Germ. 3:2 (Hanover: Library of Hanover, 1954), 105, chapter 57, clause 4. Meanwhile, Chilperic's Capitulary IV reads:

> | | |
> |---|---|
> | *Et si subito filii defuncti fuerint, filia simili modo accipiat terras ipsas, sicut et filii, si uiui fuissent, habuissent.* | And if the sons are suddenly dead, a daughter in a similar way may receive those lands just as the sons, if they were alive, would have held them. |

Pactus Legis Salicæ, 262, chapter 108, clause 2. Translations mine. Katherine Fischer Drew, *The Laws of the Salian Franks* (Philadelphia: University of Pennsylvania Press, 2012), 45, 149; James, *Origins*, 86.
25 François Hotman, *Francogallia*, eds. Ralph E. Giesey and J.H.M. Salmon (Cambridge: University Press, 1972), 272; Herbert H. Rowen, *The King's State: Proprietary Dynasticism in Early Modern France* (New Brunswick: Rutgers University Press, 1980), 38–39, 65.
26 Rowen, *King's State*, 7; Edouard Perroy, *The Hundred Years War*, trans. W.B. Wells (London: Eyre & Spottiswoode, 1951), 71.
27 François Olivier-Martin, *Histoire du Droit Français des origines à la Révolution* (Paris: Domat Montchrestien, 1948), 39.
28 Theodore Evergates, "Pariage," in *Medieval France: An Encyclopedia* (New York: Garland Publishing, 1995), 697–698; James, *Franks*, 169–182.
29 Wood, *Merovingian*, 60.
30 Wood, *Merovingian*, 56, 57.
31 Wood, *Merovingian*, 255ff.
32 Rosamond McKitterick, *Charlemagne: The Formation of a European Identity* (Cambridge: University Press, 2008), 71, 77, 98.
33 Timothy Reuter, *Germany in the Early Middle Ages, 800–1056* (London: Longman, 1991), 23; Pierre Riché, *The Carolingians: A Family Who Forged Europe*, trans. Michael Idomir Allen (Philadelphia: University of Pennsylvania Press, 1993), 99, 132.
34 Riché, *Carolingians*, 160–169.
35 Riché, *Carolingians*, 197–199.
36 Bührer-Thierry and Mériaux, *La France*, 413.
37 Bührer-Thierry and Mériaux, *La France*, 414, 416.
38 Riché, *Carolingians*, 216–219.
39 Reuter, *Germany*, 135; Riché, *Carolingians*, 231.
40 Reuter, *Germany*, 183–191.
41 Florian Mazel, *Féodalités, 888–1180* (Paris: Belin, 2014), 21.
42 Mazel, *Féodalités*, 22.
43 Mazel, *Féodalités*, 22.
44 James, *Origins*, 184.
45 James, *Origins*, 185.
46 James, *Origins*, 185.
47 James, *Origins*, 185.
48 Rowen, *King's State*, 15.
49 Elizabeth M. Hallam and Judith Everard, *Capetian France, 987–1328*, second edition (Harlow: Longman, 2001), 83, 90.
50 James, *Origins*, 186.

51 Andrew W. Lewis, *Royal Succession in Capetian France: Studies on Familial Order and the State* (Cambridge, MA: Harvard University Press, 1981), 24, 44, 56.
52 Lewis, *Royal Succession*, 37.
53 Ralph E. Giesey, *Le rôle méconnu de la Loi Salique: La succession royale, XIVe–XVIe siècles* (Paris: Les Belles Lettres, 2007), 27, 35.
54 See Figure 22.1.
55 Giesey, *Le role méconnu*, 27.
56 Maurielle Gaude-Ferragu, *Queenship in Medieval France, 1300–1500*, trans. Angela Krieger (London: Palgrave Macmillan, 2016), 82.
57 Giesey, *Le role méconnu*, 35.
58 Giesey, *Le role méconnu*, 36.
59 Gaude–Ferragu, *Queenship*, 82; Giesey, *Le role méconnu*, 40.
60 Giesey, *Le role méconnu*, 43–47.
61 Gaude–Ferragu, *Queenship*, 82.
62 Giesey, *Le role méconnu*, 60–68. Parisian customs supported Edward's right to the throne, see Olivier Martin, *Histoire de la coutume de la prévôté et vicomté de Paris*, vol. 1 (Paris: Ernest Leroux, 1922), 305–306. For contemporary depictions of this discussion, see Jules Viard, ed., *Les Grandes Chroniques de France*, vol. 9 (Paris: Librairie Ancienne Honoré Champion, 1937), 72 n2, 73, 330.
63 Rowen, *King's State*, 20.
64 Perroy, *Hundred Years War*, 71.
65 Éliane Viennot, *La France, les femmes et le pouvoir: L'invention de la loi salique (Ve–XVIe siècle)* (Paris: Perrin, 2006), 316.
66 For a full discussion on the legal aspects of this topic, see Craig Taylor, "Edward III and the Plantagenet Claim to the French Throne," in *The Age of Edward III*, ed. James Bothwell (Woodbridge, UK: Boydell & Brewer, 2001): 155–169.
67 Perroy, *Hundred Years War*, 75; Paul Viollet, "Comment les femmes ont été exclues en France de la succession à la couronne," *Mémoires de l'Académie des inscriptions et belles-lettres* 34, no. 2 (1893): 48.
68 Françoise Autrand, *Charles V: Le sage* (Paris: Fayard, 1994), 279–284.
69 Autrand, *Charles V*, 207, 270.
70 See Autrand, *Charles V*, 221–390.
71 Bührer-Thierry and Mériaux, *La France*, 575.
72 Richard Lescot, "Genealogia aliquorum regum Francie," in *Chronique de Richard Lescot, religieux de Saint-Denis (1328–1344) suivie de la continuation de cette chronique (1344–1364)*, ed. Jean Lemoine (Paris: Librairie Renouard, 1896), 173–178.
73 Beaune, *Birth*, 251.
74 Lescot, "Genealogia," 178.
75 Gaude-Ferragu, *Queenship*, 84.
76 Beaune, *Birth*, 251.
77 See Giesey, *Le rôle méconnu*.
78 Viennot, *La France*.
79 See, among other works, Tracy Adams, *Christine de Pizan and the Fight for France* (University Park, PA: Pennsylvania State University Press, 2014); Daisy Delogu, *Allegorical Bodies: Power and Gender in Late Medieval France* (Toronto: University Press, 2015); Sarah Hanley, "Identity Politics and Rulership in France: Female Political Place and the Fraudulent Salic Law in Christine de Pizan and Jean de Montreuil," in *Changing Identities in Early Modern France*, ed. Michael Wolfe (Durham, NC: Duke University Press, 1997): 78–94; and Craig Taylor, "The Salic Law, French Queenship and the Defence of Women in the Late Middle Ages," *French Historical Studies* 29, no. 4 (2006): 187–207.
80 Viennot, *La France*, 347–348.
81 See Jonathan Sumption, *The Hundred Years War*, vol. IV: Cursed Kings (Philadelphia: University of Pennsylvania Press, 2015), and Françoise Autrand, *Charles VI: Le folie du roi* (Paris: Fayard, 1986).
82 See Juliet Barker, *Conquest: The English Kingdom of France 1417–1450* (London: Little, Brown, 2009).

83 Barker, *Conquest*, 28–29, 61.

84 Delogu, *Allegorical Bodies*, 134.

85 The Latin and French versions of this treatise are included in Jean de Montreuil, *Opera*, vol. 2: L'œuvre historique et polémique, eds. Nichole Grévy-Pons, Ezio Ornato, and Gilbert Ouy (Turin: G. Giappichelli, 1975), 91–149.

86 This treatise is available in Jean Juvénal des Ursins, "Tres crestien, tres hault, tres puissant roy," in *Écrits politiques de Jean Juvénal des Ursins*, ed. Peter S. Lewis, vol. II, 1–178 (Paris: Librairie C. Klincksieck, 1985).

87 Juvénal des Ursins, "Tres crestien," 21–22.

88 Juvénal des Ursins, "Tres crestien," 159–160; Taylor, "Introduction," 3.

89 Taylor, "Introduction," 5. This treatise is available in Craig Taylor, ed., "Pour ce que plusieurs," in *Debating the Hundred Years War. . .*, Camden Fifth Series 29 (Cambridge: University Press, 2006), 53–134.

90 Taylor, "Pour ce que plusieurs," 59. The glossed edition reads:

Nulla portio hereditatis de terra salicqua *qui est interpretandum de regali dominio quod a nullo deppendet nec alicui subicitur, ad differenciam aliarum terrarum que in alodio conceduntur* mulieri veniat, sed ad virilem sexum tota hereditas perveniat. [Gloss in *Italics.*]	No portion of the inheritance of the Salic land, *which is interpreted as the royal demesne, which is neither dependent nor subject to anybody, differentiating it from other lands that as alodes submit,* goes to the woman; but to the virile sex all the inheritance belongs.

91 Taylor, "Introduction," 18.

92 Taylor, "Introduction," 18–19.

93 Juvénal des Ursins, "Tres crestien," 22.

94 Beaune, *Birth*, 255.

95 Sarah Hanley, "The Salic Law," in *Political and Historical Encyclopedia of Women*, ed. Christine Fauré (New York: Routledge, 2003), 9, 11.

96 Delogu, *Allegorical Bodies*, 148; Lewis, *Royal Succession*, 51–52, 60, 155–156.

97 Jacques Krynen, *Idéal du prince et pouvoir royal en France a la fin du moyen age (1380–1440): Étude de la littérature politiques du temps* (Paris: Éditions A. et J. Picard, 1981), 304, 306.

98 Giesey, *Le rôle méconnu*, 130–132.

99 Krynen, *Idéal du prince*, 305.

100 Lescot, "Genealogia," 178.

101 Beaune, *Birth*, 254.

102 See Beaune, *Birth*, 70–89, and Chris Jones, *Eclipse of Empire? Perceptions of the Western Empire and its Rulers in Late-Medieval France*, Cursor Mundi 1 (Turnhout: Brepols, 2007), 145–182, 340–352.

103 Bruno Krusch, ed., *Liber Historiae Francorum*, MGH SS rer. Merov. II (Hanover: Library of Hanover, 1888), 244.

104 Beaune, *Birth*, 254.

105 Beaune, *Birth*, 246–247.

106 Taylor, "Introduction," 1, 29, 31.

107 Giesey, *Le rôle méconnu* 125.

108 Jules Viard, ed., *Les grandes chroniques*, vol. 1 (Paris: Société de l'histoire de France, 1920), 19–20.

109 Frederic J. Baumgartner, *France in the Sixteenth Century* (Basingstoke: Macmillan Press, 1995), 21. See Figure 22.2.

110 Baumgartner, *France*, 27.

111 Hanley, "Salic Law," 13.

112 Delogu, *Allegorical Bodies*, 138.

113 Beaune, *Birth*, 263; Baumgartner, *France*, 24, 30–32.

114 Baumgartner, *France*, 222.

115 Baumgartner, *France*, 288.

116 Robert J. Knecht, *The French Wars of Religion, 1559–1598* (New York: Longman Publishing, 1996), 66, 72–73. See also Frederic J. Baumgartner, "The Case for Charles X," *The Sixteenth Century Journal* 4, no. 2 (1973): 87–98.

117 Knecht, *French Wars*, 71–72.

118 Knecht, *French Wars*, 75, 78.

119 Knecht, *French Wars*, 96; Baumgartner, *France*, 235.

120 Raphael Holinshed, *The Third Volume of Chronicles. . .* (London: Signe of the Starre, 1587), 545.

121 Hotman, *Francogallia*, 272, 274; Rowen, *King's State*, 26; Viennot, *La France*, 584.

122 "Constitution de 1791," Conseil Constitutionnel, www.conseil-constitutionnel.fr/conseil-constitutionnel/francais/la-constitution/les-constitutions-de-la-france/constitution-de-1791.5082.html (accessed 9 January 2017), chapter 2, section 2, article 1.

123 Munro Price, *The Fall of the French Monarchy: Louis XVI, Marie Antoinette and the baron de Breteuil* (London: Macmillan, 2002), 343, 344.

124 Price, *Fall*, 344. See Figure 22.3.

125 Price, *Fall*, 344.

126 Price, *Fall*, 344; H.A.C. Collingham, *The July Monarchy: A Political History of France 1830–1848* (London: Longman, 1988), 55; Jean Barbey, Frédéric Bluche and Stéphane Rials, *Lois fondamentales et succession de France*, second edition (Paris: Diffusion–Université–Culture, 1984), 31.

127 Collingham, *July Monarchy*, 29.

128 "Charte constitutionnelle du 14 août 1830," Conseil Constitutionnel, www.conseil-constitutionnel.fr/conseil-constitutionnel/francais/la-constitution/les-constitutions-de-la-france/charte-constitutionnelle-du-14-aout-1830.5104.html (accessed 13 January 2017), article 65; Collingham, *July Monarchy*, 26, 34.

129 Collingham, *July Monarchy*, 412.

130 Barbey, Bluche and Rials, *Lois fondamentales*, 25–26, 31.

131 Gerald Brenan, *The Spanish Labyrinth: An Account of the Social and Political Background of the Civil War* (Cambridge: Cambridge University Press, 1960), 204; Giesey, *Le role méconnu*, 266; *Novísima Recopilacion de las Leyes de España* (Madrid: NP, 1805), Tomo II, Libro III, Tituolo I, Ley V (4–6).

132 Brenan, *Spanish Labyrinth*, 203–204.

133 See Mark Lawrence, *Spain's First Carlist War, 1833–40* (Basingstoke: Palgrave Macmillan, 2014).

134 Rowen, *King's State*, 167.

135 Barbey, Bluche and Rials, *Lois fondamentales*, 42; John Van der Kiste, *A Divided Kingdom: The Spanish Monarchy from Isabel to Juan Carlos* (Stroud: Sutton Publishing, 2007), 168.

136 Van der Kiste, *Divided Kingdom*, 182, 187, 225.

137 Richard Herr, "Flow and Ebb 1700–1833," in *Spain: A History*, ed. Raymond Carr (Oxford: University Press, 2000), 174.

138 "Costitutione di Sicilia (1812)," in *Le Costituzioni Italiane*, eds. Alberto Aquarone, Mario D'Addio and Guglielmo Negri (Milan: Edizioni di Comunità, 1958), §3 (421); "Costituzione del Regno di Napoli del 1815," in ibid., Titolo III, Articolo 32 (384).

139 Herr, "Flow and Ebb," 174; "The treaty of Aix-la-Chapelle, 1748," in *A Collection of Treaties between Great Britain and Other Powers*, vol. 1, ed. George Chalmers (London: John Stockdale, 1790), 431.

140 "Constitution de l'An XII – Empire – 28 floréal An XII," Conseil Constitutionnel, www.conseil-constitutionnel.fr/conseil-constitutionnel/francais/la-constitution/les-constitutions-de-la-france/constitution-de-l-an-xii-empire-28-floreal-an-xii.5090.html (accessed 23 January 2017), 18 May 1804, titre ii, article 3.

141 "Constitution de 1852, Second Empire," Conseil Constitutionnel, www.conseil-constitutionnel.fr/conseil-constitutionnel/francais/la-constitution/les-constitutions-de-la-france/constitution-de-1852-second-empire.5107.html (accessed 23 January 2017), Sénatus-consulte du 7 novembre 1852, article 2. See also ibid., Sénatus-consulte du 21 mai 1870, titre ii, article 2.

142 Michael Broers, *Europe Under Napoleon 1799–1815* (London: Arnold, 1996), 62–63.

143 See Judith J. Hurwich, "Inheritance Practices in Early Modern Germany," *The Journal of Interdisciplinary History* 23, no. 4 (1993): 699–718.

144 Broers, *Europe*, 87–93.

145 Heinrich August Winkler, *Germany: The Long Road West – Vol. I: 1789–1933*, trans. Alexander J. Sager (Oxford: University Press, 2006), 46.

146 Christine Alice Corcos, "From Agnatic Succession to Absolute Primogeniture: The Shift to Equal Rights of Succession to Thrones and Titles in the Modern European Constitutional Monarchy," *Michigan State Law Review* 5 (2012), 1591–1592.

147 Winkler, *Germany*, 330, 340.

148 Corcos, "From Agnatic Succession," 1628.

149 Corcos, "From Agnatic Succession," 1630–1631.

150 Corcos, "From Agnatic Succession," 1591–1593.

151 "Hausgesetsz des Fürstlichen Hauses Lichtenstein vom 26. Oktober 1993," *Liechtensteinisches Landesgesetzblatt* 100 (1993): Artikel 12, www.gesetze.li/konso/pdf/1993100000 (accessed 23 January 2017).

Key works

Corcos, Christine Alice, "From Agnatic Succession to Absolute Primogeniture: The Shift to Equal Rights of Succession to Thrones and Titles in the Modern European Constitutional Monarchy," *Michigan State Law Review* 5 (2012): 1587–1670.

Giesey, Ralph E., *Le rôle méconnu de la Loi Salique: La succession royale, XIVe–XVIe siècles* (Paris: Les Belles Lettres, 2007).

James, Edward, *The Origins of France: From Clovis to the Capetians, 500–1000* (Houndmills: Macmillan Education, 1987).

Lewis, Andrew W., *Royal Succession in Capetian France: Studies on Familial Order and the State* (Cambridge, MA: Harvard University Press, 1981).

Rowen, Herbert H., *The King's State: Proprietary Dynasticism in Early Modern France* (New Brunswick: Rutgers University Press, 1980).

Taylor, Craig, ed., "Pour ce que plusieurs (La Loy Salique)," in *Debating the Hundred Years War: Pour ce que plusieurs (La Loy Salique) and A declaration of the trew and dewe title of Henrie VIII.* Camden Fifth Series, vol. 29. (Cambridge: University Press, 2006), 53–134.

23

A FAMILY AFFAIR

Cultural anxiety, political debate and the nature of monarchy in seventeenth-century France and Britain

Jonathan Spangler

In February 1613, as part of the extravagant celebrations held in London to celebrate the wedding of Princess Elizabeth and the Elector Palatine, a recent play by Shakespeare was staged: *The Tempest.* In the play, we learn of the history of Prospero, duke of Milan, who had been overthrown by his brother Antonio, with the help of the king of Naples, Alonso, who himself is nearly betrayed by his younger brother Sebastian (plotting with Antonio). Sebastian remarks: 'I remember / You did supplant your brother Prospero.' Antonio responds: 'True. / And look how well my garments sit upon me, / Much feater than before. My brother's servants / Were then my fellows, now they are my men.'[1] In a sense, the play's title reflected some of the feeling of unrest of the time, a tempest of passions, not just in England, but across Europe. Russia was deep in the midst of its 'Time of Troubles' after the disappearance of its ruling house in 1598; Habsburg rule in Portugal continued to be contested by pretenders; King Henry IV of France was assassinated by a fanatical Jesuit in 1610 and his widow's rule was challenged by senior males from the late king's family; and, in a scenario most reminiscent of Shakespeare, Emperor Rudolf II had been deposed by his own brothers in 1611. It has been suggested that *The Tempest* was mounted in 1613 in conjunction with the Stuart-Palatine wedding as a means of contrasting the situation of chaos in Europe with the dynastic calm of Stuart England, having peacefully transitioned from the reign of the childless Elizabeth I to that of the family man, James I.[2] To underline this point, in the play's conclusion, harmony and 'legitimate' dynastic rule are re-established in both Milan and Naples through a wedding, that of Alonso's faithful son Ferdinand and Prospero's daughter, Miranda.

While in late sixteenth-century England, the issue had been a fear of not enough heirs, in France the opposite was true, and younger members of the ruling family were straining against new centralization policies of the French monarchy. Their frustrations can be read in the declarations or manifestos published and circulated among the entire political community. The younger brother of King Henry III, the duke of Alençon, for example, issued a public declaration in September 1575 that proclaimed his right, in fact his duty as a prince of the blood, to defend the ancient laws of the kingdom in demanding the expulsion of foreigners from the king's council, and calling for toleration while a national settlement was reached on the question of religion. He claimed he had a mandate for his rebellion in answering an appeal from many 'nobles, clergy, citizens and bourgeois' of the kingdom, and proclaimed for himself the title of 'King's Governor-General and Protector of Liberty and the Public Good of France'.[3] A generation later, Henri de Bourbon, prince of Condé, issued a manifesto protesting his treatment by King Henry IV (whose heir he had been until the birth of a dauphin). He too proclaimed that it was his 'devoir de révolte' as a prince of the blood, against the tyranny of a first minister, as his way of serving the state which he perceived to be in disorder ('I should, as a scion of my house, and as each regarding his own affairs should do, take my part in the care for and discovery of the causes of these disorders').[4] Similar language was used by Gaston, duke of Orléans, the younger brother of Louis XIII, who justified his own rebellion in May 1631, by warning his brother against the ambitions of his first minister, Cardinal Richelieu, and justifying his actions after witnessing the poverty of the ordinary people of France with his own eyes. As before, he felt he was obliged to act in this manner because of the condition of his birth.[5] But it must not be overlooked that Gaston had his own interests as well – he was still the heir to the throne after more than fifteen years of his brother's sterile marriage.

Historians have long recognized that the last decades of the sixteenth century and the first years of the seventeenth were particularly anxious times, especially in terms of dynastic politics.[6] We can see this reflected in the themes of popular drama in both England and France. Shakespeare's plays are full of fratricidal strife, from plays describing fairly recent history, such as *Richard III* – in which the duke of Gloucester murders his older brother, Clarence, and then his nephews in order to become king – to more distant histories, such as *Hamlet, Macbeth* or *King Lear*. Across the Channel, the titles of popular French plays also reveal the anxieties of the theatre-going public: *L'Escossoise, ou le Desastre* (1601), by Antoine de Montchrestien, about Mary, Queen of Scots; and the plays by Pierre Matthieu, whose works can be seen as criticisms of the monarchy veiled in Classical allegory: *Clytemnestre* and *Esther* (both 1589) – the subtitle of the latter is particularly indicative: *Histoire tragique en laquelle est représentée la condition des Rois et Princes sur le theatre de fortune.*[7] People in the early seventeenth century became obsessed with order, as seen in carefully choreographed court masques and public festivals. They sought an end to the chaos of the previous religiously and politically charged century. In Protestant states in particular, the role of the sovereign was now fused with religion, so there needed to be one head, not multiple, following the biblical model of the head of the body politic. Across Europe there was an increased desire to put all power into one set of hands. But historians such as Nicholas Henshall caution us from going too far in applying labels such as 'absolutism', as consultative bodies continued to exist all over the continent, even in Louis XIV's France.[8] The theorist Jean Bodin himself argued that an ideal monarch should both monopolize sovereignty *and* share it with a representative body.[9] I will argue here that there was also a strong sentiment that monarchs needed to share power with the other members of their family.

At the heart of this early modern anxiety, as expressed through politics and drama alike, are two intertwined issues: the succession of dynasties, one to the next, which is often accompanied by turmoil; and the division of power within dynasties, as brothers (and sometimes mothers and sisters) struggle to stay relevant in the changing power structures of an ever-centralizing monarchical system. Across the sixteenth century, monarchies all over Europe were adopting new structures and regulations that increasingly centralized power into the hands of one ruler, thus excluding others of his (or her) extended kin group. In the past, this latter group had derived much of this power due to their consanguinity – they shared blood with the monarch – and this was now being threatened. This change had been a long time coming, however, as monarchical practices in Europe had developed and changed over several centuries.[10] But there were many myths circulating about how kings were selected and how much power junior members of dynasties had enjoyed in previous centuries. François Hotman's *Francogallia* (1573), for example, stressed the ancient manner of choosing French kings, whereby the nobility selected candidate from amongst the royal lineage, and placed the crown upon the chosen man's head.[11] This chapter will look back at some of the ancient traditions being drawn upon (real or imagined) at the turn of the seventeenth century, notably the development from elective, clan-based monarchy to primogeniture, and the development of the apanage system to recompense the loss of power to cadet members of the dynasty. It will then look at how this system foundered in the early seventeenth century, with the increasing tightening of French 'absolutism', and how subsequent younger siblings in France modified their behaviour to resituate themselves into a new form of centralized 'modern' monarchy.

Anxieties reflected in the arts

Before turning to the deep roots of European monarchy, it is pertinent to examine closely a few more examples of contemporary political anxieties reflected in the arts, to reveal that not everything was as rosy as the official line wished to portray. In England, the transition from Tudor to Stuart in 1603 was not without its fears. Even before her death, Elizabeth I's courtiers displayed a strong desire to see her reign forever. This was not mere sycophancy, but revealed a real fear of the unknown. It has been pointed out by musicologists that the extravagant set of twenty-five madrigals published to coincide with Elizabeth's 68th birthday by Thomas Morley, Gentleman of the Chapel Royal, demonstrated a clear desire for Elizabeth's reign to never end: each and every one of the madrigals ends with the chorus, 'Long live fair Oriana'.[12] And this nostalgia for Elizabeth and her supposed 'Golden Age' only grew as the reign of James turned out to be less stable than expected.[13] As pointed out recently by James Shapiro, Shakespeare's *Macbeth* appeared at the same time as the trials following the Gunpowder Plot of 1605.[14] King James retaliated with a staging of the extravagant masque *Hymenaei* by Ben Jonson at the Banqueting House, in January 1606, to show that even after the plot, the monarchy was strong. The theme, as with *The Tempest*, was that harmony is achieved by bringing dynastic disputes to an end through marriage (in this case, two rival court factions Howard and Devereux). It also attempted to lay the ghost of Elizabeth to rest by celebrating marriage: the monarch is now married, with children. The Stuarts have a future, while the childless Elizabeth does not.[15] James emphasized this further by arranging the reburial in Westminster Abbey of queens Elizabeth and Mary together, as reconciled sisters, but unproductive, with no heirs. In obvious contrast, he also reburied his mother Mary (whom he hardly knew, and whose policies he certainly would have scorned) in a tomb that is much bigger and more resplendent than her Tudor cousins. Furthermore, he placed her not off to one side, like Elizabeth and Mary, but centrally, right next to Henry VII's mother, Margaret Beaufort, the mother of a dynasty.[16] The message is clear and is reiterated with the Palatine Wedding of 1613: the Stuarts are a united family ready to rule a united Britain.

But James I did not have the problem of a younger brother to contend with. There were no other royal Stuarts. In France, where Bourbon princes were more numerous and where censorship was much stronger, we do not see the equivalent offerings of plays or music that reflect the very real strife between Louis XIII and his younger brother, Gaston, duke of Orléans. Excluded from power at every turn, Gaston spent much of the 1620s and 1630s involved in conspiracies and outright rebellions against his brother. Like his princely forebears, Gaston felt it was his right as a member of the royal blood-line to share in some form the power of the crown, an idea heightened even further by recent writings on the mystical divinity of royal blood, not merely the office of king.[17] He was raised to think so by his father, who believed all his children were equal, and particularly by his mother, Marie de Medici, who favoured him over his older brother and encouraged his independence, and he made sure he was portrayed as such, on horse-back, in regal style. So did his powerful cousin, Henri de Bourbon, prince of Condé, who also spent much of the period in rebellion against the crown, notably during the civil war known as the second Fronde in the 1650s. By the end of that decade, both Gaston and Condé were reconciled with the crown, and from this point on presented a unified front, agreeing to play their part in the construction of the image of the most typically 'absolutist' king, Louis XIV.[18] The next generation is represented as blissfully unified in an allegorical representation of the Bourbon dynasty as Olympian gods, by Jean Nocret. It was commissioned not for the palace of the king, but for that of his younger brother, Philippe, duke of Orléans. The ballets of the 'roi soleil' were purpose-fully choreographed to demonstrate total fidelity of every subject, including members of the royal family, who danced as satellites submitting to the pull of the sun.[19]

Yet even amid this domestic bliss of the 1660s, we can take note of a play by Jean Racine, *La Thébaïde* (1664), performed only three years after the death of the king's uncle, Gaston d'Orléans. The play is subtitled 'Les frères ennemis', and the main theme of the play is about how royal power should not be divided. Eric Heinze has recently analysed this play in the light of the political situation in seventeenth-century France, but curiously draws no parallels with contemporary events in French history (Gaston is never mentioned), but instead relies on more familiar (to Anglophone readers) English history and the writings of Shakespeare.[20] In this play, twin brothers Eteocles and Polynices struggle over their father's throne in Thebes. At his death, King Oedipus had decreed they would share the throne, ruling in turn, one year each. Eteocles takes power first and insists on absolute rule, rejecting any regime of divided or alternating sovereignty. As pointed out by Heinze, playwrights like Shakespeare or Racine did not espouse any particular political stance, but explored options, discourses relevant to their times. Here it is the discourse about absolutism, and it is, fittingly, given the context of the 1660s in France, the voice of the twins' uncle, Creon, who declaims most strongly the desire for absolutism and undivided rule: 'The State's best served when just one king's in charge, / Who will apply the laws consistently / To commoners and to nobility.'[21] Is this the voice of young Louis XIV's own uncle, Gaston, having learned from past transgressions?

There are two different means of validating monarchical rule at play in the *Thébaïde* and in contemporary thought: Polynices claims the throne by lineal descent. Eteocles claims it by the will of the people who appreciate his merit, his fitness to rule. Polynices lost this popular support by allying with the enemy of Thebes (Argos) and even using their troops to invade his own country, stoking fears that he might rule merely as the puppet of his allies – he even married the enemy's daughter to gain support for his claims.[22] The parallels with Gaston d'Orléans are striking: not only had he rebelled with support of France's enemy, Spain, he had married the sister of one of the chief allied princes in Spanish service, Duke Charles IV of Lorraine, an avowed personal enemy of Gaston's brother, Louis XIII. To audiences viewing Racine's play in 1664, it is inconceivable that the similarity would go unnoticed. The court of Louis XIV from the outside may have looked happy and unified, but the almost continual domestic squabbles and sexual scandals involving the king, his brother, Philippe, and his sister-in-law (Philippe's wife), Henriette-Anne, reveal far more cracks in the façade and a continued need to address the issue of how to deal with younger members of any royal house. How had previous monarchical traditions dealt with this issue?

A history of royal successions

The relationship between a sovereign and his or her dynasty fluctuated across time and varied from place to place. In general, however, most European monarchical systems shifted from a form of 'corporate monarchy', in which power was shared by members of a ruling clan, to a more unitary system, whereby authority was consolidated within a single person or lineage, to the exclusion of the wider kin group. The former system is known to historians of the later Classical era and early Middle Ages as prevalent among the Germanic and Celtic tribes of northern and western Europe, while the latter system was developed by the Mediterranean societies and gradually diffused northwards through the efforts of Christian missionaries. The Germans and the Celts supposedly chose their rulers as the strongest among a kin group through election, while the Romans and Christians limited this choice to the son of a king, born in legitimate marriage. A short survey of some of the vast literature on this topic helps us to see that this issue is in fact more complex.

As far back as 1941, Philip Grierson warned against accepting the prevailing Romantic-Nationalistic viewpoint that the early Germanic 'folk' elected their kings from among a royal kin group, as a sign of their noble virtue and commitment to democratic and egalitarian values (popular, if contradictory, ideas in the late nineteenth century).[23] In his survey of three groups (Ostrogoths, Visigoths, Lombards) he found instead that strong kings were able to create hereditary dynasties, and weak kings were replaced by election as needed. And when the newer system (monogamy and distaste for illegitimacy brought in by Christianity) was introduced to one of these groups (the Lombards), the result was a weakening of the pool of leadership and the collapse of the monarchy. This idea is supported by more recent scholarship on other similar groups, for example the medieval Norwegian monarchy, or the kingdom of the DálRiata in what is now southwest Scotland. In both cases, the system of selection from among a wider kin group was preferable in societies that were thinly spread across a large geographical region and relied on strength and experience to defend the community against persistent enemy attack. In the Norwegian case, even after the introduction of Christianity in the mid-twelfth century, the older tradition persisted. As Jenny Jochens points out, from the ninth to the thirteenth century all kings were adulterous, and almost all contenders for the throne (of which there were no fewer than forty-six between 1130 and 1240) were illegitimate.[24] In the case of the DálRiata, Ian Whitaker argues that the Irish system of tanistry, that is, the operation of a circulating succession whereby kingship passes back and forth between lineages descended from a common ancestor, served both to keep the segments of a lineage apart and also to maintain the solidarity of the dynasty within a dispersed group.[25] This system can also be found in a much later society, that of the Ottomans in early modern Europe, or even in some modern Arab monarchies today (such as Saudi Arabia), where succession is governed by seniority, the eldest male, and not father to son.

But we must not assume that this was naturally a progression from a 'barbaric' system to a more efficient 'modern' one. As Frederick Biggs has explained in a recent analysis of the epic poem *Beowulf*, contemporaries writing at the time of the change from pagan to Christian customs in the Germanic world were aware of the flaws in both succession systems: the problem of too many heirs in the former, leading to violence and civil war, and the problem of too few in the latter, leading to dynastic extinction or weak or child rulers.[26] Looking more specifically at France, Jochens has summarized the changing relationship between legitimacy and religion in the Merovingian and Carolingian dynasties: numerous offspring made it possible for the first Frankish dynasty, the Merovingians – ignoring the demands of churchmen to favour monogamy and legitimacy for royal succession – to sustain dynastic rule for 300 years, from the fifth to the eighth century. Their successors, the Carolingians, replaced polygyny with serial monogamy, facilitated by easy divorce and combined with extramarital sexual activities. Nevertheless, as the church took greater hold over society from the mid-eighth century, a tendency emerged to sift the candidates through a screen of legitimacy. In principal, illegitimacy was not an unsurmountable barrier, but it required a special act from the king and approval from the leaders of the country.[27] Across the Channel, Anglo-Saxon kings were also serial monogamists, and both legitimate and illegitimate could succeed. This all changed, ironically, after the conquest by William 'the Bastard' in 1066. A real signal of the change occurs in 1120, when King Henry I, in default of a legitimate son, named his daughter, Matilda, as his sole heir, and not his very able bastard son, Robert of Gloucester.[28]

This change from a horizontal, clan-based system of succession to one that is more vertical, based on a more nuclear family or dynasty, reflects changes occurring in the monarchies of Capetian France and Norman England. These kingdoms were strengthening the rule of a single lineage or dynasty through the establishment of primogeniture, whereby the eldest son inherits all, and by the practice of associative monarchy, where the king associates his throne with his eldest son within his lifetime, allowing the son to succeed unquestioned. This system was designed to avoid civil wars between siblings or cousins, and to consolidate power in a single lineage rather than continuing to divide the patrimony into smaller and smaller polities as Germanic custom had previously dictated. Even if this system did sometimes produce weak kings (children or insane), its benefits outweighed the disadvantages. This is the classic view as delivered in older texts, such as Robert Fawtier's *Capetian*

Kings of France (987–1328) from 1960,[29] but has been challenged more recently by historians like Andrew W. Lewis. He argued that this system was neither completely new, nor was it an innovation of the Capetians, but a practice being developed by contemporary magnates all across the region, including the Germans, who, according to traditional orthodoxy, were supposedly left behind in this innovation and thus failed to centralize and create a viable state – the classic nineteenth-century *étatiste* point of view.[30] The older argument had been that the Capetians developed the system of associative kingship in order to defend their rule against other rival dynasties, but Lewis demonstrates that the only serious challenges to royal successions in tenth- and eleventh-century France came from within the dynasty, by younger sons eager for a chance to share in royal power.[31] Similarly, it is a mistake to attribute to the Capetians any sense of conscious state-building by refusing to divide the royal patrimony like their predecessors (again, following a nationalist myth), as recently explained by Nicholas Henshall: 'The urge for dynastic acquisition, regardless of strategy or territorial logic, constantly cut across the possibility of any internal cohesion.'[32] Even a great state builder like the 'Great Elector', Friedrich Wilhelm of Brandenburg, famously the instigator of the rise of Prussia, in his will of 1688 adhered to traditional Germanic custom and divided up his territories between his sons (though this was nullified at his death).[33]

Sibling rivalries and the apanage

This brings us back to the question of the younger son, the sibling's desire for power, and the idea of 'corporate' or collective monarchy. While consolidation of rule over the throne itself prevailed in France from the tenth and eleventh centuries, especially in ideology and formal representation, nevertheless both countries in practice continued to have a symbolic leader who wore the crown, supported and advised by the other senior members of his family: the queen mother, the royal uncles, and so on. As Lawrence Bryant has pointed out, the uses of ceremonial in medieval and renaissance monarchy in France served to strengthen links between the crown, the royal family and the elites through 'imaging politics', creating spectacles (coronations, entries, opening of estates general, funerals) to formulate and display a collective identity by association with the royal body and not simply to exalt a single ruler. It is only late in the period (the seventeenth century) that the monarch is established as the sole political embodiment of ritual and 'national' identity.[34]

For this reason, it was important for medieval monarchies in France (and in its neighbours, England, Castile, Portugal) to create a system whereby younger sons of kings were included in the overall sense of dynastic glory and authority, yet were not a threat to the actual wielding of power by the head of the family, the king. They had to be both powerful and not too powerful. As we have seen, the earlier Germanic system of dividing up the state at the death of each successive monarch caused fragmentation and dissent. The early Capetians instead held on to their power by embracing primogeniture, and, while seeing the necessity to provide an income for younger sons, encouraged them to provide for themselves, to add to the overall glory of the dynasty by marrying wealthy heiresses or conquering foreign lands. And some did this very well: Philippe, second son of Philippe II, was given very little but married the heiress of the wealthy counts of Boulogne; Robert, fifth son of Louis IX, was given the small county of Clermont but enlarged his holdings by marrying the heiress of the lords of Bourbon. Good examples of early conquering cadets include Pierre de Courtenay who set out to claim the Latin empire of Constantinople in 1216, or Charles de France, count of Anjou, who successfully conquered the kingdom of Sicily in 1266.

The system of granting much larger portions of the royal domain to younger sons got underway with the deathbed settlement made by Louis VIII (1225), which involved granting nearly one-third of the entire domain to his sons: Artois for Robert, Anjou and Maine for Jean (later Charles), and Poitiers and Auvergne for Alphonse. At this point, the monarchy was not so concerned with the details of these land grants and it was mostly through luck that Poitou, Auvergne and ultimately Anjou soon returned to the crown in default of heirs; this was not to be the case with Artois, however, which was effectively lost to the dynasty for four centuries, until the Treaty of the Pyrenees in 1659! Older ideas of encouraging foreign conquest persisted. Philip III gave the county of Valois to his son Charles, a modest gift, as he was expecting great victories from him in claiming the kingdom of Aragon, and later his even wilder aspirations in Byzantium and the Holy Roman Empire. When these failed, however, Charles's apanage was augmented by his elder brother (now King Philip IV), with the rich lands of Anjou, Maine, Alençon and Chartres.[35]

Philip IV and his immediate successors also recognized the need to delineate more carefully the honours and the restrictions of the junior princes as *apanagistes*. Between 1297 and 1328, all apanages were created with peerages attached, thereby associating all such princes formally (not just by tradition) with both the ceremonial aspects of the state (notably the coronation) and the more administrative functions of government, as members of the highest law courts in the kingdom.[36] More specifically, appearing for the first time in the grant of an apanage in 1297, a specific clause reserved for the king 'superioritas et resortum': sovereignty and appellate jurisdiction, meaning these provinces could not evolve into independent sovereignties. And crucially, from 1314, most creations specified *male only* succession.[37] As Robert Fawtier has pointed out, this system also had the added benefit of aiding the dynasty in acquiring or assimilating new territories into the royal domain. The county of Toulouse was conquered and given to Alphonse, younger brother of Louis IX, in 1249, and when he died in 1271 with no heir, the French crown easily took over. The same process was used to amalgamate the rich county of Champagne via its acquisition through marriage by Philip IV of France. More theoretically, the qualities of the dynasty could be extended to its members to raise the status of the entire clan – the king of France could not do homage to anyone, and so too claimed his brothers. Alphonse held important lordships in the county of Poitiers but would not do homage for them to bishop of Poitiers, thus they too became by default part of the royal domain.[38] The age of major apanage creations came in the middle of the fourteenth century, with the creation of major princely lineages in Anjou (1360), Berry (1360), Burgundy (1363) and Orléans (1392). Again, these were encouraged to spread out and conquer: Anjou in Provence, Lorraine and Naples-Sicily; Burgundy in the Low Countries; and Orléans in Milan. But did this satisfy the ambitions of the princes of the blood with regard to their feeling that they were, by birth, entitled to a share in the internal affairs of the French kingdom? Not at all, as can be seen by the nearly constant state of civil war and cousinly vendetta that characterizes the fifteenth century in France.[39]

Across the Channel, we can see a similar development of the apanage with the granting of earldoms to younger sons (notably Cornwall in 1225 to the second son of King John), and the encouragement of others to marry great heiresses of earldoms (Lancaster, Leicester, Derby, Norfolk, Kent). In an interesting case of parallel development, at the same time as the major apanages were created for French cadets, Edward III created a series of royal dukedoms for his own younger sons: Clarence for Lionel and Lancaster for John in 1361; and York for Edmund and Gloucester for Thomas in 1385.[40] This system is different from the French system, however, in that none of these duchies were compact territorial units in the way the French apanages were, and the rights of the apanagists were never as extensive. Here too, it is fairly obvious that this system of regulating princely ambitions did not create lasting peace and harmony, but instead generated a bloody feud now known as the 'Wars of the Roses'. Looking further afield, we can see similar dynastic disunion and bloody conflict in the kingdoms of Iberia (where similar apanage systems existed). Less so in the empire, where Germanic custom was stronger and apanages created for second sons continued to develop into nearly separate states, as in Saxony, Bavaria, or Austria. In the latter, for example, the junior lines continued to be separated from the main line as late as the sixteenth and seventeenth centuries (in Styria, in Tirol), and were only held together by a House strategy of keeping all of the dynastic territories within one of the Imperial Circles (the 'Austrian Circle'), and with only singular representation, not multiple, at the Imperial Diet. Again, it was only through dynastic luck that these lines eventually died out, and Habsburg lands were reunited in the person of Emperor Leopold I in 1665.[41]

The inter-dynastic strife in both England and France had the unplanned benefit of reducing some of the pressures on the royal house to provide for younger sons or junior branches of the dynasty. In England, there were no legitimate patrilineal branches of the Plantagenet House left standing (though agnatic kin lines would of course remain to haunt the reigns of the Tudors), and one by one the collateral branches of the House of France died out, leaving only one, the Bourbons, to contest the authority of the senior Valois line after 1525. Nevertheless, the idea of granting apanages to younger sons remained unquestioned, and by the series of edicts issued at Moulins in 1566, Charles IX not only continued to create apanages for his younger brothers (Anjou for Henri, Alençon for François), he augmented some of their powers that had been uncertain, for example the power to appoint parish priests and local judicial officers, or to collect taxes on fief holders in default of heirs or those of foreign birth.[42]

The issue is wider than simply intra-familial; it touched on debates concerning the wider political society and the nature of the monarchy itself and its relationship with its people. J. Russell Major has written about one of the last cases in which the rights of royal blood versus popular will was debated. On the death of Louis XI in 1483, the King's will indicated his desire that his young son, Charles VIII, would be governed by his elder sister, Anne de Beaujeu. But the late king's cousin, Louis, duke of Orléans, challenged this as the closest male in the family and was supported by most of the French magnates. The Regent Anne summoned an Estates General, where her client, Philippe Pot, Seigneur de la Roche, made a speech about how power derived from the people, and that it was the job of the Estates therefore to place the government in the most trustworthy hands. He evoked the ancient historical practice of the

Frankish kings being elected by 'the sovereign people', and concluded that if the rule of the commonwealth 'devolves neither upon any one prince, nor upon several princes, nor upon all of them together, it must of necessity return to the people from whom it came'.[43] The duke of Orléans' challenge failed in the Estates, but he took to the field in armed rebellion instead.

Conclusions: from revolt to accomodation

The tradition of rebellion and the claims of the dukes of Alençon and Orléans and the prince of Condé mentioned at the start of this chapter were therefore part of a long tradition of such statements. All three followed a similar trajectory of leaving the court to demonstrate their dissatisfaction, and residing for a time at the court of a foreign power, almost always in Brussels. Gaston, duke of Orléans, in particular did this, more than once, in the period when his position as member of the royal family was most challenged – despite being the heir until the birth of the dauphin in 1638.[44] But later in life, Gaston changed, transforming his 'duty to revolt' into a duty to act the part of a royal prince through patronage rather than politics. Instead of a constant rebel, he became instead one of the greatest patrons of the arts (painting, poetry, ballet, theatre, architecture) of the middle of the seventeenth century.[45] This conversion from rebel to maecenas was witnessed and emulated by Gaston's nephew and successor as duke of Orléans, Philippe, the younger brother of Louis XIV. He and younger brothers who followed would follow a different path for self-representation of their princely status through the arts rather than through rebellion.[46]

And even though the parallel cannot be seen with such intensity in Britain, where James I had no younger brother, neither did Charles I (though he was himself a second son until the death of his older brother in 1612), by looking once more at contemporary concerns reflected in the theatrical works of Shakespeare, we can see that the notions of primogeniture versus division within the royal family were still present in the public discourse of early seventeenth-century Britain. When King Lear decides to divide his kingdom between his daughters, there is protest from members of his family and other members of the nobility. Ronald Colley has recently pointed out that these concerns were not merely fictional but were rooted in very real concerns of the day: would James I try to unify England, Scotland and Ireland into one centralized union? Or would he perhaps offer one of these three crowns to a younger son? James had in fact made clear his desire to hold together all three crowns, as he advised his eldest son Henry in his *Basilicon Doron*: 'make your eldest sonne Isaac, leaving him all your kingdoms: and provide the rest with private possessions: Otherwayes by deviding your kingdoms, yee shall leave the seed of division and discord among your posteritie.'[47] But Lear says the opposite, who misguidedly hopes 'that future strife / May be prevented' by the division of his kingdom.[48]

Was primogeniture really the best system of passing on a succession to the benefit of an entire dynasty? Joan Thirsk has observed that 'The temper of the literature [on primogeniture] changed noticeably in the middle of James I's reign, and subsequently developed into a more serious debate on the disadvantages of primogeniture for society as a whole.'[49] Cooley demonstrates that political tracts from the period testify to the potentially treasonous resentment often attributed to younger sons, as in John Earle's early seventeenth-century *Micro-cosmographie* which included a character 'Younger

Brother', who 'loves not his country for this unnatural custome [primogeniture], and would have long since revolted to the Spaniard, but for Kent onely which he holds in admiration', Kent being the one county in England in which partible inheritance (called *gavelkind*) prevailed.[50] This of course has an interesting parallel with the actions of the prince of Condé and Gaston d'Orléans entering Spanish service to protest their own exclusion from the government of France in this same period.

The conclusions to be drawn are not definitive. While we do see that second sons in the major monarchies of Europe acted as fiercely loyal adjuncts to their elder brothers by the end of the century – with clear examples offered by Philippe, duke of Orléans or James, duke of York – we also see upsets and continued strainings for power, for example in the cabal of the grand dauphin, waiting and waiting for the aging Sun King to pass on; or more extremely, in the willingness of William of Orange to overthrow his uncle and father-in-law in the 'Glorious Revolution' of 1688. And although certainly no European monarchy in the later early modern period allowed for princely brothers to rule as co-sovereigns, some did divide up territory to provide for younger sons (notable examples include the secundogenitures for the Bourbons in Naples from 1734, or for the Habsburgs in Tuscany from 1765), and some bitter divisions remained between branches of cousins (the Orléanists as leaders of the opposition in Louis XVI's France), or between siblings (Louis XVI often clashed with his younger brother, the comte de Provence). In the nineteenth century, civil wars were fought between rival branches of the houses of Bourbon in Spain or Bragança in Portugal. The issue of the apanage also resurfaced in the nineteenth century, when the count of Artois, younger brother of the restored Louis XVIII, was given a financial settlement rather than the restoration of his lands and feudal powers.[51] The question of the exercise of power by someone sitting so close to, though not on, the throne persisted until the very end of the age of monarchy.

Notes

1 *The Tempest*, Act II, scene i, lines 270–274, *The Riverside Shakespeare*, second edition, ed. G. Blakemore Evans (Boston and New York: Houghton Mifflin, 1997), 1671.

2 Ann Kronbergs, "The Significance of the Court Performance of Shakespeare's *The Tempest* at the Palatine Wedding Celebrations," in *The Palatine Wedding of 1613: Protestant Alliance and Court* Festival, eds. Sara Smart and Mara R. Wade (Wiesbaden: Harrassowitz Verlag, 2013), 339–352.

3 "Declaration de Monseigneur le duc d'Alençon, Dreux, 17 septembre 1576," Bibliothèque nationale de France, Manuscrits Français, 3342, fols. 5–6.

4 "Lettre, en forme de manifeste, de M. le Prince de Condé à tous les princes, seigneurs et gentilshommes de la France, sur son absence et éloignement de la cour, 1609," printed in full as an annex in Caroline Bitsch, *Vie et Carrière d'Henri II de Bourbon, prince de Condé (1588–1646). Exemple de comportement et d'idées politiques au début du XVIIᵉ siècle* (Paris: Honoré Champion, 2008), 441–448 (here 442).

5 *Lettre escrite au Roy par Monsieur (Nancy, 30 mai 1631), et par luy envoyée à Messieurs du Parlement pour la presenter à Sa Majesté* (Paris: Antoine Vitray, 1631).

6 See the various chapters by leading scholars in this area in Robert von Friedeburg, ed., *Murder and Monarchy: Regicide in European History, 1300–1800* (New York: Palgrave Macmillan, 2004).

7 See Louis Lobbes, "P. Matthieu, dramaturge phénix," *Revue d'histoire du théâtre* 3 (1998): 207–236.

8 Nicholas Henshall, *The Zenith of European Monarchy and its Elites: The Politics of Culture, 1650–1750* (Basingstoke: Palgrave Macmillan, 2010), 86–87.

9 Bodin, as cited in G.H. Sabine, *A History of Political Theory*, third edition (London: Harrap, 1963), 107–111.

10 This issue has been examined recently in its widest global context by Jeroen Duindam in his *Dynasties: A Global History of Power, 1300–1800* (Cambridge: Cambridge University Press, 2017), particularly chapter 2, "Dynasty: Reproduction and Succession."

11 Discussed by J. Russell Major, *From Renaissance Monarchy to Absolute Monarchy: French Kings, Nobles and Estates* (Baltimore: Johns Hopkins University Press, 1994), 54.

12 Jeremy L. Smith, "Music and Late Elizabethan Politics: The Identities of Oriana and Diana," *Journal of the American Musicological Society* 58 (Fall 2005): 508–558.

13 See Michael Dobson and Nicola J. Watson, *England's Elizabeth: An Afterlife in Fame and Fantasy* (Oxford: Oxford University Press, 2002); and Susan Doran and Thomas Freeman, *The Myth of Elizabeth* (Basingstoke: Palgrave Macmillan, 2003).

14 James Shapiro, *The Year of Lear: Shakespeare in 1606* (New York: Simon & Schuster, 2015), 152–153, 199. Shapiro adds that the play in fact alludes to the plot, a dangerous thing to do, but it was acceptable since the rightful succession is restored in the end through Banquo, who will hold three sceptres, an allusion to the unification of England, Scotland and Ireland, a project close to James's heart (208–209).

15 Shapiro, *The Year of Lear*, 137–145.

16 John Guy, *"My Heart is my Own": The Life of Mary Queen of Scots* (London: Fourth Estate, 2004), 504.

17 David Sabean, "Descent and Alliance: Cultural Meanings of Blood in the Baroque," in *Blood and Kinship: Matter for Metaphor from Ancient Rome to the Present*, eds., D. Sabean, C. Johnson, B. Jussen and S. Teuscher (Oxford: Berghahn Books, 2013), 144–174. See also Richard A. Jackson, "Peers of France and Princes of the Blood," *French Historical Studies* 7, no. 1 (1971): 27–46.

18 For overviews of the rebellions and reconciliations of these princes, see Pierre Gatulle, *Gaston d'Orléans. Entre mécénat et impatience du pouvoir* (Seyssel: Champ Vallon, 2012); and Katia Béguin, *Les Princes de Condé: Rebelles, courtisans et mécènes dans la France du Grand Siècle* (Seyssel: Champ Vallon, 1999).

19 See Ellen McClure, *Sunspots and the Sun King: Sovereignty and Mediation in Seventeenth-Century France* (Chicago: University of Illinois Press, 2006); and Georgia Cowart, *The Triumph of Pleasure: Louis XIV and the Politics of Spectacle* (Chicago: University of Chicago Press, 2008).

20 Eric Heinze, "'This power isn't Power if it's Shared': Law and Violence in Jean Racine's *La Thébaïde*," *Law and Literature* 22, no. 1 (Spring 2010): 76–109.

21 Racine, *La Thébaïde*, 1.5.242–244, in *Oeuvres complètes*, ed. Georges Forestier (Paris: Gallimard, 1999).

22 Heinze, "'This power isn't power'," 93–94. Eteocles presents undivided rule as the people's preference. In response, Polynices denigrates the will of the people as a legitimate form of choosing a government, in a passage eerily echoing sentiments expressed by Hillary Clinton following the US election of 2016 : "Shall I be judged by fickle men whose vices / Tie them to this usurper, make him proud? / Fine reason never steers a lowly crowd. / I've seen how base our Theban folk can be. / They chased me once; of course they don't want me. / They cannot tell the tyrant from the victim." [Racine, *La Thébaïde*, 2.3.535–542].

23 Philip Grierson, "Election and Inheritance in Early Germanic Kingship," *Cambridge Historical Journal* 7, no. 1 (1941): 1–22. For a more recent discussion of these issues, see the essays in the collection *Making and Breaking the Rules: Succession in Medieval Europe, c.1000–c.1600*, eds. Frédérique Lachaud and Michael Penman (Turnhout: Brepols, 2008).

24 Jenny M. Jochens, "The Politics of Reproduction: Medieval Norwegian Kingship," *The American Historical Review* 92, no. 2 (April 1987): 327–349 (333, 340).

25 Ian Whitaker, "Regal Succession Among the Dálriata," *Ethnohistory* 23, no. 4 (Autumn 1976): 343–363.

26 Frederick M. Biggs, "The Politics of Succession in *Beowulf* and Anglo-Saxon England," *Speculum* 80, no. 3 (July 2005): 709–741.

27 Jochens, "Politics of Reproduction", 329–330; but see also a different view in Régine Le Jan, "La sacralité de la royauté mérovingienne," *Annales. Histoire, Sciences Sociales* 58, no. 6 (2003): 1217–1241.

28 Chris Given-Wilson and Alice Curteis, *The Royal Bastards of Medieval England* (London: Routledge and Kegan Paul, 1984), 74–77. For a more recent study of this topic, see Sara McDougall, *Royal Bastards: The Birth of Illegitimacy, 800–1230* (Oxford: Oxford University Press, 2017), particularly chapter 4, "Maternal Lineage and Anglo-Norman Succession, *c.*950–*c.*1150."

29 Robert Fawtier, *The Capetian Kings of France: Monarchy & Nation (987–1328)* (London: Macmillan, 1960).

30 Andrew W. Lewis, "Anticipatory Association of the Heir in Early Capetian France," *American Historical Review* 83, no. 4 (Oct. 1978): 906–927; see also his *Royal Succession in Capetian France: Studies in Familial Order and the State* (Cambridge, MA: Harvard University Press, 1981).

31 Lewis, "Anticipatory Association," 908–909.

32 Henshall, *Zenith of Monarchies*, 9–10.

33 Ferdinand Schevill, *The Great Elector* (Chicago: University of Chicago Press, 1947), 394–399.

34 Lawrence Bryant, *Ritual, Ceremony and the Changing Monarchy in France, 1350–1789* (Farnham: Ashgate, 2010), 1–2.

35 Fawtier, *Capetian Kings of France*, 165–167.

36 The peers formally acclaimed the monarch as 'the choice of the nation'. They also sat by right in the Parlement of Paris. On French peers, see Christophe Levantal, *Ducs et pairs et duchés-pairies laïques à l'époque moderne, 1519–1790* (Paris: Maisonneuve et Larose, 1996).

37 There are few recent studies of the institution of apanage. A scholarly website that brings together a great deal of excellent information is François Velde's "Heraldica": www.heraldica.org/topics/france/apanage.htm (accessed 27 March 2019).

38 Fawtier, *Capetian Kings of France*, 82, 123–124.

39 For an overview, see Graeme Small, *Late Medieval France* (Basingstoke: Palgrave Macmillan, 2009).

40 Charles Given-Wilson, *The English Nobility in the Late Middle Ages: The Fourteenth-Century Political Community*, second edition (London: Routledge, 1996), 43–47.

41 Thomas Winkelbauer, "Separation and Symbiosis: The Habsburg Monarchy and the Empire in the Seventeenth Century," in *The Holy Roman Empire, 1495–1806: A European Perspective*, eds., R.J.W. Evans and Peter H. Wilson (Leiden: Brill, 2012), 167–175.

42 "Edit sur l'inalienabilité du domaine de la couronne," printed in Isambert, Decrusy and Taillandier, eds., *Recueil général des anciennes lois françaises, depuis l'an 420, jusqu'à la révolution de 1789* (Paris: Belin-Leprieur, 1829), vol. XIV, part 1, 185–189.

43 Speech quoted in Jehan Masselin, *Journal des états généraux de France tenus à Tours en 1484*, ed. A. Bernier (Paris: Imprimerie Royale, 1835), 146–151.

44 For a good overview of the reasons for, and the resolutions of, Gaston's periods of rebellion, nearly continuous between 1626 and 1638, see Georges Dethan, *La Vie de Gaston d'Orléans* (Paris: Fallois, 1992).

45 This is the main theme of the biography by Pierre Gatulle, *Gaston d'Orléans. Entre mécénat et impatience du pouvoir* (Seyssel: Champ Vallon, 2012), reflected clearly in his choice of the book's three main subdivisions, which in English are roughly: 'The Dream of a Possible Sovereignty, or the Apprenticeship of Submission'; 'The Impatience for Power'; and 'The Prince as Man of Character and the Burlesque Prince'.

46 See this author's, "Expected, then Passed Over: Second Sons in the French Monarchy of the Seventeenth Century," in *Unexpected Heirs in Early Modern Europe: Potential Kings and Queens*, ed. Valerie Schutte (New York: Palgrave Macmillan, 2017), 179–203. This is a major theme in my forthcoming monograph on the second son in the French monarchy in the early modern period. For Philippe as collector, see Paul Micio, *Les Collections de Monsieur, frère de Louis XIV* (Paris: Somogy, 2014).

47 "Basilicon Doron," in *King James VI and I: Political Writings*, ed., J. Sommerville (Cambridge, Cambridge University Press, 1994), 42

48 *King Lear*, I.i.44–45, as quoted by Ronald Cooley, "Kent and Primogeniture in *King Lear*," *Studies in English Literature, 1500–1900* 48, no. 2 (Spring 2008): 327–348, at 332.

49 Joan Thirsk, "Younger Sons in the Seventeenth Century," *History* 54, no. 182 (October 1969): 358–377, at 361.
50 Cooley, "Kent and Primogeniture," 329.
51 Philip Mansel, *The Court of France, 1789–1830* (Cambridge: Cambridge University Press, 1988), 179.

Key works

Bryant, Lawrence, *Ritual, Ceremony and the Changing Monarchy in France, 1350–1789* (Farnham: Ashgate, 2010).
Gatulle, Pierre, *Gaston d'Orléans. Entre mécénat et impatience du pouvoir* (Seyssel: Champ Vallon, 2012).
Henshall, Nicholas, *The Zenith of European Monarchy and its Elites: The Politics of Culture, 1650–1750* (Basingstoke: Palgrave Macmillan, 2010).
Lachaud, Frédérique and Michael Penman, eds., *Making and Breaking the Rules: Succession in Medieval Europe, c.1000–c.1600* (Turnhout: Brepols, 2008).
Major, J. Russell, *From Renaissance Monarchy to Absolute Monarchy: French Kings, Nobles and Estates* (Baltimore: Johns Hopkins University Press, 1994).

24

WHAT'S IN A NAME?

Dynasty, succession and England's queens regnant (1553–2016)

Sarah Betts

'Dynastic periodization was of course natural to eighteenth- and nineteenth-century historians. Its widespread persistence into the twentieth century, not only in the English case, may perhaps be ascribed to institutional inertia'.[1] Thus declared C.S.L. Davies in an article propounding his findings that although 'the word "Tudor" is used obsessively by historians . . . it was almost unknown at the time', cautioning against the ingrained 'insidious and misleading' popular and academic use of concepts like 'Tudor era' or 'Tudor monarchy'. His argument against using dynastic nomenclature was essentially two-fold: that it implies a social, cultural and political hegemony over a vast number of years through which the only unifying factor was the genetic relationship of the reigning monarchs, and that it implies a conscious *and contemporary* self-promoting and public acceptance of linear connections between the policies and events of each successive reign within the grouping, which in fact can only be (questionably) elucidated through retrospective organization by historians.[2] While Davies' arguments in relation to the labelling of concurrent social legislation are hard to disagree with, this is not so clearly the case with regard to the history of monarchy itself, both in Britain and the wider world. Dynastic appellations *have* been convenient solutions to inevitable necessities of periodization in historical writing, but recent work has also illustrated that dynasty is both an identifiable component of past elite societies and a useful analytical dimension through which to study royal identity. As Jeroen Duindam observes, 'almost all peoples across the globe until very recently accepted dynastic rule as a god given and desirable form of power'.[3] This chapter suggests that dynastic periodization is still a 'natural' and valuable way in which to analyse the history of the monarchy in England, in terms of both individual monarchs and the institution as a whole of both monarchical self-fashioning and external representations. For case studies, it will take the six queens regnant, Mary I (r.1553–8), Elizabeth I (r.1558–1603), Mary II (r.1688–94), Anne (r.1702–14), Victoria (r.1837–1901) and Elizabeth II (r.1952–). This chapter does not intend to examine the now well-studied minutiae of female succession and rule, but to use the complication of royal dynastic identity brought about by each of their reigns (partly through the nature of female identity in a patriarchal society, partly because of their peculiar accessional circumstances) to highlight uses of dynastic continuity and/or change within the mechanics of monarchy as the institution's role has evolved since the 1500s.

Monarch, family, nation

'Dynasty' is basically recognized as a succession of rulers of one family, but nonetheless remains indivisible from an archaic but related denotation of power or 'lordship'. Thus, the first working definition of the term here will be as 'the family in power'. However, even identifying said family is complex. Michael Hicks has observed that the concept of a '*royal* family' as we understand it today emerged in England in the later Middle Ages following the promotion by Edward III and Richard II of all the former's sons to ducal wealth and status, formalizing the elevation of 'royal blood' among the English nobility.[4] Meanwhile, historians of more recent western monarchies have highlighted a sense of royal family based upon a Europe-wide genealogical network.[5] Liesbeth Geevers and Mirella Marini have rightly argued that although genetic kinship alone does not unequivocally equate to 'dynasty', it does provide the basic 'biological hardware' on which a dynasty could be projected.[6] This chapter will start at the genetic family of the monarch, nuclear and extended, but will also consider implications of theoretical and representational understandings of monarchy itself to the concept of royal dynasty in England.

Monarchy scholars today are familiar with the 'two bodies' theory: traceable to classical times, that a king has both a 'body natural', mortal flesh like the 'natural bodies of other people', and a 'body politic' of God-given lordship 'of [and for] the public weal' that transcends the individual human lifecycle, seamlessly passing from king to king.[7] The merging of these two bodies in the current sovereign gives them a special status, 'embodying "the Crown"', a collective notion of prerogatives and traditions seen and/or marketed as a natural and desirable vessel of consistency and continuity.[8] In this context, dynasty should be read as the present temporal monarch's stake in the perpetuity of monarchy, binding the individual to the institution past and future. Key to this definition is dynasty's potential for ensuring stability, thus a/the 'royal family' has become increasingly central to monarchical imagery, advertising security and certainty of succession, *and* highlighting the institution's changing role and relationship to 'the nation' as the indigenous 'family of families, at once dynastic and domestic, remote and accessible, magical and mundane'.[9] The role of 'family' and of 'nation' will be central to this consideration of the past, present and future monarchy appropriated, practised and promised by each of England's queens regnant.

Past and present

As Howard Nenner noted, '[the] need for a fixed and certain rule of monarchical succession ... proceeded from a larger need for political stability', and in England, times of considerable political upheaval naturally bred increasing displays and acceptance of dynastic strength and integrity from a hereditary monarchy.[10] Highlighting royal lineage could endorse 'rights' to the throne, emphasizing continuity, peace and maintenance of ancient laws and traditions. Both the Tudors and Stuarts emphasized descendance from Henry VII and Elizabeth of York, and in this respect, Davies is right in dismissing the modern significance of a 'Tudor' identity, for they were predominantly portrayed not as a new line but as the continuation of the now reunified Plantagenet one.[11] Even Victoria, in her 1857 journal, described a performance of *Richard II* as one 'in which all my ancestors figured', clearly associating her own blood and bloodline with both branches of the medieval dynasty.[12] Lineage and the past, both recent and ancient, were a crucial part of both the public face of monarchy and any privately held sense of duty and/or destiny. The easiest way to achieve this blood bridge between kings past and present was through unbroken and indisputable patrilineal descent. The mortality of the family underpinning a monarchical dynasty inevitably complicated this ideal.

Practising male-preference primogeniture renders the accession of any queen regnant unusual. The accession of each of England's queens was still more so. Only Elizabeth II directly succeeded her late father in lieu of a male sibling. Mary I, Elizabeth I and Anne each inherited from a sibling (Anne's succession was further complicated by her widowed brother-in-law's intermediary reign). Elizabeth I and Victoria were both conceived specifically to combat immediate dynastic crisis, while Mary II, Anne and Elizabeth II ultimately became heirs of childless uncles.[13] Mary II and Elizabeth II both reigned during the lifetimes of a previous occupant of the throne, and Mary and her sister, Anne, in opposition to an exiled rival. In addition to these individual circumstances, the queens' immediate families also had chequered histories of succession and rule; like all monarchs, they, and their subjects, had to choose which elements of monarchical and family history to accept and/or forget. The monarch's 'two bodies' required balancing, as while succession rights in hereditary monarchy were derived from the native royal bloodline, the body natural unites the heritage of two parents: two potentially competing or conflicting dynastic identities.

For the sixteenth-century queens, the most pressing dynastic concern was with the very recent past and legitimation of their rule. Although England's throne had not been directly *and successfully* claimed by a woman before, recent historians have rightly observed that Mary and Elizabeth's bastardy was technically more of a barrier to their monarchical inheritance than their sex as, by English law and tradition, a bastard had no parents or material past.[14] As Mary Hill Cole argues, the restoration of the official parentage and 'dynastic utility' of his daughters in Henry VIII's will was negated, not only by the will of his successor, Edward VI, but also by the very fact that it publicly enshrined their bastardy.[15] Once queen, Mary immediately worked to expunge this. To avoid admission or impression of doubts over her succession's legality and dynastic inevitability, she held her coronation, steeped in the traditions of her predecessors, her household dressed in the standard colours favoured by her father, *before* summoning parliament to legally confirm her status.[16] The Act of the Queen's Title (1553) restored the validity of her parents' marriage and consequently her own legitimacy.[17] Henry VIII's responsibility for the family breakdown was tempered through attacks upon Anne Boleyn and Archbishop Cranmer as architects of divorce and Reformation, and, taking for her personal motto 'Truth the Daughter of Time', Mary set about reinstituting the old royal dynasty and religion of her childhood. Throughout her reign she viewed Elizabeth as symbolic of that old life's destruction and a threat to the survival of her now carefully reconstructed one, even going so far as to question her sister's paternity and deny any shared royal lineage.[18]

Criminalization and execution of Elizabeth's mother by her father rendered similar retrospective familial reconstitution impossible. So too did her recognition of Mary's succession rights on the death of their brother, for, as family history could not be rewritten to recognize both the Aragon and Boleyn marriages, acceptance of Mary's rule implicitly accepted their father's will as the basis for her claim. She therefore adopted what Cole describes as a bifold approach, reasserting her descent from her father separately from rehabilitating the reputation of her mother (and Boleyn heritage) without specifically addressing the question of their marriage.[19] As queen, Elizabeth built upon moves made throughout her youth to cement her image as part of her father's complex compound-nuclear family, and rested her role and heritage as monarch upon that.[20] She claimed her throne as Henry VIII's daughter and as sister of her immediate predecessors, but also associated herself with her paternal grandparents, particularly her grandmother and namesake, Elizabeth of York, and thus implicitly with the long line of kings she entailed.[21] She drew upon her paternal lineage for a regality and confidence which later underpinned her 'Gloriana' image of anointed and immortal sovereignty. However, her maternal lines were not forgotten. Her unusually native bloodline, her prized English/Celtic looks and her origins as symbolic and literal daughter of the break with Rome and establishment of the Church of England helped foster her image as devoted to, and representative of, her realm, in stark contrast to her Romish, half-Spanish predecessor.[22] As Karen Bundesen has illustrated, her maternal dynasty also provided practical and emotional support for her throughout her reign. Unlike her paternal relations, they held no threatening claim or interest in the throne beyond what their kinswoman, Elizabeth herself, might bestow upon them from it, and she played an active part in the affairs of their extended family network and was generous in conferring offices, moneys, affection and trust upon them.[23]

The next two reigning queens were full siblings of undisputed legitimacy of birth. Their mother, Anne Hyde, was also an English commoner (rather than foreign princess) and, like Elizabeth, they consequently compared favourably in popularity to any heirs born to their Catholic father, James, duke of York, and their Italian-papist stepmother. Brought up under the influence of their politically savvy uncle, Charles II, and their Hyde relatives, the two princesses were seen as the promised safeguard against the permanent destruction of the English church by the now seemingly inevitable reign of their father. Such was the fear that the duke might one day sire a son and a new Catholic dynasty to displace his elder daughters that it has recently been convincingly argued that the Hydes, from political, religious and dynastic motivations, may have deliberately allowed Anne to fatally infect her infant half-brother in 1677.[24] The birth of a healthy Prince of Wales in 1688 led the sisters to denounce the baby's legitimacy and, with Mary's husband, William III, to depose their (now reigning) father in 'Glorious Revolution' later that year. Claiming their immediate royal heredity was challenging. Their father and half-brother were still alive, and the establishment of parliamentary consent at the heart of the new constitutional monarchy made any legacy as Charles I's granddaughters inconvenient. Instead the new regime made frequent allusions to Charles II and associations with the still popularly mythologized Elizabeth.[25] Moreover, in spite of the new constitutional mode of succession, they were keen to embrace the concept of the mystically hereditary body politic of eternal monarchy in order to retain 'crown property'.[26] Jacobite propaganda railed at the hypocrisy of Mary claiming royal connections, particularly to her uncle, while disowning the father in whom her connection to the monarchy and dynasty originated, and berated both daughters as 'unnatural' and sinful for rebelling against their father particularly when their Hyde blood had weakened the royal 'race' of the natural monarchs of her father's 'great bloods' ('Bourbon and Plantagenet').[27] The dynastic split created political and military division, unrest and instability into the next generation – royal dynastic politics and propaganda still played a part in the era of an increasingly constitutional monarchy.

By Victoria's accession in 1837, the Jacobite threat was over, and Stuart heritage was something she was willing, even eager, to embrace. Victoria frequently sojourned in their ancestral kingdom of Scotland, once commenting that she contemplated, with 'reverence':

> [t]he very scenes made historical by P[cc] Charles's[28] wonderings! . . . in this most beautiful country, which I am proud to call my own, where there was such devoted loyalty to my ancestors. For Stewart blood is in my veins & I am now, their representative & the people are as devoted and loyal to me, as they were to that unhappy Race.[29]

Despite referring to them as her 'ancestors', and to Scotland and specifically Holyrood as an ancestral home, Victoria's relationship with the Stuarts was complex.[30] Like her uncle, George IV, she found the 'unhappy race' and their political troubles romantic and relatable, but in an era where the balance of power within the constitutional monarchy was shifting evermore towards parliament, it would be unwise to identify so closely with the reviled arbitrary rule of the ultimately deposed Stuart dynasty.[31] There were also genealogical difficulties with claiming Stuart descent. While descended from James VI & I, Victoria was not directly descended from the later Stuarts, but eventual benefactress of the Hanoverian inheritance through Sophia, youngest daughter of Charles I's sister, that same Hanoverian line which had fought and ultimately crushed romantic 'P[cc] Charles' and his Scottish supporters. In claiming both her 'Stuart blood' and her 'own country' of Scotland, Victoria embraced a monarchical dynasty wider than her immediate family branch, one stretching back to ancient times and a natural affinity with the kingdom(s) she ruled. She spent more time in Scotland than the English Stuarts themselves had done, she adopted tartan and royal tartan dress, and built her highland retreat, Balmoral, in the romantic Scots baronial style. She even gave her son the regal middle name of Duncan 'as a compliment to dear Scotland'.[32] In England, she embraced popular medievalism, she and Albert starring in their medieval costume ball as Edward III and Queen Philippa, christening her daughter Alice Maud two 'old English name[s]', and commissioning a sculpture of herself and Albert in Anglo-Saxon dress.[33]

Was she then rejecting her own House of Hanover? Traditional historiography has seen Victoria's monarchy as the forge of current forms of constitutional monarchy, ignited by the queen's personal desire to break 'completely and irrevocably with the immediate Hanoverian past', and certainly she publicly distanced herself from the profligacy and philandering of her Hanoverian uncles, and avoided highlighting similarities with her grandfather, George III, that could lead to inferences of hereditary lunacy. However, as David Cannadine observed, she was not entirely successful and was in many ways 'Hanoverian' in looks, temperament and monarchical outlook.[34] She had been specifically bred to resolve the dynastic crisis brought about by the death of George III's only legitimate grandchild, Princess Charlotte of Wales. Victoria's father, Edward, duke of Kent, was anxious to bind her to both family and kingdom from birth, insisting that she be born (ideally, he hoped upon the king's birthday) and raised in England, regardless of his own living circumstances and the inhospitality of his eldest brother, the Prince Regent.[35] Furthermore, Kent wished to endow her with the family names of Georgina, Charlotte and Augusta, but the regent ultimately vetoed these choices, essentially obstructing his brother's aims to mark his daughter as dynastic inheritrix.[36] Victoria herself, though never choosing traditional English or Hanoverian royal names for her children, did turn to her paternal family for middle names, most notably in the choice of Adelaide after the queen dowager for her eldest daughter, and Edward after her own father for her eldest son. Even so, foreshadowing what was to be a perpetual problem for Victoria and her family, her friend and former prime minister, Lord Melbourne cautioned against her choice of Albert *before* Edward for the Prince of Wales writing, 'Edward is a good English appellation, and has a certain degree of popularity attached to it from ancient recollections. Albert . . . has not been so common nor so much in use since the Conquest.'[37]

Of her paternal relations, those of whom Victoria seems to have been the fondest (or held the *memory of*) were Queen Adelaide, who, as William IV's German wife, was not a direct Hanoverian dynast; Kent, who died when she was a child; and Princess Charlotte, the regent's daughter, whose death had ultimately propelled Victoria into existence and onto the throne, and who, crucially for Victoria's sense of family association, had died in childbirth, the wife of Victoria's maternal uncle, Leopold. So far as her immediate family history was concerned, her maternal family played a far greater role in Victoria's sense of dynastic identity. Leopold, as a widower in England, and later as king of Belgium, was her constant adviser, confidante and father-figure. His family, minor German (Coburg) royalty, were nicknamed by Bismarck, the 'stud farm of Europe' for marrying and fathering rulers across Europe most notably including Leopold himself, the king *jure uxoris* of Portugal and Victoria's own husband, Albert, a match strongly encouraged by their mutual uncle, Leopold himself.[38] Albert's encouragement helped to heal a difficult relationship between Victoria and her mother, bringing the duchess of Kent firmly into the sphere of familial influence. Both Victoria and Albert kept in close and affectionate contact with their extended Coburg family, particularly Leopold and Albert's brother Ernst, duke of Saxe-Coburg and Gotha. The British royal family regularly visited Coburg, and Victoria delighted in the aesthetic of her children in Coburg peasant dress on special family occasions.[39] Victoria continually assured Leopold in letters that she was his 'devoted Niece and Child', and in 1853 Victoria wrote to him that they were naming their new son Leopold as 'a mark of love and affection . . . recall[ing] the almost only happy days of my sad childhood.'[40] Such was Leopold's influence that despite her political seniority to all her relatives, and being already widowed four years, only when Leopold died did her daughter write to her, 'Now you are head of all the family!'[41] In Britain, Victoria's intense connection to her German relatives did not go unnoticed. By the time her daughter Louise married, she was forced to look for a son-in-law among the native aristocracy to mollify anti-German feeling among her subjects.[42]

For Victoria's descendants, the tension between their immediate family's Germanic roots and the need to be embraced as a traditionally English/British institution intensified as the monarchy's executive role diminished in favour of cultural symbolism. Anti-German, patriotic fervour during the World War I prompted George V, as head of the dynasty of his 'grandmother, Queen Victoria, of blessed and gracious memory', to renounce on behalf of all dynasts who were 'subjects of these realms' all German 'appellations'. Victoria and Albert's descendants, the central trunk of the monarchy, were rebranded from Albert's House of Saxe-Coburg-Gotha into the 'House and Family of Windsor'.[43] 'Windsor' was a significant choice, referencing the great fortressed-palace which dominated the Thames valley landscape, 'associated longer than any other Royal residence with the fortunes and lives of the Kings and Queens of England . . . back to William the Conqueror' and still advertised today as 'family home to British kings and queens for over 1000 years'.[44] It also echoed a public association of the castle with George's proclaimed dynastic matriarch, Victoria, known popularly as the 'Widow of Windsor' for her long seclusion there after the death of her husband. This simple change distanced the monarchy from embarrassing German heritage and symbolically associated it with a long and indigenous past. As Cannadine has argued, George in many ways innovated modern constitutional monarchy, which became increasingly about grand public ceremonial, often hinging upon performance of 'traditions' that, though long discontinued, or even unprecedented, were practised with rehearsal and persistence of ceremony and formula which conveyed an air of ancient custom and continuity.[45]

Within this formula, George V and his consort, Mary, utilized dynasty in their practice of monarchy in two key ways. First, they formalized a traditional pattern of use for the royal residences, a pattern which, in the footsteps of George III and Queen Victoria, included both public, state occupation and private retreat, creating a scenic portfolio of historic (in actuality and/or appearance), dynastic *seats*, which were at once family homes and royal *manors*. That summers at Balmoral and Christmases at Sandringham (the Norfolk home originally purchased in 1862 for Edward VII, then Prince of Wales) had become integral to monarchical culture was illustrated during the abdication crisis of 1936. When George and Mary's second son, Bertie, became King George VI, he automatically inherited 'crown property', including Buckingham Palace, and Windsor castle, which, by his 'body politic', was tied to the incumbent sovereign. Balmoral and Sandringham had been the private property of Edward VII and then George V, consequently passing on the latter's death to his eldest son, the outgoing, but living, Edward VIII. To retain these seats of monarchy within the realms of the dynasty's reigning branch, George VI purchased them from his brother, allowing both himself and his daughter to perpetuate dynastic patterns of monarchical seasons.[46]

Second, they extended the notion of the working royal family beyond the exclusivity of the monarch. While the dynastic extent of 'the crown' may have been contentious from the introduction of the Civil List in 1760, and previous monarchs may have shared (by will, force or necessity) power and/or duties with their spouses, children or other relatives, George V formalized and traditionalized the process. The enormity of his empire and the improved transportation technologies ever increased the need for members of his family to travel and act as representatives of the king. In 1911, with king and consort about to embark for India, further than any reigning predecessor had ever ventured, the process of officially including the wider family in state business began with the introduction of 'Counsellors of State', officially named individuals who could be called upon by letters patent to physically deputize for the monarch. Later, the 1937 Regency Act legally required these counsellors to be, in addition to the consort, the first four people in the line of succession over the age of 21. Not only did this provide some official duty for the heir to the throne, but it also enabled inclusion of older generations of the king's family into the business of the future monarchy. When George's granddaughter, Elizabeth, ascended in 1952, his own children, the Duke of Gloucester and Princess Mary, numbered among her counsellors, as did, at various points in her reign, her Kent, Gloucester and Harewood cousins. Beyond practical function, the extended nuclear royal family was incorporated into public ceremonial programmes. Royal weddings, once quiet affairs in private chapels and backrooms of palaces, relocated to public venues and received ever-increasing press attention (including photographs). Regular balcony appearances became an integral part of both royal engagement with historic occasions (e.g. the beginning/end of the World Wars), and the display of ceremony at key 'royal family' lifecycle moments, thus associating events of dynastic significance with those of national importance. Close to both kings, Elizabeth II continued the new 'traditions' and dynastic style of her father and grandfather.

The nature of monarchical succession in Britain entails that a reigning monarch, however young, would only ever be under the direct living influence of a non-reigning parent, and when Elizabeth came to the throne in 1952, she had living, and UK-domiciled, both previous queens consort, Queen Elizabeth (the Queen Mother), and her paternal grandmother, Queen Mary. As monarch, the new queen was officially head of the royal family and the Windsor dynasty. In practice this was inevitably more complicated. Often foreign, and brides of convenience or alliance, queens consort had been traditionally viewed as dynastic interlopers, at least until producing an heir, which gave them a vested genetic/maternal interest in their marital dynasty as much as, or over, their natal one. Both Mary of Teck and Elizabeth Bowes-Lyon came from noble (and in Mary's case royal) backgrounds, but both alliances, even the earlier, arranged one, were personal rather than political. Moreover, both queens held a strong sense of affiliation towards the monarchy and the family, readily adopting its heritage as their own through enthusiastic collection of historical artefacts with royal connections, creating 'homes' within traditional royal residences, and actively shaping its future in their meticulous performance of ceremony and duty.[47] Queen Mary's matriarchal role was central to the 'family of families' image she and George V had cultivated. Throughout the 1936 'year of three kings' crisis, she was the one constant queen, and when her younger son was crowned the following year, she broke with tradition, attending the coronation for moral support, flanking the king with her daughter-in-law in the photographs. But her influence as head of the family was more than representational. After her husband died, her daughter-in-law wrote that 'the Family, as a family, will now revolve round you . . . as a central point, because without that point it might easily disintegrate', sentiments she frequently reiterated throughout 1936 ultimately resolving that both family and nation required *Mary's* 'leadership . . . to get the country back' to its former pre-abdication stability.[48]

Throughout her letters, Elizabeth apparently distinguished between 'family', in terms of genetic relationship and affection, and *the* 'family' embodying the business of monarchy. These important distinctions were demonstrated in the contrast of her response to a 1945 visit of the *former* king, now Duke of Windsor, which she characterized as a 'private' family affair (and thus unsuitable for press attention), with her assertion that '"the Monarchy" really embraces [the public presence of] the whole Royal family'.[49]

Although largely retired from public life in the 1940s, Queen Mary remained an influential presence in the personal lives of her family. Mary's role as non-genetic dynast at the head of her reigning child's dynasty, envisaged by her daughter-in-law, was one which, Queen Elizabeth herself would ultimately fulfil for half a century of her own daughter's reign, highlighted (as with Mary) by her presence at the coronation. Following George VI's death, *The Times* confidently assumed that 'the Government will obviously wish to amend' The Regency Act to allow the Queen Mother to be appointed as a counsellor of state for her daughter declaring that 'Everyone will want to see the name of the Queen Mother included'.[50] The appointment was made and Queen Elizabeth represented her daughter both at home and abroad into old age, sometimes literally holding the monarchical fort such as in 1973 when she wrote to her grandson:

> We seem to be very short of Counsellors of State, at the moment there is only Anne[51] & me to do the papers & receive the diplomats.[52]

The Queen Mother remained close to her daughter and played an active part in the private upbringing of her grandchildren, and in royal pageantry and ceremony. Her residual popularity from World War II drew affection towards the monarchy, providing a reassuring sense of continuity. In 2000, she very publicly celebrated her 100th birthday, and a contemporary portrait encapsulates her role as both representative of the monarchy's past and anchor of its future. John Wonnacott's *The Royal Family: A Centenary Portrait* hangs in the National Portrait Gallery amid centuries of royal portraiture, and places her at the heart of both her family and *the* family. A celebration of *her* mortal longevity, she is seated at the piece's centre, but the title makes clear the significance of her role within the family, associating this longevity with that of the monarchy itself. They are *her* dynasty, not that of Elizabeth II, a blood-dynast of the royal house, who is very much a subsidiary figure. Wonnacott turned for inspiration to John Lavery's 1913 *The Family of George V*, which was set in the same room of Buckingham Palace (itself echoing Winterhalter's 1846 Victoria family portrait), but he also felt that 'the young Prince William, our future King, needed to be very large, at the front of the picture – he's lifesize'.[53] The Queen Mother bridges this contrast between past and future, becoming the dynastic present. Her link to the reigning dynasty is accentuated by featuring in this celebration of her matriarchy of only her eldest daughter and her husband, and the family of the Prince of Wales, i.e. the nucleus of the monarchical line rather than *all* of her descendants.

Present and future

Although remaining personally close to her Bowes-Lyon relatives, the Queen Mother, like her mother-in-law before her, successfully subsumed her natal dynastic identity to that of her marital, whole-heartedly adopting and promoting her husband's family. Consummate consorts, they enhanced (both physically and representationally) the monarchical family without creating conflicts of interest with those of themselves and their natal families. Partly because of this, when Elizabeth II became queen in 1952, taking the mantle directly from her own father, she was the first queen regnant of England to be *unchallenged* and *unashamedly* the dynastic inheritrix of her immediate predecessors. Any residual threat posed by the Duke of Windsor was nullified by his familial and geographical exile, and by his failure to reproduce, to cement a dynastic future. Contrastingly, Elizabeth, already mother-of-two, had been seen within the family as the dynastic future of the monarchy since childhood, her ailing grandfather apparently hoping his 'eldest son w[ould] never marry and have children, and that nothing w[ould] come between Bertie and Lilibet and the Throne'.[54] Even so, the 1952 succession was not entirely dynastically uncomplicated. Female succession remained an anomaly which challenged the two core tenets of dynastic longevity in England: the consolidation, cohesion and consequent security of 'the crown' in terms of rights, lands and wealth; and production of a new generation of dynasts to carry the monarchy forward.

Male-preference primogeniture, the intermarriage of ruling families and the notion of a 'body politic' supposedly guaranteed perpetual power and wealth within the senior dynastic branch. It also supposedly safeguarded against the infighting of royal brothers and branches disintegrating into civil war as had happened in the medieval period due to the gavelkind-style succession of the Normans, and the dissemination of influence and riches among *all* his many sons by Edward III. As noted earlier, safeguarding hereditary 'crown property' after the Glorious Revolution helped bolster the prestige and viability of the new constitutional monarchy, and George VI later took steps to bind 'family' properties to the sitting sovereign. In 1937, one MP asked 'whether it is proposed to introduce legislation to amend the Act of Settlement with a view to making clear that the Princess Elizabeth is the sole heir to the Throne and does not share it jointly with her sister on the analogy of Peerage Law?'[55] The first modern occasion when it was envisioned that a reigning monarch would leave multiple daughters but no sons, that legislators would want assurance that crown properties, titles and functions should not be subject to the division of inheritance customary in noble families in this situation, is noteworthy. So too is the Home Secretary's response that there was 'no reason to do so . . . [as there was] no doubt that in present circumstances . . . Princess Elizabeth would succeed to the Throne as sole heir'.[56] Not only was the prospect of future female rule accepted, but the crown was (or should be) considered distinct from the general aristocracy. The 'throne' was widely recognized as a specific and cohesive amalgamation of prerogatives, titles and material assets. In spite of these attitudes and public speculation to the contrary, Elizabeth was never created Princess of Wales. However unlikely it became that her parents would displace her with a son, she remained only heir presumptive, not apparent, a distinction referenced in parliamentary discussion of the Civil List and royal annuities, as it had been during the childhood of her predecessor, Victoria.[57] Although universally accepted as future queen, the most official connection she was given to Wales, traditional realm of heirs to the throne since Edward I, was her admission as Bard of the Gorsedd (as 'Elizabeth o Windsor') and opening of the 1946 Eisteddfod.[58] After her son's birth in 1948,

The Times painstakingly detailed that although an exception was made for the baby in terms of a 'royal highness' styling, in recognition of the Elizabeth's 'unique position as heiress-presumptive', the succession position of both would remain tenuous until George VI's death.[59] While displacement by a younger brother remained a possibility, a female heir remained essentially a dynastic vessel between a past and present future.

Although by 1952 she had already performed her dynastic duty by providing both an heir and a spare, her integrity as a dynast was fundamentally challenged by her gender in a society which preferenced patrilineal descent. Shortly after her accession, her husband's uncle was heard boasting 'that the House of Mountbatten now reigned', prompting immediate action from the royal family and the cabinet, long fearful of the 'dangerous' Mountbattens, 'determined to be the power behind the throne'.[60] The 1917 proclamation of George V did not cater for the eventuality that the sovereign would be a woman, and consequently it could be assumed that as 'a female descendant who had married', Elizabeth had taken the name and dynastic identity of her husband, which would now descend to the future monarchy.[61] The cabinet discussed the issue as two-fold, first in establishing the nomenclature of the 'Royal House and Family' and second in identifying the personal surname of the queen and her descendants. Once again, the link and/or distinction between *dynasty* and legal and genetic *family* is crucial. It was argued that royal titles negated the use of a surname. Members of such families were identified by location of origins and holdings, it was 'not clear that a queen need have any surname herself'.[62] It was also argued that the exception for married female descendants outlined in 1917 applied only to the section discussing the use of a personal surname and not to the reigning 'House and Family' of George V and his descendants.[63] However, the very fact that George V had formally created a surname for the royal family, the choice of regally and nationally significant 'Windsor' at a time when it was essential for the monarchy to be seen as ancient and native, and the fact that personal surnames were more relatable to the general population than dynastic titles, meant it was deemed advisable to retain the name of Windsor for all significant royal descendants. As the Lord Chancellor argued:

> Permanence and continuity are valuable factors in the maintenance of constitutional monarchy and the name of the Royal House should not be changed if change can be avoided . . . in confirming what was clearly the intention of Her father and grandfather . . . [she]would be acting in accordance with the sentiments and desires of all Her peoples. Nothing could shake their loyalty and devotion to the queen and this is personal to Her Majesty; but behind it lies their grateful memory of Her father and grandfather who immeasurably strengthened the institution of monarchy and have given to the name of Windsor a significance that should not be lost.[64]

Consequently, the queen proclaimed that the royal family would remain 'the House and Family of Windsor', the surname 'Windsor' being used by any male-line descendants who required one.[65]

Dynastic consequences of female sovereigns marrying and procreating were a key problematic in accepting female rule in England. The integral role of a 'Prince of

Wales' in propaganda of dynastic security and longevity was awkwardly undermined when the sitting monarch had no son and, consequently, any designated or recognized heir could one day be replaced. But Elizabeth II was not the first queen regnant accepted as the dynastic future for some years prior to accession. Charles Beem has partially attributed Mary I's ultimately successful accession, despite Edward VI's will, to the fact that 'for the first 17 years of her life, Mary [had] enjoyed . . . *traditional* . . . recognition of heir, without any statutory backing, [but even going so far as] . . . function[ing] for a time as a de facto Princess of Wales', when she was sent by her father, in the footsteps of recent former heirs, to reside in and rule the Principality.[66] Mary's potential marriage was an ever-present facet of Henry VIII's foreign policy, but, as would happen when her sister Elizabeth became sole legitimate heir, Henry was unwilling to relinquish control of her upbringing or person while viewing them as his only dynastic future.[67] Even once an indisputably legitimate son arrived, Henry continued to recognize the possible eventuality of his daughters' succession, and the role any future marriage would have in his dynasty's future direction. Attempting to negate his heiresses marrying into the English aristocracy at the expense of the primacy and stability of the monarchy, his will explicitly designated their marriage the Privy Council's prerogative, and the question remained unresolved throughout the reign of the young, unmarried and childless Edward VI.[68] When Mary became England's first universally recognized female monarch, the subject of her marriage was key to her dynastic self-definition. In marrying Philip of Spain, son of her mother's nephew, Charles V, Mary reinvoked the happier and less complicated days of her parent's marriage and her own tenancy as her father's undisputed legitimate heiress. It wistfully indulged her childhood 'love' and ambitions for marriage with Charles V.[69] It renewed the old Anglo-Spanish alliances of Henry VII and Henry VIII and bound her more closely with her mother's family and countrymen, her long-time political allies through the dark days of her brother's reign. Most importantly, as she strove for Catholic restoration in England, Philip represented a confessionally sound and prestigious father for an heir of her own body to continue this work after her death.

Although generally expected and accepted as a possibility, accepting potential consequences of Mary's marriage was straightforward for neither queen nor country. While turning to her Habsburg relatives seemed natural for Mary, many of her subjects were horrified by the idea of a Spanish king, and the match was vigorously protested.[70] The key complication was the traditional and legal subordination of wives' property, rights and bodies, *their very persons*, to their husbands, and although Mary resisted rescinding her choice of husband upon her subject's demands, she too was conscious that a distinction had to be made between her marriage as queen regnant and that of a princess elevated to consort. Echoing allusions at her coronation to her 'kingly' status, and legislation reaffirming her role as the true and 'desirable' sovereign addressed, as Louis Montrose argued, the:

> [u]rgent need to assert . . . [her embodiment of] the English crown['s] . . . precedence over her foreign consort, *despite* the inferiority of her gender . . . [and, as queen in her own right] . . . the influence of her foreign husband upon the queen's rule would be tempered by [her own] counsel . . . [of] trusted men who were her natural subjects.[71]

The marriage treaty thus protected Mary's own status and powers. Despite conferring him co-monarch, it also limited Philip's role, blocking his patronage within the 'realm of England, and the dominions thereunto belonging . . . [of anyone not a subject] of the said most noble queen of England'. Furthermore, his tenure was limited to Mary's lifetime, whereby if predeceased, he was committed to freely 'permit[ting] the succession thereof to come unto them to whom it shall belong and appertain by the rights and laws of the said realm', and not removing any wealth from that realm.[72]

Significantly, although both sides of the treaty recognized that the union added England to the Habsburg 'fraternity' of kingdoms, the native integrity of the reigning dynasty of England was to be preserved even in the event of a Habsburg succession. Philip already had a son by his first wife, so, to avoid succession disputes, any children of the English marriage would yield their claims to the Spanish and Italian lands and titles of their father to their elder half-brother, 'and to the children and heirs of him descending, as well females as males'.[73] This preserved any Anglo-Spanish children as *Mary*'s heirs, consolidating their investment in English national interests, undiluted by divided affiliation with those of other, more remote Habsburg lands. Philip was prevented from removing either his pregnant wife or any potential children from England where it was expected he must 'suffer them to be nourished and brought up, unless it shall be otherwise thought good by the consent and agreement of the nobility of England'.[74] Despite the queen's affinity to her mother's family, and her confessional rather than purely nationalistic ambitions, Mary's potential family tree was essentially anglicized, cementing her as matriarch to a renewed English dynasty firmly rooted in the lineage of *her* forefathers.

Ultimately, the marriage was barren, but limitations on Philip's powers as an absentee and then widowed king did mean that the throne passed, as it would have done on the death of a childless king, to Mary's half-sister, retaining the throne within her father's nuclear family, rather than ceding it to the transcontinental dynastic empire of her husband. Xenophobia towards foreign husbands for regnant queens was a complication which had to be negotiated by all of Mary's successors. Her half-sister, Elizabeth, used her bridal *potential* as a powerful diplomatic tool in her early reign, but factional fears of the various alternative princes available were a consistent barrier to completing any of the tendered marriages.[75]

Mary II and Anne's marriages were arranged by their uncle, Charles II, but with consideration of their position as likely heiresses to the crown. Mary was married to the Stadtholder of the Netherlands, William, Prince of Orange, to conclude peace among the northern Protestant powers. There was also a dynastic dimension to the match. William was also Charles II's nephew, and next familial heir after the sisters anyway. Even so, he was viewed as a foreigner, and although officially welcomed as king in 1688, Catriona Murray rightly observes that it was *Mary* who was essentially the popular face of the co-monarchy, building on her image as England's dynastic and protestant future, nurtured throughout her childhood and early marriage.[76] Experiencing a Dutch king, his absenteeism and wars to further his alien interests, left its mark on the form of English constitutional monarchy. Future foreign regnant kings were prohibited from embroiling their British subjects, financial or military resources in the affairs of territories outside the specific domains of the English crown, or from leaving their British kingdoms without parliamentary consent.[77]

The role of Anne's husband, Prince George of Denmark, was totally unlike those of his predecessors, and became the ultimate precedent for the role and status of the husbands of Victoria and Elizabeth II. Never titularized king, Beem has described George as a constitutionally ignored, 'informal consort', 'appear[ing] by the side of his sovereign wife, both cheerful and deferential . . . [and] excel[ing] so much so [in this] that the experience hardened into what appears to us today as a curious yet durable precedent'.[78] George's 'foreignness' was negated partly by his low-key, submissive role in Anne's tenures as both heiress and queen. It was also significantly nullified by the couple's lack of surviving children, or real prospects of any more, at Anne's accession. As a dynastic presence in the future British monarchy, George was a spent force. Not so for Princes Albert and Philip, marrying young queens (or future queens), of childbearing age. Here, their foreign interests and influences were a cause of anxieties. Both were sons of impoverished minor European prince-lings, both came with natal-dynastic connections with potential to drag Britain into foreign controversies, and both marriages had been advanced by dynastically ambi-tious patriarchs whom factions in the royal family, court and society mistrusted.[79]

These were the fears of dynastic takeover occasioned by the marriage of a female sovereign which impacted England's regnant queens' marriages and images. The role of procreation in the dynastic dimension of monarchical perpetuation still needs to be considered through the lens of the dynastic legacy left or promised by each. The first three queens were all childless. This certainly left dynastic ambitions unfulfilled for Mary I, forced to leave the throne to a Protestant half-sister she was still reluctant to acknowledge. For Elizabeth I and Mary II this was not quite so. Elizabeth I's stake in the English crown's future was, in the production of a direct heir, invested in her own cult of personality and power.[80] By connecting her body with her royal lineage and the eternal mantel of sovereignty as discussed earlier, by emphasizing her 'one-ness' with her kingdom and employing, and being alluded to in, symbolism, such as the pelican or the phoenix, she created for herself a role as a quasi-mystical matriarch for the future prosperity and security of her people and by extension the monarchy itself. Indeed, so powerful was this image of her that her successors reused it to bolster their own positions and reputations as her dynastic inheritors.[81] Mary II's death from smallpox in 1694 was swift and unexpected, but, still childless at the age of thirty-two and after seventeen years of marriage, hopes for the Protestant succession and lon-gevity of the Glorious Revolution had already turned towards her younger sister. As if sealing the fate of the new regime and succession laid out in the Bill of Rights, in July 1689, Anne delivered a prince, William, duke of Gloucester, and unlike her pre-vious and future offspring, Gloucester survived infancy. Keenly aware of her status as heir and mother to the only future generation of the settlement, Anne soon fell out with her sister and brother-in-law, but both William and Mary demonstrated inter-est and affection for Gloucester, apparently happily adopting him as their own heir. After Mary's death, William and his supporters fully acknowledged him, in practice and representation, as William's eventual successor, using him in what Murray has described as a propaganda war of heirs between Williamite and Jacobite rivals. Both William and Anne were personally and politically devastated by Gloucester's death in 1700.[82] Thus, when Anne acceded in 1702, the Act of Settlement was already enacted to preserve the Protestantism of the crown by passing it, in lieu of any (unlikely) heirs of Anne's, to the Hanoverians. Although it was touted that Anne might seek to restore the Jacobite line as her nearest blood family, there is no evidence that Anne ever had such intentions, and indeed, she seems to have sought and accepted a different mode of dynastic affiliation and identity.[83]

Unlike either Mary I or II, Anne did not impale her coat of arms with that of her husband, using instead the unadulterated royal arms inherited from her great-grandfather, James I, and carried by the males of her line. Thus, in addition to having diluted her dynastic ties to her father's descendants of her father by not recognizing them as her heirs, she nullified the traditional pre-eminence of her marital dynasty, linked herself to her successors through association with their common ancestor, and prioritized national symbols as her badges of lineage over specific familial insignia, creating a crown dynasty that was in some ways above near-blood relationship. For her motto she copied Elizabeth I's *semper eadem*, and in adopting imagery which echoed that of the Virgin Queen, even overtly identifying as a second Elizabeth, she cemented Elizabeth's role as the mystic perpetual crown dynast and preserver of the Protestant faith of her subjects, and simultaneously sought the like for herself. Anne's coat of arms for the United Kingdom became the pattern for her successors, ultimately becoming fixed by the next queen regnant, Victoria, the first Hanoverian monarch whose royal arms were not emblazoned with the escutcheon of the kingdom of Hanover.

Victoria's succession was a key moment for the Britishness of the crown. The Salic laws of Hanover fully separated the two kingdoms, Victoria's uncle, the Duke of Cumberland, becoming king of Hanover upon William IV's death. Once Victoria and Albert's production of multiple heirs rendered the split permanent, Albert made it clear that cultivating a 'British' image of the royal family and the apparent preservation of the primacy of British interests was of paramount importance. When his childless brother, Ernst, whose ducal heir was Albert's second son, wished his nephew to spend more time in Germany, and questioned the relevancy of a naval career for the future ruler of land-locked Coburg, Albert wrote, 'Alfred's education must not be for Coburg alone' for his place in the British succession would take priority if necessary and 'we have to consider that there are only two eyes between him and the throne. If we make a German of him, it might be very difficult' if he ultimately succeeded Victoria.[84] Albert determined to be the model 'English gentleman' in his image and pursuits, and that his family should follow suit.[85] Nevertheless, he remained publicly unpopular, while privately both Albert and Victoria were delighted by the idea of Alfred inheriting Coburg, and Albert clearly cherished hopes of building a dynastic political network across Germanic Europe.[86] The children were taught German language and culture, and the schema Albert drew up for their marriages clearly aimed, as Jane Ridley has argued, 'to weld together a liberal, anti-Russian Anglo-German bloc'.[87] While the changing political situation in Germany, Albert's death, and political pragmatism at home prompted Victoria to semi-abandon such grand-scale marital ambitions, she did continue to act, publicly and privately, as the genetic, matriarchal glue binding together a transnational association of monarchies. She organized grand gatherings for familial occasions and family portraits including the huge 1887 Lurits Tuxen painting depicting fifty-five figures of Victoria and her descendants, 'through matchmaking ... nicknames ... letter-writing and her extra-ordinary intelligence network of ladies-in-waiting and doctors whom she posted all over the European courts'.[88] Victoria's descendants still occupy many of

Europe's surviving thrones, but reigning dynasties have become increasingly nuclear and national, rather than cosmopolitan associations of extended genetic ties.[89] As mentioned earlier, the arms of the monarch have become fixed, tied to office rather than individual. Albert's arms as Victoria's consort were a hereditary anomaly, uniquely incorporating his wife's. The submersion of his own dynastic history and identity accelerated when his eldest son, Albert, abandoned both the Saxon arms of his father, which had featured in his arms as Prince of Wales, and his patronymic Christian name upon accession as Edward VII. This was completed by 1917's family name change.

Like Albert, Prince Philip has not passed his arms onto his descendants as his children all use differentiated versions of the queen's. However, the issue of the 'Mountbatten' name has been repeatedly raised. Ten years after declaring the house and family would remain 'Windsor', Elizabeth, now expecting her third child, amended the decision to reflect both Philip's feelings and concerns raised by lawyer, Edward Iwi, that by accepted law and tradition ascribing the maternal family name to a child was the 'badge of bastardy' and consequently totally irregular in contemporary society. She now declared that while the reigning line would remain 'Windsor', untitled descendants who did not carry an H.R.H. and who may need a surname, except those in the direct line of succession, would use Mountbatten-Windsor.[90] The changing perceptions of society with regard to family names has been reflected in public interest in, and attitude towards, the question which still caused some comment and confusion at the times of the Prince of Wales's investiture (1969), and Princess Anne's marriage (1973), but has passed without particular comment during more recent royal events.[91] By the 2010s, when the future succession order was being changed to absolute primogeniture regardless of gender, amid speculation and observations that any daughters of Prince William would not be superseded by any future younger brothers and consequently female succession would no longer be anomalous, there was no discussion or consideration of any consequent change to the name of the royal house and family.

Dynasty today

Of Prince Charles's alleged intention to formally embrace Mountbatten-Windsor as the royal house upon accession, historian Andrew Roberts wrote:

> With the monarchy in its present predicament, the last thing it needs today is to divest itself of the honourable name which saw it victorious through two world wars.[92]

Chiefly objecting to the apparent tribute to the late and controversial Lord Mountbatten, whose personal and dynastic influence had loomed so threateningly in 1952, Roberts's words highlighted a common 1990s perception of the monarchy's perilous image problem among journalists and scholars .[93] Increasingly seen as remote, archaic and morally lapsed (even debauched) as three royal marriages collapsed, this crisis culminated in the aftermath of Diana, Princess of Wales's death in 1997. Her death and subsequent cultural beatification, Cannadine suggested, would see Diana ultimately achieve dynastic takeover of the monarchy, investing her memory and popularity into her children, raising their public image above their *royal* relations and branding her physical, spiritual and inspirational matriarch of the future reign and dynasty of her son.[94] However, the family has since recovered much popularity, and while Diana's sons' maturing and charisma has clearly contributed to this, so too have efforts to rehabilitate the image of Prince Charles and his second wife, and, significantly, the increasingly renewed centrality of the queen's personal image within the institution's public face. While on her coronation day, she identified 'in my parents and grandparents an example I can follow with certainty and with confidence', others were already conceiving of her within a more abstract but long-term dynastic framework, the true inheritrix, almost reincarnation of her queenly forbears, particularly Victoria and Elizabeth I.[95] Her shared Christian name with the Tudor queen had been noted even in her childhood, and upon her accession Churchill proclaimed:

> Now that we have a second Queen Elizabeth also ascending the throne in her twenty-sixth year, our thoughts are carried back nearly 400 years to the magnificent figure who presided over and in many ways embodied and inspired the grandeur and genius of the Elizabethan age.[96]

As Elizabeth II has become first the oldest and then the longest reigning sovereign in English history, this idea of a 'new Elizabethan' age has been periodically revived, and 'traditional' ceremonies of monarchy have increasingly focused on celebrating the longevity and endurance of the present monarch rather than the recent or ancient dynastic past.

However, the British monarchy is still invested in an idea of perpetuity beyond individual mortality. The wider family and a sense of dynasty play a role in both ceremonial practice and popular understanding. The royal family's surname may no longer be a subject of national attention, but as has been repeatedly noted in this chapter, fore and regnal names are also significant in a dynastic context. Ridley identifies continual cross-generational 'replication of the names Victoria and Albert' as an integral glue in constructing an extended familial network of influence across Europe, and the recent arrivals of the Duke and Duchess of Cambridge's children have highlighted the endurance of such dynastic glue in both royal and popular mindsets.[97]

In both 2013 and 2015, intense public and media speculation about name choices for the royal babies were united in the belief that the Cambridges would pick traditional 'royal' names and/or the names of close genetic family. Echoing Cannadine's predictions, on both occasions the height of speculation was around the possibility of a new princess (or even queen) Diana. In the end, 'Diana' was used only as Princess Charlotte's middle name, even then, taking third place after 'Elizabeth'. In naming his son and heir with the regnal name of the queen's much-beloved father (and grandfather), Prince William clearly associated himself and his descendants with his grandmother's line. Moreover, although Diana's legacy is ever-present in discussions of William's current popularity and his role as the 'future of the monarchy', as he has taken on increasing public and ceremonial duties he and his wife have clearly positioned themselves as much following the model of his royal grandparents as injecting the new-blood style of public life of his mother. The queen meanwhile clearly still considers her family as integral to her reign and identity as she did in 1953 when arguing that she did not 'feel at all like my great Tudor forbear, who was blessed with neither husband nor children, who ruled as a despot, and was never able to leave her native shores'.[98] Elizabeth II has embraced her role as neutral political overseer, dispenser of charity and goodwill ambassador abroad, and she has also relied on her family to represent her in these tasks. The role of the wider royal family and their consequent rights to public funds has been increasingly controversial as the executive role of government has passed from monarchy to parliament, and it is widely believed that Prince Charles intends 'slimming-down' the public family to a core branch in direct line to the throne, jettisoning the families of his siblings as they slip down the succession order.[99] Recent years have seen this begin with Prince Charles and his own descendants taking an increasingly central role and even monopolizing royal balcony appearances which would previously have been populated by the extended clan. The queen seems to be content with this arrangement, herself concentrating upon this core public branch, emphasizing her private joy in their flourishing in her Christmas broadcasts surrounded by photographs of the Cambridge wedding and babies, and publishing four-generational photographs of the monarchy for events such as Prince George's christening and her own ninetieth birthday. Nonetheless, her own public image as the heart of the monarchy still positions her as part of that wider family, something well demonstrated by the release of three official photographs by Annie Leibovitz on Elizabeth's ninetieth birthday (2016). All three were taken at Windsor Castle. One shows Elizabeth the matriarch of both Family and family, the sole adult among the younger generation, *all* her great-grandchildren and her two youngest grandchildren. The second is an intimate portrait of Elizabeth the mother with one of her own children, not the immediate heir to the throne, but her daughter Princess Anne who ranks ever-lower in the succession, but remains, for the queen, an integral figure in the current monarchy. The final portrait shows Elizabeth alone with her corgis on the ramparts of Windsor Castle, relaxed and at home within the history of the English monarchy, stretching back to medieval times, a true daughter of the House of Windsor in the spirit in which her grandfather founded it.

This chapter has demonstrated that to some extent dynastic identification was, and still is, a key component of monarchical image in England, and one which is particularly highlighted when the monarch is female. The ways in which this component has been negotiated by individual sovereigns and family branches, at and through changing sociopolitical contexts throughout the past thousand years, has both reflected and helped shape the relationship between monarch, monarchy, parliament and nation. Consequently, dynastic periodization is a useful organizational *and* analytical tool to study the history of both the monarchy and its chronologically contextual history.

Notes

1 C.S.L. Davies, "Tudor: What's in a Name?" *History* 97, no. 325 (2012), 32, n. 31.
2 Davies, "Tudor: What's in a Name?", 24–42.
3 Jeroen Duindam, *Dynasties: A Global History of Power, 1300–1800* (Cambridge: Cambridge University Press, 2016), 2; Karen Hearn, *Dynasties: Painting in Tudor and Jacobean England* (London: Tate Publishing, 1995); Kevin Sharpe, *Selling the Tudor Monarchy: Authority and Image in Sixteenth-Century England* (New Haven: Yale University Press, 2009); Liesbeth

Geevers and Mirella Marini, eds., *Dynastic Identity in Early Modern Europe: Rulers, Aristocrats and the Formation of Identities* (London: Ashgate, 2015), especially 6–9.

4 Michael Hicks, *English Political Culture in the Fifteenth Century* (London: Routledge, 2002), 34–35.

5 Daniel Schönpflug, "One European Family? A Quantitative Approach to Royal Marriage Circles 1700–1918," in *Royal Kinship: Anglo-German Family Networks 1815–1918*, ed. Karina Urbach (Munich: Saur, 2008), 25.

6 Liesbeth Geevers and Mirella Marini, "Introduction: Aristocracy, Dynasty and Identity in Early Modern Europe, 1520–1700," in Geevers and Marini, eds., *Dynastic Identity*, 13.

7 Ernst H. Kantorowicz, *The King's Two Bodies: A Study in Medieval Political Theology* (Princeton: Princeton University Press, 7th paperback edition, 1997), 7, 497–498.

8 Philip Hall, *Royal Fortune: Tax, Money and the Monarchy* (London, Bloomsbury, 1992), xi.

9 Simon Schama, "The Domestication of Majesty: Royal Family Portraiture, 1500–1850," *The Journal of Interdisciplinary History* 17, no. 1 (1986): 183. See also Linda Colley, *Britons: Forging the Nation, 1707–1837*, second edition (New Haven: Yale University Press, 2005), 209–241; Laura Lunger Knoppers, *Politicizing Domesticity from Henrietta Maria to Milton's Eve* (Cambridge University Press, Cambridge, 2011); Catriona Murray, *Imaging Stuart Family Politics: Dynastic Crisis and Continuity* (London: Routledge, 2017).

10 Howard Nenner, *The Right to be King: The Succession to the Crown of England 1603–1714* (Basingstoke: Macmillan, 1995), 8

11 Jacqueline Johnson, "Elizabeth of York: Mother of the Tudor Dynasty," in *The Rituals and Rhetoric of Queenship: Medieval to Early Modern*, eds. Liz Oakley-Brown and Louise J. Wilkinson (Dublin: Four Courts Press, 2009), 51, 54; Anne Mearns, "Unnatural, Unlawful, Ungodly and Monstrous: Manipulating the Queenly Identities of Mary I and Mary II," in *The Birth of a Queen: Essays on the Quincentenary of Mary I*, eds., Sarah Duncan and Valerie Schutte (New York: Palgrave Macmillan, 2016), 208.

12 Royal Archives, RA VIC/MAIN/QVJ (W), 5th February 1857, 43, 39.

13 In terms of legitimate offspring.

14 Anne McLaren, "Memorialising Mary and Elizabeth," in *Tudor Queenship: The Reigns of Mary and Elizabeth*, eds. Alice Hunt and Anna Whitelock (Basingstoke: Palgrave Macmillan, 2010), 17. Mary Hill Cole, "The Half-Blood Princes: Mary I, Elizabeth I, and Their Strategies of Legitimation," in Duncan and Schutte, *Birth of a Queen*, 72–73, 75.

15 Cole, "Half-Blood Princes," 74.

16 Cole, 'Half-Blood Princes," 76. Sarah Duncan, *Mary I: Gender, Power, and Ceremony in the Reign of England's First Queen* (London: Palgrave Macmillan, 2012). Hilary Doda, "Lady Mary to Queen of England: Transformation, Ritual, and the Wardrobe of the Robes," in Duncan and Schutte, *Birth of a Queen* 51, 55, 57–62.

17 Included in A. Luders et al., eds., *The Statutes of Realm* (London, 1810–1828, IV, 1), 200–201.

18 Cole, "Half-Blood Princes," 77–79.

19 Ibid., 80–83.

20 Susan Frye, "Elizabeth When a Princess: Early Self-Representations in a Portrait and a Letter," in Regina Schulte, ed., *The Body of the Queen: Gender and Rule in the Courtly World 1500–2000* (Oxford: Berghahn, 2006), 43–57.

21 Cole, "Half-Blood Princes," 84; Johnson, "Elizabeth of York," 52–54.

22 Mearns, "Unnatural, Unlawful," 202

23 Karen Bundesen, "Lousy with Cousins: Elizabeth I's Family at Court," in Oakley-Brown and Wilkinson, *Rituals and Rhetoric*, 74–89.

24 Troy Heffernen, "Protecting England and its Church: Lady Anne and the Death of Charles Stuart," *The Seventeenth Century* 31, no. 1 (2016): 57–70.

25 Mearns, "Unnatural, Unlawful," 204; Carole Levin, "Elizabeth's Ghost: The Afterlife of the Queen in Stuart England," *Royal Studies Journal* 1 (2014): 1–17.

26 Hall, *Royal Fortune*, 4–5.

27 Mearns, "Unnatural, Unlawful," 204–209.

28 'Bonnie Prince Charlie'.

29 Royal Archives, RA VIC/MAIN/QVJ (W), 12th September 1873, 62, 297–298.

30 Royal Archives, RA VIC/MAIN/QVJ (W), 23rd August 1888, 88, 50.

31 Kathryn Barron, "'For Stuart blood is in my veins' (Queen Victoria): The British Monarchy's Collection of Imagery and Objects Associated with the Exiled Stuarts from the Reign of George III to the Present Day," in *The Stuart Court in Rome: The Legacy of Exile*, ed. Edward Corp (Aldershot: Ashgate, 2003), 149–155.

32 Queen Victoria, *The Letters of Queen Victoria Volume II 1844–1853* (London: John Murray, 1908), 443.

33 Queen Victoria, *The Letters of Queen Victoria Volume I 1837–1843* (London: John Murray, 1908), 480.

34 David Cannadine, "The Last Hanoverian Sovereign? The Victorian Monarchy in Historical Perspective, 1688–1988," in *The First Modern Society: Essays in English History in Honour of Lawrence Stone*, eds. A.L. Beier, David Cannadine and James M. Rosenheim (Cambridge: Cambridge University Press, 1989), 160–164, 130.

35 Erskine Neale, *The Life of Field-Marshal His Royal Highness, Edward, Duke of Kent* (London: Richard Bentley, 1850), 266–268.

36 Alison Plowden, *The Young Victoria* (London: The History Press, new edition, 2007), 36–38.

37 Victoria, *Letters*, Vol. I, 364–365.

38 Jane Ridley "'Europe's Grandmother': Queen Victoria and her German Relations," in *Hannover, Coburg-Gotha, Windsor: Problems and Perspectives of a Comparative German-British Dynastic History from the 18th to the 20th Century*, eds. Frank-Lothar Kroll and Martin Munke (Berlin: Duncker and Humblot, 2015), 244.

39 Royal Archives, RA VIC/MAIN/QVJ (W), 24th May 1844, 17, 166.

40 Victoria, *Letters*, Vol II., 445.

41 Ridley, "Europe's Grandmother," 249.

42 Ibid., 243.

43 The National Archives, CO 323/745/46. "Proclamation declaring that the name of Windsor is to be borne by [the king's] royal house and family and relinquishing the use of all German titles and dignities, 17th July 1917."

44 Anon., "Royal House of Windsor," *The Times*, Wednesday 18 July 1917, 6. Things to do, Windsor Castle, www.windsor.gov.uk/things-to-do/windsor-castle-p43983 (accessed 27 July 2017).

45 David Cannadine, "The Context, Performance, and Meaning of Ritual: The British Monarchy and the 'Invention of Tradition' c.1820–1977," in *The Invention of Tradition*, eds. Eric Hobsbawm and Terence Ranger, twentieth edition (Cambridge: Cambridge University Press, 2012), 101–164.

46 Hall, *Royal Fortune*, 75–76.

47 Barron, "Stuart Blood," 156–157. William Shawcross, *Counting One's Blessings: The Collected Letters of Queen Elizabeth the Queen Mother* (London: Pan, 2013), 456.

48 Shawcross, *Letters*, 216–217, 221–223, 225, 229.

49 Ibid., 386, 249.

50 *The Times*, "Regency Act to be Amended," 23 July 1953, 8. *The Times*, "Royal Affairs," 24 July 1953, 8.

51 Princess Royal.

52 Shawcross, *Letters*, 551.

53 John Wonnacott, "35 Years of Portraits of the Queen from the Royal Society of Portrait Painters, *The Telegraph*, www.telegraph.co.uk/news/uknews/the_queens_diamond_jubilee/9208836/35-years-of-portraits-of-the-Queen-from-the-Royal-Society-of-Portrait-Painters.html?image=9 (accessed 20 June 2017).

54 Sarah Bradford, *Elizabeth: A Biography of Britain's Queen*, revised edition (New York: Riverhead Books, 1997), 49.

55 House of Commons Sitting of Thursday 28th January 1937, Hansard, Fifth Series, Volume 319.

56 Ibid.

57 *The Times*, "The Heiress Presumptive," 12 February 1944, 5. "Civil List," House of Commons Sitting of Wednesday 17th December 1947, Hansard, Fifth Series, Volume 445. "Princess Elizabeth's and the Duke of Edinburgh's Annuities Bill," House of Commons Sitting of Tuesday 20th January 1948, Hansard, Fifth Series, Volume 446. "Provision for the Duchess of Kent," 9th August 1831, *Journals of the House of Commons* 86

(1831). "The Duchess of Kent's Annuity Bill," 10th August 1831, *Journals of the House of Commons* 86 (1831).

58 From Our Own Correspondent, "Princess Elizabeth in Wales," *The Times*, Wednesday 7 August 1946, 7.

59 *The Times*, "A Son Born to Princess Elizabeth," 15 November 1948, 4. *The Times*, "Ducal Cornwall," Tuesday 11 July 1950, 5.

60 Giles Brandreth, *Philip and Elizabeth: The Portrait of a Marriage* (London: Century, 2004), 254–255.

61 The National Archives, CO 323/745/46. "Proclamation declaring that the name of Windsor is to be borne by [the king's] royal house and family and relinquishing the use of all German titles and dignities, 17 July 1917."

62 Davies, "What's in a name?" 24–42. The National Archives, London, LCO 2/8111, Surname of the Royal Family: Declaration by the Queen that she and her children shall be styled and known as the House and Family of Windsor.

63 LCO 2/8111.

64 LCO 2/8111.

65 LCO 2/8111.

66 Charles Beem, "Princess of Wales? Mary Tudor and the History of English Heirs to the Throne," in Duncan and Schutte, *Birth of a Queen*, 13–14, 21–22.

67 Beem, "Princess of Wales?" 20–21. Susan Doran, *Monarchy and Matrimony: The Courtships of Elizabeth I* (London: Routledge, 1996), 13–14.

68 Doran, *Monarchy and Matrimony*, 15–16.

69 Anna Whitelock, *Mary Tudor: England's First Queen* (London: Bloomsbury, 2009), 30, 204–205.

70 Ibid., 202–203, 208–209.

71 Louis Montrose, *The Subject of Elizabeth: Authority, Gender and Representation* (Chicago: University of Chicago Press, 2006), 45–46.

72 Anyusha Devendra, "Act for the Marriage of Queen Mary to Philip of Spain; 1554," http://rbsche.people.wm.edu/H111_doc_marriageofqueenmary.html (accessed 11 April 2017).

73 Ibid.

74 Ibid.

75 Doran, *Monarchy and Matrimony*.

76 Murray, *Imaging Stuart Family Politics*, 120–133, 170.

77 Christopher Kampmann, "Blessing or Burden for the Personal Union? On the Inherent Contradictions of the 'Act of Settlement'," in Kroll and Munke, eds., *Hannover, Coburg-Gotha, Windsor*, 58–59.

78 Charles Beem, "Why George of Denmark Did Not Become a King of England," in *The Man Behind the Queen: Male Consorts in History*, eds. Charles Beem and Miles Taylor (London: Palgrave Macmillan, 2014), 87–88.

79 Karina Urbach, "Prince Albert: The Creative Consort," in Beem and Taylor, *The Man Behind the Queen*, 146; Edward Owens, "Love, Duty and Diplomacy: The Mixed Response to the 1947 Engagement of Princess Elizabeth," in *Royal Heirs and the Uses of Soft Power in Nineteenth-Century Europe*, eds. Frank Müller and Heidi Mehrkens (London: Palgrave Macmillan, 2016), 225–226; Cannadine, "The Last Hanoverian Sovereign?" 131, 149, 155.

80 Roy Strong, *The Cult of Elizabeth: Elizabethan Portraiture and Pageantry* (London: Pimlico, 1999); Montrose, *The Subject of Elizabeth*.

81 Levin, "Elizabeth's Ghost"; Maureen Waller, *Sovereign Ladies: The Six Reigning Queens of England* (London: John Murray, 2007), 283–284.

82 Murray, *Imaging Stuart Family Politics*, 57–69, 98–104, 170; Edward Gregg, *Queen Anne*, new edition (New Haven: Yale University Press, 2001), 120–121.

83 Gregg, *Queen Anne*, 363–391; Daniel Szechi "Jacobite Politics in the Age of Anne," *Parliamentary History* 28, no. 1 (2009), 41–58.

84 Hector Bolitho, *The Prince Consort and His Brother: Two Hundred New Letters* (London: Cobden, 1933), 167–171.

85 Urbach, "Prince Albert"; Hall, *Royal Tax*, 11.

86 Bolitho, *New Letters*, 172–174. Royal Archives, RA VIC/MAIN/QVJ (W), 23 May 1857, 43, 148–150.

87 Ridley, "Europe's Grandmother," 243–244.

88 Ibid., 245, 249, 252–253, 257.

89 For more on monarchy and nationalism, see Milinda Banerjee, Charlotte Backerra and Cathleen Sarti, eds., *Transnational Histories of the 'Royal Nation'* (London: Palgrave Macmillan, 2017).

90 *The Times*, "Obituary: Mr Edward Iwi," 9 June 1966, 12, 16.

91 *The Illustrated London News*, "The Royal Investiture," 5 July 1969, 15–19; Patrick W. Montague-Smith, "Royal Surnames," *The Times*, 4 December 1973, 17.

92 Andrew Roberts, "A Name That Must Not Taint the Windsors," *Daily Mail*, 24 October 1994, 8.

93 See, for example, Alan Mitchell, "A Royal Relaunch for the Family Firm," *The Times*, 26 October 1994, 23; Charles Carlton, "Tudors to Windsor: An Early Modern Monarchy in a Post-Modern Britain," in *State, Sovereigns and Society in Early Modern England: Essays in Honour of A.J. Slavin*, eds. Charles Carlton, Robert Woods, Mary L. Robinson and Joseph S. Block (Stroud: Sutton Publishing, 1998), 137; David Cannadine, *History in Our Time* (New Haven: Yale University Press, 1998), 82–85.

94 Cannadine, *History in Our Time*, 74, 85.

95 Her Majesty the Queen, "A Speech by the Queen on Her Coronation Day, 1953," www.royal.uk/coronation-day-speech-2-june-1953 (accessed 21 June 2017); *The Sydney Morning Herald*, "Full Text of Churchill's Tribute to King George VI," 9 February 1952, 2.

96 E. Thornton Cook, *Royal Elizabeths: The Romance of Five Princesses 1464–1840* (London: John Murray, cheap edition, 1930), v; "Churchill's Tribute to King George VI," 2.

97 Ridley, "Europe's Grandmother," 257.

98 Her Majesty the Queen, "Elizabeth II Christmas Broadcast Speech, 1953," www.royal.uk/christmas-broadcast-1953 (accessed 19 June 2017).

99 Hall, *Royal Fortune*; Richard Kay and Geoffrey Levy, "Princes at War: How Charles' Plans for a Slimmed-Down Monarchy Have 'Driven a Dagger through Andrew's Heart' – and Sparked a Palace Power Struggle," *Daily Mail Online*, www.dailymail.co.uk/news/article-2180012/Princes-war-How-Charles-plans-slimmed-monarchy-driven-dagger-Andrews-heart–sparked-Palace-power-struggle.html (accessed 28 July 2017).

Key works

Cannadine, David, "The Last Hanoverian Sovereign? The Victorian Monarchy in Historical Perspective, 1688–1988," in *The First Modern Society: Essays in English History in Honour of Lawrence Stone*, eds. A.L. Beier, David Cannadine and James M. Rosenheim (Cambridge: Cambridge University Press, 1989), 127–166.

Davies, C.S.L., "Tudor: What's in a Name?" *History* 97, no. 325 (2012): 24–42.

Doran, Susan, *Monarchy and Matrimony: The Courtships of Elizabeth I* (London: Routledge, 1996).

Duncan, Sarah and Valerie Schutte, eds., *The Birth of a Queen: Essays on the Quincentenary of Mary I* (New York: Palgrave Macmillan, 2016).

Hall, Philip, *Royal Fortune: Tax, Money and the Monarchy* (London, Bloomsbury, 1992).

Kroll, Frank-Lothar and Martin Munke, eds., *Hannover, Coburg-Gotha, Windsor: Problems and Perspectives of a comparative German-British Dynastic History from the 18th to the 20th Century* (Berlin: Duncker and Humblot, 2015).

Murray, Catriona, *Imaging Stuart Family Politics: Dynastic Crisis and Continuity* (London: Routledge, 2017).

25

FEMALE PHARAOHS IN ANCIENT EGYPT

Aidan Norrie

Mentioning the pharaohs of ancient Egypt generally invokes images of pyramids, impressive statues and mummies.[1] These three images, however, are often associated with distinctly *male* pharaohs. Indeed, it is not unreasonable to claim that the only female ruler to come to mind is Cleopatra, Egypt's *last* pharaoh. Between the uniting of Upper and Lower Egypt by Narmer in *c.*3000 BCE and the annexation of Egypt by Augustus in 30 BCE, Egypt was ruled by hundreds of pharaohs. Significantly, and despite their absence in both the scholarship and in popular culture, at least four of these pharaohs were women.

The pharaoh played a role of immense importance in Egypt that went far beyond simple administration and defence.[2] He was the living embodiment of the god Horus, one of the most significant gods of the Egyptian pantheon, who himself was descended from Atum – the creator-god who was known as the 'father of the gods and the king'.[3] Because of his descent from the gods, the pharaoh served as the intermediary between the gods and the people. The pharaoh's primary task, however, was maintaining *maat*: the divine order.[4] Should the pharaoh preserve *maat*, Egypt would prosper because the gods were pleased; should *maat* fail to be preserved, chaos would reign in Egypt. The pressure to maintain *maat* – which for a pharaoh included officiating in the various temples, keeping Egypt safe from both internal and external threats, building new temples for the gods, and ensuring that justice was delivered through the courts – meant that Egyptians desired to have a healthy and youthful man on the throne: a man who was the son of the preceding pharaoh, who could sire future pharaohs and who could successfully lead Egypt's armies.[5] As is the case with monarchies across the globe, this ideal, however ardently it is upheld, is invariably thwarted. Pharaonic Egypt was not exempted from succession crises caused by necessary deviations from this ideal. This chapter focuses on one important way that this 'ideal' succession deviated: when a woman was pharaoh.

Using the reigns of the four known female pharaohs as case studies, this chapter argues that Egyptians understood that the *office* of pharaoh was distinct from the *person* of the pharaoh, meaning that women could, under the right circumstances, succeed to the throne. Much like the (probably fictional) legal concept of the king's two bodies that Ernst Kantorowicz made famous,[6] Egyptians drew a distinction between the *hem* – the 'person' of the king – and the office of king.[7] This distinction was important due to the king's embodiment of Horus: from birth, he was imbued with a degree of divinity – after all, he was the son of a god – but he did not become divine until his accession and the coronation.[8] This separation of the body politic from the body natural allowed Egypt's *maat* to be preserved: an elderly, infant, disabled, or female pharaoh was not an issue, as long as there was a pharaoh on the throne. This is because once the pharaoh 'had undergone the correct coronation rituals he, or she, acquired a veneer of divinity that would allow him, or her, to function as a proper king'.[9] Nevertheless, while the sex of the pharaoh may not preclude accession, the pharaoh's gender – that is, 'a social category imposed on a sexed body' – certainly impacted the way a female pharaoh ruled, and this impact is thus the focus of this study.[10]

In a monarchy that was depicted as masculine and generally conceived of as being male, there were changes to the depictions of these female pharaohs visible in both their titulary and the surviving material culture. Some female pharaohs adopted masculine artistic standards and political conventions; some continued to present themselves as ruling women; and others combined the two styles. By focusing on the way that female pharaohs reigned and how they presented themselves and their reign, this chapter presents the first scholarly analysis of the reigns of the four female pharaohs of Egypt – Sobekneferu, Hatshepsut, Tausret and Cleopatra VII – and as such, focuses on the way they legitimized their rule by accentuating their royal status and the way their gender impacted their reign and legacy.

Thanks to the rise of Egyptology in the nineteenth century, Egypt and its pharaohs have been the subject of sustained study from academics and of unrelenting interest from the public.[11] What is absent from many of these academic works on the Egyptian monarchs is sustained scholarly analysis of the female pharaohs. The limited evidence of their rule – compared to the many male pharaohs – makes detailed studies more challenging, and the lives of the female pharaohs are often only revealed in popular histories.[12] Indeed, this chapter provides one of the few academic studies that analyses the lives and reigns of the female pharaohs together, and treats their reigns as a distinct historical phenomenon. This chapter builds on the works of Joyce Tyldesley and Catharine H. Roehrig, who have provided thoroughly researched and well contextualized studies of Hatshepsut's reign,[13] as well as the collections of essays edited by José M. Galán, Betsy M. Bryan and Peter F. Dorman, and Richard H. Wilkinson – both collections adding greatly to the scholarship on female rule in Egypt.[14] By building on these works, this chapter is well situated in terms of the scholarship and thus provides a gender-aware history of these women.

Space constraints mean that this chapter will not engage with the potential reigns of heavily contested female pharaohs or female co-regencies. As such, the (potentially apocryphal) pharaohs Khentkawes, Nitocris and Neferneferuaten will not be discussed here, neither will the reigns of the co-regents Arsinoe II, Berenice III, Berenice IV or Cleopatra VI be included. These women certainly exercised royal authority, but there is uncertainty surrounding their lives, and the circumstances in which they assumed the throne leaves too much to speculation.[15] Sobekneferu, Hatshepsut, Tausret and Cleopatra VII form a stronger set of examples to explore the dynamics of female rule in Egypt during the pharaonic period and have thus been selected as the focus for this case study.

Queen or female king?

In the more gender conscious scholarship on medieval and early modern Europe, women who ruled as queens regnant are increasingly referred to, or conceptualized as, female kings – thanks in part to the work of William Monter.[16] While this shift in description is useful and more reflective of the way that monarchs were conceived of by their subjects, I contend that the term is most applicable in pharaonic Egypt. Unlike most European societies, Egyptian women of all classes were full citizens under the law. Thus, men and women of equal social standing were equivalent under the law, and both could trade and inherit property, sue and be sued in court, and conduct business transactions.[17] This legal equality gave greater sociopolitical legitimization for the accession of women in Egypt than many European female kings in the medieval and early modern periods.

Unlike in European monarchies where, as Theresa Earenfight has observed, an adjective was usually added to the title of queen to denote which 'type' of queen she was – that is, regnant, consort, regent, or dowager – *pharaoh* was not gendered.[18] Indeed, in Egypt, the queen's title, *Hmt nswt* (sometimes rendered in English as *hemet nesw*), literally translates as 'king's wife'.[19] Any royal woman referred to as queen, therefore, was, or had been, the wife of a king. In thinking about the way that these women exercised their authority then, it is essential that these women be understood as female pharaohs and not as queens. Hatshepsut, Sobekneferu and Tausret were all pharaohs, just like Ramses the Great, Tutankhamen and Amenhotep III.

Sobekneferu

As previously indicated, the ideal monarchical succession in Egypt was when the male pharaoh died, he would be succeeded by his eldest son who was the child of his principal wife. History demonstrates, however, that this ideal succession was often not possible. Indeed, the tradition of the pharaoh having more than one wife, with sons from these secondary wives also able to succeed, acknowledges this reality. In the Twelfth Dynasty (*c.*1938–*c.*1755 BCE), women became central to the succession issue for the first time.

Beginning in the Eleventh Dynasty (*c.*2080–*c.*1938 BCE), and in an attempt to stabilize the succession, pharaohs instigated the use of co-regents. This anticipatory succession – where the king would choose his successor and have him crowned, and the two would rule together until the older king died, at which time the other king would become the sole ruler – is an example of an attachment to the 'ideal' succession. Its appearance across the globe (such as the case of Henry the Young King in twelfth-century England, or in Muscovy, which is the subject of Russell Martin's chapter in this volume) attests to its political and social utility.[20] This trend continued into the Twelfth Dynasty, where the founder of the dynasty, Amenemhat I, had his son, Senusret I, crowned as co-regent in the twentieth year of his reign.

The penultimate pharaoh of the Twelfth Dynasty was Amenemhat IV (r.*c.*1770–*c.*1760 BCE). He reigned as co-regent for two years with his predecessor, Amenemhat III, who, depending on how the inscriptions are translated, was his father, grandfather or step-father.[21] However, as Amenemhat's mother, Hetepi, lacks the title of 'king's wife' in her mortuary titulary, it is likely that he was Amenemhat

III's step-son, rather than his biological son.[22] Amenemhat IV is unlikely to have had any children; thus, when he died, the throne passed to his closest living royal relative: Sobekneferu.

Sobekneferu (also Neferusobek or Skemiophris, r.c.1760–c.1755 BCE) was the daughter of Amenemhat III and was thus either the sister or step-sister of Amenemhat IV. Virtually nothing is known about her accession, but she is certainly the first female pharaoh in Egypt who is named in the contemporary king lists.[23] She is included in Manetho's king list – appearing as Skemiophris – who gives her a reign of four years,[24] and the Turin King List – a list of the pharaohs of Egypt compiled during the reign of Ramses the Great (r.c.1279–c.1213 BCE) – gives her a reign of three years, ten months and twenty-four days. She is also included in the Saqqara King List in position twenty-two, following Amenemhat III and Amenemhat IV, who are numbered twenty and twenty-one respectively.[25]

Her name – which means 'Beauty of Sobek' – refers to the crocodile god Sobek, and Sobekneferu was the first of at least eight other pharaohs who would later link themselves with the god variously associated with pharaonic power, the Nile, military prowess and fertility.[26] In demonstrating her association with Sobek, she continued the (upward) shift in the god's status that her father and grandfather had instigated. Faiyum was established during the Twelfth Dynasty, and the city was the home of the cult of Sobek – hence its Greek name, Krokodilopolis. Sobekneferu's association with the cult anticipates the important place the cult would hold for pharaohs of the Thirteenth Dynasty (c.1755–c.1630 BCE).

As the first woman to rule as pharaoh, Sobekneferu asserted her authority in unique ways. There can be no doubt that she assumed the full royal titulary, albeit with the titles sometimes gendered feminine.[27] The royal titulary, known as the 'five names', were the official titles adopted by the pharaoh on their accession: the Horus name was the name adopted by the pharaoh when he or she ascended the throne; the Nebty name linked the pharaoh to Nekhbet and Wadjet, the goddesses of Upper and Lower Egypt, respectively; the Golden Horus (sometimes called the Golden Falcon) name indicated the divine status of the pharaoh; the nomen name linked the pharaoh to the god Re and was enclosed in a cartouche; and the prenomen name, which was also enclosed in a cartouche, was probably the pharaoh's birth name. Sobekneferu's five names – 'The one beloved of Re' as her Horus; 'The daughter of the powerful one [i.e. Amenemhat III] is now Mistress of the Two Lands' as her Nebty; 'Stable of appearances' as her Golden Horus; 'The very *ka* [soul] of Sobek-Re' as her prenomen; and 'Sobek is perfect' as her nomen – provide unequivocal proof of her status as a female pharaoh.[28]

The gender ambiguity of Sobekneferu's titles is visible in the various inscriptions that invoke her titles: a bead, likely from Faiyum, calls her 'King of Upper and Lower Egypt', as does an inscription on a seal located in the Cairo Museum; she is referred to variously both as the *Son* and *Daughter* of Re; sometimes her Golden Horus name was gendered male – and this gender-switching sometimes occurred on the same object, such as the inscription that calls her 'the *female* Horus, *Lord* of Action'.[29]

Despite some of the older scholarship that sought to downplay Sobekneferu's rule – often based on this gender ambiguity in her titles – her rule is unequivocally attested in the limited surviving material culture from the period. The locations where many of Sobekneferu's various statues have been found – Tell el Dab'a, Hawara and

Herkleopolis – are sites where archaeological evidence of important temples and royal tombs have been found.[30] These locations – many of which are associated with famous male pharaohs, including Amenemhat III and Mentuhotep II – emphasize her exercise of pharaonic power, particularly the pharaoh's role in maintaining *maat*. The most important evidence that Sobekneferu ruled as a female pharaoh, however, is a cylinder seal that is inscribed with her five names, which is held by the British Museum.[31] The seal uses a male Horus for her Golden Horus name, potentially demonstrating the genderless office of king.

Sobekneferu, as Hatshepsut would also do, often sought to emphasize her descent from her father. A fragment of a column, now in the Cairo Museum, displays both Amenemhat III and Sobekneferu. The column had 'propaganda value' for Sobekneferu: not only had her father already been deified by the time the column had been erected, but it also visually linked her with a god, especially given that her father's Horus is extending her the sceptre of power.[32] Sobeknerferu's name also appears on three red-granite columns in the Harawa pyramid complex: Flinders Petrie, who first excavated the site in the late-nineteenth century, noted that her name appears as many times as Amenemhat III's.[33] Most importantly, Amenemhat IV's name does not appear, meaning that it was Sobekneferu, not her predecessor, who completed the famous labyrinth at Hawara, which was written about by Herodotus: 'I have seen this building, and it is beyond my power to describe . . . the pyramids are astonishing structures . . . but the labyrinth surpasses them.'[34]

The damage many of the surviving artefacts have sustained does make it difficult to fully assess the various ways the first positively identified female pharaoh was depicted. For example, a damaged statue in the Metropolitan Museum of Art depicts a woman – likely Sobekneferu – wearing a *heb sed* cloak (a ceremony that celebrated the continued rule of a pharaoh). The regalia and headwear is unusual and potentially unique, and while the style is typical of similar statues of Middle Kingdom male pharaohs, the figure is clearly a woman. Most importantly, it is the only known example of a female ruler wearing a *heb sed* garment in the entire pharaonic period.[35]

One of the most important pieces of evidence of Sobekneferu's rule is not related to statuary or any 'official' propaganda: it is a graffito of her name on the Second Cataract (or Great Cataract) of the Nile. The cataracts were sections of the Nile that were only navigable during a flood, because they were where the river was normally shallow and rocky. In the third year of her reign, officials marked that the flood level only reached 1.83 metres, which may have caused economic difficulties for Sobekneferu.[36] As the graffito served no 'official' purpose – it was for localized record keeping, mainly – her name's survival demonstrates that her reign was accepted outside elite court circles.

Three, almost life-size, fragmentary basalt statues of Sobekneferu survive from Tell El-Dab'a: one shows her kneeling on a rectangular plinth, and the other two depict her sitting on a throne. These statues, which demonstrate Sobekneferu's authority as a female pharaoh, very closely resemble statues made for Hatshepsut shortly after her coronation, indicating that Hatshepsut's were likely modelled on them.[37] The minimal, and sometimes unconfirmed, amount of material evidence for her reign has meant that she is overshadowed by Cleopatra and Hatshepsut. Nevertheless, there can be little doubt that Sobekneferu not only ruled as a female pharaoh but that her reign also paved the way for later female pharaohs to legitimize their own reigns.

Sobekneferu was the last ruler of the Twelfth Dynasty, which Egyptologists have long considered the high point of the Middle Kingdom (*c*.2010–*c*.1630 BCE). She had no children and is unlikely to have been married. Despite her lack of a biological heir, it is unclear what her relationship with the pharaohs of the Thirteenth Dynasty was, as there is no evidence of a break between rulers that usually characterizes dynasty changes.[38] Her tomb has not yet been positively identified.

Hatshepsut

Excepting Cleopatra, Hatshepsut is arguably the most well known of the female pharaohs. Hatshepsut (r.*c*.1473–*c*.1458 BCE) is perhaps most remembered because she embarked on one of the most ambitious building programmes of any pharaoh – male or female – and her mortuary temple at Deir el-Bahri was so impressive that successive pharaohs built around it and emulated its design. In spite of these impressive achievements, Hatshepsut has also suffered from negative assessments based solely on her gender. As a woman ruling in a traditionally masculine society, Hatshepsut has been tarnished in the scholarship with the wicked step-mother stereotype;[39] it has taken more recent, revisionist scholars – such as Gae Callender and Joyce Tyldesley – to demonstrate that Hatshepsut did indeed rule as a female pharaoh and that her exercise of authority was just as legitimate as any male pharaoh's.[40]

Unlike Sobekneferu, Hatshepsut did not ascend the throne by descent alone; instead, like Tausret after her, she forged her own path to the Horus throne, making use of her royal blood and her family connections. Her father was the third pharaoh of the Eighteenth Dynasty, Thutmose I (r.*c*.1493–*c*.1481 BCE), and her mother was Thutmose's principal wife, Ahmose. Thutmose and Ahmose had two daughters (Hatshepsut and Nefrubity), so on his death, Thutmose was succeeded by a son from a secondary wife, who reigned as Thutmose II (r.*c*.1481–*c*.1479 BCE).[41] Hatshepsut married Thutmose II (her half-brother) and reigned as his queen. As the marriage only produced one daughter, Neferure, Thutmose II was also succeeded by a son from a secondary wife when he died, after a reign of less than three years.[42] Thutmose III, however, was an infant at his accession – probably around two years old – so Hatshepsut, the daughter, sister and wife of pharaohs was installed as regent.

The evidence indicates that the first years of the regency operated as was traditional: with Thutmose III as pharaoh, and Hatshepsut as 'Mistress of the Two Lands'.[43] Then, in the seventh year of the regency, Hatshepsut was crowned pharaoh and assumed the five names.[44] The reasons for this sudden change have long been debated: perhaps external affairs required an adult monarch's intervention, or there were worries over the legitimacy of the boy-pharaoh whose links to the dynasty's founder were rather tenuous.[45] Whatever the reason, Hatshepsut was now pharaoh, and Thutmose III was sidelined.

The changing nature of Hatshepsut's artistic depictions seem to mirror her increasing political authority. During the early years of her regency, Hatshepsut was depicted as would be expected of a royal woman; after her coronation, she was depicted as a woman wearing the clothing of a king; later she was depicted as a man, dressed in the ruling regalia of a king.[46] Interestingly though, her royal titles are less clear, as throughout her reign she continued to use both masculine and feminine forms of the royal titulary.[47] However Hatshepsut assumed the throne, she certainly ruled as pharaoh. Though she reigned for approximately twenty years, there is no evidence that anyone ever attempted to remove her from power, including Thutmose III.[48]

As the only surviving child of Thutmose I and his principal wife, Hatshepsut claimed to be the true heir of the widely loved pharaoh. Like Sobekneferu before her, Hatshepsut continually linked herself with her father, and claimed the dual divinity afforded to pharaohs at their coronation and the divinity that came from being the daughter of a god-pharaoh: as Thutmose I was declared 'the very image of Amun', Hatshepsut claimed to be the 'Daughter of Amun'.[49] Hatshepsut also procured a (probably fabricated) oracle from Amun that not only confirmed her as his daughter but also declared that his daughter was pharaoh.[50]

Hatshepsut is most famous for her massive mortuary temple at Deir el-Bahri – which depicts Hatshepsut at the end of her reign, when she was indisputably ruling as pharaoh – and many of the statues I discuss later come from this temple. The temple's placement linked her to Mentuhotep II (r.c.2010–c.1960 BCE), the pharaoh who successfully reunited Egypt after the First Intermediate Period (c.2125–c.2010 BCE) and was subsequently heralded as the progenitor of a golden age in Egypt's history – Hatshepsut visibly demonstrating her desire to usher in the next golden age of Egypt.[51] The temple was built according to Hatshepsut's own plans and as her *Djeser-djeseru* (holy of holies) was intended to function as the cult that would ensure her eternal life. The story of Hatshepsut's 'divine' conception and birth is recorded on the walls – Hatshepsut was conceived when her mother was visited by Amun-Re (in the guise of Thutmose I). Various scenes of the pharaoh ensuring *maat* – such as offerings to Amun-Re, the subjugation of Nubia and a sphinx-Hatshepsut tramping and smiting 'generic' Asiatic invaders – all depict Hatshepsut as male and wearing various pharonic crowns.[52] During her reign, Hatshepsut led military missions to Lebanon, and she embarked on a highly successful and well-known trade mission to the land of Punt (which returned with thirty-one live myrrh trees; an endeavour that is the first recorded attempt to transplant foreign trees) – events that are depicted on the temple walls as demonstrations of the keeping of *maat*.[53]

Hatshepsut's shifting gendered depiction is most pronounced in her ornaments and statutory. I would argue, too, that the very ability to shift iconographic depictions so noticeably over a relatively short period of time demonstrates an understanding of the separation of the person of the pharaoh from the office of pharaoh. A badly damaged life-size statue from the beginning of her reign shows her in female garb and wearing a *khat* headdress – a royal, rather than pharaonic, item. Likewise, a sphinx from the joint reign with Thutmose combines feminine features, such as her face being painted yellow (the colour used for women), with the traditional kingly style, including a mane.[54] Interestingly, one of the sphinxes uses masculine pronouns, the other feminine. Herbert Winlock convincingly argues that if the sphinxes were placed atop posts at the head of the ramp between the lower and middle terraces at Deir el-Bahri (as is likely), they would have served a welcoming, or greeting function (rather than the defensive guardianship the outdoor sphinxes portrayed), and their use of both masculine and feminine pronouns is further evidence of Hatshepsut's adoption of both masculine and feminine trappings of pharaonic power.[55] Both, however, are inscribed: 'Maatkare [Hatshepsut's prenomen], beloved of Amun, given life forever.'[56] The gender ambiguity of Hatshepsut's image is generally associated with smaller pieces, which were probably produced during the early part of her reign when her role as pharaoh was somewhat in flux.

Following her coronation, however, Hatshepsut the woman became merged with the office of pharaoh. It is thus unsurprising that the woman who had served as wife and regent to male pharaohs chose to have the colossal external statutory of her temple depict her unambiguously as Osiris – the *god* of the underworld. Other statues from later in her reign demonstrate Hatshepsut's adoption of masculine depictions. A larger than life-size statue features her wearing the *nemes* headcloth of the pharaoh (the same as the famous gold and blue-glass funerary mask of Tutankhamun), and her torso is demonstrably male, although she lacks a fake beard. Her primary titles are rendered masculine ('King of Upper and Lower Egypt'), although she retains her feminine prenomen.[57] In an offertory statute from her temple, she offers *maat* to Amun as a king, complete with *nemes* headdress, fake beard and *shendyt* kilt.[58] Another similar statue depicts an offering of plants to Amun – not only is she wearing the false beard and kilt, but she also wears the white crown of Upper Egypt, which unequivocally proves her rule as a female pharaoh.[59] The inscription is badly damaged, but what has been recovered include her Horus name, *Wosretkau*, inside a *serekh* (a kind of royal crest), and both her throne name and birth name appear in cartouches.

While her temple at Deir el-Bahari is the most famous example of her architectural authority, she also instigated a temple-building project in every major Egyptian city. In addition to her mortuary temple, she was responsible for the Red Chapel at Karnak, the Netjery-menu (Divine of Monuments), various obelisks – one of which was the largest obelisk ever constructed in the ancient world – and the Temple of Mut-in-Isheru at north Karnak.[60] These temples all reinforced her relationship with Amun and were part of the increased prominence Amun was attaining in Egypt – much like Sobekneferu's association with Sobek heralded that god's increasing prominence.

Hatshepsut died in *c.*1458 BCE after around twenty years on the throne, and Thutmose III reigned for a further thirty. Near the end of his reign, Thutmose began a programme to erase evidence of Hatshepsut's reign. Her cartouches and images were chiselled off walls, her statues were pulled down and he usurped her temples and monuments for himself.[61] Thutmose's programme was so successful that Hatshepsut's name was left off many official king lists. When Egyptologists rediscovered Hatshepsut – especially her temple at Thebes – it was assumed that she was the subject of *damnatio memoriae*, with the intention of causing her a second death in the afterlife. This led to the rise of the standard historical approach that Thutmose III attempted to erase Hatshepsut's memory because he was furious at his step-mother's usurpation of his throne. Recently, the lack of evidence for the *damnatio memoriae*, coupled with the delayed and inconsistent implementation of it after Hatshepsut's death, has been reassessed by scholars including Gae Callender, Joyce Tyldesley and Cathleen Keller, and all three conclude that Thutmose was instead likely intimidated by the success of his step-mother, and his failure to live up to her legacy meant that in a fit of jealousy, he tried to eradicate his competition.[62] Thus, rather than relying on the wicked step-mother trope, it is instead likely that Hatshepsut's successful reign meant that her male successor felt the need to remove her impressive legacy so that it did not overshadow his own.

Tausret

The third of the women to rule Egypt as pharaoh was Tausret – also rendered Tawosret and Twosret – who reigned *c*.1198–*c*.1190 BCE as the last pharaoh of the Nineteenth Dynasty (*c*.1292–*c*.1190 BCE). Tausret's path to the throne mirrors Hatshepsut's: granddaughter of Ramses II (Ramses the Great) and daughter of Merneptah (r.*c*.1213–*c*.1204 BCE) she was married to Seti II (r.*c*.1204–*c*.1198 BCE), served as the regent of his infant son, Siptah, and in the absence of any other male heir, ruled in her own right after the boy's death.[63] Tausret is given a seven-year reign by Manetho, although recent archaeological discoveries could put it as long as ten years.

The prenomen Tausret chose on her accession – 'Daughter of Re, beloved of Amun' – leaves no doubt that she ruled as pharaoh.[64] Likewise, her Horus name – 'Victorious bull, beloved of Maat, and possessor of beauty as king like Atum' – links her closely to Ramses, whose own Horus name was 'Victorious bull, beloved of Maat'.[65] Her relatively short reign, coupled with the way most of her monuments 'were altered, partially erased, or covered over in succeeding reigns' means details of her reign and the surviving material culture are often subject to speculative interpretation.[66]

Evidence survives for her role as regent for Siptah, including a damaged statue likely depicting Siptah sitting in her lap, and in a small temple dedicated to Amun and Re-Horakhty at Amada, in Nubia. Tausret is carved into the right side of the doorframe, facing left, and holding two *sistra* (a sacred instrument) in front of her. Dressed as a queen, the inscription identifies her as the 'God's Wife of Amun, the King's Great Wife, Lady of the Two Lands, Tausret-beloved-of-Mut, justified.'[67]

The only surviving statue that depicts Tausret as pharaoh was found at Medinet Nasr. While the statue is missing its head, the inscriptions identify the figure as Tausret. The almost life-size statue depicts her seated on a throne, and the remains of a *nemes*-headcloth are visible. While the figure is clearly a woman – her breasts are visible – the attire is mostly masculine, but she is not 'pretending' to be a man. She is instead 'wearing the costume appropriate for the accoutrements of a king'.[68] The inscriptions around the base identify her as pharaoh and list her various names and epithets – although the names and titles mix genders. In the inscription on the right side of the base, Tausret is declared: 'Living Horus Strong-bull-beloved-of-Maat, Beautiful lord as king like Atum, King of Upper and Lower Egypt, Daughter-of-Re-beloved-of-Amun, Son of Re, Tausret, chosen-of-Mut, beloved of Hathor-lady-of-the-red-mountain.'[69] Comparing this inscription with the one made in the temple at Amada while she was regent demonstrates her distinct reign as a female pharaoh. Tausret, like Hatshepsut, had to distinguish her reign as pharaoh from her time as regent – something Sobekneferu did not have to do.

As pharaoh, Tausret constructed a temple in western Thebes. This 'strip' of desert had been used for royal temples since the early Eighteenth Dynasty, and Tausret placed her 'Temple of Millions of Years' – so called because they honoured and preserved a person's spirit throughout all time – midway between the temples of her father Merneptah and Thutmose IV (Hatshepsut's great-great-great nephew, r.*c*.1400–*c*.1390 BCE).[70] The monument was completed, or very nearly finished, but was quarried for its stone soon afterwards (a not-uncommon ending for monuments in pharaonic Egypt), which means other than a basic floorplan, we know nothing of the temple's decoration.[71] Despite the lack of evidence from the temple, its plan closely follows the great Ramesseum (built by Ramses the Great), further linking the dynasty's last monarch with its greatest, and its very construction and placement demonstrates Tausret's full assumption of pharaonic authority.[72]

Tausret had no (surviving) children, and she was either succeeded (when she died) or overthrown by Sethnakhte, the first and founding pharaoh of the Twentieth Dynasty.[73] Her mummy has also not been conclusively identified. As befits her rise to the throne, her tomb was commenced during the reign of her husband; it was then enlarged while regent and then enlarged again during her own reign. In a tradition dating to the reign of Ramses I, queens were buried in a separate valley to kings, which has led to the existence of what is now known as the Valley of the Queens and the Valley of the Kings.[74] Tausret's political power – even before her accession – is demonstrated by the fact that her tomb was begun during the second year of her husband's reign in the Valley of the Kings. As Catharine Roehrig perceptively argues, 'The fact that her husband planned a burial for Tausret in what had become exclusively a king's cemetery suggests that very early on she played a more significant role in the court than that of most principal queens.'[75] Her successor, Sethnakhte, usurped the tomb as his own, and her sarcophagus was reused by Prince Amenherkhepshef, the son of Ramses IV. Despite the absence of a tomb, her reign is well attested in images and ephemera that have been found across Egypt. As pharaoh, she oversaw an expedition to the turquoise mines in Sinai, and her status as pharaoh is supported by ephemera found bearing her name in Lebanon, Palestine and Nubia.[76] Her *nebty* name, 'Who has founded Egypt and subdued foreign countries' (which is rendered masculine), hints that foreign incursions may have been behind her assuming the throne.[77] Like Hatshepsut before her, Tausret, the daughter and wife of pharaohs, was able to effectively fulfil the role of pharaohs – even when that meant defending Egypt's borders to preserve *maat*.

As was mentioned at the beginning of this chapter, there are similarities and differences in the ways that the three female pharaohs discussed thus far succeeded the throne. All three women combined masculine and feminine styles in their artistic and iconographic representations, although Tausret retained greater femininity in her depiction than Hatshepsut.[78] Both Hatshepsut and Tausret had been royal wives before their succession, and their path to the throne was via the regency of a young pharaoh who was not their son. Unlike Hatshepsut, Tausret was never co-regent with Siptah, neither did she attempt to subsume his reign into her own. Finally, the Horus name Tausret adopted – 'Victorious Bull, beloved of Maat' – demonstrates the undisputable authority she exercised: neither Hatshepsut nor Sobekneferu adopted a Horus name that was previously the marker of the most successful male pharaohs and Egyptian gods.[79]

Cleopatra

It is no exaggeration to suggest that Cleopatra is not only the most well-known woman ruler of Egypt, but also the most well-known Egyptian pharaoh. Indeed, the fact that she is known mononymously as Cleopatra – despite being the seventh woman to bear that name – emphasizes her renown.[80] The plethora of scholarship on Cleopatra, as well as the fact that the vast majority of evidence we have from her reigns comes from Roman sources that focus on her relationships with Julius Caesar and Marc Antony, means that her analysis here will be somewhat curtailed and will instead be focused on the material cultural evidence of her pharaonic rule. Nevertheless, while Cleopatra reigned during a period where several other Hellenistic cultures had female rulers – such as Artemisia of Halicarnassus – these reigns were usually restricted to 'moments of power for ruling women between husbands'.[81] Thus, it is without hyperbole that Duane Roller has argued 'there was no one like Cleopatra VII, ruling for 22 years and married only in name', and that her 'theory of rule' was 'influenced by the handful of indigenous Egyptian queens, most notably Hatshepsut'.[82]

Cleopatra, the sixteenth and final ruler of the Ptolemaic dynasty (303–30 BCE), was born in 69 BCE as the second daughter (and child) of Ptolemy XII and Cleopatra V.[83] The details of her accession(s) to the throne are unclear and sometimes contradictory. It is possible that while her father was in exile in Rome, Cleopatra and her mother ruled Egypt as co-regents between 57 and 55 BCE.[84] The situation of the succession after Ptolemy's death in 51 is also unclear: certainly, Cleopatra was crowned pharaoh and succeeded him. However, there is conflicting evidence as to whether she ruled alone and was later forced into a co-regency with her brother, Ptolemy XIII, or whether they were crowned together (as was stipulated in their father's will).[85] Ptolemy was killed in a sea battle in 48 BCE; soon after, in 47 BCE, another brother, Ptolemy XIV, was crowned co-regent. Interestingly, while Cleopatra's Horus name is confirmed – 'The great one, possessor of perfection and splendid of shrine' – neither Ptolemy XIII nor Ptolemy XIV appear to have adopted any royal titulary; certainly, none is attested in the hieroglyphs.[86] Cleopatra had two other names – a second Horus name, 'The great one and the (very) image of her father', and an added epithet to her prenomen, 'The goddess, beloved of her father' – both of which demonstrate her royal descent and the authority she drew from invoking her father.[87]

After the death of Caesar in 44 BCE, Cleopatra murdered her brother, Ptolemy XIV. She then elevated her son by Caesar – Caesarion – to co-regent as Ptolemy XV.[88] These convoluted co-regencies, interspersed with periods of sole rule, make characterizing Cleopatra's reign difficult. Likewise, the Roman *damnatio memoriae* against Cleopatra was certainly effective, removing many traces of her rule. What can be said of her reign, however, was that she was a clever political operator who was continually reshaping her rule to ensure she remained in power.

It is well known that she was the first Ptolemaic pharaoh to learn hieroglyphs, and one of her most astute political moves was to ally herself culturally with the Egyptians. Cleopatra demonstrated her commitment to Egyptian culture by restoring traditional religious rites and cults (many of which had been denigrated by her own family).[89] To make herself (and her family) more popular, she decreased taxes. In a taxation decree dating from 41, and found at Herkleopolis, Cleopatra asserts her authority over her son, although the survival of only the Greek version prevents us from knowing how her rule was expressed in hieroglyphs. Regardless, she is mentioned first, and her Horus name is referred to: 'Queen Cleopatra, Father-loving Goddess, and king Ptolemy, who is also Caesar, Father-loving, Mother-loving God.'[90]

The most important evidence for Cleopatra's rule comes from the reliefs on the temple of Hathor at Dendera. The temple, which was constructed on her orders, depicts her as the goddess Hathor. She stands to the left of Ptolemy XV, who is wearing the double crown of Egypt, the traditional symbol of Egyptian kingship. However, Cleopatra wears a *hepty* crown, which features two falcon feathers and a disc. This crown signifies kingship and symbolizes 'the dignity of the goddess [Hathor] as a female king'.[91] This iconography, combined with the fact that Cleopatra is referred to as the 'Ruler and Mistress of the Two Lands' inside the temple – while Ptolemy is not – demonstrates her rule as a female pharaoh. Like Hatshepsut, Cleopatra is depicted as Hathor, the cow who gave birth to and protected the pharaohs: she did not abdicate the throne in favour of her son – he was the junior monarch in their joint reign. Also, at Dendera, Cleopatra is depicted wearing the crown of Arsinoe II, the powerful co-ruler of Ptolemy II, which served to emphasize her royal and divine descent (given that Arsinoe had been defied and was still worshipped in cults around the Mediterranean).[92]

Despite the evidence examined here, the intrigues that surround Cleopatra, particularly concerning her death, have often obscured the fact that she successfully ruled as a female pharaoh, in an increasingly unstable geo-political context. Unique of the four pharaohs analysed here, Cleopatra had a child – a son and heir – who could be used to increase her own political and iconographic power. Drawing on the increasingly interconnected Hellenistic world, Cleopatra identified herself with the Hellenized goddess Isis, allowing her to be depicted as a divine mother, an identity, Joyce Tyldesley argues, 'that would be instantly recognizable to both her Egyptian and her Greek subjects'.[93] As the living embodiment of Isis, Cleopatra was 'a mother, a healer, and a powerful magician', and this embodiment further linked her to her father, Ptolemy XII, who had been revered as a new Dionysus.[94] Of the four female pharaohs analysed here, however, Cleopatra appropriated fewer of the artistic trappings of male kingship: as she is often depicted alongside her son, he was generally the one given masculine attributes. Nevertheless, Cleopatra, like Hatshepsut and Tausret, was memorialized as the 'Ruler and Mistress of the Two Lands', and ensured the continuation of *maat* by defending Egypt's borders and building temples to properly worship the gods.

The (after)lives of the female pharaohs

Thanks to the burgeoning field of queenship studies, the reigns of women who exercised monarchical authority across the globe are increasingly being given due attention by scholars. These women were not 'usurpers' or 'temporary regents' but were legitimate rulers who reigned over their subjects. Egypt, the land of mummies, pyramids and pharaohs, was one of the first societies to allow women to exercise supreme political authority. Between the uniting of Upper and Lower Egypt in *c.*3000 BCE and the Roman annexation of Egypt in 30 BCE, four women – Sobekneferu, Hatshepsut, Tausret and Cleopatra VII – succeeded to the Horus throne and ruled indisputably as pharaohs.

The four pharaohs discussed here perpetuated their rule in similar and distinctive ways. Sobekneferu is unique among the female pharaohs discussed here as she succeeded to the throne without serving as (co-)regent. Her success in securing her position meant that both Hatshepsut, and Tausret to a lesser extent, emulated many of her material and propagandistic endeavours. As Sobekneferu linked herself to her famous father, Amenemhat III, Hatshepsut emphasized her popular father, Thutmose I; Tausret linked herself to Ramses the Great; and Cleopatra's second Horus name invoked her father, Ptolemy XII. Nevertheless, all four women are depicted as pharaohs in their own right – sometimes as women depicted in the (masculine) regalia of a pharaoh – and their titles, no matter their gendered rendering, demonstrate their assumption of the Horus throne. In these cases, it is clear that despite the 'youthful male' ideal, blood trumped gender.

While the concept of the king's two bodies and its influence on the reigns of the female kings in England is well known, it has a history that stretches back 3,000 years before the first woman was crowned queen in her own right in western Europe. In drawing a distinction between the person of the king – the *hem* – and the office of the king, Egyptians paved the way for female pharaohs to be crowned 'King of Upper and Lower Egypt'. Nevertheless, the existence of only four women across more than 3,000 years who ruled as pharaoh demonstrates that the monarchy of Egypt did not resemble modern monarchies that practise absolute primogeniture. Thus, the fact that details of these female pharaohs' reigns can be recovered is significant. As Catharine Roehrig has observed:

> To the ancient Egyptians, a female ruler, however long or short her reign, would have been extraordinary – someone worthy of stories to be passed on by word of mouth . . . Perhaps this is why both rulers [i.e. Hatshepsut and Tausret] have a place in the history of Egypt written by Manetho in the time of the first Ptolemies, some eight hundred years after Tausret's death.[95]

Many places today – museums, textbooks, websites and even some academic publications – still fail to acknowledge the existence of these female pharaohs. Nevertheless, these women ruled millennia before the first female king ascended the throne in Europe, and it is thus vital that we continue to examine how these women ruled as pharaoh in a civilization that considered their monarch to be the earthly embodiment of the *male* god Horus.

Notes

1 Dates for reigns and dynasties in Egypt are approximate, and different publications offer different dates. For consistency, all dates in the chapter – which are BCE – will follow the chronology given in *The Egyptian World*, ed. Toby Wilkinson (London: Routledge, 2007), xvii–xxiv. For an overview of the chronology of pharaonic Egypt, see the timeline and period summary available on the companion website. This chapter has greatly benefitted from discussions with Robert Norrie, Jo Oranje and Joseph Massey, and I am grateful for the research assistance provided by the University of Otago library.

2 As Aidan Dodson notes, 'The term "pharaoh" is today used as a general term to describe a king of ancient Egypt'. Derived from *pr-ʿ3* (*per-aa*), the word literally means 'Great House'. The term eventually became a metonym for the occupier of the palace – like The White House is for the President of the United States – with this first known usage dating from the Eighteenth Dynasty, during the reign of Thutmose III (*c.*1458–*c.*1425 BCE). Sheshonq I (*c.*945–*c.*925 BCE), first king of the Twenty-Second Dynasty, is the first to use *per-aa* as a title.

As both scholars and non-scholars use the term widely, it will be used as a synonym for king throughout this chapter. Aidan Dodson, "Pharaoh," in *The Encyclopedia of Ancient History*, eds. Roger S. Bagnall, Kai Brodersen, Craige B. Champion, Andrew Erskine and Sabine R. Huebner (Oxford: Wiley Blackwell, 2012), 5224–5225.

3 Richard H. Wilkinson, *The Complete Gods and Goddesses of Ancient Egypt* (London: Thames and Hudson, 2003), 99, 201.

4 For more on *maat*, and particularly a pharaoh's relationship with is preservation, see Emily Teeter, *The Presentation of Maat: Ritual and Legitimacy in Ancient Egypt* (Chicago: The Oriental Institute of The University of Chicago, 1997).

5 Joyce Tyldesley, "Foremost of Women: The Female Pharaohs of Ancient Egypt," in *Tausret: Forgotten Queen and Pharaoh of Egypt*, ed. Richard H. Wilkinson (Oxford: Oxford University Press, 2012), 6.

6 Ernst Kantorowicz, *The King's Two Bodies: A Study in Mediaeval Political Theology* (Princeton: Princeton University Press, 1957). See also Carole Levin and Charles Beem, "*Itinerarium ad Windsor* and English Queenship," in *The Name of a Queen: William Fleetwood's "Itinerarium ad Windsor"*, eds. Charles Beem and Dennis Moore (New York: Palgrave Macmillan, 2013), esp. 169–171.

7 Katja Goebs, "Kingship," in *The Egyptian World*, ed. Toby Wilkinson (London: Routledge, 2007), 292.

8 Goebs, "Kingship," 292.

9 Tyldesley, "Foremost of Women," 7.

10 Joan W. Scott, "Gender: A Useful Category of Historical Analysis," *The American Historical Review* 91, no. 5 (December 1986): 1056.

11 Currently, the best and most accessible History of Egyptology is Jason Thompson's *Wonderful Things: A History of Egyptology – Volume I: From Antiquity to 1881*; and *Volume II: The Golden Age, 1881–1914* (Cairo: The American University in Cairo Press, 2015).

12 See, for example, Kara Cooney, *The Woman Who Would Be King: Hatshepsut's Rise to Power in Ancient Egypt* (New York: Crown Publishers, 2014); and Joyce Tyldesley, *Chronicle of the Queens of Egypt: From Early Dynastic Times to the Death of Cleopatra* (London: Thames and Hudson, 2006).

13 See Joyce Tyldesley, *Hatchepsut: The Female Pharaoh* (London: Penguin, 1996); and Catharine H. Roehrig, ed., *Hatshepsut: From Queen to Pharaoh* (New York: The Metropolitan Museum of Art, 2005).

14 See José M. Galán, Betsy M. Bryan and Peter F. Dorman, eds., *Creativity and Innovation in the Reign of Hatshepsut* (Chicago: The Oriental Institute of The University of Chicago, 2014); and Richard H. Wilkinson, ed., *Tausret: Forgotten Queen and Pharaoh of Egypt* (Oxford: Oxford University Press, 2012).

15 See James K. Hoffmeier and Jacobus Van Dijk, "New Light on the Amarna Period from North Sinai," *The Journal of Egyptian Archaeology* 96 (2010): 191–205; Chris Bennett, "The Chronology of Berenice III," *Zeitschrift für Papyrologie und Epigraphik* 139 (2002): 143–148; and Linda M. Ricketts, "A Dual Queenship in the Reign of Berenice IV," *The Bulletin of the American Society of Papyrologists* 27 (1990): 49–60.

16 William Monter, *The Rise of Female Kings in Europe, 1300–1800* (New Haven: Yale University Press, 2012).

17 Tyldesley, "Foremost of Women," 5.

18 Theresa Earenfight, "Without the Persona of the Prince: Kings, Queens and the Idea of Monarchy in Late Medieval Europe," *Gender and History* 19, no. 1 (April 2007): 1.

19 Tyldesley, "Foremost of Women," 7.

20 Wolfram Grajetzki, "Middle Kingdom, Egypt," in *The Encyclopedia of Ancient History*, eds. Roger S. Bagnall, Kai Brodersen, Craige B. Champion, Andrew Erskine and Sabine R. Huebner (Oxford: Wiley Blackwell, 2012), 4490. On Henry the Young King, who was crowned during the reign of his father Henry II, see Matthew Strickland, *Henry the Young King, 1155–1183* (New Haven: Yale University Press, 2016).

21 Aidan Dodson, "Amenemhat I–VII," in *The Encyclopedia of Ancient History*, eds. Roger S. Bagnall, Kai Brodersen, Craige B. Champion, Andrew Erskine and Sabine R. Huebner (Oxford: Wiley Blackwell, 2012), 357.

22 Dodson, "Amenemhat I–VII," 358.
23 Robyn Gillam, "Sobeknefru," in *The Encyclopedia of Ancient History*, eds. Roger S. Bagnall, Kai Brodersen, Craige B. Champion, Andrew Erskine and Sabine R. Huebner (Oxford: Wiley Blackwell, 2012), 6296.
24 Manetho was an Egyptian high priest at Heliopolis in the early Ptolemaic period (*c.*300 BCE). He wrote a history of Egypt that recorded the names of the pharaohs and divided them up into the dynasties we still use today. While often inaccurate, he is an important starting point for Egyptian chronologies.
25 Alan Gardiner, *Egypt of the Pharaohs: An Introduction* (Oxford: Clarendon Press, 1961), 141.
26 Gillam, "Sobeknefru," 6296.
27 Jeffrey Spencer, *The British Museum Book of Ancient Egypt* (London: British Museum Press, 2007), 84–85.
28 Ronald J. Leprohon, *The Great Name: Ancient Egyptian Royal Titulary* (Atlanta: Society of Biblical Literature, 2013), 60.
29 Gae Callender, "Materials for the Reign of Sebekneferu," in *Proceedings of the Seventh International Congress of Egyptologists*, ed. C.J. Eyre (Leuven: Uitgeverij Peeters, 1998), 233; Gae Callender, "What Sex was King Sobekneferu? And what is known about her reign?" *Kmt: A Modern Journal of Ancient Egypt* 9, no. 1 (Spring 1998): 51. My italics.
30 Tyldesley, "Foremost of Women," 11–12.
31 British Museum object EA16581. The seal can be viewed online through the British Museum's website.
32 Callender, "Materials for the Reign of Sebekneferu," 233. Callender includes an image of the column on page 234.
33 Callender, "Materials for the Reign of Sebekneferu," 230.
34 Herodotus, *The Histories*, trans. Aubrey de Sélincourt (London: Penguin, 2002), 156 (*Histories* 2.148).
35 Callender, "Materials for the Reign of Sebekneferu," 236.
36 Callender, "Materials for the Reign of Sebekneferu," 232.
37 Callender, "Materials for the Reign of Sebekneferu," 230.
38 Gillam, "Sobeknefru," 6296.
39 This trope, its appearance across the globe and the increasing reassessment it is being subjected to, is discussed in Elena Woodacre and Carey Fleiner, eds., *Royal Mothers and their Ruling Children: Wielding Political Authority from Antiquity to the Early Modern Era* (New York: Palgrave Macmillan, 2015); and Carey Fleiner and Elena Woodacre, eds., *Virtuous or Villainess? The Image of the Royal Mother from the Early Medieval to the Early Modern Era* (New York: Palgrave Macmillan, 2016).
40 Callender, "What Sex was King Sobekneferu?" 46. Concerning this gender bias, Callender writes that scholars used 'words or phrases, the overtones of which conjure up unfavourable images (e.g. calling Hatshepsut "the stepmother of Thutmose III," whereby "stepmother" evokes one's childhood memories of fairy-tale "wicked" stepmothers).'
41 Uroš Matić, "(De)queering Hatshepsut: Binary Bind in Archaeology of Egypt and Kingship Beyond the Corporeal," *Journal of Archaeological Method and Theory* 23, no. 3 (2016): 813.
42 Matić, "(De)queering Hatshepsut," 813.
43 Tyldesley, "Foremost of Women," 14.
44 Leprohon, *The Great Name*, 98. Hatshepsut adopted 'Powerful of *kas* [souls]' as her Horus, 'Flourishing of years' as her Nebty, 'Divine of appearances' as her Golden Horus, 'The true one of the *ka* of Re' as her prenomen, and 'United with Amun, foremost of noble women' as her nomen.
45 Tyldesley, "Foremost of Women," 14.
46 Dimitri Laboury, "How and Why Did Hatshepsut Invent the Image of Her Royal Power?" in *Creativity and Innovation in the Reign of Hatshepsut*, eds. José M. Galán, Betsy M. Bryan and Peter F. Dorman (Chicago: The Oriental Institute of The University of Chicago, 2014), 50.
47 Tyldesley, "Foremost of Women," 14.
48 Laboury, "How and Why Did Hatshepsut," 88.
49 Tyldesley, "Foremost of Women," 14–15.
50 Laboury, "How and Why Did Hatshepsut," 91.

51 Ann Macy Roth, "Hatshepsut's Mortuary Temple at Deir El-Bahri: Architecture as Political Statement," in *Hatshepsut: From Queen to Pharaoh*, ed. Catharine H. Roehrig (New York: The Metropolitan Museum of Art, 2005), 147.

52 Roth, "Hatshepsut's Mortuary Temple at Deir El-Bahri," 148–150.

53 Matić, "(De)queering Hatshepsut," 813.

54 The Metropolitan Museum of Art, accession number 31.3.94. See the MMoA web catalogue for images and further description.

55 H.E. Winlock, *Excavations at Deir El Bahari: 1911–1931* (New York: Macmillan, 1942), 171–173.

56 Cathleen A. Keller, "Hatshepsut as a Maned Sphinx," in *Hatshepsut: From Queen to Pharaoh*, ed. Catharine H. Roehrig (New York: The Metropolitan Museum of Art, 2005), 166.

57 MMoA 27.3.163.

58 MMoA 29.3.1.

59 MMoA 30.3.1.

60 Vivianne Callender, "Hatshepsut," in *The Encyclopedia of Ancient History*, eds. Roger S. Bagnall, Kai Brodersen, Craige B. Champion, Andrew Erskine and Sabine R. Huebner (Oxford: Wiley Blackwell, 2012), 3079.

61 Tyldesley, "Foremost of Women," 16.

62 Callender, "What Sex was King Sobekneferu?" 46; Tyldesley, "Foremost of Women," 16; Cathleen A. Keller, "The Joint Reign of Hatshepsut and Thutmose III," in *Hatshepsut: From Queen to Pharaoh*, ed. Catharine H. Roehrig (New York: The Metropolitan Museum of Art, 2005), 97.

63 Richard H. Wilkinson, "The Queen Who Would Be King," in *Tausret: Forgotten Queen and Pharaoh of Egypt*, ed. Richard H. Wilkinson (Oxford: Oxford University Press, 2012), 1–2.

64 Richard H. Wilkinson, "Tausret," in *The Encyclopedia of Ancient History*, eds. Roger S. Bagnall, Kai Brodersen, Craige B. Champion, Andrew Erskine and Sabine R. Huebner (Oxford: Wiley Blackwell, 2012), 6544.

65 Leprohon, *The Great Name*, 114, 125.

66 Catharine H. Roehrig, "Forgotten Treasures: Tausret as Seen in Her Monuments," in *Tausret: Forgotten Queen and Pharaoh of Egypt*, ed. Richard H. Wilkinson (Oxford: Oxford University Press, 2012), 49.

67 Roehrig, "Forgotten Treasures," 52.

68 Roehrig, "Forgotten Treasures," 55.

69 Roehrig, "Forgotten Treasures," 57.

70 Roehrig, "Forgotten Treasures," 60.

71 Richard H. Wilkinson, "The 'Temple of Millions of Years' of Tausret," in *Tausret: Forgotten Queen and Pharaoh of Egypt*, ed. Richard H. Wilkinson (Oxford: Oxford University Press, 2012), 102–103.

72 Wilkinson, "Tausret," 6545.

73 Wilkinson, "Tausret," 6544.

74 Roehrig, "Forgotten Treasures," 49.

75 Roehrig, "Forgotten Treasures," 50.

76 Gae Callender, "Female Horus: The Life and Reign of Tausret," in *Tausret: Forgotten Queen and Pharaoh of Egypt*, ed. Richard H. Wilkinson (Oxford: Oxford University Press, 2012), 41.

77 Leprohon, *The Great Name*, 125.

78 Roehrig, "Forgotten Treasures," 66.

79 Callender, "Female Horus," 47.

80 Indeed, the fact that she is the only Cleopatra to have an entry in *The Oxford Encyclopedia of Ancient Egypt* is telling.

81 Duane W. Roller, *Cleopatra: A Biography* (Oxford: Oxford University Press, 2010), 80.

82 Roller, *Cleopatra*, 81.

83 Robert Steven Bianchi, "Cleopatra VII," in *The Oxford Encyclopedia of Ancient Egypt*, ed. Donald B. Redford (Oxford: Oxford University Press, 2001), 273.

84 Bianchi, "Cleopatra VII," 273.

85 Manfred Clauss, "Cleopatra VII," in *The Encyclopedia of Ancient History*, eds. Roger S. Bagnall, Kai Brodersen, Craige B. Champion, Andrew Erskine and Sabine R. Huebner (Oxford: Wiley Blackwell, 2012), 1571.

86 Leprohon, *The Great Name*, 187–188.
87 Leprohon, *The Great Name*, 188.
88 Bianchi, "Cleopatra VII," 273.
89 Shelley P. Haley, "Cleopatra VII," in *The Oxford Encyclopedia of Women in World History*, ed. Bonnie G. Smith (Oxford: Oxford University Press, 2008), 417.
90 E.R. Bevan, *The House of Ptolemy* (London: Methuen Publishing, 1927), 371.
91 Barbara A. Richter, *The Theology of Hathor of Dendera: Aural and Visual Scribal Techniques in the "Per-Wer" Sanctuary* (Atlanta: Lockwood Press, 2016), 87.
92 Elizabeth Donnelly Carney, *Arsinoë of Egypt and Macedon: A Royal Life* (Oxford: Oxford University Press, 2013), 106–107.
93 Tyldesley, "Foremost of Women," 24.
94 Tyldesley, "Foremost of Women," 24.
95 Roehrig, "Forgotten Treasures," 66.

Key works

Callender, Gae, "Materials for the Reign of Sebekneferu," in *Proceedings of the Seventh International Congress of Egyptologists*, ed. C.J. Eyre (Leuven: Uitgeverij Peeters, 1998), 227–236.

Callender, Gae, "Female Horus: The Life and Reign of Tausret," in *Tausret: Forgotten Queen and Pharaoh of Egypt*, ed. Richard H. Wilkinson (Oxford: Oxford University Press, 2012), 25–47.

Clauss, Manfred, "Cleopatra VII," in *The Encyclopedia of Ancient History*, eds. Roger S. Bagnall, Kai Brodersen, Craige B. Champion, Andrew Erskine and Sabine R. Huebner (Oxford: Wiley Blackwell, 2012), 1569–1571.

Dorman, Peter F., "Hatshepsut: Princess to Queen to Co-Ruler," in *Hatshepsut: From Queen to Pharaoh*, ed. Catharine H. Roehrig (New York: The Metropolitan Museum of Art, 2005), 87–91.

Tyldesley, Joyce, "Foremost of Women: The Female Pharaohs of Ancient Egypt," in *Tausret: Forgotten Queen and Pharaoh of Egypt*, ed. Richard H. Wilkinson (Oxford: Oxford University Press, 2012), 5–24.

26

NEITHER HEIR NOR SPARE

Childless queens and the practice of monarchy in pre-modern Europe[1]

Kristen L. Geaman and Theresa Earenfight

Perpetuation of the dynasty was of vital concern in hereditary monarchies, but not every royal couple could produce the much-needed heirs without substantial delay – if at all. Conventional wisdom in the Middle Ages was based on statements such as that of Alcuin, adviser to Emperor Charlemagne, in 793: 'The king's virtue equals the welfare of the whole people, victory by the army, good weather, fertility, male off-spring, and health.'[2] He was emphatic that without a queen to bear children, there would be no question of fertility, and therefore no male offspring, and by extension, nothing but humiliating defeat, bad weather and poor health. Alcuin's comment highlights the fundamentally heteronormative attitudes towards sexuality that priv-ileged childbearing as inherent to the institution of monarchy. Scholarly work on queens, notably that of John Carmi Parsons, has prioritized the importance of mar-riage and motherhood, a vital task for all married women in a pre-industrial society that depended on heirs to both secure the family line and increase household labour output. Other work argues that queenship can be seen as a type of motherhood, whether that involved physically bearing a child or metaphorically representing the realm as a family.[3] For English queens, maternal duty was part of the coronation oath (as was intercession, which was explicitly linked to maternity). Janet Nelson argues that royal maternity was the matrix of future kings, with the pregnant queen the guarantor of the realm's survival and integrity and so of peace and control. Without a queen who provided an heir to give licit proof of his powers' survival, a Christian monarch had no legitimate way to manifest his authority.[4] Charles Wood, looking a little further afield than the British Isles, argues that medieval society allowed greater political leeway to a royal mother than a wife, citing Eleanor of Aquitaine, Blanche of Castile and Isabella of France as queens with greater authority as mothers than as wives.[5] For regnant queens, such as Isabel I of Castile, emphasizing the feminine aspects of motherhood could offset the masculine practice of governance that stirred anxieties among their subjects.[6]

Because maternity mattered, childlessness – or its near-equivalent, the failure to conceive a son – could end poorly for a queen. Catherine of Aragon, first wife of Henry VIII (r.1509–47), was pregnant often, perhaps as many as six times, but only one child lived to adulthood, a daughter, Mary, who later ruled as Mary I (r.1553–8).

Catherine was hardly childless, but the evidence for her difficult pregnancies is either nonexistent or vague, leading scholars to speculate retrospectively, without credible evidence, about what caused her to have no children. Some argue that Catherine was anorexic or that Henry carried Kell's antigen, which could have caused a fatal genetic mismatch.[7] Catherine's first pregnancy ended on 31 January 1510, when she gave birth to a stillborn child presumed to be seven months old. On 1 January 1511, she gave birth to a son, who died on 22 February, perhaps of an infection. In September 1513, she gave birth to another son who was either stillborn or died immediately after delivery. In June 1514, or November or December, she gave birth to a son who may or may not have been christened on or shortly after the third day after birth: uncertainty reveals how hard it is to know precise details. At last, on 18 February 1516, Catherine gave birth to Mary. After that, she may have been pregnant in 1517 but there is no evidence for this. It comes only from rumour among the diplomats, but we are fairly certain that on 18 November 1518 she gave birth a last time, to a son or daughter who was stillborn. Shortly after that, on 15 June 1519, Henry's mistress Elizabeth Blount, gave birth to a son, Henry Fitzroy, who lived until 1536. The rest is well known. Henry argued that his marriage to Catherine violated church regulations on consanguinity, his relationship with Anne Boleyn prompted a divorce and she, too, was unable to carry a healthy baby boy to term and lost the office of queenship.[8]

The experiences of the six wives of Henry VIII show the enduring power of the idea that queens consort needed to produce sons or face consequences. But, in fact, despite Alcuin's dire predictions, childlessness did not necessarily spell doom for a queen, although it could result in the end of the marriage. In the Crown of Aragon, Isabel of Castile (1283–1328), was married for three years to Jaume II (r.1291–1327), king of the Crown of Aragon; their childless marriage was annulled. Jaume must have been very grateful to his second wife, Blanca of Naples, for the ten children she bore but neither his third wife, Marie of Lusignan, nor his fourth wife, Elisenda de Montcada, had children. But Jaume did not end these marriages because he already had children and the burden of reproduction was removed from these women as Blanca's fertility had taken care of this issue.[9]

The evidence reveals that pre-modern queenship was a complex cultural and political institution, that it was never just about having heirs and that maternity clearly is not the sole determinant of a queen's 'success'.[10] The vast majority of childless queens, or those who did not bear sons, were not necessarily repudiated by their husbands. There were many childless queens, and not all suffered a dire fate. Anne of Bohemia (1366–94), wife of Richard II of England (r.1377–99), and Joan of the Tower (1321–62), who married King David of Scotland (r.1324–71), in 1328 were childless. This is not to say that infertility was ignored, but it was poorly understood in medical terms, and modern scholars struggle to interpret imprecise medieval terminology such as 'fever' (of unknown duration or severity) or 'indisposed' (to mean she was ill in bed) that described symptoms in general terms used to explain the circumstances. Queens and kings deployed an arsenal of medical and spiritual remedies in their quests to continue their dynasties. From bleeding to compound medicines to pilgrimages, royalty tried a host of treatments, but only some couples met with success.

This chapter explores various aspects of the non-reproductive aspects of queenship, starting with the personal, religious and medical factors that resulted in childlessness.

Then it examines the coping mechanisms in which childless monarchs (or those who wrote about them) attempted to explain away the lack of heirs through insinuations of chaste marriage or diffuse the situation by portraying childless queens as non-biological mothers. Finally, it examines the importance of intercession, cultural patronage and caring for other's children that could provide avenues to power and successful fulfilment of the role of queen in the absence of children. Throughout it all, these childless queens did not lose their title or status, emphasizing that queenship was a vital aspect of a complete monarchy and not just its reproductive element.

Chance or choice? Infertility, chastity, miscarriages and the problem of medieval medical knowledge

The difficulty of studying childless queens stems in large part from medieval medical literature concerning the maternal health of women, which was concerned mostly with tending to contraception, pregnancy, miscarriage and stillbirth.[11] Miscarriage is difficult to discern, was often not publicly discussed and much less recorded, and was often attributed to emotional causes. Philippa of Lancaster (daughter of John of Gaunt) and wife of João I of Portugal, had a miscarriage with her first child not long after her marriage in 1387. The chronicler Fernão Lopes who records this suggests that it was the shock of her new husband's serious illness that caused her to lose her child.[12]

However, some treatises exist that touch on the subject. For example, in 1444, Pierre André de Pulcro Visu, master of arts and medicine at the University of Toulouse, dedicated a treatise on fertility and childbirth to Gaston IV Count of Foix (b.1423, r.1436–72). This work, the *Pomum Aureum*, focuses on how to bring a baby to full term and takes up questions such as how a child is formed in the womb, why some couples produce more males and some produce more females, why some children look like one parent or another, how to detect a pregnancy, and a range of practices such as abortion, midwifery and childrearing.[13] The text alludes to infertility but it is frustratingly vague, stating that the woman's contribution is the seed, menstrual blood and womb, and that the man contributes natural heat and the life-giving form. It indicates a clear understanding of the connection between the need for mixing 'seeds' to create a child and the indication of their failure if the menstrual blood appears. But it does not suggest any understanding of why women and men who had sex sometimes had no children. Scholars are left to infer from oblique evidence, allusions in letters or diplomatic memoranda, and rarely, records from court physicians to discern possible causes of royal childlessness.

There are any number of reasons why queens did not have children at all and may never have been pregnant. When all else failed, explaining away their childlessness as the result of a chaste marriage (a non-consummated union) was a way to deflect criticism. For example, Edith of Wessex had a self-described chaste marriage with Edward the Confessor (r.1042–66) and their lack of a child paved the way for the conquest of England by William, Duke of Normandy in 1066.[14] Rather than trying but failing to have children, the couple had neglected earthly, hereditary concerns for spiritual success. At times, monarchs themselves promoted these holy narratives; sometimes others did it for them. The anonymous author of *The Life of Edward Who Rests at Westminster* (*c*.1067), a historical narrative commissioned by Edith, wife of

Edward the Confessor, originated the idea that she and Edward had a chaste union, thereby softening the blow their childlessness had partially caused: the end of the line of Anglo-Saxon kings.[15] Although the chastity is simply hinted at, the author largely credits Edith with virginity;[16] perhaps the queen, as patron, even suggested this in order to deflect her 'failure' to produce children who would inherit the realm. Later works, however, ignored Edith and rewrote what was once the couple's virginity into Edward's virginity. The 1163 text *Life of St Edward King and Confessor* by Aelred of Rievaulx was the earliest to state explicitly that Edward lived as a virgin and that he instigated their chaste union.[17] That virginity played a major role in Edward's canonization, effectively turned a failure to reproduce into the success of sainthood.

A lack of biological children, however, did not mean a queen could not be a mother. Mothering was a socially constructed activity which allowed both childless women and men to participate in maternal practices such as spiritual and nurturing motherhood.[18] Within *The Life of Edward Who Rests at Westminster*, Queen Edith was exalted as a spiritual mother, courtesy of her support of Wilton Abbey. A 'metaphorical' accolade to the queen within *The Life* thus addressed Edith in overtly Marian terms on the occasion of the dedication of Wilton Abbey:

> Hail, peerless mother, blessed babes to bear,
> Conceived immaculate from any sin,
> And at whose bringing forth you'll feel no pangs.
> Nor will you grieve at scanty progeny,
> Nor will one fashioned in your womb expire:
> But you will make chaste marriage vows, and lie
> In the sweet arms of everlasting God;
> Whose heavenly seed, in your womb cast, returns
> A crop from his life-giving Holy Ghost.[19]

The queen was praised for her spiritual motherhood, which had allowed her to remain a virgin and still give birth to numerous children. As Monika Otter has suggested, this veneration was designed to console Edith for her childlessness and convince her that spiritual, surrogate motherhood was preferable to the biological variety.[20] One did not have to bear children biologically to nurture spiritual children through good works. A queen such as Edith could achieve maternity through the care she took for her subjects – in her case, the nuns of Wilton Abbey.

The marriage of Emperor Henry II (d.1024) and Cunigunde was similarly remade as a chaste marriage decades after they died childless, ending the Ottonian dynasty. While no one suggested the royal couple had a virginal union during their lifetimes, the *Vita Heinrici II*, written around the time of Henry's 1146 canonization, stated the royal couple did.[21] Henry and Cunigunde's chaste marriage was thus created by the bishop of Bamberg, which supported and promoted the emperor's cult (he was buried in Bamberg Cathedral). The claim of chaste marriage could thus turn dynastic failure into saintly success in the right circumstances. While this coping mechanism reflected the need to explain away the problem of childlessness, it hints at the wider role of the queen as a partner in monarchy, whether formally governing (as regent) or informally (as patron, intercessor and manager of the royal household, for example).

King Richard II of England unsuccessfully attempted to recast his childless marriage to Anne of Bohemia as chaste. After Anne's death in 1394, Richard became increasingly attached to the cult of Edward the Confessor, who, by that time, was primarily known for his virginal union with Edith.[22] Although Richard went so far as to impale his arms with the mythical arms of Edward, placing the two in a heraldic marriage, contemporaries did not see Richard's marriage as chaste. Philippe de Mézières, in his *Letter to King Richard II* (1395), wrote somewhat sorrowfully that Richard could no longer claim the highest state of virginity:

> Old Solitary [Mézières], then, considering that of the three estates aforesaid you are deprived, though without sin, of the chief, that is, of virginity, for this reason is emboldened at this moment, for what it is worth, to recommend that state of chastity.

In essence, Richard should remarry because he was no longer a virgin.[23] If Mézières had heard rumours that Richard's first marriage was unconsummated, he evidently did not believe them.[24]

Some queens clearly never were pregnant for reasons we will never understand. María of Castile (1401–58) and her husband, Alfonso V 'the Magnanimous', king of the Crown of Aragon (b.1396, r.1416–58) were married for forty-three years but were considered a dynastic failure because they had no children. They lived together for the first eleven years of the marriage, enough time for her to become pregnant, but then they were separated for over two decades when he conquered and ruled the kingdom of Naples. She may never have been pregnant, although Alfonso had three illegitimate children. Yet they never divorced, the realm remained intact, she governed the Spanish realms and Alfonso's brother Juan succeeded him. María had her first menstrual period at the age of sixteen, which meant that María and Alfonso were forced to delay consummating their marriage. She also suffered from a variety of health problems throughout her life which may have affected her fertility, but the term used to describe what happened ('accidentes') is imprecise and could mean a sign or symptom, a manifestation of an illness, something serious or merely a fainting spell. But their Catalan subjects thought the problem was due to the king's neglect of his wife. In 1438, the town council of Barcelona appealed to Alfonso's marital duty ('lo gran deute de matrimoni') in order to persuade him to leave Italy, reunite with María and produce an heir, not specifying their preference for a son or a daughter.[25] The case of María of Castile demonstrates clearly that kings needed queens for more than just reproduction. Alfonso needed her for more than just childbearing and recognized her talent for governance. She was a vital partner in the institution of monarchy who governed ably for an absent king.

Medical remedies

Queens looked to a variety of medical remedies for childlessness. England's queen Anne of Bohemia, for instance, purchased compound medicines such as *rosata novella* and *trifera magna*, both of which were claimed to increase fertility through their purgative properties.[26] According to a Venetian ambassador, England's Mary I suffered from 'menstruous retention and suffocation of the matrix', for which the queen was 'blooded either from the foot or elsewhere', apparently with enough frequency that it kept the queen looking 'pale and emaciated'.[27] For both of these queens, the medicinal remedies sought to balance the humours and promote menstruation.

Other queens, particularly in later centuries, sought out curative spas. In 1583, Henri III of France and his wife Louise of Lorraine visited Bourbon-Lancy to take the waters. Henri's mother, the dowager queen Catherine de Medici, explicitly linked the visit with hopes for offspring, writing that 'If it pleases God to bring them back with a child in the queen's belly, it would help us overcome all our other ills.'[28] From September to 6 October 1687, Queen Mary of Modena, wife of England's James II, was in Bath. Although her trip was due to general ill health after the death of her mother, Mary certainly desired a child, as all her previous children had died very young. According to Agnes Strickland, Victorian biographer of royal women, the waters at Bath were used by married women who desired to have children.[29] In fact, the queen must have become pregnant right around the time of her trip – her son was born in June 1688.

Spiritual remedies

Spiritual recourse, such as pilgrimages, was especially popular. María of Castile travelled to the monastery of Montserrat, well known as a place where women would go to pray for a sick child or soul of a dead child, and she may have gone there to pray to the Virgin for help in conceiving. If so, she had good company. Anne Rudloff Stanton argues that the Queen Mary psalter, with its images of holy mothers, particularly St Anne, and their children may have been commissioned for a royal woman expected to bear children.[30] Louis XI of France (r.1461–83) and his wife Charlotte of Savoy, in their quest for a son, went on multiple pilgrimages of both petition and thanksgiving to Notre-Dame du Puy to offer at the shrine of St Petronilla, patroness of the dauphins of France.[31] In August 1582, Henri III of France, with Jesuits and two dukes in tow, also went on pilgrimage to Notre-Dame du Puy, seeking the Virgin Mary's intercession for a child.[32] When that proved unsuccessful, Henri III sent the Duc de Joyeuse on pilgrimage in his stead, seeking intercession for himself and his queen from the Virgin in Loretto, Italy.[33]

In England, multiple queens visited Our Lady of Walsingham in Norfolk, the most important shrine to the Virgin Mary and a popular pilgrimage destination for women to visit when requesting conception or safe childbirth.[34] Anne of Bohemia and Richard II went on pilgrimage to Walsingham in May and June of 1383.[35] Margaret of Anjou donated a valuable gold and jewelled tablet in January 1453 to the shrine and went in either 1452 or 1453. If the latter date is correct, this was possibly a pilgrimage of thanksgiving as Margaret gave birth in October 1453.[36] Edward IV and Queen Elizabeth Woodville planned to depart for Walsingham in May 1469, perhaps to petition for a son.[37] The couple had several daughters by 1469, but no son until November 1470, suggesting the 1469 pilgrimage might have been spurred by concerns about fertility for a male heir.

Catherine of Aragon also visited Walsingham on several occasions. In September 1513, she wrote to her husband Henry VIII that I 'now go to Our Lady at Walsingham that I promised so long ago to see'.[38] Catherine was pregnant at this time, so the pilgrimage was probably for a safe delivery and the child's health.

In March 1517, Catherine returned to Walsingham.[39] Although the queen had delivered the future Mary I, her first and only child to live more than a few weeks, in February 1516, Catherine still had no son. Petitioning for a son was almost surely one reason for Catherine's second pilgrimage.

As for prayers, the prayer book (now Newberry Library MS 83) of Anne of Brittany, twice queen of France, contains a number of prayers relevant to childbearing, such as those commemorating the conception of the Virgin Mary and a suffrage to St Margaret.[40] Of particular interest, though, is a prayer said to be by St Leonard, who helped Clothilde, wife of Clovis, first king of the Franks, have children. According to the preface to the prayer, when the Frankish queen 'was not succeeding in bringing to full term and was not able to produce children', the prayer was 'of very great power whenever it is read piously and listened to attentively when a woman is in course of bearing children'.[41] The prayer itself references the miraculous fertility of Abraham and Sarah, the virgin birth of Jesus, and ends with beseeching God the father, son and Holy Spirit 'that the assistance of your holiness may come upon this woman who is groaning because of the difficulty of giving birth in order that she, having been released from immediate danger may be able along with us to praise your name'.[42] This prayer for safe childbirth was also used to help enhance fertility; other childbirth prayers might have served dual functions as well.

In some cases, the line between the presumed efficacy of prayer and medical knowledge is indistinct. There is a case of miscarriage (not a queen) in William of Canterbury's *Miracula S. Thomae*, written in the 1170s. The woman had suffered a nosebleed and the foetus had died but could not be expelled; the woman's life was in danger until she prayed to Thomas Becket. In a frustratingly brief note, William of Malmesbury informed his readers that St Benignus had powers to help 'women too who carried dead fetuses in their wombs'. The belt belonging to Gilbert of Sempringham helped stave off premature labour.[43]

Queenship is more than biological motherhood

Being a queen consort was not just about providing heirs. Queens, whether mothers or not, had a vital place in the body politic as intercessors, patrons and stand-ins with governmental authority.[44] Intercession was one such well-established and much-appreciated role for a consort in thirteenth- and fourteenth-century England; often queens interceded on their coronation day as Eleanor of Provence (queen of England's Henry III) did in 1236.[45] Queenly intercession, of course, was not limited to coronation day but continued throughout a queen's life. Eleanor of Provence was an active intercessor, especially in the latter portion of her husband's reign (in particular after the civil war of 1258–65, which gave her the opportunity of reconciling the king with many of his former opponents) and during the reign of her son, Edward I.[46] Eleanor's successor Eleanor of Castile was not a particularly active intercessor (recording only thirty-six acts of intercession in thirty-six years), but Edward's second queen, Margaret of France, was a vigorous mediator. In her seven years and ten months as queen, she interceded with Edward I in sixty-eight cases.[47] The same was true of Margaret's niece and successor, Isabella of France, wife of Edward II. Isabella handled a steady stream of petitions from 1308 to 1321, engaging in eighty acts of intercession in those thirteen years.[48] Philippa of Hainault was also an active intercessor, interceding fifty-six times as an individual and twice as a member of a larger group during her forty-one years as queen (1328–69).[49] By the 1300s, intercession was an established part of a queen's duties.[50]

Anne of Bohemia took to intercession with gusto. According to the calculations of Helen Lacey, Anne individually interceded for pardons on seventy-one occasions and an additional three times as part of a group during her thirteen years as queen.[51] The previous statistics relate only to pardons, which were just one aspect of intercession. Queens also petitioned to help subjects secure lands, grants, preferment and other signs of royal favour. For instance, Anne of Bohemia interceded with Richard in 1392 for him to restore Margery, daughter and heir of John Spenser of Kent, to her father's forfeited tenement (Spenser had been executed for his role in an uprising).[52] According to Lisa Benz, who has examined the chancery rolls (patent, close, charter and fine rolls) for queens' acts of intercession, Anne has more recorded acts than Margaret, Isabella of France or Philippa of Hainault.[53] In terms of average intercessions per year, Margaret had 3.15, Isabella 3.57 and Philippa 2.2. Anne, however, averaged 4.1.[54] Anne devoted more of her energies to intercession than did previous queens, perhaps indicating that Anne turned her focus to other duties since she did not have children. Whatever the reason, Anne's intercessory activities endeared her to her English subjects. While derided as a 'tiny scrap of humanity' for whom the king had overpaid on her arrival,[55] she was called the 'most gracious queen of England'.[56] Despite never having borne an heir, Anne was considered a good queen.

Rather like Queen Edith, Anne of Bohemia practised nurturing motherhood through her work as a queenly intercessor. Scholar John Carmi Parsons argued that intercession was a way for queens to regain influence lost through childlessness, in part because they could enact a different type of motherhood – nurturing rather than biological.[57] Anne was a noted intercessor, and after her death, Richard II promoted Anne as a mother through her epitaph. Anne and Richard's joint tomb was built and completed within Richard II's lifetime, so the king presumably approved of the sentiments expressed therein.[58] Anne's epitaph is below:

> Under this wide stone lies Anne now buried,
> While living in this world married to Richard II,
> Devoted to Christ, she was noted for good deeds:
> Always prone to render her gifts to paupers:
> She settled quarrels and relieved pregnant women,
> With beautiful body and beautiful, meek face,
> Supplying solace to widows, medicine to the sick
> She departed to heaven June 7 1394.[59]

Anne was depicted as a pious woman who engaged in acts of charity and interceded on behalf of her people. Anne's intercession was explicitly highlighted in the line 'She settled quarrels and relieved pregnant women' (*Iurgia sedavit et pregnantes relevavit*).[60] In fact, this line echoes sentiments expressed in greater length in the verse eulogy 'Anglica Regina', which praised Anne because she 'allayed disputes, pacified the quarrelsome' and 'visited pregnant women in their suffering'.[61] This line thereby commemorates Anne's fulfilment of her queenly duty of intercession as well as one of her more notable works of mercy. But the decision to highlight Anne's intercession and assistance to pregnant women in the same line might not have been simply due to space constraints. Pregnancy, along with motherhood, had links with intercession, giving 'added emotional tinge' to an interceding queen's words.[62] Placing intercession and pregnancy in the same line of the epitaph signalled a connection between the two activities. The epitaph noted how Anne had engaged in intercession and surrogate motherhood. She had helped pregnant women, perhaps as a way to partake of the trials and rituals of childbirth. The joint mention of intercession and helping pregnant women made Anne's intercession more powerful.[63]

In her memorializations, Anne's intercessions and charity to pregnant women were highlighted – sometimes even side by side. Rather than a failed biological mother, Anne was remembered as a successful and beloved nurturing mother in a different sense. To a certain extent, this put a positive spin on Anne and Richard's childlessness. As van Dussen noted:

> The eulogies of Anne of Bohemia aimed to explain away the problem of succession by creating a royalist version of Anne's devotion which would justify her childlessness in terms of known paradigms for piety, particularly the piety of queens and holy mothers.[64]

Anne was a holy woman, for whom (rather like St Elizabeth of Hungary) biological motherhood was of secondary importance.[65] Intercession, however, as one of the signature traits of the Virgin Mary and Esther, fulfilled an important role – it provided excellent examples of the queen acting as a nurturing mother. What might once have been solely seen as political acts could be recast as the pious exertions of a nurturing, maternal queen. Motherhood, like queenship, was a category with room for variety.

Centuries later, Catherine of Braganza turned to cultural patronage to construct a successful queenship. Wife of England's licentious Charles II, Catherine's political role was hampered both by her childlessness and her husband's many mistresses, especially English-born ones such as Lady Castlemaine. As Lady Castlemaine's influence and the queen's fertility waned in the late 1660s and early 1670s, Catherine promoted Italian music and painting in opposition to the French culture already influential at court and represented by Charles's newest mistress, Louise de Kéroualle.[66] Although Charles II had brought in Italian musicians in 1660, the queen employed Italians at her chapel, listened to them at court and helped change the musical tastes of Londoners from French to Italian.[67] Catherine also patronized the Italian painter Benedetto Gennari, who was subsequently hired by Charles II, the duke of York and a variety of other aristocrats.[68] As Edward Corp sums it up, 'By substituting cultural for sexual politics Catherine found an alternative method of attracting the attention of her husband and countering the influence of the favorite mistresses at court.'[69] When Catherine could not bear an heir, she found other avenues of influence, so that she was still a player in court life.[70]

A queen did not need to be a mother to govern alongside the king, as the political career of María of Castile makes abundantly clear. As previously discussed, she took up the office of the queen-lieutenant when Alfonso V left the Crown of Aragon for Naples in 1420. This office was an innovation of the Crown of Aragon devised to govern various of the far-flung realms while the king was absent. Of the six queens-lieutenant, one, María of Castile, was childless and Alfonso entrusted the realms to her during his frequent absences from the peninsular realms of Aragón and Valencia, the principality of Catalunya and the island of Mallorca. For twenty-eight years, she capably governed as lieutenant general with full governmental powers over the kingdoms. The rationale for her authority was in no way connected to maternity. Her powers were equivalent to those of the king. She had the authority to rule independently with full sovereign power over all civil and criminal jurisdictions in all four realms, including the army and the military orders. Her authority superseded all the royal, seigneurial, regional and local officials; provincial governors; prelates and religious orders; the nobility, townspeople, peasants and all other subjects regardless of status. She had the authority to summon, convoke and preside over the Corts, the regional parliamentary assemblies. Her authority was equivalent to the king's in the realms stipulated by the *privilegio*, but he nevertheless retained the ultimate authority. She governed, but he held dominion. As queens-lieutenant, they were the embodiment of the king's personal authority and custodian of the realm, a co-ruler with an adult king, fully capable of ruling, who, for any number of reasons, could not govern a particular territory or territories. Although chancellors and governors performed very specific tasks, often for a specific length of time, at the king's command, they were still subject to his will. They worked for the king. As queen-lieutenant, on the other hand, María worked in place of the king. Her intimate association with the king's body was not linked to her reproductive functions, and this meant that she could take the place of that body and that her term expired when the king died.

As a childless queen, it is significant that María of Castile was ostensibly vulnerable but faced no serious opposition to her tenure as lieutenant general. When her Catalan subjects complained, they admonished the king for leaving the realms in a state 'like a widow' and for failing to return to his wife. The heart of the dispute was the constitutional and jurisdictional definition of the legal boundaries of the authority of the king and the queen-lieutenant. The Catalans were not overly troubled by rule by a woman and that a childless queen as lieutenant general was acceptable because the presence of a fully competent adult king reassured the Catalan elites that the social order would not be disrupted. To María's Catalan and Aragonese subjects, the fact that she had no children may have prompted sympathy and some concern for the succession (Alfonso was succeeded by his brother, Juan, in 1458), but at no point did it have any effect on her work as queen. In fact, it is likely that she devoted herself to her work, much like a mother would to a child. Her subjects were foremost in her mind when she fiercely advocated on behalf of the peasants seeking manumission and the Jews who faced persecution.[71] And she practised a foster motherhood for Isabel de Villena (1430–90), the illegitimate daughter of Manuel de Villena. She was orphaned as a child when her father died, and María raised her at the court in Valencia and probably encouraged her to become a nun.[72]

Whether as an intercessor, patron, or temporary replacement for an absent king, it is clear that queenship entailed far more than maternity. Queens were essential partners in the smooth management of an effective monarchy.

Conclusion

The childless queen calls into question our assumptions about the power of patrilineage. Intelligence, diplomatic skills, tact, shrewdness, even tenacity are hard to measure and vitally important to the success of a monarchical partnership without children. It is impressive that childless queens were able to manoeuvre skilfully to build and maintain the prestige and power of queenship through acts of intercession, patronage and political governance through the lieutenancy. Queens could also tap into broader ideas about motherhood, nurturing their subjects rather than myopically focusing on biological parenthood. Queenship and motherhood both transcended biological reproduction, despite the constraints of hereditary monarchy.

As Bagerius and Ekholst discuss in their chapter on marital sexuality in this volume, monarchy was predicated on a privileging of heteronormative sexuality. Thus, a king's lack of sexual intercourse could be used by political opponents or unfavourable chroniclers to denigrate a monarch's manliness and authority, and the inability to impregnate his wife as a sign of God's disfavour. Yet childlessness, a sign of a potential lack of sexual activity, did not always doom a royal couple. Childlessness also forces scholars to reconsider queenship as a composite of subtle but important variations of power. A queen's latent or potential power required only that she be born to an influential family and be young enough to bear children. This power is evident in her status as princess, or simply as a highly desirable diplomatic prize for royal families jockeying for political advantage. Her dynastic power is an obvious expression of queenship seen in marriage and is a clear expression of queenship predicated on her understanding of the power of a dutiful wife and mother of an heir. This power fluctuated significantly over the course of her life, but the lack of children did not necessarily constrain her real talent for governmental power as the king's close adviser, as regent or queen-lieutenant, and in her management of the reginal estates. A childless queen could display cultural and intellectual power as patron of art, scholarly works, literature, scholars and promoter of women's education. She could still exert diplomatic and political power in the strategic use of influence to stabilize and pacify diplomatic relations. Many queens, childless or not, possessed a deep well of charismatic power as the beloved wife of the king whose subjects adored her and whose loyalty sustained her. One of the most public displays of her religious power as devout Catholic is evident in her patronage of shrines dedicated to saints believed to aid in pregnancy and childbirth. Finally, queens showed the very real power of resistance to a king, his advisers and any subjects who sought to replace her with a fecund new young woman.

Monarchy is an institution whose operation depended not only on kings but also on queens. It is important to think more broadly about what patriarchy and its counterpart, matriarchy, mean in the context of monarchy. The success of Anne of Bohemia, María of Castile and many other childless queens depended much on their personalities, their talent for governance and their natal families. Just because a queen had no children does not necessarily mean that she did not draw power from her gender and her awareness of and ability to exploit cultural expectations of a woman. To function well, monarchy needed both the masculine and the feminine, as justice and mercy or ruler and lieutenant. Monarchy was more than a dynasty, and the king and queen were much more than a ruler and his reproductive mate.

Aside from broadening our ideas about queenship, the successes of childless queens remind us that dynasty is a broad term, encompassing many royal relatives. It might not have been as easy or convenient to identify the heir of a childless monarch, but someone was there. Perhaps medieval and early modern rulers (aside from Henry VIII) saw the royal family in broad terms and recognized that individual childlessness would not upset the whole enterprise. Dynasties move horizontally as well as vertically, so that there was no crisis when Alfonso V of the Crown of Aragon was succeeded by his brother, Juan II.

Queenship without children also questions the association of dynasty with monarchy. Dynasty is not strictly the patriarchal lineage through a single male; it encompasses the wider family and collateral lines of inheritance. A childless queen does not necessarily signal the end of a dynasty, but rather a shift from one conjugal pair to another in the same family.

Notes

1 Kristen Geaman would like to thank the USC Provost's Fellowship Program and the Schallek Awards, sponsored by the Richard III Society and the Medieval Academy of America, for their funding and support of her dissertation, in which some of this material appeared and some of the ideas were initially developed. Theresa Earenfight thanks the National Endowment for the Humanities Summer Seminar at the Wellcome Institute, London, and Monica Green, Rachel Scott and the colleagues at that Seminar whose valuable insights into women's health were instrumental in shaping my understanding of medieval medical knowledge of pregnancy and childbirth.

2 *Alcuini Epistolae*, ed. E. Dummler in *Monumental Germanica Historia (MGH) Epistolae* vol. 4, Berlin: 1895, no. 18; translated in John Carmi Parsons, "The Pregnant Queen as Counsellor and the Medieval Construction of Motherhood," *Medieval Mothering*, eds. John Carmi Parsons and Bonnie Wheeler (New York: Garland, 1996), 39–61, at 44.

3 Miriam Shadis, "Blanche of Castile and Facinger's 'Medieval Queenship': Reassessing the Argument," in *Capetian Women*, ed. Kathleen Nolan (New York: Palgrave Macmillan, 2003), 137–161, esp. 149.

4 Janet Nelson, "Inauguration Rituals," in *Early Medieval Kingship*, eds. P.H. Sawyer and I.N. Wood (Leeds, 1977), rpt. in Nelson, *Politics and Ritual in Early Medieval Europe* (Ronceverte: Variorum, 1986), 304.

5 Charles T. Wood, "The First Two Queens Elizabeth, 1464–1503," in *Women and Sovereignty*, ed. Louise Fradenburg (Edinburgh: University of Edinburgh Press, 1991), 121–131.

6 Elizabeth Lehfedlt, "Ruling Sexuality: The Political Legitimacy of Isabel of Castile," *Renaissance Quarterly* 53 (2000): 31–56.

7 Giles Tremlett, *Catherine of Aragon, Henry's Spanish Queen: A Biography* (London: Faber and Faber, 2010), 168–171; Allan C. Barnes, "Diagnosis in Retrospect: Mary Tudor," *Obstetrics and Gynecology* 1, no. 5 (1953): 585–590; John Dewhurst, "The Alleged Miscarriages of Catherine of Aragon and Anne Boleyn," *Medical History* 28 (1984): 49–56; and Catrina Banks Whitley and Kyra Kramer, "A New Explanation For the Reproductive Woes and Midlife Decline of Henry VIII," *The Historical Journal* 53, no. 4 (2010): 827–848.

8 Dewhurst, "The Alleged Miscarriages of Catherine of Aragon and Anne Boleyn," 49–56; Tremlett, *Catherine of Aragon*, 168–175, 216, 224–225.

9 R. Sablonier, "The Aragonese Royal Family Around 1300," in *Interest and Emotion: Essays on the Study of Family and Kinship*, eds. H. Medick and D.W. Sabean (Cambridge: Cambridge University Press, 1984), 210–239.

10 Pamela Sheingorn, "Appropriating the Holy Kinship: Gender and Family History," in *Interpreting Cultural Symbols: Saint Anne in Late Medieval Society*, eds. Kathleen Ashley and Pamela Sheingorn (Athens: University of Georgia Press, 1990), 169–198.

11 Monica Green (ed. and trans.), *The Trotula: An English Translation of the Medieval Compendium of Women's Medicine* (Philadelphia: University of Pennsylvania Press, 2010).

12 Iona McCleery, "Medical 'Emplotment' and Plotting Medicine: Health and Disease in Late Medieval Portuguese Chronicles," *Social History of Medicine* 24, no. 1 (2011): 125–141.

13 Paris, Biblioteque National de France, MS lat. 6992, ff. 79r–90v.

14 Pauline Stafford, *Queen Emma and Queen Edith: Queenship and Women's Power in Eleventh Century England* (Oxford: Blackwell, 1997).

15 Monika Otter, "Closed Doors: An Epithalamium for Queen Edith, Widow and Virgin," in *Constructions of Widowhood and Virginity in the Middle Ages*, eds. Cindy L. Carlson and Angela Jane Weisl (New York: St. Martin's Press, 1999), 63–92, at 63–66, 68.

16 J. Huntington, "Edward the Celibate, Edward the Saint," in *Medieval Virginities*, eds. A. Bernau, S. Salih and R. Evans (Toronto: University of Toronto Press, 2003), 119–139, at 123.

17 Huntington, "Edward the Celibate, Edward the Saint," 120–123, 131. See also Dyan Elliott, *Spiritual Marriage: Sexual Abstinence in Medieval Wedlock* (Princeton: Princeton University Press, 1993), 119–123.

18 John Carmi Parsons and Bonnie Wheeler, "Introduction," *Medieval Mothering*, ix–xvii, at x.

19 Otter, "Closed Doors," 69 (her translation). 'Inclita mater, aue, prolem paritura beatem, / quam dum concipies, nulla maculabere culpa, / . . . / sed iungere tuo per federa casa marito, / eterno sociata deo complexibus almis; / cuius fusa tua sata celica germen in aluo / uiuificante suo reddunt de flamine sancto'. The quotation from 'And at whose . . . womb expire' is from Frank Barlow, ed. and trans. *The Life of King Edward Who Rests at Westminster*, second edition (Oxford: Oxford University Press, 1992), 73 (his translation). Original Latin on page 72: 'in cuius partu nullum patiere dolorem, / nec numero rara merebis de geniture, / intereatue tuo quisquam de uentre creates'; the song was a 'typicum epitalamium'.

20 Otter, "Closed Doors," 70.

21 Elliott, *Spiritual Marriage*, 119–120.

22 Katherine J. Lewis, "Becoming a Virgin King: Richard II and Edward the Confessor," in *Gender and Holiness: Men, Women and Saints in Late Medieval Europe*, eds. S.E.J. Riches and S. Salih (London: Routledge, 2002), 86–100.

23 Philippe de Mézières, *Letter to King Richard II, A Plea Made in 1395 for Peace between England and France*, trans. G.W. Coopland (Liverpool, 1975), 35.

24 Lewis, "Becoming a Virgin King," 90 argued that in Mézières' work, Richard was 'being perceived as and appealed to within the paradigm of the virginal (or at least chaste) childless ruler'. She does not, however, believe that Mézières thought Richard was a virgin.

25 Theresa Earenfight, *The King's Other Body: María of Castile and the Crown of Aragon* (Philadelphia: University of Pennsylvania Press, 2010); Lluis Comenge I Ferrer, *La medicina en el reinado de Alfonso V de Aragón* (Barcelona: Espasa, 1903), 26, 34; Instructions from the Consell de Cent to the Catalan ambassadors in Naples, Arxiu de la Catedral de Barcelona, 24 July 1438, doc. 131, José Madurell Marimón, *Mensajeros Barceloneses en la corte de Nápoles de Alfonso V de Aragón, 1435–58* (Madrid: Consejo Superior de Investigaciones Científicas, 1963), 191–194.

26 Kristen L. Geaman, "Anne of Bohemia and Her Struggle to Conceive," *Social History of Medicine* 29, no. 2 (May 2016), 224–244, at 234–235.

27 C. H. Williams, ed., *English Historical Documents, 1485–1558* (Oxford: Oxford University Press, 1967), 400.

28 Robert J. Knecht, *Hero or Tyrant? Henry III, King of France, 1574–89* (Farnham: Ashgate, 2014), 138 (translation); Gustave Baguenault de Puchesse, *Lettres de Catherine de Médicis*, vol. 8: 1582–1585 (Paris, 1901), 142: 'si plaisoit à Dyeu les ramener avec un enfant au ventre de la Royne, ce seroit pour nous reconforter de tous nous maux'.

29 Martin Haile, *Queen Mary of Modena: Her Life and Letters* (London: J.M. Dent & Co., 1905), 166–168. Hailes notes some of his information is from Strickland.

30 Anne Rudloff Stanton, "From Eve to Bathsheba and Beyond: Motherhood in the Queen Mary Psalter," in *Women and the Book: Assessing the Visual Evidence*, eds. Lesley Smith and Jane H.M. Taylor (Toronto: University of Toronto Press, 1997), 172–189. For apt comparisons of elite London women and queens, see Katherine L. French, "The Material Culture of Childbirth in Late Medieval London and its Suburbs," *Journal of Women's History* 28, no. 2 (2016): 126–148.

31 Elizabeth L'Estrange, *Holy Motherhood: Gender, Dynasty and Visual Culture in the Later Middle Ages* (Manchester: Manchester University Press, 2008), 44; Jean Cluzel, *Anne de France: fille de Louis XI, duchesse de Bourbon* (Paris: Fayard, 2002), 28; and Legaré, "Charlotte de

Savoie's Library and Illuminators," *Journal of the Early Book Society*, 4 (2001), 32–87, at 39. For Petronilla, see www.catholic.org/saints/saint.php?saint_id=1034 (accessed 2 July 2018).

32 Knecht, *Hero or Tyrant?* 215–216.

33 Knecht, *Hero or Tyrant?* 134.

34 J.C. Dickinson, *The Shrine of Our Lady of Walsingham* (Cambridge: Cambridge University Press, 1956), 9, 13–14. See this same work for the early history of Walsingham. Susan Signe Morrison, *Women Pilgrims in Late Medieval England: Private Piety as Public Performance* (London: Routledge, 2000), 73, 142.

35 *Westminster Chronicle 1381–1394*, eds. L.C. Hector and B.F. Harvey (Oxford: Clarendon Press, 1982), 42.

36 There is disagreement over when Margaret's pilgrimage took place. For 1452, see Carole Rawcliffe, "Richard, Duke of York, the King's 'Obeisant Liegeman': A New Source for the Protectorates of 1454 and 1455," *Historical Research* 60, no. 142 (June 1987), 232–239, at 237. For 1453, see Helen E. Maurer, *Margaret of Anjou: Queenship and Power in Late Medieval England* (Woodbridge: Boydell, 2003), 43. On the jewels, see A.R. Myers, "The Jewels of Queen Margaret of Anjou," in *Crown, Household and Parliament in Fifteenth Century England* (London: Hambledon Press, 1985), 211–229, at 222.

37 *Paston Letters and Papers of the Fifteenth Century*, ed. N. Davis, two volumes (Oxford, 1971–1976), Vol. II, 397. The letter is from Jakys Hawte to John Paston II.

38 H. Ellis, *Original Letters Illustrative of English History*, vol. 1 of 3 (London: Harding, Triphook and Lepard, 1824), 89 'now goo to Our Lady at Walsyngham that I promised soo long agoo to see'.

39 Dickinson, *The Shrine of Our Lady of Walsingham*, 44.

40 L'Estrange, *Holy Motherhood*, 237–238.

41 L'Estrange, *Holy Motherhood*, 238, 261 (quotes).

42 L'Estrange, *Holy Motherhood*, 261–262 (quote from 262).

43 Hilary Powell, "The 'miracle of childbirth': The Portrayal of Parturient Women in Medieval Miracle Narratives," *Social History of Medicine* 25, no. 4 (2012), 795–811.

44 Joanna L. Laynesmith, *The Last Medieval Queens: English Queenship 1445–1503* (Oxford: Oxford University Press, 2004).

45 See John Carmi Parsons, "The Queen's Intercession in Thirteenth-Century England," in *Power of the Weak: Studies on Medieval Women*, eds. Jennifer Carpenter and Sally-Beth MacLean (Urbana: University of Illinois Press, 1995), 147–177; Parsons, "The Pregnant Queen as Counsellor," 39–61; Paul Strohm, "Queens as Intercessors," in *Hochon's Arrow: The Social Imagination of Fourteenth-Century Texts* (Princeton: Princeton University Press, 1992), 95–119; Lois L. Huneycutt, "Intercession and the High-Medieval Queen: The *Esther Topos*," in Power of the Weak, 126–146; Carolyn P. Collette, *Performing Polity: Women and Agency in the Anglo-French Tradition, 1385–1620* (Turnhout: Brepols, 2006), 116. For a coronation day example, see John Carmi Parsons, "Ritual and Symbol in English Medieval Queenship to 1500," in *Women and Sovereignty*, ed. L.O. Fradenburg (Edinburgh: Edinburgh University Press, 2002), 60–77, at 64.

46 Parson, "The Intercessory Patronage of Queens Margaret and Isabella of France," in *Thirteenth Century England VI*, eds. Michael Prestwich et al. (Woodbridge: Boydell Press, 1995), 145–156, at 149 and 149 note 9.

47 Parsons, "The Intercessory Patronage," 150.

48 Parsons, "The Intercessory Patronage," 153 and Lisa Benz St. John, *Three Medieval Queens: Queenship and the Crown in Fourteenth-Century England* (New York: Palgrave Macmillan, 2012), 171.

49 Helen Lacey, *The Royal Pardon: Access to Mercy in Fourteenth-Century England* (York: York Medieval Press, 2009), 207.

50 Intercession was perhaps especially prominent from the time of Eleanor of Provence, but it was nothing new even then. Earlier queens, such as Eleanor of Aquitaine, had served as intercessors and even been monetarily rewarded for it. See Kristen Geaman, "Queen's Gold and Intercession: The Case of Eleanor of Aquitaine," *Medieval Feminist Forum*, 46, no. 2 (2010), 10–33.

51 Lacey, *The Royal Pardon*, 213.

52 *CPR, Richard II*, Vol. V: 1391–1396, 75.
53 St John, *Three Medieval Queens*, 34, 100, 210 note 33, relying on Lacey, *The Royal Pardon*, 45 and Collette, *Performing Polity*, 115–116.
54 St John, *Three Medieval Queens*, 173. The average for Anne was taken from the personal notes of Lisa Benz St John. There is some confusion over the exact number of intercessions Anne made. St John provided fifty-eight instances from the patent rolls alone; Lacey supplied seventy-one pardons. There must be some overlap, but the exact number has not been counted by one scholar. According to St John's table of intercessory acts (*Three Medieval Queens*, 171–172), Margaret had sixty-three acts of intercession (slightly fewer than Parsons counted); Isabella had an astonishing 182; and Philippa a respectable ninety-one. Isabella, however, only had ninety-six intercessions while queen consort, so Anne might have had a larger total of intercessions (St John's numbers combined with Lacey's come to 129; even assuming fairly substantial overlap, a total of ninety-seven or more intercessions is possible).
55 *Westminster Chronicle*, 24/25. 'nam non modicam pecuniam refundebat rex Anglie pro tantilla carnis porcione'. This was probably because Anne came without a dowry and Richard had given her half-brother Wenceslas IV a large loan. An alliance with Anne's family, the Luxemburgs, proved to be in name only, mainly because of the Luxemburgs' dynastic interests in Hungary and their inability to completely wean themselves from cooperation with France. See Nigel Saul, *Richard II* (New Haven: Yale University Press, 1997), 90–91 and Anthony Tuck, "Richard II and the House of Luxemburg," in *Richard II: the Art of Kingship*, eds. Anthony Goodman and James L. Gillespie (Oxford: Clarendon Press, 1999), 205–229.
56 Adam Usk, *The Chronicle of Adam Usk, 1377–1421*, ed. and trans. Chris Given-Wilson (Oxford: Clarendon Press, 1997), 4–5 (translation). Latin on page 4: 'reginam benignissimam'.
57 Parsons, "The Queen's Intercession," 151; "Pregnant Queen as Counsellor," 53; "The Intercessory Patronage," 149.
58 Mark Duffy, *Royal Tombs of Medieval England* (Stroud: Tempus, 2003), 168 and van Dussen, "Three Verse Eulogies of Anne of Bohemia," 236 citing Philip Lindley, "Absolutism and Regal Image in Ricardian Sculpture," in *The Regal Image of Richard II and the Wilton Diptych*, eds. Dillian Gordon et al. (London: Harvey Miller, 1997), 60–84 and 288–296.
59 Duffy, *Royal Tombs of Medieval England*, 172. My translation.

Sub petra lata nunc Anna iacet tumulata,
Dum vixit mundo Ricardo nupta secundo.
Christo devota fuit hec factis bene nota:
Pauperibus prona semper sua reddere dona:
Iurgia sedavit et pregnantes relevavit.
Corpore formosa vultu mitis speciosa.
Prebens solamen viduis, egris medicamen:
Anno milleno ter C, quarto nonageno
Junii septeno mensis, migravit ameno.

60 Strohm, "Queens as Intercessors," 106.
61 Michael van Dussen, "Three Verse Eulogies," *Medium Aevum*, 78, no. 2 (2009), 231–260, at 252 (lines 5 and 25).
62 Parsons, "The Pregnant Queen as Counsellor," 45. See Strohm, "Queens as Intercessors," 99–102 for a discussion of intercession, pregnancy and Philippa of Hainault.
63 During her lifetime, Anne had assisted some pregnant women by interceding for pardons on their behalf. The first instance occurred in 1383, when Anne secured a pardon for Agnes Martyn, sentenced to die for larceny but committed to prison because she was pregnant. In 1391 Anne interceded for Juliana Gylle, condemned for theft and assault while pregnant. Both of these women owed their stays of execution to their pregnancies; possibly Anne also secured their pardons because they were pregnant. See *CPR, Richard II*, Vol. II: 1381–1385, 243 and *CPR, Richard II*, Vol. V: 1391–1396, 8.
64 van Dussen, "Three Verse Eulogies," 243.

65 Elizabeth of Hungary was well known for her nurturing, maternal behaviour, yet she failed to lavish this on her biological children, whom she largely abandoned on her path to sainthood. For a wide-ranging discussion of religion and maternity, see L'Estrange, *Holy Motherhood.*

66 Edward Corp, "Catherine of Braganza and Cultural Politics," in *Queenship in Britain, 1660–1837: Royal Patronage, Court, Culture, and Dynastic Politics*, ed. Clarissa Campbell Orr (Manchester: Manchester University Press, 2002), 53–73, at 53–56.

67 Corp, "Catherine of Braganza and cultural politics," 60.

68 Corp, "Catherine of Braganza and cultural politics," 63.

69 Corp, "Catherine of Braganza and cultural politics," 64.

70 According to Anthony Hamilton, *Memoirs of Count Grammont*, trans. Sir Walter Scott (London: Bickers and Sons, 1870), 103, Catherine 'was far from appearing with splendor in the charming court where she came to reign; however, in the end she was pretty successful'.

71 The other queen-lieutenants in the Crown of Aragon were Blanca of Naples, wife of Jaume II, in 1310; Teresa d'Entença, wife of Alfonso III, lieutenant 1324–7; Violant de Bar, third wife of Joan I, 1388–95; Maria de Luna, first wife of Martí, 1396–1401; Margarida of Prades, second wife of Martí, 1412–21; and Juana Enríquez, second wife of Juan II, 1461–77. Theresa Earenfight, *The King's Other Body*, esp. pp. 1–4, 41–42, 46–52.

72 Rosanna Cantavella, "Introduction to *Protagonistas femenines a la 'Vita Christi*," eds. Rosanna Cantavella and Lluïsa Parra (Barcelona: La Sal, 1987), viii–ix; José Enrique Ruiz-Domènec, *El depertar de la mujeres: la Mirada femenina en la Edad Media* (Barcelona: Ediciones Península, 1999), 307.

Key works

Corp, Edward T., "Catherine of Braganza and Cultural Politics," *Queenship in Britain, 1660–1837: Royal Patronage, Court, Culture, and Dynastic Politics*, ed., Clarissa Campbell Orr (Manchester: Manchester University Press, 2002), 53–73.

Dewhurst, John, "The Alleged Miscarriages of Catherine of Aragon and Anne Boleyn," *Medical History* 28 (1984): 49–56.

Earenfight, Theresa, *The King's Other Body: María of Castile and the Crown of Aragon* (Philadelphia: University of Pennsylvania Press, 2010).

L'Estrange, Elizabeth, *Holy Motherhood: Gender, Dynasty and Visual Culture in the Later Middle Ages* (Manchester: Manchester University Press, 2008).

Otter, Monica, "Closed Doors: An Epithalamium for Queen Edith Widow and Virgin," in *Constructions of Widowhood and Virginity in the Middle Ages*, eds., Cindy L. Carlson and Angela Jane Weisl (Basingstoke: Macmillan, 1999), 63–92.

Parsons, John Carmi, "The Pregnant Queen as Counsellor and the Medieval Construction of Motherhood," in *Medieval Mothering*, eds., John Carmi Parsons and Bonnie Wheeler (New York: Garland Publishing, 1996), 39–61.

27

HAREM POLITICS

Royal women and succession crises in the ancient Near East (*c.*1400–300 BCE)

Lloyd Llewellyn-Jones

The two remarkable scenes in the Hebrew bible cited below (separated by only a chapter) focus on Bathsheba, King David's infamously beautiful, infamous and favourite (but by no means highest-ranking) wife:

> Bathsheba bowed down, prostrating herself before king [David] . . . She said to him, 'My lord, you yourself swore to me [that] Solomon your son shall be king . . . But now Adonijah has become king . . . My lord . . . as soon as my lord the king is laid to rest . . . I and my son Solomon will be treated as criminals.
>
> When Bathsheba went to King Solomon to speak to him . . . the king stood up to meet her, bowed down to her and sat down on his throne. He had a throne brought for the king's mother, and she sat down at his right hand.[1]

The first scene shows her hard at work at the bedside of her dying husband attempting to manoeuvre her son, Solomon, into the role of David's heir. By drawing on earlier promises the king had (supposedly) made to her and by making it explicit that if Solomon's elder half-brother, Adonijah, became king, then her life, alongside Solomon's, was in real danger, she gets what she wants and her son is proclaimed as David's successor.

The king's reluctance to appoint an heir from among his brood of (at least) nine sons had brought about this unfortunate life-or-death situation, but it was in no way a unique occurrence in antiquity, given that primogeniture was not a practice adopted by any of the great royal dynastic houses of the Near East. Rather than appoint a first-born son as heir to the throne and train him in the arts of rulership, kings of the Near East, like David, preferred to hedge their bets on destiny and wait to appoint any one of the (potentially) many sons born to the any number of women belonging to the royal harem.

For her part, a royal mother would work assiduously at promoting the advancement of her son, for it was only with a son's accession to the throne that her future was assured. And what a future that might be: as Bathsheba's second scene reveals, a king's mother ranks supreme at court, second only to the king. He himself never forgets the debt he owes his mother and, in Solomon's case, he ceremoniously rises from his throne to greet his mother and bows before her, before enthroning her at his righthand side, the place of honour. The benefits of being a queen mother were profuse.

But why did ancient rulers play this form of dynastic Russian roulette and refuse to adopt the simple system of appointing the first-born son as the heir as a means of quelling any threats of murder and mayhem? The rationale for disregarding primogeniture could have had a practical basis, of course, for in an age of high infant mortality rates even among the aristocracy, it might be considered prudent for a father to hold off on making decisions on appointing an heir until his sons began to reach maturity. Even then, there was no guarantee of long life. The long-lived pharaoh Ramses II, for instance, witnessed the death of at least twelve of his first-born sons and was eventually succeeded by prince Merneptah, the thirteenth son who only came to power because all his older brothers had died. Merneptah was probably the fourth child of Isetnofret, one of the two 'Great Royal Wives' of Ramses II, a woman who, by all accounts, languished in Ramses' affections behind her co-wife, Nefertari who had indeed given Ramses his first-born and much-loved son, Prince Amun-her-khepeshef. He was crown prince of Egypt for the first twenty-five years of Ramses II's reign, but eventually predeceased his father in regnal year 25. The pharaoh did aspire to rank his children in order of their birth, and it was Ramses II's second oldest son, Prince Ramses, who then succeeded him as crown prince for another twenty-five years.[2] But thereafter the appointment of an heir apparent was a chaotic affair, and Merneptah would only assume the office of crown prince in regnal year 67, the year of Ramses II's death. Even the plans of a god-king, it appears, could be thwarted by disease or simple bad luck.

Warfare too could have a detrimental impact upon any aspirations towards primogeniture which a Near Eastern monarch might have harboured. In Assyria, Sennacherib's eldest son, Aššur-nadin-šumi, who seems to have been primed to be future king, disappeared and presumably died in a military campaign. In fact, Assyrian evidence confirms neither Sargon II, Esarhaddon, nor Aššurbanipal were first-born sons. In the court of Israel, as we have noted, biblical writers show that King David was succeeded by Solomon the son of Bathsheba, but that Solomon had many older half-brothers born of different mothers.

Other reasons for rejecting the notion of primogeniture could operate on a more personal level. Kings might wait to see which of his sons showed the most potential for rulership, or simply display characteristics which he himself recognized as desirable or engaging. Anthony Dolphin Alderson's frank assessment of Ottoman succession issues is apt for the ancient Near East too: 'Far from there being any theory of primogeniture . . . the law of succession may well be described as a "free-for-all," in which the strongest of the sons inherited the throne, while the others . . . suffered death.'[3]

Moreover, the relationship between a king and his women, the birth-mothers of potential heirs, could dictate a prince's future. It was common that favoured women were shown preference through the monarch's championing of their sons. As Jeroen Dunidam perceptively puts it:

> Between the sheets, crown and sceptre lost their spell. And no one could get closer to the royal ear. Wives and mistresses (and for different reasons mothers and sisters) were therefore influential . . . the confident served as a broker of the king's [power].[4]

Beyond this, however, there was active lobbying for the rights and status of sons by ambitious wives and concubines who sometimes worked with courtiers and dignitaries to promote the aspirations of their male off-spring. The large harems of the Near Eastern empires meant that, 'the presence of numerous . . . women stressed the stature of patrilineal decent' and, again as Duindam notes, 'Succession adhered to certain rules and prohibitions connected to the ideals of rulership, but it left room for the intervention of ruling elites, and notably for those at the heart of power at court.'[5]

Discord created through tensions between birth-rank and favouritism was marked in the male-dominated dynastic systems of antiquity. Succession traditions which did not include a clear preference for the eldest son (such as existed in Christian Europe and, indeed, imperial China) often led to violent contests of power, sometimes resulting in fratricide and regicide. Such tensions, a feature of the later eastern courts too, were often propounded by competition among royal women. This chapter looks at the roles played by women in the politics of the succession, exploring how the harem functioned as both a site of ancestral continuity and as a locale of dynastic disharmony. Of necessity, the evidence offered here is selective and I draw on case studies of examples from ancient Egypt, Assyria, Israel, Syria and Iran to offer some thoughts on the variability of roles which different types of women found themselves playing in the politicking of the Near East.

Dismissing the existence of the women of the harem or seeing the harem institution only as an invention of the Orientalist imagination damages our understanding of the nature and functioning of absolutist forms of dynastic government, since the harem was a central tenet in the policies of Near Eastern absolute monarchy. I am conscious that in writing this chapter I am drawing on a broad range of evidence from several successive Near Eastern societies across a wide span of time, but I do this for a purpose – to expose the realia of the use and abuse of women in dynastic politics and to counteract any disparaging attempts among scholars to regard female participation in succession issues, or in the broader politics of rule, as abnormal and the products of hostile historiography.[6] Pierre Briant has suggested that the reports of intrigues, factions and insurgences at the ancient courts are more literary motifs than authentic records of actual events,[7] but it is more likely that the conservative nature of the courts themselves truly engendered repetitive actions on the part of frustrated courtiers. As Arthur Keaveny astutely notes:

> Monarch after monarch was surrounded by thrusting officials and relatives. Given that this circumstance did not change we need not . . . wonder if, in reign after reign, they led to the same . . . consequences. It is the unchanging nature of court life over a long period rather than a *reprise de motifs littéaires* which led to the repetitious nature of the tales.[8]

Corralling evidence from across Near Eastern antiquity helps normalize harem participation in dynastic life. Harem politicking at the Near Eastern courts precipitated intense domestic rivalries among the royal women, and this (theoretical) wrangling had a direct impact upon imperial policy as wives and mothers went head-to-head with one another out of jealously over rank and status or, predominantly, to solidify the status of their sons. The sons themselves frequently united with their mothers, whom they saw as their champions, and turned upon their siblings as competition for the throne mounted.

Sex as politics

Duindam is correct to emphasize that, 'the male ruler's sex-drive was never the sole explanation of polygyny'.[9] Women were gathered together in ancient court societies to fulfil important social, cultural and ritual roles and to undertake (it was hoped) vital functions in dynastic continuity as mothers. The political impact which the women of the harem might have on a dynasty's development was profound. In the early Achaemenid period in Iran (*c*.540–485 BCE), for instance, the possession of a royal predecessor's women ensured the successor's hold on the throne; the control of the harem gave a new ruler the potential to legitimize his reign through the physical possession of a former monarch's household. This is why, upon his succession to the throne of Persia, Darius I married numerous princesses of the royal line. In this Darius was *seemingly* following a common ancient practice: the Egyptian pharaoh Akhenaten inherited his father's wives and concubines when he succeeded Amenhotep III to the throne and, a century later, Ramses II routinely inherited the women belonging to the harem of his father Seti I as a demonstration of dynastic longevity. But Darius I's acquisition of the women of his predecessors was anything but routine; he had seized the throne of the Teispids (the family of Cyrus the Great) and had proclaimed the birth of a new dynasty – the Achaemenids – with himself as the head. In his bid for power Darius had married all the available royal women of the line of Cyrus, incorporated them into his harem, and established them as the highest-ranking of all his pre-existing wives. He quickly fathered children by his new acquisitions and promoted his sons born in the purple above those born before his accession. We have no idea how the Teispid women themselves regarded the usurpation of power, or even if they went willingly to Darius' bed, but it must have been apparent to them that their family bloodline and their potential fecundity made them political agents in a world in which women were otherwise without direct power.

The possession of a predecessor's harem of women ensured the successor's hold on the throne, and the control of the harem gave a new ruler the potential to legitimize his reign through the physical possession of a former monarch's household – and the potential for sexual command over the women of any former ruler must not be overlooked here. For its part, the Achaemenid dynasty's own downfall was confirmed in 331 BCE when Alexander of Macedon defeated Darius III in battle and subsequently captured his harem, including his esteemed mother, Sisygambis. Alexander even promoted the idea that the defeated king's mother was now *his* champion. A tradition preserved in Quintus Curtius Rufus says that Sisygambis could never forgive Darius for abandoning his family post-battle and that when she was called upon to mourn his death, she was reported to have said, 'I have only one son [Alexander] and he is king of all Persia.'[10] The story (alongside that of Sisygambis starving herself to death following Alexander's death) is probably apocryphal and was coined as pro-Alexander spin to justify his takeover of Iran, but what is certain is that Alexander married Sisygambis' granddaughter, Stateira II, in 324 BCE to stamp his hold on Persia. For the Achaemenids, the Macedonian king's seizure of the Persian royal harem *en masse* and his marriage into the family heralded the end of their dynastic rule. Alexander's appropriation of the reproductive capabilities of the women of the inner court immediately nullifed the legitimacy of Darius III's reign and brought 300 years of successful empire-building crashing down.

In much the same vein, although less internationally resonant, upon his military victory and subsequent accession to the throne of Israel, King David claimed all the females of the harem of his opponent, King Saul.[11] Solomon inherited his father's harem of women and servants although, as we will explore, challenges to both David and Solomon came in the form of rebellions within the royal house when two of David's sons rebelled against the Israelite kings and attempted to win the royal concubines and incorporate them into rival royal harems. The threat of having royal women fall into the hands of opponents was very real. In the Hebrew bible, Yahweh threatened David with the prophecy that, 'I will take your women before your eyes' – and that menace resonated deeply with all the kings of the ancient Near East. Sennacherib's account of his successful 701 BCE campaign against the western princelings of his empire trumpets the fact that Hezekiah, king of Judah, 'was overwhelmed by the awesome splendour of my lordship, and he sent to me after my departure to Nineveh, my royal city . . . his daughters (and) his palace women'.[12] In other words, Hezekiah showed his acquiescence to the king of Assyria by offering Sennacherib the reproductive capabilities of the women of the Judean royal house.

In her ground-breaking study of the Ottoman harem, Leslie Peirce makes a vital observation on the nature of absolute monarchy:

> Sex for . . . any monarch in a hereditary dynasty, could never be purely pleasure, for it had significant political meaning. Its consequences – the production of offspring – affected the succession to the throne, indeed the very survival of the dynasty. It was not a random activity . . . Sexual relations between the [ruler] and chosen women of the harem were embedded in a complex politics of dynastic reproduction.[13]

Taking this logical idea very seriously, it is clear that any trivialization in which the harem is viewed as a brothel-like pleasure-palace fails to do justice to its central role in the political milieu of a royal court or, indeed, of empires at large.

A harem Who's-Who

The royal harem was a large and diverse community. The women who made up the harem varied in age from little girls to adolescents, mature mothers and widows of dead kings. Widowed or divorced sisters and aunts were also part of the harem's makeup, alongside stewardesses, female servants who performed the household chores, female slaves, female administrators, eunuchs and high-ranking males, like doctors, who might operate within the harem only temporarily. Behind references to 'the harem', therefore, there lies a hierarchically structured royal household of considerable complexity.

So, who made up the female members of royal harems of Egypt, Assyria, Israel and Persia? It is difficult to be precise since numbers of women found in royal harems varied with time and space. In Mari (Syria) a king named Yasmah-Addu is recorded as having forty-four royal women (and their staff) in his palace. His successor, Zimri-Lim, had a harem of 232 women. This is thanks mainly to his military victories. We must concede then that harem size related directly to military ambitions and the territorial gains of monarchs. The following inventory of female captives from Nineveh, dated to the latter part of the reign of Esarhaddon, constitutes a good observation point in that it articulates the nexus between military prowess and reproductive potential:

> 36 Aramean women; 15 Kushite women; 7 Assyrian women, maids [of theirs]; 4 replacements . . .; [x] 3 Tyrian women; [n] Kassite women (break of some 4 lines) . . . [n] female Corybantes; 3 Arpadite women; 1 replacement; 1 Ashdodite woman; 2 Hittite women and [n] [-ean] women: in all, 94 women and 36 maids of theirs. Grand total, of the father of the Crown Prince: in all, 140 (women) . . . [Furthermore] 8 female chief musicians; 3 Aramean women; 11 Hittite women; 13 Tyrian women; 13 female Corybantes (?); 4 women from Sah[. . .]; 9 Kassite women: in all, 61 female musicians.[14]

In most historical contexts the harem was headed by a chief queen, usually the king's mother or, in her absence, the most favoured (or influential) wife who gathered about her the other royal and noble women – secondary wives, sisters, daughters and others. Beneath those favoured women ranked the concubines, then the female administrative personnel and, at the lowest level, the female slaves. However, the harem hierarchies of antiquity must have been in a state of continual flux as, for instance, wives gave birth to sons rather than daughters and thereby gained some hierarchical cachet, or a concubine suddenly became a favoured companion of the monarch.

While a king might have many wives or concubines, he could only have one biological mother, so it is not hard to grasp the notion that the king's mother held the highest place of authority among the court ladies.[15] Of equal prestige to her position as the monarch's birth-mother was her role in connecting two generations of rulers. In the Near East, while the king's mother was not expected to exercise official power, she might gain political clout through the careful maintenance of her son's favour as a consequence of her own ambitions and personal skill. In other words, the king's mother's power was indirect although she could influence her son in his policy-making. The actual power that the king's mother could wield was limited and she acted only with the consent of the king, although strictly within the domestic sphere she may have been given *carte blanche* to take decisions on her own. Evidence also suggests that the king's mother could be independently wealthy and own private estates, and it is clear that influential royal mothers could amass personal property often gifted to her by the crown.

Near Eastern kings were polygamous, although it appears that in most societies they took only local noble-born women as wives of the highest rank. They took multiple wives so that they could beget numerous heirs, and Near Eastern literature is replete with acknowledgements of the significance of children to a man's social position:

Inanna will make for you a passionate wife to lie with you!
She will give you strong-shouldered sons!
She will create a place of happiness . . .
To marry is human.
To beget children is divine.[16]

The pressure felt by kings to father many children was tantamount to their success and reputation as mighty monarchs, and heartfelt royal pleas to the gods – such as one which Kirta, the childless king of Ugarit in Syria, pours forth:

What do I care for silver, or even the flash of gold,
Together with land wealth, and slaves in abundance?
Teams of chariot horses
From the stable of the son of a slavegirl?
Let me make sons!
Let me create a brood![17]

Although Kirta had seven wives, they had all either died in childbirth or of disease or else had deserted him, and Kirta had no surviving children. His own mother had borne eight sons although Kirta was the only one to survive childhood, and now that he had no family members to succeed him he saw that his dynasty's demise was inevitable. To prevent this type of dynastic catastrophe, the wives and concubines of Near Eastern monarchs were expected to be fertile sexual partners. They were responsible for a dynasty's promulgation given that royal power was transmitted through the wombs of the family. As Ruby Lal writes, 'Such women's lives were not for themselves, but for creating other lives; they were required to keep intact the illustrious past and secure the future of the generations to come by working upon the present ones.'[18]

Concubines were also expected to provided monarchs with children. These women might be gifted to a king by foreign potentates or be acquired as war booty; they were supposed to be physically appealing since the arousal of desire in the ruler was essential. The childless King Kirta, for example, set his mind on the idea that a brood of sons would follow on from his acquisition of beautiful aristocratic war-captured concubines. With that goal in mind he raised an army against the kingdom of Udum, demanding of its King Pubala his attractive daughter (likened by Kirta to a goddess in terms of loveliness) as a concubine:

What is not in my house you must give me: You must give me Lady Huraya,
The fair-one, your firstborn child, Who is as fair as the goddess Anat, Who is
as comely as [the goddess] Astarte . . . Who will bear a son for Kirta![19]

This practice of harem recruitment, which ensured that fertile young women entered into court service, was widespread. The Greek historian Herodotus confirms that the most beautiful girls of Ionia were dragged from their homes and sent to the Persian court, and the bible story of Esther begins with an empire-wide search for beautiful virgins who are brought to the palace at Susa.[20] The system was still operating in later royal institutions across Asia and the Middle East.[21] Yet in spite of the twin pillars of beauty and sexual allure upon which royal concubinage was built, it would be wrong to think of royal concubines as women of the demi-monde, and they should not be classed as even 'reputable disreputable' women. In no way should these women be confused with courtesans, prostitutes or mistresses. Nonetheless, in legal terms, it is doubtful that concubines were formally 'married' to a king; there were, as far as we know, no vows or financial transfers of brideprice or dowry and no ceremony or banquet of celebration. As T.M. Sharlach notes:

> When a grey-haired monarch selected a twentieth girl, perhaps from amongst the daughters of the harem-women of a conquered neighbour or the dancers, as his latest love-interest, was this really a marriage? Perhaps the concubine symbolized a stable relationship with one man (in this case, the king), so that the concubine's children could be acknowledged as his; however, a concubine (unlike a wife) did not have the same status socially or legally as her mate.[22]

Peirce notes that the Ottoman concubines had one single duty to perform: to bear a son. This event actually terminated the concubine's sexual relationship with the ruler, even if their relationship was one of passion, because tradition dictated that she give him no more children. If she produced a series of daughters then the sexual relationship could continue, but once the couple were blessed with a son, sexual congress ceased and the ruler moved on to a new concubine. From there on in, the singular purpose of the concubine-mother was to work towards her son's political advancement.[23] It is difficult to know for certain if the Ottoman-style custom operated in the Near Eastern courts of antiquity too, but it is tempting to think so given that ancient kings who are known to be the sons of concubine-mothers do not seem to have had full-blood brothers. While the official take was, perhaps, that sons born to concubines were regarded as inferior to any child born to a royal wife, the history of the succession of numerous Near Eastern kings told another story. Not infrequently the son of a concubine ascended his way to the throne. For instance, Darius II of Persia, the son of a Babylonian concubine, was crowned king on the death of his father, Artaxerxes I; the powerful pharaoh Thutmose III was the son of Iset, a concubine, and even the great 'Sun King' of Egypt, Amenhotep III, was born of a concubine-mother, Mutwemwiya, who is never even attested in the inscriptions of her husband, Thutmose IV (himself the son of a 'faceless concubine' named Tiaa).[24] Mutemwiya's pre-eminence came in the early years of her son's reign when Amenhotep promoted her to semi-divine status, advertising that his birth had been a miraculous coupling between Mutwemwiya and the god Amun.

Such facts prove that concubinage was not a dormant institution. Duindam points out that in Qing China 16% of all imperial consorts had started court life as palace maids or concubines and that in the Ming period, 64% of women had begun their careers in this humble state.[25] Of course, in the harem status system the child of a concubine always outranked its mother, since the child took its eminence (and the blood royal) from its father, but the reality of the harem was that circumstance or personal ambition could change the hierarchy, and with it the course of dynastic politics.

Within the female household, status was dependent upon gaining and maintaining the king's favour. One text, quite unparalleled in Assyrian history, shows a king, Sennacherib, clearly smitten by one of his wives:

As for Tašmetum-šarrat . . . my beloved wife, whose features [are] perfect above all women, I had a palace of loveliness, delight and joy built . . . May she be granted days of health and happiness . . . May she have her fill of well-being.[26]

Women who had sexual relations with the king would have had (even if only temporarily) greater status than those who had no access to his bed, and therefore we can speculate how competition to attract and keep the king's sexual attention could be intense. The title 'favourite of the king', found with intermittent regularity in the sources, suggests that some women – but not *all* women – were recognized as having a particular significance in the king's affections.

Love and sexual attraction aside, in the cut and thrust world of the harem, it is increasingly clear that the position of a primary wife was not necessarily a stable one given that the king might prefer the son of a lesser wife or a concubine to become his successor. Thus, as Zafrira Ben-Barak is keen to emphasize:

Women . . . had . . . to plan and establish a sophisticated power-base capable of justifying and backing their sons in their bid for power. To this end they gathered supporters to their sons' side from various political strata in the realm and recruited religious elements in order to obtain for their sons the legitimacy of divine election to kingship.[27]

Elena Woodacre makes some valuable observations, however, noting the significant cost this might mean for mothers who launched a bid for power:

[a] mother's personal ambition – and others' fear of it – could undermine her relationship with her offspring. In cases where the political situation in the realm was stable and the order of the succession was clear and secure without threat of alternative claimants, a mother's desire to see her child accede to the throne might be easily realized. However, when political instability was present in the realm or when the field of potential claimants was diverse and challenging, a mother often struggled to realize her ambition for them to rule.[28]

Despite their best efforts, some son-promoting mothers were unsuccessful in their bids for power. But the fact that we know of thwarted attempts at accessing power proves that for many mothers and sons, the power game was worth playing.

Mother love and sibling rivalry

Generally in the ancient Near East, gender ideologies adhered to an understanding of human reproduction which insisted that women were primarily receptacles of the male seed and that, as a consequence, women were only important as producers of children. In a royal context this meant that the woman who produced the son who eventually became king was automatically regarded as having the highest status among all other women, having performed best her natural duty to state and gods. The best evidence of powerful women in the Near East relates, therefore, to king's mothers rather than wives or concubines. The Neo-Assyrian kings were conscious of the role played by their mothers in their God-given progress to the throne, as Sennacherib writes in one of his inscriptions: 'The mistress of the gods, the mistress of creation, looked favourably in the womb of the mother who bore me', while, after his official recognition as crown prince, Aššurbanipal wrote a letter in which he lauds the virtues of his deceased mother: 'Aššur and Šamaš decreed for me the Crown Princeship of Assyria on account of her righteousness.'[29] This concept is located in Israelite royal ideology too: 'For you created my innermost being; you knit me together in my mother's womb. I praise you because I am . . . wonderfully made.'[30] In Persia, in the so-called 'Harem Inscription', a text recalling his succession to the throne, Xerxes carefully allies himself to his father's memory and designates himself *maθišta* (literally, 'the greatest'):

> Darius had other sons, but – thus was [the god] Ahuramazda's desire – my father Darius made me the greatest [*maθišta*] after him. When my father Darius went away from the throne, by the grace of Ahuramazda I became king on my father's throne.[31]

Xerxes' text is full of confidence and bravado, but is perhaps more hyperbole than reality, at least if we choose to follow the story of Darius' succession as told by Herodotus who reports of a 'violent struggle' which erupted between Darius' many sons. Xerxes, born to Darius after he had ascended the throne, emerges victorious because he plays the 'porphyrogeniture card' and thereby pulls rank over his brothers, the sons born to Darius while he was still a private man.[32] In the Harem Inscription Xerxes makes no mention of his mother, Atossa, and it is left to Herodotus to note how she, as Cyrus the Great's eldest daughter, 'had all the power' and manoeuvred to secure the throne for her first-born son, a facet of the story we should take seriously. Although Herodotus' foregrounding of Atossa's power and influence does not sit well with the scant mentions of her in authentic Persian sources (only two texts from Persepolis refer to 'Udusana' – Atossa – and they can both be dated before Xerxes' birth to *c*.500/499 BCE), it is probable that she only rose to real prominence after the accession of Xerxes when she became the undisputed head of the harem. Before that time she, like many other royal women before and after her, must have spent a considerable time operating behind the scenes. However, when a younger son ascended the throne he would, in a way, owe his position to his mother, for it was she who had received the king's seed and it was thus through her that he achieved legitimacy to the throne, regardless of his mother's rank. The fact that his mother had been the sexual companion of the king bestowed a dynastic legitimacy on the offspring of that union. As Sarah Melville states, a 'woman's association with the king as his wife and receptacle of his seed gives her son status, but only in retrospect, after he is chosen heir. Mothers gain prestige only when their sons are chosen for kingship'.[33] Upon the king's death, however, mothers gained the highest court status. Widowhood propelled the royal mother into untouchable authority.

In systems of absolute government, succession issues were the primary concern of the king. Having many children certainly assured that the throne would stay within the dynasty, and the advantages of having many sons to be potential heirs and to act as governors and military leaders and having numerous daughters to use as marriage pawns were clear. The drawback, however, was that the large number of male heirs increased the chance of rebellion and civil war. Competition between siblings was, it appears, part of the fabric of daily life at court.

In Israel a major rebellion erupted against King David when his son Absalom decided to break from his father and establish a rival royal court in Hebron. The catalyst for this revolt had been the rape and deflowering of Princess Tamar by her half-brother Prince Ammon. Absalom, determined to avenge his full blood-sister had Ammon murdered and for this action, he was sent into exile in Hebron by his doting and heartbroken father.[34] The whole account of Ammon's heinous crime and of the family feud that quickly escalated into civil war is fuelled by the presence of Tamar. Her rape and shame meant that the princess could have no future role to play in the politics of her father's royal house since her sexual violation rendered her valueless in the political ambitions of David. As Amy Kalmanofsky notes, 'Tamar . . . can never marry nor have children. She can never become a mother in her husband's house. Instead . . . Tamar is condemned to represent her father's troubled house and embody its distress.'[35]

Sometime later, when Absalom captured and publicly raped ten of his father's concubines in a wilful act of political revenge (the biblical chronicler describes the act as a 'stench'), the message sent to David was vividly clear: like other ambitious claimants to other thrones, Absalom was stamping his desire to rule onto the bodies of his father's women.[36] When Absalom was killed in battle, the ten concubines were reclaimed by David but, now tainted by the rape of Absalom (and with the possibility that any one of them might be carrying his child), the king ceased to have sexual relations with them (and presumably moved on to new concubines):

> Then David came to his house at Jerusalem, and the king took the ten women, the concubines whom he had left (there), and placed them under guard and provided them with sustenance, but did not go in to them. So they were shut up until the day of their death, living as widows.[37]

The disgrace within the house of David, in which a blood princess and ten concubines are rendered dynastically worthless, compromised the whole kingdom, since the sexual indiscretion of one son and the violence, sexual degeneracy and blind ambition of the other, reflected badly on the inability of the father to keep his house in order. In the context of a society in which there was no disconnect between the virtue of the ruling house and the virtue of the state as a whole, this was bound to have grave consequences. The salient point here in the ancient Near Eastern context is that the actions of the royal family profoundly impacted on the dominions over which they ruled. Dishonour brought to the women of a royal household reverberated with dynastic consequences.

In 1167 BCE Egypt was thrown into utter turmoil when Ramses III was murdered in a rebellion originating in the royal harem (scans of the royal mummy have revealed a deep cut in Ramses throat, probably made by a sharp knife). The king's murder resulted in a lengthy trial and punishment by death of those responsible, and a multitude of surviving texts describe how a group of women from the king's harem, headed by one called Teya, organized his murder so that Pentawere, Teya's only son, could ascend the throne.[38] The plan, crafted by the mother and son, involved a faction made from all walks of court society, from nobles, military men and administrative personnel to sorcerers (magic played a major role in the coup) and slaves. Susan Redford has argued that Teya must have held a high rank within Ramses III's harem, probably as one of his chief wives, otherwise, she asks, why would chief courtiers throw in their lot with the aspirations of Teya if her son were not already in a feasible position to become heir?[39] But this is not necessarily the case, and we have noted already that the sons of concubines were in no way debarred from the succession, nor lacked the required ambition to reach the throne. Quite clearly that the 'harem conspiracy' failed in its goal of crowning Pentawere. The conspirators were arrested, and some of them, including Pentawere, were compelled to commit suicide. It is not known what happened to Teya.

The Assyrian royal family too was torn apart when in 683 BCE, several of the sons of Sennacherib rebelled against their father and killed him following his unexpected appointment of a crown prince – a younger prince, Esarhaddon, the son of a foreign concubine named Zakûtu.[40] The older brothers were motivated to kill their father for this snub in order to take the throne for one of their number, although Esarhaddon managed to secure the throne and defeated his brothers' factions in a six-week civil war. He then had his brothers' families and associates executed and confirmed his legitimacy on the throne with the creation of several inscriptions which clearly outlined the events that led him to power: 'My brothers went mad. They drew their swords, godlessly, in the middle of Nineveh . . . All the gods looked with wrath on the deeds of these scoundrels, brought their strength to weakness and humbled them beneath me.' While Esarhaddon's inscription tells the basic story, it is not the whole one since it appears that, after Sennacherib announced his choice of heir and the brothers made clear their displeasure, Zakûtu sent Esarhaddon into hiding for his safety until the time was right for his return.

Esarhaddon never forgot his mother's role in safeguarding his life and helping him gain the crown, and in his later years, when he appointed one of his own younger sons, Aššurbanipal, as his successor, he was determined to avoid a repeat of the events that had thrust him into power and asked his elderly but venerable mother to oversee her grandson's safe accession. When Esarhaddon died, Zakûtu honoured her son's request and issued the so-called Loyalty Treaty (c.670 BCE) which compelled the Assyrian court and those territories under Assyrian rule to accept and support the reign of Aššurbanipal:

> Anyone who (concludes) this treaty which Zakûtu, the queen dowager . . . on behalf of Aššurbanipal, her favourite grandson, anyone who should . . . lie and carry out a deceitful or evil plan or revolt against Aššurbanipal, king of Assyria, your lord; in your hearts plot evil intrigue (or) speak slander against Aššurbanipal; in your hearts contrive (or) plan an evil mission (or) wicked proposal for rebellion (and) uprising . . . or conspire with another for the murder of Aššurbanipal . . . and if you hear and know that there are men who agitate or conspire among you –whether his brothers or royal relatives – should you hear or know, you shall seize and kill them and bring them to Zakûtu.

Here Zakûtu comes across rather as 'an active party in a mutually beneficial negotiated power relationship and, from a heterarchical perspective, it can be suggested that the son and the (grand)mother legitimize each other, both gaining status from each other'.[41]

When acting with wisdom and energy, royal mothers can be seen as dynastic guard dogs, carefully policing the continuity of the family and preventing internal strife, and while the championing of her son meant advancement for her own status, the underlying agenda of queen mothers was 'dynastic security at all costs'. The actions of Bathsheba to promote her son Solomon to the throne can be read in this light. She wasted no time, in David's dying days, in gathering the support of prominent members of the clergy, the administration and the army in supporting her son against the claims of his elder brother, Adonijah, David's fourth son by his wife Haggith, who in anticipation of his father's imminent death, had proclaimed himself king of Israel.

We might assume that upon taking the throne Adonijah would set about eliminating any rivals or opposition to his rule. This explains Bathsheba's creation of a court faction and her death bed scene reminder to David of his promise to make Solomon king (see the opening quotation at the head of this chapter). Bathsheba persuades David to give orders that Solomon should immediately be proclaimed king, and as this is done, the elder prince fled the court.[42] But Adonijah attempted to gain the throne once more early in the reign of Solomon when he tried to incorporate one of the late king David's best-loved concubines, the young and beautiful Abishag of Shunem, into his own harem. Adonijah's bold effort at appropriating the reproductive capability of his father's possession was a deliberate act intended to jeopardize the legitimacy of Solomon's rule, as Bathsheba was quick to recognize. For this (potential) act of treason, Adonijah was swiftly put to death.[43]

Less understandable are the accounts of royal mothers deliberately churning up fraternal strife and forwarding dynastic disharmony. In Persia, Darius II's influential sister-wife, Parysatis, had more than fulfilled her dynastic duty and had produced numerous healthy sons and daughters, but the two eldest sons, Prince Arses and Prince Cyrus (named after his illustrious ancestor and known to history, therefore, as Cyrus the Younger), got the bulk of the parental attention. Parysatis had a particular fondness for Cyrus, but King Darius favoured Arses and began to train him for the throne. Deciding to keep Arses close to him at court for training in kingship, Darius sent the younger brother to Ionia to act as the royal overseer of the troublesome area. Once established in the west, Cyrus bought the services of Greek mercenary soldiers and when, in the autumn of 405 BCE Darius II became ill and summoned Prince Cyrus to rejoin the court at Babylon, Cyrus arrived with 300 hoplites as a show of his new-found military prestige. Upon Darius' death the throne passed to the eldest son who took the throne-name of Artaxerxes II, but the court was immediately plunged into chaos when Cyrus was found to be plotting to usurp the throne. Artaxerxes immediately had his brother arrested and imprisoned. Parysatis quickly intervened, however, and begged Artaxerxes for Cyrus' life and persuaded by Parysatis of his innocence, the new king sent Cyrus back to Ionia to take up his duties once more. Safely ensconced in his palace on the western frontier of the empire, Cyrus, now encouraged by his mother through correspondence, began plotting to oust Artaxerxes from the throne once and for all. In 401 BCE the impetuous twenty-three-year-old Cyrus assembled his troops at Cunaxa in Babylonia. In the midst of a ferocious battle against his brother, Cyrus was mortally wounded and died. His decapitated head was sent to Babylon to be displayed to the court. Utterly devastated by the death of Cyrus, the grieving Parysatis systematically hunted down and destroyed many individuals connected to his death.

Why did Parysatis pervert the role of royal mother in this way, encouraging strife between her sons and even setting her younger son in opposition to his father? It can only be explained (from the evidence available to us at least) as a blind love for Cyrus coupled with, perhaps, a clash of personalities with her eldest son. Her devotion to Cyrus overwhelmed Parysatis' vision of dynastic circumspection. The Greek author Xenophon, who served in Cyrus' mercenary army, was clear on this point: 'Darius and Parysatis had two sons born to them ... [The younger] had ... the support of Parysatis, his mother, for she loved him better than the son who was king.'[44] Cyrus, we are led to believe, was named by Parysatis for his illustrious ancestor but also because, Xenophon (mistakenly) insists, the name meant 'sun' in Persian. Cyrus was literally his mother's ray of sunshine.

Conclusion

Ellen Weber Libby's sociological study of the bond between mothers and favourite sons exposes some interesting factors which we can see clearly operating within the gender-segregated world of ancient harem societies. Favourite sons, she argues, tend to fill the voids in their mothers' emotional lives created by husbands who are literally or emotionally absent or preoccupied; these women train their favoured sons to replace these older, adored men. Emerging from the erroneous belief that they have replaced their fathers, mothers' favourite sons tend to grow up vulnerable to sociopathic behaviours and are egocentric and comparatively ill-prepared for the trials of real life.[45] They rely on their mothers all the more.

Harem-politicking could be a dark occupation, and the world of the inner-court was one in which intense feelings of hatred, intolerance or, conversely, loyalty, and overwhelming affection, had a direct impact upon imperial policy. Women went head-to-head with one another or with the men who surrounded them to secure their own positions and to solidify the status of their sons. Executions, punishments, mutilations and even revenge killings were commonplace. Within harem societies all women were potential political players, but it is mothers (wives and concubines) who emerge as the skilled political operators and impassioned dynastic guardians. Parysatis' vendettas against the individuals who had been involved in Prince Cyrus' death is proof of the deeply felt devotion she had for her favourite son and of the commitment she had made to securing the throne for him. History judges her as misguided in her actions, but her instincts were, to her, right and justified. The murder of Ramses III marks the nadir of the dangers of harem politics, but Teya too no doubt had rationalized her thoughts and concluded that gambling upon Pentawere's succession was a risk worth taking. The biblical narrative depicts Bathsheba as a wily political practitioner who realizes that her safety completely lies with her son's accession to the throne and that only his smooth succession would bring peace to the house of David, an institution so long at war with itself. Zakûtu's loyalty-oath is a demonstration of how much the Assyrian monarchs valued female intercession in the safeguarding of the royal house and the quelling of insurrection. The Assyrians recognized that succession periods were always times of crisis and that royal mothers had an ability to bring potential dynastic chaos to a quick and effective end. Throughout the ancient Near East effective mothers of successful heirs were willing to commit themselves to playing the long game of politics; along the way a little blood might be spilt, of course, but for the continuity of the dynasty, this was a small price to pay.

Notes

1 1 Kings 1:16–20, 2:19.
2 Aiden Dodson and Dyan Hilton, *The Complete Families of Ancient Egypt* (London: Thames and Hudson, 2004), 164–177.
3 Anthony Dolphin Alderson, *The Structure of the Ottoman Dynasty* (Oxford: Clarendon Press, 1956), 13.
4 Jeoren Dunidam, *Myths of Power: Norbert Elias and the Early Modern European Court* (Amsterdam: Amsterdam University Press, 1994), 155.
5 Jeroen Duindam, *Dynasties: A Global History of Power, 1300–1800* (Cambridge: Cambridge University Press, 2016), 154.
6 See, for instance, Helene Sancisi-Weerdenburg, "Exit Atossa: Images of Women in Greek Historiography on Persia," in *Images of Women in Antiquity*, eds. A. Cameron and A. Kuhrt (London: Routledge, 1983), 20–33 and "Decadence in the Empire of Decadence in the Sources? From Source to Synthesis: Ctesias," in *Achaemenid History I: Sources, Structures and Synthesis*, ed. H. Sancisi-Weerdenburg (Leiden: Nederlands Instituut voor het Nabije Oosten, 1987), 33–45. See further, Maria Brosius, *Women in Ancient Persia (559–331 BC)* (Oxford: Oxford University Press, 1996), contra. Lloyd Llewellyn-Jones and James Robson, *Ctesias' History of Persia. Tales of the Orient* (London: Routledge, 2010) and Lloyd Llewellyn-Jones, *King and Court in Ancient Persia 559–331 BCE* (Edinburgh: Edinburgh University Press, 2013), 96–122. See also Janett Morgan, *Greek Perspectives on the Achaemenid Empire: Persia Through the Looking Glass* (Edinburgh: Edinburgh University Press, 2016), 189–221.
7 Pierre Briant, *From Cyrus to Alexander: A History of the Persian Empire* (Winona Lake: Eisenbrauns, 2002), 322.
8 Arthur Keaveney, *The Life and Journey of the Athenian Statesman Themistocles (524–460 BC) as a Refugee in Persia* (Lampeter: Edwin Mellen Press, 2003), 123.
9 Duindam, *Dynasties*, 132.
10 Waldemar Heckel, *Who's Who in the Age of Alexander the Great: A Prosopography of Alexander's Empire* (Oxford: Wiley Blackwell, 2008), sv. 'Sisygambis'.
11 2 Samuel 12:8.
12 Oriental Institute Prism, cited in Mark Chavalas, ed., *The Ancient Near East* (Oxford: Blackwell, 2006), 345–347.
13 Leslie Peirce, *The Imperial Harem: Women and Sovereignty in the Ottoman Empire* (Oxford: Oxford University Press, 1993), 3. See further Leslie Peirce, "Beyond Harem Walls: Ottoman Royal Women and the Exercise of Power," in *Servants of the Dynasty. Palace Women in World History*, ed. Anne Walthall (Berkeley: University of California Press, 2008), 81–94.
14 Frederik Fales and Nicholas Postgate, *Imperial Administrative Records. Part 2* (Helsinki: State Archives of Assyria, 1992), 24 lines 20–27.
15 See especially, Elena Woodacre, "Introduction: Royal Mothers and their Ruling Children," in *Royal Mothers and their Ruling Children: Wielding Political Authority from Antiquity to the Modern Era*, eds. Elena Woodacre and Carey Fleiner (London: Palgrave Macmillan, 2015), 1–8; and Carey Fleiner and Elena Woodacre, eds., *Virtuous or Villainess? The Image of the Royal Mother from the Early Medieval to the Early Modern Era* (London: Palgrave Macmillan, 2016). On royal mothers in antiquity see further, Lloyd Llewellyn-Jones and Alex McAuley, *Sister-Queens in the High Hellenistic Period: Kleopatra Thea and Kleopatra III* (London: Routledge, forthcoming).
16 Trans. Lloyd Llewellyn-Jones. See also a translation by Bendt Alster, *Proverbs of Ancient Sumer* (Bethesda: Capital, 1997), 29–30.
17 Trans. Lloyd Llewellyn-Jones. See also a translation by Simon Parker, *Ugaritic Narrative Poetry* (Atlanta: Society of Biblical Literature, 1997), 13–14.

18 Ruby Lal, *Domesticity and Power in the Early Mughal World* (Cambridge: Cambridge University Press, 2005), 85.

19 Trans. Lloyd Llewellyn-Jones. See also Parker, *Ugaritic Narrative Poetry*, 23.

20 Herodotus, *Histories*, 6.32, see also 4.19; 9.76; Plutarch, *Moralia*, 339e. Esther 2:5–7. The Persian practice of taking concubines as war booty is corroborated by a report in a Babylonian chronicle in which, following the Persian sack of Sidon in 345 BCE, Artaxerxes III transferred to his Babylonian palace large numbers of Phoenician women; see Llewellyn-Jones, *King and Court*, 191. Of course, not all captive women were bound for the privileges of the royal harem at all and most of them would have disappeared into the huge regiment of domestic staff who worked throughout the palaces as *arad šari* ('royal slaves') and *arad ekalli* ('palace slaves').

21 Keith McMahon, *Women Shall Not Rule: Imperial Wives and Concubines in China from Han to Liao* (Lanham: Rowman and Little, 2013) and *Celestial Women: Imperial Wives and Concubines from Song to Qing* (Lanham: Rowman and Little, 2016); Russell E. Martin, *A Bride for the Tsar: Bride-Shows and Marriage Politics in Early Modern Russia* (Dekalb: Northern Illinois University Press, 2012); Cecilia S. Seigle and Linda H. Chance, *Ōoku: The Secret World of the Shogun's Women* (Amherst: Cambria Press, 2014); Shawkat Toorawa, ed., *Ibn Al-Sa'i: Consorts of the Caliphs – Women and the Court of Baghdad* (New York: New York University Press, 2015); Matthew Gordon and Kathryn Hain, eds., *Concubines and Courtesans: Women and Slavery in Islamic History* (Oxford: Oxford University Press, 2017); Hugh Kennedy, *The Court of the Caliphs* (London: Weidenfeld and Nicolson, 2004).

22 T.M. Sharlach, *An Ox of One's Own: Royal Wives and Religion at the Court of the Third Dynasty at Ur* (Berlin: De Gruyter, 2017), 59.

23 Leslie Peirce, *Empress of the East: How a Slave Girl Became Queen of the Ottoman Empire* (New York: Basic Books, 2017), 6–7.

24 Arielle P. Kozloff, *Amenhotep III. Egypt's Radiant Pharaoh* (Cambridge: Cambridge University Press, 2012), 3 and 21–24 for Mutemwiya; see also Dodson and Hilton, *Complete Families*, 130–141.

25 Duindam, *Dynasties*, 116.

26 Sherry Lou Macgregor, *Beyond Hearth and Home: Women in the Public Sphere in Neo-Assyrian Society* (Helsinki: Neo-Assyrian Text Project, 2017), 85.

27 Zafrira Ben-Barak, "The Queen-Consort and the Struggle for Succession to the Throne," *Orientalia Lovaniensia Periodica* 17 (1986): 85–100, at 93. See also Hennie J. Marsmann, *Women in Ugarit and Israel* (Leiden: Brill, 2003), 345–370.

28 Woodacre, "Royal Mothers," 2.

29 Macgregor, *Hearth and Home*, 105.

30 Psalm 139:13–16.

31 XPf §4–5 = Xerxes, Persepolis Inscription f, lines 4–5.

32 Herodotus, *Histories*, 7.2–3.

33 Sarah Melville, "Neo-Assyrian Royal Women and Male Identity: Status as a Social Tool," *Journal of the American Oriental Society* 124, no. 1 (2004): 37–57, esp. 56.

34 2 Samuel 13:21–22.

35 Amy Kalmanofsky, *Dangerous Sisters of the Hebrew Bible* (Minneapolis: Fortress Press, 2014), 112.

36 2 Samuel 16:22–24. See Elna K. Solvang, "Guarding the House. Conflict, Rape, and David's Concubines," in *Sex in Antiquity*, eds. Mark Masterson, Nancy Sorkin Rabinowitz and James Robson (London: Routledge, 2015), 50–66; Keith Bodner, *The Rebellion of Absalom* (London: Routledge, 2014).

37 2 Samuel 20:3.

38 Susan Redford, *The Harem Conspiracy: The Murder of Ramesses III* (Delkab: University of Northern Illinois, 2002), 16. See also Dodson and Hilton, *Complete Royal Families*, 190, 193–194.

39 Redford, *Harem Conspiracy*, 35.

40 Texts also name her Naq'ia; see Macgregor, *Hearth and Home*, 97–98.

41 Saana Svärd, "Women, Power, and Heterarchy in the Neo-Assyrian Palaces," in *Organization, Representation, and Symbols of Power in the Ancient Near East*, ed. G. Wilhelm (Winona Lake: Eisenbrauns, 2012), 507–518, at 511.

42 1 Kings 1:5–53. See also Marsmann, *Women in Ugarit and Israel*, 363–365.
43 1 Kings 2:13–25.
44 Xenophon, *Anabasis*, 1.1.1–4.
45 Ellen Weber Libby, *The Favourite Child* (New York: Prometheus Books, 2010).

Key works

Ben-Barak, Zafrira, "The Queen-Consort and the Struggle for Succession to the Throne," *Orientalia Lovaniensia Periodica* 17 (1986): 85–100.

Duindam, Jeroen, *Dynasties: A Global History of Power, 1300–1800* (Cambridge: Cambridge University Press, 2016).

Llewellyn-Jones, Lloyd, *King and Court in Ancient Persia 559–331 BCE* (Edinburgh: Edinburgh University Press, 2013).

Macgregor, Sherry Lou, *Beyond Hearth and Home: Women in the Public Sphere in Neo-Assyrian Society* (Helsinki: Neo-Assyrian Text Project, 2017).

Sharlach, T.M., *An Ox of One's Own: Royal Wives and Religion at the Court of the Third Dynasty at Ur* (Berlin: De Gruyter, 2017).

Svärd, Saana, "Women, Power, and Heterarchy in the Neo-Assyrian Palaces," in *Organization, Representation, and Symbols of Power in the Ancient Near East*, ed. G. Wilhelm (Winona Lake: Eisenbrauns, 2012), 507–518.

28

CHILD KINGS AND GUARDIANSHIP IN NORTH-WESTERN EUROPE, *C*.1050–*C*.1250

Emily Joan Ward[1]

Child kingship was not an unusual problem for hereditary dynasties to face in the central Middle Ages (*c*.1050–*c*.1250), even if it was an infrequent occurrence.[2] Yet modern historians often treat child kings in isolation, focusing on a period of minority only to understand the king's later adult reign.[3] This chapter instead looks comparatively at the arrangements made when children under the age of fifteen succeeded to the thrones of Germany, France and England. Individuals who acted on a child king's behalf until he came of age are usually called 'regents', but this terminology is anachronistic for the central Middle Ages. It was not until the later fourteenth century that the vocabulary of 'regency' and 'regents' emerged, and contemporaries did not commonly use these terms until much later.[4] Instead, in the earlier period on which this chapter focuses, a range of language appeared to express the many responsibilities of a child king's guardian(s): administrative duties, governance and rule, nurturing and educating the young king, giving counsel and advice, and defending the kingdom. Contemporaries often described the men and women alongside boy kings in similar terms to aristocratic guardianship, and the legal vocabulary of wardship (*ballo*, *cura*, *custodia*, or *tutela*) regularly appeared in narrative sources and royal records to describe their charge of protecting a king's physical body and governing his kingdom. Taking a comparative approach to guardianship allows us to assess and contrast the legitimacy of the provisions made for child kingship across several kingdoms.

Queen mothers and magnates are the two groups of guardians singled out for more in-depth consideration in this chapter. In the eleventh century, Empress Agnes of Poitou (*c*.1024–77) was guardian for her son Henry IV (1050–1106) in the German realm and, contemporaneously in France, Anne of Kiev (*c*.1024–75) had a similar role alongside her son Philip I (1052–1108). Male magnates replaced Anne and Agnes as guardians before their sons came of age. A dramatic kidnap attempt in April or May 1062 removed Henry IV from Agnes's care. Archbishop Anno of Cologne (1056–75) lured the eleven-year-old boy onto a barge on the river near the royal palace of Kaiserswerth and then superseded Henry's mother in administering the kingdom.[5] Adalbert, archbishop of Hamburg-Bremen (1043–72), later supplanted Anno.[6] In France, although Anne's remarriage in 1062/3 ended her vice-regal guardianship of king and kingdom, she remained prominent at court. Count Baldwin V of Flanders (*c*.1012–67), Philip's uncle by marriage, became his 'tutor' and the protector of the kingdom, 'procurator regni'.[7] The thirteenth-century French queen Blanche of Castile (1188–1252) stands out from the earlier queen mothers in successfully maintaining a guardianship position until her son, Louis IX (1214–70), came of age. Including Blanche in this study provides an opportunity to examine how attitudes to guardianship and gender were evolving over the central Middle Ages. Queen mothers elsewhere in north-western Europe were overlooked as guardians in cases of child kingship in the first half of the thirteenth century. In England, Isabella of Angoulême (*c*.1188–1246) was never considered as a potential guardian for her son Henry III (1207–72). Instead, King John (d.1216) entrusted his eldest son and the kingdom to the papacy and the papal legate, Guala Bicchieri (d.1227). William Marshal, earl of Pembroke (*c*.1146–1219), became guardian of king and kingdom while the bishop of Winchester, Peter des Roches (d.1238), kept the young boy in his custody.[8]

Despite their prominent roles as mothers and guardians for underage kings, Agnes, Anne and Blanche have not benefited from a direct comparison with their magnate counterparts.[9] It is central to our understanding of the political and constitutional history of minority kingship that we integrate an analysis of their ability to rule for their sons, and contemporary perceptions of their suitability to do so, alongside men with similar responsibilities for a child king's care. Similar questions arise in each case. How did a guardian legitimize their position? Did a guardian's gender affect contemporary views of his or her role? How did the king's childhood affect a guardian's involvement in royal actions? These questions will be answered here by considering three themes: first, a guardian's appointment; second, perceptions of their suitability; third, a guardian's participation in affairs of justice and warfare, and their involvement in securing magnate fidelity to the king. Placing Agnes, Anne and Blanche in direct comparison with the magnates who followed them as guardians and with contemporary parallels in other kingdoms demonstrates how, although the legitimacy of guardianship could be intimately linked to gender, contemporary notions of suitability affected all those acting on a child king's behalf, not only queen mothers. Nevertheless, over time, fundamental shifts in notions of lordship and kingship created additional problems and challenges for women as guardians in situations of minority rulership.

Appointment and guardianship

Views of the provisions required to compensate for the 'problem' of a monarch's youth and incapability were relatively consistent. The need to provide for the body of the king ('rex') and the administration of the kingdom ('regnum') distinguished child kingship from absentee kingship, which only necessitated provision for the kingdom until a ruler returned from crusade or pilgrimage, or was ransomed and restored to the throne.[10] Philip I succeeded to the French throne as an eight-year-old boy after his father's death in 1060. Early in his reign, when making a gift to the monastery of Saint-Germain-des-Prés, the young king conceded that both he and his kingdom ought to be under tutelage.[11] Chroniclers across north-western Europe likewise accepted a dual purpose to guardianship. Lampert of Hersfeld, writing in the

1070s, acknowledged that Empress Agnes provided for Henry IV's upbringing and administered the kingdom while he was underage.[12] A few years after the succession of the English king Henry III in October 1217, the Anonymous of Béthune described William Marshal as the guardian of both Henry and the realm.[13] The title William used in royal documents, 'rector regis et regni', demonstrated that the earl himself recognized his twofold responsibility.[14] While the perceived objectives of vice-regal guardianship were similar – to care for the monarch and his kingdom – disparities in how contemporaries legitimized the appointment of a child king's guardian reveal gendered differences in guardianship even from nomination.

Queen mothers did not automatically become guardians for their sons; their legitimacy to act in this way depended on the authority of their husband's dying wish and the support of at least some of the kingdom's magnates or prelates. In Germany, with the end of his life fast approaching, Emperor Henry III (1017–56) relinquished his five-year-old heir, Henry IV, to the care of Pope Victor II to ease his wife's acceptance as their son's guardian.[15] Although Victor was German by birth and held the bishopric of Eïchstatt in plurality with his papal see, he could not stay away from Rome and his care of the young boy was never intended to last until Henry came of age. Instead, in the absence of Henry's 'worldly father', Victor, the child's 'spiritual father', facilitated the process by which the German princes consented to Agnes of Poitou's rule with her son.[16] Gathering bishops and secular princes to an assembly, the pope handed the kingdom to Henry IV before he left Germany early in 1057.[17] It was probably at this meeting that the magnates formally accepted Agnes as guardian.[18] Just under two centuries later, in France, ecclesiastical men acted in a comparable mediating role when Blanche of Castile became guardian for her eleven-year-old son, Louis IX. Shortly after the death of Blanche's husband, Louis VIII (d.1226), Walter Cornut, archbishop of Sens, and the bishops of Chartres and Beauvais recorded the king's intentions that his wife should be guardian for the son who succeeded him in the kingship, for the kingdom itself, and for all their other children until they came of age or died.[19] The prelates attached their seals to this record and professed that they had been present and listened to the king's deathbed intentions, indicating the authority of the dying king's recommendation. Since Louis VIII died on his return from fighting in the south of France, Blanche was not present at his deathbed, unlike Agnes, who had been at her husband's side in 1056.

Changing circumstances of royal death by the thirteenth century affected a queen mother's presence at her husband's deathbed, but it did not alter the process by which she confirmed her position as guardian.[20] Blanche, like Agnes, relied on ecclesiastical men to support her right to care for her son and his kingdom after her husband's death. The letter confirming Blanche's guardianship clearly asserts the legitimacy of her position in terms of her titles of lordship, queenship and motherhood ('domina', 'regina', 'genitrix'). Additionally, the bishops used the vocabulary of Roman and customary law to emphasize the legal basis for Blanche's 'guardianship and tutelage' of king and kingdom, something which had not been considered necessary for earlier queen mothers.[21] From the later twelfth century, customary legal texts prioritized a lord's right to guardianship of an underage child over the claims of their mother or kin.[22] Naturally, a child king had no lord and these customs did not apply to him in the same way as to other children. Nevertheless, the circulation of these ideas among the aristocracy ensured that references to lordship and law in the justification of a queen mother's position became increasingly important in the thirteenth century.

In contrast to the royal approval provided to support a queen's guardianship, there is little evidence in this period that kings ever intended royal authority to be exercised by a single magnate when their young sons succeeded. The king's deathbed maintained an enduring political significance, but its importance for a magnate's appointment as guardian was more the construct of medieval chroniclers than a reality. Later authors, entirely ignoring Anne of Kiev's more prominent role, fabricated the story that Henry I of France, on his deathbed, nominated Count Baldwin to care for his son Philip. Contemporary authors never connected the Flemish count's guardianship to Henry's deathbed, and royal acts do not show Baldwin as guardian before 1063 at the earliest.[23] It was the twelfth-century chronicler William of Malmesbury who conjured up a scene in which Henry bestowed his son and kingdom upon Baldwin as he lay dying.[24] This was evidently not the case, and William's story challenges the reliability of later monastic sources who recorded twelfth-century deathbed expectations rather than mid-eleventh-century realities.

There is significant evidence from thirteenth-century England that kings even deliberately avoided appointing a secular magnate as their child's guardian, instead preferring more collaborative arrangements. As King John lay dying in October 1216, he entrusted his kingdom and heirs to the protection of Pope Honorius III and the church.[25] The claim of William Marshal's biographer that John selected the earl of Pembroke to take charge of Henry III and govern the English kingdom is yet another fabrication.[26] William was not present at John's deathbed, and no extant record confirms the king's nomination of William, demonstrating a crucial contrast to Blanche of Castile's appointment in France a decade later. John's testament only named William as one of thirteen 'arbiters and administrators' who were asked, among other things, to provide support to John's sons, Henry and Richard, 'towards obtaining and defending their inheritance'.[27] William's biographer intended his record of the dying king's nomination to further legitimize the earl's guardianship but, in reality, John never planned for William to have sole control of his son and kingdom. William's ability to assert his position quickly and secure custody of Henry was far more imperative, as was the support 'by common counsel' of royalist magnates at an assembly in November.[28]

The case studies of Count Baldwin and William Marshal, although geographically and chronologically distinct, both warn against accepting chronicle accounts at face value when they claim a secular magnate's deathbed appointment as a child king's guardian.[29] Royal selection was not inconsequential for magnates, but it was more likely to be asserted either by later authors writing without full command of the facts or contemporaries seeking to legitimize a magnate's promotion as guardian retrospectively. Queen mothers relied more on the king's deathbed nomination to legitimize their position than did secular magnates. As the circumstances of royal death changed over the central Middle Ages, making it less likely that queens would be at their husbands' sides when they died, this increased the likelihood that royal women would be pushed out of guardianship arrangements by men better placed to act quickly. Gender alone was never sufficient grounds to prevent a queen mother from receiving support to act as her son's guardian. Nevertheless, once a queen became guardian, there is no doubt that monastic historians used her gender to express doubts about her suitability.

Suitability and opposition

A queen mother's prominence in exercising royal power for her son easily attracted hostility. Adam of Bremen, writing in the mid-1070s, recorded indignation from the German princes because the authority of a woman (Agnes of Poitou) constrained them, and because a boy ruled over them.[30] Similar worries surfaced in thirteenth-century France in respect to Blanche and Louis IX.[31] Although at least one eleventh-century author suggested gendered attacks aimed at a mother's involvement in royal governance were unreasonable since 'one may read of many queens who administered kingdoms with manly wisdom', women inevitably faced opposition to their legitimacy to act for a child king based simply on their sex.[32] Magnates were aware of the vulnerabilities of women in power and knew what allegations would most undermine their authority: apart from gender it was their foreign origin. In the eyes of Meinhard, *magister scholarum* at Bamberg cathedral, Agnes of Poitou's age, sex, nature and native land ('patria sua') were reasons to mistrust her.[33] Agnes's foreign (French) birth was the apogee for Meinhard's misgivings, outdoing even the fact that she was a woman. The schoolmaster's comments underline the ingrained societal opposition to a woman in power among some members of the German ecclesiastical community. Similar opposition had been directed at the Empress Theophanu, mother of the child king Otto III (980–1002).[34] Likewise, in France, hostile baronial propaganda against Blanche of Castile used her natal origins to attack her management of the kingdom. A poem from the initial years of Louis's minority claimed that she dipped into the royal treasury for her Spanish family.[35] A queen's 'foreign' identity may have come under more scrutiny after her husband's death, but we must avoid exaggerating this aspect without solid evidence. No contemporary sources substantiate André Poulet's claim that Anne of Kiev was pushed out of a role alongside her son because her command of the French language was 'suspect', so this claim should be rejected.[36]

Slurs of sexual transgressions with magnate advisers were another common trope used against queen mothers but not against magnate guardians. Authors who reported these stories often openly acknowledged them as rumours, but a more serious anxiety from men at court regarding hierarchy and preferential treatment underlined these illicit tales. Agnes of Poitou's reliance on the intimate advice of Bishop Henry of Augsburg attracted rumours of a scandalous liaison. Lampert of Hersfeld rationalized the offence felt by the German princes, 'for they saw that, because of private affection for a single individual, their own authority – which should have been the most powerful in the State – had been almost obliterated'.[37] Other authors confirm Bishop Henry's prominence in Agnes's counsels without any sexual innuendo.[38] In France, jealousy among the princes at Blanche's close relationships with the papal legate Romanus Frangipani and Count Theobald of Champagne, son of her cousin Blanche of Navarre, led to allegations of the queen's carnal relations with both men.[39]

Although it was the gender of the king's guardian which enabled stories to be circulated about queen mothers and their close advisers, the underlying concerns regarding preferential access to royal authority were common worries when a child was king. In 1063, while Henry IV was under Anno's guardianship, disputes over ecclesiastical hierarchy led to fighting in the king's presence in Goslar church, presenting one of the most serious tests to royal authority.[40] Later in Henry's reign, German bishops refused to provide him with their customary 'servicia' because they perceived Adalbert to be usurping the power of the kingdom and isolating the king from other advisers.[41] That the princes had similarly denied royal services out of protest against Agnes's guardianship suggests that Adam of Bremen was a little too quick to blame the empress's gender alone for magnate dissension.[42] In England, William Marshal was afraid that the barons would squabble among themselves for the prime position as guardian after his death.[43] He, like King John, decided on his deathbed to entrust Henry III and the kingdom to the pope and to Guala's replacement as papal legate, Pandulph.

Doubts regarding suitability for the task of guardianship affected men as well as women, even if a mother's involvement in royal governance was more likely to be disputed. Contemporary misgivings concerning Anno of Cologne's legitimacy to act as Henry IV's guardian centred on the way in which he secured his position through violently kidnapping the king from his mother.[44] One chronicler claimed Anno succeeding in 'usurping' the government of the royal court over several years.[45] Accusations of usurping a position as the king's guardian were serious charges only levelled at male magnates. In Anno's case, other German bishops feared his assumption of the guardianship would be entirely self-serving rather than for the good of the kingdom. He had to make concessions of authority to placate the disgruntled episcopate.[46] In England, William Marshal's successful appropriation of Henry III's guardianship did not go entirely unchallenged. A party representing the interests of Ranulf (III), earl of Chester, approached the papacy casting doubts on William's fitness for office based on his old age.[47] Pope Honorius III relayed their worries to the legate Guala in July 1217, although he left their suggestion that Ranulf be appointed as co-guardian to Guala's deliberation.

Vice-regal guardianship, by its very nature, was never a permanent arrangement, whether the role was filled by the child's mother or by secular or ecclesiastical magnates. While most contemporary opposition towards queen mothers predictably had a gendered (and, in some cases, clearly misogynistic) basis, uncertainty surrounding a child on the throne heightened concerns in all cases as to who gained access to, and thus control over, royal authority.

Acting for the king

Similar ideas of good kingship across Germany, France and England led contemporaries to expect rulers to work to maintain peace, to uphold justice, good customs and the law, and to use military force to defend the kingdom when needed. These were, of course, the promises of good governance made at a king's coronation, and child kings were not exempt from upholding these pledges. The memorandum of Philip I's inauguration in 1059 recorded that the seven-year-old French king promised before God 'to maintain and defend, as far as I am able, the canon law, the customary law, and justice for the churches throughout the kingdom'.[48] Henry III of England swore in 1216 to observe honour, peace, and reverence towards

God and his church, to observe strict justice, and to abolish bad laws and customs while upholding good ones.[49] A child king's immaturity unavoidably compromised his ability to safeguard these promises. Guardians, counsellors and officials had to advocate for his royal authority and maintain systems of governance. By considering a guardian's involvement in royal justice and military leadership – two aspects of medieval rulership often gendered as predominantly, if not exclusively, 'male' – we can see how gender did not exclude women from participating in these duties. In fact, a queen's gender and royal status sometimes even worked explicitly in her favour since they allowed her, as her son's guardian, to be included in actions of royal lordship from which male magnates were naturally excluded.

Despite the dubious means by which William Marshal seized his position as Henry III's guardian, and some contemporary doubts regarding his suitability, he ultimately justified his position as protector of king and kingdom through his actions.[50] William was, in many ways, the archetypical vice-regal guardian. The large number of royal instructions issued by his hand attest to his embodiment of royal authority. The earl used his own communications to carry out government business and applied his personal seal to royal letters until Henry had his own.[51] William's extensive military experience was put to good use in mustering royal troops, conducting siege warfare and leading men into battle at Lincoln in 1217.[52] Later that year, William helped negotiate the terms of the Treaty of Lambeth which finally brought Louis, son of the French king Philip Augustus (d.1223), and the rebel English barons to peace.[53] The earl also presided over the reinstatement of the general eyre, restoring the judicial procedures for royal appeals.[54] Of course, William was not acting alone. He had the support of the legate Guala, the bishop of Winchester and many other men who sat in the chancery, exchequer and king's bench. Yet contemporaries praised the earl's actions in defending the kingdom and securing support for the boy king. The centralized nature of thirteenth-century English royal government produced record evidence in far greater quantity than elsewhere in north-western Europe. Geographical disparities in evidence mean that we lack such extensive records for the participation of queen mothers in royal governance. Nonetheless, since it was his deeds which truly legitimized William's position as Henry III's guardian, we must similarly look at the involvement of other vice-regal guardians in royal governance.

Royal documents from eleventh-century Germany and France show that mothers and magnates acted alike as intermediaries between petitioners and the child king while providing their support, advice and confirmation to royal actions. Yet Agnes of Poitou's visible role in royal justice alongside her underage son distinguished the empress from the archbishops who replaced her.[55] Agnes's intervention and petition enabled Bishop Herrand of Strasburg to request arbitration from her son Henry in October 1059 in a dispute over rights in an episcopal forest.[56] Later the same month, in Augsburg, Agnes's involvement compelled another bishop and count to settle their quarrel.[57] Insights into Agnes's judicial participation may be few and far between, but they reveal the queen mother's significant role in supporting her son's actions as judge. A lawsuit to settle an encroachment onto the property of St Michael's monastery in Bamberg was held and adjudicated in the presence of the king, his mother and the princes of the kingdom.[58] Agnes's inclusion in the documentary record of royal justice is exceptional in comparison to the archbishops who later acted as Henry IV's guardians. Neither Anno nor Adalbert administered justice alongside the king in the same way. In fact, Anno seems to have devolved judicial responsibility to the localities when he decreed 'that any bishop in whose diocese the king was residing at that particular time . . . should have a special responsibility for the cases that were referred to the king'.[59] In France, records of appeals to royal justice during Philip I's minority are even rarer. The scarcity of sources for Anne of Kiev's brief years as guardian means we cannot be certain of her involvement in the exercise of justice. Anne's husband had included her in settling a legal dispute between the monastery of Saint-Thierry and the archbishop of Reims earlier in the 1050s, but there is no evidence that Anne participated in dispute settlement during her son's minority.[60] It was Count Baldwin of Flanders, not Anne, who was alongside the child king when, in 1063, Philip confirmed a sentence pronounced in the royal court in favour of the abbot of Saint-Bertin. The case had been heard 'in the presence of the renowned count Baldwin and king Philip, who is still a child'.[61] Philip and Baldwin both assented to the charter and subscribed their names to it. Explanations for why some vice-regal guardians participated in the administration of royal justice while others did not should focus more on geographical or political explanations than on the gender of the individual in question. Even so, gender may have influenced contemporary opinion as to a woman's legitimacy to involve herself in secular justice.

Canon law had prohibited female involvement in secular jurisdiction for several centuries.[62] At the turn of the thirteenth century, Pope Innocent III banned women from administering justice in principle although he made exceptions for 'eminent women', with particular reference to the queen of France in her capacity as ruler.[63] Blanche of Castile provides a near-contemporary example that even legal promulgations did not necessarily affect a queen mother's ability to act for her young son in secular law. Geoffrey of Beaulieu, writing at papal request in the latter half of the thirteenth century, explicitly credited Blanche with having administered, protected and defended the laws of the kingdom. Royal justice triumphed due to Blanche's clever foresight and her embodiment of feminine reasoning and a masculine mind.[64] Geoffrey's purpose in writing was to assert Louis IX's sanctity, but the later author's claims regarding Blanche's involvement in the administration of justice should not be written off as a hagiographer's *topos*. Lindy Grant has recently drawn attention to judicial cases where Blanche was alongside her son, such as the settlement in August 1227 by which Lambert Cadurc was released from prison.[65] Although Blanche was not always represented alongside her young son in legal decisions, she was certainly not excluded because of her gender. Gender had more of a practical effect on contemporary perceptions of a queen's ability to act as military leader and thus her legitimacy to provide for the defence of her son's realm.[66]

When the king was a child and hitherto untested as a soldier, although diplomatic action could help to pre-empt and avoid conflict, his guardian was expected to provide military leadership on his behalf. Matthew Strickland has shown how the effectiveness of a king's presence in warfare could depend on his personal military reputation.[67] For child kings yet to make their name in the field of war, their image and reputation depended on others, especially their guardians. The military reputation of magnate guardians was far from rhetorical. Men such as Baldwin V, Adalbert and William Marshal were familiar with campaigning and leading armies. Adam of Bremen, although a little disparaging regarding the propriety of a cleric acting as a war counsellor, claimed that Adalbert had experience of subduing enemies.[68] This military expertise was invaluable on Henry IV's first military expedition into Hungary in 1063.[69] In the eyes of monastic authors and a child king's *fideles*, it would have been questionable whether a queen mother could provide similar military leadership, despite notable royal and aristocratic exceptions such as Matilda of Tuscany (d.1115), Matilda of Boulogne (d.1152) and Countess Blanche of Champagne (d.1229).[70] Warfare was undeniably a masculine activity but, when required, women prepared for military engagements or acted in military affairs. Before becoming queen, Blanche of Castile canvassed for funding from her father-in-law and helped to raise reinforcements for her husband's campaign in England.[71] During Louis IX's minority, Blanche acted in the role of military commander between 1227 and 1231, accompanying Louis on campaigns most years.[72] One author claimed that it was jointly due to Louis and Blanche that an invasion by Henry III of England was unsuccessful.[73]

Criticism of a queen mother's ability as guardian to fight in defence of her son's kingdom came under greater scrutiny in the thirteenth century. Changing attitudes to military kingship over the central Middle Ages directly affected child kings. Whereas in the mid-eleventh century Philip I and Henry IV were knighted several years into their reigns, aged fourteen or fifteen, knighting in the early thirteenth century became a prerequisite to a child's coronation in England and France. Henry III and Louis IX were ceremonially recognized as able to bear military arms before they succeeded. Greater emphasis on the recognition of a child king as military leader, as well as the knowledge that both these kings' fathers had died on military campaigns, brought to the fore the issue of a guardian's legitimacy to bear arms themselves. Hugh of la Ferté, in a poem addressing the young king Louis, encouraged him to avoid women and instead surround himself with armed men.[74] Thus far, we have seen how a position as a child king's guardian involved some queen mothers in both royal justice and military leadership, much as their male counterparts. We have also observed how contemporary attitudes may not have been favourable to women acting in these ways, especially by the thirteenth century. Yet, as we will now see, the queen's gender could allow her incorporation into networks of lordship and fidelity alongside her son.

The acceptance of queen mothers in affirmations of fidelity to the child king provides evidence of a striking departure from contemporary male guardians who were never associated with the king in oaths of loyalty. Historians have often doubted the accuracy of accounts which specify the queen's presence at these oaths or downplayed their significance. However, since it was not unusual for aristocratic women to receive homage or fidelity in a lordship capacity, we should not discount the idea that a queen mother's royal status and guardianship of her son allowed her to be associated in a similar way.[75] Although pre-thirteenth-century evidence is sparse, pledges of fealty to the queen mother and child king were an active acceptance of her guardianship position. In 1076, Pope Gregory VII recalled an oath, 'iuramentum', the princes swore to Agnes of Poitou in case her son died before she did, possibly a guarantee of fidelity to Agnes's involvement in choosing a royal successor.[76] The date of this oath was not given, but the early years of Henry's reign would be its most likely dating. Two centuries later, the Ménestrel of Reims, probably writing in the 1260s, suggested that the French nobles performed homage to Louis IX and

Blanche because she held her son's guardianship.[77] The Ménestrel, a notoriously unreliable source, is the only author to mention homage being performed to the queen, but Matthew Paris, a more reliable witness, similarly suggested that she was present alongside Louis when he received homage.[78] Shortly after Louis's accession to the throne, during agreements for the release of one of Blanche's Iberian cousins Ferdinand, count of Flanders, several French and Flemish lords, and urban communities in Flanders, confirmed in writing that they would faithfully adhere to and support the lord king, the lady queen (his mother) and her other children.[79] Other oaths of fidelity were made to Louis and Blanche together to last until he reached a lawful age.[80] These records never claimed that men performed homage to Blanche but, since the magnates promised fidelity to the mother and child(ren) together, they recognized her right as guardian and queen mother to act in a lordship capacity alongside her underage son.

The Ménestrel's assertion that French barons performed homage to Blanche remains unconfirmed, but the author's claim that this action aroused great envy from the barons provides a valuable insight into contemporary attitudes. Queens attracted secular magnates' hostility and jealousy when their gender allowed them, as vice-regal guardians, to behave in a way not permitted to the magnates. Queen mothers could accept fidelity alongside their sons without challenging the social hierarchy of lordship and kingship. It would have been a dangerous precedent to allow a similar level of equality to a secular lord who himself owed allegiance to the king. Oaths of fidelity to a child king and his mother did not necessarily prevent challenges to her guardianship, but they reinforced her legitimacy by providing a clear assertion of the queen's place with her son in acts of kingship.

Conclusion

Greater similarity appears in the provision of guardianship arrangements for child kings in north-western Europe when we look beyond the vitriolic layer of misogyny which was a common propaganda tool wielded against many powerful women during the Middle Ages. First, magnate support was crucial to legitimizing any individual's claim to act for an underage king. Right from the start of a child's reign, both mothers and magnates depended on the collaboration and cooperation of princes and prelates to be accepted as guardian, although these relationships could later come under pressure or break down entirely. Second, while some strategies, such as rumours of sexual affairs, were confined to occasions of maternal guardianship, queen mothers were not alone in facing doubts regarding their suitability to rule for a child king. The composition of the king's intimate circle was always of concern to magnates since having the king's ear helped advance political careers and brought material gains. Finally, a guardian's gender did not necessarily negatively affect their ability to act to uphold royal promises such as the provision of justice or defence of the kingdom. In fact, a woman's position as anointed queen and the king's mother sometimes permitted her to participate in demonstrations of royal authority more intimately, as with Blanche's central role in securing allegiances to Louis IX, while the necessity of working within permissible spheres of lordship and kingship limited the actions of secular magnates such as William Marshal. Contemporary expectations of royal rule affected all those in a guardianship position.

Despite these similarities, gender predictably influenced the way contemporaries viewed a queen mother's legitimacy to act for her underage son. By 1250, queens faced more pronounced challenges to their appointment as guardians and to the range of their actions. The greater likelihood that a thirteenth-century king would die without his wife and eldest son at his side meant that the absent queen mother relied on the men at the royal deathbed to support her guardianship. Magnate support was more imperative than ever before. Furthermore, an increasing emphasis on the military nature of kingship attracted gendered criticism of a mother's incapacity to bear arms, and new legal promulgations regarding female involvement in the execution of justice may have similarly fortified opposition to a queen mother acting as vice-regal guardian. Given these further challenges to a queen mother's rule, Blanche of Castile's guardianship of her son Louis IX from his succession well into his adolescence appears even more remarkable. Blanche's success was not only due to the force of her personality. The queen mother and her ecclesiastical supporters recognized that aristocratic attitudes to maternal guardianship had shifted and took this into consideration when attempting to legitimize her role. Representing Blanche's guardianship of king and kingdom in legal terms of aristocratic wardship was a crucial first step. Just as important was the queen mother's repeated emphasis on her position alongside her son in networks of lordship and magnate loyalty. New legal and martial influences on kingship, as well as changing concepts of lordship, meant that queen mothers in the thirteenth century had to become more creative to secure and maintain a place as guardian alongside the child king.

Notes

1 This chapter is based on research for the author's doctoral thesis, "Child Kingship in England, Scotland, France, and Germany, *c.*1050–*c.*1250," (Unpublished PhD thesis, University of Cambridge, 2018). The author would like to extend her grateful thanks for funding from the AHRC, the Institute of Historical Research, and Emmanuel College, Cambridge. Heartful gratitude must also go to Liesbeth van Houts for her helpful comments on an initial draft.

2 Thomas Vogtherr, "'Weh dir, Land, dessen König ein Kind ist'. Minderjährige Könige um 1200 im europäischen Vergleich," *Frühmittelalterliche Studien* 37 (2003): 293. Vogtherr estimates there were about eighty boy kings across Europe between the eleventh and fifteenth centuries.

3 For some notable exceptions, Theo Kölzer, "Das Königtum Minderjähriger im fränkisch-deutschen Mittelalter. Eine Skizze," *Historische Zeitschrift* 251 (1990): 291–323; Thilo Offergeld, *Reges pueri: das Königtum Minderjähriger im frühen Mittelalter* (Hanover: Hahn, 2001); Christian Hillen, "The Minority Governments of Henry III, Henry (VII) and Louis IX Compared," *Thirteenth Century England* 11 (2007): 46–60; Charles Beem, ed., *The Royal Minorities of Medieval and Early Modern England* (New York: Palgrave Macmillan, 2008).

4 Maria Teresa Guerra Medici, "La régence de la mère dans le droit médiéval," *Parliaments, Estates and Representation* 17 (1997): 2.

5 Lampert of Hersfeld, "Annales," in *Lamperti monachi Hersfeldensis opera*, ed. Oswald Holder-Egger, MGH SS rer. Germ. 38 (Hanover: Hahn, 1894), 79–80; Tilman Struve, "Lampert von Hersfeld, der Königsraub von Kaiserswerth im Jahre 1062 und die Erinnerungskultur des 19. Jahrhunderts," *Archiv für Kulturgeschichte* 88 (2006): 251–278.

6 Edgar N. Johnson, "Adalbert of Hamburg-Bremen: A Politician of the Eleventh Century," *Speculum* 9 (1934): 147–179.

7 Maurice Prou, ed., *Recueil des actes de Philippe Ier, roi de France* (Paris: Imprimerie nationale, 1908), nos. 18, 25, 27.

8 David A. Carpenter, *The Minority of Henry III* (London: Methuen, 1990).

9 These women tend to be studied alone or only in comparison with other women, Mechthild Black-Veldtrup, *Kaiserin Agnes (1043–1077): quellenkritische Studien* (Cologne: Böhlau, 1995);

Roger Hallu, *Anne de Kiev, reine de France* (Rome: Università cattolica ucraina, 1973); Miriam Shadis, "Blanche of Castile and Facinger's 'Medieval Queenship': Reassessing the Argument," in *Capetian Women*, ed. Kathleen Nolan (New York: Palgrave Macmillan, 2003), 137–161; Lindy Grant, *Blanche of Castile, Queen of France* (New Haven: Yale University Press, 2016).

10 Félix Olivier-Martin, *Les régences et la majorité des rois sous les Capétiens directs et les premiers Valois (1060–1375)* (Paris: Recueil Sirey, 1931). Olivier-Martin compares child kingship with absentee kingship.

11 'in quorum tutela et nos et regnum nostrum esse decebat', Prou, *Recueil*, no. 13.

12 'Imperatrix, nutriens adhuc filium suum, regni negocia per se ipsam curabat', Lampert, "Annales," 79; Ian S. Robinson, trans., *The Annals of Lampert of Hersfeld* (Manchester: Manchester University Press, 2015), 80.

13 Francis Michel, ed., *Histoire des ducs de Normandie et des rois d'Angleterre* (Paris: J. Renouard, 1840), 180, 194.

14 Thomas D. Hardy, ed., *Rotuli litterarum clausarum in turri Londiniensi*, 2 vols. (London: Eyre and Spottiswoode, 1833–44), 1.293.

15 Edmund von Oefele, ed., *Annales Altahenses maiores*, MGH SS rer. Germ. 4 (Hanover: Hahn, 1891), 53. Otto III's succession as a three-year-old boy in 983 – an earlier precedent only slightly out of living memory for those at Henry III's court – had demonstrated the necessity for a mother's presence at the deathbed if she was to gain immediate control of her son. For Otto III and his mother, the empress Theophanu, see Karl Leyser, "*Theophanu divina gratia imperatrix augusta*: Western and Eastern Emperorship in the Later Tenth Century," in *The Empress Theophano: Byzantium and the West at the Turn of the First Millennium*, ed. Adelbert Davids (Cambridge: Cambridge University Press, 1995), 1–27.

16 Dietrich von Gladiss and Alfred Gawlik, eds., *Diplomata regum et imperatorum Germaniae. Die Urkunden Heinrichs IV*, MGH DD reg. imp. Germ. 6, 3 vols. (Weimar: Böhlau, 1941–78), vol. 1, no. 2. Henry, granting a confirmation through Agnes's intervention, addresses Victor as 'noster spiritualis pater'.

17 D.G. Waitz, ed., *Chronicon Wirziburgense*, MGH SS 6 (Hanover: Hahn, 1844), 31.

18 Berthold of Reichenau, *Die Chroniken Bertholds von Reichenau und Bernolds von Konstanz*, ed. Ian S. Robinson, MGH SS rer. Germ. N. S. 14 (Hanover: Hahn, 2003), 182; Robinson, trans., *Eleventh-Century Germany: the Swabian Chronicles* (Manchester: Manchester University Press, 2008).

19 Alexandre Teulet, ed., *Layettes du trésor des chartes: de l'année 1224 à l'année 1246* (Paris: Plon, 1866), no. 1828. Olivier-Martin, *Régences*, 49–52, who dispelled earlier historiography arguing that the document was a later creation. Grant, *Blanche*, 77, 80.

20 In England, Blanche's close contemporary, Isabella of Angoulême, Henry III's mother, was similarly absent from John's side due to his military campaigning.

21 'sub *ballo sive tutela* karissime domine nostre B. (Blanche) regine, genetricis eorum', Teulet, *Layettes*, no. 1828 (my italics).

22 Ernest-Joseph Tardif, ed., *Coutumiers de Normandie*, 2 vols. (Rouen: E. Cagniard, 1881), 1.10–12.

23 Philip Grierson, ed., *Les annales de Saint-Pierre de Gand et de Saint-Amand* (Brussels: Palais des académies, 1937), 27; Prou, *Recueil*, no. 17; Emily J. Ward, "Anne of Kiev (*c.*1024–*c.*1075) and a Reassessment of Maternal Power in the Minority Kingship of Philip I of France," *Historical Research* 89 (2016): 435–453.

24 William of Malmesbury, *Gesta regum Anglorum*, eds. R.A.B. Mynors, Rodney M. Thomson and Michael Winterbottom, 2 vols. (Oxford: Clarendon Press, 1998–9), 1.436–437.

25 Nicholas Vincent, ed., *The Letters and Charters of Cardinal Guala Bicchieri, Papal Legate in England, 1216–1218* (Woodbridge: The Boydell Press, 1996), 105–106.

26 A.J. Holden, ed., *History of William Marshal*, trans. Stewart Gregory, 3 vols. (London: Anglo-Norman Text Society, 2002–6), 2.260–261; David Crouch, *William Marshal*, third edition (London: Routledge, 2016), 158–160.

27 'sustentacione prestanda filiis meis pro hereditate sua perquirenda et defendenda', Stephen Church, "King John's Testament and the Last Days of His Reign," *English Historical Review* 125 (2010): 516.

28 'ex communi consilio', *Memoriale fratris Walteri de Coventria*, ed. William Stubbs, Rolls Series 58, 2 vols. (London: Longman, 1872–3), 2.233. Crouch, *William Marshal*, 160. Crouch downplays the role of magnate consent.

29 Philippe Buc, "Noch einmal 918–919: Of the Death of Kings and of Political Rituals in General," in *Zeichen – Rituale – Werte: internationales Kolloquium des Sonderforschungsbereichs 496 an der Westfälischen Wilhelms-Universität Münster*, ed. Gerd Althoff (Münster: Rhema, 2004), 151–178, who considers some problems encountered in sources dealing with royal death, such as the 'ritualization' of death and ornamentation of political messages.

30 'Indignantes enim principes aut muliebri potestate constringi aut infantili ditione regi', Adam of Bremen, *Gesta Hammaburgensis ecclesiae pontificum*, ed. Bernhard Schmeidler, MGH SS rer. Germ. 2 (Hanover: Hahn, 1917), 176; Francis J. Tschan, trans., *History of the Archbishops of Hamburg-Bremen* (New York: Columbia University Press, 2002), 141.

31 'Regno etenim Franciae sic in manu mulieris et pueri derelicto', Michel-Jean-Joseph Brial, ed., *Ex chronico Turonensi: auctore anonymo, S. Martini Turon. canonico*, Recueil des historiens des Gaules et de la France 18 (Paris: Imprimerie Royale, 1879), 318 (hereafter, series cited as RHGF).

32 Theodor E. Mommsen and Karl F. Morrison, trans., *Imperial Lives and Letters in the Eleventh Century*, ed. Robert L. Benson (London: Columbia University Press, 1962), 106; Latin in Wilhelm Eberhard, ed., *Vita Heinrici IV imperatoris*, MGH SS rer. Germ. 58 (Hanover: Hahn, 1899), 13.

33 Carl Erdmann and Norbert Fickermann, eds., *Briefsammlungen der Zeit Heinrichs IV*, MGH Briefe d. dt. Kaiserzeit 5 (Weimar: Böhlau, 1950), 118–119.

34 Gerd Althoff, *Otto III* (Darmstadt: Wissenschaftliche Buchgesellschaft, 1996), 54–72. See also Otloh of St Emmeram, *Liber Visionum*, ed. Paul Gerhard Schmidt, MGH Quellen zur Geistesgeschichte des Mittelalters (Weimar: Böhlau, 1989), Visio 17, 91–92. Otloh, writing during Henry IV's minority, recalled with some negativity the 'Greek' habits Theophanu had brought to the Ottonian court.

35 Leroux de Lincy, *Recueil de chants historiques français, depuis le XIIe jusqu'au XVIIIe siècle*, 2 vols. (Paris: C. Gosselin, 1841–2), 1.166. Grant, *Blanche*, 80–82.

36 André Poulet, "Capetian Women and the Regency: The Genesis of a Vocation," in *Medieval Queenship*, ed. John C. Parsons (Stroud: Alan Sutton, 1994), 106. None of the sources Poulet cites says anything about Anne's competency in French. Miriam G. Büttner, "The Education of Queens in the Eleventh and Twelfth Centuries" (PhD dissertation, University of Cambridge, 2003): 167–187. Büttner discusses the language learning of royal women.

37 Robinson, *Annals*, 81; Lampert, "Annales," 79.

38 Berthold, *Chroniken*, 185; Otto of Freising, *Chronica sive historia de duabus civitatibus*, ed. Adolf Hofmeister, MGH SS rer. Germ. 45 (Hanover: Hahn, 1912), 302.

39 Leroux de Lincy, *Recueil*, 1.155–159, 171. Grant, *Blanche*, 80, 86, 94–95, 99.

40 Robinson, *Annals*, 84–86; Berthold, *Chroniken*, 196.

41 Robinson, *Annals*, 109; Lampert, "Annales," 100.

42 Adam of Bremen, *Gesta*, 176.

43 Holden, *History*, 2.404–405.

44 Bruno of Merseburg, *Brunos Buch vom Sachsenkrieg*, ed. Hans-Eberhard Lohmann, MGH Dt. MA 2 (Leipzig: Karl W. Hiersemann, 1937), 13; Berthold, *Chroniken*, 194.

45 'regalis curiae providentiam sibi per annos aliquot usurparet', Wilhelm Wattenbach, ed., *Triumphus Sancti Remacli Stabulensis de coenobio Malmundariensi*, MGH SS 11 (Hanover: Hahn, 1854), 435.

46 Lampert, "Annales," 80; Robinson, *Annals*, 82.

47 'iam gravioris aetatis affectus', Walter W. Shirley, ed., *Royal and Other Historical Letters Illustrative of the Reign of Henry III*, 2 vols. (London: Longman, Green, Longman and Roberts, 1862–6), 1.532.

48 *Ordines coronationis Franciae: Texts and Ordines for the Coronation of Frankish and French Kings and Queens in the Middle Ages*, ed. Richard A. Jackson, 2 vols. (Philadelphia: University of Pennsylvania Press, 1995–2000), 1.227–228.

49 Roger of Wendover, *Liber qui dicitur flores historiarum*, ed. Henry G. Hewlett, 3 vols., Rolls Series 84 (London: Longman, 1886–9), 2.197–198.

50 Carpenter, *Minority*, 50–127.

51 For select examples, David Crouch, ed., *The Acts and Letters of the Marshal Family: Marshals of England and Earls of Pembroke, 1145–1248* (Cambridge: Cambridge University Press for the Royal Historical Society, 2015), 101; Carpenter, *Minority*, 52; G.J. Turner, "The Minority of Henry III. Part I," *Transactions of the Royal Historical Society* 18 (1904): 268. For William's seal, *Patent Rolls of the Reign of Henry III, A. D. 1216–1225* (London: HMSO, 1901), 1.

52 Holden, *History*, 2.300–303, 308–355; Roger of Wendover, *Flores historiarum*, 2.211–213; Crouch, *William Marshal*, 163–167.

53 Michel, *Histoire*, 203–204; Roger of Wendover, *Flores historiarum*, 2.223–224. Carpenter, *Minority*, 45. Carpenter discusses later hostility directed at William's leniency to Louis.

54 Carpenter, *Minority*, 96–101.

55 David Bates, "The Representation of Queens and Queenship in Anglo-Norman Charters," in *Frankland: The Franks and the World of the Early Middle Ages: Essays in Honour of Dame Jinty Nelson*, eds. Paul Fouracre and David Ganz (Manchester: Manchester University Press, 2008), 300. Bates highlights the queen's important role as judge.

56 Gladiss and Gawlik, *Urkunden*, vol. 1, no. 59.

57 Georg H. Pertz, ed., *Annales Augustani*, MGH SS 3 (Hanover: Hahn, 1839), 127.

58 'praesente supra dicto rege et matre eius Agnete imperatrice et principibus regni', Gladiss and Gawlik, *Urkunden*, vol. 1, no. 7. Amalie Fößel, *Die Königin im mittelalterlichen Reich: Herrschaftsausübung, Herrschaftsrechte, Handlungsspielräume* (Stuttgart: J. Thorbecke, 2000), 153–156.

59 Robinson, *Annals*, 82; Lampert, "Annales," 80.

60 Frédéric Soehnée, ed., *Catalogue des actes d'Henri Ier, roi de France (1031–1060)* (Paris: H. Champion, 1907), no. 89. Talia Zajac, "Gloriosa Regina or 'Alien Queen'? Some Reconsiderations on Anna Yaroslavna's Queenship (r. 1050–1075)," *Royal Studies Journal* 3 (2016): 35–36, 58.

61 'coram inclito marchione Balduino et rege adhuc puero Philippo', Prou, *Recueil*, no. 17.

62 Burchard of Worms, *Decretum*, Patrologia Latina Database 140, lib. 8, cap. 85, col. 808. David J. Hay, *The Military Leadership of Matilda of Canossa, 1046–1115* (Manchester: Manchester University Press, 2008), 216–218.

63 'feminae praecellentes', *Innocentii III Romani pontificis regestorum sive epistolarum liber quintus*, Patrologia Latina Database 214, no. 98, col. 1095. René Metz, *La femme et l'enfant dans le droit canonique médiéval* (London: Variorum Reprints, 1985), 103–105.

64 Geoffrey of Beaulieu, *Vita et sancta conversatio piae memoriae Ludovici quondam regis Francorum*, eds. Pierre C.F. Daunou and Joseph Naudet, RHGF 20 (Paris: Imprimerie royale, 1840), 4.

65 Teulet, *Layettes*, nos. 1937–8. Grant, *Blanche*, 303–307.

66 Megan McLaughlin, "The Woman Warrior: Gender, Warfare and Society in Medieval Europe," *Women's Studies* 17 (1990): 193–209; Ursula Vones-Liebenstein, "Une femme gardienne du royaume? Régentes en temps de guerre (France-Castille, XIIIe siècle)," in *La Guerre, la violence et les gens au Moyen Age*, eds. Philippe Contamine and Olivier Guyotjeannin, 2 vols. (Paris: Editions du CTHS, 1996), 2.9–22.

67 Matthew Strickland, "Against the Lord's Anointed: Aspects of Warfare and Baronial Rebellion in England and Normandy, 1075–1265," in *Law and Government in Medieval England and Normandy: Essays in Honour of Sir James Holt*, eds. George Garnett and John Hudson (Cambridge: Cambridge University Press, 1994), 70.

68 Tschan, *History*, 139.

69 Adam of Bremen, *Gesta*, 186; *Annales Altahenses maiores*, 62; *Annales Augustani*, 127; Johnson, "Adalbert," 166.

70 Hay, *Matilda of Canossa*, esp. 4–11 and chap. 5. Heather Tanner, "Queenship: Office, Custom, or Ad Hoc? The Case of Queen Matilda III of England (1135–1152)," in *Eleanor of Aquitaine: Lord and Lady*, eds. Bonnie Wheeler and John C. Parsons (New York: Palgrave Macmillan, 2002), 140.

71 Henry R. Luard, ed., "Burton Annals," in *Annales Monastici*, 5 vols., Rolls Series 36 (London: Longman, Green, Longman, Roberts and Green, 1864–9), 1.224; Michel, *Histoire*, 198;

Holden, *History*, 2.358–359; Natalis de Wailly, ed., *Récits d'un ménestrel de Reims au treizième siècle* (Paris: Renouard, 1876), 157.

72 Brial, *Ex chronico Turonensi*, 319; Aubri of Trois-Fontaines, *Chronica*, MGH SS 23, ed. Paul Scheffer-Boichorst (Hanover: Hahn, 1874), 924.

73 Joseph-Daniel Guigniaut and Natalis de Wailly, eds., *Extraits de la chronique attribuée à Baudoin d'Avesnes*, RHGF 21 (Paris: Imprimerie Impériale, 1855), 162.

74 'Rois, ne créés mie / Gent de femenie, / Mais faites ceus apeler / Qui armes saichent porter', Leroux de Lincy, *Recueil*, 1.174.

75 Theodore Evergates, "Aristocratic Women in the County of Champagne," in *Aristocratic Women in Medieval France*, ed. Theodore Evergates (Philadelphia: University of Pennsylvania Press, 1999), 78, 83, 109. Kimberley A. LoPrete, "Women, Gender and Lordship in France, c.1050–1250," *History Compass* 5/6 (2007): 1921–1941.

76 Erich Caspar, ed., *Das Register Gregors VII*, second edition, 2 vols. (Berlin: Weidmannsche Buchhandlung, 1955), vol. 1, no. 4.3; H.E.J. Cowdrey, ed., *The Register of Pope Gregory VII, 1073–1085: An English Translation* (Oxford: Oxford University Press, 2002), 213; Ian S. Robinson, *Henry IV of Germany 1056–1106* (Cambridge: Cambridge University Press, 1999), 28.

77 'elle tenroit le bail', De Wailly, *Récits*, 176; Robert Levine, trans., *A Thirteenth-Century Minstrel's Chronicle: A Translation and Introduction* (Lampeter: Mellen, 1990), 82. Olivier-Martin, *Régences*, 67–72.

78 Matthew Paris, *Chronica maiora*, ed. Henry R. Luard, 7 vols., Rolls Series 34 (London: Longman, 1872–83), 3.123.

79 Teulet, *Layettes*, no. 1831. Nos. 1832–94 are in the same form. Shadis, "Blanche," 140. Since the documents refer only to fidelity, Shadis is wrong to claim these documents as evidence for homage being given to Blanche.

80 'ad legitimam devenerit etatem', Teulet, *Layettes*, no. 2060.

Key works

Carpenter, David A., *The Minority of Henry III* (London: Methuen, 1990).

Grant, Lindy, *Blanche of Castile, Queen of France* (New Haven: Yale University Press, 2016).

Hillen, Christian, "The Minority Governments of Henry III, Henry (VII) and Louis IX Compared," *Thirteenth Century England* 11 (2007): 46–60.

Olivier-Martin, Félix, *Les régences et la majorité des rois sous les Capétiens directs et les premiers Valois (1060–1375)* (Paris: Recueil Sirey, 1931).

Poulet, André, "Capetian Women and the Regency: The Genesis of a Vocation." In *Medieval Queenship*, ed. John C. Parsons (Stroud: Alan Sutton, 1994), 93–116.

Ward, Emily J., "Anne of Kiev (*c.*1024–*c.*1075) and a Reassessment of Maternal Power in the Minority Kingship of Philip I of France," *Historical Research* 89 (2016): 435–453.

29

CREATING CHIEFS AND QUEEN MOTHERS IN GHANA

Obstacles and opportunities

Beverly J. Stoeltje

Politics raises questions of authority and access to power, introducing the potential for change, whereas monarchy stands for continuity and stability, maintaining authority through time. Though in reality these two models can be modified and manipulated, the two systems operate with quite different procedures for succession to the seat of power and authority; it is, then, to succession that we turn if we want to identify the distinctive features and the difficulties posed by either of these two models.

Chieftaincy in Ghana

In contemporary Ghana, a modern country located on the coast in West Africa, we find monarchy embodied in the indigenous system known as chieftaincy. It flourishes alongside the state, a government run by elected officials. Chieftaincy commands a great deal of public attention in Ghana, one reason being its popularity and another being the many individuals who hold the titles, *chief* and *queen mother*. Unlike countries or empires in which chieftaincy is defined by one monarch, in Ghana the various ethnic and cultural groups have their own chiefs. Further, the several Akan societies replicate leadership from the top of a hierarchical model through a level of paramount chiefs and queen mothers and into the next level of the hierarchy, towns and villages. Each location has its own chief and queen mother, and each one has a position in the hierarchy. Moreover, among the Akan, who are matrilineal in kinship, leadership is defined as a dual gender system; every chief is paired with a queen mother.[1] Increasingly, other ethnic groups, those that are patrilineal in kinship and who have not had queen mothers in the past, are adding the position through the duties that are defined by each specific group.

Among the Akan, when a chief's stool becomes vacant, it is the queen mother who nominates an individual to assume the position of chief because she knows who the qualified individuals are. This succession process involves a complex set of rules and procedures, some of which are mentioned below. As my ethnographic research for the past twenty years has concentrated on chieftaincy affairs in Asante, much of the data that follows is concerned with the Asante. However, the government of Ghana maintains a cabinet appointment for chieftaincy, an indication of the fact that chieftaincy is widespread throughout Ghana. Although each ethnic/cultural group in Ghana has its own language and history, they also have different kinship systems and other differences that affect how chieftaincy and succession are defined. However, the many national and international influences functioning in Ghana at the present time are affecting chieftaincy throughout Ghana in very similar ways, as numerous scholars have noted.

An important distinction in Ghana is the recognition of chieftaincy by the state. In a chapter on chieftaincy, the Constitution of Ghana not only recognizes and 'protects' chieftaincy but establishes Regional Houses of Chiefs and a National House of Chiefs; in those institutions chiefs representing all of the ethnic groups come together to deal with chieftaincy issues. Queen mothers are also defined as chiefs in the chapter on chieftaincy. (In the *Twi* language [spoken by the Asante] the terms for chief and queen mother are *ohene* for chief and *ohemaa* for queen mother, also indicating that queen mothers are chiefs.) As specified in the constitution, chiefs and queen mothers are prohibited from participating in electoral politics, but chiefs are expected to serve on government committees and boards of public institutions and to provide advice to government officials.[2]

An institution of major influence, chieftaincy has constituted the social and political organization for the numerous cultural groups in Ghana for centuries, and, as indicated earlier, it has been integrated into the modern state. Today, many chiefs and some queen mothers are well-educated individuals with international experience who have willingly served the national government, bringing their knowledge of the local populations to bear on national matters. George P. Hagan, senior scholar at the Institute of African Studies, University of Ghana, explains that they have stepped onto the national stage to play key advocacy roles in national development – in education, health, population management and the protection of the environment. They are engaged in conflict resolution and are offering leadership in civil society nationwide. Among international funding agencies, chiefs appear more credible as agents of change than the democratically elected governments of their countries.[3]

H.E. John Agyekum Kufour, President of Ghana for two terms from 2000 to 2008, recognized the significance of chieftaincy when he stated: 'One of the most important challenges facing governance in this nation and on the continent is the role that chiefs can play in the political process.'[4]

In recognizing continuity and the authority it sustains, we can argue that chieftaincy has contributed to stability in Ghana because it provides grass roots leadership that is recognized by the population. Moreover, having remained in place for centuries, it is familiar, offering a clear identity to those who participate in custom and chieftaincy affairs as well as a site for the resolution of conflict, oversight of land management and traditional religious practices. These, as well as other matters, fall under the responsibility of chiefs and queen mothers. Nevertheless, it would be incorrect to suggest that chieftaincy is a stranger to politics and to controversy. Some would describe it as an ongoing drama that consumes the interest of some and offends that of others. A significant percentage of the population does not participate in chieftaincy at all for a wide variety of reasons. Another percentage does not participate in chieftaincy affairs but maintains contact with family members who do, attends important funerals involving chieftaincy and pays visits privately to those involved. Very lively debates have been underway since before independence and continue today in the halls of power and through popular discourse, especially online, regarding the value of chieftaincy and whether or not it should be supported, relegated to a tourist attraction, or abolished entirely.

While these debates revolve around many different arguments, ranging from the effects of having a monarchy in a democratic state to the particulars of specific instances involving corruption or special interests, at the heart of these issues is succession. At one level, succession raises the issue of inherited positions of authority, and some have argued that chieftaincy should be an elected position. In fact, in the United States and some European countries, Ghanaian diaspora groups have established chiefs and queen mothers as leaders, and they are elected. At another level, succession becomes an issue in specific instances when the procedure for selections and installation of a chief or queen mother is not followed, or problems arise that cannot be resolved. One can be certain that when there is a vacancy, ambiguities and vulnerabilities in the system will become apparent, possibly creating a crisis that leads to litigation or one that produces long-range conflicts.

Because positions of leadership are endowed with authority and linked to power, they attract both those with noble and ignoble motivations, some with qualifications and others without. Because leaders and potential leaders are rarely individuals acting alone but have followers, supporters and organized forces behind them – whether those are visible or not – questions of succession can engage and in some instances divide a family, a town or an entire society. Yet, succession rests on a structure and a process, though it is often assumed rather than codified. Nevertheless, we are reminded through history, literature and popular discourse that succession is laced with ambiguities and vulnerabilities.

The Asante

The Asante are an influential people and many in number, who belong to the larger ethno/linguistic group known as the Akan. The Asante are identified with Kente cloth, gold and an illustrious history. As the Asante people are very active participants in chieftaincy affairs, the discussion below will mention their complex political-legal system and the process of succession they follow.[5]

The Asante state's power endured from 1701 to 1874, stretching beyond the boundaries of contemporary Ghana. Like the Asante, the several other Akan societies are matrilineal. The political system of the Akan defines leadership as dual: every separate location has a chief and a queen mother. Located in the Ashanti region of southern Ghana where Kumasi, their precolonial capital, continues to be a thriving city, the Asante are widely known for their participation in custom and events involving chieftaincy.

The structure that has successfully sustained this political system through several centuries is hierarchical; moreover, this system is shaped like a pyramid. At the top is the position of the king and queen mother of the Asante who are invested with the greatest authority and power in Asante. They are located in separate palaces in Kumasi on a hilltop known as Manhyia. In *Twi* (the language of the Asante) their titles are the *Asantehene* (the king) and the *Asantehemaa.* (the queen mother). Paramount chiefs and queen mothers make up the next category in the hierarchy, those whose authority is centred in a specific town but covers the surrounding region, including smaller towns and villages. In addition to their paramountcy, they also exercise power and influence as a group within Asante and at the Regional and National Houses of Chiefs. Division chiefs and queen mothers oversee smaller domains. Each town and village has its leaders as well, and their titles are *odikro* for the male and *oba panyin* for the female. Each location is linked to the next larger unit and through it to the larger Asante confederacy, as it is sometimes named today.

Like 'the throne' in European monarchies, 'the stool' represents authority in Asante. Each chief and queen mother occupies their own stool and has separate responsibilities, though they are expected to work together in the interests of the people in their domain. Each of them must be members of the royal family in that location. In a few instances the queen mother is or has been the biological mother of the chief; in most locations, however, the relationship is aunt and nephew, uncle and niece, sister and brother, or cousins. They are never married to each other, but they have spouses.

When placed in the position of authority it is said that they have been enstooled; if a chief or queen mother violates the standards, he or she can be destooled, or removed from the office. A chief and queen mother must be from the royal family of their particular location and will be members of a specific clan. The royal family in other towns will be members of a different clan. It is generally thought that the origin of the royal family in each location was determined in the distant past by which family was the founder of the town or of the early state that existed before the Asante state unified the existing chiefdoms in the region in 1701.[6]

The Asante people identify a wide range of activities with *custom*: a broad umbrella term that incorporates indigenous beliefs, practices and chieftaincy. While not an abstract phenomenon, the performance of custom and chieftaincy generates social relations and sets the stage for the negotiation of power. Through ritual events including the installation of new chiefs and queen mothers and large outdoor funerals, ordinary people known as commoners come together with those known as royals in activities that express and display gender ideology, customary law, traditional religion, mythology and history, and also serve as an informal platform for politics. Widely recognized and invested in performing their culture in these various events, dressed in African cloth and accompanied by drumming and song, commoners and royals come together in one large field that defines reality.

In spite of having a clear and orderly procedure for selecting a new chief, in contemporary Asante (and throughout Ghana as well) individuals spend an inordinate amount of time and energy working through the processes of succession. The following discussion describes the complex procedure, noting variations and the ambiguities they create, which at times invite controversy.

Succession and the queen mother

R.S. Rattray, the early British anthropologist of the colonial era who spent ten years with the Asante, described the process of succession as follows:

Moreover, in olden times when a chief had to be chosen it was the Queen Mother who had most to say in the choice to be made. She would summon her clan mates, male and female, and they would discuss the matter apart from the sub-chiefs and elders belonging to other clans. Having chosen the chief, the Queen Mother sends a message to the sub-chiefs and elders who now discuss the nominee, and when they have agreed, as I am told they generally do – no one can be put upon the stool against whom the Queen Mother gives her veto – the Queen Mother is informed.[7]

Though changes and variations have developed since that time, the fundamental procedure has remained. Foundational to the process in Asante is the *Ohemaa* (queen mother). The *Ohemaa* is considered to be the mother of the clan in her political unit and, therefore, the mother of her chief whether she is the biological mother or other relative. As the mother of the clan, she embodies knowledge about the clan, the lineages and political dynamics. Through her leadership she is expected to impart wisdom to the chief and her elders. The *Offinsohene*, a paramount chief, explained this relationship to me in 1990 with a metaphorical statement:

The King sucks the breast of the Queenmother.

The proverb is a metaphor expressing an analogy to motherhood. In Asante, motherhood is perceived as nurturing, and breast milk is the essential means of nurturing; thus the proverb compares the nurturing power of a mother's breast milk to the wisdom that a queen mother provides to the chief.

This knowledge and wisdom linked to the concept of the mother is what legitimizes her authority and defines the functions of the queen mother. These functions and the source of their legitimacy are described as follows by the *Juabenhene*, a paramount chief whose queen mother was his biological mother from the time he became a chief at the age of twenty-six years until she passed on. He explains her authority in relation to the chief. She is: '1) the Advisor [to the chief] on matters of tradition and religion, insuring that taboos are not breached; 2) the Advisor [to the chief] on secular affairs of state; 3) the Nominator of the chief; 4) the Procreator'.

Especially important in her body of knowledge is the genealogy of the royal family. When a chief's stool has been vacated, either through death or destoolment, the queen mother nominates a person to become the new chief. She is responsible, therefore, for knowing the individuals who are descended from the royal ancestress of the clan, distinguishing them from others, especially anyone who might have been incorporated into the family as full members whose ancestors were slaves or strangers. As a chief or queen mother must be descended through the royal family of each specific political unit, and the queen mother knows the genealogy, she knows who is qualified to occupy the chief's stool. This knowledge and her role as nominator of the chief constitute the moment in which she asserts her greatest authority.

Sources agree that she should consult with the elders of the royal family as she identifies and nominates a candidate from among those qualified. She then presents the nominee to the elders of the royal family (sometimes known as the 'the king-makers') or in some cases to the traditional council of the paramountcy for their approval. If the candidate is not acceptable to the kingmakers or the traditional council, she then has two more opportunities to nominate a candidate who will be acceptable. If the queen mother and the other authorities cannot agree on a candidate after she provides three nominations, the council or kingmakers can then nominate an individual. Some sources believe that the queen mother must still approve the candidate as qualified for the stool, while others do not – an ambiguity that often leads to conflict.

In the queen mother's deliberations, she is expected to be familiar with the character of the individuals who qualify and to nominate the one among those whose character is best suited for the stool. The many and varied political units have different opinions about the guidelines the queen mother and her elders should follow in choosing; these differences can lead to confusion and conflict, as the authorities can be influenced by financial factors, political standings, kinship relations, education and more.

The ambiguities mentioned earlier coupled with variations in the procedure among the many locations and the changes that occur through time, all contribute to the difficulties in maintaining peaceful transitions. A serious complication has been the changes, such as those colonialism introduced, that have altered and created confusion in the succession process. Compounding those changes has been the method for passing knowledge through time regarding these procedures. Knowledge has been handed down by oral tradition. In each paramountcy are oral poets who can recount the history of that particular stool. Important also are a host of linguists whose title in Twi is *okyeame* (sing.) or *akyeame* (pl.) who are spokespersons for the chief or queen mother, recognized as powerful figures in the circle of authority; also powerful can be the elders of the royal family and sub-chiefs of a specific location (sub-chiefs are chiefs of the commoners: those who are not members of the clan of the royal family of the town in which they reside; yet, in another town the clan of these commoners might be the royal family in that town). Any and all of these categories of participants in chieftaincy may be knowledgeable about procedures, but they may also be well or badly informed about the circumstances surrounding succession and thus eager to influence the ultimate decision.

A major issue related to variation and change is whether a queen mother can be the biological mother of the chief. Some groups have simply ruled this out while occasionally a few others attempt to place them both on the stool at the same time, usually leading to difficulties. Successful exceptions do exist, however. An especially prominent example is the king of Asante whose queen mother was his biological mother until her passing in 2017. The paramountcy of Juaben also demonstrates this practice. It has long been a tradition in Juaben that the queen mother could be the biological mother of the chief, and indeed when the paramount chief of Juaben, the Juabenhene, was enstooled in 1971, the queen mother was his biological mother. When she passed on, the sister of the chief became the queen mother of Juaben.

What is noteworthy throughout Asante, however, is that variations do occur from one place to another in the succession procedure, and it is these that are most likely to invite controversies and conflicts. In response to the widespread disputes and multiple variations that have long characterized chieftaincy, a Supreme Court Justice published a 700-page volume in 2008 that codifies the laws of chieftaincy: *The Law of Chieftaincy in Ghana*, S.A. Brobbey. This comprehensive text is designed to clarify these ambiguities and therefore reduce conflict.

Instances occur in which a queen mother and a traditional council can disagree about a candidate for the chief's stool. In 1976 the queen mother of Akim Abuakwa and the Traditional Council failed to agree on the nomination for chief. The Council asked the queen mother for her approval of a candidate, but she refused, and the Council destooled her. She took the case to the high court in Korforidua to quash destoolment. The high court ruled in her favour, ruling that the destoolment was wrong and that the queen mother is a chief.[8]

In today's Ashanti region, however, there is general consensus that the queen mother is the nominator of the chief, a powerful position, consistent with her role as queen mother. When the queen mother's stool is vacant, the elders of the royal family and the chief come together and agree on who of the qualified candidates (a member of the royal family) is the one best suited for the stool. Often a queen mother who was especially strong and effective designated an individual to succeed her before her passing or perhaps her retirement due to health, and the chief and elders would have been aware of her choice. In other cases, a strong chief will determine who will be his new queen mother, and the royal family will agree or perhaps not. Most sources lean towards the opinion that the chief has the power to select the queen mother. However, if the chief is engaged in a dispute or has generated controversy, then his selection of a queen mother can lead to further controversies.

Disputes and dramas in Ghanaian chieftaincy

Though the political-legal system of chieftaincy in Ghana has adapted to the modern nation-state and is now recognized and protected by the constitution, it nevertheless suffers from its popularity. The politics of self-interest frequently become entangled with chieftaincy, the results of which have been described by George Hagan as, 'wasteful litigation, factional strife and destruction of the peace of communities'.[9] Challenges increasingly swirl around succession, encroaching on monarchy, more so as the economy has improved in recent decades. Quite often succession evolves into what is known as a 'chieftaincy dispute', which generally leads to litigation through the channels set up within chieftaincy. A regular feature in Ghanaian society today, I have chosen to call them chieftaincy dramas when members of a community become involved in a dispute and form factions. The driving force of these dramas can be access to power, the display of status, or the perceived potential of financial gain.

In his chapter on "Litigation on Chiefs and Chieftaincy" Justice Brobbey's comments are enlightening. He offers three reasons for this litigation, beginning with the position that the litigation landscape involves chieftaincy at centre stage because the people of Ghana cherish chieftaincy and value their chiefs, and 'people are more prone to contest what will bring them honour and glory. So it is with chieftaincy too'. Second, some people foment litigation merely to make money out of it, and they are disparagingly dubbed 'chieftaincy contractors'. The third reason concerns property acquisition, the property (land, gold ornaments for adornment and more) that is believed to belong to a stool that some may want to protect or to exploit.[10]

The attraction of money and acquisition of property are especially relevant because economic conditions in Ghana have been improving gradually since a serious decline in the 1980s. However, since the late 1990s, the economic expansion has been dramatic, visible today in the capital city, Accra. It has developed high rise office buildings, condos, beachfront luxury hotels, gated communities, coffee shops and other signs of a twenty-first-century economy influenced by neo-liberal policies. Along with these changes, value has been added to chieftaincy. Individuals who discounted chieftaincy in years past now find it attractive. Hagan tells us that chiefships have acquired such added value that: 1) the wealthy have begun to contest for the office of chief, whether or not they have a claim or title to the office; 2) competition among legitimate royals is so intense that they become divided over who can occupy the position, and communities develop permanent and intractable election disputes; and 3) because a chief or queen mother is placed on the stool for life, there are royals who are impatient to occupy a stool and will lay charges against the occupant of the stool to try to remove them.[11] Moreover, in less prestigious locations, individuals of lesser status who do not have a legitimate claim are often attempting to be enstooled as well, at times promising funds to individuals in return for becoming a chief. A third kind of person who does not have a claim is someone who is descended from a slave. In Ghana, slaves were often incorporated into the family in which they served, and over time the status of slave was forgotten. As mentioned earlier, however, in Asante a family history may reach far into the past and will retain that knowledge of the ancestry. Even though an individual might have independent finances which could be used to support the stool, and even though such a person might be of good character, he would, nevertheless, be prevented from being placed on the stool due to his ancestral status, known to the queen mother. In such a situation, the persons supporting the individual who could be a candidate for chief might challenge the queen mother; depending on the strength of the argument on all sides, the issues could become a dispute, but, alternatively, the individual at the centre of the issue might choose to drop the matter rather than have it become a public discussion.

Though complications and disputes are not new in the affairs of chieftaincy, in contemporary Ghana, the source of these complications in the twenty-first century is the status with which chieftaincy is viewed; elites as well as others are attracted to chieftaincy and are employing the politics of self-interest to the institution, manipulating the procedures for succession.

National and international influences

National and international conditions of the twentieth and twenty-first centuries have created new pressures which motivate some individuals to exploit the ambiguities and loopholes available in the political systems of which chieftaincy is a part. As this discussion shifts to these larger forces, it continues to note effects in Asante, but it also changes the focus to include the entire field of chieftaincy in Ghana. The impact of these forces is generally directed at and felt in the process of succession as it provides access to the power and authority of chieftaincy in any ethnic group. Therefore, when external forces have an interest in chieftaincy, they will be concerned with succession and those who are on the stool.

The forces identified as major external influences are listed below. Each of them deserves a full, serious study, and certainly many lengthy studies have addressed these influences from the perspective of democracy in Africa, culture and customs, chieftaincy as an institution, economic studies, languages spoken, and much more, but rarely does a study focus on the relationship of one of these influences to chieftaincy itself. Moreover, scholars and researchers concerned with these influences often disregard chieftaincy, considering it irrelevant or perhaps too controversial to explore in depth. This regard is changing, however, especially within Ghana as scholars of the twenty-first century are increasingly interested in chieftaincy affairs. The hefty volume on chieftaincy edited by Irene Odotei and Albert Awedoba, mentioned earlier, is a welcome addition to scholarship that integrates issues of the indigenous political system with the forces of postcolonialism and modernity.[12]

The discussion below identifies selected external influences and comments briefly on their impact on chieftaincy. Due to spatial limitations, these comments are limited.

British colonialism

Some policies and practices of a dominating force, especially those involving institutions, will have a residual effect on social and political life long after that force has left. The British were engaged in trade with the Gold Coast from the sixteenth century, so they were quite familiar with the potential resources of the region – the natural resources, especially gold, the people and their chieftaincy system, which the British compared favourably to their own monarchy at times. As the colonial power in Ghana, the British chose to dominate the Gold Coast, Ashanti and Northern Territories with a system known as 'indirect rule'. Through this system the British appointed chiefs whom they expected to cooperate with them, especially in the matter of collecting taxes from the population. In this they totally disregarded the indigenous political system of selecting leaders. Especially egregious for the Akan groups, the British ignored the queen mothers.

As described earlier, the queen mother has the most powerful role in the succession process of the Akan groups. She is the pivot around which all succession decisions are negotiated. Not only is she the designated individual who identifies the candidate(s) for the position of chief, but her decision is based on specialized knowledge and wisdom. To abolish her power is to leave the way clear for any individual to manipulate his way onto the stool under colonial power.

After his many years in Asante, R.S. Rattray devoted an entire chapter to matrilineal descent in his volume, *Ashanti*, where he discussed the role of the queen mother and the unfortunate colonial policy of according political recognition to the chiefs only. He explained:

> To-day the Queen Mothers are unrecognized by us and their position and influence are rapidly passing away. Many of us have only been made conscious of her presence by her 'troublesome' activities in stool palavers; so . . . Official recognition she has none . . . I have asked the old men and women why I did not know all this – I have spent very many years in Ashanti. The answer is always the same: 'The white man never asked us this; you have dealings with and recognize only the men; we supposed the European considered women of no account, and we know you do not recognize them as we have always done.'[13]

Perhaps the most devastating act of British colonialism for the Asante was the exile of the Asantehene, his queen mother and their entire entourage to the Seychelles in 1896. In spite of the efforts of English speaking Asante ambassadors who were sent to London to negotiate a peace, the British Governor Maxwell demanded of the Asantehene, Agyeman Prempeh I, a payment of 50,000 ounces of gold and then arrested the Asantehene, his queen mother, father, brother and eight other office holders, and sent them into exile under armed guard. The Asantehemaa passed on while in exile, and sixty-seven babies were born in the Seychelles. The Asantehene and his entourage were returned in 1924, twenty-eight years after the British exiled them.[14]

Elementary and secondary schools along the coast were established by missionaries, and some few females were allowed to attend but not to continue onto any higher education. (Relatively few of these schools were located in the Ashanti region.) Having an interest in creating an educated elite who would then work for them, managing their interests in Ghana, the British encouraged some young men to pursue higher education in England. Young men from the coast went to England for further education, especially in law. John Mensah Sarbah studied law in England and returned as the youngest barrister in the country; more importantly, when he returned, he consistently resisted British efforts to claim the land and impose authority over Ghanaians.[15] Queen mothers were not included in educational efforts or political affairs. As men increasingly acquired education, dealing with the British and accruing authority, queen mothers continued to be ignored even as women became educated but were not expected to assume positions in public. This condition marginalized queen mothers, contributing to the widespread opinion that they were simply outdated, uneducated old women who had no place in modern society, an attitude I encountered in 1990 when I initiated my research.

When Ghanaian independence was declared in 1957, a compromise between Kwame Nkrumah, the incoming president, and the opposing political party led to the establishment of the Regional Houses of Chiefs. The result of Nkrumah's hostility to chieftaincy, he was persuaded that he could contain chiefs through these meeting houses in each region.[16] After Nkrumah's overthrow, a subsequent government established the National House of Chiefs. Although these modern institutions that gather chiefs together to represent their regions benefit chieftaincy, neither the Regional Houses nor the National House of Chiefs includes queen mothers. And, no parallel House for queen mothers has ever been established. Thus, the legacy of the British lives on – chiefs are privileged and queen mothers ignored.

Government interference and the constitution

J.J. Rawlings ruled Ghana as a military dictator, and then as president, for a total of nineteen years. Chieftaincy, and the Asante in particular, made him very uncomfortable. And he made people in Asante very uncomfortable. During those years, the oral tradition in Kumasi frequently circulated stories reporting on 'spies in university classrooms' sent out by Rawlings, 'accidents' on the highway involving ancient trucks hauling enormous logs, bizarre events and mysterious deaths, all attributed to Rawlings' agency.

Though no evidence could be found for these happenings, no one doubted that he and his cabinet did interfere in chieftaincy affairs. Chiefs had to be 'gazetted' by the government when newly enstooled, and the government could refuse to accept a chief if it chose to do so. As in most dictatorships, it was clear who supported the government and who did not, and how those who supported the government benefitted. This was as true for chiefs as for others.

In one specific chieftaincy dispute involving a great many people on all sides, a chief had pocketed significant money intended for the benefit of his town. Not his first offence, leaders from the town brought him to trial; however, due to the government's influence, he was found innocent of all charges. This chief was rebelling against the conventions of chieftaincy, portraying himself as the victim of chiefs senior to him. Consequently, the government and chiefs who supported the government defended him at every opportunity. The government was persistent, however. A well-informed sub-chief was leading the effort to destool the chief and gaining support among others to file destoolment charges. A representative from the government met with him and attempted to pay him off if he would cease his efforts. When that failed, the government sent an investigator to arrest him and kept him imprisoned for two weeks with no charges.[17] In spite of the government's efforts, the twenty-one destoolment charges were filed, and eventually, when there was a change in the government and after seemingly endless court appearances, the chief was destooled.

Like the long-range effects of colonialism, corruption in government, especially in a dictatorship which by definition has no restrictions or regulations, has long-lasting effects. Ghana continues to struggle with corruption through each successive government. While the cause of corruption cannot be completely laid at the feet of the Rawlings government, nineteen years is a long period during which not only corruption and abuse of government power grows but suspicion is planted in the minds of the populace and tensions grow into hostilities, all of which are difficult to delete.

Ironically, the Rawlings government created a women's organization, led by his wife, Nana Konadu Agyeman-Rawlings, called the December 31st movement. It had branches throughout Ghana and proposed to advance women's position in the world. In a second effort to benefit women, the Rawlings government proposed that queen mothers be admitted to the Regional and National Houses of Chiefs. A vote was held, and the proposal was defeated. Unfortunately, many people saw these efforts as poorly disguised strategies for gaining women's votes and infiltrating the Houses of Chiefs, setting back any gains in queen mothers' status.

On the positive side, the 1992 constitution not only contains a chapter on chieftaincy, guaranteeing and protecting it, but in multiple places it specifies that a chief will serve on specific boards and committees and will also advise the president of the country. In this, a bridge between the state and chieftaincy has been established, transcending previous hostilities, enabling the government to benefit from the knowledge and expertise some chiefs can offer. No mention of queen mothers appears, however, except that they are considered chiefs.

The economy

Perhaps the most serious and pressing cause of difficulties involving succession today is the economy, especially the neo-liberal economic system. To explore this issue requires a brief reflection on precolonial history. Throughout the Asante state (and other precolonial political units) a traditional economy provided tribute for the various stools. This tribute then provided support for the chief, one-third of which was designated for the queen mother.

Scholars have shown that the Asante were not simply passive recipients of tribute but were active in trade and were encouraged by the Asantehene to accumulate wealth. T.C. McCaskie described the importance of wealth in the precolonial state and mentions the special category of the wealthy:

> Wealth and surplus – in gold (the *ur* substance), and in food, and also in people, in goods and in artefacts – were located in Asante experience . . . that societal and individual achievement was, and historically always had been, built upon assiduously pursued processes of accumulation . . . Hence, the accumulation of wealth as imperative and as yardstick . . . were abiding and central features of Asante life, history and self-knowledge . . . Moreover, the most successful entrepreneurs were awarded with a title (ObirEmpon) and recognized with a complex ritual.[18]

The arrival of the British brought a major upheaval in the economy, ultimately questioning sustainability in chieftaincy. With colonialism came a modern capitalist economic system based on wages and salaries, debts and profits, and heavy taxes and profits handed over to the British, all of which replaced the indigenous economy that provided tribute for the stools and trade opportunities for many.

Some stools today have recovered resources, especially if their domains include gold, timber, palm oil or another resource that can be marketed in the global economy. Also, some stools have benefitted from the business acumen of their chief as is the case in Juaben where the paramount chief of Juaben has brought development to his town and his region (roads, hospital, schools, market, jobs and a bank).[19] Others, however, are without resources. In such a case if the chief's stool has become vacant and the town has little money, a candidate who promises money for the stool or for jobs may emerge. If unqualified according to the genealogy, the queen mother will likely turn down the candidate who has presented himself; the supporters of the candidate who want to enstool him will challenge the queen mother and a serious conflict can develop. Many disputes involving succession have this issue at the core of the problem.

A queen mother suffers an additional disadvantage because her only source of income, according to the traditional system, is a one-third portion of the 'tribute' that comes to the chief. Today, many chiefs ignore that directive, and, unfortunately, some chiefs from small towns or villages have no 'tribute' to share. Moreover, few queen mothers are married, as most men are reluctant to marry a woman who has more authority than they have, so it is rare for a queen mother to have a husband who will provide support. Further, usually a queen mother has several children; the society expects a queen mother to have children as it exhibits her motherhood (it is not necessary that she be married). Depending on their age and education, some of those children will be a financial burden until they become adults, but even then, there is no guarantee that they will have sufficient funds to support their queen mother. As a result, queen mothers generally have few resources unless they have developed a trading network or cultivated a career before becoming queen mother. These conditions have a profound effect on a queen mother's status and power.[20]

Though not all groups have the same political and economic structure as the Akan, chieftaincy and queen mothers in any group often face economic difficulties.

The diaspora

Throughout Europe and the United States, Ghanaians cluster together, creating communities that sponsor Ghanaian festivals and elect chiefs and queen mothers. In frequent gatherings, groups share information about their home towns, chieftaincy affairs and other relevant news. Social media makes it possible to remain up to date, and international calling has facilitated communication as well.

Because Ghanaians tend to have multiple siblings and multiple sisters and brothers through their clans, they have many relatives in the diaspora. In addition, home town organizations and graduates of private schools have been meeting together in Ghanaian cities long before there was a diaspora. Those home town gatherings have been transported to international sites and are often expanded to an all Ghana gathering or festival.

When a chief or a queen mother from Ghana comes to visit relatives and supporters in the diaspora, Ghanaians from that particular town will come together to honour him or her, providing dance, music, food and socialization. Most importantly, if there is a dispute underway or a project being planned, perhaps the enstoolment of a new chief or queen mother, then this will be explained and contributions raised.

Succession problems involving the diaspora can become complicated. Individuals from a specific town may be spread from Dallas to Washington, and from London to Amsterdam and every city in between. Some of these Ghanaians are royals in graduate school who may return to Ghana when their programme is complete and become a nominee for the position of queen mother or chief. Others may be studying to be bankers or businessmen or women. Others may become residents or citizens and are driving taxis – a common occupation in Dublin, Chicago and New York City. Even though communication can be rapid with social media, news of a complicated dispute is likely to become simplified and personalized when it travels across continents and oceans, through networks representing one view or the opposite. Consequently, the diaspora can be a hidden and unidentified influence on succession issues – until diaspora Ghanaians arrive at a funeral in Ghana showing their support for a position and proudly revealing their identity.

Conclusion

Chieftaincy rates quite highly in Ghana in the twenty-first century if we are to judge the eagerness with which individuals, especially elites, are attempting to occupy the position of chief or queen mother. While the question of how this will eventually develop and to whose benefit remains unanswered, it is apparent that the question of succession is the point at which any investigation should begin. An investigation would be wise to examine the process of succession. Should it change to become a democratic process? Is it possible to curtail corruption in the succession process, especially if the queen mother in Akan societies is not respected? Or, should the criteria continue to include the defining feature that one must be a member of the royal family? Could the criteria be changed to require a level of education, a level of financial security, a level of knowledge about the system, and if so, should it be different for different levels of chiefs and queen mothers? Should chiefs and queen mothers still be prohibited from running for political office? How can queen mothers be organized in ways that enhance their communication and ability to work together? Should they have a National House of Queen Mothers, or should they be integrated into the National House of Chiefs?

Some individuals would simply vote to abolish chieftaincy. If a serious conversation is taking place, that voice should be included as well, if only to generate the articulation of fundamental issues.

This brief study has suggested that the institution of chieftaincy in Ghana would benefit from an examination of the succession process in each and every cultural group to identify the ambiguities and vulnerabilities that invite exploitation and controversies. Equally important, the institution would benefit from identifying where the gains and losses are if the external influences affecting chieftaincy were carefully studied and their influence traced as it is played out.

Certainly, it is not a secret that all political systems have vulnerabilities, and the leaders in every system, whatever labels they wear, are capable of falling prey to the hungry vultures that circle around every site of power and authority. Some moments in time shimmer with opportunity, equally attractive to the noble and the ignoble. It is most important that, at those moments, the ones who have been appointed guardians of the public interest exercise their responsibilities.

Chieftaincy has served Ghanaians well as a system of authority that has continuity; it is sustainable. Together the two political systems can bring great gains to Ghana in this moment of opportunity. To ensure good leadership in that moment means to examine critically the process of succession in both systems.

Notes

1 Beverly J. Stoeltje, "Asante Queenmothers: A Study in Female Authority," in *Queens, Queen Mothers, Priestesses, and Power*, ed. Flora Kaplan (Baltimore: Johns Hopkins Press, 1997), 41–71.
2 *Constitution of the Republic of Ghana* (Accra: Ghana Publishing Corporation, 1992), 164–168.
3 G.P. Hagan, "Epilogue: The Way Forward – New Wines and Broken Bottles," in *Chieftaincy in Ghana*, eds. Irene K. Odotei and Albert K Awedoba (Legon, Accra: Sub-Saharan Publishers, 2006), 663–664.
4 H.E. John Agyekum Kufour, "Address," in *Chieftaincy in Ghana*, eds. Irene K. Odotei and Albert K. Awedoba (Legon, Accra: Sub-Saharan Publishers, 2006), 678.
5 See also Kwame Arhin, *Traditional Rule in Ghana* (Accra: Sedco Publishing Ltd, 1985); T.C. McKaskie, "Agyeman Prempeh before the Exile," in *The History of Ashanti Kings and the Whole Country Itself*, eds. A. Adu Boahen, Emmanuel Akyeampong, Nancy Lawler, T.C. McCaskie and Ivor Wilks (New York: Oxford University Press, 2003), 3–20; Christianne Owusu-Sarpong, "From Words to Ritual Objects," in *Ghana: Yesterday and Today*, eds. Christiane Falgayrettes-Leveau and Christiane Owusu-Sarpong (Paris: Musee Dapper, 2003); Ivor Wilks, *Asante in the Nineteenth Century* (Cambridge: Cambridge University Press, 1975).
6 See Stoeltje, "Asante Queenmothers."
7 R.S. Rattray, *Ashanti* (London: Oxford University Press, 1923), 82.
8 1977: Part 3. 9–77.
9 Hagan, "Epilogue," 664.
10 S.A. Brobbey, *The Law of Chieftaincy in Ghana* (Accra: Advanced Legal Publications, 2008), 217–218.

11 Hagan "Epilogue," 664.
12 Irene Odotei and Albert Awedoba, eds., *Chieftancy in Ghana: Culture, Governance and Development* (Accra: Sub-Saharan Publishers, 2006).
13 Rattray, *Ashanti*, 84.
14 See McCaskie, "Agyeman."
15 John Mensah Sarbah, *Fanti National Constitution* (London: Frank Cass and Co. Limited, 1906).
16 Richard Rathbone, *Nkrumah and the Chiefs* (Oxford: James Curry, 2000).
17 He worked closely with me on my research, and I had first-hand information from him.
18 T.C. McCaskie, *State and Society in Pre-colonial Asante* (Cambridge: Cambridge University Press, 1995), 37–42.
19 Beverly J. Stoeltje, "Disentangling Modernity in Ghana: The Cosmopolitan Chief," *West African Review* 22 (2013): 9–25.
20 Beverly J. Stoeltje, "Asante Queenmothers: Precolonial Authority in a Postcolonial Society," *Research Review* 19, no. 2 (2003): 1–19.

Key works

Hagan, G.P., "Epilogue: The Way Forward – New Wines and Broken Bottles," in *Chieftaincy in Ghana*, eds. Irene K. Odotei and Albert K. Awedoba (Legon, Accra: Sub-Saharan Publishers, 2006), 663–673.

McKaskie, T.C., "Agyeman Prempeh before the Exile," in *The History of Ashanti Kings and the Whole Country Itself*, eds. A. Adu Boahen, Emmanuel Akyeampong, Nancy Lawler, T.C. McCaskie and Ivor Wilks (New York: Oxford University Press, 2003), 3–20.

Odotei, Irene and Albert Awedoba, eds., *Chieftancy in Ghana: Culture, Governance and Development* (Accra: Sub-Saharan Publishers, 2006).

Rattray, R.S., *Ashanti* (London: Oxford University Press, 1923).

Stoeltje, Beverly J., "Asante Queenmothers: A Study in Female Authority," in *Queens, Queen Mothers, Priestesses, and Power*, ed. Flora Kaplan (Baltimore: Johns Hopkins Press, 1997), 41–71.

30

DEPOSITIONS OF MONARCHS IN NORTHERN EUROPEAN KINGDOMS, 1300–1700

Cathleen Sarti

The often presumed 'normal' way of succession to the throne in premodern Europe was by inheriting it after the death of the father. The heir was usually the oldest legitimate son after a system called agnatic primogeniture, which favoured sons before daughters. Dynastic rules of inheritance came into play to determine the next heir in the absence of legitimate sons. Nonetheless, the inheritance of a throne was considered the usual way of succession, even in electoral monarchies like the Holy Roman Empire or Poland-Lithuania in which dynasties of the Habsburg or the Vasa managed to establish a nearly unbroken line of election to the throne.[1]

Taking a closer look at the changing of monarchs reveals, however, that for the period between *c.*1300 and 1700 depositions, that is the removal of a monarch from their throne against their wishes, were a common occurrence. Depositions of monarchs and the installation of a new monarch or ruler were the case in roughly 30% of all changes of rulership in the kingdoms of northern Europe.[2] This chapter focuses on these kingdoms, that is Scotland, England, Denmark, Norway and Sweden, because of a similar political culture based on a shared history, a system of (mostly) common or Nordic law, and – in the later centuries – the Protestant confession and the break from Rome. Nonetheless, the different ideas about depositions as political conflicts and about diverse elements necessary in these events can provide the starting point for research into depositions in other geographical regions, or at other times.

Depositions are possible in theory from three different positions of the deposers: from below, from the same level, or from above. The deposition from above, for example by the pope or the emperor, was – theoretically – possible in monarchies who acknowledged the dominion of either pope or emperor. Depositions from the same level are actually a very fancy way of talking about conquests. They present a different kind of political conflict with a focus on international relations rather than a domestic conflict, as with depositions from below. The focus of this chapter lies on depositions from below, that is from the inhabitants of a kingdom who turned against the monarch to whom they may have sworn allegiance and obedience. Additionally, these monarchs were – according to widespread belief – supported on their throne by divine right, or at least were supposed to rule until their natural death according to custom.[3]

The analysis of depositions from below allows an approach to questions of rulership, especially on different forms of royal rule, what was considered a good or a bad monarch, when the beginning and the end of a rule was, and how a monarchy worked in times of crisis. This topic therefore touches the fields of royal studies, rulership, right of resistance, political history, legitimacy, state-building and political culture regarding the question of how different groups form the politics of a monarchy.[4] A study of depositions reveals the complicated structure of premodern kingdoms in which all inhabitants, from the monarch to the peasants, were necessary for the reign of a monarch. As such, this analysis adds to the growing historiographic discussion on how premodern, royal rule was actually imagined, discussed and executed. In Great Britain, Michael J. Braddick edited a volume on the question of how power in early modern Britain was negotiated, and more recently, Kevin Sharpe's trilogy on Tudor and Stuart rule changed the way we think about royal authority.[5] In Germany, research concepts on consensual rule by Bernd Schneidmüller, or on the impact of representation and discourses by Barbara Stollberg-Rilinger and others, have enhanced our understanding of the inner workings of governmental authority.[6] In Sweden, scholars like Mats Hallenberg and Johan Holm looked at the influence of peasants and how they used legal opportunities, e.g. the right to petition the crown.[7]

Premodern societies did not want any disturbances to the political order. This presented a problem when subjects of the realm saw depositions which were neither allowed, or even covered, by law as the only way out left for them in a political crisis. This chapter will expand on who deposed monarchs, their reasons and the different forms of depositions, and contextualize these occurrences of the changing of a throne into the broader context of premodern northern Europe. While a thorough analysis of all aspects of even one deposition is not possible on just a few pages, never mind all twenty-five monarchs who were deposed thirty-four times in total in northern Europe between 1300 and 1700 (some of these twenty-five monarchs were deposed more than once), it gives an overview of depositions as a specific form of the succession to the throne and should encourage the reader to expand further on this topic. The cases which form the basis for this chapter can be further explored through the companion website of this volume. Six sections will analyse 1) who deposed the monarchs; 2) the reasons for the depositions; 3) how allegiance could be taken away from a monarch; 4) how one deposition caused even more depositions; 5) what ways were found to pretend a deposition did not occur; and finally 6) discuss the most extreme forms of depositions, the explicit deposition and the killing of monarchs, the regicide. The conclusion will bring together this discussion of depositions of monarchs in premodern northern Europe by highlighting different results on questions of rulership, authority, political conflict and state formation.

Political elites and royal dynasties

Domestic political conflict which ended with the ruling monarch unwillingly leaving their throne and (most times) a new monarch taking over, occurred on a scale: renouncing allegiance in a semi-legal way was the most moderate form, forced abdication required much more (illegal) violence against the monarch, and the most radical forms were official deposition and regicide. Regicides were, however, a last resort of the political actors. Most depositions took place long before a political conflict had become so severe that regicide was seen as the only way forward. The political elite of a kingdom usually played the decisive role in determining when the rule of a monarch was in danger of ending in severe political conflict.

Institutions like royal councils, parliaments and legal assemblies (especially the Scandinavian law *tings*), but also individual jurists and legal seminars at universities, played an important role as a space for the political elite to discuss the problems in the kingdom with each other and with the reigning monarch, and – if necessary – also as a space where alliances against the monarch were formed, oaths of allegiance were retracted and depositions were legitimized *ex post facto*.[8] While political and legal institutions representing the political elite remained influential from the fourteenth until the seventeenth century, the role of certain institutions changed during this time. In the later Middle Ages and the early sixteenth century, councils with representatives from high nobility and high clergy were the most important factor both in Scandinavia and in the British Isles. The deposition of Jane Grey in England in 1553 marks a turning point in this aspect: while Jane Grey had the formal support of the council and the officials in London, her opponent, Mary Tudor, mobilized the gentry and population outside of London, forcing members of the council to switch allegiance pretty quickly. In Sweden, the depositions of Christian II (1523) and of Erik XIV (1569), in which parliaments legitimized the change of rulership after it was pushed through by force, show the growing importance of parliament. However, the most obvious change occurred in the 1590s when the opponent of the reigning monarch called several (illegal) parliaments and used them to challenge the king. The importance of parliaments in the seventeenth century (in the depositions of Charles I and James VII & II) confirmed that these assemblies were the most influential political institutions aside from the crown and represented a broader population than councils.[9]

Other than the support of institutions with their increasing officiality, formality and influence, successful depositions needed a reliable opponent to the reigning monarch. This opponent, the rival candidate, should have his or her own strong claim to the throne according to the rules of succession of the realm in question. In the British Isles, the rules of succession depended on hereditary right, which was the right of the oldest son to rule before his younger brothers and sisters. At the same time, in the Scandinavian electoral monarchies, hereditary succession still played a role, but the idea that the successor should be the best candidate out of all children of the old monarch was much more influential. Regardless of the exact rules of succession, the rival candidate in depositions usually had a claim as first, second, or third in line to the crown. This also means, that – aside from a few exceptions like Charles VIII and Gustav I in Sweden, or Oliver Cromwell in England – the opponent and successor of the reigning monarch was a close relative and often from the same dynasty.

Reasons for deposing a monarch

Although most opponents and successors of deposed monarchs were from their own close family, it does not mean that depositions were simply power struggles within dynasties. Rival candidates needed the political elite as well as broader support to enforce a change of rulership. This meant that different groups of subjects all needed to have their own good reasons why they wanted to depose the monarch, and risk disturbances to the political order.

Fears that the politics of the monarch in question would lead to tyranny was such a reason. Political thinkers and poets since Antiquity like Plato, Aeschylus, Sophocles, Augustine, John of Salisbury, Thomas Aquinas, Shakespeare and Machiavelli among many others have warned against the dangers of tyranny.[10] Since only one person ruled in a monarchy, the dangers of tyranny, an illegal, illegitimate and cruel form of the one-person-rule, were especially high. The problem was to reach a consensus on what was considered 'illegal' in a time before written constitutions made traditions into law. 'Illegitimate' was an equally contested term since competing legitimacies were at the basis of many conflicts.[11]

The analysis of depositions and the discussions surrounding these events showed that contemporaries mostly understood tyranny as a rule not according to the political culture of the kingdom, which – of course – was also not a fixed term. This arbitrary construction of what was seen as tyranny is an often-used argument against a ruler in one of the many personal unions[12] in premodern Europe. In particular, the deposers accused the monarch of breaking traditions and laws of the land, and using foreign officials instead of native ones. Such a problem with foreign officials exercising power also shaped the union of Kalmar, the personal union between all three Scandinavian kingdoms from 1397 to 1523.[13] In its 126 years of official existence, only 60 were under one rule. While the first monarch of the Kalmar Union, Eric of Pomerania, was deposed in all three kingdoms, later depositions occurred mostly only in Sweden and were led by Swedish elites against union kings perceived to be too Danish. In the six depositions of the Kalmar Union, the Swedish council legitimated their renouncing of allegiance with the monarch's breaking of Swedish law, acting against Swedish interest, or being a foreigner and bringing in men, who were 'foreigners, slaves, and criminals'.[14] At the end of the sixteenth century, not much had changed in this regard. The official deposition of Sigismund of Sweden (1599) stated explicitly his 'foreign rule with violence and tyranny'.[15]

The accusation of tyranny and being unfit to rule, moreover, was not only confined to foreign rulers acting against the (supposed) political culture of the realm. It was also used against a monarch who did not correspond with common expectations of rulership. Monarchs who risked and lost crown territory in wars, who had a bad reputation (Mary Stuart), who were insane (Erik XIV), who were otherwise obviously punished by God (Charles I, 'that man of blood'), or who did not act as a just ruler in regard to his own subjects (Christian II, James II) lost their legitimate right to the crown in the eyes of many of their subjects – they became *tyrannus exercitio*.

Renouncing of allegiance and rival kings

Even though northern European kingdoms had a similar political culture, the different preferred forms of depositions in the British Isles and in Scandinavia reveal slight differences in political culture. Scandinavians could more easily legitimize their depositions than the British. Except for Norway, the monarchs ruled over elective kingdoms in which, according to the political and legal tradition, the council of the realm decided on a new ruler. Although once elected monarchs should rule until their death, the idea of deposing the monarch and, more concretely, the idea of having the right to renounce allegiance and give it to someone else, never lost its impact in these kingdoms. Even after the introduction of hereditary monarchy (Sweden in 1544, Denmark in 1665), the Swedish political elite proved the long impact of this idea by deposing Erik XIV in 1569 and Sigismund in 1599 by renouncing allegiance.

The practice of renouncing allegiance was closely connected to the organization of political representation. From the fourteenth until the beginning of the sixteenth century, the council of the realm was the deciding element, which was often supported by regional councils. In a typical Scandinavian deposition, the council first renounced allegiance, as in the case of Birger Magnusson (1319), Magnus VII and Haakon (1364), Eric of Pomerania (1434, again in 1436 and in 1439), Charles VIII (1457) and John II (1501), and afterwards, regional councils (*tings*) withdrew their oath of allegiance as well. In cases like the deposition of Christian II (1523), these different renouncings of oath occurred over a longer period. In April 1522, the *ting* in Dalarna was the first to withdraw their support, but it was not until 6 June 1523 that Christian II was completely deposed by declaring Gustav I king of Sweden. In the sixteenth century, the only thing that changed was the role of the parliament which acted in the depositions of Eric XIV and of Sigismund instead of the council. Military conflicts broke out all over the realm at the same time as these formal and ritualized acts until the former monarch was forced out of the kingdom.[16] Magnates of the realm used the renouncing of allegiance in Sweden as an instrument of power. In this sense, Sweden – very much like Scotland in the late Middle Ages – was more a royal aristocracy than a monarchy.

Looking at depositions raises the question as to which conflicts to declare as depositions. Such a disputed case occurred in Denmark in the 1320s and 1330s. King Christopher II had problems fulfilling the conditions the Danish council demanded in exchange for their acceptance of his rule in 1319, written down in a so-called *handfæste*, an electoral capitulation. In 1326, he had to flee the country and a new child-king, Valdemar III, was installed to legitimize the rule of the powerful magnates from Denmark and neighbouring Holstein. However, there was never a renouncing of allegiance. Instead a rival king was raised. And again, three years later in 1329, when Christopher came back to Denmark after having reached an agreement with the Danish and Holstein magnates, Valdemar III was not formally deposed in any way, but one of the Danish *tings* elected Christopher to the throne. Nonetheless, magnates dominated his rule, and his death in 1332 resulted in an interregnum until 1340. This interregnum could possibly still have been under the official rule of Valdemar III due to some missing formal documents.[17] Since 1326, diverse Danish and Holstein magnates executed the actual power, so could a deposition really be a deposition if the deposed monarch did not actually rule over anything, but only had the title? Following on from this, what really constitutes a monarch – their actual power, formal acts like coronations, or continuous acceptance by his subjects? Or, maybe a mixture of all these criteria? The answer, of course, is dependent on a historian's question and methodology used. Since depositions were defined as the removal of a monarch from their throne against their will, for the purposes of this chapter, the events in Denmark in the 1320s are considered to be depositions. In both the deposition of Christopher II in 1326 and the deposition of Valdemar III in 1329, these took the form of the raising of a rival king. This practice of raising rival kings was also dominant in the conflict between the Swedish magnates, King Charles VIII, and the union-king Christian I in the 1450s and 1460s, in which falling from power, exile, raising a rival king, interregnum, banishing kings, and also formal renouncing of allegiance took place. Nonetheless, looking closely at the circumstances of depositions and the formal actions (e.g. renouncing of allegiance) highlights how authority and power were formed, executed, discussed and changed over time. The problem of answering a seemingly simple question like when exactly was the start of a royal rule, shows the complexity of premodern, monarchical rule.

Chains of depositions in English history

A chain of depositions dominated English politics in the period between 1399 (the deposition of Richard II) and 1485 (the death of Richard III), signalling a severe power struggle, mostly due to Edward III having too many sons, namely five, who reached adulthood and had issue themselves, and – after the first deposition – competing legitimacies. While the first deposition could easily be viewed as usurpation, later depositions were legitimized by trying to restore the original dynastic order of succession. The practice of establishing rival kings marked this chain of deposition, similar to the events in the 1320s and 1330s in Denmark, or the 1450s and 1460s in Sweden. However, in Scandinavia, different political institutions (*tings*, council, parliament) participated in the decision of who ruled, while the events in England were dynastic conflicts over the correct legitimacy of a monarch. Never mind that the specific conditions of any legitimate rule were the topic of intense discussion – what constituted tyranny, concepts of bad or good rulership, political and legal traditions and laws, including hereditary laws – and were not even a little agreed on, as Howard Nenner pointed out in 1995:

> A selective review of the record could demonstrate persuasively that English princes took their thrones by hereditary right – or that they did not; that, in England, conquest was a legitimate path to the throne – or that it was not; that crowns were given to English monarchs by their parliaments and their people – or that they were not. The problem, then, did not derive from any want of opinion about there being a definable rule of monarchical succession. It was rather that in times of political crisis there were multiple opinions invariably in conflict and consequently leading to confusion.[18]

In 1399, with the deposition of Richard II by Henry (IV), a chain of depositions started, based not only on the problem that there was a deposition in the first place but mostly due to the problem that Richard II was deposed not by the next-in-line for the throne (at this time, this would have been the eight-year-old Edmund Mortimer, the heir to the line of Richard's oldest uncle, Lionel of Antwerp), but by Henry, heir to the branch of Richard's second oldest uncle, John of Gaunt.[19]

Rival kings, though a sign for contentious legitimacy, usually only occur in conjunction with other reasons for deposition. The problem of these different branches started in 1399 with the deposition of Richard II, and while at this time there was not enough overall support in the country for successful rebellions against the new king Henry IV, the basic conflict remained at the back of politics during the fifteenth century.[20] The competing claims to the throne once again were used as legitimations for several depositions in the 1450s and 1460s. First, Edward IV deposed Henry VI in March 1461; second, the faction surrounding Henry VI, who was hardly more than a puppet lost in bouts of insanity by this time, deposed Edward IV in October 1470 by military defeat; and third, Edward IV reclaimed the throne in March and April 1471 by entry into London and taking possession of the city, including the tower and the former king, Henry VI, within.[21] This chain of depositions finally ended when Richard III (who deposed the son of Edward IV, Edward V, in 1483) was defeated (and killed) in the battle of Bosworth by Henry VII. Henry VII succeeded in starting anew, helped in no small part by the deaths of most of the nobles involved during more than thirty years of battle for the English crown and more than 100 years of fighting for the French crown.

Declaring a rival king in the British Isles could only be done when the legitimate rule of the monarch could be disputed, as in the cases of the competing lines of Lancaster and York, or as in the cases of the very short rules of Edward V and Jane Grey. Other than in the Scandinavian depositions, the most important actors here were the rival candidates who led a supporting party against the ruling monarch to assert their own claim to the throne. This was a power struggle in which different concepts of what constituted the legitimate ruler were just one part of the arsenal. After military means enforced their claim, the battle for legitimacy began and is still somewhat fought today in historiography. This is most obvious in the case of Mary Stuart, where Antonia Fraser and Jenny Wormald are representatives of two lines viewing the deposition as either legitimated or unjust usurpation. But also the case of Jane Grey remains questionable. Was her deposition rightful, or a usurpation by Mary Tudor, as Eric Ives stated: 'We have to turn tradition on its head and recognize that it was not Mary but Jane who was the reigning queen; her so-called "rebellion" against Queen Mary was, in reality, the "rebellion of Lady Mary" against Queen Jane.'[22]

In some ways, the practice of rival kings and changing of allegiance can also be seen in medieval Scotland, although the various power struggles between Scottish nobles usually stopped (except in the few cases discussed here) shortly before deposition. Kings were imprisoned, fought against, threatened, kept out of government, or left in England's prisons without losing their crown. If they managed to restore themselves to power, they were again accepted as Scottish kings until the next power struggle. As such, rivals were only rivals, not rival kings, and Scotland – though full of political conflict with their rulers – had not nearly as many depositions as the English despite having as many kings who have fallen from power as the other kingdoms.[23]

Deposition without deposing: forced abdications

A form of deposition specific to the British Isles, in particular to England, but less frequently also used in Scotland, was the cloaking of a forced removal from the throne as a willingly agreed decision to abdicate.[24] The first English deposition of the fourteenth century, Edward II in 1327, was an example of this, as was Richard II's in 1399 which started a chain of depositions. After 1500, Mary Stuart's deposition as Queen of Scotland in 1567 and James II's deposition in England in 1688/89 – though not in the same year in Scotland – were further examples.

The discussion of the deposers and their reasons for choosing to present *de facto* depositions as *de jure* abdications indicate several legal and political problems. First, depositions were not considered possible in the unwritten constitutions, traditions and laws of the kingdoms. Not even the English Magna Carta allowed this. The relevant article 61 allows a consortium of twenty-five barons to 'distrain and distress us [the monarch] in all ways they can', but 'when it [the transgression in question] is redressed, they shall obey us as they did before'.[25] Second, there was no consensus or model that could depose the monarch. Scholarly discussions among the so-called Monarchomachs on the right of resistance in the sixteenth and seventeenth centuries brought forward ideas of ephors (e.g. Johannes Althusius in *Politica*, 1603) or other bodies who would have the power and right to control the monarchs. Even though the radicality of such ideas against monarchical rule has attracted the interest of modern scholars like Glenn Burgess, Robert von Friedeburg, or Luise Schorn-Schütte, these discussions remained strictly academic and lacked a consensus among different political thinkers.[26] Third, since there was neither a legal basis for deposition nor a consensus of who could be a deposer, there was also not an established form or ritual, which differs from the Scandinavian cases where the renouncing of allegiance is practised so often that it can be used as legitimization.[27] Altogether, these challenges to depositions presented would-be deposers with the serious problem of how exactly to depose a monarch. In four British cases, the answer to that question was to force the monarch to abdicate. This way, nothing would disturb the political order, since the 'deposer' would be the monarch themselves.

Nonetheless, the problem remains of how to force the monarch to abdicate their throne. A common sequence of events shows the political conflict turn violent between the monarch and several different groups of subjects, who were often a mixture of political elite and commonalty. Forced abdications followed a military conflict, as was the norm in most depositions, which took the actual power away from the monarch and left it in the hands of the nobles at the head of the opposition. In 1326, Edward II was imprisoned and his opponents discussed his deposition. However, since his intended successor, his son Edward (III), was among the magnates insisting on a regular procedure of enthronement, a forced abdication seemed to be the only possible solution.[28] The deposition of Edward II and the power struggle between English magnates and the crown was also the background to the forced abdication of Edward II's great-grandson, Richard II, in 1399. Since 1397, Richard II took revenge against several magnates who limited his monarchy for most of the first twenty years of his reign. Unfortunately for him, he took it too far, and further opposition, led by his cousin, managed to overpower him and force him to abdicate in the summer of 1399.[29]

Captivity was often a prerequisite of a forced abdication. Mary Stuart was taken into custody by the Confederate Lords of Scotland after the meeting of the armies on the battlefield near Carberry Hill. Even though imprisoning the legitimate monarch was hardly a novelty in Scottish politics and usually led to a new compromise between monarch and political elite, Mary resolutely withstood all attempts to negotiate a new truce as a basis for her rule.[30] Not knowing what to do in such a case, and considering that the Scottish Lords had already expressed their fear that Mary's behaviour would fall back on the kingdom and be seen as 'sklanderous and abhominabill to all nationis', these Lords faced the typical conflict of depositions: there was no future imaginable with this queen, but she was also an anointed monarch with the right to rule until her natural death.[31] This latter problem forced several Scottish nobles to change course, realizing that Mary could not be persuaded to agree to their terms. These so-called Loyal Lords, however, also did not have an answer on how to solve the first problem when Mary resisted any compromise. Their answer was mostly to withdraw from the capital, spend the summer on their estates in the countryside, and just wait. This was, moreover, a strategy also employed by many from the political elite during the critical months in the winter of 1648/9 before the trial and execution of Charles I. In the meantime, the more radical minority of the Confederate Lords used Mary's weak position in prison to force her to sign a prepared letter of abdication on 24 July 1567.[32] The very quick coronation of Mary's legitimate, one-year old son, James VI, completed this deposition masked as abdication.

This confusion on what to do, which also characterizes several other depositions, is also very clear in the discussions of the convention parliament of 1689, when James II left England after retreating from William III's army on 23 November 1688. This flight in a critical moment when a foreign army was standing right in the middle of the kingdom, and violent riots had broken out in the capital, however, disappointed even the most staunch supporters of James.[33] In long discussions they decided to understand his flight as an abdication, even though James II had written several letters from his exile in France to different lords to explain his reasoning and enforce his monarchical rule.[34]

The most radical forms of deposition: depositions and regicides

Somewhat ironically, the rarest form of deposition was the actual deposing of the monarch. Depositions were sold as abdications, as an assumed right to renounce allegiance, by declaring for a rival monarch (and usually ignoring the monarch who was deposed by this action), or by skirting around the problem and questioning the legitimacy of a monarch. But they were hardly ever called depositions. In fact, the only deposition between 1300 and 1700 in northern Europe which stated this fact explicitly was the deposition of James VII of Scotland in 1689. While the same James was pretended to have abdicated by his actions in England, the Scottish parliament was clearer, and declared: 'whereby he hath forfeited the right to the crown, and the throne is become vacant'.[35]

If actual depositions were the rarest form of depositions in premodern Europe, regicides were certainly the most radical and scandalous way of deposing an unwanted monarch.[36] They posed the greatest threat to the order and peace of a monarchical realm and were also pretty rare between 1300 and 1700.[37] Even taking into account a wider European context, the assassinations of Henry III (1589) and Henry IV (1610) of France were the exception, also because they were done by political outsiders.[38] One other case of assassination was the Scottish king James I, who was murdered in 1437 by a conspiracy of Scottish nobles led by Walter Stewart, earl of Atholl and uncle of James I. Walter Stewart was one of the many children of the Scottish king, Robert II (grandfather to James I), which was not only the reason for several branches of the House of Stewart but also for long-lasting disputes and conflict over which branch was the legitimate heir to the throne (comparable to the English cases presented earlier).[39] In contrast to the exceptions of Henry III and Henry IV of France, this

Scottish assassination was, like many other depositions, carried out by members of the political elite, and especially by nobles who had their own claim to the throne.

Aside from the assassination of the Scottish king James I, the killing of a monarch still wearing their crown without trial was not practised in northern Europe between 1300 and 1700. Regicide as a practised form of deposition seems to have had its high-days before 1200 and after 1789 until the middle of the twentieth century.[40] Killing a monarch after he had already lost his crown, however, was an established English praxis, giving them a reputation as 'king-slayers'.[41] The emphasis on the idea that the monarch, especially the anointed monarch, was only judgeable by God, and the view of the monarch standing on top and outside of the political community, in addition to practical problems of the monarch usually being the supreme judge and law-maker not being subjected to anyone's will, made regicide nearly unthinkable.[42] Because of this, accusing, condemning and executing the Scottish queen Mary Stuart in 1587 was already considered highly controversial by contemporaries.[43] The regicide of Mary Stuart then indeed was a trigger for the sailing of the Spanish Armada against England. Although the conflict between Spain and England had been building for quite some time, the regicide left the sympathies of Catholic monarchies with Spain and could be used as a legitimization. Furthermore, Mary's case was not 'only' the trial of an already deposed queen, not even by her own subjects (who deposed her in 1567), but a trial by another kingdom in which she supposedly tried to commit treason by deposing the legitimate monarch herself.

Even more disturbing to the order of society was the trial and execution of Mary's grandson, Charles I in 1649. This monarch of England, Scotland and Ireland managed to make everything even worse in an already difficult time.[44] The dynamics in the ever wider spreading conflict between parliament and king, Scottish Covenanters and Charles I, and finally one half of the British kingdoms against the other half, led in the end to the imprisonment of Charles I by the New Model Army. Charles's refusal to compromise in any way, or even to abdicate, combined with the radicalization of the other parties, which had occurred over the time of the British civil wars, left only one way open – the blaming of the monarch for the political disorder as 'that man of blood',[45] the accusation as 'public enemy to the Commonwealth',[46] and finally his execution. The uncontrollable dynamics of the 1640s in England, and in the British Isles more generally, were also the reason why this deposition was the only one until the deposition of Louis XVI in 1792 which changed the form of government. Deposing monarchs to establish a republic is a modern practice – before 1789, depositions were not against monarchy, but against a specific person occupying the throne.

Conclusions

Depositions viewed in a longue durée showed that in premodern kingdoms royal rule was dependent on the consensus of the political elite and (later) even on the consensus of the majority of a kingdom's inhabitants. Moreover, the times of depositions indicate times of political crisis or of changing contexts of royal rule. The question of what constitutes a good, legitimate monarch was raised in depositions, and either solved in various ways or not solved, which then mostly led to another deposition a few years later, as in the case of the Swedish and English depositions in the fifteenth century.[47]

The political discussions surrounding depositions were about the concept of good rulership, limitations to the monarchy, tyranny and right of resistance, and on the conditions of monarchical rule in a certain kingdom, thereby contributing to pre-modern state-formation.[48] As a specific form of domestic political conflict, depositions formed states by forcing the negotiation of a new consensus of royal rule.

Notes

1 See also the chapter in this volume by Matthias Schnettger on the Holy Roman Empire.

2 For the purpose of giving a rough estimate, the list of monarchs from Michael F. Feldkamp, *Regentenlisten und Stammtafeln zur Geschichte Europas: Vom Mittelalter bis zur Gegenwart* (Stuttgart: Reclam, 2002) will suffice. A more detailed account of this list is available on the companion website of this volume. Michael F. Feldkamp counted twenty-two monarchs for England for the period 1300–1700. Nine of them lost their throne prematurely by being deposed by their subjects. In Scotland sixteen monarchs ruled and four monarchs could be considered to have been deposed. In Denmark seventeen kings rules, of which four were deposed. Also in Norway seventeen monarchs ruled, and three were deposed. The absolute record holder in Europe for depositions is, however, Sweden with fifteen monarchs of which eleven were deposed. All in all, this makes thirty-one deposed monarchs among the eighty-seven northern monarchs between 1300 and 1700. Since some of the monarchs were deposed by several countries, e.g. Christian II in Denmark, Sweden and Norway, the number of deposed monarchs is actually twenty-five. Some of the monarchs like Charles VIII or Henry VI were deposed more than once in the same kingdom, raising the total number of unique depositions to thirty-four.

3 The idea that a monarch ruled by divine right was especially forced in the seventeenth century, partly in response to texts on the right of resistance, see also Robert von Friedeburg, "Introduction," in *Murder and Monarchy. Regicide in European History, 1300–1800*, ed. Robert von Friedeburg (Basingstoke: Palgrave Macmillan, 2004), 14 and 16–37 for an overview of the changing legitimations of monarchical rule.

4 In regard to some of the terms used here, I would like to thank the participants of a lively discussion in the Royal Studies Facebook group about the difficulties when using 'kingship' while also meaning 'regnant queenship'. Mostly it was agreed, and this will be used in this chapter in this way, that 'rulership' also includes some understanding of royalty and means the quality and value of being a royal ruler. However, an unambiguous term including both genders and concentrating on the quality of being a monarch while excluding regents, political leaders, etc., is still missing.

5 Michael J. Braddick and John Walter, eds., *Negotiating Power in Early Modern Society: Order, Hierarchy and Subordination in Britain and Ireland* (Cambridge: Cambridge University Press, 2001). Kevin Sharpe, *Selling the Tudor Monarchy: Authority and Image in Sixteenth-Century England* (New Haven: Yale University Press, 2009); Kevin Sharpe, *Image Wars: Promoting Kings and Commonwealths in England, 1603–1660* (New Haven: Yale University Press, 2010); Kevin Sharpe, *Rebranding Rule. The Restoration and Revolution Monarchy, 1660–1714* (New Haven: Yale University Press, 2013).

6 Bernd Schneidmüller, "Konsensuale Herrschaft: Ein Essay über Formen und Konzepte politischer Ordnung im Mittelalter," in *Reich, Regionen und Europa im Mittelalter und Neuzeit. Festschrift für Peter Moraw*, eds. Paul-Joachim Heinig et al. (Berlin: Duncker & Humblot, 2000), 53–87. Barbara Stollberg-Rilinger et al., eds., *Spektakel der Macht: Rituale im alten Europa 800–1800* (Darmstadt: WBG, 2008). Barbara Stollberg-Rilinger, Tim Neu and Christina Brauner, eds., *Alles nur symbolisch? Bilanz und Perspektiven der Erforschung symbolischer Kommunikation* (Cologne: Böhlau, 2013).

7 Mats Hallenberg, "For the Wealth of the Realm: The Transformation of the Public Sphere in Swedish Politics, c.1434–1650," *Scandinavian Journal of History* 37, no. 5 (2012): 557–577. Mats Hallenberg and Johan Holm, *Man ur huse: Hur krig, upplopp och förhandlingar påverkade svensk statsbildning i tidigmodern tid* (Lund: Nordic Academic Press, 2016).

8 On the influence of jurists and legal seminars in depositions, see Helmut G. Walther, "Der gelehrte Jurist als politischer Ratgeber: Die Kölner Universität und die Absetzung König Wenzels 1400," in *Die Kölner Universität im Mittelalter. Geistige Wurzeln und soziale Wirklichkeit*, ed. Albert Zimmermann, Miscellanea Mediaevalia 20 (Berlin: de Gruyter 1989), 467–487.

9 See further on the development of parliaments for Sweden, Michael F. Metcalf, ed., *The Riksdag: A History of the Swedish Parliament* (New York: St Martin's Press, 1987) and more generally, Michael A.R. Graves, *The Parliaments of Early Modern Europe* (Harlow: Longman, 2001) and Maija Jansson, ed., *Realities of Representation. State Building in Early Modern Europe and European America* (Basingstoke: Palgrave Macmillan, 2007).

10 One of the best recent works on the history of tyranny and its scholarly reception is by Mario Turchetti, *Tyrannie et tyrannicide de l'Antiquité à nos jours* (Paris: Presses universitaires de France, 2001). The recent bestseller by Timothy Snyder, *On Tyranny: Twenty Lessons from the Twentieth Century* (London: The Bodley Head, 2017), shows the never-ending importance of this topic and the interest it manages to attract.

11 Howard Nenner, *The Right to be King: The Succession to the Crown of England, 1603–1714* (Basingstoke: Macmillan, 1995) shows this for the right of the English succession, and Colin Rhys Lovell, *English Constitutional and Legal History: A Survey* (New York: Oxford University Press, 1962) more generally for English law. The same is true for Scandinavian law, cf. Armin Wolf, *Gesetzgebung in Europa: 1100–1500: Zur Entstehung der Territorialstaaten*, 2, rev. and exp. edition. (Munich: Beck, 1996), esp. 314. Wolfgang Reinhard, *Geschichte der Staatsgewalt: Eine vergleichende Verfassungsgeschichte Europas von den Anfängen bis zur Gegenwart* (Munich: Beck, 1999), 304 states the eighteenth to the twentieth century as the time of codification in most European states.

12 See: Charlotte Backerra, "Personal union, composite monarchy and 'multiple rule'", 89–111 in this volume.

13 As an introduction to and overview of Scandinavian history, see Byron J. Nordstrom, ed., *Dictionary of Scandinavian History* (Westport: Greenwood Press, 1986) and Knut Helle, ed., *The Cambridge History of Scandinavia: Prehistory to 1520*, vol. I (Cambridge: Cambridge University Press, 2003).

14 O.S. Rydberg, ed., *Sverges traktater med främmande magter jemte andra dit hörande handlingar: Tredje Delen, 1409–1520*, 4 vols. 3 (Stockholm: P.A. Norstedt & Söner, 1895), document 565, 486–489. The quote is taken from the deposition document of Christian II in Denmark, "Opsigelsesbrev til Christian 2," in *Kampen om Danmark: Dansk politik på reformationstiden 1513–1536*, ed. Carsten E. Knudsen (Herning, 1984), http://danmarkshistorien.dk/leksikon-og-kilder/vis/materiale/opsigelsesbrev-til-christian-2-ca-20-januar-1523/ (accessed 15 February 2016).

15 Anders Anton Stiernman, *Alla Riksdagars och Mötens Besluth: samt arfföreningar / Regements-Former, Försäkringar och Bewillningar / som / på allmenna Riksdagar och Möten / ifrån år 1521. intil år 1727. giorde / stadgade och bewiljade äro; med the för hwart och ett Stånd utfärdade all-menna Resolutioner* (Stockholm, 1728), 481.

16 The rituality of depositions is discussed by Frank Rexroth, "Tyrannen und Taugenichtse: Beobachtungen zur Ritualität europäischer Königsabsetzungen im späten Mittelalter," *Historische Zeitschrift* 278, no. 1 (2004): 27–53.

17 For Christopher II and Valdemar III, see Charlotte Rock, *Herrscherwechsel im spätmittelalterlichen Skandinavien: Handlungsmuster und Legitimationsstrategien*. Mittelalter-Forschungen 50 (Ostfildern: Jan Thorbecke Verlag, 2016), 40–49. Charlotte Rock argues that because of missing technicalities these events should not be considered depositions, ibid. 46.

18 Nenner, *The Right to be King*, 1.

19 See also David Hipshon, *Richard III*, Routledge Historical Biographies (London: Routledge, 2011), 49–50.

20 Christopher Allmand, "Opposition to Royal Power in England in the Late Middle Ages," in *Königliche Gewalt: Gewalt gegen Könige – Macht und Mord im spätmittelalterlichen Europa*, ed. Martin Kintzinger and Jörg Rogge, Zeitschrift für historische Forschung Beiheft 33 (Berlin: Duncker & Humblot, 2004), 61.

21 Hipshon, *Richard III*, 85–86.

22 Eric Ives, *Lady Jane Grey: A Tudor Mystery* (Chichester: Wiley-Blackwell, 2011), 2.
23 Michael Lynch, ed., *The Oxford Companion to Scottish History* (Oxford: Oxford University Press, 2001) is an excellent introduction to and overview of Scottish history.
24 See further on voluntary abdications the volume by Susan Richter and Dirk Dirbach, eds., *Thronverzicht: Die Abdankung in Monarchien vom Mittelalter bis in die Neuzeit* (Cologne: Böhlau, 2010). See also on the rituals used to cloak a deposition as abdication, Rexroth, *Tyrannen und Taugenichtse*, 41–49.
25 The 1215 version of the Magna Carta used here is edited and translated in David Carpenter, *Magna Carta* (Harmondsworth: Penguin Books, 2015), 36–69, at 65.
26 An overview of these writings by the so-called Monarchomachs is given by Günter Stricker, *Das politische Denken der Monarchomachen: Ein Beitrag zur Geschichte der politischen Ideen im 16. Jahrhundert* (Heidelberg, 1967). Important recent works on the right of resistance in the sixteenth and seventeenth centuries are by Glenn Burgess, *British Political Thought, 1500–1660: The Politics of the Post-Reformation* (Basingstoke: Palgrave Macmillan, 2009); Robert von Friedeburg, ed., *Widerstandsrecht in der frühen Neuzeit: Erträge und Perspektiven der Forschung im deutsch-britischen Vergleich*, Zeitschrift für historische Forschung Beiheft 26 (Berlin: Duncker & Humblot, 2001); Luise Schorn-Schütte, *Gottes Wort und Menschenherrschaft: Politisch-theologische Sprachen im Europa der Frühen Neuzeit* (Munich: Beck, 2015).
27 See further on the importance of establishing a process which then can be used to legitimize political changes, Barbara Stollberg-Rilinger and André Krischer, eds., *Herstellung und Darstellung von Entscheidungen: Verfahren, Verwalten und Verhandeln in der Vormoderne*, Zeitschrift für historische Forschung Beiheft 44 (Berlin: Duncker & Humblot, 2010). Their study adapts Niklas Luhmann's work for premodern societies, Niklas Luhmann, *Legitimation durch Verfahren* (Frankfurt am Main: Suhrkamp, 1983). Christine Carpenter, "Resisting and Deposing Kings in England in the Thirteenth, Fourteenth and Fifteenth Centuries," in Friedeburg, *Murder and Monarchy* argues for the establishment of such a process in late medieval England.
28 Dieter Berg, *Die Anjou-Plantagenets: Die englischen Könige im Europa des Mittelalters (1100–1400)* (Stuttgart: Kohlhammer, 2003), 214. See also William Huse Dunham Jr. and Charles T. Wood, "The Right to Rule in England: Depositions and the Kingdom's Authority, 1327–1485, " *The American Historical Review* 81, no. 4 (1976), 740–741.
29 Berg, *Die Anjou-Plantagenets*, 274–275, and Dunham Jr. and Wood, "The Right to Rule in England," 747–748.
30 The behaviour of Mary Stuart in this situation is, as many others of her actions, a topic of open debate, e.g. in the studies of Retha M. Warnicke, *Mary Queen of Scots* (New York: Routledge, 2006) and John Guy, *Queen of Scots: The True Life of Mary Stuart* (Boston: Houghton Mifflin, 2004).
31 John H. Burton, ed., *The Register of the Privy Council of Scotland: [1. Series] 1: 1545–1569* (Edinburgh: H.M. General Register House, 1877), 519.
32 Keith M. Brown, ed., *The Records of the Parliaments of Scotland to 1707* (2007–2014), www.rps.ac.uk/trans/1567/7/25/1 (accessed 28 March 2019).
33 David L. Jones, "Introduction," in *A Parliamentary History of the Glorious Revolution*, ed. David L. Jones (London: Her Majesty's Stationery Office, 1988), 5–6, or Robert Beddard, "Introduction: The Dynastic Revolution," in *A Kingdom Without a King: The Journal of the Provisional Government in the Revolution of 1688*, ed. Robert Beddard (Oxford: Phaidon, 1988), 36.
34 Robert Beddard, ed., *A Kingdom Without a King: The Journal of the Provisional Government in the Revolution of 1688* (Oxford: Phaidon, 1988), 159–160.
35 Andrew Browning, ed., *English Historical Documents: 1660–1714* (London: Eyre & Spottiswoode, 1966), document 248, 635–639, at 636.
36 Cf. Robert von Friedeburg, ed., *Murder and Monarchy: Regicide in European History, 1300–1800* (Basingstoke: Palgrave Macmillan, 2004), especially the chapter by Jean P. Genet, "Murdering the Anointed," in Friedeburg, *Murder and Monarchy*.
37 Manuel Eisner, "Killing Kings: Patterns of Regicide in Europe, AD 600–1800," *The British Journal of Criminology* 51, no. 3 (2011), 563, table 2, counted 227 of 1,513 monarchs between 600 and 1800 who were either executed after a trial or murdered. However, the

distribution of these numbers across the centuries shows peaks in the seventh and the eleventh centuries, after which there is a constant decline in numbers, see ibid., 569, figure 2.

38 Manuel Eisner calls them 'politically radicalized outsiders', instead of part of the political elite, ibid., 565–566.

39 An overview of the royal Stewarts (becoming Stuarts later) is given by Oliver Thomson, *The Rises and Falls of the Royal Stewarts* (Stroud: History, 2009). More detailed information can be found in Lynch, *The Oxford Companion to Scottish History*.

40 Eisner, "Killing Kings."

41 See Carpenter, "Resisting and Deposing Kings," 99 for a discussion on the English as 'king-slayers'.

42 See also the chapter by Matthias Range in this volume.

43 See, e.g. Guy, *Queen of Scots*, 9.

44 See further on the complexity of the British civil wars, Austin Woolrych, *Britain in Revolution, 1625–1660* (Oxford: Oxford University Press, 2004); Martyn Bennett, *The Civil Wars in Britain and Ireland, 1638–1651* (Oxford: Blackwell, 1997); Michael J. Braddick, ed., *The Oxford Handbook of the English Revolution*, Oxford Handbooks in History (Oxford: Oxford University Press, 2015); Charles W. Prior and Glenn Burgess, eds., *England's Wars of Religion, Revisited* (Farnham: Ashgate, 2011). Especially the crisis in the mid-seventeenth century, see John H. Elliott, "Revolution and Continuity in Early Modern Europe," *Past & Present* 42 (1969).

45 Keith Lindley, ed., *The English Civil War and Revolution: A Sourcebook* (New York: Routledge, 1998), 167. See also Clive Holmes, "The Trial and Execution of Charles I," *The Historical Journal* 53, no. 2 (2010), and Patricia Crawford, "Charles Stuart, 'That Man of Blood'," *Journal of British Studies* 16, no. 2 (1977).

46 Samuel R. Gardiner, ed., *The Constitutional Documents of the Puritan Revolution 1625–1660*, third edition (Oxford: Clarendon Press, 1906), 378–379.

47 See also Allmand, "Opposition to Royal Power", 64–66 and 69–70 for similar observations about the English depositions.

48 Similar also Dunham Jr. and Wood, "The Right to Rule in England," 760 about depositions in late medieval England. The prolific research on the right of resistance is reviewed by Friedeburg, "Introduction." For more on early modern state-formation, see e.g. Wim Blockmans, André Holenstein and Jon Mathieu, eds., *Empowering Interactions: Political Cultures and the Emergence of the State in Europe, 1300–1900* (Farnham: Ashgate, 2009).

Key works

Carpenter, David, *Magna Carta* (Harmondsworth: Penguin Books, 2015).

Dunham Jr., William Huse and Charles T. Wood, "The Right to Rule in England: Depositions and the Kingdom's Authority, 1327–1485," *The American Historical Review* 81, no. 4 (1976): 738–761.

Helle, Knut, ed., *The Cambridge History of Scandinavia: Prehistory to 1520*, vol. I (Cambridge: Cambridge University Press, 2003).

Reinhard, Wolfgang, *Geschichte der Staatsgewalt: Eine vergleichende Verfassungsgeschichte Europas von den Anfängen bis zur Gegenwart* (Munich: Beck, 1999).

Schubert, Ernst, *Königsabsetzung im deutschen Mittelalter: Eine Studie zum Werden der Reichsverfassung* (Göttingen: Vandenhoeck & Ruprecht, 2005).

PART IV

EXERCISING AUTHORITY AND EXERTING INFLUENCE

INTRODUCTION

Zita Eva Rohr

This part, 'Exercising authority and exerting influence', adopts a *longue dureé* approach to shed light upon the activity of a multiplicity of actors within the wider framework of monarchy. Applying cross-disciplinary thinking and methodologies, the chapters in this part combine to scrutinize the mechanisms of sovereignty and legitimacy. In tackling the ways in which monarchies across time have sought to exercise authority and exert influence, the contributors to this part confront, problematize and elaborate upon pivotal themes raised across the entirety of this collection – themes such as power, law, religion, the use of ceremony, display and representation, and dynasties, courts and realms.

I have argued elsewhere that while authority reposing in a king or queen presents many opportunities to the individual in possession of it, the exercise of it is by no means a simple undertaking.[1] The exercise of monarchical authority demands both power and personality (charisma).[2] Taking the latter of these two intangibles into consideration, in her introduction to this collection, 'Understanding the mechanisms of monarchy', Elena Woodacre points to Max Weber's contention that charisma is linked to the divine.[3] In his examination of authority and charisma, Weber argues succinctly that charisma is 'a certain quality of an individual personality by virtue of which he is set apart from ordinary men'.[4] I sense, however, that while charisma is undoubtedly essential to the exercise of authority and the attainment and maintenance of sovereignty, it is *power* – the capacity to impose one's will upon others – that is the fundamental prerequisite for the exercise of authority and exertion of influence. In defining the essence of power, Michel Foucault asserts that 'power is neither given or exchanged, or recovered, but rather exercised . . . it exists only in action . . . [it] is above all a relation of force' – and an intangible force at that.[5] If we take Foucault's definition as our point of departure, it might be understood that power manifests itself a lot like electricity (itself a power source). We cannot see electricity – or power – but we are able to witness the work they do. Both are phenomena rather than tangible objects or concepts. In lamenting the difficulties of arriving at a scholarly understanding of power, David Cannadine echoes Foucault's ideas, observing that 'Power is like the wind: we cannot see it, but we feel its force . . . The invisible and the ephemeral are, by definition, not the easiest subjects for scholars to study', which should not, however, prevent us from examining its role in politics and diplomacy. Indeed, Natalie Zemon Davis offers us exciting and subtle ideas to explore by pithily defining the intangible, alluring and sometimes fugacious phenomenon of power, asserting that it 'can lodge in dangerous nooks and crannies . . . It can be informal, unpredictable, unaccountable, frittered away, or saved for important occasions. *It needs to be examined in its full complexity*'.[6] It is this very complexity that has attracted me to the study of premodern power in all its manifestations and contexts, and I am not alone in this. In his recent essay on Machiavelli's *Prince*, Thomas E. Cronin demonstrates his subtle grasp of Machiavelli's very specific conception of power, one well worth considering when turning our minds to questions of authority, power, and influence:

> Effective princes must have a finely tuned understanding of power. They must know what power is – hard as well as soft power – and how to acquire and exercise it. They must know how to play one interest off against another. Their own success and the success of their state trump conventional pieties about moral character.[7]

The exercise of authority and exertion of influence, as well as the full complexity of the power upon which these rest – and wherein their effectiveness resides – are far more fascinating ideas to excavate and examine than the mere possession of acknowledged authority and a very nice crown, and the usual accoutrements to indicate who is nominally in charge. Power is one of the most useful lenses by which to approach ideas of authority and influence, and this very useful tool – or lens – is effectively deployed by the contributors to this part as they examine a wide diversity of monarchical practices in the various geographical and temporal contexts to which they have chosen to turn their attention.

While this part covers the more traditionally studied geographies of northern and western Europe, it also harvests innovative inter-disciplinary scholarship stretching into less studied areas. Although the Crusader States and their individual kings consort have been studied quite deeply, Stephen Donnachie's comparative and longitudinal study is rather unique. The same can be said of Kim Bergqvists's contribution examining the activities of kings and nobles on the fringes of Christendom, and indeed Frank Jacob's chapter revealing the agency of a nineteenth-century Korean empress whose influence upon foreign policy hampered Japanese imperial expansion on the Korean Peninsula. This ultimate section of *Routledge History of Monarchy* advances our understanding of the importance of the masculinities and sexualities of male monarchs and kings consort from the aforementioned Crusader States of the Latin east to the European kingdoms of England, Sweden, and into the early modern period of pre-Revolutionary France. Moreover, the seven contributors to this part bring to bear a number of innovative lenses reflecting wider trends in the field of historical study *viz.* emotions, sexuality studies, gender and masculinities, and diplomacy and counsel. While the bulk of the chapters in this part fall into the traditionally studied 'comfort zones' of medieval and early modern Europe, the research contributions of Bagerius and Ekholst, Donnachie and Jacob combine to give the reader a very different perspective in terms of period and place. Susan Broomhall's meticulous comparative study, 'Ruling emotions: affective and emotional strategies of power and authority among early modern European monarchies', introduces ground-breaking scholarship of the history of emotions, pointing to the importance of affective and emotional strategies when considering the exercise of power and authority in early modern European monarchies.

In keeping with Davis's overriding concern that 'we should be interested in the history of both men and women',[8] with our goal being 'to understand the signifi-cance of the *sexes*, of gender groups in the historical past',[9] several of the chapters in this part combine to examine how the maintenance (as well as the not infrequent inversion or subversion) of a 'proper' gender order defined the complementary roles of the king and queen, providing security and continuity to realms in times of upheaval and transformation. Their contributions dovetail with Davis's sound counsel regarding the ductile zones of transition between apparently fixed gen-dered boundaries of power and influence, our aim determinedly being 'to explain why sex roles were sometimes tightly prescribed and sometimes fluid, sometimes markedly asymmetrical and sometimes more even'. This part also draws heavily upon the important work of Theresa Earenfight who has built upon and refined Davis's understanding of sex roles and gendered performance as well as Foucault's understanding of power in her research on the institution of queenship within the edifice of monarchy.[10] 'Exercising authority and exerting influence' highlights that the personality, education, experience, networks and political stamina of monarchs were – and remain – just as important as access to an officially constituted authority to rule.[11] With all of this in mind, the new scholarly perspectives put forward in this part on the significance of the ties that bound royal dynasties to their aristocrats are worthy and essential contributions to current trends in the scholarship of monar-chy, as are those dealing with the necessity of targeted advice and sound counsel to ruling and aspirant dynasties in a variety of geopolitical contexts in medieval and early modern Europe.

The Crusader States on the frontiers of Christendom, protecting Christianity's holiest landscape, faced major challenges to their very existences. Added to the obvi-ous challenges requiring warfare and diplomacy were dynastic crises in the kingdom of Jerusalem and the principality of Antioch, where the ruling male lines frequently petered out with female heiresses remaining to do the heavy lifting of buttressing dynastic continuity. Stephen Donnachie examines this phenomenon in the opening chapter of this part. He explains why and how it was that, time and again, the bar-ons of these Christian outposts were called upon to seek out suitable male consorts in the Latin west for female heiresses in the Latin east to fill vacant royal posts. The masculine sphere of medieval kingship – especially in these contested Crusader States – needed male consorts who were willing and able to travel eastwards to ful-fil masculine roles of warfare and virile diplomacy. The fact that these men were the 'mere' consorts of their regnant female spouses meant that very often female 'intrusion' into their male sphere threw up the need for what Joan-Lluís Palos terms 'gender and cultural adaption'.[12] This begs the question as to whether or not 'it was particularly problematic for men to adapt to cultural and political conditions that made them subordinate'[13] to their regnant wives – a question Donnachie explores in his chapter. With his comparative overview of their tenures, Donnachie brings these male consorts back into the traditional narrative of monarchy, placing women equally at the helm. He conceives of the construction of sovereignty as gendered, demonstrating the unique challenges these monarchs faced in their efforts to exert authority and exercise influence.

There has been a marked shift in early modern political history away from the study of the formal or professional sphere of institutions and office bearers towards informal political spheres, such as the non-institutional and domestic. Recent scholarship has demonstrated that all modern political systems have been produced within an informal political arena alongside government.[14] The chapters in this part build further upon this more contemporary understanding of the mechanisms of authority and influence, providing more evidence – if any were needed – that the dichotomy between formal and informal authority, power and influence simply does not hold. In his examination of the case of kings and nobles on the fringes of Christendom, Kim Bergqvist adds to this burgeoning body of evidence, taking a comparative perspective on monarchy and aristocracy in Europe in the Middle Ages. He focuses upon the relationship between kingship and nobilities in areas that have been frequently overlooked or dismissed as being peripheral to medieval western Europe. Bergqvist presents us with an extended relational case study of Iberia and Scandinavia from the twelfth to the fifteenth centuries. During the European Middle Ages, the king's authority was founded upon his ability to control military resources and other means of force; amass economic assets; and exert authority legally as well as symbolically. Bergqvist scrutinizes the ways in which the secular and clerical nobility and the aristocracy were indispensable to a king's exercise of power. Naturally, and as was so often the case, this gave ambitious players just the opening they needed to exert their influence over the king and his policies. While the birth and growth of the state in medieval Europe and its process of centralization led to an initial surge in monarchical authority in several kingdoms during the high Middle Ages, nobles soon found ways to form ideologically vested agenda for their own involvement in statehood and its concomitant institutions. Aristocrats and nobles needed their own theatres in which to exert influence over their monarchs to push for and implement their respective political views and, while official and public representative institutions gained momentum in the late Middle Ages, private and informal means of influence also became increasingly important.

Bergqvist reveals that recent research concerning ideological expressions in medieval Scandinavian texts from the high to late medieval periods, as well as research on the monarchy as an area of conflict in medieval Iberia, have much to offer us, not least because their particularities come to the fore in relation to the Iberian Reconquista and the Baltic Crusades. Bergqvist notes that, while certain fundamental aspects of noble influence upon royal authority – such as the right to offer counsel – was in some respects constant throughout the period, it was often contested and challenged and that the forms of the expression of such influence were transformed in accordance with overall societal change. His chapter synthesizes some of the most important developments in contemporary research on kingship and nobilities in these very different contexts that seldom, if ever, have been discussed in scholarly exchanges. Bergqvist aims to remove silo-thinking and, in so doing, contributes to informed scholarly dialogue by offering comparative analyses and new insights into the varied and constantly shifting circumstances that guided the political life within high and late medieval European monarchies on the fringes of Christendom.

With their collaboration, Henric Bagerius and Christine Ekholst remind us that in medieval society the royal marriage worked to construct social order, an order wherein every woman, in theory at least, lovingly accepted her subordination to a man. Their chapter presents interesting points of comparison with Donnachie's contribution whose royal couples also endured many crises, as they too were obliged to struggle in order to wield power together and negotiate their personal and political partnerships. The royal household stood as an ideal for all other marriages and was meant to be loving, reproductive and hierarchical. Sexuality played an important part in the construction of these idealized royal unions. In medieval society, sexual intercourse – the conjugal debt – was conceived of as an act one person (the male) did to another (the female). It was not conceptualized as a mutual act, it was interpreted instead as reflecting and reinforcing a divine and natural order in society. Sex between husband and wife helped to maintain the proper gender order, and it might be understood from this that the (hetero)sexual act symbolically reflected that the husband was the master of his house and therefore was responsible for his subordinate wife. This was even more the case when it came to a royal marriage – the queen was, theoretically and potentially, a powerful woman who needed to be kept firmly under masculine control. Bagerius and Ekholst's contribution examines the politically motivated criticism directed at six medieval royal couples in the diverse polities of England, Castile and Sweden.

Bagerius and Ekholst first draw our attention to the fraught English couplings of Edward II and Isabella of France, and Henry VI and Margaret of Anjou, thence shifting our attention northwards to the Swedish-Norwegian king, Magnus Eriksson and his wife, Blanche of Namur. They continue their scrutiny, taking the reader on a scholarly journey to Castile where they pause to examine Enrique IV and his wives, Blanca of Navarre and Juana of Portugal, before moving on to the revealing case study of Juan II and his wives, María of Aragon and Isabel of Portugal. For Bagerius and Ekholst, it is not so much the case histories of these individual couples that has piqued their scholarly interest, but rather the political critiques directed against the couples concerned. They argue cogently that clear patterns emerge from propagandistic sources, and that the couples' critics used the potency and salaciousness of sexual allegations to undermine the sovereignty – the authority – of the king to rule. His actions – or indeed inactions – in this nominally intimate marital sphere could render him unmanly and therefore unfit to rule.

Bagerius and Ekholst argue convincingly that sexuality was fundamental both to the construction of the royal marriage and in helping to define and manifest the 'proper' roles of the king and his queen. They posit that this went well beyond the need to produce heirs, spares and marriageable daughters for the reigning dynasty. The sexual allegations levelled against late medieval kings and queens were highly gendered and reveal to us the anxieties held that the balance of power would be overturned should the king and queen cease to have intercourse with one another. While obsessing on a fairly constant basis about the sexual reputations, behaviours and appetites of queens, chroniclers were also much troubled when it appeared that a king might be spending rather too much time with his male favourites. I have recently put forward the hypothesis that this is precisely why some royal wives tolerated females – mistresses – in the post of royal favourite.[15] This should give one pause to ponder, especially when one takes into account the level of tolerance afforded by royal wives such as Queen Marie of Anjou towards her king-husband's favourite, Agnès Sorel – the first official female French royal favourite. Before *la belle* Agnès sashayed onto the scene, Charles VII had succumbed to the influence of a particularly odious string of male favourites who determinedly usurped his royal authority to enrich themselves and exert almost unchecked power and influence over the king. By the same token, a queen could be, and not infrequently was, charged with unruliness when she was no longer being subdued sexually, and therefore socially, by her royal spouse. Attacks upon a royal woman's regency were framed in much the same way – widowed, or left at the helm of the ship of state – she was reimagined as power hungry, greedy and adulterous. Yet another reason, if one were needed, for queens and female regents to fashion themselves a spotlessly chaste and pious persona.[16] The other side of the coin, a lack of marital sexuality on the part of the king became linked to passivity and unmanly behaviour – ultimately working to undermine his authority and regnal sovereignty. If the king were not master in his own marriage, how could he hope to be master of the realm?

Following on from Bagerius and Ekholst's contribution, the part turns its attention to the reign of the Tudors, which one historian describes as a time when 'England was economically healthier, more expansive, and more optimistic . . . than at any time in a thousand years'.[17] Joanne Paul, in collaboration with Valerie Schutte, rises to the challenge of teasing out the relationship between counsel and the Tudor crown, arguing convincingly that understanding this very particular relationship is essential if we are to grasp both the ways in which counsel influenced sovereignty in the early modern period and the political operations of the Tudor regime. Paul pays particular attention to the fundamental shift between the 'humanist' discourse of counsel in the early decades of the sixteenth century to the 'Machiavellian' discourse of the middle of the century, which would lay the foundation for the Reason of State tradition of political counsel in the second half of the sixteenth century. To demonstrate this, Paul provides us with two case studies – one from the first half of the sixteenth century during the reign of Henry VIII (r.1509–47), the other from the second half of the sixteenth century during the reigns of his children Edward VI (r.1547–53), Mary I (r.1553–8) and Elizabeth I (r.1558–1603). By focusing upon these comparative case studies, Paul is able to reveal the shift in conciliar strategies between the two halves of the sixteenth century and the complex ways in which they interacted with monarchical authority.

From the busy and sometimes turbulent Tudor courts, Susan Broomhall shifts our gaze to the wider theatre of early modern European monarchy – to the successful territorial monarchies that transformed themselves into what we would eventually recognize as the modern state. Broomhall brings to bear the emerging scholarship of the history of emotions on the exercise of power in the early modern period. She lays bare how emotional rhetoric and affective display were integral components of the construction of rule for both male and female monarchs, monarchs who operated within culturally and gender-specific practices of both feeling and rule. Broomhall examines and analyses how carefully constructed emotional rhetoric worked to underpin sovereignty in edicts, letters and other textual forms, and how power and authority were expressed through controlled emotional labour and calculated displays of corporeal feeling, captured in eye-witness reports, portraits, ceremony, entries and ritual practices. Drawing upon examples from across western Europe, Broomhall uncovers how socialities and sociabilities were grounded in particular emotional expressions and practices, and how they were key to the maintenance of power. Studying these in the context of gift exchange processes, art and architectural commissions, and courtly practice surrounding the monarch, Broomhall demonstrates the vital importance of emotional content to the power of the monarchy as a system of rule.

In his chapter, Chad Denton draws our attention to the ways in which the biographies of the last three reigning kings of France's Bourbon dynasty – all of whom were helpfully named Louis – reveal striking contrasts in their intimate relationships and how their relationships with women were received by the French public. While these individual monarchs have received considerable attention over the years, Denton's contribution offers the reader an intensive and scholarly comparison that gives a fresh perspective on these men. From the standpoint of their subjects, Louis XIV's sexual comportment was regarded as normal, Louis XV's as unworthy, and Louis XVI's as ridiculously chaste. In the case of Louis XVI, while he determinedly constructed a model of royal domesticity, he ultimately came to be regarded as an impotent king married to a corrupt nymphomaniac and extravagant queen. Denton argues that a comparison of attitudes towards the sexual behaviours of these final reigning Bourbon kings of France evinces a pronounced shift, even within different genres 'from the songs and broadsheets fresh off the streets of Paris to the memoirs of the most respected nobles at the royal court'. Denton stresses that while we should not neglect factors such as the kings' individual personalities and behaviours, he is right to focus on how the kings' sexual lives were understood by their respective publics. He makes the compelling observation that differing ways of discussing the sex lives of these three kings Louis 'provide important lenses by which to assess the broad changes unfolding in early modern France, including religious and moral discourses, gender and women's freedom, and ideas about marriage'. These factors transformed what were regarded initially as harmless romantic *galanteries* into scandals that undermined and potentially destroyed the reputation of a once popular king.

The final chapter in this section is Frank Jacob's contribution, which explores the influence of a nineteenth-century Korean empress upon Korean foreign policy between 1876 and 1895. Empress Myeongseong – Queen Min as she was known in the west – was probably the most influential woman in the modern history of Korea. As the first empress of the Korean empire, she established her influence upon the politics of Korea at a very early stage and was a decisive force in attempts to check Japan's imperial ambitions on the Korean Peninsula. In addition to her foreign policy agenda, she stimulated domestic social change by supporting limited reform in the education sector and peripherally elsewhere. Jacob supplies the reader with a brief biographical introduction to assist those of us who might find themselves in unfamiliar territory – enabling us to better appreciate the geographical and chronological background of events. He highlights Empress Myeongseong's role in the development of a strong anti-Japanese foreign policy, one which eventually – and perhaps inevitably – led to her assassination by Japanese agents in 1895. Jacob asserts that it is important to understand how Myeongseong ruled the country, and how she was able to secure the necessary influence to challenge Japanese ambitions in Korea. He places special emphasis upon her foreign policy during the years leading to her assassination and focuses upon how she contemplated alliances – using Russia to check Japanese ambitions – to try to understand what her real political agenda might have been. Jacob homes in on Myeongseong's case, examining her role in considerable detail as a means by which to demonstrate the ways that this woman, well positioned by her marriage to the emperor, had the power to exercise her authority and profoundly influence regional and international politics. Myeongseong's agency is best presented as a form of indirect rule whereby a woman was able eventually to take over the business of running the state. Here once more, informal authority and power come into play. Jacob not only highlights the political interconnection between Japan and Korea in the last third of the nineteenth century but also provides the reader with an analysis of Empress Myeongseong's role with regards to this shared political history.

With this part, the major themes raised in Woodacre's introduction, and indeed the entire collection, have come full circle. Theories and concepts of monarchy have been examined alongside the realities of the practice of monarchy in a variety of contexts.[18] The contributors to 'Exercising authority and exerting influence' have considered what monarchies needed to function successfully and, when they failed or stumbled, they have shed light upon some of the reasons for their respective shortcomings.[19] They have highlighted the threats, both internal and external, which not infrequently undermined the institution of monarchy and individual rulerships. They have demonstrated the ways in which power – not just authority – was one of the most fundamental aspects defining a monarch's success and efficacy. They have addressed sexualities, masculinities and gender – Woodacre's elephant in the room – taking into account Earenfight's reconsideration of gender and power to accord both men and woman their rightful places in the historical narrative of power, authority and influence.[20] As Woodacre anticipates, this part brings together all the elements of monarchy described by her in her introduction to this collection, and it does so by focusing upon the activities of particular agents across time within the framework of monarchy.[21] The exercise of authority and influence is intimately and consistently associated with any examination of the monarchy and monarchs. The monarch, for whatever reason, was not, however, always the most powerful and important individual in the realm, because the theory of sovereignty and regnant authority did not always accord with the reality of ruling.[22] Taken as whole, the chapters in this final part provide the reader with an insight into the variety of ways in which some monarchs, as well as their spouses and entourages, exercised authority and exerted influence. As discussed earlier, in some cases, monarchs were unable to do so – particularly with regards to the exercise of sanctioned and sanctified sovereignties. Each in their own way, the chapters in this part combine to raise many questions for the reader to ponder, problematizing the notion that a monarch – whether male or female – was all powerful *semper et ubique* (always and everywhere). Monarchy is a slippery concept, as is the way in which individual monarchs have sought to rule – and not just to reign – in the practical exercise of their sanctioned authorities and in the ways they were forced to confront those who sought to influence and sometimes usurp their regal sovereignties. The Church, their counsellors, their assemblies, their nobility and aristocracies, their relatives and, of course, their spouses and mistresses, frequently had their own agenda to push – and their projects did not always accord with the wishes and priorities of their sovereigns.

Notes

1 Zita Eva Rohr, "Introduction," in *Yolande of Aragon (1381–1442), Family and Power: The Reverse of the Tapestry* (Basingstoke and New York: Palgrave Macmillan, 2016), 1–11.
2 Ibid., 10.
3 Elena Woodacre, "Understanding the Mechanisms of Monarchy," 4–5 in this volume.
4 Max Weber, *On Charisma and Institution Building*, ed. S.N. Eisenstadt (Chicago: University of Chicago Press, 1968), 48.
5 Michel Foucault, Colin Gordon et al., eds and trans., *Power/Knowledge: Selected Interviews and Other Writings, 1972–77* (New York: Pantheon, 1980), 89–90.
6 Natalie Zemon Davis, "'Women's History' in Transition: The European Case," *Feminist Studies* 3, nos. 3–4 (1976), 83–104, at 90 (emphasis is mine).
7 Thomas E. Cronin, "Machiavelli's *Prince*: An Americanist's Perspective," in *Machiavelli's Legacy: The Prince After Five Hundred Years*, ed. Timothy Fuller (Philadelphia: University of Pennsylvania Press, 2016), 127–155, at 136.
8 Davis, "Women's History," 90.
9 Ibid.
10 Theresa Earenfight, "Without the Persona of the Prince: Kings, Queens and the Idea of Monarchy in Late Medieval Europe," *Gender & History* 19, no. 1 (April 2007): 1–21.
11 See Zita Eva Rohr, "Lessons for My Daughter: Self-Fashioning Stateswomanship in the Late Medieval Crown of Aragon," in *Self-Fashioning and Assumptions of Identity in Medieval and Early Modern Iberia*, ed. Laura Delbrugge (Leiden and Boston: Brill, 2015), 46–78; Núria Silleras-Fernández, *Power, Piety, and Patronage in Late Medieval Queenship: Maria de Luna* (Basingstoke and New York: Palgrave Macmillan, 2008); Núria Silleras-Fernández, *Chariots of Ladies: Francesc Eiximenis and the Court Culture of Medieval and Early Modern Iberia* (Ithaca: Cornell University Press, 2015).
12 Joan-Lluís Palos, "Introduction: Bargaining Chips – Strategic Marriages and Cultural Circulation in Early Modern Europe," in *Early Modern Dynastic Marriages and Cultural Transfer*, eds. Joan-Lluís Palos and Magdalena S. Sánchez (Farnham: Ashgate, 2016), 1–18, at 8.
13 Ibid.
14 Cf. Giorgio Chittolini, "'The 'Private', the 'Public', the 'State'," *The Journal of Modern History* 67, Supplement: The Origin of the State in Italy, 1300–1600 (December 1995): S34–S61; Stanley Chojnacki, *Women and Men in Renaissance Venice: Twelve Essays on Patrician Society* (Baltimore: Johns Hopkins University Press, 2000); Theresa Earenfight "Introduction: Personal Relations, Political Agency, and Economic Clout in Medieval and Early Modern Royal and Elite Households," in *Royal and Elite Households in Medieval and Early Modern Europe: More than Just a Castle*, ed. Theresa Earenfight (Leiden and Boston: Brill, 2018), 1–14; Zita Eva Rohr, "Rocking the Cradle and Ruling the World: Queens' Households in Late Medieval and Early Modern Aragon and France," in *Royal and Elite Households*, 309–337; J.P. Haseldine, "Friendship Networks in Medieval Europe: New Models of a Political Relationship," *Amity: The Journal of Friendship Studies* 1, no. 1 (2013), 69–88; and Simon Hodson, "The Power of Female Dynastic Networks: A Brief Study of Louise de Coligny, Princess of Orange, and Her Stepdaughters," *Women's History Review* 16, no. 3 (2007): 335–351.
15 Zita Eva Rohr, "No Job for a Man: The Position of Royal Favourite During the Reign of Charles VII" (unpublished conference paper presented at the Royal Studies Network Kings and Queens Conference 7: 'Ruling Sexualities, Gender, and the Crown', The University of Winchester, UK, July 10, 2018); see also Rohr, *Yolande of Aragon*, 264–265, n. 155.
16 See Anne de France, *Enseignements à sa fille suivis de l'Histoire du siège de Brest*, in eds. and trans. Tatiana Clavier and Eliane Viennot (Saint-Etienne: Publications de l'Université de Saint-Etienne, 2006). For an English translation, consult Anne de France, *Anne of France: Lessons for My Daughter*, ed. and trans. Sharon L. Jansen (Cambridge: D.S. Brewer, 2004); Symphorium Champier, *The Ship of Virtuous Ladies*, ed. and trans. Todd W. Reeser (Toronto: Iter Press, 2018). See also Silleras-Fernández, *Chariots of Ladies*.
17 John Alexander Guy, *Tudor England* (Oxford: Oxford University Press), 1990.

18 Woodacre, "Understanding the Mechanisms of Monarchy," page 1–3 in this volume.
19 Ibid., page 13–14.
20 Ibid., pages 2–3.
21 Ibid., page 2.
22 Ibid., 1–2

Key works

Cannadine, David and Simon Price eds., *Rituals of Royalty: Power and Ceremonial in Traditional Societies* (Cambridge: Cambridge University Press, 1987).

Cronin, Thomas E., "Machiavelli's *Prince*: An Americanist's Perspective," in *Machiavelli's Legacy: The Prince After Five Hundred Years*, ed. Timothy Fuller (Philadelphia: University of Pennsylvania Press, 2016), 127–155.

Davis, Natalie Zemon, "'Women's History' in Transition: The European Case," *Feminist Studies*, 3, nos. 3–4 (1976): 83–104.

Earenfight, Theresa, "Without the Persona of the Prince: Kings, Queens and the Idea of Monarchy in Late Medieval Europe," *Gender & History*, 19, no. 1 (April 2007): 1–21.

Foucault, Michel, *Power/Knowledge: Selected Interviews and Other Writings, 1972–77*, eds. and trans. Colin Gordon et al. (New York: Pantheon, 1980). Weber, Max, *On Charisma and Institution Building*, ed. S.N. Eisenstadt (Chicago: University of Chicago Press, 1968).

31

MALE CONSORTS AND ROYAL AUTHORITY IN THE CRUSADER STATES

Stephen Donnachie

The European polities founded in the Levant in the wake of the First Crusade (1095–9), commonly known as the Crusader States, were remote islands of Latin Christian civilization surrounded by a wider Islamic world. Conflict with their Muslim neighbours was a consistent feature of these states' existence, which demanded the leadership of capable rulers experienced in military affairs to maintain their security. However, the dynasties founded in the Latin East by the first generation of crusaders consistently failed in the male line, as men fell as casualties in the recurrent warfare, or through accident of birth, where only daughters were born or survived into adulthood. Consequently, these realms witnessed the repeated succession of women to the highest positions of political power.[1] Across the twelfth and thirteenth centuries, succession to two of these states, the Latin kingdom of Jerusalem and the principality of Antioch, regularly fell to heiresses. While the hereditary principles on which these women succeeded their male kin were acknowledged in both law and custom, the dominant patriarchal paradigms of medieval society were hard pressed to view these women as independent rulers in their own right, but rather characterized them as transmitters of legitimacy to their husbands or sons.[2] An heiress could act as a vessel to transfer royal authority, but she could not reign alone when the threat of conflict required a monarch to take an active military leadership role. The need for skilled commanders in the Latin East was paramount, but such overtly masculine activities lay outside of a queen's traditional duties, and the chronicler William of Tyre lamented the death of the prince of Antioch in 1149 and the capture of the count of Edessa in 1150, because their lands were abandoned to feminine rule.[3] Suitable husbands had to be found for these heiresses, and the barons of Jerusalem and Antioch repeatedly turned to their co-religionists in the Latin West to provide them with the men they needed. The Crusader States, therefore, were frequently ruled by male consorts who reigned as monarchs through the merit of their marriages (Figure 31.1). However, how these men exercised their royal authority as consorts, and the challenges it presented to their kingship, have not been suitably examined.

Despite the growth of Crusader studies in recent decades, and the field of gender within it, the place of these atypical ruling male figures remains a void in the

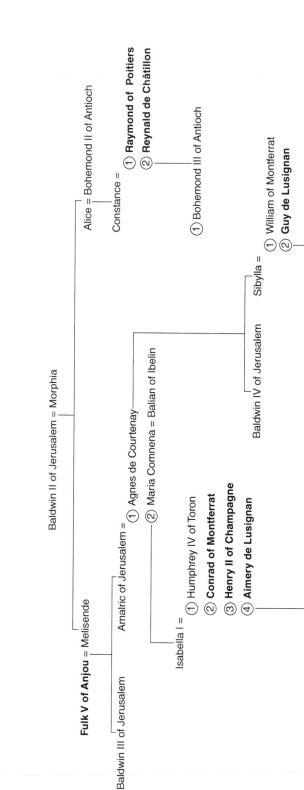

Figure 31.1 The male consorts of Jerusalem and Antioch

current historiography.[4] This lacuna is more notable given that during the 192-year existence of the kingdom of Jerusalem (1099–1291), over sixty years fell under the reigns of seven king consorts, while the principality of Antioch (1098–1268) experienced twenty years under the rule of two prince consorts in the mid-twelfth century.[5] These men's roles as consorts are frequently acknowledged, but the impact their position had upon their rule, the conduct of their reigns and the nature of their kingship is rarely explored.[6] Moreover, the reigns of these consorts have not been sufficiently compared, and common methods in their approaches to ruling have not been identified. Not all consorts were of the same social status or possessed the same personal resources which they could use to aid their rule and substantiate their royal authority. The Jerusalemite consorts Guy de Lusignan (1186–92) and John of Brienne (1210–25) were younger sons of the middling French nobility, and therefore of lesser rank than the final king consort of Jerusalem, the German emperor, Frederick II Hohenstaufen (1225–43), who was the premier magnate of the Latin West. How did their reigns compare to each other, and did their different statuses affect the actions they took as monarchs?

Additionally, scholars often separate consorts from the role of their wives, even though their authority to rule as monarchs was derived from their marriages. Heiresses are crucial to the narrative that explains how consorts came to power, but their influence on the rest of a consort's reign is not always assessed. For example, the Jerusalemite heiress Isabella I was married four times, but any influence she exerted upon her husbands' reigns is largely ignored.[7] In part, this is a consequence of the marginalization of heiresses within narrative sources across the twelfth and thirteenth centuries, but a dearth of surviving charter material for these heiresses in comparison to their consorts is also problematic.[8] The majority of charters that exist for the Jerusalemite heiress Sibylla predate her reign and marriage to her consort, Guy de Lusignan, while none remains for the reign of her half-sister Isabella I. Consequently, the reigns of these consorts have been examined independently, with little consideration given to the influence their wives had upon their royal authority. Yet medieval kings and queens did not act in isolation from each other, but rather operated as a pair of complementary elements within a monarchical system.[9] In the case of the male consorts of the Crusader States, it is essential to reunite them with the home with whom they ruled.

The concentration of male consorts in the Latin East offers an excellent opportunity to investigate the role of these very particular royal figures within medieval society. While it is not within the scope of this chapter to provide an in-depth study of every consort's reign, it will provide an overview of the subject and identify common actions that they undertook to consolidate and exercise their authority as monarchs. An examination of these consorts' reigns demonstrates that the creation of networks of loyal supporters, often drawn from their own lands in the Latin West, was crucial to asserting their authority in the Latin East. Furthermore, the political influence of their wives could not be easily ignored once they had acceded to power. Though consorts assumed the dominant governing position in their new realms, cooperative approaches to ruling with their wives were frequently essential features of their kingship. This cooperation was brought about partly by the circumstances of each consort's reign, but also through the challenges that were inherent in the position of male consorts ruling as monarchs.

Indeed, male consorts were unusual monarchical figures in the medieval world. On the one hand, they were highly desirable because they could secure political alliances, administer government and continue a ruling dynasty, while avoiding any internal dissension that marriage to a member of the native nobility could create. In the case of the Crusader States, they also provided vital western connections, money and manpower that were needed to bolster the defences of the Latin East.[10] However, they could also be objects of suspicion, reviled by the native aristocracy who resented the interference of foreigners in the politics of the realm. Indeed, the very first king consort of Jerusalem, Count Fulk V of Anjou (1131–43), faced a rebellion from the native Jerusalemite baronage after the influx of Angevins into the realm's key offices and lordships, while the second king consort of Jerusalem, Guy de Lusignan, was criticized because of his foreignness.[11]

Though consorts were crowned and anointed as kings, their authority did not arise from any natural sources, such as inheritance through a dynastic line, but rather through the rights of their wives. Patriarchal models of medieval society emphasized men's role as the dominant spouse in a marital relationship, but consorts had to exercise their political authority through their wife, as that authority was ultimately dependent upon her. Indeed, the opening clauses of consorts' royal charters were a consistent reminder that their power devolved to them through their wives, as they regularly stated that they acted with their assent. If the female ruler were to die, or if the couple were to divorce, then a consort's claim to royal authority ended. If the marriage had produced any children, then in accordance with the laws of the Latin East a widowed male consort could expect to act as regent for the child until they came of age.[12] This could temporarily preserve his ruling position, but any attempt to continue his kingship was open to challenge as his royal authority had died with his wife. Such was the situation encountered by John of Brienne when his wife, Queen Maria of Jerusalem, died in 1212. With the loss of his queen, John faced baronial challenges to his continued reign despite acting as regent for his infant daughter, the heiress Isabella II.[13]

Furthermore, the process of selecting a suitable consort was often undertaken with the involvement of the native aristocracy who provided their counsel and consent in choosing candidates. It had been 'with the universal counsel of all the princes' that Fulk of Anjou had been chosen as consort in 1127, while in 1206, a letter issued collectively by the barons of Jerusalem called upon King Peter II of Aragon to accept the kingdom's crown.[14] This undermined a consort's authority by indebting him to the very barons who had raised them to power and over whom they now had to rule. Moreover, if the baronage had the ability to raise consorts to power, then there was the possibility that they could depose those who proved to be unpopular or inept. Guy de Lusignan led Christian forces to a calamitous defeat at the battle of Hattin in 1187, which saw the kingdom of Jerusalem almost annihilated and much of the Latin East permanently lost to Islam.[15] Following the death of his wife, Queen Sibylla, and their daughters in 1190, the disgruntled baronage quickly replaced Guy as king, raising a rival consort, Conrad, marquis of Montferrat (1190–2), to power by hastily marrying him to the kingdom's sole remaining heiress, Sibylla's half-sister, Isabella I.[16] In a more extreme case, the king consort of Cilician-Armenia, Philip of Antioch (1222–4), was so detested by his barons that he was overthrown, imprisoned and assassinated by them in 1224.[17]

Even if consorts enjoyed amicable relations with their barons, it was still necessary to exercise authority over them. A consort's relocation to the Latin East isolated him from his traditional powerbases, deprived him of his networks of allies and made him dependent upon the resources of his new possessions to enforce his political will. The vicissitudes of the Crusader States' conflicts with their neighbours made the territorial resources available to a consort highly variable. The loss of territory following the battle of Hattin, including much of the kingdom of Jerusalem's royal demesne, exacerbated the situation considerably. Those consorts who reigned after 1187 were denied resources available to their earlier twelfth-century counterparts, limiting their options to enforce their authority as monarchs over their barons. Therefore, consorts were dependent upon the goodwill of the baronage to enforce their royal will, but that dependency could be exploited to control a consort. Such was the experience of Ralph, count of Soissons, in 1243. Ralph was a western magnate who had arrived in the Latin East on crusade and had been granted the regency of the kingdom of Jerusalem after marrying one of its claimants, Alice of Champagne, dowager queen of Cyprus. However, Ralph was forced to retire from the kingdom because he lacked the resources to enforce his will over the native barons, who held so much power that Ralph appeared to be nothing more than a shadow.[18]

The men who ruled as consorts in the Latin East encountered a host of limitations to their rule, and though they may have expected to wield their authority like any other medieval monarch, the foundations to their reigns were anything but secure. Indeed, the increasing study of male consorts has shown the comparable challenges that they consistently faced as monarchs and indicates that the experiences of consorts in the Latin East were no different to their counterparts who ruled in medieval Navarre, Tudor England, or eighteenth-century Sweden. In Navarre, the domineering rule and foreign attitudes of consorts were highly resented, while attempts to rule beyond the death of their wife encouraged periods of civil conflict.[19] In Tudor England, there was great concern over the number and influence of the Spanish courtiers of the consort Philip of Habsburg (1554–8), and efforts were made to foster goodwill between English and Spanish nobles to avert violence.[20] In eighteenth-century Sweden, the native aristocracy took steps to limit the power of the monarchy in agreeing to the accession of the king consort Frederick I (1720–51), because they feared a return to absolutism under his rule.[21] A consistent theme that emerges from these studies, is that for consorts to act as monarchs effectively, they frequently had to share power with their wives. This did not always require an equal division of royal authority, but some measure of cooperative rulership was needed. In Navarre, the ambitions of some consorts benefited from the separation of royal duties with their wives, while in Tudor England, attempts to integrate English and Spanish households eased Philip of Habsburg into the position of consort and helped develop a co-regency. Frederick I of Sweden's elevation to king consort came about through the unceasing efforts of his queen against aristocratic opposition. Accordingly, we should not find it unusual that similar power-sharing dynamics also appear among many of the consorts who reigned in the Latin East in the twelfth and thirteenth centuries. The most potent demonstration of this power-sharing relationship can be seen in the reign of the kingdom of Jerusalem's first king consort, Count Fulk V of Anjou.

Fulk of Anjou, having received an embassy from the Latin East in 1128, arrived in the Latin kingdom of Jerusalem in 1129 to marry its heiress, Melisende, the daughter of King Baldwin II (1118–31). To secure Melisende's succession and to make her marriage more attractive to a western magnate, Baldwin had increasingly associated his daughter with his rule by having her appear in his royal charters as his designated heir.[22] However, just before his death in 1131, Baldwin jointly conferred the governance of the kingdom upon Fulk and Melisende in front of the assembled baronage.[23] There is some debate over whether Fulk and Melisende's joint rule had always been Baldwin's intention, or if his deathbed declaration was designed to preserve his daughter's share in the kingdom, because he feared that Fulk might set aside Melisende and establish his own Angevin dynasty.[24] Whatever Baldwin's intentions, Fulk was an experienced political operator who had ruled authoritatively in Anjou since 1109, where power was firmly centralized under the control of the count.[25] It was unlikely that he would accept any unwarranted interference from Melisende in the governance of his new realm, and he soon tried to exclude her from power.

Fulk's efforts began with his coronation. Fulk and Melisende were crowned together in Jerusalem, in the Church of the Holy Sepulchre, on 14 September 1131.[26] This was the feast of the Exaltation of the Cross, which celebrated the relic of the True Cross, its seventh-century return to Jerusalem from pagan possession and the consecration of the Holy Sepulchre. Until this point, kings of Jerusalem had been crowned on Christmas day in the Church of the Nativity in Bethlehem, associating their rule in the nascent kingdom of Jerusalem with the establishment of Christ's own earthly reign.[27] Moreover, these early kings had refused to be crowned with gold in the holy city where once Christ had been crowned with thorns. While Fulk and Melisende's joint coronation publicly affirmed Baldwin II's wishes for them to rule the kingdom together, the alteration to the kingdom's traditional coronation practices for its first king consort heralded a change in its direction and enabled Fulk to deliver a powerful message emphasizing his new kingship. By moving his coronation to Christianity's most sacred location, the site of the crucifixion and resurrection, and by breaking with established royal customs, Fulk declared his reign to be superior to those of his predecessors and associated his temporal rule with the more powerful image of Christ's own heavenly kingship.[28] Furthermore, his coronation associated him with the Holy Sepulchre and the return of the True Cross to Jerusalem from pagan bondage. This allowed Fulk to present himself as a new defender of Jerusalem and its sacred geography, enabling him to infuse his reign with crusading prestige and forge a crusading pedigree that connected him to the kingdom's founders.[29] Moreover, such militaristic connotations emphasized his role as king and excluded Melisende, because those traits did not fall under the auspices of a queen. Fulk was a consort of high status, and his experience as count of Anjou no doubt informed his attitude towards ruling in Jerusalem. But with Baldwin II's deathbed declaration on the succession of royal power in the kingdom, it was necessary for Fulk to demonstrate to the realm that his authority as king was distinct to that which he derived through his marriage to Melisende.

As Fulk was isolated from his traditional sources of power in Anjou, it was essential for him to build a new powerbase in the Latin East so that he could more effectively exercise his royal authority. Fulk soon replaced royal officials in the kingdom of Jerusalem with his own Angevin followers, or promoted other men loyal to his rule to positions of influence. These included the royal butler, the kingdom's chancellor, the viscount of Jerusalem and the royal castellan of Hebron. Even the new grandmaster of the Templars, Robert de Craon, was a figure with whom Fulk had been familiar from his time as count of Anjou.[30] In addition to these new men, Fulk also established connections with members of the native baronage. Two such figures were William of Buris, prince of Galilee and constable of Jerusalem, and Guy Brisebarre, brother to the lord of Beirut. Both had been part of the 1128 embassy to Fulk responsible for negotiating his position as consort. William of Buris had been an important figure under Baldwin II and continued to appear with regularity as a witness in Fulk's royal charters, suggesting his presence as a member of Fulk's ruling circle.[31] Under Fulk, Guy Brisebarre replaced his brother as the lord of Beirut, and it is possible that Guy had come to an independent arrangement with Fulk during the 1128 negotiations, whereby he provided support for the future consort in return for control of the lordship.[32] By appointing new officials and promoting his supporters to power, Fulk acquired the very tools he needed to exercise his authority in his new realm, and he steadily began to reorient the political hierarchy of the kingdom about himself. Such methods would regularly be taken up by other consorts in the Latin East.

In addition to putting his own men into power, Fulk also attempted to exclude Melisende from government. No charters issued by Fulk for the kingdom of Jerusalem from the early years of his reign have survived, but one issued by William of Buris donating property to the Holy Sepulchre in 1132 is suggestive.[33] Fulk's approval of the charter is declared in its opening lines, and he is also included among the charter's witnesses, but there is no mention of Melisende. While her omission from the charter could have been an act by William of Buris as one of Fulk's supporters, that the charter's beneficiaries, the canons of the Holy Sepulchre, did not demand her presence is indicative of her exclusion from power. As the charter's beneficiaries, the canons had an interest in ensuring its legitimacy in case of any legal disputes, and the attestation of the realm's leading figures, which included the king, the patriarch and its principal barons, granted the charter greater validity. Melisende's absence, despite having previously appeared in her father's charters and being one of the kingdom's joint rulers, is striking. That Melisende does not appear in the charter suggests that Fulk's authority alone was considered sufficient to validate it and that Melisende's approval was not required.

Such methods by Fulk to promote his ruling position and exercise his authority independently of Melisende must have met with some success, because in 1134 he faced a rebellion by the native barons in support of Melisende against the dominance of his Angevin party. Though the revolt was defeated, hostilities continued as Melisende marshalled her influence to her faction's advantage by asserting her authority over the royal court, expelling Fulk's supporters and even putting Fulk in fear of his own life. How long the queen's animosity lasted is not clear, but it may have been a factor in encouraging Fulk to leave the kingdom for longer than was necessary in 1135, when he went to Antioch to oversee the principality's affairs as regent for its young heiress.[34] That Melisende achieved this, despite being excluded from power, suggests her considerable influence within the kingdom, and though the revolt had failed, it did encourage Fulk to act more uxoriously towards Melisende so that he consulted her upon all matters. From 1135 onwards, Fulk and Melisende appear alongside each other in royal charters and continued to do so until Fulk's death in 1143.[35]

To understand Fulk's change of attitude from seeking independence to cooperative rule with his wife, despite his victory against the 1134 revolt, a comparison with Melisende's younger sister, Alice of Antioch , should be drawn. Alice was the widowed princess of Antioch who attempted to rule as regent for her young daughter, Constance, after the death of her husband, Prince Bohemond II (1126–30), in 1130. In the absence of a prince, the barons of Antioch invited Baldwin II, and then Fulk, to act as regents for the principality. Alice gathered her own party of Antiochene nobles and repeatedly rebelled against the Jerusalemite regency, forcing Baldwin II and Fulk to intervene in the principality's affairs. By 1134, Alice's faction was openly operating a rival independent government from her dower lands in Latakiah to the Jerusalemite regency in Antioch.[36] Alice's claims to authority in Antioch were tenuous and untested, but Melisende was an anointed queen and the recognized heiress of Jerusalem. Her position was considerably stronger. If Melisende was like her sister, then she could present a serious challenge to Fulk's authority with the possibility of further revolts. Compromise with Melisende was critical, because Fulk could not attend to the affairs of Jerusalem or Antioch while leaving such a threat unresolved. Fulk had attempted to rule alone, brushing aside Melisende's rights and excluding her from government, but Melisende could not be ignored indefinitely, and it was crucial for him to cooperate with her if his reign was to proceed without further interruption. Fulk could take steps to bolster his authority by establishing his own party of supporters in power and symbolically stressing his abilities as king, but sharing power with his wife was essential for a successful reign.

However, the situation was quite different for Fulk's contemporary, the first prince consort of Antioch, Raymond of Poitiers (1136–49). Raymond was the second son of Duke William IX of Aquitaine who arrived in the Latin East in mid-1136 to marry the eight-year-old heiress Constance, having been selected as prince consort on the advice of Fulk and the barons of Antioch. While Raymond lacked his own western lands, he was from a prestigious family and very experienced in military affairs.[37] Though Raymond was a non-inheriting second son and therefore of lesser standing than Fulk, he was able to exercise his authority much more independently. Much like Fulk, Raymond installed his western companions to office, placing his own men in the posts of marshal, constable and the castellan of Antioch. A fellow Poitevin, Aimery of Limoges, became patriarch of Antioch, while Raymond's kinsmen, perhaps half-brothers, Baldwin and Reynald, acquired the strategically important frontier lordship of Marash.[38] Raymond's charters also indicate that he attempted to diminish Constance's role in the governance of the realm, just as Fulk had done with Melisende. Though he did issue charters where she appeared alongside him as his wife, the opening clauses did not always state that they had been granted with her consent, while some charters excluded her entirely and mention him as the son-in-law of Bohemond II. This omission allowed Raymond to circumvent Constance and transcend the position of prince consort to designate himself as Antioch's rightful heir.[39] That the barons of Antioch participated in the creation and verification of these charters indicates that they were willing to accept Raymond's presumptive authority, much like their counterparts in Jerusalem had for Fulk. Though a consort's right to rule was predicated on their marriage, that they were able to issue official documents that were considered legally binding without reference to their wife, suggests that the right to exercise their authority as monarch once in power was not.

Unlike Fulk, Raymond faced no major revolts in response to bypassing his wife's position or the promotion of new men to power, and he was able to operate much more freely and exert his authority more independently than Fulk because the situation in Antioch was much more favourable to his rule. The kingdom of Jerusalem had witnessed a relatively smooth transition of power from Baldwin II to Fulk and Melisende, but Antioch had been without a prince since 1130. This deprived it of the male leadership it required at a time when the growing rival powers of neighbouring Cilican-Armenia and Zengid Aleppo, who both exploited Antiochene weakness to raid the principality in 1135, made it absolutely vital.[40] Furthermore, Constance was only a child with no experience of ruling. Unlike Melisende, she could not enforce her regnal rights against her husband to make him share power with her, and would not be of an age or position to do so for many years to come. Only the barons could limit Raymond's authority on her behalf, but in light of external threats to the principality and the divisions caused by Alice's regency, there was little inclination for them to do so, and they granted their support to the new prince consort because the situation required it. Consequently, unlike Fulk in Jerusalem, there was no need for Raymond to pursue a more collaborative approach to ruling in Antioch, and he had little reason to closely involve Constance in the principality's governance.

However, the circumstances of later king consorts of Jerusalem were much less favourable than those encountered by Fulk or Raymond in the earlier twelfth century, because the foundations of their reigns were much less secure. The second king consort of Jerusalem, Guy de Lusignan, was a younger son of the lord of Lusignan from Poitou who had come to the Latin East by 1180, and had risen to prominence after marrying Sibylla, the sister of King Baldwin IV (1174–85).[41] As a foreign parvenu who quickly achieved an exalted position, Guy was an unpopular figure with the native baronage who considered him unsuitable for the crown, and attempts were soon made to exclude him from royal succession.[42] However, in 1186, Sibylla acceded to the crown as queen of Jerusalem, and while there were expectations that she would divorce Guy, she defied baronial opposition to bring her husband to power. During her coronation, when asked to choose a consort, she bestowed a crown directly upon Guy and named him as her husband and king of Jerusalem.[43] Guy had been crowned and anointed as king, but the very nature of his coronation publicly reinforced the fact that his legitimacy as monarch derived solely from Sibylla. Moreover, he had not come to power with the wider approval of the baronage, and his authority was dealt a blow when prominent barons rejected his rule and refused to do him homage.[44] His position was further undermined by his catastrophic defeat at the battle of Hattin in 1187, which demonstrated his lack of military acumen that was a critical royal trait.

Following Hattin, Guy found his reign contested by Conrad, marquis of Montferrat, a powerful northern Italian noble of much greater status who had arrived in the Latin East shortly after the battle and successfully defended the city of Tyre. Arriving before Tyre in 1189, Guy attempted to assert his authority as king over the city, but was rebuffed by Conrad who denied him entrance.[45] The death of Sibylla and her daughters in 1190 removed Guy's claim to royal authority, and Conrad was quickly raised as a rival consort by Guy's baronial opponents through his marriage to the heiress Isabella I. However, Isabella had previously been married to a native baron, Humphrey IV, lord of Toron. Isabella was forcibly divorced from Humphrey, as he was considered unsuitable to be king, and remarried to Conrad.[46] The legality of

Isabella's divorce was questioned by her contemporaries, and so long as Humphrey lived, it continued to cast doubt over the validity of her later marriages to other consorts.[47] In April 1192, Conrad was elected king and Guy was forced to concede his crown to his rival. However, Conrad's was never crowned as he was assassinated within the month. To prevent Guy's return to power, anti-Lusignan barons hastily remarried Isabella, pregnant with Conrad's posthumous daughter Maria, to Count Henry II of Champagne (r.1192–7). Henry was one of the premier magnates of the Latin West, a nephew of the kings of France and England, who had arrived in the Latin East as part of the Third Crusade (1189–92).[48] Henry took command of the kingdom and ruled until his death in 1197, whereupon the barons of Jerusalem selected Aimery de Lusignan (1197–1205), Guy's brother and king of Cyprus, to become king of Jerusalem as Isabella's fourth and final husband. It was only with her marriage to Aimery that Isabella was actually crowned queen.[49]

Much like the consorts who reigned before them, charter material suitably highlights the cadres of loyal baronial supporters that these men fashioned about themselves and through whom they wielded their authority. Guy de Lusignan surrounded himself with men from Poitou. This included his brother Aimery de Lusignan, who acted as his constable, another brother, Geoffrey de Lusignan, who was a participant of the Third Crusade and to whom Guy granted the important lordship of Jaffa following its recapture in 1191, as well as another Poitevin, Hugh Martin, who occupied the office of marshal from 1191. Guy even sought to arrange the marriage of yet another brother, William of Valence, to a prominent Jerusalemite heiresses, who was the daughter of his close baronial ally, Joscelin III, count of Edessa, to further secure his ruling position.[50] Conrad initially surrounded himself with trusted men from his own entourage who had accompanied him to the Latin East in 1187. These included his seneschal Hubert Nepos, his chamberlain, Henry de Canelli, an individual called Bandini who acted as his chancellor, and Ansaldo Buonvicino whom Conrad promoted to be the castellan of Tyre by 1190. But Conrad also drew extensively upon the support of the native barons who were opposed to Lusignan rule. Leading baronial figures such as Pagan, lord of Haifa, Reynald, lord of Sidon, and Balian, lord of Ibelin, dominate the witness lists of Conrad's charters after the death of Queen Sibylla in 1190.[51]

When Henry of Champagne acquired the crown of Jerusalem after Conrad's death, he needed his own loyal party of barons to counter any potential Lusignan revanche, and he found one ready made in Conrad's former circle who went on to form the core of his new ruling cadre. Henry gathered Balian of Ibelin, Reynald of Sidon, along with many other native barons about him, while a Champenois contingent that included Milo Breban, who had been the treasurer of Champagne, and Villain d'Aulnay, whose brother had been the marshal of Champagne, also assumed a prominent role in the kingdom.[52] Henry also relied upon other new migrants to the Latin East who were similarly isolated and therefore dependent upon the crown for patronage. These included Thierry de Dendermonde, Thierry d'Orgue and Aymar de Lairon, who were all frequent witnesses to his royal charters from 1193 onwards, and who through marriage and Henry's largesse respectively acquired the important lordships of Adelon, Arsuf and Caesarea.[53]

While the creation of loyal parties of supporters continued to be a key method by which consorts exercised their authority, these later consorts had to seek other means to bolster their positions as monarchs in the Latin East. Guy de Lusignan had been an unpopular consort, responsible for an unprecedented military disaster, whose claims to rule had been stripped away by Sibylla's death, while the nature of Isabella's questionable divorce cast doubt on the legitimacy of his successors. Consequently, consorts sought additional support from external bodies to substantiate their reigns and validate their authority as monarchs. Conrad of Montferrat was a cousin to the king of France, the German emperor and the duke of Austria. The arrival of some of these great western magnates in the Latin East, as part of the Third Crusade, significantly enhanced Conrad's candidacy for the Jerusalemite crown. In 1190 Conrad appealed to his kinsman Duke Frederick VI of Swabia, son of the German emperor and commander of the German crusaders. The approach of Duke Frederick caused such apprehension in the Lusignan camp that even Muslim chroniclers became aware of it.[54] Furthermore, King Philip II of France and Duke Leopold V of Austria featured among witnesses to a charter issued by Conrad in May 1191. This charter named Conrad as 'rex electus', and its confirmation by these western magnates indicates their endorsement of his royal title, presumptive though it was for no formal election process had yet occurred.[55]

It was only through the backing of King Richard I of England, the commander of the Third Crusade, count of Poitou and therefore suzerain to the Lusignans, that Guy's royal aspirations were kept alive after Sibylla's death. However, when Richard announced his intentions to return to the Latin West in April 1192, Guy's position crumbled. Even Richard had to accept Conrad's claims to rule as he was elected by the Jerusalemite baronage as their king.[56] Henry of Champagne was a prestigious western magnate whose status was far greater than Guy's, but it was only after he received the approval of his uncle, Richard I, that he agreed to marry Isabella and assume the crown of Jerusalem.[57] Even John of Brienne sought to extend his reign as king of Jerusalem by appealing to the German emperor, Frederick II, in 1225. Frederick had married John's daughter and heiress to the kingdom of Jerusalem, Isabella II, thereby becoming its new king. It was during Isabella II's marriage negotiations that John sought to retain his crown by gaining Frederick's approval for his continued authority in the Latin East.[58] Fulk of Anjou had been endorsed by the papacy as a potential consort in 1128, but he had not made such appeals to external powers to legitimize his authority directly, because unlike the later Jerusalemite consorts, the circumstances of his reign did not require it. A consort's right to rule stemmed from the sovereign authority of his wife, but it appears that his right to exercise his authority as monarch could be drawn from elsewhere.

However, while these consorts did seek external sources to legitimize their authority as monarchs, they could not afford to disassociate themselves from any authority that they derived from their wives, as Fulk of Anjou and Raymond of Poitiers had done. While the source material is less plentiful in describing the actions undertaken by Sibylla and Isabella I during their reigns in comparison to their grandmother Melisende, the limited evidence does suggest that these royal women continued to be involved in their husbands' reigns and that some measure of cooperative rulership was employed. Sibylla had been instrumental in bringing Guy to power in 1186, and her consistent appearance in his charters indicates that she remained close to him until her death in 1190.[59] Indeed, in the summer of 1189, she wrote to the German emperor and crusader, Frederick I Barbarossa, to advise him of the political developments in the region, suggesting that she was privy to the highest levels of information and a part of the realm's government.[60] However, Sibylla's assent to Guy's charters is not always declared. This suggests that Guy attempted to present their ruling relationship as one of relative equals, and that his authority was not entirely subject to uxorial limitations. Even so, Sibylla's presence was still a necessity. Sibylla had accompanied Guy to Tyre in 1189, and he had invoked their authority as monarchs jointly in his bid to assert dominion over the city.[61] That Sibylla also accompanied Guy to the siege of Acre thereafter, rather than seek safety away from the frontlines, demonstrates her importance to him as a physical symbol of his royal authority. Guy was king, but he could not exercise his authority without the presence of his queen. Henry of Champagne similarly needed Isabella's symbolic presence to assert his authority over the former Lusignan-held cities of the kingdom as he processed through his new realm following their marriage in 1192.[62]

Like Sibylla, Isabella appears consistently in the charters of her husbands, Conrad of Montferrat, Henry of Champagne and Aimery de Lusignan, and her assent is stated with regularity. She is also named as the daughter of the illustrious King Amalric (1163–74). Such associations for these consorts emphasized their connection through Isabella to the unquestionable legitimacy of her father, and their wife's dynastic line, to reinforce their authority as monarchs. Aimery even went so far as to include reference to Amalric and Baldwin IV in his 1198 coronation oath. Through bypassing the reigns of the two previous uncrowned consorts, and the controversial reign of his brother, Aimery was able to connect himself to the undeniable authority of the earlier kings of Jerusalem and the political order they represented.[63] Indeed, the creation of the *Livre au Roi*, the kingdom of Jerusalem's first written body of secular law, under Aimery's reign, stressed this connection further. The *Livre au Roi* jointly presents both the king and queen as enactors of the law and depicts them as equals in their roles as ruling monarchs. This suggests that Isabella occupied a more central position in the politics of Jerusalem under Aimery, and that an expectation of more cooperative royal rule by consorts had developed by the beginning of the thirteenth century.[64]

The men who reigned as consorts in the Latin East employed a variety of techniques to exercise their royal authority in their new realms. The appointment of loyal supporters, especially from a consort's own western lands, to positions of power and influence reoriented the native political hierarchy and created new powerbases that consorts could call upon to exert their influence. Appeals to native ruling practices, past monarchs and external bodies were also made to help strengthen their ruling position and the authority they wielded. Though some consorts aspired to rule independently as monarchs and limit the involvement of their wives in the governance of their new realm, the circumstances of their reigns meant that this was not always possible, and their wives' legitimizing presence could not be ignored. It was, therefore, frequently necessary for consorts to share power with their wives and pursue more cooperative forms of monarchical rule for their reigns to be a success.

Notes

1 King Baldwin II of Jerusalem had no sons but four daughters, while Queen Isabella I of Jerusalem was survived by five daughters. Sylvia Schein, "Women in Medieval Colonial Society: The Latin Kingdom of Jerusalem in the Twelfth Century," in *Gendering the Crusades*, eds. Susan B. Edgington and Sarah Lambert (Cardiff: University of Wales Press, 2001), 141.

2 Lois Huneycutt, "Female Succession and the Language of Power in the Writings of Twelfth-Century Churchmen," in *Medieval Queenship*, ed. John Carmi Parsons (Stroud: Sutton Publishing, 1998), 191–196; Sarah Lambert, "Queen or Consort: Rulership and Politics in the Latin East, 1118–1228," in *Queens and Queenship in Medieval Europe*, ed. Anne J. Duggan (Woodbridge: Boydell, 1997), 151–169.

3 William of Tyre, "Chronicon," in *Corpus Christianorum: Continuatio Mediaevalis* 63, ed. R.B.C. Huygens, 2 vols. (Turnhout, 1986) (hereafter cited as WT), 774–775, 780.

4 For a summary of the historiography, see Deborah Gerish, "Gender Theory," in *Palgrave Advances in the Crusades*, ed. Helen Nicholson (Basingstoke: Palgrave Macmillan, 2005), 130–147.

5 The king consorts for the kingdom of Jerusalem were Fulk V, count of Anjou (1131–43); Guy de Lusignan (1186–92); Conrad, marquis of Montferrat (1190–2); Henry II, count of Champagne (1192–7); Aimery de Lusignan (1197–1205); John of Brienne (1210–25); and the German emperor, Frederick II Hohenstaufen (1225–43). The prince consorts of Antioch were Raymond of Poitiers (1136–49) and Reynald de Châtillon (1153–60).

6 Individual issues such as entourages have been explored, but no general assessment of these consorts' reigns has been undertaken. Bernard Hamilton, "King Consorts of Jerusalem and their Entourages from the West from 1186 to 1250," in *Die Kreuzfahrerstaaten als multikulturelle Gesellschaft*, ed. H.E. Mayer (Munich: Oldenbourg, 1997), 13–24.

7 Traditional historiography has described Isabella as being weak and feckless. Bernard Hamilton's examination of the twelfth-century queens of Jerusalem ignores her reign, while his assessment of Sibylla's reign is overshadowed by the actions of her mother, Agnes of Courtenay. Steven Runciman, *A History of the Crusades*, vol. 3, *The Kingdom of Acre* (London: Penguin, 2002), 104; Bernard Hamilton, "Women in the Crusader States: The Queens of Jerusalem, 1100–1190," in *Medieval Women*, ed. Derek Baker (Oxford: Blackwell, 1978), 163–174.

8 Lambert, "Queen or Consort," 165–169.

9 Theresa Earenfight, "Without the Presence of the Prince: Kings, Queens and the Idea of Monarchy in Late Medieval Europe," *Gender and History* 19 (2007): 7–8.

10 Husbands for heiresses were a central part of the Latin east's diplomacy. See Johnathan Philips, *Defenders of the Holy Land: Relations between the Latin East and West 1119–1187* (Oxford: Clarendon Press, 1996).

11 Hans Mayer, "Angevins versus Normans: The New Men of King Fulk of Jerusalem," *Proceedings of the American Philosophical Society* 133 (1989): 1–25; William of Newburgh, "Historium Rerum Anglicarum," in *Chronicles of the Reigns of Stephen, Henry II, and Richard I*, vol. 1, ed. Richard Howlett (London: Longman, 1884), 256.

12 Myriam Greilsammer, *Le Livre au Roi* (Paris: L'Académie des Inscriptions et Belles-Lettres, 1995), 147–150.

13 Guy Perry, *John of Brienne: King of Jerusalem, Emperor of Constantinople, c.1175–1237* (Cambridge: Cambridge University Press, 2013), 68–71.

14 WT, 618; H.E. Mayer, ed., *Die Urkunden der lateinischen Könige von Jerusalem*, 4 vols. (Hannover: Hahnsche Buchhandlung, 2010) (hereafter cited as D. Jerus.), vol. 3 no. 645.

15 For the background to Hattin, see Bernard Hamilton, *The Leper King and his Heirs* (Cambridge: Cambridge University Press, 2000).

16 "L'Estoire de Eracles empereur et la conqueste de la terre d'Outremer," in *Recueil des Historiens des Croisades: Historiens Occidentaux*, vol. 2 (Paris, 1859) (hereafter cited as Eracles), 151–152; William Stubbs, ed., *Chronicles and Memorials of the Reign of Richard I*, vol. 1, *Itinerarium Peregrinorum et gesta Regis Ricardi, auctore, ut videtur, Ricardo Canonico Sanctae Trinitatis Londoniensis* (London: Longman, 1864), 342–343.

17 Eracles, 347–348.

18 Eracles, 420.

19 Elena Crislyn Woodacre, "The King Consorts of Navarre: 1284–1512," in *The Man Behind the Queen: Male Consorts in History*, eds. Charles Beem and Miles Taylor (Basingstoke: Palgrave, 2014), 11–31.

20 Sarah Duncan, "'He to be Intituled Kinge': King Philip of England and the Anglo-Spanish Court," in Beem and Taylor, *Man Behind the Queen*, 55–80.

21 Fabian Persson "From Ruler in the Shadows to Shadow King: Frederick I of Sweden," in Beem and Taylor, *Man Behind the Queen*, 93–102.
22 Hans Mayer, "The Succession to Baldwin II of Jerusalem: English Impact on the East," *Dumbarton Oaks Papers* 39 (1985): 144; D. Jerus., 1: nos 105, 153.
23 WT, 625.
24 Hans Mayer has argued that in accordance with the marriage negotiations of 1128, Baldwin II had initially intended for Fulk to rule Jerusalem alone, but fearing Fulk would replace Melisende, altered his position. Bernard Hamilton has suggested that Fulk and Melisende were always meant to rule jointly and that the 1128 marriage negotiations were not incompatible with Baldwin's dying wishes. Hans Mayer, "Studies in the History of Queen Melisende of Jerusalem," *Dumbarton Oaks Papers* 26 (1972): 99–102; Hamilton, "Women in the Crusader States," 149–150.
25 Jean Dunbabin, *France in the Making, 843–1180* (Oxford: Oxford University Press, 1985), 184–190, 333–340.
26 WT, 633–634.
27 WT, 463, 562.
28 Ernst Kantorowicz, *The King's Two Bodies: A Study in Mediaeval Political Theology* (Princeton: Princeton University Press, 1997), 42–86.
29 For the importance of crusading to royal authority, see James Naus, *Constructing Kingship: The Capetian Monarchs of France and the Early Crusades* (Manchester: Manchester University Press, 2016).
30 D. Jerus., 1: nos 131, 132, 135, 138, 139, 141, 146; Mayer, "Angevins versus Normans," 7–21.
31 D. Jerus., 1: nos 132, 135, 138–140; Mayer, "Angevins versus Normans," 12–15.
32 Hans Mayer, "The Wheel of Fortune: Seigneurial Vicissitudes under Kings Fulk and Baldwin III of Jerusalem," *Speculum* 65 (1990): 860–877.
33 D. Jerus., 1: no. 128.
34 Mayer, "Studies in the History of Queen Melisende," 107; Natasha Hodgson, *Women, Crusading and the Holy Land in Historical Narrative* (Woodbridge: Boydell, 2007), 135.
35 WT, 654–656; D. Jerus., 1: nos 131, 132, 135–141.
36 Thomas Asbridge, "Alice of Antioch: Female Power in the Twelfth Century," in *The Experience of Crusading Vol. 2*, eds. Peter Edbury and Jonathan Philips (Cambridge: Cambridge University Press, 2003), 33–42.
37 WT, 657–659.
38 Reinhold Röhricht, ed., *Regesta Regni Hierosolymitani, MXCVII–MCCXCI* (Innsbruck, 1893), nos. 195, 197, 228; Andrew Buck, *The Principality of Antioch and its Frontiers in the Twelfth Century* (Woodbridge: Boydell, 2017), 29, 90, 103, 113.
39 Buck, *Antioch*, 74–75.
40 Buck, *Antioch*, 22–32.
41 WT, 1007–1008.
42 Elena Woodacre, "Questionable Authority: Female Sovereigns and their Consorts in Medieval and Renaissance Chronicles," in *Authority and Gender in Medieval and Renaissance Chronicles*, eds. Juliana Dresvina and Nichola Sparks (Newcastle-Upon-Tyne: Cambridge Scholars Publishing, 2012), 393–397.
43 Hamilton, *Leper King*, 216–221.
44 These were Count Raymond III of Tripoli and Baldwin, lord of Ramla. Eracles, 32–34.
45 Eracles, 123–124.
46 Woodacre, "Questionable Authority," 398–399.
47 Alan V. Murray, "Women in the Royal Succession of the Latin Kingdom of Jerusalem (1099–1291)," in *Mächtige Frauen? Königinnen und Fürstinnen im europäischen Mittelalter (11.–14. Jahrhundert)*, ed. Claudia Zey (Ostfildern: Thorbecke, 2015), 154–155.
48 Stubbs, *Itinerarium*, 342–343.
49 Eracles, 222–224.
50 D. Jerus., 2: nos. 475–480, 482, 485, 486, 488; Hamilton, "King Consorts," 13–14.
51 D. Jerus., 2: nos. 519–526, 529, 530, 533; Stephen Donnachie, "Crown and Baronage in the Latin Kingdom of Jerusalem after the Battle of Hattin, 1187–1228," *Medieval Prosopography* 32 (2017): 94–99; Hamilton, "King Consorts," 14.

52 D. Jerus., 2: nos. 568–570, 572, 573, 575, 576, 581; Donnachie, "Crown and Baronage," 105; Hamilton, "King Consorts," 15.
53 D. Jerus., 2: nos. 572, 575–580; Hamilton, "King Consorts," 14–16.
54 Baha al-Din, *The Rare and Excellent History of Saladin*, trans. D.S. Richards (Aldershot: Ashgate, 2001), 128.
55 D. Jerus., 2: no. 530.
56 Stubbs, *Itinerarum*, 334–337.
57 Stubbs, *Itinerarum*, 342–343.
58 Perry, *John of Brienne*, 122–141.
59 D. Jerus., 2: nos. 472–474, 476–480, 482.
60 Röhricht, *Regesta*, no. 681.
61 Eracles, 123–124.
62 Stubbs, *Itinerarium*, 349; Hodgson, *Women*, 82.
63 D. Jerus., 2: nos. 529–530, 568–573, 575–581, 609–614, 620–621; Geneviève Bresc-Bautier, *Le Cartulaire du Chapitre du Saint-Sépulcre de Jérusalem* (Paris: Librairie Orientaliste Paul Geuthner, 1984), no. 172.
64 Greilsammer, *Livre au Roi*, 136, 138, 141, 151, 201, 209, 213, 217, 264, 283.

Key works

Beem Charles and Miles Taylor, eds., *The Man Behind the Queen: Male Consorts in History* (Basingstoke: Palgrave, 2014).

Earenfight, Theresa, "Without the Presence of the Prince: Kings, Queens and the Idea of Monarchy in Late Medieval Europe," *Gender and History* 19 (2007): 1–21.

Hamilton, Bernard, "King Consorts of Jerusalem and their Entourages from the West from 1186 to 1250," in *Die Kreuzfahrerstaaten als multikulturelle Gesellschaft*, ed. H.E. Mayer (Munich: Oldenbourg, 1997), 13–24.

Lambert, Sarah, "Queen or Consort: Rulership and Politics in the Latin East, 1118–1228," in *Queens and Queenship in Medieval Europe*, ed. Anne J. Duggan (Woodbridge: Boydell, 1997), 151–169.

Mayer, Hans, "Angevins versus Normans: The New Men of King Fulk of Jerusalem," *Proceedings of the American Philosophical Society* 133 (1989): 1–25.

Perry, Guy, *John of Brienne: King of Jerusalem, Emperor of Constantinople, c.1175–1237* (Cambridge: Cambridge University Press, 2013).

Woodacre, Elena, "Questionable Authority: Female Sovereigns and their Consorts in Medieval and Renaissance Chronicles," in *Authority and Gender in Medieval and Renaissance Chronicles*, eds. Juliana Dresvina and Nichola Sparks (Newcastle-Upon-Tyne: Cambridge Scholars Publishing, 2012), 367–406.

32

KINGS AND NOBLES ON THE FRINGES OF CHRISTENDOM

A comparative perspective on monarchy and aristocracy in the European Middle Ages[1]

Kim Bergqvist

In medieval Europe, representatives of monarchy and aristocracy vied for supremacy, often in open conflict. Nevertheless, their relationship was also one of interdependence and, occasionally, symbiosis. During the high Middle Ages (the eleventh through to the thirteenth century), the rights of kings, supported by the Church, came to signify something more than being the first among equals of the great landholders of a region. Kings increasingly challenged nobles' rights to taxation and jurisdiction by displacing lordly local power through centralization and institutions of statecraft.[2] Thus, magnates' influence was curtailed by the growing sphere of royal authority, and the powerful lords sought new ways of participating in the practice of power and politics. The king's authority in the medieval period was founded upon his ability to control military resources and means of violence, amass economic assets, and exert legal and symbolic authority. The secular aristocracy of these realms was indispensable to the king's exercise of power, both because of the lack of a monarchical institutional basis on a local level before the late Middle Ages, and not least because any major military operation by the crown depended on the cooperation of nobles and the contribution of their hosts of soldiers to the war effort.[3] This gave nobles the opportunity to exert their influence on the king and his policies – unduly in the opinion of some. In times of regal minorities, some advanced from positions as councillors of the king to regents, essentially governing the realm in the absence of an adult king. This led repeatedly to civil strife – after the regency of Tyrgils Knutsson for King Birger Magnusson of Sweden 1290–1304, in the years following the election of the young king Magnus Eriksson (c.1319–22), and during the minority of the Castilian kings Fernando IV (1295–1301) and Alfonso XI (1312–25) – a fact that has left numerous traces in the historiography of the period.

This chapter on the relationship between kingship and nobility focuses on the kingdoms of Castile-León and Sweden during the thirteenth and fourteenth centuries. The rationale behind this comparative study is to demonstrate that structural similarities and parallel events characterize the situation in Iberia and Scandinavia, and that – though they are often considered peripheral or seen as part of the fringes surrounding the European core – there is also a general correspondence between these cases and several central and western European kingdoms. Differences exist, of course, due to dissimilarities in political systems and because of particular political circumstances, which are examined later.

The growth of the state in medieval Europe and its process of centralization created a surge in monarchs' authority during the high Middle Ages, but nobles soon established ideologically invested agendas for their own involvement in statehood and its concomitant institutions. John Watts regards this as a form of lordly capitulation to the king; the lords' participation in representative assemblies signifies for him the equation of their political role within the kingdom with being 'counsellors, servants, representatives in someone else's *regnum*'.[4] In certain cases, however, the nobility allowed itself to speak for the community of the whole realm, and thus to give voice to the greater good of the kingdom. While the greater part of the thirteenth century saw the growth of state institutions and monarchical authority through legal developments in Sweden, as well as in Castile-León, the late thirteenth and early fourteenth centuries represented, in part, a reaction against this development.[5] Sweden has been characterized by a leading historian as an 'aristocratic republic' in the fifteenth century, when royal power was often physically absent during the union with Denmark, but the process began much earlier, and nobles' control of the judicial organization throughout the Middle Ages allowed them to make strong claims for power.[6] Castile experienced 'aristocratization' under Sancho IV (r.1284–95), which would not be countered until Alfonso XI (r.1312–50) reached his majority. Sancho thus privileged those noble lineages that had supported his claim for power and his rebellion against his father. This can be compared to the notion that England in the thirteenth century experienced a time of 'aristocratic self-confidence and strength'.[7] Today, scholars generally reject the idea of the aristocracy as a homogeneous and cohesive social group. Part of this rejection stems from the questioning of older paradigms that privileged national narratives. Monarchy and nobility were far from two distinct actors always in conflict; the aristocracy was heterogeneous and often divided on the grounds of which contender for the throne a faction supported.

Nobles needed arenas in which to exert influence on monarchs in order to implement their political views, and while public representative institutions gained momentum in the late Middle Ages, informal means of influence (such as royal favouritism) also became increasingly important.[8] Proximity to the king was accordingly important for those aristocrats who wanted to sway the king by influencing his decisions. Friendships and other informal alliances had been essential for political culture during the early Middle Ages and would remain so throughout the period.[9] Such alliances could garner authority and legitimacy by their formalization and written documentation, as was the case with the Spanish *hermandades*, brotherhoods that bound together peers with shared objectives by sworn oaths of mutual protection. These were an outlet for the political voice of the nobility, but sometimes had the expressed approval of the crown.[10]

Whereas most of the general knowledge of – and recent research on[11] – medieval kingship and its relationship to the lay aristocracy builds on English, French and German empirical findings, recent research on political culture and ideological expressions in medieval Scandinavia and Iberia has much to offer the general reader of medieval European history. Though the process of centralization and institutionalization of the state took place later in Castile and Sweden, and they thus display partially different patterns of power dynamics, there are aspects of the experience of these kingdoms that are relevant to the study of the European Middle Ages in general. While some scholars see Scandinavia and Iberia as being all too different to be productively compared with the European core, both the differences and the many similarities make for a fruitful comparison. This chapter will contribute to research on kingship and nobility in these contexts – ones that seldom take part in the same scholarly dialogues – with a comparative analysis of the varied and shifting political circumstances of medieval European monarchies.

Nobility on the Iberian Peninsula and in Scandinavia

In Iberia, military activity became the principal *raison d'être* of the noble and the knightly classes, and thus the main legitimation of their privileges.[12] The particular military, social and economic landscape created by the Christian conquest of Muslim Spain is at least a partial explanation for this. While many Castilian nobles gathered large tracts of land as patrimonies, they were dependent on their kings' leadership for the further expansion of their territories. In contrast to the current view of the European Middle Ages in general, where it is assumed that nobles and kings clashed over jurisdiction, taxation and other privileges from the inception of kings as something above powerful lords, the Castilian nobility were indebted to the kings for these rights. Though nobles independently owned their lands, the right of the king to 'national' jurisdiction and taxation was recognized. In a similar vein, Edward I of England (r.1272–1307) made the lords accept, in the 1290 statute of *quo warranto*, that the authority they held over their lands was delegated from the crown, rather than earned by right of conquest.[13]

Although the military function of the nobility became its principal occupation in Europe in general, this change seems particularly marked in the Iberian Peninsula, where even kings were judged above all according to the degree to which they successfully carried out their military duties. Some striking examples are to be found among the first kings of Portugal: Afonso Henriques (r.1139–85), granted the title of king because of his successful conquests, and Sancho II (r.1223–48), who was deemed a useless king (*rex inutilis*) by Innocent IV because of his failure to protect his lands against his Muslim enemies, and who was deposed and exiled after a civil war.[14] Naturally, the peninsula was for almost the entire medieval period a frontier zone between Christian and Muslim polities, characterized by military struggle, resettlement and colonization, and between fragmented Christian polities whose borders were equally contested. This affected the position, composition and outlook of the nobility and consolidated a prestigious military elite, not least in Portugal.[15]

The clash between the nobility and the crown in later medieval Castile was caused by the replacement in the fourteenth and fifteenth centuries of the high nobility in the royal administration by professional *letrados*, educated officials of lower birth, and the reconceptualization of monarchy of which this process was but one expression. This process was a conscious attempt on the king's part to restrict the influence of the magnates.[16] With time, it would contribute to the displacement of the old nobility and the ascent of the new.[17] Much the same happened even earlier in Portugal, where Afonso Henriques promoted a new generation of nobles that would be entirely indebted to him for their positions, and in post-conquest England.[18]

In the Scandinavian kingdoms developments were largely similar. Noble titles were imported from continental Europe but applied to magnates and nobles who had long been powerful. In Norway, the titles of baron (*barún*) and knight (*riddari*) were used to designate the followers of the king serving in his retinue (*hird*), his house-hold men. In 1280, Magnus (III) Birgersson (r.1255–75) introduced to Sweden by royal ordinance a legal stipulation of tax exemption for a mounted knight's military service. The purpose appears to have been to gather a modern military resource under the helm of the king. It was connected, almost certainly, to the idea that the king had to make war against the enemies of the realm and that every subject was responsible to serve him in order to successfully perform that task. In practice, it created a functional definition of the *frälse* (those exempt from royal taxation) and a fluidity in the social group for those who were granted this privilege. The ability to present a properly outfitted mounted warrior and charger was regularly overseen, and the privilege could easily be lost. Many who belonged to this group would have been comparable to the category of *caballeros villanos* or *caballeros de cuantía* in the Crown of Castile in the thirteenth and fourteenth centuries. In Castile, the need for repopulation and defence in the newly conquered areas, Extremadura (the fron-tier regions south of the Duero River) and Castilla la Nueva (New Castile), created possibilities for knights without noble lineage to take advantage of tax exemptions and rise within the social hierarchy, beginning in the twelfth century.[19] Once they amassed humble fortunes, these urban knights would start dressing and acting sim-ilarly to the noble *hidalgos*, trying to erase the dividing lines that the high nobility would enforce by conspicuous consumption and cultural production.

Contrary to the often repeated assertion that the Swedish aristocracy was 'young' around the year 1300, because of the equation of a legally stipulated tax exemption and an aristocratic social group, some families had held extensive property and been influential in the circle surrounding the kings for generations. They were affected by cultural trends emanating from central and western Europe, where some of them had studied at universities or had visited princely courts on diplomatic missions. Their attempts to appear as Christian European knights are evident in material evi-dence, such as seals, from the twelfth century onwards. The change actually implied by the Alsnö ordinance of 1280 was more of a military, political and economic nature: the king needed to be able to summon a supply of well-armed mounted warriors, and he needed to control the size of armed hosts riding through his king-dom. Thus, the aristocracy was granted legal exemption from royal taxation while the king secured high-profile military resources for his own ends. It was a step in the process of making sure that the king's rights were expanded and universally recog-nized within the realm, by legal means, with inspiration taken from Roman law.[20] Undoubtedly, the regulation formed part of an overarching process of formalization of political practice in thirteenth-century Sweden. During this period, new adminis-trative offices came into use, and customary law and royal ordinances were written down and disseminated.

Similarly, the first legal stipulations regarding the knighthood in medieval Castile were promulgated by Alfonso X *el Sabio* (r.1252–84), though hierarchical divisions within the nobility had been in place since at least a century before that. Alfonso attempted to control noble violence and subsume all knights into the shared nat-ural bond to the king, guided by the virtue of loyalty.[21] The Swedish and Castilian legal stipulations can be read as an attempt to join as many of the most resourceful men as possible to the king's service, by promoting the idea that proximity to the king entailed political influence. In Norway, the core of the aristocracy was the men in the king's direct service, and serving the king became a prerequisite for aristocratic status.[22]

In Castilian territories, the large tracts of newly conquered land were in dire need of Christian repopulation, and the king was forced to grant generous privileges to those who would settle there. This created the foundation for strong noble centres of power away from the royal court, which magnates amassed in the later Middle Ages. As opposed to England after the Norman Conquest, nobles seem to have enjoyed a more prominent position in overseeing local government throughout the medieval period in both Sweden and Castile.[23]

In early fourteenth-century Sweden, an unknown poet composed the *Erikskrönika* (The Chronicle of Duke Erik, *c.*1320), a voluminous verse chronicle and the first original domestic literary creation in Old Swedish, which gives insight into the worldview and aspirations of the medieval Swedish aristocracy.[24] The Swedish nobles are presented as chivalric and courtly knights proficient in tournament, well mannered and refined at feasts, as well as *milites Christi* who did not hesitate to use deadly force when needed. In a manner similar to that found among the French nobility in the thirteenth century by Gabrielle Spiegel, the Swedish aristocracy used history writing as a means to affirm their position and standing. While the strengthened monarchy threatened their traditional political roles and military organization, the lack of any fixed boundaries in the social hierarchy – which at least theoretically allowed for social movement – was a further cause for concern. Together, these created the need for a glorification of the aristocracy, its past and its historical importance for the kingdom.[25] Similarly, Castilian chronicles discuss the relative importance of the nobility and the kings in the Reconquest, seeking to legitimize certain practices in the present by means of historical discourse.[26]

Royal minorities: questionable authority

The question of the relative authority of the nobility in relation to the crown came to the fore particularly during periods of the minority of young kings, when the issue of regency was often disputed. Prolonged and destabilizing royal minorities were experienced both in Castile and in Sweden several times during the Middle Ages. When the given candidate to kingship was not old enough to exert authority, a vacuum of power arose that attracted the attention of power-hungry candidates. Unless the late king had named a regent, a candidate to temporarily fulfil the role the king – a child – could not handle by himself, there was no undisputed way in which to tackle the problem. The *Siete partidas* of Alfonso X tried to resolve the issue by stipulating that, if the late king had not already chosen a regent, an assembly of leading noblemen and clerics would come to a decision and choose loyal men who would safeguard the common good of the realm as its regents.[27] A boy king was an important strategic piece to hold in negotiations, and royal minorities were periods when magnates saw themselves as legitimately speaking and negotiating on behalf of the kingdom, and when members of the nobility attempted to exert maximum authority. We see this happening both in the form of contention for the regency and in the formulation of clearly aristocratic policies by members of regnal representative assemblies, such as the Swedish Council of the Realm.

During the reign of Fernando IV (r.1295–1312), the *Cortes*, the representative assembly of Castile-León, was summoned to Valladolid in 1307. Here, the high nobility managed to replace the royal officials with their own trusted men.[28] The political programme of the magnates met with no real resistance when there was no strong king at hand. The minority of King Alfonso XI has been called a period of anarchy, and his childhood years also coincided with a more general crisis in the kingdom. During that period, bands of noble lineages would compete for the tutorship of the king, and the chronicles are rife with descriptions of how the immoderate magnates ravaged and ransacked the lands.[29] Partly, this anti-noble discourse originates in biased historical narratives promoted by the monarchy in order to present royal rule as a stabilizing force, a safeguard for justice and the common good, while nobles are represented as power-hungry vultures. Such leanings are betrayed both by the great historiographical project of Alfonso X, the *Estoria de Espanna* (1270s), and its continuations in the royal chronicles composed by Fernán Sánchez de Valladolid in the 1340s at the behest of the learned king's namesake, Alfonso XI. Simon Doubleday's insistence that we examine the attempts at self-aggrandizement and power accumulation of kings as well as nobles in a more balanced and objective manner, are important to keep in mind.[30]

There is a particularly striking number of parallels to be found between the situation in Sweden and Norway under King Magnus Eriksson (r.1319–64) and Castile-León under Alfonso XI. The former was elected king of Sweden in the summer of 1319 at age three, and declared hereditary king of Norway a couple of months later. A regency, greatly influenced by the king's mother Ingeborg Håkonsdatter (1301–61), controlled the government until the king was declared of age a dozen years later in 1331. Norwegian nobles protested and a rebellion ensued, though the rebels ultimately submitted to the king's authority in 1333. The latter was proclaimed king after his father, Fernando IV, died in 1312, leaving a one-year-old heir. The government was entrusted to close relatives as tutors and regents, but a decisive influence and, in the end sole regent, was the king's grandmother, María de Molina (*c*.1265–1321), wife of the late Sancho IV. Alfonso was declared of age in 1325.

Both of these kings would rule their kingdoms for several decades and make important legal and administrative innovations, most notably the national law code *Magnus Eriksson's Landslag* (*c*.1350) and the *Ordenamiento de Alcalá* (1348) promulgated by Alfonso XI. The relationship between the monarchy and the respective aristocracies of these kingdoms was fraught in both contexts. Both kings were especially determined in their attempts to strengthen the position of the monarchy, and as such met resistance from the high nobility, representatives of which were mindful of their privileges and felt their positions threatened. They also had to face the question of how to respond to the period of rule that preceded their coming of age. In these cases, the perceived misrule of the regencies prompted the restructuring and reorganization of major political and administrative institutions.

There is evidence to suggest that Magnus Eriksson was highly dissatisfied with the way the kingdom's finances had been handled during the years of his minority. These accusations were a powerful weapon in the hands of the young king, who wanted to shift blame for the disastrous economic situation in which Sweden found itself away from himself.[31] Alfonso, ready to take the reins of power at age fourteen, would immediately go on to suppress the *malfetrías*, the abuse perpetrated by the powerful during his minority, and to reinstate order and justice in the kingdom. His attempts at dominating and replacing the old nobility had to be carried out by degrees, however, since he needed their military might to fight outward enemies.[32]

Rebellion: challenging authority

The question of whether rising against an unjust king and deposing him was justified was debated by political and religious thinkers throughout the Middle Ages, and put into practice by rebellious noblemen. Given the contexts at hand, who then sought to entice or represent the voice of the people, the commonalty of the realms being examined in this chapter? Clearly, the nobility or aristocracy of these kingdoms had the strongest political voice as well as the authority to make valid and reasonable claims for political reform or change. The situation in Sweden, as an elective monarchy, was partly different compared to hereditary kingdoms. In several cases during the thirteenth and fourteenth centuries, it became clear that the nobility perceived it as their right to depose kings who were guilty of misrule. Such was the case of King Birger Magnusson (r.1290–1318) of Sweden, against whom his brothers rebelled; King Magnus Eriksson, whose eldest son turned against him; and Alfonso X of Castile and León, who was opposed by his second-born son, Sancho (IV) – all these with the aid and support of major segments of the nobility. On what grounds did such uprisings rest? Surely, not all insurrections were aimed at deposing kings? The basic principle, recognizable from the English case of baronial revolt, was that strategic violence could be an instrument for reform.[33]

In 1272, Alfonso X of Castile and León faced a rebellion whose protagonists belonged to the highest echelons of the nobility. These magnates, the *ricos omnes*, belonged to prominent families that combined illustrious genealogies with large patrimonies and a long tradition of elevated service and important offices within the royal administration.[34] In the rising against Alfonso, a number of complaints were voiced by the magnates, most of them based on the idea that the king had ruptured tradition by his economic and legal reforms, therefore straying from good customary practice as it had been exercised under previous kings. Supplementary taxes, innovations in law ('national' codes to replace local customary *fueros*) and perhaps, above all, the *fecho de imperio*, Alfonso's costly and protracted attempt to be elected and anointed Holy Roman Emperor, were regarded as ill advised by his noblemen.[35] In contrast to what happened a century later, in the dynastic change that led to the rule of the first Trastámara king, Enrique II (r.1369–79), when new noble lineages replaced the old in positions of power, the succession of Sancho IV (r.1284–95) did not entail such a drastic transformation.[36] In the face of his questionable legitimacy and the contested status of his marriage to María de Molina, he felt a pressing need to secure the loyalty of the powerful noble lineages in order to safeguard the succession.

Of course, the magnates were not a uniform group in constant opposition to the monarchy. In disputes over succession, the Castilian magnates often divided into factions that supported one or other claimant to the throne, and the same occurred in Sweden. This was the case after Alfonso X's second-born son Sancho disputed the claim of his late older brother Fernando de la Cerda's eldest son to succeed the aging Alfonso. That conflict, between the future Sancho IV (and later his wife María de Molina and their son Fernando IV) and Alfonso de la Cerda (the Disinherited), would carry on until more than half a century after Fernando's death, with the magnates representing the principal Castilian noble families found on either side of that dividing line. Famously, the Lara family came into direct confrontation with the king during no fewer than four consecutive reigns. This is not to say that ideological assumptions did not run contrary to these lines. Leonardo Funes has argued in favour of the ideological homogeneity of the Middle Ages, contending that the sociopolitical conflicts should not deceive us into believing that we stand before two opposing ideologies, which would have been inconceivable in the medieval political imagination. Rather, all the actors involved in this confrontation were convinced of having the same worldview and scale of values.[37] Nonetheless, there were surely differences between a centralist monarchical ideology and the views of proponents of decentralized or constitutional rule. It has been suggested that the monarchical ideology known as the *molinismo* (pertaining to the queen regent María de Molina, Sancho IV's widow, and her followers) was promoted not just by the queen and her closest collaborators but by a greater part of the nobility that considered the rule legitimate. While the nobility on the whole surely held some ideological notions that underscored the importance of its position and function in society, all nobles were not contrarian towards the centralizing tendencies of the Alfonsine political agenda. To suggest that the nobility was a purely conservative force for the decentralization of power is clearly an oversimplification. Those who opposed Alfonso X acted out of different motivations. Some must have felt personally encroached upon as regards economic or legal privileges (and pragmatic in their responses), while some may have had ideological points to make that related more to political thought as such. Some scholars, of course, judge the thirteenth and fourteenth centuries to precede any concrete construction of a noble or aristocratic ideology whatsoever.[38] The fact that the nobility often presented itself as the voice of the people is often passed over by scholars, but it is an important aspect of ideology formation and the new ways in which nobles engaged with the framework of state and realm.

The monarchical reinforcement and ideological renewal undertaken by Alfonso XI met similar resistance to those projects commenced by his great-grandfather, though the younger man would be more successful in his retort.[39] Possibly, this had something to do with his relentless and ruthless rule; he did not hesitate to execute powerful enemies. In 1332, Alfonso had to subjugate the rebellion instigated by Juan Alfonso de Haro (d.1334), *señor de los Cameros*, the Castilian nobleman who was executed by order of the king. Alfonso XI transferred many important offices into the hands of lesser nobility and learned commoners, which did not please the Castilian magnates. He would confer the highest knightly status to nobles of secondary rank in order to secure their loyalty and to have a solid foundation from which to challenge the power of the magnates.[40] Undoubtedly, it was a mark of the ambitions of the magnates that the appointment of royal offices, in the chancery, treasury and other important institutions, was of such great concern to them. It had become commonplace among the high nobility that they were both great landowners and held high offices within the royal administration.[41]

In mid-fourteenth-century Sweden, Saint Birgitta (1303–73) espoused the view that a rebellion against King Magnus Eriksson would be legitimate. In an extant autograph of a section of her *Revelations*, Birgitta reports a vision of the Virgin Mary telling her that another king would come forth after the deposition of King Magnus. The appeal is directed towards four people (whose names were erased from the manuscript at a later date), who are urged to exhort the knighthood to action.[42] Several accusations are levelled against the king, but the most serious ones in relation to the welfare of the realm are that he has robbed the lands and estates of the crown and handed over the southernmost region of the kingdom to the Danish king. The inalienable status of the whole of the territory of the kingdom is an essential principle in the political landscape of both Sweden and Castile from the thirteenth century onwards. King Magnus was later harshly criticized for favouring foreigners, though of course a king privileging one of his men over all others created indignation among the nobility all through the Middle Ages.[43]

The *Erikskrönika* also contains complaints against kings for favouring foreigners and giving them important positions in Sweden. The chronicle tells of the uprising of the Folkung faction[44] against King Magnus Birgersson, his favouring Danish noblemen above the Swedes being presented as the primary motivation. More specifically, the chronicle has the dissatisfied noblemen complain of the king handing over castles to foreigners and giving them influence at court, above and beyond that of Swedish men. Such complaints go hand in hand with the rights defended in the so-called Charter of Liberties (*Frihetsbrevet*), issued in 1319, which attempted to retain certain privileges for men born within the Swedish realm. It was rhetorically grounded in the support of traditional practices and values, the defence of the realm and the common good, and the need to keep new taxes to a minimum. It has been compared to the English *Magna Carta* of 1215 and resembles the Danish medieval *håndfæstninger* (electoral capitulations) – the first of which King Erik V Klipping (r.1259–86) had to agree to in 1282.[45] In these documents, the king swore to uphold some principles that in practice diminished his authority and safeguarded the magnates' right to participate in the government of the realm and the regular summoning of the representative assembly (the *Danehof*).

In 1356, the eldest son of King Magnus Eriksson launched a rebellion against his father. The eighteen-year-old, in line for the throne of Sweden, had in the past year seen his younger brother Haakon confirmed successor to the royal throne of Norway, and the elevation of the king's favourite, Bengt Algotsson, to the rank of duke. This title had since its importation to Sweden a century previously, been reserved for sons of the king.[46] Though the strong favouritism of any single person was guaranteed to provoke envy, suspicion and mistrust in the rest of the nobility, it seems as if such symbolic acts as the granting of unprecedentedly high rank were particularly galling to rivals. Likewise, the elevation by King Sancho IV of his *privado* don Lope Díaz de Haro to the rank of count (*conde*) – which had fallen out of use – sparked the aversion felt towards him by his contemporaries.[47] As their contemporary, Don Juan Manuel wrote in the first *enxiemplo* of his *Conde Lucanor* (1335): 'There was a king who had a favourite in whom he trusted very much. And it cannot be that men who fare well are not envied by others.'[48]

The developments must have worried Erik Magnusson, who as of yet had no independent position of power, and so sparked the rebellious initiative. Erik was projected to inherit the Swedish crown, although as a legally elective monarchy, Sweden did not usually confirm a successor until after the last king's death. However, some scholars have disregarded Erik and seen the young heir principally as a puppet in the hands of the aristocracy. Dissatisfaction with the rule of Magnus Eriksson would have been the cause of the noble uprising, for which Erik came to act as a rallying point. Scholars have identified a dividing line between the king and his supporters, on the one hand, and the high nobility or council aristocracy, on the other. The political values that had been threatened by King Magnus' actions were those that had been famously espoused in the Charter of Liberties issued by the Council of the Realm in 1319, at the beginning of the regency for the boy king Magnus. The alliance between Erik Magnusson and the nobles can be seen as logical, due to their common understanding of the actions of King Magnus as detrimental to the crown and the common good, and to their own interests. In the final analysis, the conflict would then have centred on the distribution of power within the realm, on the territorial integrity of the kingdom and – again – on the ancient privileges and liberties (*omnia antiqua libertate*) of the nobles, which they were allowed to keep in the final settlement agreement with the king.[49] In this, there are several parallels with the political programme espoused by the Castilian magnates in their conflicts with Alfonso X in 1272. Some have argued that these conflicts in the Iberian context, with its less well-developed national identity, presupposed nobles acting out of the interests of their own class, protecting privileges against royal infractions. That is to say the revolt did not include reform measures intended to benefit the whole of the population, as was partly the case with the Swedish Charter of Liberties of 1319.[50] In both contexts, noble displeasure over the kings' disastrous economic and fiscal policies also arrived centre stage. Similar claims were made by French nobles – notably the Leagues of 1314–15 and in the mid-fourteenth-century crises (1346–7, 1356–7) – who opposed onerous taxation and interference in provincial custom, and levelled criticism against evil counsellors and other royal officials.[51] Nevertheless, the effects of these revolts and insurrections ultimately depended on the relative power and influence of the current king, the nobility and other estates, and of course on the political system on the whole. These revolts did not contribute to creating or shaping a community of the realm in all cases; in France they appear to have augmented conflict between different social groups.[52] In the magnates' rebellion against Alfonso, we see again how the concrete military reality of the *Reconquista* affected the practice of politics. By reference to the demands exerted by the Muslim presence in southern Iberia, nobles could question any loftier or idealistic aims of the Castilian king, such as his attempt to win the imperial title for himself, as a futile fool's errand and a cause for further ruin to the realm.

Conclusion: comparisons and contingencies

Though the cases studied demonstrate structural similarities between Sweden and Castile, they also display the cohesion among European nobilities in general in the period. A formation as a social and political class was still in process in several realms. The principle of access to the king, domestic versus foreign influence, and magnates versus upstarts or new men, were important to the power dynamics of most European societies of the time. Whereas the origin and disposition of the nobility in the Swedish and Castilian crowns may arguably have been more similar to those of their respective neighbours (Norway and Denmark, Aragon and Portugal) than to each other, their self-image, their roles in the government of the realm, their respective involvement in military affairs and their ideological development resonate strongly with each other. The need to seek new means to exert influence beyond the local sphere was a preoccupation felt by magnates in many European realms.

The recurrent periods of royal minority in Sweden and Castile were times when the nobility or aristocracy had the opportunity to implement their own political agendas. Rebellions broke out at times when the reasonable limits of monarchical authority were perceived to have been overstepped. Rebellious noblemen often used the weight of the past, tradition and custom, to explain their displeasure with royal policies. References were made to legal usage that was practised since long before the current king's rule and to which he had to conform. In both of these contexts, the sons and brothers of kings – in Sweden dukes (*hertigar*), in Castile *infantes* – played an important role on the political stage, situated as they were in an intermediary position between kings and nobles, being magnates, landowners and office-holders in their own right. Their claims to power were often at the forefront of conflicts in both realms. They demonstrate that medieval politics was a matter of debate – not a mere physical struggle but rather a discursive battle for the priority of interpretation and symbolic victories.[53]

While often seen as disruptive, rebellious movements and aristocratic revolts in medieval Europe sometimes contributed to stressing the importance of representation in weighty matters such as taxation and warfare. Revolts that involved issues that mattered to several sectors of society, or where other social groups apart from the nobility were well represented, also contributed to the shaping of the idea of a community of the realm. Underlining the processual character of political developments will open up new facets for understanding the interdependence of monarchical and aristocratic authority. In contrast to the German empire in the same period, where emperors such as Frederick II (r.1220–50) would coax and incite princes to share in the burden of government, Swedish and Castilian kings were restrictive in sharing power and seem to have preferred to employ men of lower standing or foreigners in order to outmanoeuvre the domestic lords, in the case of Magnus Eriksson even leaving the highest offices unoccupied for a time.[54] In stressing the importance of aristocratic cooperative government, both Sweden and Castile were more similar to England than to either France or the German empire. Thus, rather than local jurisdiction and decentralized power, the struggle came to revolve around access to positions in the central administration and state governmental institutions.[55] A concept such as loyalty could hence implicate very different things in different contexts.[56] In England, magnates were reminded in the thirteenth century that 'effective royal rule was both necessary and desirable',[57] and likewise the goal for the Swedish Council of the Realm in 1319 or the rebellious Castilian noblemen in the early 1270s was not to create an aristocratic republic but to restore a rightful and legitimate monarchy, supported by a domestic aristocracy with legally defined rights.[58]

In this chapter, it has been demonstrated that both Sweden and Castile share common traits with contemporary kingdoms in western and central Europe, and that a comparative perspective is profitable in order to make connections between seemingly disparate contexts. The principal differences identified seem to depend on variations in political systems – elective vs. hereditary monarchy, frequency and model of representative assemblies, among other aspects. In the end, the distance between these two cases and the distinctive character of the respective historiographies allows for the discovery of previously unfamiliar parallels between them, as well as new inferences to be made.

Notes

1 *A Jaume 'Santi' Aurell, con mucho afecto.*
2 Constance Brittain Bouchard, *'Strong of Body, Brave and Noble': Chivalry and Society in Medieval France* (Ithaca: Cornell University Press, 1998), 31–34.
3 Fernando Arias Guillén, *Guerra y fortalecimiento del poder regio en Castilla. El reinado de Alfonso XI (1312–1350)* (Madrid: Ministerio de Defensa/CSIC, 2012), 129; John Watts, *The Making of Polities: Europe, 1300–1500* (Cambridge: Cambridge University Press, 2009), 219–224
4 Watts, *Making of Polities*, 93–94.
5 Simon Doubleday, *The Lara Family: Crown and Nobility in Medieval Spain* (Cambridge, MA: Harvard University Press, 2001), 62.
6 Helle Vogt and Kim Esmark, "Introduction to Part Two," in *Disputing Strategies in Medieval Scandinavia*, eds. Kim Esmark, Lars Hermanson, Hans Jacob Orning and Helle Vogt (Leiden: Brill, 2013), 143–160, at 148.
7 Herman Schück, "Sweden as an Aristocratic Republic," *Scandinavian Journal of History* 9 (1984): 65–72; José Luis Villacañas Berlanga, *La monarquía hispánica* (Madrid: Espasa, 2008); Jean Gautier-Dalché, « L'histoire castillane dans la première moitié du XIVe siècle," *Anuario de Estudios Medievales* 7 (1970–71): 239–252; David Crouch, *The English Aristocracy, 1070–1272: A Social Transformation* (New Haven: Yale University Press, 2010), 83; Andrew M. Spencer, *Nobility and Kingship in Medieval England: The Earls and Edward I, 1272–1307* (Cambridge: Cambridge University Press, 2014), 262–265.
8 Watts, *Making of Polities*, 153–157.
9 Hans Jacob Orning, *Unpredictability and Presence: Norwegian Kingship in the High Middle Ages* (Leiden: Brill, 2008), 189–194; Antonella Liuzzo Scorpo, *Friendship in Medieval Iberia: Historical, Legal, and Literary Perspectives* (Farnham: Ashgate, 2014).
10 Watts, *Making of Polities*, 102–103.
11 See e.g. Björn Weiler, *Kingship, Rebellion and Political Culture: England and Germany, c.1215–c.1250* (Basingstoke: Palgrave Macmillan, 2007); Spencer, *Nobility and Kingship in Medieval England*.
12 Julio Valdeón Baruque, *Alfonso X el Sabio: La forja de la España moderna*, second edition (Madrid: Planeta, 2011), 89.
13 Spencer, *Nobility and Kingship in Medieval England*, 263.
14 For Portugal see Stephen Lay, *The Reconquest Kings of Portugal: Political and Cultural Reorientation on the Medieval Frontier* (Basingstoke: Palgrave Macmillan, 2009); S.T. Ambler, *Bishops in the Political Community of England, 1213–1272* (Oxford: Oxford University Press, 2017), 54; Cf. María Fernanda Nussbaum, *Claves del entorno ideológico del Poema de Alfonso XI* (Zaragoza: Pórtico Librerías, 2012), 395–397.
15 Anne J. Duggan, "Introduction: Concepts, Origins, Transformations," in *Nobles and Nobility in Medieval Europe: Concepts, Origins, Transformations*, ed. Anne J. Duggan (Woodbridge: The Boydell Press, 2000), 1–14, at 6.
16 Doubleday, *Lara Family*, 119–120.
17 Salvador de Moxó, "De la nobleza vieja a la nobleza nueva: La transformación nobiliaria castellana en la Baja Edad Media," *Cuadernos de Historia* 3 (1969): 1–209.
18 Maria João Violante Branco, "The Nobility of Medieval Portugal (XIth–XIVth Centuries)," in *Nobles and Nobility*, 230–233.
19 José Sánchez-Arcilla Bernal, *Alfonso XI, 1312–1350* (Palencia: Diputación Provincial de Palencia, Editorial La Olmeda, 1995), 14.
20 This stipulation followed the introduction of the king's right to unclaimed territories, fines for serious crimes, the death penalty for *lèse majesté*, etc.

21 Georges Martin, "Control regio de la violencia nobiliaria: La caballeria según Alfonso X de Castilla (comentario al titulo XXI de la Segunda partida)," *Annexes des Cahiers de linguistique et de civilisation hispaniques médiévales* 16 (2004): 219–234.

22 Sverre Bagge, *From Viking Stronghold to Christian Kingdom: State Formation in Norway, c. 900–1350* (Copenhagen: Museum Tusculanum Press/University of Copenhagen, 2010), 325.

23 Spencer, *Nobility and Kingship in Medieval England*, 264.

24 The chronicle was recently made available to an Anglophone readership by Erik Carlquist and Peter C. Hogg, *The Chronicle of Duke Erik: A Verse Epic from Medieval Sweden* (Lund: Nordic Academic Press, 2012).

25 Gabrielle M. Spiegel, *Romancing the Past: The Rise of Vernacular Prose Historiography in Thirteenth-Century France* (Berkeley: University of California Press, 1993), 3–4.

26 Pablo Enrique Saracino, "Apuntes para una lectura ideológica de la cronística medieval: el caso de la *Crónica de tres reyes*," *Anclajes*, 21, no. 1 (2017): 84–86.

27 *Las Siete Partidas del rey Don Alfonso el Sabio*, vol. I–III, eds. Real Academia de la Historia (Madrid: Real Academia de la Historia, 1807): second part, title XV, law III.

28 Nussbaum, *Claves del entorno ideológico*, 274, 302.

29 César González Mínguez, *Poder real y poder nobiliar en la Corona de Castilla (1252–1369)* (Bilbao: Universidad del País Vasco, 2012), 119.

30 Doubleday, *Lara Family*, 9–10; Miguel Ángel Ladero Quesada, *Los señores de Andalucía: Investigaciones sobre nobles y señoríos en los siglos XIII a XV* (Cádiz: Servicio de Publicaciones de la Universidad de Cádiz, 1998), 124–127.

31 Hans Torben Gilkær, *The Political Ideas of St. Birgitta and her Spanish Confessor, Alfonso Pecha: Liber Celestis Imperatoris ad Reges: A Mirror of Princes*, trans. Michael Cain (Odense: Odense University Press, 1993).

32 González Mínguez, *Poder real y poder nobiliar*, 133–147.

33 Claire Valente, *The Theory and Practice of Revolt in Medieval England* (Aldershot: Ashgate, 2003), 28–30.

34 Valdeón Baruque, *Alfonso X el Sabio*, 89.

35 Isabel Alfonso, "*Desheredamiento* y *desafuero*, o la pretendida justificación de una revuelta nobiliaria," *Cahiers de linguistique et de civilisation hispaniques médiévales* 25 (2002): 99–129; Jillian M. Bjerke, "A Castilian Agreement and Two English Briefs: Writing in Revolt in Thirteenth-Century Castile and England," *Journal of Medieval Iberian Studies* 8, no. 1 (2016): 75–93; Julio Escalona, "Los nobles contra su rey. Argumentos y motivaciones de la insubordinación nobiliaria de 1272–1273," *Cahiers de linguistique et de civilisation hispaniques médiévales* 25 (2002): 131–162; Manuel Hijano Villegas, "Fuentes romances de las crónicas generales: el testimonio de la *Historia menos atajante*," *Hispanic Research Journal* 12, no. 2 (2011): 118–134, at 130; Valdeón Baruque, *Alfonso X el Sabio*, 95–99.

36 José Manuel Nieto Soria, *Sancho IV, 1284–1295* (Palencia: Diputación Provincial, Editorial La Olmeda, 1994), 192.

37 Leonardo Funes, "Dos versiones antagónicas de la historia y de la ley: una visión de la historiografía castellana de Alfonso X al Canciller Ayala," in *Teoría y práctica de la historiografía hispánica medieval*, ed. Aengus Ward (Birmingham: University of Birmingham Press, 2000), 8–31: 'Todos los actores de esta contienda tenían la convicción de participar de una misma cosmovisión, de una misma escala de valores'.

38 E.g. Bernard F. Reilly, *The Medieval Spains* (Cambridge: Cambridge University Press, 1993), 183–184: 'The nobility had no program against the crown except a passive one. They wanted to be left alone to enjoy their traditional dignities'. Cf. Miguel Ángel Ladero Quesada, "La Corona de Castilla: Transformaciones y crisis políticas, 1250–1350," in *Poder político y sociedad en Castilla, siglos XIII al XV: selección de estudios* (Madrid: Dykinson, 2014), 150, and, similarly, González Mínguez, *Poder real y poder nobiliar*, 216–217.

39 Carlos Estepa, "The Strengthening of Royal Power in Castile under Alfonso XI," in *Building Legitimacy: Political Discourses and Forms of Legitimacy in Medieval Societies*, eds. Isabel Alfonso, Hugh Kennedy and Julio Escalona (Leiden: Brill, 2004), 179–222.

40 Doubleday, *Lara Family*, 107–108

41 Valdeón Baruque, *Alfonso X el Sabio*, 89–92.

42 Olle Ferm, "Heliga Birgittas program för uppror mot Magnus Eriksson. En studie i politisk argumentationskonst," in *Heliga Birgitta: budskapet och förebilden*, eds. Alf Härdelin and Mereth Lindgren (Stockholm: Kungl. Vitterhets Historie och Antikvitets Akademien, 1993), 125–143, at 129.

43 For the early medieval period, see Gerd Althoff, *Family, Friends and Followers: Political and Social Bonds in Early Medieval Europe* (Cambridge: Cambridge University Press, 2004), 111.

44 This noble faction should not be mistaken for the royal dynasty of the same name, the so-called false Folkungar, the descendants of Earl Birger Magnusson, the first king of which was Birger's son Valdemar.

45 Vogt and Esmark, "Introduction," 153.

46 Gilkær, *The Political Ideas of St. Birgitta and her Spanish Confessor*, 198–199.

47 Nieto Soria, *Sancho IV*, 88.

48 Juan Manuel, *Obras completas*, eds. Carlos Alvar and Sarah Finci (Madrid: Fundación José Antonio de Castro, 2007), 33: 'vn rey era que avia vn priuado en que fiaua mucho. Et por que non puede seer que los omnes que alguna buena andança an, que algunos otros non ayan envidia dellos'.

49 Gilkær, *The Political Ideas of St. Birgitta and her Spanish Confessor*, 199–201.

50 Escalona, "Los nobles contra su rey"; Valente, *Theory and Practice of Revolt in Medieval England*, 250–251.

51 Luke Sunderland, *Rebel Barons: Resisting Royal Power in Medieval Culture* (Oxford: Oxford University Press, 2017), 79.

52 Valente, *Theory and Practice of Revolt in Medieval England*, 251–252.

53 Cf. Weiler, *Kingship, Rebellion and Political Culture*, 177.

54 Göran B. Nilsson, "Vad man bör veta om Yngre Västgötalagen," *Kungl. Vitterhets historie och antikvitetsakademiens årsbok* (2014): 104.

55 Weiler, *Kingship, Rebellion and Political Culture*, 39–42.

56 Weiler, *Kingship, Rebellion and Political Culture*, 96; Orning, *Unpredictability and Presence*, 224–226.

57 Spencer, *Nobility and Kingship in Medieval England*, 262.

58 In both these cases, alliances were also sought outside of the immediate regnal context. The Castilian nobles sought the aid of Nasrid Granada, while the prevalence of cross-border alliances in medieval Scandinavia was equally commonplace. This is an area of investigation that will most likely yield fruitful results in the future.

Key works

Doubleday, Simon, *The Lara Family: Crown and Nobility in Medieval Spain* (Cambridge: Harvard University Press, 2001).

Gilkær, Hans Torben, *The Political Ideas of St. Birgitta and her Spanish Confessor, Alfonso Pecha. Liber Celestis Imperatoris ad Reges: A Mirror of Princes*, trans. Michael Cain (Odense: Odense University Press, 1993).

González Mínguez, César, *Poder real y poder nobiliar en la Corona de Castilla (1252–1369)* (Bilbao: Universidad del País Vasco, 2012).

Spencer, Andrew M., *Nobility and Kingship in Medieval England: The Earls and Edward I, 1272–1307* (Cambridge: Cambridge University Press, 2014).

Valdeón Baruque, Julio, *Alfonso X el Sabio: La forja de la España moderna*, second edition (Madrid: Planeta, 2011).

Valente, Claire, *The Theory and Practice of Revolt in Medieval England* (Aldershot: Ashgate, 2003).

Weiler, Björn, *Kingship, Rebellion and Political Culture: England and Germany, c.1215–c.1250* (Basingstoke: Palgrave Macmillan, 2007).

33

FOR BETTER OR FOR WORSE

Royal marital sexuality as political critique in late medieval Europe

Henric Bagerius and Christine Ekholst

Introduction

The fourteenth and fifteenth centuries were times of crisis for many European monarchies.[1] England was no exception; during his reign in the early 1300s, Edward II faced numerous rebellions, warfare with the Scots, and he was furthermore accused of letting his favourites gain too much power. Eventually, Edward II was imprisoned and his favourite, Hugh Despenser the Younger, was put on trial and executed.[2] According to French chronicler Jean Froissart, Despenser was also castrated for being 'a heretic and a sodomite, even, it was said, with the king, which was why the king had driven the queen away' at the favourite's suggestion.[3] During the trial in 1326 there were many allegations launched against Edward's favourite; a recurring one was that he had come between the king and the queen. The accusers claimed that Despenser had even put Queen Isabella's life in jeopardy when he convinced the king to abandon her and her entourage during the war with the Scots. The allegations end by declaring Despenser a traitor and 'always disloyal' because he had sown discord between the king and the queen.[4] An attempt to ruin the royal couple's marital relations could thus be considered an act of treason, which demonstrates that the relationship between the king and the queen was of great societal and political importance. This chapter examines how the relationship between the king and the queen reflected on the king's authority in the late medieval era. We will argue that the royal marriage symbolized the state of the kingdom, and that marital issues, not least those of a sexual character, were used to express concern with how the kingdom was ruled.

Many late medieval kings struggled with rebellious aristocrats who wanted a bigger share of political power. Many also faced riots and uprisings from peasants and urban workers who protested against high taxes. In turn, these taxes were required to pay for the extensive warfare that characterized the period: wars with other countries as well as internal conflicts.[5] With this as a backdrop, it can come as no surprise that many sources written during this time period are biased or partisan. Contemporary texts launched criticism against kings, queens and the king's counsellors and favourites; several of these critical voices suggested that the king and queen had marital problems.

Our analysis focuses on a number of late medieval royal couples that in one way or another were described as experiencing marital difficulties. The couples this chapter takes as its examples are the English King Edward II (r.1307–27) and his wife Isabella of France; Norwegian and Swedish King Magnus Eriksson (r. Norway 1319–55, Sweden 1319–64) and his wife Blanche of Namur; Castilian King Juan II (r.1406–54) and his wives María of Aragon and Isabel of Portugal; English King Henry VI (r.1422–61 and 1470–1) and his wife Margaret of Anjou; and Castilian King Enrique IV (r.1454–74) and his wives Blanca of Navarre and Juana of Portugal. The focus here is not on the couples per se – they have been studied in great detail before – but on a comparison of the narratives surrounding them. All, or most, sources we discuss are to be regarded as political critique, and there is often reason to question the sources' veracity. The critics came from various backgrounds. Some were part of the opposition and actively supported rival dynastic claims; this is likely the case for Magnus Eriksson and Blanche of Namur's critics.[6] The same applies to some of Henry VI and Margaret of Anjou's critics, and many sources for this time period are described as pro-Yorkists to denote their partisan character.[7] In the same way, chroniclers that were highly critical of Enrique IV's reign are at times called pro-Isabelline because their writings were part of a process to justify Enrique's half-sister Isabel's succession to the throne.[8] It has also been suggested that Isabella of France, after the deposition of Edward II, commissioned Robert of Reading to write a chronicle denouncing her husband's kingship.[9] However, in many cases, it is not possible to determine who the authors of these texts were, let alone their intentions. To give but one example, a royal clerk likely wrote the *Vita Edwardi Secundi*, an important source to Edward II's reign, and, while the chronicle probably was meant to serve as an exemplum, it is unknown for whom he was writing.[10] We, therefore, cannot tell why he was so opposed to the king and what he intended to achieve with his chronicle. In addition, critical depictions tend to change over time, often becoming more outspoken or adjusted to current political realities. The outcome of conflicts would frequently determine which stories survived and would become the dominant narratives.[11]

While these source-specific nuances, as well as the particularities of the various regimes, deserve scholarly attention, it is not the purpose of this chapter to examine them; neither is it our goal to discuss whether these royal couples had actual marital crises. We are interested in the constructed image of the royal marriage as it appears in strongly partisan and often competing and contradictory sources. In the 'sea of histories', to use Richard Kagan's expression, critics made use of shared discourses and narrative tropes that can be found all over medieval Europe.[12] Our aim is to expose reoccurring discursive patterns in chronicles, annals and other sources that describe the royal couples' marital lives. Our purpose is to uncover those critical discourses that built on perceptions of gender and sexuality.

These discourses could be explicit and direct, but more often they were implicit and built on insinuations or associations. They demonstrate that medieval authors regarded seemingly private matters (according to modern sensibilities) as public and political and, therefore, used them to explain why a rulership had failed. More specifically, this chapter will explain why some medieval writers found it problematic that the king did not have sexual intercourse with his wife. It argues that allegations of impotence or same-sex desire highlighted that the king lacked the masculine authority needed to rule. In turn, many sources imply that, due to this, the queen had become unruly. Descriptions of an independent and politically active queen further suggested that the king had lost control over his household. In this way, the authors connected the royal couple's perceived or invented marital problems to the crisis in the kingdom; one thing could explain the other. Critics thus used gendered and sexual allegations to provide explanations as to why a king had to be dethroned or why the succession had been altered. In turn, these negative descriptions reveal norms for kingly and queenly behaviour. This chapter aims to further our understanding of how medieval authors construed rulership and highlights the fact that ideas of gender and sexuality can be found at the core of medieval monarchy.

Gender, sexuality and rulership

Many of the events discussed in this chapter are directly related to the crises and developments that the monarchies went through towards the end of the Middle Ages. This tumultuous period was also a time of intense state formation, and many kingdoms experienced important constitutional changes. Power became more centralized, and the king was expected to govern with a council and a parliamentary assembly. As can be expected, many aristocrats protested against this centralization, which effectively removed power from the local lords and gave it to the king and his council.[13] Part of the problem was that power and governance still depended to a very high degree on personal relationships. The king did not rule alone, and a well-functioning government depended on the king's relationships with his councillors, with his courtiers, with his favourites; and with his queen.[14] The relationship between the king and the queen was thus crucial. The queen was the link between the king and his subjects; a symbol for how the royal dynasty could create social unity and order.[15] Indeed, the union of the king and the queen symbolized the social contract, and the royal marriage represented the bond between the king and his subjects. It also epitomized the societal relationship between men and women. According to John Carmi Parsons, the successful marital life of the king and the queen symbolized a peaceful coexistence where the woman lovingly submitted to the man.[16] It re-enacted the God-given hierarchical gender order and it helped create that order.[17]

Theresa Earenfight argues that, in order for scholars to understand how medieval monarchies functioned, we need to break up the dichotomies between the political and the personal, between public and private. Medieval monarchies were complex and alternated between the personal and the political; they made the personal political in coronations and funerals. They made the political personal when they confirmed alliances through marriages. We also need to break up the dichotomy between king and queen. Earenfight encourages us to see the king and the queen as a corporate unit. She uses the term *rulership*, which incorporates both the king and queen as well as potential favourites that gained influence and power. The king and the queen were understood to complement each other; from a gender perspective, they embodied masculinity and femininity respectively.[18]

Several scholars have examined the importance of masculinity and femininity for pre-modern rulership. Cynthia Herrup has argued that in order to rule well kings or queens regnant needed to incorporate and make use of both masculine and feminine traits when governing.[19] They needed to be able to declare war and send troops into battle, but they were expected also to conclude peace treaties. They needed to punish traitors harshly, but also show mercy and leniency. This balancing act could be difficult to achieve; if a king displayed too many feminine traits he would be criticized. Any excesses could in fact be interpreted as feminine, so while strength and harshness were seen as masculine, cruelty would have been regarded as feminine. In such cases, a king might even have been regarded as a tyrant.[20] Kings clearly needed to keep their feminine characteristics under strict control.

This could be more easily achieved if a king had a queen by his side. Herrup provides some examples of when queens influenced kings to be more lenient and show mercy. The most illustrative example is the fictionalized description of English Queen Philippa, pregnant and on her knees, begging her husband Edward III to show mercy towards a conquered town.[21] As Helen Maurer puts it, the queen's intercession allowed the king to 'bend without appearing weak, to change his mind without seeming foolish and to moderate harshness without forfeiting credibility'.[22] A king could therefore show determination, toughness and self-control and, if he needed to compromise or show leniency, he could utilize his wife, who represented the feminine and 'softer' sides of rulership. Mark Ormrod refers to this as the informal division of duties between the king and the queen.[23]

The division of roles between king and queen also allowed the royal couple to express the hierarchy between masculinity and femininity. While scholarly work on masculinity has flourished over the last decades, it is only recently that scholars have started to examine kings from a gender perspective.[24] As Katherine Lewis writes, the masculinity of kings has remained largely invisible and was only brought up when gendered criticism formed a ground for deposition.[25] But, of course, a king's masculinity was central to how he was perceived as a ruler. As Lewis points out, Edward III's outstanding kingship was entwined with, and enabled by, his exceptional manhood.[26] Masculinity is culture-dependent and will vary over time. However, central features for kingly masculinity were strength, dominance and control. A king was meant to control others and himself.[27] He was also expected to act vigorously, with concern for honour and would not hesitate to use violence if needed; his actions were based on reason and moderation.[28]

By contrast, a medieval queen consort epitomized the household and the family. She was meant to be a role model for other women and was expected to be pious and chaste. Like any wife of the time, she was required to present herself as subordinate and obedient to her husband.[29] Naturally, this did not mean that she was without power; many queens consort exercised great power and influence. Her close presence to the king gave her influence at the court. In addition, she had the ability to affect politics and political relationships directly through patronage and intercession.[30] In some cases queens consort also functioned as regents. This could happen if their husbands were unable to rule due to mental disabilities or illness; this could also occur when the king was at war or was required to reside in his other kingdoms.[31]

Notwithstanding, in general a medieval queen consort's power was informal: her political influence depended on specific circumstances such as her personality and inclinations, her husband-king's personality, their relationship, her natal family's status and the state of the kingdom. Medieval queenship was inherently paradoxical, and the unclear norms for the king's wife made her an easy target for criticism.[32] A queen who was seen as too politically active and powerful, and thereby exhibiting masculine behaviour, was often harshly criticized. Indeed, it was imperative that the power balance between the king and the queen appeared to be stable. It was crucial that they upheld the 'royal equilibrium' which highlighted a hierarchical and seemingly benevolent patriarchal relationship between king and queen.[33]

It is evident that sexuality was a key part of the monarchical system. Most monarchies, including the ones who elected their kings, were hereditary. A queen's most important duty was to provide the kingdom with a male heir; her role and influence were intimately linked to her sexual body. It was in the marital bed that the queen had the greatest access to the king; it was there that she could influence him and convince him to intercede on her behalf.[34] However, royal sexuality was important also for other reasons; it implicitly demonstrated the hierarchy between the king and the queen. Ruth Mazo Karras posits that sexual intercourse in the Middle Ages was not necessarily conceptualized as a mutual act; it was seen instead as something that one person did to another. Penetration symbolized power, as Karras has it. The sexual act involved one person who penetrated, who was seen therefore as the dominant, active and masculine partner, and one person who was penetrated, who was regarded as subordinate, passive and feminine (or feminized if a man).[35] This does not suggest that women could not initiate sexual activity or feel lust; many medieval texts describe women as being inherently more lustful than men.[36] Moreover, some authorities thought that sexual intercourse between men and women was necessary to keep a woman happy and healthy.[37]

The importance of marital sexual intercourse was established in canon law. Canonists declared marital coitus a mutual obligation and described it as a conjugal debt. Each party owed this obligation to the other; and both husband and wife had the right to payment on demand.[38] The reasoning behind this idea of conjugal debt was based upon St Paul's statement that it was better to marry than to burn; if a person could not abstain from sex then marital sex would protect her or him from worse sins. Medieval authors argued that if a wife declined to have sex with her husband, he could become an adulterer or worse: a sodomite. The same applied to women; if women were not provided with a sexual outlet within marriage, they could seek sexual satisfaction elsewhere.[39]

Sexual activity and fatherhood were furthermore core parts of medieval aristocratic masculinity.[40] There could be severe repercussions if a man was unable to have sexual intercourse; impotence was a cause for marital annulment or divorce and might lead to questions about a man's masculinity.[41] For kings, this had wider implications since they were expected to produce an heir to the throne. Even if medieval authors usually blamed the woman if a couple failed to conceive, sources could also imply that the king was not able or willing to have intercourse with his queen.[42] This was a serious allegation.

Sexual intercourse was seen as vital to the relationship between a king and his queen. It was likewise crucial in order for rulership to function well. The sexual act was necessary for a harmonious marriage wherein the queen remained happily subordinate and the king could demonstrate his masculine strength and dominance.

The incapable king

There were of course many reasons why a married couple did not have sexual intercourse, one of which was male impotence. In the Middle Ages, impotence was a cause for annulment of a marriage and this could require a formal investigation. In some cases, the court would order a group of women to determine whether the man was completely impotent or if he could achieve an erection with women other than his wife.[43] The fifteenth-century Castilian king, Enrique IV, was subjected to this type of investigation, and he is remembered in history as 'the Impotent'.[44] As a teenaged prince, he had married Blanca of Navarre and, according to the *Crónica de Juan II*, he was never able to consummate their marriage: after their wedding night, the princess was still a virgin, as untouched 'as when she was born', and this apparently 'made everybody very angry'.[45] Castilian chronicler Alfonso de Palencia asserts that Enrique 'had no devotion to marital love' and that he had even tried to persuade his wife to take a lover who could impregnate her.[46] During the humiliating examinations that led up to the annulment of their marriage, the court established that Blanca was still a virgin after many years of marriage. The court also determined that Enrique was only impotent with his wife; he was perfectly able to achieve an erection with other women. It was concluded that someone must have put a spell on him, and therefore both he and Blanca were allowed to marry again.[47] Palencia, however, doubted that Enrique had ever successfully engaged in sexual intercourse, implying that the prince had obtained his annulment by telling lies and giving false testimony.[48]

Enrique IV's reign was characterized by political chaos and, in the 1460s, rebellions would lead to a civil war between competing factions. During this time, a very curious event, now known as the Farce of Ávila, took place. Outside the town of Ávila a group of rebels staged a dethronement in effigy of Enrique IV. As retold by the Castilian chronicler Diego de Valera, the rebels put up a statue of the absent king on a throne and then read out a long list of accusations. Finally, they removed the statue's royal symbols – his crown, sceptre and sword – and kicked the 'king' off the throne with the words 'Eat dirt, male whore!'[49] Barbara Weissberger has interpreted this as a symbolic way of de-masculinizing Enrique by robbing him of all his symbols of power, and she claims that his symbolic dethronement was meant to mark the restoration of Castile's virility.[50] According to contemporary xenophobic beliefs, Castile had been weakened by foreign influence, especially by Muslim traditions. Enrique had reportedly dressed in Moorish clothes, chosen Moors as his guards, and was said to prefer Moorish customs when it came to 'other secret and more shameful excesses'.[51] This carried a very particular meaning, since sodomy – here used in its narrower meaning: sex between men – was considered very common among Muslims.[52] Castilian aristocrats had several times protested against what they perceived to be Moorish influences in the realm, claiming that the king's bodyguards were so depraved that they forced Christian men and boys to have intercourse with them.[53] That Enrique had permitted this to continue could be taken as proof that he too had allowed himself to be used sexually, and had become their 'male whore' – to use Diego de Valera's words.

Similar xenophobic sentiment – linking foreignness to sexual deviance – is to be found in the narratives surrounding Enrique's second wife. The marriage of Enrique IV to Juana of Portugal was designed to create a strong alliance between their countries. However, in political criticism targeting the queen, Juana was vilified as lascivious and adulterous and accused of spreading 'through the kingdom the flames that were to destroy it'.[54] Her Portuguese ladies-in-waiting were depicted as indecent seductresses and, allegedly, the queen had not only been seduced by the king's favourite but had also been unfaithful with one of the men who held her captive during the civil war in the 1460s.[55] Chronicler Juan de Flores went so far as to claim that no queen had been 'more offensive, defamed and debased' than Juana.[56] In 1468, when Enrique IV finally had to admit that the queen was pregnant with another man's child, it became evident that the king had failed in his husbandly duties to control his wife sexually.

Henry VI of England reigned contemporaneously with Enrique IV, and he too experienced the same type of rebellion that culminated in civil war. Almost unanimously, Henry VI has been considered an inadequate ruler.[57] The king's marriage to the French princess Margaret of Anjou was negotiated to symbolize the new peaceful relations between England and France. However, England's bargaining position was weak, and the new queen arrived with no substantial dowry as part of a short-term truce.[58] She soon came to represent England's failure and was at times regarded as an enemy – a traitor – from within.[59] In 1453, Henry VI suffered a mental breakdown, which compelled Margaret to take a more active role in governance and she would thereafter play a leading role in the Wars of the Roses.[60]

One of the initial problems for Henry and Margaret was to secure the succession. The king had no brothers, which made it even more important that the couple produce an heir. However, the royal couple failed to conceive during the first eight years of their marriage. It was only in 1453, during the king's mental breakdown, that Margaret finally gave birth to their only child, Edward. The long wait for an heir had led to speculation.[61] First, rumours spread that Edward was not Margaret's child, but eventually sources alleged that he was the queen's illegitimate son.[62] *The English Chronicle* links the queen's rulership of the realm to her reputation as an adulteress:

> The quene with suche as were of her affynyte rewled the reame as her lyked, gaderyng ryches innumerable. The office[r]s of the reme, and specially þe Erle of Wylshyre, tresorere of Engelonde, forto enryche hymself, peled the pore peple, and disheryted ryghtfull eyres, and dede meny wronges. The quene was defamed and desclaundered that he that was called prince was nat hir sone but a bastard goten in avowtry.[63]

The chronicler further claims that Margaret, fearing that her son would not succeed his father, allied with knights and squires to convince the lords of England to force the king to resign his crown to her son, but that she failed to achieve this.[64] As Joanna Laynesmith points out, allegations regarding the illegitimacy of the heir did not necessarily reflect real concerns about the queen's chastity.[65] The queen's theoretical adultery highlighted the king's inability to control his wife. As a result, the queen's dominance, her greed and the misrule of the realm could all be explained by the fact that the king had lost control of his wife. The real target of these allegations therefore was not necessarily the queen, but rather the king.[66] She was just a casualty of war and a very convenient scapegoat.

The Brut posits the situation somewhat differently. The chronicler claims that no one dared to disobey the queen who 'rewled pesibly al þat was done About þe Kyng, which was A gode, simple, & Innocent man'.[67] The chronicler highlights Margaret's unruly character by noting that the queen refused to obey a decision made in parliament, which made her enemy, the Duke of York, the legitimate heir to the throne.

She then absented herself from the king and went north. It was decided that the Duke of York should fetch back the queen and subdue those who would not obey him. This episode can be interpreted as an attempt or a wish to regain the vital masculine authority over an increasingly insubordinate queen, who 'wold nat obey such thinges as was concluded in þe parlement'.[68] Ultimately, that Margaret had become such an unruly wife could be explained by her husband's lack of guidance and failure to control her. The king's passivity in the bedchamber would reinforce this impression.

The king's biographer, John Blacman, further emphasizes the image of the king as a good, meek and pious man. In fact, he describes him more as a monk than a king.[69] Blacman claims that Henry was chaste and pure from his earliest years. He kept his marriage vow wholly and sincerely, and never dealt unchastely with any other woman, despite the queen being absent for long periods. 'Neither when they lived together did he use his wife unseemly, but with all honesty and gravity.'[70] This presumably served to explain why they only had one child. Blacman describes a king who worked actively to maintain his chastity. He avoided the sight of naked people and made 'a covenant with his eyes' to never look unchastely upon any woman. When a nobleman organized a performance featuring ladies with bared bosoms, Henry decamped angrily to his chamber. Blacman adds that the king abhorred nakedness and regarded nudity – even the sight of naked men having a bath – as a great offence.[71]

The young king viewed sexuality as a threat to his authority: he would keep careful watch through hidden windows of his chamber to make sure that no foolish impertinence by women would cause the downfall of one of his households.[72] While Blacman likely attempted to present a positive interpretation of the king's behaviour, it is still evident that Henry did not behave as a king should.[73] Throughout the text, the king is depicted as inherently different from other aristocratic men; Blacman portrays a king who is not active and dominating, but rather passive and subordinate. Overall, sources point to an incompetent king lacking in masculine strength and kingly authority. He was passive in the bedchamber and therefore a passive ruler. In keeping with other such descriptions, Margaret thereby became unruly and dominant.[74]

The neglected queen

This chapter was introduced with mention of the trial against Hugh Despenser the Younger who, among other things, was accused of sowing discord between Edward II and his queen, Isabella of France. This was not the only occasion when Edward and Isabella's marital issues were discussed publicly. Chroniclers report that, long before these events, the king had neglected his queen to spend time with his long-standing favourite, Piers Gaveston.[75] Even at their joint coronation, Edward preferred to sit with his dear friend Gaveston, rather than with Isabella. According to *Annales Paulini*, this made the new queen's uncles so upset that they left England in anger. Edward seemed to love his favourite more than he loved his wife.[76] Likewise, Ranulf Higden, the author of *Polychronicon*, states that the English king's interest in Piers Gaveston led to Edward neglecting Isabella, his queen.[77] A monk at St Albans Abbey reports that the king spent so much time with his favourite that Isabella turned to

Philippe IV, her father, to complain about the situation, with another chronicler adding that the king of France hated Gaveston because Edward, 'having married his daughter, loved her indifferently because of the aforesaid Piers'.[78]

According to their critics, Edward and Isabella's marital issues only got worse during the 1320s when there were conflicts between England and France. The situation became difficult for Isabella when the French king, her brother (who had succeeded their father to the throne), threatened to invade England.[79] Edward II confiscated Isabella's property and, according to one of the monks in Westminster Abbey, he refused to be near the queen. The monk angrily states:

> Oh! the insane stupidity of the king of the English, condemned by God and men, who should not love his own infamy and illicit bed, full of sin, and should never have removed from his side his noble consort and her gentle wifely embraces, in contempt of her noble birth.[80]

According to the monk, Isabella's French origin did not justify the king's rejection of her embraces. It is clear that the main reason Edward II abandoned his queen was because he preferred an 'illicit bed, full of sin'. It is probable that this refers to sodomy and the claim that the king neglected his queen because he preferred his favourite, even in bed.[81] According to the *Vita Edwardi Secundi* Isabella declared that Edward's favourite was the reason why her marriage had failed and why she refused to return to England from France, where she had been sent to negotiate with her brother.[82] According to *Vita Edwardi Secundi*, she stated:

> I feel that marriage is a union of a man and a woman, holding fast to the practice of a life together, and that someone has come between my husband and myself and is trying to break this bond; I declare that I will not return until this intruder is removed, but, discarding my marriage garment, shall put on the robes of widowhood and mourning until I am avenged of this Pharisee.[83]

The chronicler Geoffrey le Baker claims that the English held different opinions as to why the queen did not return with her son, the heir to the throne. Some thought that she was being held against her will. Others, however, 'guessed that she had found comfort in the unlawful embraces of Roger Mortimer, and was just as unwilling to return to England as was Mortimer and the other English exiles whom she found in France'.[84] Medieval people would see this as a natural consequence of husbandly neglect; if a woman was left to herself, she was bound to look for another man for comfort and protection.[85] Medieval gender norms were based on the hierarchical relationship between men and women. Women were seen as lustful, frivolous and controlled by emotion rather than reason; this explained why women needed to be put under the guardianship of men. Men were supposed to be dominant and in charge because women needed men to control them.

Together with Roger Mortimer, Isabella gathered an army, invaded England and defeated her husband and his favourite. In his chronicle, Geoffrey le Baker refers to Isabella as an 'enraged virago' who hunted her husband down and had him incarcerated.[86] Edward II, on the other hand, is portrayed as the victim of a most disloyal wife. However, in spite of her betrayal, Edward complained of no misfortune except that Isabella, 'whom he was not able not to love, did not want to see him, although he had lived a widower from her embraces for more than a year'.[87] He had begged her desperately for reconciliation, but according to le Baker, these words made Isabella even more furious and she feared that the Church would force her to share a bed with her husband, the man that she had repudiated. Isabella concluded that the only solution was to have him killed.[88]

As Mark Ormrod has noted, Geoffrey le Baker reinterprets the marriage between Edward II and Isabella of France, possibly in an attempt to improve the king's reputation and make him appear to be a good husband.[89] In le Baker's chronicle, Isabella is the one who abandoned her spouse, while Edward remains faithful and can love no other woman. The queen refuses to return to the marital bed and thereby rejects her legitimate position in society: at her husband's side and under his submission. It was in bed that a husband could control his wife; it was through (hetero) sexual intercourse that she would become subordinate and find happiness.

Other fourteenth-century kings allegedly spurned their queens with serious consequences. According to his critics, Magnus Eriksson, king of Norway and Sweden, experienced marital problems of the same sort. In fact, the description of Magnus Eriksson's issues is so similar to the others that it is likely that medieval writers throughout Europe, also in the far north, used similar tropes based on medieval assumptions regarding gender and sexuality. King Magnus was likewise accused of having had intercourse with men and of loving men more than his wife. Magnus too, had a favourite whom some blamed for the chaotic state of the kingdom.[90] According to the *Libellus de Magno Erici Rege*, the king refused to have sexual intercourse with his wife. Queen Blanche judged this so difficult to endure that she spoke to Magnus' counsellors to solicit their help. They tried to convince Magnus to return to the marital bed, but he declared that he would rather die than return to 'the ordinary'. While Magnus succumbed to lust by sinning against nature, the queen took decisive political action. She left Sweden for Denmark to negotiate with the Danish king regarding military support. The chronicler of the *Libellus de Magno Erici Rege* states that everyone thought it improper and suspicious that the queen had meddled in affairs of the state, while the king calmly stayed at home.[91]

Here again is a sexually rejected queen who inverts the gender hierarchy, to become dominant and usurp power. Critics highlight that Margaret, Isabella and Blanche assumed positions that were not theirs in the normal scheme of things; they upset the gender balance and the royal equilibrium. Queens often served as convenient scapegoats; Blanche was for example described as the root of all the bad things that happened in the realm.[92] However, for the late medieval mind, an unruly woman was ultimately the result of poor domestic governance. A husband who could not control the members of his household was considered weak. Unruly, neglected queens suggested that the king was incapable of controlling his household and, in turn, unable to properly exercise his authority.

The scheming intruder

It goes without saying that any individual who sought to criticize a king had to tread very gently indeed. It was often impossible to be outspoken and direct the criticism towards a king. A king's power was, after all, divinely sanctioned. It was common – and safer – to point the finger of blame at someone close to a king: his queen, his counsellors, or his favourites. By targeting a king's 'wicked advisers' it was possible to enact important political changes without directly challenging a king's authority.[93] Even Isabella of France did not criticize her husband, Edward II, directly; instead, she blamed their failed marriage on an 'intruder'.

One way to further deflect responsibility from a king, while still criticizing his actions, was to introduce allegations of magic or sorcery. Impotence and magic were connected, and witchcraft was often used as an explanation for the failure to achieve an erection.[94] As discussed, Enrique was thought to have been exposed to witchcraft, and the court believed that this explained why he was impotent with his first wife, but not with other women. This theme is also embedded within allegations of favouritism: a king had been bewitched by a favourite and was therefore not able to control himself or his actions. This was used by several critics to explain why Edward II rejected his queen. The author of the *Annales Paulini*, for example, states that the king loved a sorcerer more than his wife.[95] Likewise, Hugh Despenser must have bewitched the king – what else could explain Edward's excessive behaviour?[96]

Much in the same vein, Juan II, king of Castile, was allegedly bewitched by his favourite Álvaro de Luna, who functioned as constable of Castile and grand master of the Order of Santiago. There is no denying that Luna attained a remarkably powerful position in Castile, a position that he managed to hold on to for thirty years. It is therefore perhaps not strange that Luna was vilified, often by making reference to his low birth or his Aragonese origins.[97] His opponents suspected that the constable had bound the king's bodily and intellectual powers 'through magic and diabolic spells' and in this way ruled the kingdom.[98]

According to the Castilian poet, Fernán Pérez de Guzmán, Álvaro de Luna was in complete control of the realm and of the king's household. His power was so great that Juan II was not even allowed to decide when to have intercourse with María of Aragon, his queen:

> One might find it even more astounding – and, indeed, it has been said – that even concerning natural functions, the King followed the orders of the Constable. Although the King was a young man of healthy constitution and had a young and beautiful queen, if the Constable would tell him not to, the King would not sleep in the Queen's chambers, nor would he give his attentions to other women even though he was, by nature, quite inclined to do so.[99]

This pattern continued into Juan's second marriage to Isabel of Portugal, wrote Pérez de Guzmán. In fact, he claims that Álvaro de Luna did everything he could to prevent the king from approaching his new wife: 'The Constable did not even allow the King to be with his wife, the second queen, or to have relations with her when he wanted to.'[100] Juan II's obedience to his favourite was a mystery to Pérez de Guzmán. The king behaved as a son would with his father, or a monk with his abbot. His 'very special love' for, and 'excessive confidence' in, Álvaro de Luna was beyond comprehension.[101]

Juan II's son, Enrique IV, would also be accused of favouritism. According to his critics, he was just as devoted to his favourites, as his father had been. He bestowed them with expensive gifts and prestigious titles, and he cared for them more than he cared for either of his wives. Soon after his remarriage to Juana of Portugal, Enrique made the young Beltrán de la Cueva his principal counsellor. Cueva became more and more important to the king, to the point that, claims the chronicler Alfonso de Palencia, the king 'asked him to be the principal master of his household' and even 'of his marriage bed'.[102] These chroniclers suggested that Juan II and Enrique IV were so powerless and de-masculinized that they were unable to exert control over their marital beds. Enrique would allegedly take this even further; he actively invited someone to replace him in the bedchamber.

Palencia reports that, from the very beginning of their marriage, Enrique IV avoided his new wife and her bedchamber – the king had only married her to hide the fact that he was impotent. Since he was unable to provide the realm with an heir to the throne himself, he tried to convince Queen Juana to have an extramarital affair. Enrique found that neither flattery nor threats could convince her to be unfaithful so he decided to try to make her jealous by courting one of her ladies-in-waiting. Palencia doubted that the king actually had sexual intercourse with his mistress, but she did gain considerable influence over the king. This enraged the queen, but she still refused to break her marriage vows. At this point, Enrique convinced Beltrán de la Cueva – to whom he 'showed an inordinate love' – to seduce the queen.[103] Enrique's favourite wooed the queen so intensely that eventually she surrendered and agreed to become his mistress. In the fall of 1461, Juana was pregnant with Cueva's child; and the king was delighted.[104]

Alfonso de Palencia was not the only one to claim that Beltrán de la Cueva was the queen's lover. The author of *Crónica anónima de Enrique IV* stated that Cueva 'was the one that the king preferred to all others and who spent most of his time with the queen'. According to the chronicler, it was widely believed that Cueva was the father of her child. Likewise, another chronicler, Fernando del Pulgar, was sure that Cueva had had a sexual relationship with the queen.[105] There is nonetheless reason to doubt the veracity of these accounts. All of them wrote their chronicles after Enrique IV's death at which point his half-sister Isabel the Catholic had succeeded to the throne. As a consequence, Queen Juana's daughter – who would become known as Juana la Beltraneja – was never allowed to succeed her father Enrique IV.[106] It was in the interest of the new ruler, Isabel I, that the girl was regarded as illegitimate. Sexual allegations were an efficient weapon in the game of thrones.

Conclusions

This chapter has traversed centuries and very complex historical contexts in order to expose common traits in the political criticism directed against kings and queens. Such criticism was built up over time; and, this study has aimed to point to different chronicles and other sources as part of a pattern wherein royal couples' relationship problems were linked to larger political issues. Gender and sexuality were used – implicitly or explicitly – to criticize how a kingdom was ruled. While marital and sexual issues might seem parenthetical, private and unimportant compared to other issues of state, for the medieval authors they captured the essence of what was wrong in certain polities. Sexual matters were used deliberately to highlight fundamental shortcomings in how a country was being governed.

A king's inability to be sexually active indicated a lack of masculine authority. The reasons why he was unable to have sexual intercourse were not always important. What mattered was that penetration symbolized power, while the inability or unwillingness to have sex was interpreted as a flaw in the king's manhood. In other words, kingly masculinity and dominance were closely linked, and an effeminate king was an unthinkable proposition. In addition, since the king and queen were regarded as a unit, his behaviour would impact how she was judged. A passive and incapable king neglected his wife sexually, and his failure to control his wife represented a serious fault in the rulership. Moreover, a king's lack of masculinity threatened to unleash the dangerous power that lay within queenship itself. A queen was a woman in a powerful position; nothing was more important than keeping her subject to her king. A subordinate and well-behaved queen required a dominant and masculine king by her side. The king was meant to be the master of his household; if he failed in this, his patriarchal authority and ability to rule could be called into question.

Notes

1 J.H. Burns, *Lordship, Kingship, and Empire: The Idea of Monarchy, 1400–1525* (Oxford: Clarendon Press, 1992), 1–15.

2 On the reign of Edward II see Roy Martin Haines, *King Edward II: His Life, His Reign, and Its Aftermath, 1284–1330* (Montreal: McGill-Queen's University Press, 2003); Seymour Phillips, *Edward II* (New Haven: Yale University Press, 2010). The relationship between Edward II and his most beloved favourites is discussed in Natalie Fryde, *The Tyranny and Fall of Edward II 1321–1326* (Cambridge: Cambridge University Press, 1979); J.S. Hamilton, *Piers Gaveston, Earl of Cornwall, 1307–1312: Politics and Patronage in the Reign of Edward II* (Detroit: Wayne State University Press, 1988); Pierre Chaplais, *Piers Gaveston: Edward II's Adoptive Brother* (Oxford: Clarendon Press, 1994). See also Arnd Reitemeier, "Günstlinge und ihre Wahrnehmung am englischen Hof des 14. Jahrhunderts," in *Der Fall des Günstlings: Hofparteien in Europa vom 13. bis zum 17. Jahrhundert*, eds. Jan Hirschbiegel and Werner Paravicini (Ostfildern: Thorbecke, 2004), 191–207; Jochen Burgtorf, "'With My Life, His Joyes Began and Ended': Piers Gaveston and King Edward II of England Revisited," in *Fourteenth Century England 5*, ed. Nigel Saul (Woodbridge: Boydell Press, 2008), 31–51.

3 Jean Froissart, *Chroniques*, vol. 1, ed. Siméon Luce (Paris: Renouard, 1869), 34. Froissart took the description from Jean le Bel, whose work he was strongly influenced by. Compare Jean le Bel, *Chronique*, vol. 1, eds. Jules Viard and Eugène Déprez (Paris: Renouard, 1904), 27–28. See also Claire Sponsler, "The King's Boyfriend: Froissart's Political Theater of 1326," in *Queering the Middle Ages*, eds. Glenn Burger and Stephen F. Kruger (Minneapolis: University of Minnesota Press, 2001), 143–167; Danielle Westerhof, "Deconstructing Identities on the Scaffold: The Execution of Hugh Despenser the Younger, 1326," *Journal of Medieval History* 33 (2007): 87–106; Zrinka Stahuljak, "The Sexuality of History: The Demise of Hugh Despenser, Roger Mortimer, and Richard II in Jean Le Bel, Jean Froissart, and Jean d'Outremeuse," in *Violence and the Writing of History in the Medieval Francophone World*, eds. Noah D. Guynn and Zrinka Stahuljak (Cambridge: D.S. Brewer, 2013), 133–147.

4 G.A. Holmes, "Judgment on the Younger Despenser, 1326," *The English Historical Review* 70 (1955): 265–266.

5 Richard W. Kaeuper, *War, Justice, and Public Order: England and France in the Later Middle Ages* (Oxford: Clarendon Press, 1988), 381–392. As Steven Gunn points out, the late medieval and early modern process towards standing armies and permanent taxes was by no means a linear, direct one. Steven Gunn, "War and the Emergence of the State: Western Europe, 1350–1600," in *European Warfare, 1350–1750*, eds. Frank Tallett and D.J.B. Trim (Cambridge: Cambridge University Press, 2010), 53–54.

6 Henric Bagerius and Christine Ekholst, "En olydig sodomit: Om Magnus Eriksson och det heteronormativa regentskapet," *Scandia* 73, no. 2 (2007): 7–38; Henric Bagerius and Christine Ekholst, "The Unruly Queen: Blanche of Namur and Dysfunctional Rulership in Medieval Sweden," in *Queenship, Gender, and Reputation in the Medieval and Early Modern West, 1060–1600*, eds. Zita Eva Rohr and Lisa Benz (New York: Palgrave Macmillan, 2016), 99–118.

7 See, for example, the introduction to Keith Dockray, *Henry VI, Margaret of Anjou and the Wars of the Roses: A Source Book* (Stroud: Sutton Publishers, 2000), ix–x. As Katherine Lewis points out, the extent to which the sources are partisan has not always been fully acknowledged in scholarship on Henry VI. Katherine J. Lewis, *Kingship and Masculinity in Late Medieval England* (London: Routledge, 2013), 57.

8 Richard L. Kagan, *Clio and the Crown: The Politics of History in Medieval and Early Modern Spain* (Baltimore: Johns Hopkins University Press, 2009), 28–45. See also Barbara F. Weissberger, *Isabel Rules: Constructing Queenship, Wielding Power* (Minneapolis: University of Minnesota Press, 2003).

9 Antonia Gransden, "The Continuations of the *Flores Historiarum* from 1265 to 1327," *Mediaeval Studies* 36 (1974): 488–489; Antonia Gransden, *Historical Writing in England*, vol. 2: *C. 1307 to the Early Sixteenth Century* (London: Cornell University Press, 1982), 17–22; Chris Given-Wilson, *Chronicles: The Writing of History in Medieval England* (London: Hambledon and London, 2004), 154–155.

10 Given-Wilson, *Chronicles*, 167–171

11 Kagan, *Clio and the Crown*, 45; Lewis, *Kingship and Masculinity in Late Medieval England*, 45.

12 Kagan, *Clio and the Crown*, 42.

13 Michael North, *The Expansion of Europe, 1250–1500* (Manchester: Manchester University Press, 2012), 14–15.

14 Theresa Earenfight, "Without the Persona of the Prince: Kings, Queens and the Idea of Monarchy in Late Medieval Europe," *Gender & History* 19 (2007): 8.

15 Theresa Earenfight, *Queenship in Medieval Europe* (Basingstoke: Palgrave Macmillan, 2013), 6.

16 John Carmi Parsons, "Family, Sex, and Power: The Rhythms of Medieval Queenship," in *Medieval Queenship*, ed. John Carmi Parsons (Stroud: Allan Sutton, 1994), 4.

17 Earenfight, *Queenship in Medieval Europe*, 7.

18 Earenfight, "Without the Persona of the Prince," 9–10.

19 Cynthia Herrup, "The King's Two Genders," *Journal of British Studies* 45 (2006): 498.

20 Herrup, "The King's Two Genders," 498–499. See also Louise Olga Fradenburg, "Introduction: Rethinking Queenship," in *Women and Sovereignty*, ed. Louise Olga Fradenburg (Edinburgh: Edinburgh University Press, 1992), 1–3.

21 Herrup, however, notes that complaints of too powerful female intercessors were more common than positive stories of successful persuasion. Herrup, "The King's Two Genders," 507. Philippa of Hainault's intercession is discussed in, for example, John Carmi Parsons, "The Pregnant Queen as Counsellor and the Medieval Construction of Motherhood," in *Medieval Mothering*, eds. John Carmi Parsons and Bonnie Wheeler (New York: Garland, 1996), 40–41.

22 Helen E. Maurer, *Margaret of Anjou: Queenship and Power in Late Medieval England* (Woodbridge: Boydell Press, 2003), 11.

23 W.M. Ormrod, "Monarchy, Martyrdom, and Masculinity: England in the Later Middle Ages," in *Holiness and Masculinity in the Middle Ages*, eds. P.H. Cullum and Katherine J. Lewis (Cardiff: University of Wales Press, 2004), 175.

24 Examples of scholars who have done important work in the field of kingly masculinity are Christopher Fletcher, Mark Ormrod and Katherine Lewis. In addition, several queenship scholars, such as Helen Maurer and Joanna Laynesmith, base their analyses on the idea that the king and queen were a unit and that the king's masculinity would affect the queen. For a discussion of this scholarship see Lewis, *Kingship and Masculinity in Late Medieval England*, 9–12.

25 Lewis, *Kingship and Masculinity in Late Medieval England*, 4.

26 Lewis, *Kingship and Masculinity in Late Medieval England*, 2.

27 Lewis, *Kingship and Masculinity in Late Medieval England*, 26.
28 Christopher Fletcher, "Manhood, Kingship and the Public in Late Medieval England," *Edad Media: Revista de Historia* 13 (2012): 123–142. Christopher Fletcher claims that manhood in the Middle Ages had stronger links to steadfastness, vigour and worthiness of respect than with sexual activity. We hope to show that sexual activity was linked to these characteristics and in addition to control and dominance. We agree that it was not always the sexual activities themselves that were important, but rather what they represented.
29 Joanna L. Chamberlayne, "Crowns and Virgins: Queenmaking during the Wars of the Roses," in *Young Medieval Women*, eds. Katherine J. Lewis, Noël James Manuge and Kim M. Phillips (Stroud: Sutton, 1999), 49–54.
30 Paul Strohm, *Hochon's Arrow: The Social Imagination of Fourteenth-Century Texts* (Princeton: Princeton University Press, 1992), 95–119; Lois L. Huneycutt, "Intercession and the High-Medieval Queen: The Esther Topos," in *Power of the Weak: Studies on Medieval Women*, eds. Jennifer Carpenter and Sally-Beth MacLean (Urbana: University of Illinois Press, 1995), 126–146; John Carmi Parsons, "The Queen's Intercession in Thirteenth-Century England," in *Power of the Weak*, 147–177; John Carmi Parsons, "The Pregnant Queen as Counsellor and the Medieval Construction of Motherhood," in *Medieval Mothering*, 39–61; John Carmi Parsons, "Intercessory Patronage of Queens Margaret and Isabella of France," in *Thirteenth Century England* 6, eds. Michael Prestwich, Richard Britnell and Robin Frame (Woodbridge: Boydell & Brewer, 1997), 145–156; Lisa Benz St John, *Three Medieval Queens: Queenship and the Crown in Fourteenth-Century England* (New York: Palgrave Macmillan, 2012), 33–63.
31 Theresa Earenfight, "Absent Kings: Queens as Political Partners in the Medieval Crown of Aragon," in *Queenship and Political Power in Medieval and Early Modern Spain*, ed. Theresa Earenfight (Burlington: Ashgate, 2005), 33–51.
32 János M. Bak, "Queens as Scapegoats in Medieval Hungary," in *Queens and Queenship in Medieval Europe: Proceedings of a Conference held at King's College London April 1995*, ed. Anne J. Duggan (Woodbridge: Boydell Press, 1997), 223–233. See also J.L. Laynesmith, *The Last Medieval Queens: English Queenship 1445–1503* (Oxford: Oxford University Press, 2004), 4.
33 Bagerius and Ekholst, "The Unruly Queen," 131–133.
34 Benz St John, *Three Medieval Queens*, 35. John Carmi Parsons, "Ritual and Symbol in the English Medieval Queenship to 1500," in *Women and Sovereignty*, 67–68.
35 Ruth Mazo Karras, *Sexuality in Medieval Europe: Doing unto Others*, second edition (London: Routledge, 2012), 3–4, 30.
36 Karras, *Sexuality in Medieval Europe*, 4.
37 Vern L. Bullough, "On Being a Male in the Middle Ages," in *Medieval Masculinities*, eds. Clare A. Lees with Thelma Fenster and Jo Ann McNamara (Minneapolis: University of Minnesota Press, 1994), 39, 41; Joan Cadden, *Meanings of Sex Difference in the Middle Ages: Medicine, Science and Culture* (Cambridge: Cambridge University Press, 1993), 271–277.
38 James A. Brundage, "Sexual Equality in Medieval Canon Law," in *Medieval Women and the Sources of Medieval History*, ed. Joel T. Rosenthal (Athens: The University of Georgia Press, 1990), 69; Elizabeth M. Makowski, "The Conjugal Debt and Medieval Canon Law," *Journal of Medieval History* 3 (1977): 99–114; Dyan Elliott, *Spiritual Marriage: Sexual Abstinence in Medieval Wedlock* (Princeton: Princeton University Press, 1993), 148–155; Pierre J. Payer, *The Bridling of Desire: Views of Sex in Later Middle Ages* (Toronto: University of Toronto Press, 1993), 89–97. See also Dyan Elliott, "Bernardino of Siena and the Marriage Debt," in *Desire and Discipline: Sex and Sexuality in the Premodern West*, eds. Jacqueline Murray and Konrad Eisenbichler (Toronto: University of Toronto Press, 1996), 168–200.
39 Jacqueline Murray, "Historicizing Sexuality, Sexualizing History," in *Writing Medieval History*, ed. Nancy Partner (London: Arnold, 2005), 139.
40 Ruth Mazo Karras, "Knighthood, Compulsory Heterosexuality, and Sodomy," in *The Boswell Thesis: Essays on 'Christianity, Social Tolerance, and Homosexuality'* ed. Mathew Kuefler (Chicago: University of Chicago Press, 2006), 273–274; Ruth Mazo Karras, *From Boys to Men: Formation of Masculinity in Late Medieval Europe* (Philadelphia: University of Pennsylvania Press, 2003), 47–57, 165–166. See also Fletcher, "Manhood, Kingship and the Public in Late Medieval England," 131. The scholarship on medieval masculinities

is abundant. Examples of books that analyse late medieval masculine identities more comprehensively are Derek G. Neal, *The Masculine Self in Late Medieval England* (Chicago: University of Chicago Press, 2008); Isabel Davis, *Writing Masculinity in the Later Middle Ages* (Cambridge: Cambridge University Press, 2010). See also Michelle M. Sauer, *Gender in Medieval Culture* (London: Bloomsbury Academic, 2015).

41 Bullough, "On Being a Male," 41.

42 Katherine J. Lewis, "Becoming a Virgin King: Richard II and Edward the Confessor," in *Gender and Holiness: Men, Women and Saints in Late Medieval Europe*, eds. Samantha J.E. Riches and Sarah Salih (London: Routledge, 2002), 91–92. For the tendency to blame infertility on the woman, see Cadden, *Meanings of Sex Difference*, 258; Kristen L. Geaman, "Anne of Bohemia and Her Struggle to Conceive," *Social History of Medicine* 29 (2016): 2, 15. However, Catherine Rider argues that there was an awareness in medical writings that men might be capable of sexual intercourse but not able to beget a child. Although male infertility might not have been the first explanation that medieval people thought of, it was discussed as a possibility in the medical community. Catherine Rider, "Men and Infertility in Late Medieval English Medicine," *Social History of Medicine* 29 (2016): 266.

43 Jacqueline Murray, "On the Origins and Role of 'Wise Women' in Causes for Annulment on the Grounds of Male Impotence," *Journal of Medieval History* 16 (1990): 238–241.

44 On the reign of Enrique IV see José-Luis Martín, *Enrique IV de Castilla: Rey de Navarra, Príncipe de Cataluña* (Hondarribia: Nerea, 2003); Luis Suárez, *Enrique IV de Castilla: La difamación como arma política* (Barcelona: Ariel, 2013).

45 "Comienza la Crónica del serenísimo Príncipe Don Juan, segundo rey deste nombre, en Castilla y en Leon," ['Crónica de Juan II'] in *Crónicas de los reyes de Castilla desde Don Alfonso el Sabio, hasta los Católicos Don Fernando y Doña Isabel*, vol. 2, ed. Cayetano Rosell (Madrid: Rivadeneyra, 1877), 567.

46 Alfonso de Palencia, *Gesta hispaniensia ex annalibvs svorvm diervm collecta*, vol. 1, eds. Brian Tate and Jeremy Lawrance (Madrid: Real Academia de la Historia, 1998), 5.

47 Martín, *Enrique IV de Castilla*, 36–45; Suárez, *Enrique IV de Castilla*, 121–123.

48 Palencia, *Gesta hispaniensia*, vol. 1, 27.

49 Mosén Diego de Valera, *Memorial de diversas hazañas: Crónica de Enrique IV*, ed. Juan de Mata Carriazo (Madrid: Espasa-Calpe, 1941), 99. Also see Angus MacKay, "Ritual and Propaganda in Fifteenth-Century Castile," *Past & Present* 107 (1985): 3–43; M. Isabel del Val Valdivieso, "La 'Farsa de Ávila' en las crónicas de la época," in *Espacios de poder y formas sociales en la Edad Media: Estudios dedicados a Ángel Barrios*, eds. Gregorio del Ser Quijano and Iñaki Martín Viso (Salamanca: Ediciones Universidad de Salamanca, 2007), 355–367.

50 Barbara Weissberger, "'¡A tierra, puto!': Alfonso de Palencia's Discourse of Effeminacy," in *Queer Iberia: Sexualities, Cultures, and Crossings from the Middle Ages to the Renaissance*, eds. Josiah Blackmore and Gregory S. Hutcheson (Durham: Duke University Press, 1999), 301.

51 Palencia, *Gesta hispaniensia*, vol. 1, 114. Also see José Antonio Ramos Arteaga, "Homofobia y propaganda: La construcción literaria y política de Enrique IV," in *Actas del VIII Congreso Internacional de la Asociación Hispánica de Literatura Medieval (Santander, 22–26 de septiembre de 1999, Palacio de la Magdalena, Universidad Internacional Menéndez Pelayo)*, vol. 1, eds. Margarita Freixas and Silvia Iriso (Santander: Gobierno de Cantabria, 2000), 1501–1510.

52 Michael Goodich, *The Unmentionable Vice: Homosexuality in the Later Medieval Period* (Santa Barbara: ABC-Clio, 1979), 3–9; Mark D. Jordan, *The Invention of Sodomy in Christian Theology* (Chicago: University of Chicago Press, 1997), 163; Karras, *Sexuality in Medieval Europe*, 170–172.

53 Weissberger, "'¡A tierra, puto!' 301. See also Gregory S. Hutcheson, "The Sodomitic Moor: Queerness in the Narrative of Reconquista," in *Queering the Middle Ages*, eds. Glenn Burger and Steven F. Kruger (Minneapolis: University of Minnesota Press, 2001), 99–122.

54 Alonso de Palencia, *Cronica de Enrique IV*, vol. 2, ed. A. Paz y Melia (Madrid: Atlas, 1975), 194.

55 Nancy F. Marino, "How Portuguese Damas Scandalized the Court of Enrique IV of Castile," *Essays in Medieval Studies* 18 (2001): 43–52; Suárez, *Enrique IV de Castilla*, 397–407.

56 Julio Puyol, ed., *Crónica incompleta de los Reyes Católicos (1469–1476): Según un manuscrito anónimo de la época* (Madrid: Real Academia de la Historia, 1934), 198.

57 John Watts, *Henry VI and the Politics of Kingship* (Cambridge: Cambridge University Press, 1996), 10. However, as Bertram Wolffe points out, his father Henry V left behind a glorious legend and a task impossible to fulfil. Bertram Wolffe, *Henry VI* (London: Eyre Methuen, 1981; repr. New Haven: Yale University Press, 2001), 26.

58 Laynesmith, *Last Medieval Queens*, 11–15, 42–43. Ralph Griffiths points out that even those who previously had tolerated the match would have been disappointed by the short truce that would allow the French to strengthen their troops. Ralph A. Griffiths, *The Reign of King Henry VI: The Exercise of Royal Authority, 1422–61* (London: Ernest Benn Limited, 1981), 482.

59 *The English Chronicle* states ominously that the truce was meddled with treason. William Marx, ed., *An English Chronicle, 1377–1461: Edited from Aberystwyth, National Library of Wales MS 21068 and Oxford, Bodleian Library MS Lyell 34* (Woodbridge: Boydell Press, 2003), 65.

60 Alison Basil has analysed the connection between Henry VI's mental breakdown and gender disruption. Alison Basil, "Henry VI and Margaret of Anjou: Madness, Gender Dysfunction and Perceptions of Dis-Ease in the Royal Body," in *The Image and Perception of Monarchy in Medieval and Early Modern Europe*, eds. Sean McGlynn and Elena Woodacre (Newcastle upon Tyne: Cambridge Scholars Publishing, 2014), 168–182. Almost all contemporary and later sources were in fact biased against Margaret of Anjou and could not necessarily be taken as proof of her character or role. Patricia-Ann Lee, "Reflections of Power: Margaret of Anjou and the Dark Side of Queenship," *Renaissance Quarterly* 39 (1986): 206–210.

61 Kristen Geaman discusses how their failure to conceive during the first eight years of marriage impacted the rulership. Kristen Geaman, "A Bastard and a Changeling? England's Edward of Westminster and Delayed Childbirth," in *Unexpected Heirs in Early Modern Europe: Potential Kings and Queens*, ed. Valerie Schutte (Cham: Springer International Publishing, 2017), 11–33.

62 Maurer, *Margaret of Anjou*, 45–47.

63 Marx, *English Chronicle*, 78, v. 21–26. This seems to confound the rumour that Edward was a changeling with the rumour that Margaret had committed adultery. Laynesmith, *Last Medieval Queens*, 137.

64 Marx, *English Chronicle*, 78, v. 25–34.

65 Laynesmith, *Last Medieval Queens*, 135–136.

66 Lewis, *Kingship and Masculinity*, 233.

67 Friedrich W.D. Brie, ed., *The Brut or the Chronicles of England*, vol. 2 (London: Kegan Paul, Trench, Trübner & Co., 1908), 527.

68 Brie, *Brut*, vol. 2, 530.

69 M. R. James, ed., *Henry the Sixth: A Reprint of John Blacman's Memoir with Translation and Notes* (Cambridge: The University Press, 1919), 26–27.

70 James, *Blacman's Memoir*, 29.

71 James, *Blacman's Memoir*, 29–30

72 James, *Blacman's Memoir*, 30. Thomas Prendergast describes the king as a 'voyeur'. Thomas A. Prendergast, "The Invisible Spouse: Henry VI, Arthur and the Fifteenth-Century Subject," *Journal of Medieval and Early Modern Studies* 32 (2002): 310.

73 Blacman describes a man that comes close to the clerical ideal of manhood as described in Fletcher, "Manhood, Kingship and the Public," 128. For a somewhat different interpretation, see Lewis, *Kingship and Masculinity*, 201.

74 Prendergast, "Invisible Spouse," 311.

75 Lisa Benz argues that King Edward and Queen Isabella had a conventional relationship and it was only in 1325 that Isabella realized that her relationship with Edward had been fractured. Lisa Benz St John, "In the Best Interest of the Queen: Isabella of France, Edward II and the Image of a Functional Relationship," in *Fourteenth Century England 8*, ed. J.S. Hamilton (Woodbridge: Boydell Press, 2014), 38. In addition, Benz argues that, in reality, it was the dowager queen, Margaret of France, who felt threatened by Gaveston. Lisa Benz, "Conspiracy and Alienation: Queen Margaret of France and Piers Gaveston, the King's Favorite," in *Queenship, Gender and Reputation in the Medieval and Early Modern West, 1060–1600*, 119–141.

76 "Annales Paulini," in *Chronicles of the Reigns of Edward I and Edward II*, vol. 1, ed. William Stubbs (London: Longman & Co., 1882), 262.

77 Churchill Babington and Joseph Rawson, eds., *Polychronicon Ranulphi Higden Monachi Cestrensis together with the English Translation of John Trevisa and of an Unknown Writer of the Fifteenth Century*, vol. 8 (London: Longman & Co., 1882), 300.

78 "Johannis de Trokelowe Annales," in *Chronica monasterii S. Albani*, vol. 3, ed. Henry Thomas Riley (London: Longmans, Green, Reader and Dyer, 1866), 68; Joseph Stevenson, ed., *Chronicon de Lanercost, 1201–1346* (Edinburgh: n.p. 1839), 217; Herbert Maxwell, trans., *The Chronicle of Lanercost: 1272–1346* (Glasgow: MacLehose, 1913), 196. Lisa Benz claims that the chroniclers who believed Isabella had been harmed by the king's actions wrote their narratives after 1327. Benz St John, "In the Best Interest of the Queen," 24.

79 Sophia Menache, "Isabelle of France, Queen of England: A Reconsideration," *Journal of Medieval History* 10 (1984): 110.

80 Henry Richard Luard, ed., *Flores Historiarum*, vol. 3 (London: Eyre and Spottiswoode, 1890), 229. The translation is from Gransden, *Historical Writing in England*, vol. 2, 21.

81 Richard E. Zeikowitz, *Homoeroticism and Chivalry: Discourses of Male Same-Sex Desire in the Fourteenth Century* (New York: Palgrave Macmillan, 2003), 117; Aleardo Zanghellini, *The Sexual Constitution of Political Authority: The 'Trials' of Same-Sex Desire* (New York: Routledge, 2015), 81.

82 Phillips, *Edward II*, 468–479.

83 Wendy R. Childs, ed., *Vita Edwardi Secundi: The Life of Edward the Second* (Oxford: Clarendon Press, 2005), 243.

84 Edward Maunde Thompson, ed., *Chronicon Galfridi le Baker de Swynebroke* (Oxford: Clarendon Press, 1889), 20; David Preest, trans., *The Chronicle of Geoffrey le Baker* (Woodbridge: Boydell Press, 2012), 20.

85 Karras, *Sexuality in Medieval Europe*, 115. Leah Otis-Cour presents several cases where the court placed responsibility for a wife's adultery on her husband. Absences from home, mistreatment, age difference between husband and wife were all presented as mitigating causes for wifely extramarital affairs. Leah Otis-Cour, "*De jure novo*: Dealing with Adultery in the Fifteenth-Century Tolousain," *Speculum* 84 (2009): 378–379.

86 Thompson, *Chronicon Galfridi le Baker*, 20; Preest, *Chronicle of Geoffrey le Baker*, 20.

87 Thompson, *Chronicon Galfridi le Baker*, 29; Preest, *Chronicle of Geoffrey le Baker*, 28.

88 Thompson, *Chronicon Galfridi le Baker*, 29; Preest, *Chronicle of Geoffrey le Baker*, 28.

89 Mark Ormrod discusses how the political critique against Edward II changed over time. W.M. Ormrod, "The Sexualities of Edward II," in *The Reign of Edward II: New Perspectives*, eds. Gwilym Dodd and Anthony Musson (Woodbridge: York Medieval, 2006), 43–46.

90 Bagerius and Ekholst, "Unruly Queen," 133–135.

91 "Libellus de Magno Erici Rege," in *Scriptores Rerum Svecicarum Medii Ævi*, vol. 3, ed. Claudius Annerstedt (Uppsala: Edvardus Berling, 1871–1876), 14. See also Bagerius and Ekholst, "Unruly Queen," 137–139.

92 "Libellus de Magno Erici Rege," 14.

93 Joel T. Rosenthal, "The King's 'Wicked Advisers' and Medieval Baronial Rebellions," *Political Science Quarterly* 82 (1967): 595–618. The scholarship on royal favouritism is abundant. Two important anthologies are J.H. Elliot and L.W.B. Brockliss, eds., *The World of the Favourite* (New Haven: Yale University Press, 1999) and Jan Hirschbiegel and Werner Paravicini, eds., *Der Fall des Günstlings: Hofparteien in Europa vom 13. bis zum 17. Jahrhundert* (Ostfildern: Thorbacke, 2004). Klaus Oschema has analysed late medieval favourites and examined their impact on politics in "The Cruel End of the Favourite: Clandestine Death and Public Retaliation at Late Medieval Courts in England and France," in *Death at Court*, eds. Karl-Heinz Spiess and Immo Warntjes (Wiesbaden: Harrassowitz, 2012), 171–195. We have discussed how favouritism was used in political critique in Henric Bagerius and Christine Ekholst, "Kings and Favourites: Sexuality and Politics in Late Medieval Europe," *Journal of Medieval History* 43 (2017): 298–319.

94 Bullough, "On Being a Male," 42. For a more extensive analysis, see Catherine Rider, *Magic and Impotence in the Middle Ages* (Oxford: Oxford University Press, 2006).

95 "Annales Paulini," 262.

96 Thompson, *Chronicon Galfridi le Baker*, 10; Preest, *Chronicle of Geoffrey le Baker*, 10.

97 Bagerius and Ekholst, "Kings and Favourites," 300–301. On the reign of Juan II and his relationship to Álvaro de Luna, see Pedro Andrés Arboledas, *Juan II, rey de Castilla y León (1406–1454)* (Gijón: Ediciones Trea, 2009); José Manuel Calderón Ortega, *Álvaro de Luna: Riqueza y poder en la Castilla del siglo XV* (Madrid: Dykinson, 1998); José Serrano Belinchón, *El condestable: De la vida, prisión y muerte de don Álvaro de Luna* (Guadalajara: Aache, 2000). See also L.J. Andrew Villalon, "Don Alvaro de Luna and the Indictment against Royal Favoritism in Late Medieval Castile," in *The Emergence of Léon-Castile, c. 1065–1500: Essays Presented to J.F. O'Callaghan*, ed. James J. Todesca (Farnham: Ashgate, 2015), 161–183.

98 "Crónica de Juan II," 562. See also Gregory S. Hutcheson, "Desperately Seeking Sodom: Queerness in the Chronicles of Alvaro de Luna," in *Queer Iberia*, 222–249.

99 Fernán Pérez de Guzmán, "Generaciones, semblanzas é obras," in *Crónicas de los reyes de Castilla*, vol. 2, 713; Fernán Pérez de Guzmán, *Pen Portraits of Illustrious Castilians*, trans. Marie Gilette and Loretta Zehngut (Washington, DC: Catholic University of America Press, 2003), 56.

100 Pérez de Guzmán, "Generaciones, semblanzas é obras," 714; Pérez de Guzmán, *Pen Portraits of Illustrious Castilians*, 59.

101 Pérez de Guzmán, "Generaciones, semblanzas é obras," 714; Pérez de Guzmán, *Pen Portraits of Illustrious Castilians*, 56. On the relationship between Álvaro de Luna and Juan II's two wives, see Diana Pelaz Flores, "Queenly Time in the Reign of Juan II of Castile (1406–1454)," in *Queenship in the Mediterranean: Negotiating the Role of the Queen in the Medieval and Early Modern Eras*, ed. Elena Woodacre (Basingstoke: Palgrave Macmillan, 2013), 169–190.

102 Palencia, *Gesta hispaniensia*, vol. 1, 190. On Beltrán de la Cueva see María del Pilar Carceller Cerviño, *Beltrán de la Cueva, el último privado: Monarquía y nobleza a fines de la Edad Media* (Madrid: Sílex, 2011). See also María del Pilar Carceller Cerviño, "Álvaro de Luna, Juan Pacheco y Beltrán de la Cueva: Un estudio comparativo del privado regio a fines de la Edad Media," *En la España Medieval* 32 (2009): 85–112.

103 Palencia, *Gesta hispaniensia*, vol. 1, 190.

104 Palencia, *Gesta hispaniensia*, vol. 1, 138–139, 147, 180; Alfonso de Palencia, *Gesta hispaniensia ex annalibvs svorvm diervm collecta*, vol. 2, eds. Brian Tate and Jeremy Lawrance (Madrid: Real Academia de la Historia, 1999), 235–236. See also Óscar Villarroel González, *Juana la Beltraneja: La construcción de una ilegitimidad* (Madrid: Sílex, 2014), 47–77.

105 María Pilar Sánchez-Parra, ed., *Crónica anónima de Enrique IV de Castilla 1454–1474 (Crónica castellana)*, vol. 2 (Madrid: Ediciones de la Torre, 1991), 117; Fernando del Pulgar, *Crónica de los Reyes Católicos*, vol. 1, ed. Juan de Mata Carriazo (Madrid: Espasa-Calpe, 1943), 5.

106 Villarroel González, *Juana la Beltraneja*, 247–253.

Key works

Bagerius, Henric and Christine Ekholst, "Kings and Favourites: Sexuality and Politics in Late Medieval Europe," *Journal of Medieval History* 43 (2017): 298–319.

Earenfight, Theresa, "Without the Persona of the Prince: Kings, Queens and the Idea of Monarchy in Late Medieval Europe," *Gender & History* 19 (2007): 1–21.

Herrup, Cynthia, "The King's Two Genders," *Journal of British Studies* 45 (2006): 493–510.

Lewis, Katherine J., *Kingship and Masculinity in Late Medieval England* (London: Routledge, 2013).

Ormrod, W.M., "The Sexualities of Edward II," in *The Reign of Edward II: New Perspectives*, eds. Gwilym Dodd and Anthony Musson (Woodbridge: York Medieval, 2006), 22–47.

Weissberger, Barbara, "'¡A tierra, puto!': Alfonso de Palencia's Discourse of Effeminacy," in *Queer Iberia: Sexualities, Cultures, and Crossings from the Middle Ages to the Renaissance*, eds. Josiah Blackmore and Gregory S. Hutcheson (Durham: Duke University Press, 1999), 291–324.

34

THE TUDOR MONARCHY OF COUNSEL AND THE GROWTH OF REASON OF STATE

Joanne Paul with Valerie Schutte

There is a curious paradox in scholarly understandings of counsel during the Tudor period. On the one hand, political counsel is widely recognized to have been one of the central, if not *the* central, political concern of the Tudor period, as evidenced by its significance in texts such as More's *Utopia*, Elyot's *Boke Called the Governor*, Bacon's *Essays* and so on.[1] On the other hand, the two longest reigning and best-known monarchs of the period, Henry VIII and Elizabeth I, have a reputation – then and now – for being notoriously difficult to counsel, for refusing advice or being offended by the presentation of it.[2] To add further complexity, both Henry VIII and his daughter Elizabeth were products of a humanist education which stressed the importance of counsel to a monarch, and went to great lengths to *appear* as if they were recipients of educated advice.[3]

Thus, teasing out the relationship between counsel and the Tudor crown is not easy, but it is essential to understanding both the way in which counsel influenced sovereignty in the early modern period as well as the political operations of the Tudor regime. This chapter will provide an outline of the discourse of counsel during the Tudor 'monarchy of counsel', before examining in particular the fundamental shift from a 'humanist' discourse of counsel in the early decades of the sixteenth century to a 'Machiavellian' discourse from the middle of the century.[4] It will examine how this latter vocabulary became the foundation of the Reason of State tradition, which emphasizes the prioritization of the 'interest' of the state often over more moral or religious considerations.[5] These shifts are especially visible in the English, as opposed to European, context where the rule of a minor and two women in the second half of the sixteenth century shifted attention (and suspicion) onto the figure of the counsellor in a more explicit way than on the continent. The bulk of the chapter will thus focus on the Elizabethan discourse of Reason of State and how it fundamentally changed political counsel in this period.

Studying the English discourse of counsel

The 'discourse', 'problem' and 'paradox' of counsel in England during the 'monarchy of counsel' (from the end of the Wars of the Roses to the English Civil War) have received noteworthy attention of late, though significant gaps still exist in the literature. As John Watts has suggested, 'much more attention has been given to the growth of central government, the functioning of clientage networks, the changing structures of political society and the securing of compliance' than to counsel, but the study of the 'problem of counsel' has been revived in large part because of the generation of what John Guy has called the 'new political history' of Tudor England.[6] Guy was the first to attempt a categorization of two 'vocabularies' of the 'rhetoric of counsel': 'feudal-baronial' and 'humanist-classical', noting especially how they arose under the reign of Henry VIII.[7] Even more recently, attempts to understand the 'monarchy of counsel' have been led by Jacqueline Rose, whose article on 'Kingship and Counsel in Early Modern England' added a third vocabulary to Guy's two, an 'exclusively religious' language of counsel.[8]

Work has also been undertaken on counsel in particular Tudor regimes, though little has been done to compare and contrast across them. Perhaps the least explored is that of Henry VII, though work has been done on the changes he made to institutional councils during his reign, for instance by Peter Holmes, as well as Stephen Gunn, who has also drawn attention to the role of 'new men' within court and council.[9] The complexities and brevity of Edwardian and Marian rule often mean that counsel is overlooked, though Stephen Alford has explored the theme in his *Kingship and Politics in the Reign of Edward VI*, and Joanne Paul has recently attempted to draw out some of the negotiations surrounding counsel in the reign of Mary I, from under the shadow of her half-sister's reign.[10] These reigns are often passed over in favour of the more widely studied Tudor monarchs: Henry VIII and Elizabeth I.

Studies of counsel under Henry VIII tend to focus on particular writings, such as those of Thomas More,[11] Thomas Elyot,[12] or Thomas Starkey.[13] They also often isolate the role of councils, such as the Privy Council or parliament,[14] or the roles of various fora for counsel, such as plays or poetry.[15] Guy has especially noted the vocabularies and strategies of counsel in this period,[16] and Richard Rex has shown how Henry VIII used counsel as a means to consensus following the break with Rome.[17] The consensus is that humanism dominated Henrician expectations surrounding counsel-giving, which emphasized the virtue of both counsellor and monarch.

Commentary on counsel in the reign of the final Tudor monarch, Elizabeth I, contains far less consensus and remains more of a developing field than that which examines her father's reign. Generally, however, and as one might expect, it has focused on the issue of gender. Anne McLaren, in particular, has drawn attention to the way in which Elizabeth's gender, combined with humanist expectations regarding counsel, generated the need for a strong mixed monarchy and 'queen-in-parliament' model of rule.[18] Natalie Mears, contrastingly, focuses on the personal, rather than institutional, relationships and mechanisms of counsel,[19] and recently Susan Doran has argued against the widely held belief that Elizabeth and her counsellors were constantly at opposition, fighting over the reins of power.[20] None of these accounts takes seriously the context of Machiavellianism and the development of Reason of State under Elizabeth I.[21] This chapter attempts to remedy this omission, by focusing on changes in discussions and vocabularies in the discourse of counsel in the Elizabethan period in comparison with those that had existed previously.

Changing discourses of counsel

By the early modern period, political counsel had been a part of European political thinking since its earliest days in ancient Greece and was an essential part of medieval political discourse.[22] Medieval theory had placed the responsibility of giving counsel into the hands of the politically disengaged philosopher – Aristotle serving as the model[23] – as well as the political right of the noble class, as a means of ensuring that they were given a voice in the decisions of the state.[24] When this right was not respected, monarchs could be justifiably overthrown, as was the case with Richard II – Richard the 'redeless' (or adviceless) – in England in 1399.[25]

With the spread of Renaissance humanism, philosopher was combined with courtier in crafting a new kind of counsellor who tempered truthful advice with an awareness of circumstance, as evidenced in Baldassare Castiglione's *Book of the Courtier* (1528). Such a courtier-counsellor ought to combine 'knoweleage of the truth' with 'Courtliness' so 'In the wise maye he leade [the prince], throughe the toughe way of vertue (as it were) deckynge yt aout with boowes to shadowe yt and strawinge it over wyth sightlye flouers'.[26] A similar sentiment is expressed in Thomas More's *Utopia* (1516), through the character of Morus, who recommends an 'indirect approach' and a 'more civil philosophy' (*philosophia ciuilior*)[27] 'that takes its cue, adapts itself to the drama in hand and acts its part neatly and appropriately' or '*cum decoro*'.[28]

By the middle of the sixteenth century, however, such a figure became the object of deep suspicion. The reason was the rise of Machiavellianism – a political perspective based on, though not always faithful to, the writings of Niccolò Machiavelli, primarily *The Prince* (written 1513, published posthumously 1532). Machiavelli reversed the humanist model of counsel in which the prince is 'led' or 'instructed' by the prudence of his counsellor(s), instead suggesting that the prince's prudence determines the wisdom of his council.[29] Rhetoric, the tool of the humanist counsellor, was especially distrusted for its ability to 'move' or manipulate the emotions of the hearer, because in such a case, who truly ruled: prince or counsellor? For this reason, the middle of the century onwards saw an increase in the recommendation of books of history as counsellors (or counsellors who simply related the lessons of such books). Hence the popular maxim 'the best counsellors are the dead' for 'the penne is of a more free condition then the tongue'.[30]

In the later sixteenth century the rise of Reason of State literature, a phenomenon first described in print by Giovanni Botero in 1589, meant that the attention shifted to the 'observations' of neighbouring states – their geographical positions, policies and 'interests' – with the aim of advancing one's own state interest over that of the others.[31] It was, in short, a far cry from the virtuous courtiers of the humanist tradition and begins to look much more like the realist political 'science' of the modern period.

These tendencies were seen across Europe, but were especially felt in England where the discourse of counsel took on a particular importance.[32] As has been noted, from the end of the Wars of Roses to the English Civil War, counsel was such a fundamental part of English political discourse that the regime has been identified as a 'monarchy of counsel'.[33] This is, of course, a contradiction in terms, as many throughout the sixteenth century realized, revealing the 'paradox of counsel' which defined relations between counsel and command in the period. If the counsellor, as in the humanist tradition, in fact knew better than the monarch, and led or governed him or her, then what was the role of a monarch at all? How could a monarch be truly said to be ruling?

These questions were latent during the reigns of Henry VII and Henry VIII.[34] The 'tragedy of counsel' in this period encompassed not worries surrounding an overly powerful counsellor, but rather increasing absolutism in the person of the monarch. Thus much of the literature struggled with how both to speak truth to a monarch (*parrhesia*) and keep one's head; a topic epitomized by both the writing and career of Thomas More, and known as the 'problem of counsel'.

It is with the death of Henry VIII and the reign of his son, Edward VI, that attention and power shifts clearly onto the figure of the counsellor in the English court, along with a substantial level of suspicion. Importantly, this moment coincides with the growth in the Machiavellian conciliar discourse noted earlier. Machiavelli's work circulated Europe, including in England, from the 1520s. In fact, of the small number of examples of articulated responses to Machiavelli in the first half of the sixteenth century, most address an English context, and the first attempts to apply his theories to political analysis were by English writers.[35]

This convergence of changed political reality – a minor on the throne, who was followed by two queens regnant – with changes in political discourse drew further attention to the role of the counsellor, though seldom in a positive way. Both minors and women were considered to be more easily influenced by adult male counsellors (as they lacked the prudence and rationality to rule over their counsellors or know good counsel from bad).[36] At the same time, the prevalence of Machiavellian thought increased the perception of counsellors as self-interested Machiavels who would all too willingly take advantage of such inferior rulers.[37]

Queen Elizabeth I and Reason of State

It was not just Elizabeth's gender which prompted significant changes to the means, content and significance of counsel during her reign, but also the confluence of factors, noted earlier, that dramatically altered the discourse of counsel in this period.[38] Counsel in the reign of Elizabeth I became more 'practical' and outright, aiming at the preservation of the state, and less concerned with the virtue of monarch or subjects. Elizabethan counsellors were required by the expectations of the time to adapt to the goals and vocabularies of Reason of State as its primary agents.

Reason of State, as an idea, is notoriously difficult to pin down, which is why it seldom appears in scholarship on Elizabeth's reign.[39] Reason of State, put succinctly, refers to the prioritization of the good, or 'interest', of the state, as well as the means to procure that end. As Botero defines it, it is 'the knowledge [*notitia*]' of such means by which a state, a 'firm rule over a people', may be 'found[ed], conserve[d] and expand[ed]'.[40] Often it appears as the knowledge required to manage the state towards these ends in the absence of the laws and in extraordinary circumstances.[41] It was this element especially which linked it to the role of the counsellor, who was often seen as the actor to provide guidance in circumstances which the laws did not cover, or in which they had to be contravened.[42] In particular, this was often couched in the language of 'necessity' and 'occasion', the recognition that the good of the state required, in such emergency conditions, immoral or even unlawful action.[43] It was the counsellors' job to recognize these exceptional moments and act accordingly.[44] These ideas defined the discourse of counsel under Elizabeth in ways hitherto little explored.

From sixteenth-century accounts, we can pick out two distinct Reason of State traditions: 'Machiavellian' and 'Jesuit'.[45] The first develops from the spread of Machiavellian ideas from the 1530s onwards.[46] Central to Machiavellianism was the dissociation of *utile* and *honestum* – profit and honesty, often thought of as 'policy' and religion.[47] A Machiavellian account accepted that the good of the state (or the prince) might be achieved through immoral or irreligious means, overturning the Ciceronian acceptance that morality and expediency went hand-in-hand.[48] For instance, in the 1571 *Treatise of Treasons*, 'a Machiauellian State & Regime[n]t' is 'where Religion is put behind in the seco[n]d & last place: wher y^t ciuil Policie . . . is preferred before it'.[49] Botero agrees, suggesting that Machiavelli 'bases his Reason of State on lack of conscience'.[50]

The second, 'Jesuit', tradition seeks to oppose this Machiavellian discourse, advancing a 'true' Reason of State, which re-establishes the relationship between *utile* and *honestum* – policy and religion – while retaining much of the vocabulary and framework of a Machiavellian account. This is the intention of the fallen Jesuit, Giovanni Botero, in the *Della Ragione di Stato* (1589), and is repeated in the work of the English priest and (after 1614) Jesuit, Thomas Fitzherbert, who seeks to compose 'some discourse concerning the necessarie concurrence of the reason of state with conscience and religion'.[51] We might also turn to Fitzherbert's 'friend and mentor' and fellow Jesuit, Robert Persons (or Parsons), whose 1593 *Newes from Spayne and Holland* criticizes the 'councelles' of Lord Burghley for being lacking in 'iustice or co[n]science' as well as in 'humane wisdome and pollycy set downe by Machauel him selfe'.[52] Persons demonstrates that it is 'a great ouersight in reason of state' for Elizabeth to have made 'so vniuersal a change of religion' by once again rejecting the Catholic religion.[53] For Persons, Reason of State would have been aligned with God's will in steering Elizabeth to the restoration of the Catholic religion. Because they sought to oppose Machiavellian Reason of State in its own terms, these writers accepted some of its fundamental ideas. This significantly shifted expectations regarding how political counsel was given and received, and what it ought to contain.

The phrase 'Reason of State' appears seldom in Elizabethan political writing, despite Botero's assertions that Reason of State is 'mention[ed] nearly every day' in the 'courts of kings and great princes'.[54] Given its immoral and irreligious associations, we may not be surprised.[55] There are notable examples, however, which run counter to the prominent suggestion that it only permeates English political discourse in the mid-seventeenth century.[56] In a letter ascribed to Francis Bacon from the 1580s, the author suggests that the queen ought to determine 'in all reason of state' what to do about the Catholics, who threaten her rule, noting he does not see how 'either in conscience' or 'in policy' she will be able to make them content.[57] The Privy Council itself in 1601 judges a matter to do with the Lord Mayer 'according to the reason of state and good government'.[58] In short, by the end of Elizabeth's reign, Reason of State is present not only in published writings, such as those of Persons, but has entered into quotidian political parlance as well, albeit rarely.

More important than the term, however, are vocabularies and modes of political thinking associated with this new political discourse. Central to both Machiavellian and Jesuit Reason of State traditions was the emphasis on 'relations' or (later) 'observations': accounts of the 'situations' and affairs of other states.[59] Such information provides the foundation for the politic scheming essential to working out how to secure the interest of one's own state. Botero's *Relationi Universali*, first published two years after his *Ragione* (1591–6) was an almanac of sorts, detailing the state of universal relations between states. There was no contemporary English translation of the *Ragione*, but the *Relationi* went through seven print editions between 1601 and 1630, each time altered and updated to align with changing political realities and the interests of the translator.[60]

Even before Botero, counsellors inspired by Machiavelli had begun to compile precisely these sorts of accounts. For instance, William Thomas's advice to Edward VI, composed sometime in late 1551, was heavily inspired by Machiavelli; when Edward can 'not plaie the Lyon' – i.e. use overt force – Thomas tells him that 'it [is] no shame to plaie the Foxe' or, in other words, to 'worke by policie'.[61] 'Policie', Thomas suggests, 'is no vice' and is unavoidable in 'these daies' when princes commonly employ such tactics. In another short piece by Thomas, 'My private opinion tooching your Ma[ies]^ties outward affaires at this present', he gives detailed accounts of England's relations with various European nations, and the motives each nation has for various paths of action.[62] Robert Beale composes a similar account in his *Treatise of the Office of a Councellor and principal Secretarie to her Ma[jes]tie*, written in 1592. There, he recommends Thomas Smith's *De Republica Anglorum* for understanding 'the State of the whole Realme' (though in it 'ther be many defects').[63] This is not enough, however, and a secretary must also 'obtaine by dilligent readinge and observac[i]on of the histories of all Countryes' an understanding of the relationship between England and the nations with which it has dealings.[64] In this, Beale is more detailed, because 'I would wish you to followe another course w[i]th them than hath beene of maie yeares heretofore used.'[65] Some have even 'despised' this knowledge, so that the queen is 'not duelie informed how thinges passe, nor hath anye of her subiects so acquainted w[i]th forraine affaires as is fitt for her Ma[jes]tie's service'.[66] The remedy? The secretary ought to have on hand 'your Italian *Relationi*', Botero's text, which 'may stande you in some steede for the knowledge of forraigne Estates'.[67]

Beale's specific advice about affairs with other nations is rife with the language of Reason of State. In particular, Beale suggests – in reference to dealing with the Italians – *cum Cretensibus Cretisandum est*, a phrase that also appears in a letter by Burghley from 1593: *cretisare cum cretensi* or 'to deceive among deceivers', which he says is 'allowable'.[68] The phrase also appears in an earlier 1580 letter to Burghley from Thomas Radcliff, Earl of Sussex, who worries that the French *cretizare cum cretensibus*, assuming that the English are deceiving them. Like Thomas and others, Beale has accepted the necessity of occasional deception, to the end of preserving the state.[69]

Whereas appearances of the phrase 'Reason of State' and references to Botero's *Relationi*, or writings like it, are scattered, the language of 'necessity', 'occasion' and 'temporizing' is ubiquitous. These ideas, it should be said, were not new in the mid-sixteenth century. The vocabulary of occasion complete with its immoral and exceptional associations comes from the ancient concept, *kairos*, or 'the opportune moment', which had appeared in the works of various classical thinkers, including Plato, Isocrates and Plutarch, and was revived in the Renaissance.[70] The idea that such opportune moments must not be 'let slip', or else the state would face dangerous threats, appears in political discourse of the fifteenth century and early sixteenth centuries, but by the mid-sixteenth century had acquired an air of greater deception and urgency, as well as appearing more frequently. In 1549, under the reign of the young Edward VI, William Paget especially connected such language to the role of counsellors, telling Thomas Smith that 'Wherefore whenne princes be in saden [sudden] heates, and specially without certaine ground, we Secretaries must temporise the matter w^t termes convenient.'[71]

By the reign of Elizabeth, this language was pervasive. John Challoner writes to William Cecil twice in November 1559, urging him to remind the queen not to lose the 'occasion' and that 'It is good to remember that occasion serves not alwaye.'[72] It is important, these letters make clear, to take advantage of opportunity when England has it, before it shifts to England's enemies; as Ambrose Dudley, Earl of Warwick and Amias Poulet, ambassador to France, write to Robert Dudley and Cecil in 1563, 'leaving the good occasion p[re]sently offered, [Elizabeth] wold seme to kepe peace towards theym w^{ho} will not faile to make her as extreme . . . warre as they can[n] devise as sone as they shall se the tyme off [sic] advantage'.[73] Poulet writes again to Burghley in 1578, hoping that the queen is aware of this temporizing game:

> I hope her ma[jes]tie is to well acquainted w[i]th the Spaniarde to be abused w[i]th his Rhethoricke, and yt behoveth us to knowe that the loss of a daye is of greate moment in these actions. The Spaniarde knoweth yt, and therefore sekyth to wynne tyme by all meanes possible, and when his turne is served, he maye p[er]chance turne his flatteries into threatenings.[74]

Elizabeth will never escape the 'malice and cruelty' of the Spanish unless she 'make her profytt of gudde blessings, I meane [inserted: of] the tyme when it serveth, and of occasions when they are profered'.[75]

There also exists, however, a recognition that these games of opportunity are not enough. In regard to Elizabeth's opposition to Anjou over the lordship of the Low Countries, in which she had asked her ambassadors to use 'delays' against Anjou until English forces arrive, Thomas Wilson writes that 'Temporysinge hath been thought heretofore good policie', but 'There was never so da[n]gorouse a tyme as this is, and temporizinge wil no longer serue'.[76] Instead, he is glad to see that Elizabeth is now considering 'preventi[n]g against da[n]ger to be feared'.[77] In particular, this pre-vention needed to be taken against those who would seize their own opportunities against the English crown.

This language of emergency and pre-emption is clearest in the discussion of what is to be done about Mary, Queen of Scots. In 1572, reasons were laid out in the House of Commons why Elizabeth was 'bound in Conscience to proceed with Severity' against Mary, which urged Elizabeth that a new law would not be enough, as 'no Law hath any force with her' as she is 'fully minded to take her advantage upon any apt occasion offered'.[78] The willingness to seize occasion, regardless of morality and law, means these are not enough to bind someone; extra-legal measures must be embraced. In a 1587 document titled 'A discourse plainlie proveinge that as well the sentence of death latelie given against that unfortunate ladie Marie late Queene of Scotts as also the execution of the same sentence were honourable just necessarie and lawfull', the author stresses that the spread of the 'disease' presented by the threat of Mary became 'dailie more and more desperate' and so there could be no longer any 'delay'.[79] For Elizabeth's part, the author suggests she wishes 'the occasion had never bene given' to overcome Mary, and that 'the regarde of state' (a rendering of Reason of State) 'and regall administration were not so great and obligatory . . . as in troth they be'.[80] Princes, he makes clear, follow different rules than do private individuals, for they are bound by 'their office and dutie of administration' and the 'Case of the Commonwealth', in which they are guided by 'all the wiser Iudgements of the Realme and the three estates assembled in full Parliament'.[81] Every other prince, he maintains would have done the same, with 'the oportunitie so well serving for that purpose', 'even when no necessitie of the state or p[er]ill of the Prince of that dominion inforced, as nowe it did'.[82]

Elizabeth's decision was 'expedient in all good pollicy' and her reputation would have suffered had she done otherwise, for 'all great Princes and governors are then thought wisest and most worthie of their Administration when they be vigilant and lett not slipp any good and honest advantage offered them'.[83] In fact, he goes on, Elizabeth, by 'exacte pollicie' might even be expected to seek the life of the young King James VI, but 'as a most *Christian* and vertuous Princesse utterly detesteth all such manner of Pollicie, and houldeth it in great horror and abhomination and all those that would p[re]sume to give her any such advice'.[84]

The author argues that Elizabeth *did* proceed according to the law, and with the consent of parliament, though also suggests that she acted according to the 'universall Consent and uniformitie of mans opinion and will', which 'thoughe it be not properlie a iustifying lawe' it is not 'altogether not a lawe', namely 'rather to kill than be killed'.[85] And another, that 'the greater good is p[re]ferred befor the smaller, the generall before the speciall and the Cases of necessitie before those that be ^not^ necessary'.[86] In short, Elizabeth, the author maintains, did act according to the law and expectations of honour, but she *also* acted in line with the expectations of Reason of State; this alone would have been enough to justify her actions, and indeed, worse ones.

The backdrop of Reason of State rendered Elizabeth's perceived ability – already limited by gender – to judge good counsel from bad more suspect, and thus increased the apparent power of the counsellor to benefit or destroy the realm. In response, Elizabeth used delay as a political tool against the demands of her counsellors, whose emphasis on seizing occasion often proceeded from frustration at Elizabeth's irresolution. In a political culture where her gender could give her the appearance of weakness in contrast to her male counsellors, Elizabeth used her own temporizing strategies to maintain power and control.

Conclusion

Elizabeth's gender was certainly important in shaping the political culture of her reign, but there were other influences determining the nature of the discourse of counsel in the latter half of the sixteenth century. Reason of State introduced a new political language, as well as a new way of thinking about politics built on moral flexibility, the emphasis on inter-state relations and an awareness of opportunity, temporizing and necessity, even exceptionalism. This fundamentally altered the role of the counsellor and the content of political counsel in this period, with important implications for early modern political authority.

England saw a shift in councilliar strategies not only because of the rule of one minor and two women but also due in part to continental influences. The analysis of Elizabethan counsel offers a contribution to existing literature, by showing that Reason of State vocabularies were pervasive in Elizabethan politics. By the end of the sixteenth century, counsel had shifted from a rhetorical practice aimed at the achievement of virtue, to apparently straightforward (though sometimes still deceptively rhetorical) practical advice regarding the state 'interests'.

Notes

1 See Thomas More, *Utopia*, eds. George M. Logan and Robert M. Adams (Cambridge: Cambridge University Press, 1989), 13–37; Thomas Elyot, *The Book Named the Governor*, ed. S.E. Lehmberg (New York: Everyman's Library, 1962), 13, 108, 236–241; Francis Bacon, *Essaies* (London, 1612), 56–69.

2 For Henry VIII see below. See Christopher Haigh, *Elizabeth I* (London: Routledge, 2001), 200. Elizabeth's approach to receiving counsel is also evidenced in the history described by Raphael Holinshed, *The First Volume of the Chronicles of England, Scotlande, and Ireland* (London, 1577), 1777.

3 This was often accomplished through performance, see Greg Walker, *The Politics of Performance in Early Renaissance Drama* (Cambridge: Cambridge University Press, 1998), 67; W.R. Streitberger, *The Masters of the Revels and Elizabeth I's Court Theatre* (Oxford: Oxford University Press, 2016), 17, 78, 172; see also a number of contributions in the volume Jayne Elizabeth Archer, Elizabeth Goldring and Sarah Knight, eds., *The Progresses, Pageants, and Entertainments of Queen Elizabeth I* (Oxford: Oxford University Press, 2007), 4, 86, 90, 92, 99, 101–102.

4 For the 'monarchy of counsel' see J.G.A. Pocock, "A Discourse of Sovereignty: Observations on the Work in Progress," in *Political Discourse in Early Modern Britain*, eds. Nicholas Phillipson and Quentin Skinner (Cambridge: Cambridge University Press, 1993), 396.

5 These categories are not without their problems. To juxtapose the 'humanist' and 'Machiavellian' perspectives on counsel seems to overlook the fact that Machiavelli, too, was a humanist. In addition, the 'Machiavellian' discourse of counsel often had very little to do with Machiavelli's own views. However, these titles are the best available to refer to these traditions and thus will be adopted throughout this chapter. More will be said about the definition of Reason of State in what follows.

6 John Watts, "Counsel and the King's Council in England, c.1340–c.1540," in *The Politics of Counsel in England and Scotland, 1286–1707*, ed. Jacqueline Rose (Oxford: Oxford University Press, 2017), 63. The 'problem of counsel' was the subject of a number of studies in the 1950s–1970s. See Arthur B. Ferguson, "The Problem of Counsel in Mum and the Sothsegger," *Studies in the Renaissance* 2 (1955): 67–83; Stanford E. Lehmberg, "English Humanists, the Reformation, and the Problem of Counsel," *Archiv Für Reformationsgeschichte - Archive for Reformation History* 52 (1961): 74–91; J.H. Hexter, "Thomas More and the Problem of Counsel," in *Quincentennial Essays on St. Thomas More: Selected Papers from the Thomas More College Conference* (Boone: Albion, 1978), 55–66. For more on the 'new political history' of Tudor England, see John Guy, *Tudor Monarchy* (London: Hodder Education Publishers, 1997), 1–8; Stephen Alford, "Politics and Political History in the Tudor Century," *The Historical Journal* 42, no. 2 (1999): 535–548.

7 John Guy, "The Rhetoric of Counsel in Early Modern England," in *Tudor Political Culture*, ed. Dale Hoak (Cambridge: Cambridge University Press, 1995), 292–310.

8 Jacqueline Rose, "Kingship and Counsel in Early Modern England," *The Historical Journal* 54, no. 1 (2011): 47–71.

9 Peter Holmes, "The Great Council in the Reign of Henry VII," *The English Historical Review* 101, no. 401 (1986): 840–862; Stephen Gunn, *Henry VII's New Men and the Making of Tudor England* (Oxford: Oxford University Press, 2016).

10 Stephen Alford, *Kingship and Politics in the Reign of Edward VI* (Cambridge: Cambridge University Press, 2004), 46–48, 63–64; Joanne Paul, "Sovereign Council or Counseled Sovereign: The Marian Conciliar Compromise," in *The Birth of a Queen: Essays on the Quincentenary of Mary I*, eds. Sarah Duncan and Valerie Schutte (New York: Palgrave, 2016), 135–153.

11 J.H. Hexter, "Thomas More and the Problem of Counsel," in *Quincentennial Essays on St. Thomas More: Selected Papers from the Thomas More College Conference* (Boone: Albion, 1978), 55–66; Ivan Lupic, "Subjects of Advice: Drama and Counsel from More to Shakespeare" (PhD dissertation, Columbia University, 2014).

12 F.W. Conrad, "A Preservative Against Tyranny: Sir Thomas Elyot and the Rhetoric of Counsel," in *Reformation, Humanism, and 'Revolution': Papers Presented at the Folger Institute Seminar 'Political Thought in the Henrician Age, 1500–1550'*, ed. Gordon J. Schochet (Washington, DC: The Folger Institute, 1990), 191–206; F.W. Conrad, "The Problem of Counsel Reconsidered: The Case of Sir Thomas Elyot," in *Political Thought and the Tudor Commonwealth: Deep Structure, Discourse and Disguise*, eds. Paul Fideler and Thomas Mayer (London: Routledge, 2003), 77–110; Arthur Walzer, "Rhetoric of Counsel in Thomas Elyot's Pasquil the Playne," *Rhetorica: A Journal of the History of Rhetoric* 30, no. 1 (2012): 1–21; Arthur E. Walzer, "The Rhetoric of Counsel and Thomas Elyot's Of the Knowledge Which Maketh a Wise Man," *Philosophy and Rhetoric* 45, no. 1 (2012): 24–45.

13 Thomas F. Mayer, "Thomas Starkey, an Unknown Conciliarist at the Court of Henry VIII," *Journal of the History of Ideas* 49, no. 2 (1988): 207–227; Thomas F. Mayer, "Faction and Ideology: Thomas Starkey's Dialogue," *The Historical Journal* 28, no. 1 (1985): 1–25.

14 G.R. Elton, *The Tudor Revolution in Government* (Cambridge; Cambridge University Press, 1953), 316–369.

15 Greg Walker, *Writing Under Tyranny: English Literature and the Henrician Reformation* (Oxford: Oxford University Press, 2007); Greg Walker, *Plays of Persuasion: Drama and Politics at the Court of Henry VIII* (Cambridge: Cambridge University Press, 2009).

16 John Guy, "The Rhetoric of Counsel in Early Modern England," in *Tudor Political Culture*, ed. Dale Hoak (Cambridge: Cambridge University Press, 1995), 292–310; John Guy, "Ideas of Counsel Under Henry VIII: The Tudors," www.tudors.org/undergraduate/ideas-of-counsel-under-henry-viii/ (accessed 25 October 2017).

17 Richard Rex, "Councils, Counsel and Consensus in Henry VIII's Reformation," in *The Politics of Counsel in England and Scotland, 1286–1707* (Oxford: British Academy, 2016).

18 A.N. McLaren, *Political Culture Reign Elizabeth I: Queen and Commonwealth 1558–1585* (Cambridge: Cambridge University Press, 2004).

19 Natalie Mears, *Queenship and Political Discourse in the Elizabethan Realms* (Cambridge: Cambridge University Press, 2005).

20 Susan Doran, "Elizabeth I and Counsel," in *The Politics of Counsel in England and Scotland, 1286–1707*, ed. Jacqueline Rose (Oxford: Oxford University Press, 2017), 151–161.

21 The exception to this is Peter Lake, *Bad Queen Bess? Libels, Secret Histories, and the Politics of Publicity in the Reign of Queen Elizabeth I* (Oxford: Oxford University Press, 2016) which examines charges of Machiavellianism in a variety of Elizabethan libels and pamphlets.

22 This summary is also given in Helen Matheson-Pollock, Joanne Paul and Catherine Fletcher, introduction to *Queenship and Counsel in Early Modern Europe* (Cham: Palgrave Macmillan, 2018), i–xiv. For a more detailed account of the changing discourse of counsel in the early modern period, see Joanne Paul, "Counsel and Command in Anglophone Political Thought, 1485–1651" (PhD dissertation, Queen Mary University of London, 2013) and Joanne Paul, *Counsel and Command in Early Modern English Thought* (Cambridge: Cambridge University Press, forthcoming)..

23 Best evidenced by the immensely popular *Secretum Secretorum*; see M.A. Manzalaoui, ed., *Secretum Secretorum: Nine English Versions* (Oxford: Oxford University Press, 1977), ix and Steven J. Williams, *The Secret of Secrets: The Scholarly Career of a Pseudo-Aristotelian Text in the Latin Middle Ages* (Ann Arbor: University of Michigan Press, 2003), 10–28.

24 See Guy, "The Rhetoric of Counsel in Early Modern England," 292–310.

25 James M. Dean, ed., *Richard the Redeless and Mum and the Sothseggar* (Kalamazoo: Medieval Institute Publications, 2000).

26 Baldassare Castiglione, *The Book of the Courtier*, trans. Thomas Hoby, ed. Virginia Cox (London: Everyman, 1994), 338, 299. Notably, Castiglione still holds Aristotle (as well as Plato) to be an example of such a counsellor. They both 'practiced the deedes of Courtiershippe and gave them selves to this ende, the one with the great Alexander, the other with the kynges of Sicilia' (337). This is opposed to Calisthenes, 'who bicause he was a right philosopher and so sharpe a minister of the bare truth without mynglinge it with Courtlinesse, he lost his lief and profited not, but rather gave a scaundler to Alexander' (338).

27 My translation from Thomas More, *Utopia*, trans. and eds. Edward Surtz and J.H. Hexter (New Haven: Yale University Press, 1965), 99.

28 More, *Utopia*, 34–35.

29 Niccolò Machiavelli, *The Prince*, eds. Quentin Skinner and Russell Price (Cambridge: Cambridge University Press, 1988), 82.

30 Matthew Coignet, *Politique discourses upon trueth and lying*, trans. Edward Hoby (London, 1586), 69–70. See Joanne Paul, "The Best Counsellors are the Dead: Counsel and Shakespeare's *Hamlet*," *Renaissance Studies* 30, no. 5 (2016): 646–665.

31 Giovanni Botero, *Botero: The Reason of State*, ed. Robert Bireley (Cambridge: Cambridge University Press, 2017). More detail about this literature is given in what follows.

32 See Guy, "The Rhetoric of Counsel," 292–310; David Colclough, "'Parrhesia': The Rhetoric of Free Speech in Early Modern England," *Rhetorica* 17, no. 2 (1999): 177–212; Jacqueline Rose, "Kingship and Counsel in Early Modern England," *The Historical Journal* 54, no. 1 (2011): 47–71; Janet Coleman, "A Culture of Political Counsel: The Case of Fourteenth-Century England's 'Virtuous' Monarchy vs Royal Absolutism and Seventeenth-Century Reinterpretations," in *Monarchy and Absolutism in Early Modern Europe*, eds. Cesare Cuttica and Glenn Burgess (London: Pickering and Chatto, 2012), 19–31.

33 Pocock, "A Discourse of Sovereignty," 396.

34 In the case of a counsellor like Cardinal Wolsey, the fears surrounding his rise had less to do with the persuasive power of his rhetoric and more to do with his increasing direct political control.

35 Sydney Anglo, *Machiavelli: The First Century – Studies in Enthusiasm, Hostility and Tudor Politics in the Sixteenth Century* (Oxford: Oxford University Press, 2005), 102.

36 For women's perceived lack of prudence, see Leah Bradshaw, "Political Rule, Prudence and the 'Woman Question' in Aristotle," *Canadian Journal of Political Science* 24, no. 3 (1991): 563–570. Partly, this was because they could not possibly have the political experience requisite for such a virtue – women ended up excluded from politics because they had been excluded from politics – but it also had to do with a long-standing tradition of seeing women's advice on many matters as irrational, self-interested and dangerous. For a contemporary commentary on women's inability to engage with political counsel, see John Knox, *The First Blast of the Trumpet Against the Monstruous Regiment of Women* (Geneva: J. Poullain and A. Rebul, 1558), 9–10. See also Misty Schieberle, *Feminized Counsel and the Literature of Advice in England, 1380–1500* (Turnhout: Brepolis, 2014).

37 See, for instance, *Treatise of Treasons* (Antwerp, 1572), fos. 86ᵛ, 86ʳ; John Stubbe, *Gaping Gulf*, ed. Lloyd E. Berry (Charlottesville: University Press of Virginia, 1986), 12; *Leicester's Commonwealth*, ed. D.C. Peck (Athens: Ohio University Press 1985), 132, 154.

38 As described earlier.

39 See Thomas M. Poole, *Reason of State: Law, Prerogative and Empire* (Cambridge: Cambridge University Press, 2015), 2–3 for the various meanings of Reason of State across time and space. Notably, although he acknowledges its influence from the death of Machiavelli, his study begins in roughly 1650. Alessandro Arienzo, "From Machiavellian Policy to Parliamentary Reason of State: Sketches in Early Stuart Political Culture," in *Machiavellian Encounters in Tudor and Stuart England: Literary and Political Influences from the Reformation to the Restoration*, eds. Alessandro Arienzo and Alessandra Petrina (London: Routledge, 2013), ebook, focuses largely on Reason of State in the seventeenth century. Alexandra Gadja, "Tacitus and Political Thought in Early Modern Europe, c. 1530–c. 1640," *The Cambridge Companion to Tacitus*, ed. A.J. Woodman (Cambridge: Cambridge University

Press, 2009), 266, claims that 'there was no strong native equivalent of Continental "reason of state" literature'. For the origins of the term, see Conal Condren, "Reason of State and Sovereignty in Early Modern England: A Question of Ideology?" *Parergon* 28, no. 2 (2011): 13; he too has little to say about Elizabethan politics and Reason of State.

40 Botero, *Botero: The Reason of State*, 4, see fn. 2.

41 David Tucker, *The End of Intelligence: Espionage and State Power in the Information Age* (Stanford: Stanford University Press, 2014), 27; Poole, *Reason of State*, 3–4; see also Maurizio Viroli, *From Politics to Reason of State: The Acquisition and Transformation of the Language of Politics, 1250–1600* (Cambridge: Cambridge University Press, 1992), 240–241.

42 As Viroli, *From Politics to Reason of State*, 241 points out, within Reason of State logic, the only universal rule is to rely on experienced counsellors who can advise on specific circumstances (and to rule justly).

43 See Viroli, *From Politics to Reason of State*, 249; Condren, "Reason of State," 14.

44 Paul, "Counsel and Command," 120–121, 131–133, 143, 145–146, 280–312.

45 This distinction between the two traditions is my own, though Arienzo, "From Machiavellian Policy," points out that, in contrast to Machiavellianism, Reason of State *could* have a positive meaning 'distinguished from a false Machiavellian *practice*', thus allowing for the possibility of two different kinds of Reason of State: one negative and Machiavellian, the other positive and anti-Machiavellian.

46 It is also, notably, associated with Tacitus. Work has been done on the influence of Tacitus on Elizabethan thought and politics, though not always with reference to Reason of State. See John Guy, *The Reign of Elizabeth I: Court and Culture in the Last Decade* (Cambridge: Cambridge University Press, 1995), 15–16; Gadja, "Tacitus and Political Thought," 266–267; Susan Doran, *Elizabeth I and Her Circle* (Oxford: Oxford University Press, 2015), 303–308.

47 Arienzo, "From Machiavellian Policy," ebook.

48 See *Treatise of Treaons* (Antwerp, 1572), sig. a5^r.

49 [Leslie] 1572, sig. a5^r. The book is anonymous, but is usually attributed to John Leslie, Bishop of Ross; see Ethan H. Shagan, *Catholics and the 'Protestant Nation': Religious Politics and Identity in Early Modern England* (Manchester: Manchester University Press, 2005), 77.

50 Botero, *Botero: The Reason of State*, 1. Of course, much of this is actually a misreading of Machiavelli's own work, but it is consistent with how it was read in the sixteenth century.

51 Thomas Fitzherbert, *The First Part of a Treatise Concerning Policy, and Religion* (London, 1606), 36. See also Robert Persons, *Newes from Spayne and Holland* (London, 1593), 22 and Benjamin Carier, *A Treatise* (London, 1614), 30, 32.

52 Persons, *Newes from Spayne*, 22; see Höpfl, Harro, "Thomas Fitzherbert's Reason of State," *History of European Ideas* 37, no. 2 (2011): 94–101.

53 Persons, *Newes from Spayne*, 22. The later Catholic writer Benjamin Carier disagrees in his *Treatise* (1614), suggesting that 'it were necessary in reason of State' for Elizabeth to 'continue the Doctrine of Diuision' with Rome (as the daughter of Henry VIII and Anne Boleyn) (32). Reason of State and the true religion were, for a short time, indeed at odds. However, this no longer applies under James I, so Carier finds that Reason of State and the Catholic religion are realigned in his reign: he 'doe finde as little cause of holding out in reason of State, as I doe in truth of Doctrine' (30).

54 Botero, *Botero: The Reason of State*, 1; see Condren, "Reason of State," 17–18.

55 Viroli, *From Politics to Reason of State*, 252.

56 See fn. 39 above.

57 [Francis Bacon?], '[Letter of Advice to Queen Elizabeth I]' in *The Letters and Life of Francis Bacon*, ed. James Spedding (London: Longman, Green, Longman, and Roberts, 1861), 47, 48. On Bacon and Reason of State, see Vera Keller, "Mining Tacitus: Secrets of Empire, Nature and Art in the Reason of State," *British Journal for the History of Science* 45, no. 2 (2012): 189–212.

58 PC 2/26 f.493, 1601.

59 See Arienzo, "From Machiavellian Policy," ebook; Keller, "Mining Tacitus," 192.

60 See Joanne Paul and Kurosh Meshkat, "Johnson's *Relations*: Visions of Global Order, 1601–1630," *Journal of Intellectual History and Political Thought* 1, no. 1 (2013): 108–140.

61 Thomas, William, *The Works of William Thomas*, ed. Abraham D'Aubant (London: J. Almon, 1774), 136.

62 Ibid., 179–192.
63 Robert Beale, "A Treatise of the Office of a Councellor and principal Secretarie to her Ma[ies]tie," in *Mr Secretary Walsingham and the Policy of Queen Elizabeth*, vol I, ed. Conyers Read (Oxford: Clarendon Press, 1925), 428.
64 Beale, "A Treatise," 433.
65 Beale, "A Treatise," 435.
66 Beale, "A Treatise," 435.
67 Beale, "A Treatise," 435.
68 Beale, "A Treatise," 434; Bughley to Robert Cecil 1593 in Thomas Wright, "Queen Elizabeth and Her Times: A Series of Original Letters," vol. II (London, 1838), 425. The Epimenides paradox depends on the deception of Cretans and is repeated in St Paul's letter to Titus (1:12). Machiavelli sets out the necessity of deceiving among deceivers in chapter XV of *The Prince*.
69 See Francis Bacon, "Certain Observations Made Upon a Libel Published This Present Year, 1592," in *The Letters and the Life of Francis Bacon*, ed. James Spedding (London: Longman, Green, Longman and Roberts, 1861), 167–170; SP 59/10 f.42, 15 September 1565; SP 84/20 f.28, 7 January 1588.
70 See Joanne Paul, "The Use of Kairos in Renaissance Political Philosophy," *Renaissance Quarterly* 67, no. 1 (2014): 43–78.
71 SP 68/3 f.146^v, 26 June 1549
72 SP 70/8 f.122^v, 10 November 1559; SP 70/8 f.161^r, 23 November 1559.
73 SP 70/52 f.44^r, 3 March 1563.
74 SP 78/2 f.27^r, 2 April 1578.
75 SP 78/2 f.27^r, 2 April 1578.
76 SP 83/8 f.24^r, 9 August 1578.
77 SP 83/8 f.24^r, 9 August 1578.
78 Simonds d'Ewes, "Journal of the House of Commons: May 1572," in *The Journals of All the Parliaments During the Reign of Queen Elizabeth* (Shannon, 1682), 205–221.
79 Cotton Caligula D/I f. 45^v.
80 Cotton Caligula D/I f. 46^{r-v}.
81 Cotton Caligula D/I f. 46^v.
82 Cotton Caligula D/I f. 49^r, 49^v.
83 Cotton Caligula D/I f. 54^v.
84 Cotton Caligula D/I f. 77^r.
85 Cotton Caligula D/I f. 82^v.
86 Cotton Caligula D/I f. 84^r.

Key works

Anglo, Sydney, *Machiavelli: The First Century – Studies in Enthusiasm, Hostility and Tudor Politics in the Sixteenth Century* (Oxford: Oxford University Press. 2005).

Condren, Conal, "Reason of State and Sovereignty in Early Modern England: A Question of Ideology?" *Parergon* 28, no. 2 (2011): 5–27.

Guy, John, "The Rhetoric of Counsel in Early Modern England," in *Tudor Political Culture*, ed. Dale Hoak (Cambridge: Cambridge University Press, 1995), 292–310.

Paul, Joanne, "Sovereign Council or Counseled Sovereign: The Marian Conciliar Compromise," in *The Birth of a Queen: Essays on the Quincentenary of Mary I*, eds. Sarah Duncan and Valerie Schutte (New York: Palgrave, 2016), 135–153.

Rose, Jacqueline, "Kingship and Counsel in Early Modern England," *The Historical Journal* 54, no. 1 (2011): 47–71.

Viroli, Maurizio, *From Politics to Reason of State: The Acquisition and Transformation of the Language of Politics, 1250–1600* (Cambridge: Cambridge University Press, 1992).

35

RULING EMOTIONS

Affective and emotional strategies of power and authority among early modern European monarchies*

Susan Broomhall

This chapter explores how the emerging scholarship of the history of emotions might usefully inform the study of monarchy in the early modern period. Historical analysis regarding power and rule in early modern Europe has fruitfully explored and extended anthropological and sociological frameworks for analysing rituals, material culture and space as cultural and gendered forms of power.[1] More recent work has begun to consider how emotions too define the nature of power in individual expressions and collective formations. After all, authority to rule over another is a social and cultural practice that involves people as individuals and groups in relationships of domination and subordination. Various scholars have offered consideration of the ways emotions channel and become in themselves forms of power. Joanna Bourke, for example, reflects that 'emotions align people with others within social groups, subjecting them to power relations', and Sara Ahmed has explored community alignment and marginalization as the cultural politics of emotion, while Judith Butler has proposed a notion of the 'psychic life of power'.[2] This chapter likewise considers emotions as a critical aspect of the social acts and behaviour that create capacity for domination and subordination, while also recognizing that they are themselves shaped by specific cultural contexts and local understandings of race, faith and gender politics, among other considerations.[3] Furthermore, it proposes that feeling practices not only reflect modes of domination and subordination but that particular kinds of emotional expression can themselves be understood as forms and performances of power (as well as a disruption of these).[4] As such, this chapter asks what emotional expressions and practices could do for those who ruled in the early modern period, as representatives of a system and as individuals.

Analysis of historical emotions in relation to rule requires some precision of terminology. They are not self-evident but must be interpreted in the context, first of the cultures in which they were expressed, and second of the source materials in which they appear. Asking what emotions did or could do does not mean looking in past documents for 'emotion words' recognizable to us. Emotions then as now were rarely experienced or understood as singular and discrete dispositions but as complex, layered events that occurred momentarily or could be sustained for years, and as moods that set a tone for interactions, domination and subordination. Instead, this chapter examines instances in a range of sources where we can discern emotional ideas or behaviours whether purposefully or unconsciously described, and how these were interpreted by contemporaries in emotional terms. The source types available to such an investigation are many and varied, as emotional practices and rhetoric were articulated in words, visual and material culture, and through actions that could be ritualized or unexpected. Emotions could be theorized, assumed, expected, discussed and imagined as well as lived, performed, ritualized, embodied or materialized in particular times and places. Moreover, rule required consideration and regulation of both a monarch's emotions and also those in the wider dynasty, courtiers, administrators, diplomats and the wider populace who were ruled. What follows explores these questions in relation to a range of case studies of western European contexts during the early modern period, to discern patterns and specificities in how emotional expression informed the theory and practice of rule. While this relatively brief summative analysis requires firm boundaries to its exploration, its particular focus is not intended to suggest that such features of emotional expressions and its study operate only at this time; indeed, this seems unlikely. However, the meaning of emotional expression and the sources in which it can be analysed first demand interpretation in precise historical contexts. Future studies across a wider chronology and geography will help to tease out a broader history of the relationship between emotions and rule.

The emotions of statecraft

Emotions were a vital part of political discourse, as has been demonstrated from antiquity to the present.[5] This section explores how, in the early modern period, concepts and practices of love, care and friendship structured rulers' relations with subjects, and with each other, and the nature of the sources in which such expression can be located.

Rule came with paternalistic responsibilities to protect one's people. The 1559 Peace of Cateau-Cambrésis that brought an end to the long-running conflict between the Habsburg and Valois dynasties, which had played out across much of Europe, was justified in the first line of the document as a result of the recognition by Philip II of Spain and Henri II of France of responsibilities to their peoples. God, it explained, had 'touched the hearts of these two great princes' to put an end to their differences 'after so many hard wars . . . from which have resulted great evils, damages and inconveniences to the poor people on both sides . . . for the common good, solace and respite of their people and subjects'.[6] As Helen Watanabe-O'Kelly has recently observed, the contract between subjects and their monarchs entailed dependency, love and also fear. The coronation ceremony held at Westminster Abbey for James VI & I, as King of England, in 1601 spoke of expectations that he 'be feared, and loved of all Men'.[7] Scholars have argued that the expression of some strong emotions – such as anger – articulated the power of authoritative men.[8] However, when monarchs did not perform to collective expectations of rights and justice, the anger of subordinates could be expressed – either as a legitimate response from representatives of the people, or in unsanctioned riots and mob violence. These were calculated, affective responses, often ritualized in particular forms and spaces, which were likewise part of the political process and reciprocal bond founded on emotions between ruler and ruled.[9] Many examples of such emotional negotiation have been analysed at the level of local governments, but the English Civil Wars and French Revolution likewise both saw political protagonists attempting to sunder the emotional contract between subjects and rulers that enabled executions of the latter as monarchs and as individuals.

Treaties between rulers were texts of feelings that voiced friendships or love between brothers and were recorded and visualized as embodied ritual behaviours such as the kiss.[10] Philip and Henri, for example, agreed to a series of conditions that would more firmly secure 'this knot of friendship that the said Princes want to tie together'.[11] These powerful emotions were visualized for both Spanish and French populations in celebratory medals that depicted their clasped hands and in their accompanying devices signalling the 'concord between kings' that set an affective tone in celebration of 'the happiness of the times'.[12] This treaty was further symbolized by Giorgio di Giovanni and circulated to the viewing audience as a physical encounter between two men, and monarchs, locked in a warm embrace (Figure 35.1). This image was displayed in the legal and financial heart of Siena, the Biccherna, one of many territories on the Italian peninsula to be affected by the implications of these changed relations.

Monarchs' corporeal and gestural performances of emotion constituted strategic political actions and were carefully managed. Tears were multivalent fluids with enormous psychic charge. They could variously suggest the piety and mercy of a monarch in relationships with God, family members and subjects.[13] However, they could also be deemed a sign of weakness. The Spanish ambassador Francés de Alavá overheard the French Constable Anne de Montmorency advise the king in his room that he should not cry in public 'because it would be very much noticed by his subjects and foreigners and was very bad for Kings to have tears in their eyes'.[14] For women, tears of sorrow might also help to produce political agency, as they did for Catherine de' Medici, wife of Henri II, as the grieving widow who was required to manage the Valois dynasty legacy as regent for her son Charles IX. Her elaborate emphasis on tears was part of a concerted visual and material grief programme that Catherine introduced after the untimely death of Henri, who had been fatally injured in a jousting accident.[15] Similarly, the austere black habit of the widow could form part of a programme of emotional display through the body that enabled others such as Henrietta Maria, widow of Charles I of England, a strategic retreat from court to the convent in changing political and pecuniary contexts.[16]

The body of the monarch was a persuasive tool of communication, and oratory manuals encouraged rulers to harness the oratory power of their faces and bodies. Antoine Fouquelin, author of *La Rhétorique française* (1555) and tutor to the young Mary, Queen of Scots, warned that the face 'is the image of the mind, and can express all its emotions, cogitations and thoughts' and 'the eyes are indicators of it, the sadness and gaiety of which must be moderated according to the matter in question'.[17] Nonetheless, as Tilman Haug has argued, diplomats believed that provoking strong emotions in others could offer valuable insights.[18] Alavá reported to Philip II that Catherine 'burst into tears, and although she does it easily, truly' when he pressed her for an answer in May 1565 as to whether she intended to meet with an envoy from the Sultan Suleiman I.[19] Ambassadors read these emotional performances through the lens of contemporary assumptions about the bodies of men and

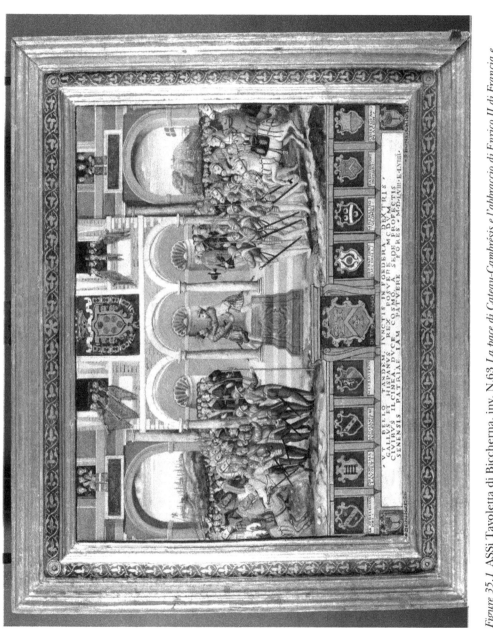

Figure 35.1 ASSi Tavoletta di Biccherna, inv. N.63 *La pace di Cateau-Cambrésis e l'abbraccio di Enrico II di Francia e Filippo II di Spagna* (1559)

women and their suitability (or unsuitability) for political engagement.[20] What Alavá interpreted as Catherine's consternation might well have been the queen mother's tactical delay in providing a response.

More broadly, monarchs set and managed the emotional tone for the court through their leisure activities. Hunting, dancing and games were all regulated by formally structuring feeling among courtiers interacting at close quarters. Catherine de' Medici recommended to her son the works of his grandfather François I:

> [t]wo things were needed to live in peace with the French and to have them love their King: to keep them happy, and to keep them busy at something. To do so, it often required combat on horseback or foot, lance throwing, and . . . other honest pastimes in which he involved himself and had them employed in.[21]

Louis XIV echoed Catherine in his memoirs, intended to instruct the dauphin, in which he explained the importance of lavish festivities in delighting his subjects and shaping their feelings for him.[22] Many kings (and some queens such as Anne of England) engaged in hunting, which encouraged exclusive sociabilities among favoured courtiers. These extended, as in the case of William III of England, not only to those who joined the king on the hunt but through his award of hunting rights to privileged followers, and the building up of royal and elite lands with hunting grounds, parks, kennels and packs as a reflection of such passions.

Moreover, emotions were often the explicit theme of courtly ballets, masques and masquerades, with late medieval and early modern choreography exploring specific emotions in complex and highly intellectual formulations that could be read at several levels. Domenico da Piacenza's fifteenth-century *ballo Gelosia* took jealousy as its central narrative, just as Cesare Negri's later treatise, *Le gratie d'amore* (1602), was an exploration of forms of love.[23] Their complex emotional content likely held different meanings for participants, spectators and those whose access to courtly dance came via printed sources. Thus, feeling rules for individual and communal emotional and social behaviours were embedded in such political leisure pursuits at court. These activities helped to constitute emotional communities of shared feeling displays and practices, which could be particularly important to quell political rivalries and religious differences among elite courtiers. And, while some pastimes risked creating inappropriate emotions, others – chess, literary composition, or embroidery – were understood to promote morality and education in these mixed-sex environments. Chess, for example, was encouraged by a succession of French queens as a mechanism through which to model desirable feeling regimes and to socialize women and men appropriately at court.[24]

Perhaps the ultimate corporeal and emotional engagement of monarchs with the exigencies of statecraft lies in intimate acts of marriage and reproduction. As Tracy Adams has argued, elite marriage was itself a form of affective diplomacy.[25] In 1559, Elisabeth, the eldest daughter of Henri II and Catherine de' Medici, was married to Philip II 'for the further consolidation of this peace and to render the friendship, union and confederation firmer and indissoluble'.[26] Furthermore, the words of the Peace of Cateau-Cambrésis elaborated further on another marriage borne of this agreement. Emanuel Philibert of Savoy, Philip's ally who had routed the French just two years earlier at Saint-Quentin, now 'begged' Henri and wished 'to more firmly establish this reconciliation, affinity and friendship that he seeks and desires of His Majesty' by marrying Henri's sister Marguerite. Indeed, the treaty operated as a more explicit declaration of Emanuel Philibert's feelings for Marguerite than it did for the soon-to-be Spanish royal couple. To have the 'most excellent princess', the treaty continued, Emanuel Philibert would 'be honoured with such a princess that he singularly desires, as much for the proximity of blood that she shares with His Majesty as for the worthy, excellent and rare virtues that are in her'. For his part, Henri was ostensibly gratified 'by the assurance that he had of the honour and good treatment that Madame his sister, whom he loved and was as dear to him as his own daughter, would receive and His Majesty all satisfaction, contentment and perfect friendship' from the union.[27]

The brotherly love expressed in treaties was therefore based in real kinship ties forged through such intermarriages. Such expressions of friendship and family between monarchs provided a useful platform when diplomatic negotiations proved challenging. In the dispute over their shared ambitions to colonize the Florida peninsula, the Spanish king Philip had his ambassador complain to the French king Charles IX, brother of his wife, Elisabeth, that a French colony would not be in keeping with the 'brotherhood' that he had with Charles.[28] Male sociabilities were also created and reinforced among ruling men through gift exchanges that reflected gendered ideas about power and the care and breeding of horses, as an aristocratic male privilege. Kings were regularly depicted on horseback and offered prize horses as gifts to leading men in their network, as did the Danish king, Frederick III, who gifted 'Frederiksborg horses', a special Danish breed.

Sometimes the dead horses of kings were preserved as a sign of affection for the human master who had been lost. For example, when the Swedish king Gustavus Adolphus died in battle in Lützen in 1632 and his mount, Streiff, died shortly after of wounds sustained in the battle, the Oldenberg stallion was returned to Sweden and his skin mounted onto a wooden frame for display in the Swedish Royal Armouries. While Streiff provided a conduit to appropriate expressions of grief for Swedes, another of Gustavus's mounts who had been shot by a cannon ball from under him earlier that year at the battle for Ingolstadt during his unsuccessful siege of the town, became a cipher for rather different feelings. This horse was similarly preserved and exhibited by the townsfolk but as a war trophy and a reminder of the king's failure to capture their town and their community's heroic resistance.

As with the medals struck after the Peace of Cateau-Cambrésis, a range of objects was employed to reflect the monarch's emotions as well as to suggest appropriate feeling states for their subjects. Material culture, from medallions to prints and pottery, enabled people to participate in an emotional community that incorporated ruler and ruled in different roles. The availability of cheap prints enabled many supporters on both sides of the Channel to engage with William III's sorrow at the death of his wife, Mary II, as they accessed a presentation of the weeping monarch's grief beside her deathbed (Figure 35.2). Simply collecting or displaying portraits of monarchs depicted at key life stages such as baptisms, marriage or in death, in prints and cheap earthenware, could create a political community of feeling, just as witnessing entries and processions and visiting royal tombs engaged the ruled in ritual emotional behaviours and performances consistent with their familial contract with the monarch.

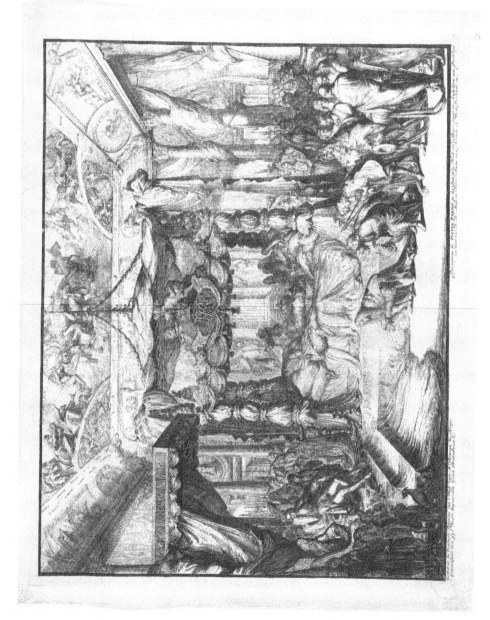

Figure 35.2 Romeyn de Hooghe and Pieter Persoy, *Queen Mary II Stuart on her Deathbed*, 1695; 1695, etching, 470mm x 591 mm. Rijksmuseum, Amsterdam, RP-P-OB-67.728.

Emotional performances of statecraft involved textual rhetoric, material and gestured corporeal practice. These were expressed in a range of sources from the correspondence of monarchs and representatives who were involved in negotiating in person and in texts on their behalf, to rituals and ceremonies, visual and material culture and elite bodies that created distinctive male and female sociabilities and friendships, and emphasized heterosexual love and desire. In these ways, the articulation of emotions by both monarchs and subjects was narrated within specific cultural frameworks concerning gendered individuals and ideologies about the social, political and emotional contract that bound ruler and ruled together.

The emotions of individuals

Monarchs were of course also individuals whose lived emotional experience sometimes coalesced with the agenda of statecraft and at other times proved problematic to it. This section explores how rulers were not only responsible to their subjects but also to parents, kin, siblings, courtiers and servants, embedded in ties of family, dynasty, friendship and proximities that entailed specific emotional demands and responsibilities and which did not necessarily align with each other or with rule. In doing so, it explores different kinds of early modern source materials in which such behaviours were articulated.

Expressions of feeling were not understood only as political rhetoric. Claims about an individual monarch's emotions might also be used strategically to subvert an undesirable political direction. For example, there was strategic value in recognizing the validity of monarchs' feelings – as mothers and fathers, as children, as love and life partners – to secure political advantages or break off marriage promises. The personal feelings of monarchs were well understood by contemporaries to drive diplomatic and military engagements as well. When the head of the French army, the constable Anne de Montmorency, was captured at the battle of Saint-Quentin in 1557 by forces fighting for Philip II, letters to the French statesmen from the king, Henri II, declared his distress:

> I beg you to believe that you are the person in the world that I love the most, and for all that, I know nothing to offer you, since my heart is yours. I think that you know well that I would spare nothing I own or nothing in my power to have the happiness to see you again.[29]

When Montmorency was released on parole to mediate between the warring monarchs, the Ferrarese ambassador Julio Alvarotti noted that Henri held the constable in an embrace lasting minutes and that the king and Montmorency shared a bed for the next two nights while they were together.[30] The king's desire to see Montmorency return to French territory was repeatedly expressed across multiple letters:

> [n]othing other than death could separate me from you, I would think myself happy and would die content when I see a good peace and the man whom I love and esteem most in the world, and so do not be afraid to set the ransom at any price, for I will spare nothing that is in my power to see you again.[31]

Knowledge of Henri's feelings among ambassadors and Philip's negotiators may well have driven up the price of Montmorency's freedom, which was secured by Henri's signing of the Peace of Cateau-Cambrésis.

Moreover, the personal attachments of rulers could prove deeply problematic if they threatened to disrupt political networks and conventional lines of authority. The deep attachment of Frederick of Hohenzollern, who later became Frederick II, king of Prussia, to a number of male retainers contributed to a deep rift between the young man and his father, Frederick William I. Frederick's sister Wilhelmine later recalled how Frederick and a young page Peter Karl Christoph Keith were so close that the Prince 'loved him passionately and gave him his entire confidence', until the young men were separated by the king.[32] A further emotional connection in 1730 with the youthful nobleman Hans Hermann von Katte drove Frederick to plan to leave for England in the company of Katte and a number of young officers. This attachment would have fatal consequences when the king learned of the plan. Frederick William ordered his son to be present at Katte's execution for treason, a compelling scene that artists and viewers sought to imagine (Figure 35.3). Frederick William then enrolled his son in a rigorous two-year scholastic programme preparing him for future military leadership and statecraft. Frederick, 'the prisoner' as he termed himself, consoled himself by corresponding with Wilhelmine, and soon after, married Elisabeth Christine von Brauschweig-Wolfenbüttel-Bevern although he had confessed to his sister: 'I do not like this princess at all; on the contrary, I feel repugnance towards her and our marriage is not worth much, there being no possibility of friendship or union between us.'[33] Frederick forged in correspondence with his sister a new and socially appropriate outlet for at least some of his emotional expression. After her

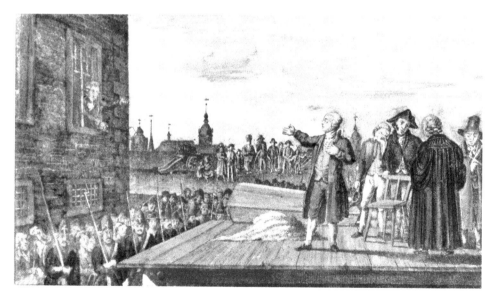

Figure 35.3 Images imagining Frederick of Hohenzollern, later Frederick II of Prussia farewelling Hans Herman von Katte at his execution, Küstrin, 6 November 1730. Copper engraving, coloured, c. 1790. © akg-images

death in 1758, this intense sibling bond found new expression in material form, when Frederick had the Temple of Friendship constructed at Sanssouci in her memory.

The role of strong, positive feelings in Frederick's marriage was evidently not considered a requirement by those negotiating the couple's fate. Yet emotions, articulated and felt, were pivotal in royal marriage arrangements.[34] The interactions between the Stuarts and the Orange-Nassaus regarding the marriage of Prince Charles, later Charles II, highlight the many roles that emotions played in rhetoric and action in such negotiations. In 1643, Frederik Hendrik, Prince of Orange, and his wife Amalia von Solms-Braunfels, approached Charles I and Henrietta Maria about a match between their daughter Luise Henriette and Charles, Prince of Wales. For the Stuarts, however, Charles' marriage was a critical mechanism to garner support for their re-establishment. By 1646, negotiator Stephen Goffe wrote to Frederik Hendrik to annul any further discussions of the match. Goffe stressed 'with what passion and sincerity the King and Queen have always hoped for a happy end to the treaty of the marriage . . . this marriage being the thing that they most wished for in all the world'.[35] The qualities of love and friendship were critical to the expression of this delicate matter that was in essence a rejection of the political value and status of the Orange-Nassau dynasty. In 1657, however, a dispossessed Charles II sought the hand of another Orange-Nassau daughter, Henriette Catherine, having exchanged letters with her for some time. Charles told his confidante, Lord Taaffe, 'The professions I receive from her every letter, are large and full as ether you do or can say.'[36] Charles declared to Taaffe that Henriette Catherine was 'the worthiest to be lov'd of the sex'.[37] When Oliver Cromwell died on 3 September 1658, improving Charles' prospects of reinstatement, he wrote to the widowed Amalia to ask whether a proposal of marriage might be entertained. However, Charles was acutely disappointed by Amalia's negative response, lamenting: 'You will permit me also to complain of my unhappiness that I have learned by your letter . . . all that can console me is the continuation of your friendship.'[38] To Taaffe, he joked that he had perhaps not paid enough attention to 'the old woman', writing 'I see now how ill an old strumpett takes it not to be f[ucked].'[39] When Charles II was restored to the throne in 1660, the Orange-Nassau family approached him secretly about the possibility of marrying their youngest daughter, eighteen-year-old Maria.[40] Charles declined. A vast range of feeling performances – love, desire, pride, anger, frustration – drove or sundered these successive negotiations, and their articulation by rulers and their delegates could be used to encourage, delay, or refuse suitors.

The personal triumphs and losses of rulers also sustained connections between far-flung members of families who understood the distinct pressures borne of promulgating dynasties. When Willem IV, Prince of Orange, and his wife Anne, suffered the sorrow of two stillborn daughters in the late 1730s, grief was shared and communicated along through gendered lines. Anne's younger sisters, Princesses Amelia and Caroline of Great Britain, wrote their consolations to Anne while Frederick II of Prussia addressed Willem's sorrow:

> I so truly feel the sorrow that such a fatal accident must have caused you, and I am stunned at the constancy of fate to pursue you. It is for you, my dear Prince, to oppose with a constancy equal to fate's own and to show that your soul is above these vulgar misfortunes.

Frederick offered the consolations of philosophy:

> All my life has been a school of adversity, so to speak, after having passed a
> thousand sorrows, I have learned that there is nothing safer than to apply
> reason to those things one cannot change and to use all your strength to
> amend those on which prudence might achieve something.[41]

Frederick and William were themselves part of a wider dynastic network with shared
faith values. Dynastic connections of this kind formed a complex dynamic for rulers, with obligations, beliefs and ambitions that pushed and pulled individuals and
needed to be managed as part of rulers' emotional lives.

Just as reproductive pressures were felt and narrated in different ways by men and
women as rulers, so too were emotions experienced in individuals' roles as partners.
Perceptions about a queen consort's feelings for her natal family and her nation
of birth fed fears and anxieties about powerful women. A culture of concern about
power in the hands of a 'foreign' queen understood that a consort's devotion to her
own natal dynasty rather than that of her husband compromised her trustworthi-
ness. These same expectations could also inform relationships within ruling families.
Just a year after Marie-Antoinette's arrival at the French court, her mother, Maria
Theresia, Empress of Austria, reminded her daughter of her particular duties of
friendship and protection for Germans at the French court:

> Give a distinct welcome to the highest ranked, and generosity to all Germans,
> especially my subjects and from the first houses, and to the lesser, those who
> do have access to the Court here, kindness, affection and protection ... It
> is not your beauty, which is hardly great, nor your talents or learning (you
> know very well that you have none), but the goodness of your heart, this
> sincerity, these attentions applied with careful judgement.[42]

Marie-Antoinette's letters in return insisted upon her warm welcome of Germans at
the French court. These missives regularly professed her respect and duty towards
her mother, and the pair continued to exchange letters twice a month from the time
of Marie-Antoinette's departure until her mother's death.

Gift objects were also drivers for, manifestations of, and responses to, many diverse
feelings between the pair. In December 1778, to celebrate the arrival of her granddaughter, Maria Theresia had sent her daughter Marie-Antoinette a *urushi* box, a
present that symbolized a mother's ongoing commitment to her married daughter in a foreign land. Marie-Antoinette compiled an extensive Japanese lacquerware
collection, much of which had been given or bequeathed to her by her mother
Maria Theresia. At Schloss Schönbrunn, the imperial summer residence that Marie-
Antoinette knew well from her childhood, there were exquisitely crafted accents
inspired by the exotic east – porcelain, lacquer panels and silk wallpapers. Maria
Theresia displayed life-sized portraits of her far-flung children, the exotic and the
domestic side-by-side, in intimate spaces to which only a few people in the palace
had access. Marie-Antoinette eventually sent her mother Élisabeth Vigée Le Brun's
1779–1780 full-length image of the French queen in court dress, to join her mother's collection there. Maria Theresia's lacquerware gifts both signalled her intimate

knowledge of her daughter's pleasures and were also a call to home. Correspondence and gift exchange reveals the complex entanglement of feelings between powerful mothers and daughters – daughters whom they wanted to see become strong and confident influences in their new homelands, but whom they also often expected to secure natal interests.

Queens' material collections could also be a source of personal anxiety for their owners in other ways. In her spiritual memoirs, Mary II of England, for instance, professed deeply mixed emotions about her involvement in building works at Kensington and Hampton Court, especially after a series of accidents occurred.[43] She interpreted the fatalities as a punishment from God and reflected later that such events had 'truly, I hope, weaned me from the vanities I was most fond of, that is ease and good lodgings'.[44] She assigned herself a moral programme of scriptural and historical readings and meditations. Shortly after Mary's death, the Hampton Court Water Gallery to which she had devoted so much attention was demolished, considered by her widower, William III, and his designers to interfere with the view of the river from the State Apartments.[45] Her extensive porcelain collection built up over many years likewise did not remain intact as a display of royal power. Instead, Daniel Defoe famously critiqued Mary's 'love of fine East-India calicoes' and 'humour, as I may call it, of furnishing houses with china-ware'.[46] Forging new sociabilities among elite men, Mary's lovingly accrued collection was redistributed almost immediately by William III as gifts, including 787 pieces at Kensington Palace given to his favourite, Arnold Joost van Keppel, first earl of Albemarle.[47]

However, material production was also understood by contemporaries to assist rulers in managing their emotional state. The embroidery of Mary, Queen of Scots during her captivity in England has been interpreted by a number of scholars for its political programme.[48] However, eyewitnesses reported distinctly different impressions of needlework's value and significance for Mary. In 1569, George Talbot, the Earl of Shrewsbury (1528–90), informed William Cecil that Mary joined his wife and ladies in waiting in needlework, in which she 'much delighteth and in devising works'.[49] By contrast, Nicholas White who had paid a visit to Mary at Tutbury in the same year, recorded for Cecil a rather more negative appraisal from Mary of her labour:

> She sayd that all the day she wrought with her needil, and that the diversitie
> of the colors made the worke seme less tedious, and continued so long at it
> till the very payn did make her to give it over.[50]

Clearly, there was a variety of evaluations of the enjoyment a queen could extract from needlework. A very public attestation of a ruler's feeling within a political programme was provided by Mary's son, James VI & I, in the dual monuments that he created at Westminster Abbey for Elizabeth I and his disgraced mother. Disinterring both their bodies to move them into his new, rehabilitative memorial environment, in which his mother's tomb was larger than that of Elizabeth, James's actions were praised by the Earl of Northampton as representing the 'piety of a matchless son'.[51] These new monuments that lay at the heart of English royal ceremonial space could thus be understood as intimate and familial gestures.

Many, though not all, of the emotional expressions examined in this section of the chapter as those of rulers as individuals occur in different kinds of sources to those analysed earlier. However, these letters, memoirs and material collections were not private documents accessible to only a few, even where they suggested varied degrees of intimacy, and were frequently open to interpretation by others. So too were individuals' bodies embedded in the very public politics of statecraft, in which not only their reproductive capacities but also their outward affective manifestations such as blushes and smiles and their desires, including sexual desires, were available for assessment by others.

Conclusions

This chapter argues that ideas about feelings defined the nature of the bond between ruler and subject. For rulers, our focus here, emotional rhetoric and affective display were integral components of the construction of power for both male and female monarchs, who operated within culturally – and gender-specific – practices of both feeling and rule. The assumption that rule was a predominantly male preserve clearly informed the manner in which regnants, consorts, regents and heirs, as men and women, conducted emotional practice, as speech, gesture, through their bodies and in material productions and gift exchange, to persuade and influence but also be considered appropriate to their sex. Power and authority were expressed through controlled emotional labour. Deliberate feeling displays of the body, captured in eyewitness reports, portraits, ceremony, entries and ritual practices and in carefully constructed emotional rhetoric, underpinned the notion of rule in edicts, letters and other textual forms. Socialities and sociabilities grounded in particular emotional expression and practice were key to the maintenance of power, as explored here in the context of gift exchange processes, art and architectural commissions, and courtly practices and activities around the monarch.

Through particular, often practised and sometimes unexpected, emotional displays, monarchs could assert their authority over subordinates and exert wide influence. They could do so as individuals and also as representatives of a system of rule. Indeed, as the examples here suggest, the imperatives of the latter could also override the feelings and desires of the individuals who were its manifestations. The personal feelings of monarchs and the emotional displays demanded by the framework of monarchy cannot be easily separated, either by the sources that remain or in the nature of how they were performed and experienced. The extent to which the strategic performance of emotional rhetoric was lived, embodied and felt in the mind and through sensations of the body of its agent is challenging to discern. It is perhaps therefore most productive to analyse these as complex ensembles with varied components of value to political processes.

Notes

* I would like to thank the editors and anonymous reviewers for their insights, as well as the Australian Research Council Centre of Excellence for the History of Emotions (CE110001011) for financial support for image reproductions.
1 Jeroen Duindam, *Myths of Power: Norbert Elias and the Early Modern European Court* (Amsterdam: Amsterdam University Press, 1995); T.C.W. Blanning, *The Culture of Power and*

the *Power of Culture: Old Regime Europe, 1660–1789* (Oxford: Oxford University Press, 2002); Anne J. Cruz and Maria Galli Stampino, eds., *Early Modern Habsburg Women: Transnational Contexts, Cultural Conflicts, Dynastic Continuities* (Farnham: Ashgate, 2013); Giora Sternberg, *Status Interaction during the Reign of Louis XIV* (Oxford: Oxford University Press, 2014); James Daybell and Svante Norrhem, eds., *Gender and Political Culture in Early Modern Europe* (London: Routledge, 2016).

2 Joanna Bourke, "Fear and Anxiety: Writing about Emotion in Modern History," *History Workshop Journal* 55, no. 1 (2003): 125; Sara Ahmed, *Cultural Politics of Emotion* (London: Routledge, 2004); Judith Butler, *The Psychic Life of Power* (Stanford: Stanford University Press, 1997).

3 Two recent collections that explore these ideas broadly in medieval and early modern societies are Susan Broomhall, ed., *Authority, Gender and Emotions in Late Medieval and Early Modern England* (Basingstoke: Palgrave Macmillan, 2015) and Susan Broomhall, ed., *Gender and Emotions in Medieval and Early Modern Europe: Destroying Order, Structuring Disorder* (Farnham: Ashgate, 2015).

4 Catherine A. Lutz, "Feminist Emotions," in *Power and the Self*, ed. Jeannette Marie Mageo (Cambridge: Cambridge University Press, 2002), 194–215.

5 Anne Vial-Logeay, "L'univers romain," and Bruno Dumézil, "Les barbares," in *Histoire des Emotions*, vol. 1, ed. Georges Vigarello (Paris: Seuil, 2016), 64–85, 93–105; and Ahmed, *Cultural Politics of Emotion*, as just three examples of the significance of emotions to power and rule in other times.

6 'après si tant et si dures guerres . . . dont sont sortiz les grands maulx, dommages et inconveniens au pauvre people de tous les deux coustez . . . toucher les cueurs de ces deux grandz princes . . . et au bien commun, soulagement et repos de leurs peuples et subjectz', cited in Bertrand Haan, *Une paix pour l'éternité: La négociation du traité du Cateau-Cambrésis* (Madrid: Casa de Velázquez, 2010), 197–198.

7 Helen Watanabe-O'Kelly, "Monarchies," in *Early Modern Emotions: An Introduction*, ed. Susan Broomhall (London: Routledge, 2016), 179.

8 Barbara H. Rosenwein, ed., *Anger's Past: The Social Uses of an Emotion in the Middle Ages* (Ithaca: Cornell University Press, 1998); Karl A.E. Enenkel and Anita Traininger, eds., *Discourses of Anger in the Early Modern Period* (Leiden: Brill, 2015).

9 See Jelle Haemers, "In Public: Collectivities and Polities," in *A Cultural History of the Emotions in the Late-Medieval, Reformation and Renaissance Age (1300–1600)*, eds. Andrew Lynch and Susan Broomhall, vol. 3 (London: Bloomsbury, 2018).

10 Randall Lesaffer, "'Amicitia' in Renaissance Peace and Alliance Treaties (1450–1530)," *Journal of the History of International Law* 4 (2002): 77–99; Klaus Ochema, ed., *Freundschaft oder "amitié"? Ein politisch-soziales Konzept der Vormoderne in zwischen-sprachlichen Vergleich (15–17 Jahrundert)* (Berlin: Duncker & Humblot, 2007); Nicolas Offenstadt, *Faire la paix au Moyen Âge: discours et gestes de paix pendant la guerre de Cent Ans* (Paris: Odile Jacob, 2007); Laurent Smagghe, *Les Émotions du Prince: Émotion et discours politique dans l'espace bourguignon* (Paris: Classiques Garnier, 2012).

11 'ce noued d'amitié que lesd. Princes veullent fermer ensemble', in Haan, *Une paix pour l'éternité*, 212.

12 "FELICITAS TEMPORUM," in Jean Leclerc, *Explication historique des principales medailles frapées pour servir à l' histoire des Provinces-Unies des Pays-Bas*, second edition (Amsterdam: Zacharie Chatelaine, 1736), 6–7.

13 Piroska Nagy, *Le don des larmes au Moyen Age: Un instrument en quête d'institution (Ve-XIIIe siècle)* (Paris: Albin Michel, 2000); Xavier Le Person, *"Practiques" et "practiqueurs": La vie politique à la fin du règne de Henri III* (Geneva: Droz, 2002), 232; Susan Broomhall, "Catherine's Tears: Diplomatic Corporeality and Gender at the Sixteenth-Century French Court," in *Fluid Bodies and Bodily Fluids in Premodern Europe*, eds. Anne M. Scott and Michael Barbezat, forthcoming.

14 'porque sería muy notado de sus vasallos y de los extranjeros y les estaba muy mal a los Reyes las lágrimas en los ojos', Alavá to Philip II, 4 July 1565. *Negociaciones con Francia*, vol. 7 (Madrid: Editorial Maestre, 1953), 517.

15 See Katherine Crawford, "Catherine de Medicis: Staging the Political Woman," *Perilous Performances: Gender and Regency in Early Modern France* (Cambridge, MA: Harvard University Press, 2004), 24–58.

16 Gesa Stedman, *Cultural Exchange in Seventeenth-Century France and England* (Farnham: Ashgate, 2013), 55.

17 'est image de l'esprit, laquelle peut exprimer toutes les affections, cogitations & pensees d'icelluy . . . ainsi les yeus sont indices d'iceluy: la tristesse & gayeté desquelz, il faudra moderer selon les choses desquelles il sera question', Antoine Fouquelin, *La Rhétorique française* (Paris: André Wichel, 1555), 129.

18 Tilman Haug, "Negotiating with 'Spirits of Brimstone and Saltpetre': Seventeenth-Century French Political Officials and Their Practices and Representations of Anger," in *Discourses of Anger*, 381–402.

19 'Aquí le saltaron las lágrimas de los ojos, y cierto, aunque ella las da fácilmente', Alavá to Philip II, 31 May 1565, *Negociaciones*, vol. 7, 365.

20 See Broomhall, "Catherine's Tears."

21 'j'ay ouy dire au Roy vostre grand-père qu'il falloit deux choses pour vivre en repos avec les François et qu'ils aimassent leur Roy: les tenir joyeux, et occuper à quelque exercise; pour cest effect, souvent il falloit combattre à cheval et à pied, courre la lance . . . avec des autres exercices honnestes èsquels il s'employoit et les faisoit employer', [8 September 1563]. *Lettres de Catherine de Médicis*, ed. Hector de la Ferrière, vol. 2 (Paris: Imprimerie nationale, 1885), 92.

22 Watanabe-O'Kelly, "Monarchies," 180.

23 Denis Collins and Jennifer Nevile, "Music and Dance," in *A Cultural History of the Emotions*, vol. 3 (London: Bloomsbury, 2019).

24 See Susan Broomhall, "The Game of Politics: Catherine de' Medici and Chess," *Early Modern Women: An Interdisciplinary Journal* 12, no. 1 (2017), 104–118.

25 Tracy Adams, "Married Noblewomen as Diplomats: Affective Diplomacy," in *Gender and Emotions in Medieval and Early Modern Europe: Destroying Order, Structuring Disorder*, ed. Susna Broomhall (Farnham: Ashgate, 2015), 51–66; see also John Watkins, *After Lavinia: A Literary History of Premodern Marriage Diplomacy* (Ithaca: Cornell University Press, 2017).

26 'pour plus grande consolation de ceste paix et render l'amitié, union et confederation plus ferme et indissoluble', Haan, *Une paix pour l'éternité*, 207.

27 'le suppliant qu'il veuille pour plus fermement establir cested. Reconciliation, affinité et l'amitié qu'il recherché et desire de Sad. M' . . . 'très excellente princesse' . . . 'l'honorer d'une telle princesse qu'il desire singulièrement, tant pour la proximité de sang dont elle attouche à S.M. que pour les dignes, excellentes et rares vertuz qui sont en elle' . . . 'l'asseurance aussy qu'il a de l'honneur et bon traictement que mad. dame sa seur, qu'il ayme et tent cher comme sa propre fille, en recevra, et Sad. M. toute satisfaction, contantement et parfaicte amitié'. Haan, *Une paix pour l'éternité*, 209.

28 'pensava no tratar mas dello pero que la hermandad que tienne con el Roy Chris^mo y la claridad y sinceridad con que a de proceder con el'. *Plainte de l'ambassadeur du Roy catholique presentée au Roy Très Chrestien sur le faict de la Floride*, Célestin Douais ed., "Lettres de Charles IX à M. de Fourquevaux, ambassadeur du roi Charles IX en Espagne, 1568–1572," *Mémoires de l'Académie des sciences et lettres de Montpellier*, Section des lettres, 2e série, vol. 2 (1897), 3.

29 'Je vous prye de croyre que vous estes la persoune de se monde que je me le plus et pour sela je ne vous saroys ryens oferyr car puys que mon ceur est a vous je croy que vous panses byen que je nepergnere mes byens ny se quy sera an ma puysanse pour avoyr set heur que de vous ravoy'. *Bibliothèque nationale de France* (BNF), ms fr 3139, 16^r.

30 Lucien Romier, *Les origines politiques des guerres de religion*, vol. 2 (Paris: Perrin, 1913), 301.

31 'autre ocasyon que sele de la mort ne me saroyt separer daueque vous la quele jestimeroys heureuse et mouroys contant quant je veroys une bonne pays et loume du monde que jayme et estime le plus et pour sela necregnes de vous mestre à ranson à quelque pris que se soyt car ie nepargnere chose quy soyt an ma puysanse pour vous ravoyr'. BNF, ms fr 3139, 5^r.

32 'qu'il l'aimoit passionnément et lui donnoit son entière confiance'. In *Mémoires de Frédérique Sophie Wilhelmine, margrave de Bayreuth soeur de Frédéric le Grand*, vol. 1 (Brunswick: Fréderic Vieweg, 1810), 131.

33 Frederick signed one letter to Wilhelmine, 1 November 1730 'le prisonnier'; 'Je n'aime point la princesse; au contraire, j'ai plutôt de la repugnance pour elle, et notre marriage ne vaudra pas grand'chose, ne pouvant y avoir ni amitié ni union entre nous', 5 September 1732. *Oeuvres de Frédéric le Grand: Correspondance*, ed. Johann David Erdmann Preuss, Premiere partie, vol. 27 (Berlin: Imprimerie royale (R. Decker), 1856), 3, 8.

34 Broomhall and Van Gent, "Courting Nassau Affections: Performing love in Orange-Nassau marriage negotiations," in *Emotions in the Premodern World*, eds. Joanne McEwan, Anne M. Scott and Philippa Maddern (Turnhout: Brepols, 2018), 133–168.

35 'avec combien de passion et sincérité le Roy et la Reine ont tousjours souhaité une heureuse fin au traité du marriage . . . ce mariage estant la chose au monde qu'ils ont souhaité le plus', Goffe to Frederik Hendrik, 9 April 1646. *Archives ou correspondance inédite de la maison d'Orange-Nassau*, ed. G. Groen van Prinsterer, series 2, IV (1642–50), Utrecht: Kemink et fils, 1859), 152–153.

36 [31 January 1657], *Charles II to Lord Taaffe: Letters in Exile*, ed. Timothy Crist (Cambridge: Rampant Lions Press, 1974), 21.

37 [February or March 1658], *Ibid.*, 29.

38 'vous me permettres aussi de me plaindre de mon malheur que i'ay apris par vostre letre . . . tout ce qui m'en peut consoler, est la continuation de vostre amitié, me faites esperer par vostre derniere', Charles II to Amalia, 21 October 1658. *Landsarchiv Oranienbaum, Abteilung Dessau*, A 7b Nr. 84, 12^r.

39 [5 March 1659], *Charles II to Lord Taaffe*, 35.

40 Lieuwe van Aitzema, *Saken van staet en Oorlogh*, vol. 4 (The Hague: Johan Veely, 1664), 875.

41 'j'entre véritablement dans les chagrins q'une ausi funeste acsident a du vous causer, et je m'étone de la constance du sort à vous poursuivre, c'est à vous mon cher Prince de lui oposér une constance égale à la siene, et de montrér que votre ame est audesus des malheurs vulgaires . . . toute ma vie n'a, pour ainsi dire, été qu'une école d'adversité, apres avoir passé par mille chagrins, j'ai experimenté q'il n'y avoit rien de plus sûr, que de se faire une raison sur toutes les choses qu'on ne sauroit changér et d'employér toute son aplication à redresser celles sur les quels la prudance peu quelque chose', 2 February 1740. *Briefwechsel Friedrich des Grossen mit dem Prinzen Wilhelm IV. von Oranien und mit dessen Gemahlin Anna, geb. Princess Royal von England*, ed. Leopold von Ranke (Berlin: Buchdruckerei der Königl. Akademie der Wissenschaften, 1869), 52–53.

42 'Faites un accueil distingué aux premiers, et des bontés à tous les Allemands, sur tout ceux de mes sujets et des premiers maisons; aux moindres, c'est-à-dire qui n'ont point d'entrée à la Cour chez nous, de bonté, d'affection et de protection . . . Ce n'est ni votre beauté, qui effectivement ne l'est pas telle, ni vos talents ni savoir (vous savez bien que tout cela n'existe pas), c'est votre bonté de Coeur, cette franchise, ces attentions, appliquées avec tant de jugement', Maria Theresia to Marie-Antoinette, 8 May 1771. *Correspondance (1770–1793)*, ed. Évelyne Lever (Paris: Tallandier, 2005), 76.

43 Ernest Law, *The History of Hampton Court Palace. Vol. 3: Orange and Guelph Times* (London: G. Bell, 1891), 24.

44 R. Doebner, ed., *Memoirs of Mary Queen of England, together with her Letters, and those of James II and William III to the Electress Sophia of Hanover* (London: David Nutt, 1886), 43–44.

45 Law, *The History of Hampton Court Palace*, 128.

46 Daniel Defoe, *A Tour through the Whole Island of Great Britain*, eds. P.N. Furbank, W.R. Owens and A.J. Coulson (New Haven: Yale University Press, 1991), 65.

47 Linda Rosenfeld Shulsky, "Kensington and de Voorst," *Journal of the History of Collections* 2, no. 1 (1990): 47–62.

48 See Margaret H. Swain, *The Needlework of Mary Queen of Scots* (Carlton: Bean, 1986), 87–88; Sarah Randles, "'The Pattern of All Patience': Gender, Agency, and Emotions in Embroidery and Pattern Books in Early Modern England," in *Authority, Gender and Emotions*, ed. Susan Broomhall, 150–167.

49 Michael Bath, *Emblems for a Queen: The Needlework of Mary Queen of Scots* (London: Archetype, 2008), 4.

50 *Ibid.*, 4.

51 Peter Sherlock, "Monuments," in *Early Modern Emotions*, ed. Susan Broomhall, 152.

Key works

Broomhall, Susan and Jacqueline Van Gent, "Courting Nassau Affections: Performing love in Orange-Nassau marriage negotiations," in *Emotions in the Premodern World*, eds., Joanne McEwan, Anne M. Scott and Philippa Maddern (Turnhout: Brepols, 2018), 133–168.

Lasaffer, Randall, "'Amicitia' in Renaissance Peace and Alliance Treaties (1450–1530)," *Journal of the History of International Law* 4 (2002): 77–99.

Le Person, Xavier, *"Practiques" et "practiqueurs": La vie politique à la fin du règne de Henri III* (Geneva: Droz, 2002).

Ochema, Klaus ed., *Freundschaft oder "amitié"? Ein politisch-soziales Konzept der Vormoderne in zwischen-sprachlichlen Vergleich (15–17 Jahrundert)* (Berlin: Duncker & Humblot, 2007).

Smagghe, Laurent, *Les Émotions du Prince: Émotion et discours politique dans l'espace bourguignon* (Paris: Classiques Garnier, 2012).

36

FROM *GALANTERIE* TO SCANDAL

The sexuality of the king from Louis XIV to Louis XVI

Chad Denton

When writing about attitudes toward the sexual behaviours of the three King Louis who reigned between the establishment of the royal court at Versailles and the French Revolution, there is a confusing spectrum of reactions. After Louis XIV (r.1643–1715) ended his long career of womanizing and tried to reform court morals under the influence of his last mistress and morganatic wife Madame de Maintenon, there was a comic verse which appeared, titled 'The Devout King Who Has Renounced Gallantry' that warmly recalled Louis XIV's sexual escapades, despairing that 'It is no longer fashionable to make love, even the King no longer finds it fun.'[1] Popular verse would be much less forgiving about the *amours* of Louis XV (r.1715–74), with one song declaring upon his death, 'This monster, who had a stomach but no guts, / Gave famine to France and the pox to Versailles.'[2] Yet, despite such vehement reactions to Louis XV's sexual excesses, Louis XVI (r.1774–92), who took no mistresses or even had any extramarital rendezvous, was pilloried in underground pamphlets as someone who was impotent both as a man and a king, cuckolded by a nymphomaniac queen.[3] While sometimes even in conflict with each other, these different perceptions of and reactions to sexual behaviours in the life of the king were fed by tumultuous shifts in attitudes about gender, marriage and religion that turned the king's harmless romantic *galanteries*, emotional and romantic dalliances with women, into scandal that could destroy the reputation of one king and lead the public to hope for a moral reformation from another.

Any discussion of the sexual behaviour of the early modern kings of France, especially the Bourbons, usually centres not around their lawful wives and queens, but rather around the *maîtresse en titre*, the titular or official mistress. She was given a prominent place at the royal court as the king's visible companion and a living fulcrum of the royal court. Modern historiography often credits Agnès Sorel (1422?–1450), the mistress of King Charles VII (r.1422–61), as being the first *maîtresse en titre*. While this may be questioned,[4] she was arguably the first royal mistress in France to have a strongly acknowledged position at the same time her lover's queen did not or could not adopt a strong public role.[5]

Certainly, in early modern France, queens, with the undeniable exception of those who because of circumstances took on the role of queen regent, seem to recede into the background. Kathleen Wellman has argued that Diane de Poitiers (1499–1566), the celebrated mistress of Henri II (r.1547–59), became the 'public face of the monarchy' while Henri's actual marriage to Catherine de' Medici (1519–89) was presented as 'merely prosaic, mundane, and pragmatic'.[6] This would become even more true for the queens of Louis XIV and Louis XV, Marie-Thérèse (1638–83) and Marie Leszczyńska (1703–68) respectively, who performed traditional acts of piety and charity, made ceremonial appearances, gambled with courtiers and, of course, gave birth to new royals, while at the same time some *maîtresses en titre* engaged in *avant garde* cultural patronage. It was not his queen Marie-Thérèse, but Louis XIV's mistress Madame de Montespan (1640–1707) who became famous for her sponsorship of various popular musicians, playwrights and artists, including La Fontaine and Molière.[7] Later Louis XV's mistress, Madame de Pompadour (1707–64), gave patronage to Voltaire, among others, and had promoted the publication of the pivotal Enlightenment achievement, the *Encyclopédie*, defending its merits to the king himself.[8]

Cultural patronage was an outward expression of a more important aspect of the position of *maîtresse en titre*. While the queen was primarily a symbol of dynastic alliance and the mother of legitimate heirs, by the Bourbon era the *maîtresse en titre* was understood as fulfilling not only the king's carnal desires outside marriage but his need for emotional and intellectual companionship. King Louis XIV himself, who had taken both *maîtresses en titre* and more casual trysts, discussed the subject of mistresses in an 'advice manual' written for his son and designated heir that spoke of 'being deeply in love',[9] not in lust. Observers often spoke of the king's relationship with the *maîtresse en titre* in monogamous terms, even though the Bourbon kings rarely if ever showed their mistresses fidelity. When describing how Louis XIV had intercourse with other women during his relationship with Montespan, Madame de Caylus wrote of the *infidélités du Roi*.[10] During the reign of Louis XV, when Madame de Pompadour's position was in apparent danger of being usurped by Madame de Choiseul, the duc de Croÿ wrote that 'the gossip of Paris was that the king had wished to commit an infidelity with the young Madame de Choiseul'.[11] The *maîtresse en titre* was not in any sense a legitimate wife – this was testified to by the fact that the mere suggestion that the king would give his illegitimate sons a place in the succession awakened fears of a political crisis and even civil war twice in Bourbon history, once in Henri IV's lifetime and again with Louis XIV's will – but she was not quite just an adulterous fling either.

The concept of the *maîtresse en titre* fit cleanly with prevailing ideas about the value of heterogeneous sociability. This was not something entirely new in seventeenth- and eighteenth-century France. In the sixteenth century, François I (r.1515–47) declared that a royal court without women is like 'a year without spring' and 'resembles the court of a satrap or Turk than that of a great Christian king'.[12] However, extending beyond court culture, the emergence in the late seventeenth century of *salons*, intellectual gatherings hosted in the homes of noble and upper-*bourgeoisie* women, cemented the reputation of women – educated and elite French women, in particular – as agents of male refinement. In 1751, Charles Pinot-Duclos remarked that even already learned men who attended *salons* 'perfected their taste, polished their wit, softened their manners, and in several cases found enlightenment that they would have not discovered in books'.[13] 'Women's very weakness predisposed her to virtue and suited her to ends higher than the physical,' Carolyn C. Lougée explains. 'She was seen as the creator and peaceful sustainer, man as the brute destroyer.'[14] Even outside France, the English journalist Joseph Addison, who once demanded a law banning from England 'French fopperies', nonetheless thought that the French had a social advantage through their custom of allowing women to socialize freely with men since 'Man would not only be an unhappy, but a rude unfinished Creature, were he conversant with none but those of his own make.'[15] With such ideas, it is no surprise that at least by the late seventeenth century, among the nobility the tacitly accepted practice of adultery became common enough that it was commented upon by multiple observers.[16] If sentimental love and fulfilling marriage could not be found within a marriage, it would be found with a mistress. A mistress, moreover, who could fulfil and exercise all the classical roles and obligations into which queens traditionally had been educated. These mistresses were now appearing to fulfil royal duties – an interesting development indeed – essentially two queens for every king.

There was no concern that an early modern French king would have need of being civilized, but the *maîtresse en titre* provided a sophisticated partner to and courtly representative of her royal *gallant*, proving his sexual virility as well as providing a locus for court culture. Wit was an essential quality prized in a *maîtresse en titre*, with Madame de Montespan keeping Louis XIV's affections in part by ruthlessly mocking other courtiers to such an extent that passing by the windows of Montespan's apartments when she and the king were present became known as 'going before the guns'.[17] Even Louis XIV's later and more uptight mistress, Madame de Maintenon, was approvingly noted by Saint-Simon to be a 'woman of much wit'.[18] Besides such natural mental assets, mistresses were also expected to be able to navigate informed conversations and engage in artistic activities. In spite of their *bourgeois* background, Pompadour's own mother, who apparently had hopes of Pompadour becoming a mistress, gave her an extensive training in not only court etiquette, but in dancing, the theatre and contemporary literature.[19] Portraits of Montespan, Maintenon and Pompadour all emphasized them as women of artistic and intellectual interests and achievements.[20] It is perhaps unsurprising that Louis XV's last *maîtresse en titre*, Madame du Barry, who came from a lower class background and was a former shop girl, tried to compensate by buying a library containing more than a thousand books.[21]

If mistresses had to a degree usurped the cultural patronage that in past eras had been the purview of queens, they also played a role that was political, if extremely limited and contested. The apex of the political influence of the 'official mistress' was undoubtedly Pompadour's direct role in the negotiations that resulted in the Treaty of Paris and the end of the Seven Years' War in 1763. The Comte d'Argenson accused Pompadour of essentially masterminding the entire treaty, but at the same time diplomats involved in the negotiations, such as the Cardinal de Bernis, the Duc de Choiseul and the Prince of Kaunitz-Rietberg, welcomed Pompadour's involvement and praised her in terms reminiscent of the complementary role women were believed to have in the lives of elite men.[22] Less controversial was when Madame du Barry, early in her tenure as *maîtresse en titre*, interceded for an aged noble couple, the Comte and Comtesse de Loüesme, who had fatally shot a bailiff during an attempt to sequester their ancestral chateau. Du Berry's plea saved the couple from execution and instead they were sentenced to imprisonment and later banishment.

This act of mercy, which was more appropriate for a woman in the shadow of older prevailing attitudes towards gender and power, delighted Louis XV and won du Barry sympathizers.[23] However ambiguous the role of the mistress might have been, there were tangible ways in which the mistress participated openly and decisively in the exercise of royal power and responsibility.

While the *maîtresses en titre* often served as *de facto* cultural ministers and advisers, another compelling reason to tolerate their legitimized adultery was that they were also reliable allies for relatives and friends in securing posts. Even Louise de Valliére (1644–1710), remembered by historians as the most 'reluctant' and modest of Louis XIV's mistresses, found employment for her relatives, who were among less affluent provincial nobility. 'I will say, once and for all, that there is not one lady of quality who would not have the ambition to be the lover of her prince,' Primi Visconti wrote about Louis XIV's court. He continued:

> Also there must be some indulgence for the King if he falls into error, with so many devils surrounding him, busy with tempting him. But the worst is that the families, the fathers, and the mothers and even certain husbands pride themselves on such affairs.[24]

All of this made the sexual inclinations of the king a matter of state. When on a night of July 1722, a group of young noblemen had an orgy at Versailles just under the windows of the apartments of the then eleven-year old King Louis XV (an act that some courtiers could apparently see from inside the palace thanks to the moonlight), the Duchesse de la Ferté suspected it was a plot to actually alter the sexuality of the king:

> [i]n the history of the loves (*galanterie*) of the kings, it has alternated one after another; Henri II and Charles IX loved women, and Henri III *mignons*; Henri IV loved the women, Louis XIII the men, Louis XIV the women, and at present the age of the *mignons* has returned.[25]

Of course, the opposite turned out to be true. The duc de Bourbon, whom Edmond-Jean-François Barbier claims arranged for Louis XV to lose his virginity during a hunting expedition in order 'to give the king a taste for women, because it is hoped that it would make him more malleable and more refined',[26] apparently succeeded where the would-be *mignons* failed. Women were also cynically deployed to dislodge a reigning *maîtresse en titre*.

> It is said that there is a great question concerning a change in mistress: the king is tired of the Marquise de Pompadour, who looks scrawny because of the bad state of her breasts . . . one often wishes to go to the other extreme, and the court is excited to test the waters with the fat comtesse de la Mark. It is true that this Sultana is eaten up with hemorrhoids and that she has been with everybody. It is the amorous who have the power of instigation and insinuation; they will keep trying for a long time.[27]

Some extent of nepotism was usually accepted, especially in a political culture where naked patronage was the norm; much less so was the alleged power mistresses had over the king's political decisions. That said, having the status of an adviser or coun-sellor intimately suggests a strong voice when it comes to making political decisions, for example Pompadour and the Treaty of Paris. Perhaps such criticisms were lev-ied against her *because* her role as an adviser meant she was directly involved in decision making. Mistresses were always a favourite scapegoat for unpopular deci-sions by the kings, such as Madame de Maintenon being blamed for Louis XIV's persecution of the Huguenots and Madame de Pompadour being held responsible for the expulsion of the Jesuits in 1764 and the provision in the Treaty of Paris that saw France surrendering virtually all of their North American holdings. There were plenty of historical precedents for such a view of the mistress, and indeed of the royal favourite in general, from Cleopatra to the Duke of Buckingham. Precisely because royal favourites were so useful for criticizing a monarch's actions without blaming the monarch themselves, it was axiomatic in political thought that the influence of favourites on politics was often disastrous. Louis XIV may have been melodramatic, but he was drawing on this widespread knowledge when he wrote to his son that because of kings slavishly following the advice of their lovers 'we see in history so many ghastly examples of houses extinct, of thrones overthrown, of provinces devastated, of empires destroyed'.[28]

What about, however, the immorality of adultery itself? After all, adultery by either the wife or the husband was unequivocally condemned in both the Old and New Testaments. Even before the time of Louis XIV, there had been tension between the existence of a *maîtresse en titre* and Christian moral tradition, even if the 'double standard' granting much greater leniency towards adultery committed by husbands was firmly rooted in law and social attitudes. At the least, the prominence granted to mistresses provoked surprised comments. For one example, an English ambassador was taken aback by François I appearing alongside his mistress, Anne de Pisseleu d'Heilly (1508–80) during the ceremonies surrounding the coronation of the new queen, Eleanor of Austria.[29] Almost two centuries later, Primi Visconti similarly noted how Louis XIV's queen received visits from the mistress and their illegitimate chil-dren. Even during Mass, Visconti noted with bemusement, the king would appear alongside his queen, Madame de Montespan, and all his legitimate and illegitimate children, praying in public view 'as if they were saints . . . What a comedy court life is!'[30] The duchesse d'Orléans recalled in 1716 another public appearance by Louis XIV alongside Montespan, when the king was inspecting a regiment of German mercenaries. Seeing Montespan, they shouted excitedly, *Konigs Hure!* ('The king's whore!'). That evening, according to Orléans, Montespan remarked to Louis that she found the Germans 'so naïve' since they 'named something by what it actually was'.[31] Whether it was a foreign visitor like Visconti commenting on the mistress and her children being allowed to occupy a sacred and public space with the legitimate royal family, or mercenaries gawking at a 'whore', the official mistress benefited from her proximity to the royal body and contributed to the public image of the monarchy, strongly suggesting that mistresses had a political voice that reached the king's ear, influencing decision making. However, the limits of her position *vis-à-vis* the king also had to be maintained – in other words, she had to know her place.

In the traditional religious politics of the French monarchy, that place was not inim-ical to the king's piety, as shown by Louis XIV's lack of reluctance to appear in church accompanied by his illegitimate family. True, half a century before Louis XIV's time,

King Charles I of England (r.1625–49), who had no extramarital affairs and was the first English king to commission portraits of the royal family enjoying basic domesticity, promoted the idea of the royal court and family as a microcosm of society at large. Moral, domesticated behaviour by the king and queen encouraged morality throughout the realm, at least according to this rather optimistic theory.[32] Louis XIV acknowledged a similar moral dimension of kingship when he wrote to his son:

> I should tell you first that since a prince should always be a perfect model of virtue, it would be desirable for him to be completely immune to the failings of the rest of mankind, all the more since he is sure that they could never be hidden . . . [but if a prince] . . . should happen to fall, in spite of ourselves . . . [there were still] . . . precautions . . . [he should take].[33]

Both Louis XIV and Montespan were indeed pious by contemporary standards. Madame de Caylus observed that Louis XIV only missed Mass twice in his life, both times because he was on a military campaign. As for Montespan, Caylus recalled that one day the duchesse d'Uzés, seeing Montespan fastidiously observing her prayers, admitted she was surprised by seeing Montespan acting so devout. 'What!' Montespan is said to have replied. 'Because I commit one sin, must I do all the others?'[34] It is perhaps important that the ideas of adulterous actions and piety were incompatible as was assumed by the duchesse d'Uzés. At any rate, there were limits to how much adultery could be legitimized in the light of religion. Before Louis XIV and Montespan, *maîtresses en titre* were either unmarried or placed in a sham marriage to a loyal courtier after they became the king's lover. Montespan was already married when she began her relationship with Louis XIV. This 'double adultery' pushed against the norms of royal adultery, but the behaviour of Montespan's husband, Louis-Henri de Gondrin de Pardaillan, who claimed he had deliberately infected himself with syphilis by going to brothels and attempted to rape his wife to infect her with the disease, at least gave Louis XIV cause to imprison Louis-Henri briefly and exile him to his estates, far away from the vicinity of Versailles.[35]

A new form of religious expression proved to be an even more potent threat to Louis XIV and Montespan's relationship than the stain of double adultery. Catholicism after the Catholic Reformation encouraged an 'internalization of religious values' and greater self-understanding and self-control of the desires motivating one's behaviour.[36] Madame de Maintenon and others would write of a *conversion* that entailed not simply a submission to Catholic doctrine and rituals but a totalizing moral transformation. Maintenon herself would write of being 'given to God', after which '[one] has sorrows, but one has a firm consolation and a peace at the bottom of the heart amidst the greatest sorrows'.[37] That the king did indeed remain loyal to Maintenon after their morganatic marriage sometime in the winter of 1684–5 and actively promoted a more austere atmosphere at court does show how much external pious behaviour was important in illuminating one's internal surrender to God.

This tension between the older and the newer views of moral behaviour and faith came to the fore in Easter of 1675. When Montespan went to confession at the chapel in Versailles, the curate Father Lécuyer refused to grant her absolution, saying, 'Is that the Madame de Montespan who scandalizes the whole of France? Well, Madame, cease your scandals and come and throw yourself at the ministers of Jesus Christ!' Sincerely distraught, she appealed personally to his superior Father Thibout, but he agreed with Lécuyer's actions, and without confession Montespan could not receive Holy Communion at the Easter Mass.[38] Louis XIV asked the dauphin's tutor, Bishop Bossuet, to settle the dispute. However, Bossuet instead lectured the king at length about the evils of adultery and wrote to urge him to end the relationship. Famously Bossuet urged the king in a letter:

> It is not a day's work, I admit it; but the more long and difficult the work is, the more it must be done . . . I do not ask, Sire, that you extinguish in an instant a flame so violent; that would be to ask the impossible; but, Sire, diminish it little by little; be afraid of nourishing it.

He urged him to undergo a 'true conversion' by forsaking Montespan.[39] Interestingly, Bossuet acknowledges the emotional component of Louis XIV's relationship and, by extension, the necessity to sublimate such emotion into a lawful marriage, rather than into an illicit relationship displeasing to God.

Louis XIV eventually consented to never see Montespan again, but the decision did not last. Still, this victory illustrated the existence of a faction in court that was invested in the moral reform of the king himself. This faction was most strongly represented in contemporaneous accounts by Bossuet and Madame de Maintenon. For them, being a virtuous Catholic monarch was incompatible with the royal body being stained by the sin of adultery, despite whatever 'precautions' Louis XIV could undertake. On another occasion, Madame de Maintenon herself took the opportunity to attempt to induce the king's 'conversion':

> When I found myself on such terms with the king that I might speak to him frankly, one day when he was holding a reception, I had the honor of walking with him, while the others were playing cards or doing something else. When we were outside of earshot I stopped and said to him, 'Sire, you are most devoted to your musketeers . . . what would you do if Your Majesty were told that one of those musketeers you hold dear had taken the wife of another man, and was living with her? I am sure that from that very evening he would be barred from the residence of the musketeers, and would no longer be allowed to sleep there, however late it might be.'

In response, the king nervously agreed.[40] In the end, it was Maintenon who succeeded where the clergy of the Catholic Church failed. She wrote triumphantly in February of 1690 to her friend Madame de Brinon, 'Those people at Versailles are good, because the King carries himself perfectly; his health and sanctity are fortified every day; piety is very much becoming *à la mode*. May God make all hearts who profess Him sincere!'[41]

Nonetheless, the new moralistic regime at Versailles was immensely unpopular, with young nobles leaving Versailles for Paris for the more relaxed court of the king's cousin, the future Regent Philippe d'Orléans, at Saint-Cloud. As the Cardinal de Bernis described it, the court under Maintenon was 'very devout, or to put it more accurately, very hypocritical'.[42] Perhaps the 'success' of this pious environment at

Versailles is best illustrated by Saint-Simon's claim that the young nobleman Louis XIV and Maintenon thought was the most pious in Versailles, Courcillon, snickered about Maintenon's piety with his friends.[43] Neither did this shift really address concerns about Louis XIV's mistresses held outside Maintenon's devout circle. Although Saint-Simon did claim that the 'scandal' of Louis XIV's mistresses 'echoed across Europe', his main complaint was not really the taint of adultery, but the 'excess of power' allegedly held by the mistresses.[44] Outside the court, at the time of his death, Louis XIV was reviled in popular song for being politically controlled by Maintenon, for his wars and for high taxation, but not for his former sexual habits.[45]

This was unlike his great-grandson and successor Louis XV, who during his reign and at the time of his own death became known for his uncontrolled sexuality. In December 1750, an officer of the royal guards had publicly erected a placard denouncing Louis XV's mistress Madame de Pompadour as a 'leech . . . without shame or fear' and 'the disgrace of the king'. Contrary to modern expectations regarding *bourgeois* values towards the end of the *ancien regime*, Louis XV did have his defenders, like the reporter of these events, the lawyer Edmond-Jean-François Barber, who criticized such reactions to royal adultery. He argued that there were nobles who committed much worse crimes, including noblemen who lived with their mistresses while ignoring their wives, and abbots who flagrantly violated their vows of chastity, and yet they were not subjected to public scrutiny and criticism. Instead the king was being held to a higher standard than his own subjects or even past kings, regardless of his own political accomplishments and service to the kingdom.[46]

Still, contemporaneous sources do suggest that criticism of Louis XV's sexual activities was a major factor that moulded contemporary and historic images of the king. Jean-Paul Guicciardi goes so far as to argue that perceptions of the sexuality of Louis XV was a significant factor in the decline of the monarchy's prestige and even in the march towards 1789.[47] At least, Jeffrey Merrick acknowledged the sexual scandals surrounding Louis XV as one of multiple causes towards what he termed 'the desacralization' of the French monarchy.[48] As John Hardman notes, when Louis XV fell ill in 1744, 6,000 candles at Notre-Dame were lit for his recovery. After the attempted assassination in 1757, it was reduced to 600. During the illness that would claim his life, it was reduced to three.[49]

There is the question of *why* Louis XV's sexuality had such political ramifications, whereas the public and prolific affairs of his predecessors had no such impact. Of course, the obvious answer may not lie in broad shifts in thought unfolding outside the enclosed spaces of Versailles, but simply in the king's personal behaviour. Louis XV broke the unspoken rules imposed on the king's extramarital sexual activities in a couple of respects. First, he established the *parc aux cerfs*, 'Deer Park', a private house where the king secretly kept lovers for casual trysts. More than Louis XV's other publicized trysts and relationships, like his having taken four sisters of the Mailly-Nesle family as his mistresses, this shattered the pretence, however hollow it was in the past, that the king's relationships with women other than the queen involved sentiment and an intellectual and emotional desire for companionship. Second, his two most famous *maîtresses en titre*, Pompadour and du Barry, were taken from the *bourgeoisie* and the urban working class, respectively, not from even minor nobility. Even Madame de Maintenon, whose father was relatively impoverished and was imprisoned at the time of Maintenon's birth, was still of noble birth.

Whatever the impact of the personal, there were changes in attitudes that made for a generally less favourable climate to the *maîtresses en titre*. Of course, suspicions about the power favourites, especially female favourites, had always been a factor, but beginning at least in the mid-eighteenth century there was an increased anxiety over the blurring of genders and women's power in the political realm. This was a time when, as Gary Keates has argued, gender stratification could be seen hardening in various fora from literature to fashion.[50] In 1758, Rousseau had already repudiated the assumption from earlier in the century that sociability with women was good for noblemen. 'Unable to make themselves into men, the women make us into women,' Rousseau notoriously complained.[51]

Some late seventeenth-century writers like Mary Astell in England and Poullain de la Barre in France had, inspired by the Cartesian separation of mind and body, argued that women's subordinate role is engineered by education and cultural forces. At most the only biological characteristic that explained women's subordinate place in European societies was men's greater physical strength. This was rejected by Rousseau and other mainstream *philosophes* in favour of the idea that gender roles are inborn and innate. Voltaire, who was generally more favourable towards women participating in social and intellectual circles than Rousseau, still expressed the assumption that women are naturally more sensitive and emotional.[52] Even the Cardinal de Bernis, who explicitly agreed that men are only dominant in society because of physical strength and superior education, bemoaned that:

> [t]oday there are women who learn to think like men; at seventeen years old, and sometimes sooner, a man enters the world; it is natural at that age to think the most important goal is to please women; at a young age a man becomes accustomed to the softness and the frivolity, he is appointed to pointless posts, and the court is filled with false principles.[53]

Instead of intellectual companions who assisted and improved their lovers, women like Pompadour, du Barry and even later Queen Marie Antoinette, became symbols of dissimulation, corruption and lack of political transparency. It was the vision of policies being shaped in bedrooms and parlours between the king and his lovers (or in the case of Marie Antoinette between her and her lovers), rather than in meetings between ministers and officials in the public eye. As Lynn Hunt summarizes the view of Rousseau and others, 'Virtue could only be restored if women returned to the private sphere.'[54]

There was one other crucial, interrelated development: changing attitudes towards marriage and how they discredited ideas of the *galant* and extramarital love. Although eighteenth-century France did not widely accept arguments for companionate marriages founded primarily on love, the social movement that William Reddy defined as 'sentimentalism' did offer a new understanding of marriage.[55] Like the older discourse pushed by Bossuet and Madame de Maintenon on the helpless Louis XIV, the new 'sentimental' understanding of marriage condemned adultery by both spouses, but it also provided a much more innate role for emotional attachment. In the traditional understanding, love and desire had been something that was not necessary for a marriage, and if it was present could easily be taken to excess and *harm* the marriage.[56] However, under the doctrine of sentimentalism love between spouses became necessary for a successful marriage and domestic life, even if such love had to be cultivated after the marriage was first established. Reddy writes, 'By 1700 . . . love within marriage takes on the status of an ideal, in which friendship and sexuality are linked, and familial affection becomes a natural model of love.'[57]

The sentimental understanding of marriage was more encompassing and could be understood in terms that were spread not by the sermon, but the novel and the salon. Also, it was deeply connected to a trend, championed by Rousseau, of 'rediscovering' motherhood. For instance, Virginia E. Swain argues that such a push may be found in not only Rousseau's philosophical writings like in his educational treatise *Émile* but in mid-late eighteenth-century works such as Jean-Baptiste Greuze's painting *The Well-Beloved Mother* and Elie de Beaumont's novel *Lettres du Marquis de Roselle*.[58]

With such an understanding of marriage, the *maîtresse-en-titre* could only be an intruder who was operating against the natural emotional order of marriage, even of royal marriages. Adultery could be accepted under the terms of Catholic penitence and religious propriety. Through the more intensive Catholicism of Madame de Maintenon as well as sentimentalism, there was no such release valve. Instead the *maîtresse-en-titre* could only be a symbol of unnatural decadence through both religious and secular discourses. If there is a tangible sign of the triumph of these new discourses over the institution of the *maîtresse-en-titre*, it was the fact that, after Louis XV's death, one of the very first official acts of the new regime of Louis XVI was to exile Madame du Barry not only from the royal court but from Versailles and Paris altogether.

The new king and queen, King Louis XVI and Marie Antoinette, were better models of this doctrine of sentimental marriage than their predecessors. Louis XV, who was characteristically depicted in the 1775 pamphlet *Anécdotes sur la comtesse du Barry*, as a lecherous old man exploited by du Barry in her campaign against good ministers,[59] was now replaced by a young man known for his chaste behaviour and interest in moral reform, Louis XVI. This was certainly the hope of Louis XIV's mother-in-law, Maria Theresa of Austria. Delighted at learning that Louis XVI had not died from smallpox as rumour reported, she hailed the 'twenty-year old king and nineteen-year old queen' who had the:

> [r]eligion, morals, so necessary to obtain the benediction of God and to guide the people, will not be forgotten . . . How in this moment I love the French! . . . I wish for them constancy and less frivolity. By correcting their morals, this will also change.[60]

In practice, Marie Antoinette embraced a model of motherhood that would have not been alien to Rousseau. She initially wanted to breastfeed her first daughter Madame Royale, something Rousseau had urged noblewomen to do because he believed breastfeeding facilitated more intimate connections between mothers and their infants. Also a facsimile of a rural village, the Hameau de la Reine, was constructed on the grounds of Versailles so that Marie Antoinette and her children could experience the 'natural ideal' praised by Rousseau. In a similar vein, portraiture depicting Marie Antoinette and her children did not strictly follow earlier Bourbon portraits of queens with their children, which tended to be set in formal, courtly settings and focused on the symbols of royal legitimacy and dynastic continuity. Instead, the portraits Marie Antoinette commissioned depicted her and her children in naturalistic settings and, while not devoid of royal symbols, emphasized domesticity. Marie Antoinette was to be shown not only as a queen but as a mother.[61]

As a wife, Marie Antoinette attempted to convey an image of a happy and intimate marriage. This was intended as a model for the court nobility, who had so long practised open adultery and separate living arrangements with their spouses. To an extent, it succeeded as one courtly writer noted:

> [t]hey went out like man and wife, the young king giving his arm to the Queen ... The influence of this example had such an effect upon the courtiers, that the next day several couples, who had long, and for good reasons been disunited, were, to the amusement of the whole court, seen walking upon the terrace with the same apparent conjugal intimacy.[62]

In his memoirs, the comte de Ségur remarked:

> Our young King, by the example of his private life, had revived decorum among us ... [gallantry] covered itself with a veil; few persons dared make a parade of vice; the language of an exaggerated sensibility ... replaced that of a licentious gallantry.[63]

However, as Carolyn Harris noted, Marie Antoinette's attempts to forge a compelling narrative of an emotionally and personally fulfilling royal marriage in a court culture where loveless, pragmatic unions and sentimental relationships outside marriage were the norm, made her appear deceitful, bourgeois and un-French. In addition to her openly discussed difficulties in conceiving an heir during the early years of the marriage, the alleged impotence of Louis XVI and her challenge in sharing her husband's interest in hunting and mechanics, were some of the reasons why such negative perceptions of her developed.[64]

Still, even on the streets, songs hailed Louis XVI as a restorer of morals to the court. A 1774 song predicted the new king would 'bring back good morals and abundance' but still reserves criticism for the nobility: 'If he wants honour and morals / what will become of our noblemen?' One song from early in his reign hailed Louis XVI as the reincarnation of the founder of the Bourbon dynasty, Henri IV, who was still celebrated in popular memory. 'He has ... the truth for a mistress', another song went. 'What will become of the courtesans? / If it is possible, honest women.' However, as Louis XVI's reign continued, songs continued to decry corruption at the court while mocking Louis XVI for his failure to father an heir: 'Everyone asks: Can the King do it? Can he not? / The sad queen has become desperate.' Even after Marie Antoinette gave birth to a new dauphin, one 1784 song ominously went, 'If the king is not a father to us / the queen is not a mother as well.'[65]

The discourse both Louis XVI and Marie Antoinette promoted, that of a queen who was a model of domestic happiness and a king who would restore morals, competed with a growing, rival model, that of Marie Antoinette as the villainous, nymphomaniac queen and Louis XVI the weak, inept ruler. In the end, the latter would win out, with unfathomable consequences for the monarchy. Carolyn Harris suggests Marie Antoinette had to carry the burden of being both the queen and the *maîtresse-en-titre*. Instead of being a political non-entity who instead was a harmless model of piety like the queens of Louis XIV and XV, she was an assertive woman with political and cultural influence in the public gaze like a mistress, a role that was now intolerable in a queen. 'A queen who exercised a dominant influence in both the king's personal and political realms had the potential to undermine both the monarch's actual and perceived sovereign authority.'[66]

This sovereign authority was under quite a lot of strain by the 1780s. The publication of the French government's financial records for the very first time in 1781 sparked what Ségur described as 'a kind of revolution in the public mind' that stirred greater public interest in France's poor economy and in potential reforms.[67] Unfortunately, Louis XVI's inability to push through such reforms, in spite of his own interest in economic reforms, was due in no small part his failure to overcome opposition from the *parlements* and to manage and fully support his ministers. Meanwhile, Marie Antoinette's reputation, already on unsteady foundations, was dealt a devastating blow in 1785 by the Affair of the Diamond Necklace, a complex incident in which a con-artist named Jeanne de Valois forged letters purporting to be from Marie Antoinette in order to trick the powerful Cardinal de Rohan into buying for Jeanne a 2,000,000 livre diamond necklace. Although Marie Antoinette was not even aware of what was happening in her name, she was undoubtedly the villain in the public eye. The circumstances of the scandal and its aftermath confirmed Marie Antoinette's taste for luxury in a time of economic crisis and her inappropriate, un-queenly behaviour. Even the Parlement of Paris's trial against the Cardinal de Rohan ended with Rohan being acquitted and Marie Antoinette rebuked in an official statement for her 'frivolity and indiscretion'.[68] Perceptions of Louis XVI's weakness and Marie Antoinette's corruption could not have possibly better fit Rousseau's warnings about women's corrupting influence in politics.

Critical and even outright pornographic *libelles* spread, taking the royal couple as a favourite theme. Typically, Louis XVI was portrayed as an impotent alcoholic while Marie Antoinette was a nymphomaniac who took her brothers-in-law and the guards as lovers.[69] The problem was not necessarily that Louis XVI was chaste, even if he was eschewing the celebrated sexual virility and sense of *joie de vivre* the French popular imagination had once granted to kings like François I and Henri IV. It was that his sexuality and masculinity were seen as stunted and how readily that fit with the narrative of an incompetent king who could not truly rule. Instead of the king revelling in sexual conquests and exercising power, it was the queen.

The story of the sexual lives of the three Louis' and how their contemporaries perceived them is one of competing discourses. Was it possible to commit adultery and still be a good Catholic, or was the sin of adultery incompatible with a true conversion? Was the king entitled to his own sexual indiscretions especially in the midst of a courtly culture that was no better at valuing marital fidelity? Were mistresses a benefit to the king and even to the realm itself, or was the influence of any mistress inevitably toxic? Were Louis XVI and Marie Antoinette models of moral domesticity or simply the apex of dissimulation, greed and ineptitude at Versailles? Such questions reflect profound and far-reaching changes in religious discourses, attitudes towards gender, and the political and intellectual landscapes unfolding far beyond the confines of Versailles. The three Louis' romantic and sexual lives were at the intersection of dynastic politics, ongoing changes in gender norms and the tension between individual desire and the immortal, sacrosanct body of the king.

Notes

1 "Sur le roi qui prenant le parti de la dévotion, renonçait à la galanterie," in Michael Strich, *Liselotte und Ludwig XIV, Historische Bibliothek: Herausgegeben von Redaktion der Historischen Zeitschrift* (Munich: R. Oldenbourg, 1912), 95.

2 *Recueil Clairambault-Maurepas: Chansonnier historique du XVIIIe siècle*, ed. Émile Raunié (Paris, 1882), 7.55.

3 Robert Darnton, *The Devil in the Holy Water, or The Art of Slander From Louis XIV to Napoleon* (Philadelphia: University of Pennsylvania Press, 2010), 143–144.

4 Tracy Adams, "H-France Review: Adams on Wellman," *Queens and Mistresses of Renaissance France*, 30 September 2015.

5 M.G.A. Vale, *Charles VII* (London: Eyre Methuen, 1974), 91.

6 Kathleen Wellman, *Queens and Mistresses of Renaissance France* (New Haven: Yale University Press, 2013), 220.

7 Lisa Hilton, *Athénaïs: The Life of Louis XIV's Mistress, the Real Queen of France* (Boston: Little, Brown and Company), 130–135.

8 Evelyne Lever, *Madame de Pompadour, A Life*, trans. Catherine Temerson (New York: Farrar, Straus and Giroux, 2002), 107–110, 168–179.

9 Louis XIV, *Mémoires for the Instruction of the Dauphin*, trans. Paul Sonnino (New York: Free Press, 1970), 246.

10 Marthe-Marguerite de Mursay, madame de Caylus, *Souvenirs*, ed. Bernard Noël (Paris: Mercure de France, 1965), 53.

11 Charles-Alexandre, duc de Croÿ, *Journal inédit*, eds. Vte de Grouchy and Paul Cottin (Paris: Ernest Flammarion, 1996), 1.189–190.

12 Quoted in Wellman, *Queens and Mistresses*, 111–112.

13 Charles Pinot-Duclos, *Considérations sur les mœurs de ce siècle* (Amsterdam, 1751), 255–256.

14 Carolyn C. Lugée, *Le Paradis des Femmes: Women, Salons, and Social Stratification in Seventeenth-Century France* (Princeton University Press, 1976), 32.

15 Joseph Addison, *The Spectator*, no. 435, 19 July 1712; no. 433, 17 July 1712.

16 Wendy Gibson, *Women in Seventeenth Century France* (Basingstoke: Macmillan, 1989), 65–66.

17 Hilton, *Athénaïs*, 87–88.

18 Louis de Rouvroy, duc de Saint-Simon *Mémoires*, ed. Yves Coirault (Paris: Gallimard, 1983), 5.548–550.

19 Christine Pevitt Algrant, *Madame de Pompadour, Mistress of France* (New York: Grove Press, 2002), 22–24.

20 Colin James, *Madame de Pompadour: Images of a Mistress* (London: National Gallery Company, 2002), 62–65.

21 Maurice Rheims, *La vie étrange des objets: histoire de la curiosité* (Paris: Plon, 1959), 313.

22 Rosamond Hooper-Hamersley, *The Hunt after Jeanne-Antoinette de Pompadour: Patronage, Politics, Art and the French Enlightenment* (Plymouth: Lexington Books, 2011), 157–166.

23 Mathieu-François Pidansat de Mairobert, *Anecdotes* (1778), 1.152.

24 Primi Visconti, *L'Histoire et Mémoires*, ed. Emmanuel de Waresuqiel (Paris: Perrin, 1988), 47.

25 Matthieu Marais, *Journal et mémoires* (Paris: Firmin Didot frères, 1863–8), 2.322. The same theory is shared in *Mémoires pour servir à l'histoire du régiment de la calotte* (Paris: n.p., 1725), 2.111–120

26 Edmond-Jean-François Barbier, *Journal d'un bourgeois de Paris sous le règne de Louis XV*, ed. Philippe Bernard (Paris: Union générale d'éditions, 1963), 80.

27 René-Louis de Argenson, *Mémoires* (Paris: P. Janett, 1857), 5.112.

28 Louis XIV, *Mémoires for the Instruction of the Dauphin*, 248.

29 *State Papers of Henry VIII*, vii. 891, quoted in R.J. Knecht, *Renaissance Warrior and Patron: The Reign of Francis I* (Cambridge: Cambridge University Press, 1994), 289.

30 Visconti, *L'Histoires et Memoires*, 121.

31 Elisabeth Charlotte, duchesse d'Orléans, *Correspondance complete*, trans. M.G. Brunet (Paris: G. Charpenter, 1857), 3 July 1716.

32 Kevin Sharpe, *The Personal Rule of Charles I* (New Haven: Yale University Press, 1992), 183–188.

33 Louis XIV, *Mémoires for the Instruction of the Dauphin*, 246–247.

34 Madame de Caylus, *Souvenirs de Madame de Caylus*, ed. Bernard Noël (Paris: Mercure de France, 1965), 45.

35 Antonia Fraser, *Love and Louis XIV: The Women in the Life of the Sun King* (New York: Doubleday, 2006), 116–118.

36 James R. Farr, *Authority and Sexuality in Early Modern Burgundy (1550–1730)* (Oxford: Oxford University Press, 1995), 41–45.

37 Madame de Maintenon, *Lettres de Madame de Maintenon*, eds. Hans Bots and Eugénie Bots-Estourgie (Paris: Honore Champion, 2009), 9 November 1702.

38 For a description of the episode, see Fraser, *Love and Louis XIV*, 161–168; Georges Minois, *Bussuet entre Dieu et le Soleil* (Paris: Perrin, 2003), 303–310; Hilton, *Athénais*, 136–144; Jean-Christian Petitfils, *Madame de Montespan* (Paris: Fayard, 1998), 123–126; and Georges Guitton, "Cas de Conscience pour un confesseur du Roi: Madame De Monespan," *Nouvelle Revue Theologique* 77 (1955), 61–70.

39 Quoted in Minois, *Bussuet*, 305.

40 Marie d'Aumale, *Memoire et lettres inédites* (Paris: Calmann-Lévy, 1896–1902), 66–68.

41 Madame de Maintenon, *Lettres*, 23 February 1690.

42 Cardinal de Bernis, *Mémoires et lettres* (Paris: Librairie Paul Ollendorf, 1903), 1.40.

43 Saint-Simon, *Mémoires*, 2.806–808.

44 Ibid., 5.548.

45 For examples, see *Chansonnier historique du XVIIIe siècle*, ed. Marie-André-Alfred-Émile Raunié (Paris: A. Quentin, 1879–84), 1.3, 1.21, 1.50, 1.51, 1.60–61 and 1.100.

46 Edmond-Jean-François Barber, *Journal d'un Bourgeois de Paris sous le Regne de Louis XV* (Paris: 10/18, 1963).

47 Jean-Paul Guicciardi, "Between the Licit and the Illicit: The Sexuality of the King," trans. Michael Murray, *'Tis Nature's Fault: Unauthorized Sexuality during the Enlightenment*, ed. Robert P. Maccubbin (Cambridge: University of Cambridge Press, 1987), 89–98.

48 Jeffrey Merrick, *The Desacralization of the French Monarchy in the Eighteenth Century* (Baton Rouge: Louisiana University Press, 1990), 20–21.

49 John Hardman, *Louis XVI* (Yale University Press, 1993), 25.

50 Gary Kates, *Monsieur d'Eon is a Woman: A Tale of Political Intrigue and Sexual Masquerade* (Baltimore: Johns Hopkins Press, 2001), 166–181.

51 Jean-Jacques Rousseau, *Politics and the Arts: The Letter to d'Alembert on the Theater*, trans. Allan Bloom (Ithaca: Cornell University Press, 1968), 100–101.

52 Vera Lee, *The Reign of Women* (Cambridge: Schenkman Publishing Company, 1975), 50–52, 72–77.

53 Bernis, *Mémoires et lettres*, 1.98, 100.

54 Lynn Hunt, *The Family Romance of the French Revolution* (Berkeley: University of California Press, 1992), 98.

55 William M. Reddy, *The Navigation of Feeling: A Framework for the History of Emotions* (Cambridge: Cambridge University Press, 2001), 158.

56 Gibson, *Women in Seventeenth Century France*, 68.

57 Reddy, *The Navigation of Feeling*, 153.

58 Virginia E. Swain, "Hidden from View: French Women Authors and the Language of Rights, 1727–1792," in *Intimate Encounters*, ed. Richard Rand (Princeton: Princeton University Press, 1997), 29.

59 [Pidansat de Mairobert], *Anécdotes sur la comtesse du Barry* (London [Paris], [1775] 1776).

60 *Marie-Antoinette Correspondance* (1770–1793), ed. Evelyne Lever (Paris: Tallandier, 2005), 16 June 1774.

61 Cécile Berly, *La Reine scandaleuse: Idèes reçues sur Marie-Antoinette* (Paris: Editions Le Cavalier Bleu, 2012), 46–47; Antonia Fraser, *Marie Antoinette: The Journey* (New York: Anchor Books, 2001), 169–170, 255.

62 Madame Campan, *Memoirs of the Private Life of Queen Marie Antoinette of France*, vol. 1 (London: Henry Colburn, 1824), 85.

63 Louis-Philippe, Comte de Ségur, *Memoires*, ed. and trans. Eveline Cruickshanks (London: The Folio Society, 1960), 173.

64 Carolyn Harris, *Queenship and Revolution in Early Modern Europe: Henrietta Maria and Marie Antoinette* (New York: Palgrave Macmillan, 2016), 107–112.
65 *Chansonnier historique*, 8.21–23, 9.32, 9.79, 10.17–18.
66 Harris, *Queenship and Revolution*, 111–112.
67 Ségur, *Memoires*, 103.
68 Caroline Weber, *Queen of Fashion: What Marie Antoinette Wore to the Revolution* (New York: Henry Holt and Company, 2006), 164–171.
69 Berly, *La Reine scandaleuse*, 103–142; Hunt, *The Family Romance*, 103–114.

Key works

Berly, Cécile, *La Reine scandaleuse: Idèes reçues sur Marie-Antoinette* (Paris: Editions Le Cavalier Bleu, 2012).

Darnton, Robert, *The Devil in the Holy Water, or The Art of Slander From Louis XIV to Napoleon* (Philadelphia: University of Pennsylvania Press, 2010).

Kates, Gary, *Monsieur d'Eon is a Woman: A Tale of Political Intrigue and Sexual Masquerade* (Baltimore: Johns Hopkins Press, 2001).

Lugée, Carolyn C., *Le Paradis des Femmes: Women, Salons, and Social Stratification in Seventeenth-Century France* (Princeton: Princeton University Press, 1976).

Merrick, Jeffrey, *The Desacralization of the French Monarchy in the Eighteenth Century* (Baton Rouge: Louisiana University Press, 1990).

Wellman, Kathleen, *Queens and Mistresses of Renaissance France* (New Haven: Yale University Press, 2013).

37

QUEEN MIN, FOREIGN POLICY AND THE ROLE OF FEMALE LEADERSHIP IN LATE NINETEENTH-CENTURY KOREA

Frank Jacob

Introduction

On 8 October 1895 Korea lost one of its most powerful female rulers. Empress Myeongseong (1851–95) – or Queen Min, as she was known to western readers at the time – was assassinated by Japanese agents in the cruellest of ways:

> The palace gates were open as usual and there were only a few soldiers guarding them, because such an attack was totally unexpected. The guards were killed, and, as planned, the attackers dashed into the queen's chamber. The Japanese attackers caught the queen before she could even realize what was happening. They stabbed her numerous times, and when she was dead, they dragged her body out to the courtyard, sprayed kerosene over it and set it afire.[1]

The queen was killed with such violence because she had been an obstacle in the path of Japan's expansionist aims. However, the assassins not only killed the Korean ruler's powerful wife, they also killed a living example of female strength in a time of change. The empress, who grew up in an impoverished family of Korean nobility, who had been chosen to be queen by her father-in-law – a man who later tried to humiliate her in every possible way – who had suffered a miscarriage and the loss of reputation as a reliable wife, but who was also able to make her way to becoming one of the leading figures of the Korean state of the nineteenth century, embodied both the strength of the 'modern' female and the new nation. Nevertheless, until recently, her case has not aroused much interest among scholars and the public more broadly.

Notwithstanding this, since the 1990s, Empress Myeongseong is one of the historical protagonists to have emerged consistently on Korean television as well as in a major musical production, arousing public interest in her in South Korea and abroad. Additionally, newspapers have featured articles about this famous queen of modern Korean history, and novels have presented her life story to the general reader. While she has since been deployed as a 'new banner of Korean nationalism',[2] her life story has become more and more vague and misunderstood. Since the late

1990s, it is the contemporary public image, burdened with national semiotics, which dominates public discourse, while the real queen seems to have all but disappeared. Mostly dealing with the Eulmi incident, that is, the assassination of the queen by Japanese nationalists in 1895, Empress Myeongseong's death overshadows her life and the role played by her in Korean politics between the 1860s and 1890s.[3] Michael Finch observes that one thing remains true: the Korean queen 'has been an ambivalent figure in Korean historiography'.[4] Moreover, her image has varied in different periods since her death, being also dependent upon the national context of specific Queen Min-related historiography. For a long time, the empress was not popular in Korea; she was instead considered an 'embodiment of all the evils of the decaying dynasty'.[5] As a consequence, the queen has been depicted 'as a reactionary force in the politics of the period, blamed for obstructing the reform programs of members of the Enlightenment party (*Kaehwadang*)', which argues that she had controlled and manipulated her weak husband to secure the rise of the Min clan during her influential years.[6] Michael Finch further emphasizes that the 'ambivalent attitudes of Korean historians . . . appear to have their origins in the queen's own Machiavellian struggle for survival within the intrigues of the Korean court',[7] and especially against her father-in-law, the Daewongun (1820–98).

For their part, Japanese historians have belittled her, referring to her by her westernized name Queen Min (*Min-bi*) and considering her an unimportant element in the Japanese-Korean relations, which were instead related to great power policies rather than being connected to a Korean royal woman. As such, she is usually only mentioned in relation to her death, which caused a political crisis for Japanese expansionist ambitions on the Asian mainland and led to tensions with Russia over Korea.[8] By way of contrast, however, Empress Myeongseong's western contemporaries largely agreed in their description of this Korean female ruler, that 'she was a woman of outstanding intelligence and ability'.[9] Regardless of the fact that she dominated Korean history for more than two decades from 1874 to 1895, unfortunately, it is 'her violent death under cover of darkness at the hands of a foreign aggressor with the collaboration of her own people [that] remains a potent symbol of Korea's own loss of sovereignty'.[10] Since 1876, Korea's modern history has been determined largely by Japanese imperialist ambitions, which led to the country's occupation between 1910 and 1945 as well as its political and geographical division in the aftermath of World War II and the Korean War. The assassination of Empress Myeongseong marks a major event in this period of history, one that led to Korea being suppressed by the Japanese empire and its expansionist ambitions on the Asian mainland. Nationalist voices in Korea tend to lump together Myeongseong's assassination with the history of the 'comfort women' (*ianfu*)[11] – a euphemistic expression for the women and girls who were kidnapped by the Japanese to serve as sex slaves for the Imperial Army, especially since Japan has never officially apologized for being involved in the assassination of the last Korean queen on 8 October 1895.[12] The incident represents a wound in Korea's historical memory, one that has been kept open by the non-conciliatory positions of the governments involved and, all the while, as described earlier, Queen Min's image has been transformed to fit specific narratives. As a result, there are several interpretations of her character, as well as of her role and influence in the years leading to the end of the Sino-Japanese War in 1895, making it hard to identify the empress's 'real' nature. In discussions of the incident, the role of the queen was rather diminished when they began to focus on the responsibilities for the assassination per se. While early Japanese accounts of those who were involved in Japan's 'Korean business' stressed the role of her father-in-law, who had plotted against Myeongseong and staged a charade that would appear to involve Japanese aggression,[13] the later Japanese historian, Yamabe Kentarō, revealed that it was in fact the Japanese Minister in Korea, Miura Gorō (1847–1926) who had been behind the assassination plans.[14] Regardless of her findings, some authors have kept the discussion about the 'real assassins'[15] alive, especially since Japanese nationalists feel offended by accepting the guilt for the events in 1895.

While most Japanese authors tend to deny the incident's importance, Korean authors stress its impact, especially since the death of Empress Myeongseong marked the beginning of Japan's aggressive imperialist course leading to the annexation of the Korean Peninsula in 1910.[16] With the powerful queen out of the way, King Kojong (1864–1907) lost political control, an event that also stimulated growing Russian ambition towards Korea, something that would later culminate in the war between Russia and Japan in 1904–5.[17] As a result, works for a Korean audience usually focused on the Japanese involvement in the fateful events of 1895.[18]

However, the queen was not only a controversial figure within national historiographies. Contemporary reports related to her person also range from admiration to demonization. That said, when reading reports published in western newspapers and journals, it should be acknowledged that many reform party members from Korea, who had been expelled previously by the queen, found sanctuary in the United States. Their contact with US journalists, interest groups and political representatives might have stimulated the specific perspective about the queen who received rather positive reports by foreign visitors to Korea.

The following descriptions of Queen Min demonstrate this phenomenon. *The Evening Dispatch* (Provo, Utah) published a characterization of Queen Min in *Demorest's Magazine* on 28 February 1895 which described her as attractive and 'every inch a queen'.[19] On the other hand, the *New York Times* portrays a corrupt ruler in constant fear of assassination, claiming that she 'ruled the King with a rod of iron'.[20] This description might have been stimulated by reports from Korean reformers, who, due to their involvement in the pro-Japanese cabinet that ruled in 1894 and 1895, were interested in painting the empress as an evil person.

Seeking to achieve reform within the country, especially as he considered the queen to be corrupt, Yu Kil-chun (1856–1914), the first Korean to study abroad before embarking on a diplomatic mission to the United States, supported Japanese rule in Korea in 1894 and 1895.[21] It was due to Korean-Japanese reform efforts that 'the expenditure of the Royal House was fixed at a sum of $500,000 a year, thus prevent[ing] the unlawful squandering of national money by the Queen for her mere selfishness'.[22] In one of his letters to his US contacts, he too describes the Korean empress in negative light as the 'worst woman the world has ever produced'.[23]

Since contemporaries were faced with conflicting reports about Myeongseong, it was difficult to determine if she was benevolent or cruel. Since either those supporting or opposing the queen were based on individual political aims, both views should be considered with caution. To better understand how these different images of the queen might have been established, it is essential to reconstruct Korean historical contexts to evaluate the role of Empress Myeongseong via a contextual lens. Before closely analysing her violent death, the first part of this chapter will provide a discussion of her queenship and what it meant in relation to traditional gender roles. Afterwards it will elaborate on the historical context that led to Queen Min's assassination in October 1895. The queen's posthumous image will then be closely examined to show how historical events were integrated into the Korean post-colonial narrative of what occurred, which became an 'invented tradition' of female heroism.

Being queen in late nineteenth-century Korea

Empress Myeongseong was not only a strong female ruler at the end of the nineteenth century, but she also deserves more considered attention because she was able to achieve such a position in a country that usually did not care much for their women in general, and for their queens in particular. It is therefore important to shed some light on her rise to power. In most cases, royal chronicles have little to say about the queens of the Korean court, especially since their lives were considered unimportant, with most entries dealing with their marriages or the birth of their children. Within the palace, a large number of former and current queens resided together after they had outlived the generally short reigns of their husbands. Although only five of the twenty-seven kings of the Yi Dynasty reached the age of sixty, their wives remained members of the court after their husbands had died and held positions as dowagers or otherwise within the royal court.[24]

Empress Myeongseong would, however, not only rise to power, but she would also witness change in the role of women in Korean society, stimulated by the work of western missionaries. Female Christian missionaries from the United States who went to Korea were very often considered 'pioneers of Korean modern womanhood', because they challenged 'hierarchical Confucian gender relations in which women had been regarded as inferior to men'.[25] The female missionaries' work threatened existing Confucian values by highlighting the 'contradiction between the new public opportunities for women and their idealized role in the private domain of the family', which of course ought not to make us believe that women were not discriminated against in contemporaneous Christian communities as well.[26] Nevertheless, as Hyaeweol Choi demonstrates: 'The majority of New Women in Korea were educated at Christian mission schools and formed the first cadre of professional women in Korea, becoming the symbol of modern womanhood.'[27] As a result, traditional gender roles, as laid out in Confucian teachings, were increasingly challenged, and initial reforms in 1894 – when Queen Min was still alive – paved the way for the achievement of a new status for women within modern Korean society. Step by step, 'Ideas about gender equality, women's education, and the role of women in society beyond the family started to gain currency as a new moral order in public discourse and literature.'[28] Such reforms, however, did not mean a change in procedures at the royal court, which was still dominated by intrigues against the possibility of female rule.

Empress Myeongseong was born to a noble family, the Min clan, in Kyongi Province on 25 September 1851. She would become the third queen in the history of the clan – two other women had ruled earlier as queens during the Yi Dynasty from 1401 to 1418 and from 1675 to 1720, respectively. By the time that the future Empress Myeongseong was born in 1851, however, the Min clan had already lost most of its influence, which is why it was rather surprising that a girl from this family should rise again to power as queen of Korea.[29] The eventual Empress Myeongseong entered the court as a consequence of royal politics. The Daewongun, in collaboration with Queen Dowager Cho (1809–90), also known as Queen Sinjong, who had been married to King Sunjo's (1790–1834) son, wanted to destroy the influence of the Andong Kim clan. When King Cheoljong (1849–63) died in 1863, Queen Cho had the right to name an heir and decided in favour of the Deawongun's twelve-year-old second son, Yi Myeong-bok, later known as King Kojong. Officially, Queen Cho ruled until 1866, but in reality the Daewongun held all the power in his hands. He orchestrated reforms, and the Andong Kims were either executed or sent into exile. Nevertheless, during these years, the Yi Dynasty 'faced the most serious crisis in its long history'.[30]

In this situation, the Daewongun, 'instead of purposely altering the political system to eliminate imperfection . . . often preferred to manipulate it'.[31] When it was time to choose a queen for his son, he thought he would prevent future trouble by selecting a girl from his own wife's lineage, who, since the Min clan was so weak at this time, would not cause any future danger to his powerbase. The description of the young girl attracted the Daewongun, who found her more than suitable to match his own aims: 'Orphaned, beautiful of face, healthy in body, level of education no less than of the most noble in the country.'[32] After a successful first meeting, a wedding ceremony took place on 20 March 1866 and the girl was introduced to the royal court before becoming queen on 4 May of that same year. What seemed to have been a good choice of the Daewongun for political reasons, however, would turn into an unfortunate one for him, because 'Queen Min proved to be the ablest female politician in the history of the dynasty.'[33]

It had never occurred to the new queen that she would find love in her marriage, and she soon realized that her husband did not hold any real power but was instead afraid of his father. She therefore steadily supported Kojong to help him to find his own way, especially since her relationship with her father-in-law was a rather poisoned one. Likewise, Queen Min also understood that she was not the only wife in the king's life, which also threatened her position. She was expected to give birth to a royal heir, which must have put enormous pressure on her. Furthermore, she could be expelled for one of 'seven evils' defined in Confucian teachings: 'disobeying parents-in-law, bearing no son, committing adultery, jealousy, carrying a hereditary disease, garrulousness, and larceny'.[34] The queen therefore correctly understood the royal palace to be a conflict zone, where intrigues and political competitions for power would decide her fate. She also realized that in such a situation the power of the Min clan needed to be reactivated to secure her own standing, which is why she began to support family members by bringing them into powerful positions, especially in the six ministries.[35]

In 1863, twelve-year-old Kojong was adopted by the former king, Cheoljong (d.1864), with the Dowager Cho instructing that his biological father, the Daewongun, be installed as regent until King Kojong could rule for himself. However:

> [t]he older man was greedy for power, keen and crafty, and not inclined to hand over the reins of government; he therefore selected a wife for his son from a family of his near friends, choosing a woman he supposed he could easily control; but he was mistaken in her character and gifts.[36]

Queen Min eventually led a plot against him, and 'the old man found himself displaced, and a new cabinet and set of advisers selected from the friends and cousins of the queen. His rage knew no bounds, and from that time forth he planned her destruction'.[37]

In 1871, Queen Min gave birth to a boy who died shortly after his birth, and it was speculated whether a 'ginseng palliative', administered by the queen's father-in-law, might have been responsible for these tragic events. Three years later, the queen was ready to seize power for her husband, having secured powerful positions for up to thirty members of her clan. It had taken her years to prepare for this move, but once all strategic preconditions had been fulfilled, she was well positioned to initiate a political struggle against her father-in-law. For his part, the latter had tried to get rid of the queen and her growing influence numerous times, but failed. When Queen Min gave birth to another son on 8 February 1874, her position with regard to the royal lineage was strengthened further, a development she deployed to increase her political power.

The context of Queen Min's rule

During the latter part of the 'long' nineteenth century,[38] Korea's history was heavily impacted by China, Japan and Russia's colonial ambitions.[39] While the Korean empire considered itself to be politically part of China's tributary system[40] – and the Qing empire accepted this dependency – the changing international relations in East Asia, as well as Japan's project of expansion based on western laws, caused a clash between traditional and modern values in the region. King Kojong had started to rule in his own name, yet he had to resist not only the ambitions of his father, the Daewongun, but also Japan's further penetration of the peninsula.[41]

The internal political issues of Korea reflected both a desire to reform the government and wider concerns about the influence of these Asian powers. In 1884, a group of reformers led by members of the Enlightenment Party tried to take over power during the Kaspin Coup.[42] Their target was to achieve complete independence from the Korean nation-state and from any other power that might have interfered with the country's internal politics. While the idea was to break Korea out of the traditional Chinese tributary system, they also advocated for the ruling family to abandon the throne and for the Daewongun to lead a new reform-oriented government. The king was responsive to these demands, but a majority of the Korean upper class and officials were unwilling to accept such drastic changes, and Koreans in favour of Confucian traditions did not wish to accept any changes to the social order. In this struggle between reformers and traditionalists, Queen Min showed herself to be successful in exploiting the conflict in order to position members of her own family in powerful and strategically important positions. Her male relatives would eventually dominate the Korean government in 1884 and, once the *coup d'état* had begun, they repressed the reform-oriented forces.[43] As China and Japan had an interest in using turmoil in Korea for their own expansionist ideas, the Kaspin Coup had important political implications. In 1884, King Kojong favoured Japan and was assured by the Tokyo government that he could rely on Japanese help should the Middle Kingdom send additional troops to the peninsula.[44] Frequently, the queen found herself between opposing factions that sought to decide upon the fate of

Korea. She had to manoeuvre between reformers and foreign powers alike and, at the same time, remember that she was not the official ruler of the peninsula but the wife of the king. That said, Queen Min always strove to find supporters for her desire to keep Korea independent and ensure that her own family remained in charge of the domestic politics of the country.

The internal antagonism between the queen and her revenge-driven father-in-law also complicated the royal position towards political change. Like King Kojong, Queen Min favoured western reforms, but she also needed to prevent anybody she could not trust from holding government positions. Consequently, as enlightened as she might have been, her image remained corrupt and reactionary, and she was caught up in a dilemma that would further strengthen opposition against her indirect rule. She could not act as freely as a reform-oriented leader should, which is why she was often accused of being an agent of reactionary conservatism. The reality was that her father-in-law was 'the avowed champion of anti-foreign (particularly anti-Russian) causes, the inveterate enemy of pro-Western Queen Min'.[45] The old man accused the queen of being responsible for the decline of the dynasty, persuading conservative forces in China and Korea alike to act against the most powerful woman in the country. Queen Min herself had to manoeuvre through dangerous times – times in which conservative and modernist forces accused her of wrongdoing and of choosing the wrong path for Korea. It seems natural therefore that she should only choose trustworthy people to hold political positions, but these decisions strengthened both parties' accusations against her, especially for being corrupt and guilty of nepotism.

The tensions at court increased in 1892, when the Min tried to have the queen's dangerous father-in-law assassinated. The Daewongun 'desperately sought ways to overcome his political enemies',[46] making overtures to the Japanese and to the Korean exiles abroad as he needed a strong ally to plan his revenge against his daughter-in-law, Queen Min, who favoured the Chinese at the time. The internal quarrel between the two factions further stimulated the queen's negative image, which, of course, was spread by her enemies and repeated by, to name just one example, Augustine Heard II, the US Minister to Seoul:

> The Min family, at the head of which is the Queen, which has seized and holds nearly all the positions of power and wealth in the Kingdom, is hated, and, if a leader of real ability were to offer himself, the elements for revolution would speedily group themselves about him.[47]

Indeed, the growing danger of the Donghak Rebellion,[48] which erupted in early 1894 to protest against the influence of foreigners and corrupt government officials, would cause trouble for Queen Min and lead her into a disadvantageous and eventually deadly political game of chess.

The political volatility in Korea was further inflamed by wider regional politics, as China and Japan had resumed hostilities and the government in Tokyo sought to free Korea from China's spell once and for all.[49] Japanese troops were sent to Korea in June 1894, and in November of that year, Prime Minister Itō Hirobumi (1841–1909) appointed Inoue Kaoru (1836–1915) to represent and secure Japanese interests in Korea.[50] The new cabinet, which had been formed under the Daewongun's leadership, would cut traditional ties with China to begin the reforms that Inoue would oversee. The king, in the presence of his wife and family, had to declare that his family members would no longer be allowed to interfere with Korean politics and, between November 1894 and June 1896, 421 proclamations and orders for major reforms were released and announced to the public.[51] As C.I. Eugene Kim and Han-Kyo Kim put it, 'By a stroke of the pen, the royal household was separated from the government, and members of the royal family . . . were forbidden to interfere in the affairs of the state'.[52] Japan's leading role in the reform process was emphasized by its three million yen loan to Korea, which would be used to finance the reforms.

Korean reformers like Pak Yŏng-hyo (1861–1939), who led the Kabo Reform Movement, started many western – or Japanese-oriented reforms – without betraying Korea, per se. The Korean reformer Pak, however, tried to act as independently as possible, promoting his own followers to key positions in the military structure and the new police system once he became home minister. As a result, he was able to influence crucial sectors and strengthen his personal power within the new government, even if he did not officially act as prime minister. Most of the new ministers were young capable men who had risen into the government from a variety of backgrounds through their own merits. Many had a foreign education or experience and favoured change, but a majority favoured westernization over Japanization because more than half of the men had had first-hand experience in the United States.

While the new ministers worked on reform-related issues, Queen Min began to devise a strategy to regain her power and tried to contact the third foreign power that had an interest in Korean affairs and might support her political comeback: Russia. While Pak emphasized his own loyalty to the throne, his reforms had eroded Queen Min's tradition-based power, which is why the queen was forced to search for alternatives to remain in power. Pak's initial wish might have been to 'promote modern reform within the framework of the monarchical tradition',[53] but he was not interested in a revolution that would alter Korea's entire social and political structure. Even so, the queen likely considered his intensive reform work as a threat to her status as the most powerful woman in Korea. Furthermore, that the Japanese also relied on the Daewongun's support made the situation appear far more dangerous than it was, especially since Japan was not interested in Korean political instability in the aftermath of an anti-royal coup.

For his part, the king supported reform and took an oath over the new constitution in January 1895, which was based on the reformist party's demands. In this legal document of high importance for Korea's modern history, the head of state declared the following as essential to the nation:

1. Affirmation of Korean independence, particularly from China
2. Separation of power between the royal court and the government with an aim to concentrate state power in the latter
3. Modernization of the financial and taxation systems
4. Modernization of the military system
5. Modernization of the educational system
6. Recruitment of officials on the basis of merit
7. Reform of the local government system
8. Reform of the judiciary system.[54]

This constitution became the legal expression and 'theoretical matrix of the reform movement in 1895'.[55] What followed in the next few months was essentially based on these targets, but these events would also weaken the royal family's position whose members would no longer be able to rule as plenipotentiaries. Instead, they would function as symbolic heads of a modern nation-state. In June 1895, Pak appointed new governors to the provinces, favouring his personal recommendations and protégés for the new positions. The Min family consequently lost more and more of its political hold, which at the same time weakened its queen, who could only rule directly by using the positions she had given to her family members. Officially, she never held authority in the political arena and, to secure her position, even against her husband, she needed friends and family to manage political business. At the same time, Japan became aware of Pak's double-crossing tactics and tried to increase its influence again, especially after the island nation's success in the Sino-Japanese War.

While Pak was initially considered a pro-Japanese counterweight to the queen's influence, he was still too loyal towards the royal court to neutralize definitively the influence of this powerful woman, who was experienced at ruling from the shadows. Queen Min was unwilling to lose her power without a fight.[56] She 'did everything she could to counter Japanese influence',[57] and, since China had lost its political weight due to its defeat in the Sino-Japanese War, she had to find new allies. This was particularly important because her political position was weakened by the reformers, many of whom disliked her for her past role in Korean politics. The above-quoted Yu Kil-chun further accused her of a Marie Antoinette-like lifestyle in the face of Korean poverty, when he detailed *verbatim* the queen's expenditure of state money:

1. *Bangitte* [banquet] at court, day after day, night after night, while the nation suffered starvation.
2. Offering things to the God of heaven and spirits of earth, mountains, rivers and millions of idols in the kingdom, begging for Her longevity, while the people in the nation cried for immediate [death] from their sufferings of torturing and [financial] squeezing.
3. Electric light in the palace while the whole nation was placed in a dark corner with not a new ray of civilization shone upon it.
4. Precious jewels, and silks for cloth, stuff for herself and her favorites . . . while all payment of soldiers and officers was stopped by her . . . Besides this, witches, fortune-tellers, singers and dancers and every kind of ignoble man thronged to the place [palace], seeking the queen's favor and to make money.[58]

Moreover, Queen Min was accused of not supporting the reform movement, having 'secret intercourse with [a] Russian minister seeking for help' and becoming 'a convert to Christianity for getting [help] from missionary men'.[59] These accusations were stimulated by the pro-Japanese position of some reformers, but the queen herself believed she had no choice but to find a new powerful foreign ally in the aftermath of the Sino-Japanese War. Since she feared Japan's increasing anti-royal position, and also because their government had initially supported her arch-enemy, Russia offered her hope for the future, especially since the Russian government 'promised protection to the Queen of Korea and members of the Min family in case of an emergency'.[60] Tokyo decided upon a policy of non-interference, but local forces would ignore the higher authorities and act against the female ruler who had so often interfered with Japanese expansionist ambitions in the past decade.[61]

Queen Min's assassination

In early 1895, a British travel writer, Isabella Bird Bishop (1831–1904), was granted an audience with the king and queen of Korea, which she later described in some detail and in a rather favourable manner, noting that 'there were a simplicity, dignity, kindliness, courtesy, and propriety which have left a very agreeable impression on me, and my four audiences at Palace were the great feature of my second visit to Korea'.[62] Bird Bishop had hoped to repeat this experience, but, by the time she returned to Korea at the end of the year, the queen had already been assassinated. Queen Min seems to have been friendly to foreigners, including foreign missionaries.[63] Contrasting with such positive encounters, Korea's female ruler was widely considered to be evil, living on the sorrow of her subordinates and spending abundant sums on witches, fortune tellers and other entertainers who were summoned to the palace. Moreover, Min family members were steadily acquiring their wealth illegally.[64]

For Lieutenant-General Miura Gorō, the queen's image went beyond all these different perceptions. For him, Empress Myeongseong was the enemy of Japan's interests in Korea. By the time he arrived in Seoul to replace the Japanese political representative in Korea, Inoue, the queen had placed a favourable faction in the cabinet and also led a pro-Russian party.[65] The pro-Japanese forces were nearly excluded from power. As a result, Gorō decided to 'take matters into his own hands' instead of '[waiting] to see Russia eclipse Japan at the Korean court'.[66] Sugimura Fukashi (1848–1906), who would act as chief of staff during the operation leading to Queen Min's assassination, likewise favoured action over observation, especially since he thought the situation in 1894 resembled the one in 1884 when the queen succeeded in overcoming political instability with foreign help from China.[67] As such, the Japanese military favoured an aggressive course against the Korean queen. To wage an attack against her, a number of *sōshi* (political 'rowdies') or, as C.I. Eugene Kim and Han-Kyo Kim refer to them, 'adventurous civilian extremists',[68] were recruited to participate in the attack against the queen's palace.

Some of these violent Japanese civilians were members of the Black Ocean Society (*Gen'yōsha*), where former samurai had found a new haven in the transformative years during and after the Meiji Restoration.[69] Considering themselves *tairiku rōnin* (masterless samurai on the Asian mainland), members of the *Gen'yōsha* would spy for the military or otherwise cause trouble, which could then be used as an excuse for a Japanese military expedition. In 1884, the Black Ocean Society wanted to send a private army to Korea to cause a war against China, but the plot was prevented by the police in Osaka. In the following years, members of the Black Ocean Society were involved in assassination attempts in Japan, as well as in the smuggling of weapons. They also provided shelter for Kim Ok-kyun after 1884.[70] The support for Kim's *Dokuritsutō* (Independence Party) also provided a possibility for the Black Ocean Society to influence Korean matters, while an offshoot of the *Gen'yōsha*, the *Katsudōtō* (Action Party), was established to organize spying in Korea, China and Mongolia after 1884.[71]

Ten years later, the Donghak Rebellion was stimulated further by a paramilitary group known as the *Tenyūkyō* (Gallant Assistance from Heaven), whose seventeen members were sent to Korea to create chaos and foster hostility with China.[72] These men were trained and were experts in sabotage, the use of dynamite, translation and much more besides. While taking over the leadership of larger Korean groups, they sought to cause confusion and chaos on the peninsula. They would attack Korean soldiers, supply lines and governmental buildings, which forced the Korean government to ask for help from China and therefore provide Japan with a trigger to send troops to the country.[73] Considering that the Donghak movement had already forced the Korean government to react shortly before the *Tenyūkyō* members arrived, it is not certain if these men were truly able to achieve their task. However, the *Gen'yōsha*'s later narratives suggested it was the actions of these brave men that stimulated later Japanese success. During the war, they would work as translators and spies for the Imperial Japanese Army and some would be recruited in 1895 to end Queen Min's attempt to draw Russia into Japan's sphere of interest. The military was willing to cooperate with these radicals, who could act harshly without much concern for future government punishment.[74] The final act against the Korean empress was decided upon when she chose to dissolve a Japanese-trained regiment of the Korean Army, and the plotters struck against her on 8 October 1895.[75]

Although 'the complicity of the Japanese Legation, no longer under the steady hand of Inoue, was proved beyond any shadow of doubt',[76] what happened, and who was involved in Empress Myeongseong's assassination, was unclear. All that could be reported in the following days' newspapers was that the Korean queen had been killed and the king had fled to a foreign embassy,[77] which would later turn out to be the Russian one. It was later reported that during the 'Butchery at the Royal Palace', Japanese soldiers had waited at the gates of the palace.[78] Later, it became known that:

> [p]ersons wearing Japanese dress and carrying Japanese swords were among the rioters who . . . attacked the royal palace in Seoul, Korea. They were first thought to be Koreans disguised as Japanese, but now it is suspected that they were Japanese *soshi*, apparently hired ruffians.[79]

It was made clear that the Japanese soldiers basically acted as bystanders while the radical civilians, accompanied by Koreans, performed the dirty work.[80] It was reported to have been:

> A crowd of Japanese civilians . . . all heavily armed . . . [which] rushed into the royal quarters . . . brandishing their weapons, but without directly attacking his person nor that of the Crown Prince,[81] . . . [before] killing fifteen women-in-waiting in a horrible manner, they secured the queen and maids, placed them in sacks and carried them outside the palace, where their bodies were slashed with knives, then placed in a roaring fire kindled for the purpose, the bodies being wholly destroyed. Large quantities of oil were placed on the fire, and the rebels danced about the flames as the remains were burned to ashes.[82]

It was later confirmed that the queen had been killed by *sōshi*, and it was reported that a pro-Japanese faction had again taken over the government in Korea after the empress's supporters fled the capital.[83] During the events, the Crown Prince was said to have 'secretly sent from the palace a statement giving a description of the assassins, by which they are identified as Japanese'.[84] The Japanese minister in Korea was also linked to the events, especially since Japan's forces were the leading force in the political arena while Queen Min, 'a friend of China', was no more.[85]

Regardless of the fact that Miura and Sugimura considered themselves successful in defending Japanese interests on the Asian mainland, their superiors in Tokyo were not only surprised but also embarrassed by the events.[86] Prime Minister Itō publicly apologized for the 'unworthy sons of Japan' who had planned and were responsible for the death of a foreign ruler's wife. Together with his supporters, Miura was later recalled from Korea and brought to trial, but not convicted, in Japan.[87] Regardless of Tokyo's statement, the government was considered to be responsible for the events, as 'Miura had been sent as the accredited minister of Japan, and his acts, though unforeseen by his superiors, could not but partake of an official character'.[88]

These events also demonstrated that civilians, who served the military in fields where specialists had not been trained before, had to be considered a dangerous risk. While the Meiji government and military circles had to rely on members of secret societies,[89] later decades would see special forces trained by the military itself to prevent uncontrollable acts by civil forces claiming to act in Japan's best interest.[90] Queen Min's death changed perspectives within Korean politics and, in later years, she would become a symbol of anti-Japanese nationalism. As such, it is worth offering here a short analysis of the queen's refashioning in Korean performative arts.

Posthumous images of Korea's female ruler

It was Japan's victory in the Sino-Japanese War and its violent aftermath in Korea that forced Russia to intervene in Korean affairs, not Queen Min's flirting or the king's escape to the Russian embassy.[91] Changes in East Asia's power structures – especially the assassination of the empress – forced the Czarist empire to act, especially in the form of the Triple Intervention, which would later stimulate the outbreak of the Russo-Japanese War in 1904.[92] While the king had been traumatized by Japan's actions (chiefly the assassination of his wife),[93] and later refused to trust anyone from Japan, his flight to the Russian embassy was only the first episode of a new wave of anti-Japanese feeling in Korea. The queen immediately became a symbol of Korean nationalism with all past accusations against her seemingly forgotten. The desecration of her body by the Japanese assassins would later resemble the 'raping' of Korea under Japanese colonial rule. More than ever, Koreans today identify with the old order Queen Min had represented, and when Japanese reformers ordered the cutting off of top knots in the country, anti-foreign sentiments against Japan grew, while protesters were united in memory of their assassinated first lady.[94]

The transformation of Queen Min's legacy was based 'on the theme of the morally upright female', strongly impacting Korea's 'cultural ideology and tradition'.[95] She became emblematic of the self-sacrificing heroine who resisted the Japanese attempt to colonize the Korean peninsula, her story becoming a 'victim narrative' that would also apply to many future national idols. The attempt to avenge Queen Min's death was also considered a 'demonstration of masculine toughness',[96] which was later transformed into anti-Japanese resistance. Furthermore, the queen had set a precedent that strong women could reign in a patriarchal society. Under the Yi Dynasty, the role of women in Korean society had been rather limited with 'a long tradition of female subordination and exclusion from public life'.[97]

In contrast to the classical gender norms under which female submission was rather common, Queen Min, who had ruled through her spousal influence upon King Kojong from 'behind the curtain', provided the image of a strong and independent woman who could only be hampered by the criminality of an imperialist power. Her self-perception might have been the reason why she supported Christian missionaries in Korea, since:

> [m]issionaries brought Korean women into contact with a number of organizations in which Christian women would be expected to be active ... and ... Christian women in Korea, then, were able to gain access to nationwide and often worldwide organizations within which broad social goals could be pursued, and social, political, and organizational skills learned.[98]

The queen might have considered the idea, that a trained corps of women might help her in supporting her claim for leadership in a reformed Korean society, yet this must remain a speculation at this point. Queen Min therefore was portrayed ambivalently when her role was redefined in later years: both that of a strong woman and a national heroine. Both of these images are intimated in the musical *The Last Empress* (1995). In this work, 'cultural texts inculcate anti-Japanese sentiment by juxtaposing a single century-old incident ... onto contemporary South Korean social contexts'.[99] The interpretation of the events in 1895 to a current South Korean audience in the form of musical theatre intentionally 'reproduces a traditional image of glorious, self-sacrificing womanhood that is intended to elevate her death to the level of national reconstruction'[100] and thereby strengthens the 'invented tradition' of modern South Korean nationalism, which reconfigures the Japanese criminal act as the initial watershed moment responsible for a long history of colonial suppression and exploitation. The death of Queen Min is appropriated to instil feelings about and an understanding of the nation's 'historical trauma', but also to display her role as an 'obstacle to Japan's imperial project of colonizing Korea'.[101] While the image of the queen before her assassination was that of a corrupt and power-hungry woman who manipulated the men around her to get what she wanted, the post-assassination image of the same woman was redefined as one of a national heroine, who tried to save her country from colonial exploitation in the future. The portrayal of her history on national and international stages was thus the 'reenaction of historical trauma', which naturally 'appeals to nationalist sentiments'.[102]

The musical, which was directed by the Korean Yun Ho-jin, focuses on the assassination of Queen Min. She is depicted as 'a strong woman of humble beginnings who married a leader, persuaded her husband to follow her advice on national policy, was both loved and hated, got carried away with her own importance and died before her time'.[103] Overall, it provides a positivistic view of the woman who supposedly ruled Korea at the end of the nineteenth century, while the finale of the musical 'functions as a ritual of resurrection, as the spectral image of the Empress crosses its theatrical boundary to become resituated as a visual of Korea's nationalistic ambition for undying power and longevity'.[104] After having been killed in the previous scene, the queen appears as a ghost and is reimagined as a martyr for Korean freedom and independence, 'embodying the notions of innocence, purity, and sacrifice'.[105] The last song of the musical, 'Rise People of Chosun' provides an appeal to Koreans' nationalist emotions and offers a powerful message. As such, the song has been compared to the power of the 'Marseillaise' or the 'Internationale'.[106] *The Last Empress* is a re-identification with a reimagined and reinstalled Queen Min, one that better serves the narrative of the national memory than its actual historical truth.

Conclusion

Queen Min's image is difficult to elaborate on, especially because it has changed throughout the last century. Historically, the empress of Korea was a powerful woman, who, in an internal political fight against the Daewongun, tried to place her family in a prominent position within existing state structures for the sake of power and security. However, she was also interested in modernization – probably for Korean women in particular – and in keeping her country sovereign and independent. Consequently, she sought to manoeuvre East Asian power structures by leaning towards China, and later Russia, to regulate the growing Japanese expansionist interest in the Korean Peninsula.

Queen Min was hated by many reformers, and by her father-in-law, because her interests seemed to always lie in what was best for her. Nevertheless, sometimes her wishes corresponded with what was best for her country. Regardless of this, since people often had to trust and support her ambitions, it is difficult to assess how much influence she truly had, especially since the male members of the Min clan framed politics according to their own influential positions in the ministries. Bribery might have led to her success, but the steady loyalty she received from reformers like Pak and her husband suggests another conclusion. In the end, one might argue that she was supposed to be a pawn in the chess game of her father-in-law, who, once emancipated from this role, developed her own strategies to reach personal goals, that is, the renaissance of the Min clan. Unfortunately, she eventually became the victim of great power policies and of Japan's thirst for expansion rather than of her own ambitions.

In her posthumous construction, memory and memorialization, Queen Min was eventually rendered a martyr for Korean freedom and the first victim of Japanese colonialism in the long and painful decades to come for the peninsula's population. She thus became a national icon whose power was created by a will for resistance and national pride in a time of suppression. Although the Queen Min on stage since the mid-1990s and the historical queen might reflect two different people, both of them might have tried to serve their nation's best interests.

Notes

1 Kenneth B. Lee, *Korea and East Asia: The Story of a Phoenix* (Westport: Praeger, 1997), 133.
2 Tatiana M. Simbirtseva, "Queen Min of Korea: Coming to Power," *Transactions of the Royal Asiatic Society-Korea Branch* 71, no. 4 (1996): 42.
3 Kim Young-Soo, "Two Perspectives on the 1895 Assassination of Queen Min," *Korea Journal* 48, no. 2 (2008): 162.

4 Michael Finch, *Min Yŏng-hwan: A Political Biography* (Honolulu: University of Hawai'i Press, 2002), 1.
5 Choe Byong Ik, cited in Simbirtseva, "Queen Min of Korea," 41.
6 Finch, *Min Yŏng-hwan*, 1.
7 Ibid., 2.
8 Nakajima Takeshi, "Ajiashugi wo kangaeru: Sangoku kanshū to Min-bi ansatsu," *Ushio* 626 (2011): 316–327.
9 Finch, *Min Yŏng-hwan*, 2.
10 Ibid.
11 For a discussion of this issue see Frank Jacob, *Japanese War Crimes during World War II: Atrocity and the Psychology of Collective Violence* (Westport: Praeger, 2018), ch. 4. (forthcoming).
12 Moon Son, "Modern Korea and Her Structural Violence in the Transformative Perspective of Religious Education," 2014 REA Annual Meeting in Chicago, *Religion and Education in the (Un)making of Violence*, https://religiouseducation.net/rea2014/files/2014/07/RIG-Son.pdf (accessed 1 May 2017), 2.
13 Miura Gorō, *Kanju shōgun kaikoroku: Denki Miura Gorō* (Tokyo: Ōzorasha, 1925), 329–341; Sugimura Shun, *Zaikan kushinroku* (Tokyo: Ajia bunkasha, 1932), 175.
14 Yamabe Kentarō, *Nikkan heigō shōshi* (Tokyo: Iwanami Shoten, 1966), 119–124.
15 Tanaka Hideo, "Min-bi ansatsu no shin-han'nin," *Rekishitsū* 17 (2012): 72–82.
16 Kim, "Two Perspectives on the 1895 Assassination of Queen Min," 161.
17 On that war and its regional as well as global impact, see Frank Jacob, *The Russo-Japanese War and Its Shaping of the Twentieth Century* (London: Routledge, 2018).
18 Choi Moon-Hyung, "Preface," in *Myeongseong hwanghu sihae sageon*, ed. Choe Mun-hyeong (Seoul: Minumsa, 1992), 6–26; Kang Chang-il, "Miura Goro gongsa-wa Minbi sihae sageon," in ibid., 31–67; Sin Guk-ju, "Myeongseong hwanghu salhae sageon-e daehan jaepyeongga," *Hanguk jeongchi oegyosa yeongu* 18 (1998): 53.
19 *The Evening Dispatch* (Provo, Utah), 28 February 1895, 1.
20 *New York Times*, 10 November 1895, 11.
21 Kwang-rin Lee, "The Letters of Yu Kil-chun," *Korean Studies* 14 (1990): 98.
22 Ibid., 112.
23 Ibid. The text is unchanged and was kept in its original language.
24 Simbirtseva, "Queen Min of Korea: Coming to Power," 41, 46.
25 Hyaeweol Choi, *Gender and Mission Encounters in Korea: New Women, Old Ways* (Berkeley: University of California Press, 2009), 1–2.
26 Ibid., 2–3.
27 Ibid., 7.
28 Ibid., 14.
29 Simbirtseva, "Queen Min of Korea: Coming to Power," 44. If not indicated otherwise, the description of Queen Min's rise to power follows Simbirtseva's description.
30 James B. Palais, *Politics and Policy in Traditional Korea* (Cambridge, MA: Harvard University Press, 1991), 1. For a detailed description of Kojong's succession, see chapter 2.
31 Palais, *Politics*, 44.
32 Simbirtseva, "Queen Min of Korea: Coming to Power," 47.
33 Palais, *Politics*, 45.
34 Simbirtseva, "Queen Min of Korea: Coming to Power," 48.
35 Palais, *Politics*, 45.
36 Ibid., 26.
37 Ibid.
38 For a discussion of the concept of a "long" 19th century, see Franz J. Bauer, *Das lange 19. Jahrhundert (1789–1917): Profil einer Epoche* (Stuttgart: Reclam, 2014).
39 For a survey on the literature related to this topic, see Andre Schmid, "Colonialism and the 'Korea Problem' in the Historiography of Modern Japan: A Review Article," *The Journal of Asian Studies* 59, no. 4 (2000): 951–976.
40 For a survey of this political structure, see John K. Fairbank, "A Preliminary Framework," in *The Chinese World Order*, ed. John K. Fairbank (Cambridge, MA: Harvard University Press, 1968), 1–19.

41 Ibid., 86.

42 The further description of the events related to this coup follows Yŏng-ho Ch'oe, "The Kapsin Coup of 1884: A Reassessment," *Korean Studies* 6 (1982): 105–124.

43 James B. Palais, "Political Participation in Traditional Korea, 1876–1910," *The Journal of Korean Studies* 1 (1979): 83.

44 Itō Hirobumi, ed., *Chōsen kōshō shiryō* (Tokyo: Hisho Ruisan Kankōkai, 1933), vol. 1, 430–467.

45 Young I. Lew, "Yüan Shih-k'ai's Residency and the Korean Enlightenment Movement (1885–1894)," *The Journal of Korean Studies* 5 (1984): 63–107, at 69..

46 Young I. Lew, "Korean-Japanese Politics behind the Kabo-Ŭlmi Reform Movement, 1894 to 1896," *The Journal of Korean Studies* 3 (1981): 39–81, at 45.

47 Cited in ibid.

48 For a survey of the rebellion, its causes and impacts, see Sun-ch'ŏl Sin et al., *A Short History of the Donghak Peasant Revolution* (Chŏnju-si: Donghak Peasant Revolution Memorial Association, 2008).

49 "Japan Had the Necessary Yen," *The Scranton Tribune* (PA), 11 August 1894, 1.

50 For the treaty see Yamabe Kentarō and Nikkan Heigō Shōshi (Tokyo: Iwanami Shoten, 1972), 106–107.

51 C.I. Eugene Kim and Han-Kyo Kim, *Korea and the Politics of Imperialism, 1876–1910* (Berkeley: University of California Press, 1967), 80–81..

52 Ibid., 81–82.

53 Ibid., 43.

54 Ibid., 46.

55 Ibid.

56 Janet Hunter, "Japanese Government Policy, Business Opinion and the Seoul-Pusan Railway, 1894–1906," *Modern Asian Studies* 11, no. 4 (1977): 573–599, at 576.

57 Daniel A. Métraux, "Frederick Arthur McKenzie on the Japanese Seizure of Korea," *Southeast Review of Asian Studies* 36 (2014): 132.

58 Lee, "The Letters of Yu Kil-chun," 113.

59 Ibid.

60 "Moving on Seoul," *The Morning Call* (San Francisco), 11 August 1894, 1. See also "Japan Had the Necessary Yen," *The Scranton Tribune* (PA), 11 August 1894, 1.

61 Kim, *Korea and the Politics of Imperialism*, 86.

62 Isabella Bird Bishop, *Korea and Her Neighbors* (New York: Fleming H. Revell Company, 1898), 260.

63 Lillias H. Underwood, *Underwood of Korea* (New York: Fleming H. Revell, 1918), 146–147.

64 Kim, *Korea and the Politics of Imperialism*, 74–75.

65 Ibid., 86. For documents related to his rule in Korea, see Yamamoto Shirō, ed., *Miura Gōro Kankei Bunsho* (Tokyo: Meiji Shiryō Kenkyū Renrakukai, 1960).

66 Kim, *Korea and the Politics of Imperialism*, 87.

67 Itō, *Chōsen kōshō shiryō*, vol. 2, 526.

68 Kim, *Korea and the Politics of Imperialism*, 87.

69 Eiko Maruko Siniawer, *Ruffians, Yakuza, Nationalists: The Violent Politics of Modern Japan, 1860–1960* (Ithaca: Cornell University Press, 2008), 53. The men also called themselves *shishi*.

70 John W. Sabey, "The Gen'yōsha, the Kokuryūkai, and Japanese Expansionism" (PhD Thesis, University of Michigan, 1972), 84.

71 Ibid., 91.

72 Gen'yōsha, ed. *Gen'yōsha shashi* (Tokyo: Gen'yōsha Shashi Hensankai, 1917), 440–441. Next to Uchida Ryōhei, the following 16 men were named as members of the group: Kuzuo Yoshiaki, Homma Kyūsuke, Shibata Kujirō, Chiba Hisanosuke, Takeda Norihide, Shimizu Kenkichi, Ōkubo Tadashi, Nishiwaki Hidesuke, Tokizawa Yūichi, Yoshikura Hiromasa, Harumoto Torakichi, Ōhara Yoshitaka, Ōzaki Masakichi, Suzuki Tengan, Inoue Fujisaburō, Tanaka Jirō. Some of the biographies of these and other men who were members of the Gen'yōsha are available in Kokūryukai, *Tōa senkaku shishi kiden*, 3 vols. (Tokyo: Hara Shobō, 1966).

73 *Gen'yōsha shashi*, 462–477.

74 Siniawer, *Ruffians*, 55.

75 Kim, *Korea and the Politics of Imperialism*, 87.

76 Hunter, "Japanese Government Policy," 577.

77 "Marines Sent to Seoul," *The San Francisco Call*, 13 October 1895, 1. Rear-Admiral Carpenter here reports the king had escaped to the US embassy.

78 "Queen of Korea Dead," *The Seattle Post-Intelligencer*, 14 October 1895, 1.

79 Ibid.

80 John A. Cockerill, "Chaos Reigns in Korea," *The Morning Times* (Washington, DC), 14 October 1895, 1.

81 Homer B. Hulbert, *The Passing of Korea* (New York: Doubleday, Page & Company, 1906), 138–139.

82 "The Killing of Korea's Queen," *The Seattle Post-Intelligencer*, 1 December 1895, 1. See also Hulbert, *The Passing*, 139.

83 "Japanese Implicated," *The Evening Times* (Washington, DC), 19 October 1895, 1 and "Slain by Japanese," *The San Francisco Call*, 14 October 1895, 1.

84 John A. Cockerill, "Assassins of the Queen," *The Morning Times* (Washington, DC), 17 October 1895, 1.

85 "Queen of Korea Dead," *The Seattle Post-Intelligencer*, 14 October 1895, 1.

86 Gaimushō, *Nihon gaikō bunsho* (Tokyo: Nihon Kokusai Rengō Kyōkai, 1953), vol. 28, pt. 1, 377.

87 Hilary Conroy, "Chōsen Mondai: The Korean Problem in Meiji Japan," *Proceedings of the American Philosophical Society* 100, no. 5 (1956): 449; "Japanese Implicated," *The Evening Times* (Washington, DC), 19 October 1895, 1; Kim, *Korea and the Politics of Imperialism*, 88.

88 Hulbert, *The Passing*, 138.

89 For a detailed evaluation, see Frank Jacob, "Der unkontrollierte Geheimdienst: Die Spionagearbeit geheimer Gesellschaften für das japanische Militär während der Meiji-Zeit, 1868–1912," in *Kampf um Wissen: Spionage, Geheimhaltung und Öffentlichkeit 1870–1940*, eds. Lisa Medrow, Daniel Münzer and Robert Radu (Paderborn: Schöningh, 2015), 179–193.

90 Stephen C. Mercado, *The Shadow Warriors of Nakano: A History of the Imperial Japanese Army's Elite Intelligence School* (Washington, DC: Brassey's, 2002), 2–6.

91 George Alexander Lensen, "Japan and Tsarist Russia: The Changing Relationships, 1875–1917," *Jahrbücher für Geschichte Osteuropas* 10, no. 3 (1962): 340.

92 Ibid., 338–339.

93 Yŏng-ho Ch'oe and Tae-jin Yi, "The Mystery of Emperor Kojong's Sudden Death in 1919: Were the Highest JapaneseOfficials Responsible?" *Korean Studies* 35 (2011): 139–140.

94 Michael E. Robinson, "Ch'oe Hyŏn-bae and Korean Nationalism: Language, Culture, and National Development," *Occasional Papers on Korea* 3 (1975): 19.

95 Diane M. Hoffman, "Blurred Genders: The Cultural Construction of Male and Female in South Korea," *Korean Studies* 19 (1995): 118.

96 Vladimir Tikhonov, "Masculinizing the Nation: Gender Ideologies in Traditional Korea and in the 1890s–1900sKorean Enlightenment Discourse," *The Journal of Asian Studies* 66, no. 4 (2007): 1040.

97 R. Darcy and Sunhee Song, "Men and Women in the South Korean National Assembly: Social Barriers to Representational Roles," *Asian Survey* 26, no. 6 (1986): 671.

98 Ibid., 672.

99 Hyun-jung Lee, "Haunting the Empress: Representations of Empress Myungsung in Contemporary South Korean Cultural Products," *Situations* 2 (2008): 93.

100 Ibid., 95.

101 Ibid.

102 Ibid.

103 Anita Gates, "The Ascent from Wife to Empress," *New York Times*, 21 August 1997, 13.

104 Lee, "Haunting the Empress," 97.

105 Ibid., 98.

106 Gates, "The Ascent from Wife to Empress," 13.

Key works

Kim, Young-Soo, "Two Perspectives on the 1895 Assassination of Queen Min," *Korea Journal* 48, no. 2 (2008): 160–185.

Lee, Hyun-jung, "Haunting the Empress: Representations of Empress Myungsung in Contemporary South Korean Cultural Products," *Situations* 2 (2008): 93–111.

Lew, Young I., "Korean-Japanese Politics behind the Kabo-Ŭlmi Reform Movement, 1894 to 1896," *The Journal of Korean Studies* 3 (1981): 39–81.

Palais, James B., *Politics and Policy in Traditional Korea* (Cambridge, MA: Harvard University Press, 1991).

Simbirtseva, Tatiana M., "Queen Min of Korea: Coming to Power," *Transactions of the Royal Asiatic Society-Korea Branch* 71, no. 4 (1996): 41–53.

Tikhonov, Vladimir, "Masculinizing the Nation: Gender Ideologies in Traditional Korea and in the 1890s–1900s Korean Enlightenment Discourse," *The Journal of Asian Studies* 66, no. 4 (2007): 1029–1065.

INDEX

9 780367 727574